Patterson's Allergic Diseases

SEVENTH EDITION

Patterson's Allergic Diseases

SEVENTH EDITION

Editors

Leslie C. Grammer, MD
Director
Ernest S. Bazley Asthma and
Allergic Diseases Center
Professor
Feinberg School of Medicine
Clinic Practice Director
Division of Allergy–Immunology
Northwestern University
Chicago, Ilinois

Paul A. Greenberger, MD
Professor
Feinburg School of Medicine
Associate Chief
Education and Clinical Affairs
Division of Allergy–Immunology
Northwestern University Medical School
Attending Physician
Northwestern Memorial Hospital
Chicago, Illinois

Wolters Kluwer | Lippincott Williams & Wilkins
Health
Philadelphia · Baltimore · New York · London
Buenos Aires · Hong Kong · Sydney · Tokyo

Acquisitions Editor: Julia Seto
Managing Editor: Leanne McMillan
Marketing Manager: Kim Schonberger
Production Editor: Julie Montalbano
Designer: Doug Smock
Compositor: Cadmus Communications

7th Edition

351 West Camden Street   530 Walnut Street
Baltimore, MD 21201   Philadelphia, PA 19106

Printed in China

9 8 7 6 5 4 3 2 1

Library of Congress Cataloging-in-Publication Data

Patterson's allergic diseases / editors, Leslie C. Grammer, Paul A. Greenberger. — 7th ed.
  p. ; cm.
  Includes bibliographical references and index.
  ISBN 978-0-7817-9425-1
  1. Allergy. I. Patterson, Roy, 1926- II. Grammer, Leslie Carroll. III. Greenberger, Paul A. IV. Title: Allergic diseases.
  [DNLM: 1. Hypersensitivity—diagnosis. 2. Hypersensitivity—therapy. WD 300 P3185 2009]
  RC584.A34 2009
  616.97—dc22   2009002318

DISCLAIMER

Care has been taken to confirm the accuracy of the information present and to describe generally accepted practices. However, the authors, editors, and publisher are not responsible for errors or omissions or for any consequences from application of the information in this book and make no warranty, expressed or implied, with respect to the currency, completeness, or accuracy of the contents of the publication. Application of this information in a particular situation remains the professional responsibility of the practitioner; the clinical treatments described and recommended may not be considered absolute and universal recommendations.

The authors, editors, and publisher have exerted every effort to ensure that drug selection and dosage set forth in this text are in accordance with the current recommendations and practice at the time of publication. However, in view of ongoing research, changes in government regulations, and the constant flow of information relating to drug therapy and drug reactions, the reader is urged to check the package insert for each drug for any change in indications and dosage and for added warnings and precautions. This is particularly important when the recommended agent is a new or infrequently employed drug.

It is with appreciation and admiration that we remember the life of Roy Patterson, the founding editor of this textbook. He spent his early years in the Upper Peninsula of Michigan, enlisted in the Navy, and served in the Pacific theater during World War II. At the University of Michigan Medical School, he became a member of Alpha Omega Alpha. After an internal medicine residency and fellowship at Michigan, he completed a research fellowship in Immunochemistry with Frank Dixon. He was appointed assistant professor of medicine at Northwestern University in 1960.

In the 40 years that followed, Roy developed the Allergy-Immunology Program at Northwestern into one of the leading centers in the world. In his role as educator, 118 allergist–immunologists trained in the Northwestern program during Roy's tenure; among those are the 2 editors and 19 authors of the current text. As an investigator, he contributed much to the specialty in terms of research that was both practical and innovative in diseases including allergic bronchopulmonary aspergillosis, drug allergies, asthma caused by low-molecular-weight chemicals, and idiopathic anaphylaxis. In addition, he was a superb clinician with an exceptional understanding of the relationships between clinical disease and molecular/cell biology.

He served on multiple committees of the National Institutes of Health. He was a strong advocate for clinical, translational, and basic research funding for asthma and related allergic diseases in his role as a member of the Board of Scientific Councilors of the National Institute of Allergy and Infectious Diseases. He was elected to membership in both the American Society for Clinical Investigation and the Association of Professors of Medicine.

Dr. Patterson became Chairman of the Department of Medicine at Northwestern University in 1973. He was one of only a very few allergist-immunologists to attain a significant administrative position in an academic institution. As such, he played an important part in maintaining the subspecialty of allergy–immunology in the mainstream of scientific medicine.

In 1972, he published the first edition of this text, and participated in every subsequent edition except the present one. He was a man of great intelligence, skill, and integrity. We are proud to have been his mentees and then colleagues. As editors of this text, we hope to continue his legacy of excellence in the clinical practice of allergy–immunology.

LCG
PAG

Preface

As we reflect on finalizing the seventh edition of Patterson's Allergic Diseases, we are struck by the fact that the first edition of this book was published in 1972, when we were still in college. This seventh edition is only the second one not lead by our mentor, Dr Roy Patterson. He was an extremely gifted clinical allergist-immunologist, investigator, and educator, a true "triple threat." We are committed to extending Roy's tradition of allergy-immunology excellence with this newest edition that we believe is replete with knowledge that continues to exponentially expand in our fascinating field.

Like every edition before it, this book is written principally as a guide for physicians and other healthcare providers. While it is intended to be oriented toward patient evaluation and management, there are also discussions of the underlying immunologic mechanisms, pathophysiology, pharmacology and diagnostic techniques. Because atopic diseases are prevalent, and becoming more so, we hope that a variety of healthcare providers will find this edition useful as they care for patients with allergic and other immunologic diseases. We have added four new chapters dealing with cough; pruritus; gastrointestinal disorders, namely, eosinophilic esophagitis and gastroesophageal reflux; and the results from the "alphabet soup" of asthma clinical trials such as CAMP, SMART, and IMPACT. This edition also includes a companion Web site with fully searchable text, as well as additional references, tables, and figures. Throughout the book, bold, italicized call-outs denote these extra web materials.

We believe that caring for patients with atopic diseases sometimes is best accomplished in collaboration with physicians from other specialties. Therefore, about one quarter of the chapters are actually written by other specialists with whom the allergist-immunologist is likely to collaborate. Those specialties include dermatology, gastroenterology, otolaryngology, psychiatry, pulmonology, and radiology. We are indebted to each of the contributing authors, and hereby express our heartfelt gratitude for their participation in this newest edition of Patterson's Allergic Diseases.

Leslie C. Grammer, MD
Paul A. Greenberger, MD

Contributor's List

Andrea J. Apter, MD, MA, MSc
Professor
Department of Medicine
Section of Allergy & Immunology
Division of Pulmonary, Allergy Critical Care
University of Pennsylvania
Philadelphia, Pennsylvania

Pedro Avila, MD
Associate Professor
Department of Medicine
Northwestern University Feinberg
    School of Medicine
Attending
Department of Medicine
Northwestern Memorial Hospital
Chicago, Illinois

Melvin Berger, MD, PhD
Professor of Pediatrics and Pathology
Case Western Reserve University School of
    Medicine
Division of Allergy/Immunology
Rainbow Babies and Children's Hospital

David I. Bernstein, MD
Professor of Clinical Medicine & Environmental
Health
Department of Internal Medicine, Division of
    Immunology
University of Cincinnati College of Medicine
Cincinnati, Ohio

Jonathan A. Bernstein, MD
Professor of Clinical Medicine
Department of Internal Medicine
Division of Immunology/Allergy Section
University of Cincinnnati College of Medicine

Michael S. Blaiss, MD
Clinical Professor
Departments of Pediatrics and Medicine
University of Tennessee, Memphis

Department of Pediatrics
Le Bonheur Children's Medical Center
Memphis, Tennessee

G. Daniel Brooks, MD
Dean Health Service
Janesville, Wisconsin

Wesley Burks, MD
Professor and Chief
Pediatric Allergy and Immunology
Duke University Medical Center
Durham, North Carolina

Robert K. Bush, MD
Professor (Emeritus), Medicine
Department of Medicine
UW School of Medicine and Public Health
University of Wisconsin
Madison, Wisconsin
Chief of Allergy
WMS Middleton VA Hospital
Madison, Wisconsin

Rakesh K. Chandra, MD
Assistant Professor
Department of Otolaryngology–Head &
    Neck Surgery
Physician, Northwestern Sinus and Allergy Center
Northwestern University Feinberg
    School of Medicine
Attending Physician
Northwestern Memorial Hospital
Chicago, Illinois

Seong Cho, MD
Division of Allergy-Immunology–Northwestern
    University Feinberg School of Medicine
Chicago, Illinois

Dennis J. Cleri, MD
Director
Internal Medicine Residency Program

Department of Medicine
St. Francis Medical Center
Trenton, New Jersey

David B. Conley, MD
Associate Professor
Division of Pulmonary and Critical Care Medicine
Department of Otolaryngology–Head & Neck
    Surgery
Physician, Northwestern Sinus and Allergy Center
Northwestern University Feinberg School of
    Medicine
Attending Physician
Northwestern Memorial Hospital
Chicago, Illinois

Thomas Corbridge, MD, FCCP
Professor
Division of Pulmonary and Critical Care Medicine
Department of Medicine
Northwestern University Feinberg School of
    Medicine
Attending Physician
Medical Intensive Care Unit
Northwestern Memorial Hospital
Chicago, Illinois

Susan Corbridge, PhD, APN, ACND
Department of Medical-Surgical Nursing
University of Illinois at Chicago
Chicago, Illinois

Jane E. DeMatte, MD, MBA
Associate Professor
Department of Medicine
Northwestern University
Associate Chief for Clinical Services
Division of Pulmonary and Critical Care Medicine
Northwestern Medical Faculty Foundation
Chicago, Illinonis

Anne Ditto, MD
Associate Professor
Division of Allergy–Immunology
Department of Medicine
Northwestern University Feinberg School of
    Medicine
Attending Physician
Northwestern Memorial Hospital
Chicago, Illinois

Tolly G. Epstein, MD
Fellow
Department of Internal Medicine, Division of
    Immunology/Allergy

University of Cincinnati
University of Cincinnati Medical Center
Cincinnati, Ohio

Jordan N. Fink, MD
Professor
Departments of Pediatrics and Medicine
Milwaukee, Wisconsin
Staff
Department of Allergy-Immunology
Medical College of Wisconsin
Milwaukee, Wisconsin

Chhavi Gandhi, MD
Fellow
Department of Allergy and Immunology
University of California, San Diego

Jackie K. Gollan, PhD
Assistant Professor
Department of Psychiatry and Behavioral Sciences
Northwestern University Feinberg School of
    Medicine
Clinical Psychologist
Department of Psychiatry
Northwestern Memorial Hospital
Chicago, Illinois

Nirmala Gonsalves, MD
Assistant Professor
Division of Gastroenterology
Department of Medicine
Northwestern University Feinberg School of
    Medicine
Attending Physician
Northwestern Memorial Hospital
Chicago

Leslie C. Grammer, MD
Professor and Director
Ernest S. Bazley Asthma and Allergic Diseases
    Center
Division of Allergy–Immunology
Department of Medicine
Physician, Northwestern Sinus and Allergy
    Center
Northwestern University Feinberg School of
    Medicine
Attending Physician
Northwestern Memorial Hospital
Chicago, Illinois

Thomas Grant, DO, FACR
Professor of Radiology
Department of Radiology

Feinberg School of Medicine
Northwestern University
Chicago, Illinois

Paul A. Greenberger, MD
Professor
Division of Allergy–Immunology
Department of Medicine
Northwestern University Feinberg School of
    Medicine
Attending Physician
Northwestern Memorial Hospital
Chicago, Illinois

Kathleen E. Harris, BS
Senior Life Sciences Researcher
Division of Allergy–Immunology
Department of Medicine
Northwestern University Feinberg School of
    Medicine
Chicago, Illinois

Ikuo Hirano, MD
Associate Professor
Fellowship Program Director
Division of Gastroenterology
Department of Medicine
Northwestern University Feinberg School of
    Medicine
Attending Physician
Northwestern Memorial Hospital
Chicago, Illinois

Mary Beth Hogan, MD
Professor of Pediatrics
Department of Pediatrics
Section Chief: Alltergy/Immunology/Pulmonary
    Medicine
University of Nevada School of Medicine
Reno, Nevada

John M. James, MD
Colorado Allergy and Asthma Centers, P.C.
Fort Collins, Colorado

Ravi Kalhan, MD
Assistant Professor
Division of Pulmonary and Critical
    Care Medicine
Department of Medicine
Northwestern University Feinberg School of
    Medicine
Attending Physician
Northwestern Memorial Hospital
Chicago, Illinois

Achilles Karagianis, DO
Assistant Professor
Department of Radiology
Northwestern University Feinberg School of
    Medicine
Chief of Head & Neck Radiology
Department of Radiology
Northwestern Memorial Hospital
Chicago, Illinois

Robert C. Kern, MD
Professor and Chairman
Department of Otolaryngology–Head & Neck
    Surgery
Physician, Northwestern Sinus and Allergy
    Center
Northwestern University Feinberg School of
    Medicine
Attending Physician
Northwestern Memorial Hospital
Chicago, Illinois

Jennifer S. Kim, MD
Assistant Professor
Department of Pediatrics
Northwestern University Feinberg School of
    Medicine
Attending Physician
Clinical Practice Director
Division of Allergy/Immunology
Children's Memorial Hospital
Chicago, Illinois

Anne Laumann, MBChB, MRCP(UK)
Associate Professor of Dermatology
Department of Dermatology
Northwestern University Feinberg School of
    Medicine
Attending Physician
Department of Dermatology
Northwestern Memorial Hospital
Chicago, Illinois

Theodore M. Lee, MD
Clinical Faculty
Department of Medicine
Division of Pulmonary, Allergy & Critical Care
Emory University School of Medicine
Peachtree Allergy and Asthma Clinic, P.C.
Atlanta, Georgia

Donald Y.M. Leung, MD, PhD
Professor
Department of Pediatrics

University of Colorado Denver Health Sciences
    Center
Aurora, Colorado
Head, Pediatric Allergy/Immunology Division
Department of Pediatrics
National Jewish Medical and Research Center
Denver, Colorado

Phil Lieberman, MD
Clinical Professor
Departments of Medicine and Pediatrics
University of Tennessee College of Medicine
Memphis, Tennessee

Umbreen S. Lodi, MD
Assistant Professor
Department of Medicine, Division of
    Pulmonology, Allergy & Critical Care
Emory University School of Medicine
Atlanta, Georgia
Department of Allergy/Immunology
Emory University/Grady Hospital
Atlanta Georgia

Kris G. McGrath, MD
Division of Allergy–Immunology
Department of Medicine
Northwestern University Feinberg School of
    Medicine
Chief
Department of Allergy–Immunology
Resurrection Health Care
Chicago, Illinois

Roger W. Melvold, PhD
Professor and Chair
Department of Microbiology and Immunology
University of North Dakota
Grand Forks, North Dakota

Michelle J. Naidich, MD
Assistant Professor of Radiology
Department of Radiology
Northwestern University Feinberg School of
    Medicine
Faculty
Department of Radiology
Northwestern Memorial Hospital
Chicago, Illinois

Sai R. Nimmagadda, MD
Assistant Professor
Department of Pediatrics
Northwestern University Feinberg School of
    Medicine

Attending Physician
Children's Memorial Hospital
Chicago, Illinois

Peck Y. Ong, MD
Assistant Professor of Clinical Pediatrics
Department of Pediatrics
Keck School of Medicine, University of Southern
    California
Attending Physician
Division of Clinical Immunology and Allergy
Childrens Hospital Los Angeles
Los Angeles, California

Anju T. Peters, MD
Associate Professor
Division of Allergy–Immunology
Department of Medicine
Physician, Northwestern Sinus and Allergy
    Center
Northwestern University Feinberg School of
    Medicine
Attending Physician
Northwestern Memorial Hospital
Chicago, Illinois

Neill T. Peters, MD
Clinical Instructor
Northwestern University Feinberg School of
    Medicine
Attending Physician
Northwestern Memorial Hospital
Mercy Hospital and Medical Center
Chicago, Illinois

Jacqueline Ann Pongracic, MD
Associate Professor and Chief
Division of Allergy–Immunology
Department of Pediatrics
Northwestern University Feinberg School of
    Medicine
Attending Physician
Children's Memorial Hospital
Chicago, Illinois

David C. Reid, MD
Resident Physician
Department of Dermatology
Feinberg School of Medicine Northwestern
    University
Chicago, Ilinois

Robert E. Reisman, MD
Clinical Professor
Department of Medicine and Pediatrics

State University of New York at Buffalo
Attending Allergist
Department of Medicine (Allergy/Immunology)
Buffalo General Hospital
Buffalo, New York

Anthony J. Ricketti, MD
Associate Professor and Chairman
Department of Medicine
Seton Hall University Graduate School of
    Medicine
St. Francis Medical Center
Trenton, New Jersey

Eric J. Russell, MD, FACR
Chairman
Department of Radiology
Northwestern University Feinberg School of
    Medicine
Northwestern Memorial Hospital
Chicago, Illinois

Carol A. Saltoun, MD
Assistant Professor
Division of Allergy–Immunology
Department of Medicine
Northwestern University Feinberg School of
    Medicine
Attending Physician
Northwestern Memorial Hospital
Chicago, Illinois

Andrew Scheman, MD
Associate Professor of Clinical Dermatology
Department of Dermatology
Northwestern University Medical Center
Attending
Department of Dermatology
Northwestern Memorial Hospital
Chicago, Illinois

William R. Soloman, MD
Professor Emeritus
Department of Internal Medicine (Allergy)
University of Michigan Medical School and
    University of Michigan Medical Center
Ann Arbor, Michigan

Rachel Story, MD
Assistant Professor
Division of Allergy–Immunology
    Department of Pediatrics
Northwestern University Feinberg School of
    Medicine
Attending Physician

Children's Memorial Hospital
Chicago, Illinois

Abba I. Terr, MD
Department of Medicine
University of California San Francisco School of
    Medicine
San Francisco, California

Stephen I. Wasserman, MD
Professor of Medicine
Department of Medicine
University of California, San Diego
La Jolla, California
Professor
Department of Medicine
University of California, San Diego Medical Center
San Diego, California

Carol Ann Wiggins, MD
Clinical Assistant Professor
Department of Medicine
Emory University School of Medicine
Piedmont Hospital
Department of Medicine
Atlanta, Georgia

Nevin W. Wilson, MD
Professor and Chair of Pediatrics
Department of Pediatrics
University of Nevada School of Medicine
Reno, Nevada

Lisa Wolfe, MD
Assistant Professor
Division of Pulmonary Critical Care Medicine
Department of Medicine
Center for Sleep & Circardian Biology
Northwestern University Feinberg School of
    Medicine
Attending Physician
Northwestern Memorial Hospital
Chicago, Illinois

Michael C. Zacharisen, MD
Professor
Department of Pediatrics
Medical College of Wisconsin
Staff Physician
Children's Hospital of Wisconsin
Milwaukee, Wisconsin

C. Raymond Zeiss, MD
Emeritus Professor
Division of Allergy–Immunology

Department of Medicine
Northwestern University Feinberg School of
    Medicine
Staff Physician
Jessie Brown VA Medical Center
Chicago, Illinois

Robert M. Zemble, MD
Fellow
Division of Pulmonary, Allergy and Critical Care
Hospital of the University of Pennsylvania
Philadelphia, Pennyslvania

Michael S. Ziffra, MD
Instructor
Department of Psychiatry and Behavioral
    Sciences
Northwestern University Feinberg School of
    Medicine
Associate
Department of Psychiatry
Northwestern Memorial Hospital
Chicago, Illinois

Acknowledgments

A volume such as this one is not produced by two editors. Rather, it is the contributions of many others that allow us to edit this text which we hope will help physicians and other health care providers deliver the best possible care to their patients who suffer from allergic, immunologic, and related diseases.

In particular we owe a debt of gratitude to all of the following for their support in producing this book:

The Ernest S. Bazley Trustees: Catherine Ryan of the Bank of America and the late Ernest S. Bazley, Jr. The Ernest S. Bazley Grant to Northwestern Memorial Hospital and Northwestern University has provided continuing research support that has been invaluable to the Allergy–Immunology Division of Northwestern University.

Our clinical colleagues, many of whom contributed chapters to this book;

Our trainees: medical students, residents, and allergy-immunology fellows whose curiosity inspires us;

Graduates of the Northwestern Allergy-Immunology fellowship training program;

Our patients, from whom we learn every day;

Our families, who've allowed us to work on this book which is a "labor of love."

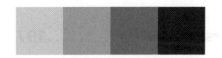

Contents

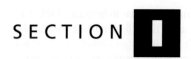
The Immune System: Biologic and Clinical Aspects

CHAPTER **1**

Review of Immunology

ROGER W. MELVOLD

Although immunology is a relative newcomer among the sciences, its phenomena have long been recognized and manipulated. Ancient peoples understood that survivors of particular diseases were protected from those diseases for the remainder of their lives, and the ancient Chinese and Egyptians even practiced forms of immunization. Surgeons have also long understood that tissues and organs would not survive when exchanged between different individuals (e.g., from cadaver donors) but could succeed when transplanted from one site to another within the same individual. However, only during the past century have the mechanisms of the immune system been illuminated, at least in part. Keep in mind that the immune system, as we usually think of it, comprises the body's second and third lines of defense. The first line of defense consists of a number of *physical* barriers, including the skin and mucous membranes, the fatty acids of the skin, the *low* pH of the stomach, enzymes and microcidal molecules secreted by a variety of cell types, resident microbial populations, and cells that act nonspecifically against infectious organisms (1).

■ THE INNATE IMMUNE SYSTEM

Pathogen-Associated Molecular Patterns, Pattern Recognition Receptors, and Stress Molecules

When microbes breach these barriers, they are confronted with the second line of defense, the innate immune system, and, if necessary, the third line, the adaptive immune system. The innate immune system is the first of these two systems to react (2). By relying on preformed receptors, the innate immune system is able to take immediate action on contact with microbial invaders. It is only in recent years that the innate immune system's vital role and its operational mechanisms have become appreciated (3). The innate system utilizes a set of receptors that are "hard-wired" into our genomes as a result of evolution and selection over the long period of divergence between the microbial world and our own. These receptors, called *pattern recognition receptors* (PRRs), are not diversified somatically within each individual by chromosomal rearrangement or junctional diversity, as are the antigen receptors of T and B

1

lymphocytes. PRRs recognize and bind two types of molecules: (a) molecules that are synthesized (often widely expressed) by microbes, but not by host cells, and (b) "stress signals" produced by infected or injured host cells. The first of these are called *pathogen-associated molecular patterns* (PAMPs) that are characteristically displayed on a broad range of microbial cells. Prominent examples among the extensive array of PAMPs include lipopolysaccharide (LPS), peptidoglycan, and flagellin. *Stress signals*, on the other hand, result from the expression of host cell genes in response to stress induced by insults such as infection, injury, and neoplastic transformation. In humans, stress signals include the MHC class I chain-related protein A (MICA) and MICB molecules (4).

PRRs can be found on external cell membranes, intracellular membranes, and even in soluble form (as in the case of certain complement components). In mammals, some PRRs belong to the group of receptors known as the *Toll-like receptors* (TLR) that are found predominantly on phagocytic cells (e.g., dendritic cells, macrophages, neutrophils) and on some other cell types including certain endothelial and epithelial cells (5). Numerous different

TLRs have been identified thus far in humans (Table 1.1), some of them located on the cell membrane and capable of detecting stimuli arriving from outside the cell, and others located on endosomal membranes within the cell and capable of detecting PAMPs derived from microbes or microbial products that are already within the cell. Some PRRs are found in soluble form, such as certain components of the complement system. All normal humans express the same array of TLRs (6,7).

Phagocytes

Binding of PAMPs to membrane-bound PRRs causes activation of those cells. Activated phagocytes enlarge, increase their production of particular cytokines (e.g., IL-1, -6, -8, -12, and TNF-α), increase their production of antimicrobial molecules, increase the rate at which they ingest and degrade microbes, and begin to actively engage in hunting down additional microbes (3,4,8). The ingested and degraded material may be recycled to the cell surface by a limited subset of phagocytes (e.g., dendritic cells and macrophages) known as

TABLE 1.1   MAMMALIAN (HUMAN AND/OR MOUSE) TOLL-LIKE RECEPTORS (TLR)

TLR	EXPRESSED BY	DETECTS AND BINDS
TLR1/ TLR2	Monocytes, macrophages, B lymphocytes, some dendritic cells; *expressed as a heterodimer on surface membrane*	Bacterial tri-acyl lipopeptides
TLR2/ TLR6	Monocytes, macrophages, mast cells, some dendritic cells; *expressed as a heterodimer on surface membrane*	Bacterial glycolipids, lipopeptides, and lipoproteins; peptidoglycan; lipoteichoic acid; HSP70; zymosan; numerous others
TLR3	Dendritic cells, B lymphocytes; *expressed as a homodimer on endosomal membranes*	Double-stranded viral DNA
TLR4	Monocytes, macrophages, mast cells, intestinal epithelium, some dendritic cells; *expressed as a homodimer on surface membrane*	Lipopolysaccharide of Gram-negative bacteria; multiple heat shock proteins of bacterial and host cell origin; host cell fibrinogen, heparan sulfate fragments, and hyaluronic acid fragments
TLR5	Monocytes, macrophages, intestinal epithelium, some dendritic cells; *expressed as a homodimer on surface membrane*	Bacterial flagellin
TLR7	Monocytes, macrophages, B lymphocytes, some dendritic cells; *expressed as a homodimer on endosomal membranes*	Synthetic compounds imidezoquinoline, loxoribine, and bropirimine
TLR8	Monocytes, macrophages, mast cells, some dendritic cells; *expressed as a homodimer on endosomal membranes*	Unknown
TLR9	Monocytes, macrophages, B lymphocytes, some dendritic cells; *expressed as a homodimer on endosomal membranes*	CpG motifs in bacterial DNA
TLR10	Monocytes, macrophages, B lymphocytes	Unknown
TLR11	Macrophages, liver, kidney, bladder epithelium. Present in humans, but not in mice.	Profilin-like molecule from *Trypanosoma cruzi*

antigen-presenting cells (APCs) (9). When "presented" appropriately on the surfaces of these cells, the degraded material can be detected and bound by the antigenic receptors on T lymphocytes. This binding, together with additional signals exchanged between the APCs and the T lymphocytes, can lead to activation of the T lymphocytes and the initiation of adaptive immune responses, a process described later in this chapter.

Natural Killer Cells

Natural killer (NK) cells appear to distinguish between normal cells and those altered by neoplastic transformation or infection by some viruses, and to preferentially kill the altered cells (10,11). They do not express the types of specific antigen receptors seen on T and B lymphocytes, but instead make this distinction by detecting the presence of stress molecules. Their activity is heightened by the presence of cytokines IFN-γ and IL-2. Using receptors called killer activation receptors (KAR), NK cells recognize and bind to infected or transformed cells expressing the MICA or MICB stress molecules. Using another set of receptors called killer inhibition receptors (KIR), they then assess the expression of class I MHC molecules on the surface of those cells. MHC class I expression can be reduced or absent on transformed cells or on those infected by certain types of viruses. If MHC I expression is subnormal, killing of the targeted cells proceeds. If, however, the MHC I levels are normal, the NK cells terminate their killing program and release the targeted cells.

The Mannose Binding Lectin and Alternative Pathways of Complement Activation

Complement is the composite term for a number of serum proteins (complement components) that can interact with one another, as well as with antibodies under some circumstances, to produce several different chemical signals and destructive responses (3,4,12). There are three pathways for activation (Fig. 1.1). The complement components act on one another sequentially (the complement "*cascade*"). The cascade begins with the binding of either component C1 to an antigen–antibody complex or of component C3 to a bacterial or other membrane surface (*without* the assistance of antibody). The *classical pathway* is initiated by the binding of certain isotypes and subclasses of antibodies (IgM, IgG$_1$, IgG$_2$, IgG$_3$) to antigen and then to complement component C1. Because of the involvement of antibodies, this pathway is usually not considered part of the innate immune system and will instead be discussed in more detail later. However, the *alternative pathway* and the *MBL* (mannose-binding lectin) *pathway* (also called the *lectin pathway*) begin with the binding of PAMPs on microbial surfaces by two molecules, C3 and mannose-binding protein (MBP), that serve as soluble PRRs. The direct binding of C3 (actually, by the C3b fragment of C3) to a microbial surface initiates the alternative pathway (involving the additional binding of components D, B, and P). The alternative pathway generates both C3 convertase that cleaves C3 itself into C3a and C3b, and serves as an amplification pathway for the generation of large amounts of fragment C3b. C3b bound to a microbial surface also serves as a potent opsonin, and phagocytic destruction of C3b-bound microbes is heightened. A third pathway for complement activation, the MBL pathway/lectin pathway, begins with the binding of MBP to mannose on bacterial cell surfaces. This pathway also leads to formation of a C3 convertase that can cleave C3 into C3a and C3b. Both the alternative and MBL pathways also result in the generation of a C5 convertase that cleaves and activates component C5 into fragments C5a and C5b. C5b can go on to bind to initiate another cascade that results in the binding of components C5b, C6, C7, C8, and C9 to a cell surface. The completion of this combination (C5b through C9) is termed the *membrane attack complex* and results in the rupture of the cell surface to which it is attached (3,4,12).

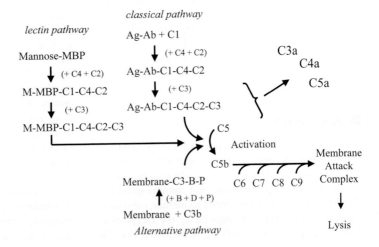

■ **FIGURE 1.1** The complement cascade.

As complement components interact with one another, each is cleaved into fragments. Some become enzymatically active to continue the cascade. The smaller fragments (anaphylotoxins) gain hormone-like functions and are important in stimulating various inflammatory reactions. C5a (a fragment of C5) attracts neutrophils and macrophages to the site of interest. C3a (a fragment of C3) increases vascular permeability and stimulates basophils, mast cells, and platelets to release histamine and other chemicals contributing to inflammation. C4a (fragment of C4) has activity similar to C5a, although less effective. C3b (the larger fragment of C3) stimulates the phagocytic uptake of the C3b-bound microbes.

Like the nervous and endocrine systems, the immune system is adaptive, specific, and communicative. It recognizes and responds to changes in the environment, and it displays memory by adapting or altering its response to previously encountered stimuli. It can detect the presence of millions of different substances (antigens) and has an exquisite ability to discriminate among closely related molecules. Communication and interaction, involving both direct contact and soluble mediators, must occur among a variety of lymphoid and other cells for optimal function.

The complexity of the immune system is extended by genetic differences among individuals. This is because the "repertoire" of immune responses varies among unrelated individuals in an outbred, genetically heterogeneous species such as our own. Furthermore, each of us, in a sense, is "immunologically incomplete" because none of us is able to recognize and respond to all of the possible antigens that exist. Several factors contribute to this: (a) genetic or environmentally induced conditions that nonspecifically diminish immune functions, (b) variation among individuals in the genes encoding the antigen receptors of lymphocytes, (c) genetically encoded differences among individuals (often determined by the highly polymorphic genes of the human leukocyte antigen [HLA] complex) that influence whether and how the individual will respond to specific antigens, and (d) the fact that each individual's immune system must differentiate between *self* (those substances that are a normal part of the body) and foreign, or *nonself*, to avoid autoimmunity. However, because self differs from one individual to the next, what is foreign also differs among individuals.

■ ANTIGENS

Antigens were initially defined as substances identified and bound by antibodies (immunoglobulins) produced by B lymphocytes. However, because the specific antigen receptors of T lymphocytes are not immunoglobulins, the definition must be broadened to include substances that can be specifically recognized by the receptors of T or B lymphocytes or both. It is estimated that the immune system can specifically recognize at least 10^6 to 10^7 different antigens. These include both substances that are foreign to the body (nonself) and substances that are normal constituents of the body (self).

The immune system must distinguish between nonself and self antigens so that, under normal conditions, it will attack the former but not the latter. Thus, the immune system should be tolerant of self but intolerant of nonself. Autoimmune diseases arise when such distinctions are lost and the immune system attacks self antigens, a phenomenon originally described by Paul Erlich as *horror autotoxicus*. Well-known examples include rheumatoid arthritis, psoriasis, systemic lupus erythematosus, and some forms of diabetes.

Antigens can be divided into three general types—immunogens, haptens, and tolerogens—depending on the way in which they stimulate and interact with the immune system (3,4,13). An immunogen can, by itself, both stimulate an immune response and subsequently serve as a target of that response. The terms *immunogen* and *antigen* are often, but inappropriately, used interchangeably. A hapten cannot, by itself, stimulate an immune response. However, if a hapten is attached to a larger immunogenic molecule (a "carrier"), responses can be stimulated against both the carrier and the hapten, and the hapten itself can subsequently serve as the target of a response so provoked. A tolerogen is a substance that, after an initial exposure to the immune system, inhibits future responses against itself.

Because of the genetic diversity among individuals, a substance that is an immunogen for one person may be a tolerogen for another and may be ignored completely by the immune system of yet another. Also, a substance that acts as an immunogen when administered by one route (e.g., intramuscularly) may act as a tolerogen when applied by a different route (e.g., intragastrically), in a different form (e.g., denatured), or following treatment of the individual with therapeutic agents.

Antigens are usually protein or carbohydrate in nature and may be found as free single molecules or as parts of larger structures (e.g., expressed on the surface of an infectious agent). Although some antigens are very small and simple, others are large and complex, containing many different sites that can be individually identified by lymphocyte receptors or free immunoglobulins. Each such individual part of an antigen that can be distinctly identified by the immune system is called an *epitope* or *determinant* (i.e., the smallest identifiable antigenic unit). Thus, a single large antigen may contain many different epitopes. In general, the more complex the molecule and the greater the number of epitopes it displays, the more potent it is as an immunogen.

Adjuvants are substances that, when administered together with an immunogen (or a hapten coupled to an immunogen), enhance the response against it. For example, immunogens may be suspended in mixtures (e.g., colloidal suspensions of mycobacterial proteins and oil) that induce localized inflammation and aid in arousal of the immune system.

■ MOLECULES OF THE ADAPTIVE IMMUNE SYSTEM

Immunoglobulin

B lymphocytes synthesize receptors (immunoglobulins) able to recognize and bind specific structures (antigens, determinants, epitopes). All immunoglobulins produced by a single B cell, or by a clonally derived set of B cells, have the same specificity and are able to recognize and bind only a single antigen or epitope (3,4). Immunoglobulin exists either as a surface membrane-bound molecule or in a secreted form by B cells that have been appropriately stimulated and matured.

The immunoglobulin molecule is a glycoprotein composed of two identical light chains and two identical heavy chains (Fig. 1.2) linked by disulfide bonds (3,4). Enzymatic cleavage of the immunoglobulin molecule creates defined fragments. Papain produces two antigen-binding fragments (Fab) and one crystallizable fragment (Fc). Pepsin produces only a divalent antigen-binding fragment termed F(ab')$_2$, and the remainder of the molecule tends to be degraded and lost.

Each chain (heavy and light) contains one or more constant regions (C_H or C_L) and a variable region (V_H or V_L). Together, the variable regions of the light and heavy chains contribute to the antigen-binding sites (Fab) of the immunoglobulin molecule. The constant regions of the heavy chain (particularly in the Fc portion) determine what subsequent interactions may occur between the bound immunoglobulin and other cells or molecules of the immune system. When the antigen-binding sites are filled, a signal is transmitted

through the immunoglobulin molecule, which results in conformational changes in the Fc portion of the heavy chain. These conformational changes permit the Fc portion to then interact with other molecules and cells. The conformationally altered Fc may be recognized by receptors (Fc receptors [FcR]) on macrophages and other cells, which allow them to distinguish bound from unbound immunoglobulin molecules (3,4), increasing their efficiency of phagocytosis. Other conformational changes in the Fc portion of bound immunoglobulin permit the binding of complement component C1q to initiate the classic pathway of complement activation. The Fab and F(ab')$_2$ fragments are useful experimental and therapeutic tools that can bind antigens without the ensuing consequences resulting from the presence of the Fc region.

Immunoglobulin light chains contain one of two types of constant regions, κ or λ. The constant regions of the heavy chains exist in five major forms (Table 1.2), each associated with a particular immunoglobulin isotype or class: Cα (immunoglobulin A [IgA]), Cδ (IgD), Cε (IgE), Cγ (IgG), and Cμ (IgM). Some of these can be subdivided into subclasses (e.g., IgG1, IgG2, IgG3, and IgG4 in humans). In the most relevant experimental animal model, the mouse, the Ig subtypes are IgG1, IgG2a, IgG2b, IgG3; however, similarly numbered subtypes in the two species are not necessarily comparable in function. Each normal individual can generate all of the isotypes. Within a single immunoglobulin molecule, both light chains are identical and of the same type (both κ or both λ), and the two heavy chains are likewise identical and of the same isotype. IgD, IgG, and IgE exist only as monomeric basic immunoglobulin units (two heavy chains and two light chains), but serum IgM exists as a pentamer of five basic units united by a J (joining) chain. IgA can be found in a variety of forms (monomers, dimers, trimers, tetramers), but is most commonly seen as a monomer (in serum) or as a dimer (in external body fluids, such as mucus, tears, and saliva). The dimeric form contains two basic units bound together by a J chain. In passing through specialized epithelial cells to external fluids, it also adds a "secretory piece," which increases its resistance to degradation by external enzymes (3,4,14).

In addition to antigen-binding specificity, variability among immunoglobulin molecules derives from three other sources: allotypes, isotypes, and idiotypes. Allotypes are dictated by minor amino acid sequence differences in the constant regions of heavy or light chains, which result from slight polymorphisms in the genes encoding these molecules. Allotypic differences typically do not affect the function of the molecule and segregate within families like typical mendelian traits. Isotypes, as already discussed, are determined by more substantial differences in the heavy chain constant regions affecting the functional properties of the immunoglobulins (Table 1.2). Finally, many antigenic

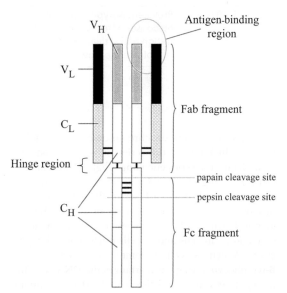

■ FIGURE 1.2   The immunoglobulin molecule.

TABLE 1.2   IMMUNOGLOBULIN ISOTYPES

ISOTYPE	MOLECULAR WEIGHT	ADDITIONAL COMPONENTS	SERUM IMMUNOGLOBULIN (%)	HALF-LIFE	FUNCTIONS
IgA					
Monomer[a, b]	160,000	—	13–19	6 d	—
Dimer[b]	385,000	J chain, secretory piece	0.3		Provides antibodies for external body fluids including mucous, saliva, and tears. Effective at neutralizing infectious agents, agglutination, and (when aggregated) activation of the alternative complement pathway. In humans, subclasses are IgA1 & IgA2.
IgD					
Monomer[a, b]	180,000		<1	3 d	Almost entirely found in membrane bound form. The function is unknown, but may be related to maturational stages.
IgE					
Monomer[a, b]	190,000		<0.001	3 d	Serum level is very low because most secreted IgE is bound to mast cell surfaces. Subsequent binding of antigen stimulates mast cell degranulation, leading to immediate hypersensitivity responses (allergy).
IgG					
Monomer[a, b]	145,000–170,000		72–80	20 d	Prevalent isotype in secondary responses. In humans, subclasses are IgG1, IgG2, IgG3, IgG4.
IgM					
Monomer[a]	—	—	—	—	—
Pentamer[b]	970,000	J chain	6–8	5–10 d	Prevalent isotype in primary responses. Effective at agglutination and activation of classic complement pathway.

[a] Membrane-bound form.

[b] Secreted form.

determinants may be bound in more than one way, and thus there may be multiple, structurally distinct immunoglobulins with the same antigenic specificity. These differences within the antigen-binding domains of immunoglobulins that bind the same antigenic determinants are termed *idiotypes*.

Generation of Antigen-Binding Diversity among Immunoglobulins

Each immunoglobulin chain, light and heavy, is encoded not by a single gene but by a series of genes occurring in clusters on chromosomes 2, 14, and 22 (3,4,15). In humans, the series of genes encoding κ light chains, the series encoding λ light chains, and the series encoding heavy chains are all located on separate chromosomes. Within each series, the genes are found in clusters, each containing a set of similar, but not identical, genes. All of the genes are present in embryonic and germ cells and in cells other than B lymphocytes. When a cell becomes committed to the B-lymphocyte lineage, it rearranges the DNA encoding its light and heavy chains (3,4,12,16) by clipping out and degrading some of the DNA sequences. Each

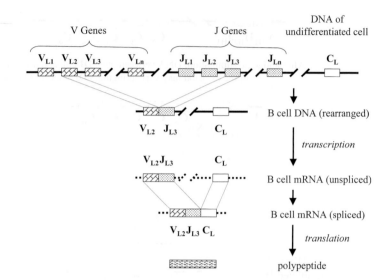

■ **FIGURE 1.3** Synthesis of immunoglobulin light chains.

differentiating B cell chooses either the κ series or the λ series (but not both). In addition, although both the maternally and paternally derived chromosomes carry these sets of genes, each B cell uses only one of them (*either* paternal *or* maternal) to produce a functional chain, a phenomenon termed *allelic exclusion.*

For the light chains, there are three distinct clusters of genes that contribute to the synthesis of the entire polypeptide: variable genes (V_L), joining genes (J_L), and constant genes (C_L) (Fig. 1.3). In addition, each V gene is preceded by a leader sequence encoding a portion of the polypeptide that is important during the synthetic process but is removed when the molecule becomes functional. The V_L and D_L genes are used to produce the variable domain of the light chain. This is

accomplished by the random selection of a single V_L gene and a single J_L gene to be united (V_L–J_L) by splicing out and discarding the intervening DNA. Henceforth, that cell and all of its clonal descendants are committed to that particular V_L–J_L combination. Messenger RNA for the light chain is transcribed to include the V_L–J_L genes, the C_L gene or genes, and the intervening DNA between them. Before translation, the messenger RNA (mRNA) is spliced to unite the V_L–J_L genes with a C_L gene so that a single continuous polypeptide can be produced from three genes that were originally separated on the chromosome.

For heavy chains, there are four distinct clusters of genes involved (Fig. 1.4): variable genes (V_H), diversity genes (D_H), joining genes (J_H), and a series of distinct

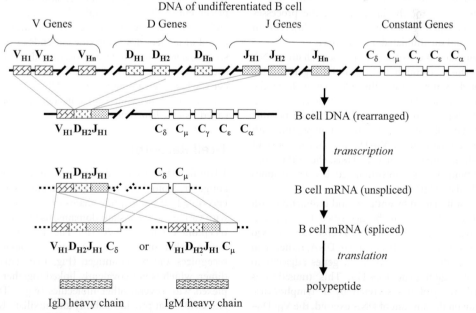

■ **FIGURE 1.4** Synthesis of immunoglobulin heavy chains.

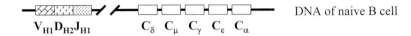

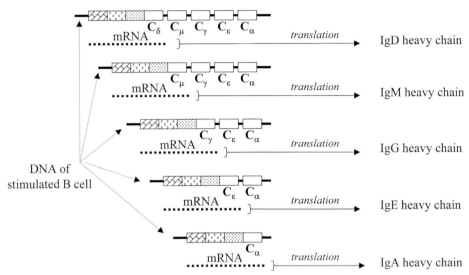

■ FIGURE 1.5 The isotype switch.

constant genes (C_μ, C_δ, C_γ, C_ε, and C_α). As with the light chain genes, each V gene is preceded by a leader sequence (L) that plays a role during synthesis but is subsequently lost. One V_H gene, one D_H gene, and one J_H gene are randomly selected, and the intervening DNA segments are excised and discarded to bring these genes together (V_H–D_H–J_H). Messenger RNA is then transcribed to include both the V_H–D_H–J_H and constant genes, but unlike for the light chains, the processes involving constant genes are distinctly different in stimulated and unstimulated B lymphocytes.

Unstimulated B cells transcribe heavy chain mRNA from V_H–D_H–J_H through the C_μ and C_δ genes. This transcript does not contain the information from the C_γ, C_ε, or C_α genes. The mRNA is then spliced to bring V_H–D_H–J_H adjacent to either C_μ or C_δ, which permits the translation of a single continuous polypeptide with a variable domain (from V_H–D_H–J_H) and a constant domain (from either C_μ or C_δ). Thus, the surface immunoglobulin of naïve unstimulated B cells includes only the IgM and IgD isotypes.

After restimulation by antigen (and interaction with certain T lymphocytes, to be described later), previously activated B cells ("memory" B cells) can undergo an isotype switch in which splicing of DNA, rather than RNA, brings the united V_H–D_H–J_H genes adjacent to a constant region gene (3,4,17). This transition is controlled by cytokines secreted by T lymphocytes. Depending on the amount of DNA excised, the V_H–D_H–J_H genes may be joined to any of the different C_H genes

(Fig. 1.5). As a result of the isotype switch, B-cell "subclones" are generated that produce an array of immunoglobulins that have identical antigen-binding specificity but different isotypes.

Two additional sources of diversity in the variable (antigen-binding) regions of light and heavy immunoglobulin chains occur (3,4,18,19). First, *junctional diversity* may result from imprecision in the precise placement of the cutting and splicing that bring V, D, and J genes together and the enzymatic addition or removal of nucleotides before the cut ends are annealed; second, *somatic mutations* may occur and accumulate in successive generations of clonally derived B lymphocytes when they undergo restimulation through later exposures to the same antigenic epitopes, a process called *somatic hypermutation*.

T-cell Receptors

T lymphocytes (T cells) do not use immunoglobulins as antigen receptors but rather use a distinct set of genes encoding four polypeptide chains (α, β, γ, and δ), each with variable and constant domains, used to form T-cell receptors (TCRs) (3,4,20,21). The TCR is a heterodimer, either an α-β or a γ-δ chain combination, that recognizes and binds antigen (Fig. 1.6). This heterodimer, which is not covalently linked together, is complexed with several other molecules (e.g., CD3, CD4, and CD8), that provide stability and auxiliary functions for the receptor (3,4,22,23). Unlike immunoglobulin,

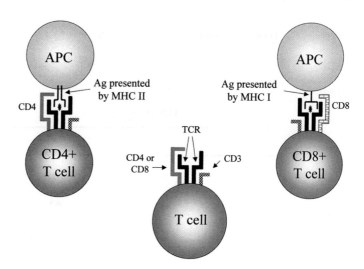

■ **FIGURE 1.6** The T-cell receptor.

which can bind to free antigen alone, TCRs bind only to specific combinations of antigen and certain self cell surface molecules. They are therefore restricted to recognition and binding of antigen on cell surfaces and are unable to bind free antigen. In humans, the self molecules are encoded by the polymorphic genes of the HLA complex (9,25,26): class I (encoded by the HLA-A, -B, and -C loci) and class II (encoded by the -DP, -DQ, and -DR loci within the D/DR region). TCRs of T cells in which CD8 is part of the TCR complex can recognize and bind antigen only when that antigen is associated with (or presented by) class I molecules, whereas those T cells in which CD4 is part of the TCR complex can recognize and bind antigen only when the antigen is presented by class II molecules. T cells do not express both CD4 and CD8 simultaneously, except briefly during their earliest stages of development in the thymus.

Like immunoglobulins, the TCR chains contain variable and constant domains. The variable domains are encoded by a series of V, J, and sometimes D (β and δ chains only) gene clusters that undergo DNA rearrangement, and the constant regions are encoded by constant genes. TCRs do not undergo any changes equivalent to the isotype switch. Junctional diversity provides an additional source of variation for the variable regions of TCR chains. Somatic mutation, so important in the diversity of immunoglobulins, does not occur in TCRs and is apparently "forbidden."

Cell Determinant Molecules

Several cell surface molecules, the cell determinant (CD) molecules, indicate the functional capacities of lymphocytes and other cells (3,4,27). The most commonly used are those distinguishing T-lymphocyte subsets.

- *CD3* is a complex of several molecules associated with the T-cell antigen receptor (22). It provides support for the TCR and is involved in transmembrane signaling when the TCR is filled. It is found on all T cells.
- *CD4* is found on T lymphocytes of the helper T cell (T_H) and delayed hypersensitivity (T_{dh}) subsets (23). CD4 molecules are found in association with the TCR and recognize class II MHC molecules on APCs. The TCR of CD4$^+$ cells are thus restricted to recognizing combinations of antigen and class II MHC.
- *CD8* is found on T cells of the cytotoxic T-lymphocyte (CTL) and suppressor T-cell (T_s) subsets (23). CD8 molecules are found in association with the TCR and recognize class I MHC molecules on APCs. The TCR of CD8$^+$ cells are thus restricted to recognizing combinations of antigen and class I MHC.

All αβ T cells express either CD4 or CD8 (although they briefly express both during their early differentiation before losing one or the other). The γδ T cells, on the other hand, develop somewhat differently and often express neither CD4 nor CD8 (21).

Human Leukocyte Antigen Molecules

The HLA is the MHC of humans (3,4,28). It is a small region of chromosome 6 containing several genes encoding proteins of three different types, called class I, II, and III MHC molecules (Fig. 1.7A).

- *Class I molecules* are membrane-bound glycoproteins found on all nucleated cells. They are a single large polypeptide (about 350 amino acids) associated with a smaller molecule (β_2-microglobulin). The HLA complex includes three distinct class I loci (HLA-A, -B, and -C), each having scores of alleles. They are expressed on all nucleated cells and are sometimes called the "classical" MHC class I molecules.

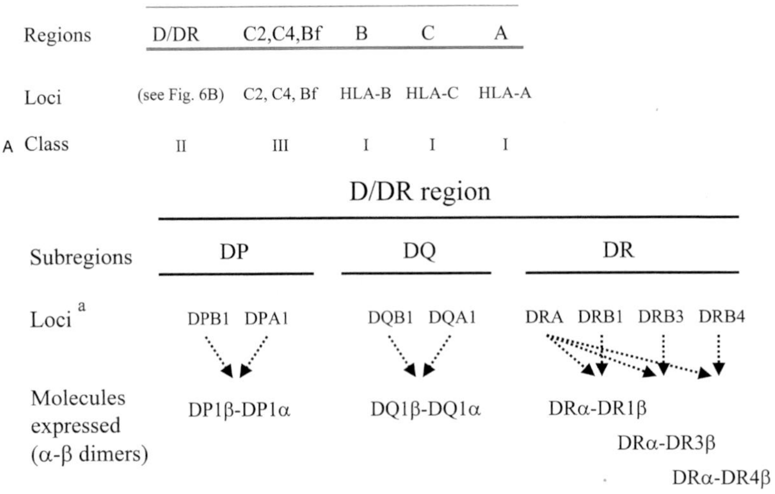

Regions	D/DR	C2,C4,Bf	B	C	A
Loci	(see Fig. 6B)	C2, C4, Bf	HLA-B	HLA-C	HLA-A
A Class	II	III	I	I	I

D/DR region

Subregions	DP	DQ	DR
Loci [a]	DPB1 DPA1	DQB1 DQA1	DRA DRB1 DRB3 DRB4
Molecules expressed (α-β dimers)	DP1β-DP1α	DQ1β-DQ1α	DRα-DR1β DRα-DR3β DRα-DR4β

■ **FIGURE 1.7 A**: The HLA complex. **B**: The D/DR region. [a] Only expressed loci are given. Loci designated "B" encode α chains; those designated "B" encode β chains. There are additional unexpressed pseudogenes (*e.g.*, DPB2, BPA2, DQB2, DQA2, DRB2 *etc.*). The number of DRB loci can vary among individuals.

There is also a set of class I-like molecules (the *class Ib* molecules) encoded by other genes (e.g., HLA-E, -F, -G, -H) located adjacent to the MHC. These class Ib molecules are expressed by only limited subsets of cells, display far less variability than the "classical" MHC class I molecules, and are involved largely in presentation of nonprotein antigens to a limited subset of T lymphocytes (29).

- *Class II molecules* are heterodimers (Fig. 1.7B) consisting of two membrane-bound, noncovalently linked chains (α and β) and show a much more limited cellular distribution than do class I molecules. The α- and β-chains are encoded separately by sets of genes within the DR, DP, and DQ regions of the HLA complex. They are expressed constitutively on B lymphocytes, macrophages, monocytes, and similar cells in various tissues (Kupffer cells, astrocytes, Langerhans cells of the skin). Some other cells (e.g., vascular epithelium) are able to express class II molecules transiently under particular conditions.
- *Class III molecules* are those complement molecules (e.g., C2, C4, Bf) encoded within the HLA complex.

Cytokines, Chemokines, and Membrane Ligands

Cytokines are short-range acting, soluble products that are important in the cellular communication necessary for the generation of immune responses (3,4,30,31). Those produced predominantly by lymphocytes or monocytes are often referred to as *lymphokines* or *monokines*, but because so many are produced by multiple cell types, the term *cytokine* has gained favor. A large number of cytokines have been identified, although the roles of many of them are not yet well understood. Many of the cytokines are crucial in regulating lymphocyte development and the types of immune responses evoked by specific responses. *Chemokines* are small molecules whose function is to attract and activate cells, including phagocytic cells. Those most basically involved in common immune responses are listed in Table 1.3.

Membrane ligands refer to cell surface molecules that bind molecules on the surfaces of other cells to transmit or receive signals critical to development or activation. Among those important for immune function are B7/CD28 and CD40/CD40 ligand. B7 on APCs binds CD28 or CTLA-4 (or both) on T lymphocytes to provide signals for activation and inhibition, respectively (33,34). CD40 ligand (CD40L) on activated T lymphocytes binds CD40 on B lymphocytes and macrophages to provide activation signals to those cells (35).

Antigen–Antibody Complexes

Binding of antigen with antibody is noncovalent and reversible. The strength of the interaction is termed *affinity* and determines the relative concentrations of bound versus free antigen and antibody. The formation of antigen–antibody complexes results into lattice-like aggregates of soluble antigen and antibody, and the efficiency of such binding is affected by the relative concentrations of antigen and antibody (3,4,36). This is best illustrated by the quantitative precipitin reaction (Fig. 1.8). When there is an excess of either antibody or antigen, the antigen–antibody complexes tend to remain small and in solution. The optimal binding, producing large aggregates that fall out of solution, occurs when the concentrations of antibody and antigen are in equivalence. The quantitative precipitin curve provides the basis of laboratory methods for determining the amount of antigen or antibody in, for example, a patient's serum.

TABLE 1.3   CYTOKINES/CHEMOKINES (AN ABBREVIATED LISTING)

CYTOKINE	ACTIVITIES	SOURCES
Interleukin-1 (IL-1)	Stimulates the synthesis of IL-2 and of receptors for IL-2 (IL-2R) by T lymphocytes; involved in inflammatory responses. Also known as *lymphocyte-activating factor* (LAF).	Activated macrophages and dendritic cells
Interleukin-2 (IL-2)	Stimulates proliferation and maturation of T lymphocytes; stimulates differentiation of B lymphocytes. Stimulates NK cells. Also known as *T-cell growth factor* (TCGF).	T cells, especially $CD4^+$ T_H1; some $CD8^+$ T cells
Interleukin-3 (IL-3)	Stimulates proliferation and maturation of T lymphocytes and of stem cells; induces IL-1 synthesis by activated macrophages.	$CD4^+$ T cells; some $CD8^+$ T cells; eosinophils
Interleukin-4 (IL-4)	Stimulates proliferation of activated B lymphocytes and of T_H2 lymphocytes; stimulates isotype switch in B lymphocytes for production of IgE and IgG1. Downregulates activities of $CD4^+$ T_H1 lymphocytes. Also known as *B-cell growth factor* (BCGF).	$CD4^+$ T_H2 T cells; mast cells
Interleukin-5 (IL-5)	Stimulates production of IgA by B lymphocytes.	$CD4^+$ T_H2 T cells
Interleukin-6 (IL-6)	Stimulates proliferation and differentiation of B lymphocytes; involved in acute-phase response.	$CD4^+T_H2$ T cells; macrophages
Interleukin-7 (IL-7)	Promotes growth of pre-T and pre-B lymphocytes.	Stromal cells
Interleukin-8 (IL-8) (chemokine; also called CXCL8)	Chemotactic/activating factor for neutrophils and basophils; some T cells, and some endothelial cells.	Activated macrophages and dendritic cells and other monocytes; eosinophils
Interleukin-10 (IL-10)	Inhibits macrophage activity, stimulates B cells and mast cells, inhibits $CD4^+$ T_H1 T cells.	$CD4^+$ T_H2 T cells
Interleukin-12 (IL-12)	Stimulates IFN-γ production by NK cells. Induces T_H1 cells.	Activated macrophages and dendritic cells and other monocytes; B cells
Tumor necrosis factor-α (TNF-α)	Has toxic activity toward tumor cells; involved in some inflammatory responses.	T cells; activated macrophages and dendritic cells; NK cells
Tumor necrosis factor-β (TNF-β)	Has toxic activity toward tumor cells. Stimulates macrophages. Also called *lymphotoxin* (LT).	$CD4^+$ T_H1 T cells; B cells
Interferon-γ (IFN-γ)	Activates macrophages, stimulates increased expression of class I and II MHC molecules, inhibits viral replication, promotes the differentiation of some B lymphocytes to promote isotype switch to IgG1, and stimulates activity of NK cells. Inhibits $CD4^+$ T_H2 T cells. Also known as *macrophage-activating factor* (MAF).	$CD4^+$ T_H1 T cells; $CD8^+$ T cells; NK cells
Interleukin-13 (IL-13)	Promotes differentiation of B cells.	$CD4^+$ T_H2 T cells
Interleukin -17 (IL-17)	Release of IL-6, PGE, G-CSF; enhances ICAM, sustains $CD34^+$ progenitors.	$CD4^+$ T cells
Interferon-α (IFN-α)	Stimulates NK cells, promotes class I MHC expression, provides antiviral effect.	Leukocytes
Interferon-β (IFN-β)	Stimulates NK cells, promotes class I MHC expression, provides antiviral effect.	Fibroblasts
Transforming growth factor-β (TGF-β)	Anti-inflammatory effect; stimulates isotype switch in B lymphocytes for production of IgA.	Monocytes and T cells

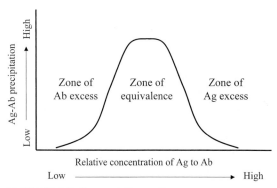

■ **FIGURE 1.8** The precipitin reactions.

The Classical Pathway of Complement Activation

The binding of C1 initiates what is termed the *classical pathway* (Fig. 1.1). The cascade begins with the binding of component C1 to an antigen–antibody complex (12). The binding of C1 initiates a cascade that subsequently includes components C4, C2, and C3. The cascade results, like the other pathways, in the formation of C3 convertase and C5 convertase. Like the alternative and MBL pathways, the classical pathway leads to production of the opsonin C3b, the anaphylotoxins (C5a, C3a, and C4a), and the cleavage of C5 to initiate the membrane attack complex.

■ MOLECULES FOR ADHESION, RECIRCULATION, AND HOMING

A number of surface molecules (adhesins, integrins, selectins) are used by various elements of the immune system to stabilize binding between cells to facilitate binding of antigen-specific receptors, to facilitate attachment of leukocytes to endothelial surfaces in order to leave the blood vessels and enter into the surrounding tissues, to identify and accumulate at sites of inflammation, and to identify organ- or tissue-specific sites (e.g., lymph nodes, intestinal mucosa) into which they must enter to undergo developmental processes or carry out other immunologic functions (3,4,37). In addition, cells often rely on chemokines to help attract and guide them to their destinations.

■ CELLS OF THE IMMUNE SYSTEM

Lymphocytes (General)

The ability of the immune system to recognize specifically a diverse range of antigens resides with the lymphocytes (3,4). The lymphocytic lineage, derived from stem cells residing within the bone marrow, includes the B lymphocytes, T lymphocytes, and null

cells. B lymphocytes mature in the bone marrow, and those destined to become T lymphocytes migrate to the thymus, where they mature. The bone marrow and thymus thus constitute the primary lymphoid organs of the immune system, as opposed to the secondary organs (e.g., spleen, lymph nodes, Peyer patches), where cells later periodically congregate as they circulate throughout the body.

The ability of the immune system to identify so many different antigens is based on a division of labor—each lymphocyte (or clone of lymphocytes) is able to identify only one epitope or determinant. During its development and differentiation, each cell that is committed to becoming a B or T lymphocyte rearranges the DNA encoding its receptors (as previously described) to construct a unique antigen receptor. Thereafter, that cell and all of its clonal descendants express receptors with the same antigenic specificity. Other surface molecules and secreted products serve to define functional subsets of lymphocytes (Table 1.4). The specificity of an immune response lies in the fact that the entry of a foreign antigen into the body stimulates only those lymphocytes whose receptors recognize and bind the determinants expressed on the antigen. As a result of this specific binding and subsequent intercellular communication, a response is initiated that includes the following distinct phases:

1. Recognition of antigen by binding to the receptors of lymphoid cells—often manifested by clonal proliferation of the stimulated cells
2. Differentiation and maturation of the stimulated cells to achieve mature functional capacity
3. Response against the antigen (molecule, cell, or organism) by any of several methods
4. Establishment of immunologic memory.

Memory resides in a portion of the activated lymphocytes that do not immediately carry out effector functions (38–40). Instead, they remain quiescent in the system, providing an enlarged pool of activated cells specific for the original stimulating epitope. As a result, subsequent exposures to that same epitope can produce faster and higher (secondary or anamnestic) responses than were seen in the initial (primary) response. Memory can persist for long periods of time and it exists for both T lymphocytes and B lymphocytes.

B Lymphocytes

Immunoglobulins recognize and bind specific antigens and determinants. Each B cell, or clonally derived set of B cells, expresses only a single "species" of immunoglobulin and is capable of recognizing and binding to only a single epitope (3,4). Immunoglobulin can be either membrane-bound or secreted, and these forms serve two different purposes:

TABLE 1.4   CELLS OF THE HUMAN IMMUNE SYSTEM: MARKERS AND FUNCTIONS

CELL	ANTIGEN RECEPTOR	DISTINCTIVE MARKERS[a]	SOLUBLE PRODUCTS	CELL FUNCTIONS
B lymphocyte	Ig	Ig Class II MHC FcγRIIB(CD32) C3R B7(CD80/CD86) CD40	Ig	Antibody synthesis/secretion Antigen processing/presentation Inhibition of B cells
T lymphocyte				
T_H1	TCR	TCR CD2 CD3 CD4 CD28 CD40L	IL-2 IL-3 IFN-γ TNF-α, -β	Delayed-type hypersensitivity Inhibition of T_H2 T cells Help for cell-mediated immunity, including inflammatory responses
T_H2	TCR	TCR CD2 CD3 CD4 CD28	IL-3 IL-4 IL-5 IL-10 IL-13 TGF-β	Help for B lymphocytes producing Ig Control of "isotype switch" Stimulation of granulocytes, mast cells, and eosinophils Inhibition of T_H1 cells
Tc	TCR	TCR CD2 CD3 CD8	IL-2[a] IFN-γ[a] TNF-α, -β [a]	Lysis, by direct contact, of cells altered by infection or malignancy
T_H17	TCR	CD28 TCR TH17R	IL-17 IL-6 IL-21	Recruitment of PMNs; chemokinesis for proinflammatory cells
T_{reg}	TCR	TCR CD4 CD25 FoxP3+ CTLA-4 GITR	TNF-α IL-10 TGF-β	Suppress T_H1 and T_H2 responses
NK cell	None	FcR KIR KAR (e.g., CD94/NKG2)	IFN-γ	Lysis of infected or transformed cells
NKT cell	TCR	TCR CD3 CD4 (some) NK1.1 [b] CD16 [b] CD56 [b]	IL-4 IFN-γ IL-2 TNF-α	Recognize and respond to lipid/glycolipid antigens presented by CD1d (a class Ib molecule)
Dendritic cell, macrophage, monocyte, dendritic cell	None	Class II MHC FCr C3R B7 CD40	IL-1 IL-6 IL-12 TNF-α, -β TGF-β	Phagocytosis, antigen processing and presentation, delayed-type hypersensitivity; acute-phase response
Mast cell and basophil	None	FcεRI	Histamine Platelet-activating factor	Immediate hypersensitivity

TABLE 1.4   CELLS OF THE HUMAN IMMUNE SYSTEM: MARKERS AND FUNCTIONS (*CONTINUED*)

CELL	ANTIGEN RECEPTOR	DISTINCTIVE MARKERS[a]	SOLUBLE PRODUCTS	CELL FUNCTIONS
Neutrophil	None		Enzymes	Pinocytosis, inflammation
Eosinophil	None		IL-3 IL-5 IL-8	Anti-parasite activity

Ig, immunoglobulin; TCR, T-cell receptor; MHC, major histocompatibility complex; IL, interleukin; IFN, interferon; NK, natural killer; FcR, Fc receptor; FcεRI, receptor for Fc of unbound IgE; C3R, C3 receptor.

[a] Some CD8 cells

[b] NK cell markers

1. When membrane-bound on a B-cell surface, immunoglobulin detects the antigen or epitope for which that particular B cell is specific. The binding of antigen to the surface immunoglobulin, together with "help" from T lymphocytes (proliferative and differentiation signals), induces the B cell to proliferate and mature either into a plasma cell that secretes large amounts of immunoglobulin or becomes a memory B cell.

2. When secreted by plasma cells, immunoglobulin binds to the antigen of interest, "tagging" it for removal or for subsequent interaction with other cells and molecules (e.g., complement or phagocytic cells). The binding specificity of the membrane-bound and secreted immunoglobulins from a single B cell or from a clonal set of B cells/plasma cells is essentially identical. However, as mentioned previously, somatic hypermutation can occur in the immunoglobulin-encoding genes of B lymphocytes undergoing proliferation after restimulation with antigen. Where the mutated immunoglobulins are capable of binding more tightly to the antigen, the cells producing those immunoglobulins are stimulated to proliferate more rapidly. In this way, an ongoing antibody response can generate new immunoglobulin varieties with higher affinity for the antigen in question, a process known as *affinity maturation*. Affinity maturation does not occur in T lymphocytes.

T Lymphocytes

T lymphocytes (T cells) also bear antigen-specific surface receptors. The TCRs of most T cells is an α-β heterodimer, complexed with other molecules (e.g., CD3, CD4, and CD8) providing auxiliary functions. As described earlier, the TCRs bind not to antigen alone, but rather to specific combinations of antigen and class I or II MHC molecules. T cells include several different functional groups:

- *Helper T cells (CD4$^+$)* initiate responses by proliferating and providing help to B cells and to other T cells (e.g., cytotoxic T lymphocytes) and participate in inflammatory responses. T-cell help consists of a variety of cytokines that are required for activation, proliferation, and differentiation of cells involved in the immune response, including the helper T cells themselves. CD4$^+$ T cells, in turn, comprise four broad categories: T_H1, T_H2, T_H17, and T_{reg} (41), which secrete different sets of cytokines. These particular subsets have been best characterized in mice, and comparable subsets are being identified in humans. All bear the CD4 marker and receptors that recognize combinations of antigen and class II HLA molecules.

- *T_H1 cells* help other effector T cells (e.g., cytotoxic T lymphocytes) to carry out cell-mediated responses (57,58). In humans, they also help B cells to undergo the isotype switches leading to production of the IgG1 and IgG3 isotypes. T_H1 cells are characterized by the production of interleukin-2 (IL-2), tumor necrosis factor-α (TNF-α), and interferon-γ (IFN-γ) (Table 1.3). They participate in delayed-typed hypersensitivity (DTH) responses, but it is unclear whether the cells doing so are a distinct subset of T_H1. In addition to its helper functions, IFN-γ also diminishes the activity of T_H2 cells.

- *T_H2 cells* cells provide help for most B cells and are characterized by the production of IL-4, IL-5, IL-6, IL-10, and IL-13 (Table 1.3). These cytokines are involved in the isotype switches that lead to production of IgG1, IgG3, IgG4, IgE, and IgA. In addition to their helper functions, IL-4 and IL-10 diminish the activity of T_H1 cells.

- *T_H17 cells* are CD4 T cells that have regulatory functions and are characterized by the secretion of IL-17. They are a distinct subpopulation from T_H1 and T_H2 CD4$^+$ T cells.

- T_{reg} are CD4$^+$ T cells that have regulatory functions and are characterized by expression of CD25 and FOXP3. They are distinct from T_H1, T_H2, and T_H17 T cells.
- *Cytotoxic T lymphocytes (CTLs)* can lyse other cells, which they identify as altered by infection or transformation, through direct contact (3,4,42) and using a short-range acting cytolysin, which does not damage the membrane of the CTL itself. These cells, which require help from T_H1 cells to proliferate and differentiate, bear CD8 molecules and TCRs recognizing antigen and class I HLA molecule combinations on the surface of antigen-producing cells (where they are first stimulated) and later on the surface of cells that they subsequently identify as targets for destruction. In order for a CTL to attack and lyse a potential target cell, it must see (on that target) the same combination of antigen and class I HLA molecule that provided its initial stimulation.
- *DTH T cells* (a subset of T_H1) mediate an effector mechanism whereby the T_{dh}, bearing CD4 molecules and triggered by specific combinations of antigen and class II HLA molecules, produce cytokines that attract and activate macrophages (2,3,43). The activated macrophages, which themselves have no specificity for antigen, then produce a localized inflammatory response arising 24 hours to 72 hours after antigenic challenge.
- *Suppressor T cells* (T_s) provide negative regulation to the immune system—the counterweight to T_H cells. These cells, which include both CD4$^+$ and CD8$^+$ T cells, are involved in keeping immune responses within acceptable levels of intensity, depressing them as the antigenic stimulation declines, and preventing aberrant immune responses against self antigens. The mechanisms by which T_s cells carry out these functions are currently a topic of intense debate, and some investigators question their existence altogether. One subset of these, the CD4$^+$CD25$^+$ Foxp3$^+$ T regulatory (T_{reg}) cells have also been implicated in some types of suppression, including the generation and maintenance of normal self-tolerance, and their possible use in disease and therapy is of great current interest (44). In addition, the mutual negative regulation of CD4$^+$ T_H1 and CD4$^+$ T_H2 cells is another example of one T-cell type inhibiting the activity of another.
- NK-like T (NKT) cells are a subset of T cells that have some properties of both T cells and NK cells in that they express both T-cell receptors and NK cell receptors (45,46). They tend to recognize and respond to nonpeptide antigen fragments presented by class Ib molecules. They are found often in the mucosal immune system. The mucosal immune system is also the site where some other atypical T cells can be found that express unusal forms of CB8 molecules or other surface markers.

Although T lymphocytes with αβ TCR also express either the CD4 or CD8 markers, those with γδ TCR usually express neither. The ontogeny, distribution, and functional roles of γδ T lymphocytes are still not as well understood as those of αβ T lymphocytes (21,47). The TCRs of T lymphocytes do not undergo affinity maturation and accumulate additional mutations, as do immunoglobulins.

Dendritic Cells, Macrophages, and Other Antigen-presenting Cells

TCRs do not usually recognize antigen alone in its natural form, but rather bind to antigen (usually peptide) that has been processed and presented on the surface of appropriate APCs. APCs internalize antigen, enzymatically degrade it into fragments (processing), and put the fragments back onto their surface in association with class I and II MHC molecules (presentation) (9). APCs (Table 1.4) include dendritic cells, monocytes, macrophages, and other related tissue-specific cells that express class II MHC molecules (e.g., astrocytes in the central nervous system, Langerhans cells in the skin, Kupffer cells in the liver, and so forth). In addition, B lymphocytes (which normally express class II) can efficiently process and present antigen. There are some other cells that are capable of transient expression of class II (e.g., vascular endothelium). In addition, a variety of other molecules on APCs and T cells serve to stabilize the contact between the TCR and combination of antigen and MHC molecule.

Null Cells

In addition to T and B cells, the lymphoid lineage includes a subset of cells lacking both of the classic lymphoid antigen receptors (immunoglobulin and TCR). This subset includes killer (K) and natural killer (NK) cells, and probably other cells, such as lymphokine-activated killer cells and large granular lymphocytes, which may represent differentially activated forms of K and NK cells. K cells bear Fc receptors capable of recognizing the Fc portion of bound immunoglobulins. If the antigen is on the surface of a cell, the K cell uses the bound immunoglobulin to make contact with that cell and lyse it by direct contact, a process termed *antibody-dependent cellular cytotoxicity* (ADCC). The K cell has no specificity for the antigen that is bound to the antibody, only for the Fc portion of the bound antibody (48). Some evidence suggests that K cells may actually be a subset of NK cells and that the distinction between them may simply reflect distinct stages of differentiation, or even simply the use of different assay systems.

Mast Cells and Granulocytes

A variety of other cells are involved in some immune responses, particularly those involving inflammation

(Table 1.4). Mast cells and basophils bear receptors (FcεRI) for the Fc portion of unbound IgE, permitting them to use IgE on their own surface as an antigen detector (49). When antigen binds simultaneously to two or more such IgE molecules on the same mast cell (called *bridging*), a signal is transmitted into the cell, leading to degranulation and release of a variety of mediators, including histamine, resulting in immediate hypersensitivity (allergic) responses (50). Neutrophils are drawn to sites of inflammation by cytokines, where their phagocytic activity and production of enzymes and other soluble mediators contribute to the inflammation. Eosinophils (51) are involved in immune responses against large parasites, such as roundworms, and are apparently capable of killing them by direct contact.

■ PRIMARY ORGANS: BONE MARROW AND THYMUS

The primordial stem cells that ultimately produce the human immune system (and other elements of the hematopoietic system) originate in the yolk sac about 60 days after fertilization. These cells migrate to the fetal liver and then (beginning about 80 days after fertilization) to the bone marrow, where they remain for life. These primordial hematopoietic stem cells give rise to more specialized stem cells, which lead to the erythrocytic, granulocytic, thrombocytic (platelet), myelocytic (e.g., macrophages and monocytes), and lymphocytic lineages.

Primary lymphoid organs consist of the bone marrow and thymus, where B and T lymphocytes, respectively, mature. B cells undergo their development, including generation of immunoglobulin receptors, while in the bone marrow. Cells of the T-lymphocyte lineage, however, migrate from the bone marrow to the thymus, where they undergo development and generation of TCRs. More than 95% of the cells that migrate into the thymus perish there, failing to survive a rigorous selection process to promote the development of those relevant to the individual's MHC genotype and to eliminate potentially self-reactive cells (52). It is in the thymus, under the influence of thymic stroma, nurse cells, and thymic APCs, that T cells receive an initial "thymic education" with regard to what should be recognized as self.

Secondary Organs: Spleen and Lymph Nodes

The secondary organs (e.g., spleen, lymph nodes, Peyer patches) provide sites where recirculating lymphocytes and APCs enter after passage through diverse parts of the body, "mingle" in close proximity for a period of time, and then leave again to recirculate. This intimate contact between recirculating cells facilitates the close interactions needed to initiate immune responses and generate appropriately sensitized cells, whose activities

may then be expressed throughout the body. Thus, most immune responses are actually initiated in the secondary organs.

■ INTERACTIONS IN IMMUNE RESPONSES

Antibody Responses

More than 99% of antibody responses are against T-dependent antigens, which require the involvement of T lymphocytes in generation of the responses. The relatively few T-independent (TI) antigens, which can provoke antibody production in the absence of T-cell involvement, fall into two general categories: TI-1 and TI-2. TI-1 antigens (e.g., a variety of lectins) are mitogenic, inducing proliferation and differentiation through binding of B-cell surface molecules other than immunoglobulins, whereas TI-2 antigens have regular repeating structures (e.g., dextran, with repetitive carbohydrate moieties) and are capable of cross-linking numerous immunoglobulin molecules on the surface of the same B cell.

Antibody responses to most antigens are T-dependent and require interactions between APCs (e.g., macrophages), T lymphocytes, and B lymphocytes, as illustrated in Fig. 1.9. Lymphocytes responding to T-dependent antigens require multiple signals for proliferation and differentiation: (a) the binding of their surface immunoglobulin by appropriate specific antigen, (b) the binding of cytokines (e.g., IL-4 and other helper factors) produced by activated helper T cells, and (c) binding of membrane ligands CD40 on B lymphocytes and CD154 on helper T cells (3,4,53). The help provided by T cells acts only over a short range; thus, the T and B cells must be in fairly intimate contact for these interactions to occur successfully. The involvement of APCs, such as macrophages or even B cells themselves, is essential for the activation of helper T cells and provides a means of bringing T and B cells into proximity.

Cellular Responses

Cellular immune responses are usually detected through detection of extensive proliferation, or through assessment of cell lysis or intensity of inflammation. For example, the mixed lymphocyte response (MLR) is an *in vitro* measure of T cell proliferation (primarily of $CD4^+$ T cells) that is often used as a measure of the initial phase (recognition and proliferation) of the cellular response. Splenic and/or lymph node T cells from the individual in question (responder) are mixed with lymphocytes from another individual (stimulator or sensitizer) against whom the response is to be evaluated. The stimulating cells are usually treated to prevent them from proliferating (e.g., with mitomycin or irradiation). The two cell populations are incubated together for 4 to 5 days, after which time a label (e.g., tritiated thymidine) is added to

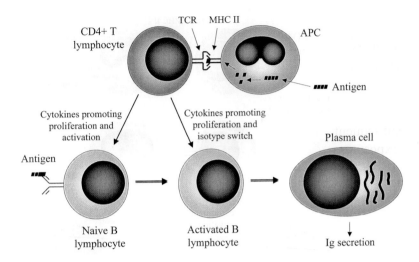

■ FIGURE 1.9 Interactions in antibody production.

the culture for a few hours. If responder cells actively proliferate as a result of the recognition of foreign antigens on the stimulating cells, increased incorporation of label (e.g., thymidine incorporation) occurs. The strongest MLR responses typically occur when the responding and sensitizing cells bear different class II MHC molecules. If the responder was highly sensitized *in vivo* before the MLR, responses to MHC class I and other non-MHC alloantigens can often be seen as well. The MLR is a subset of proliferative assays, one that is directed at genetically encoded alloantigens. The same principle can, however, be used to assess the proliferation of T cells against antigen in other forms, such as soluble antigen presented on the surface of APCs.

Cell-mediated lysis is the function of cytotoxic T lymphocytes. After appropriate stimulation (by antigen presented by class I MHC molecules on the surface of APC, together with help from T_H1 cells), CTLs proliferate and differentiate to become capable of binding and destroying target cells through direct cell–cell contact (Fig. 1.10). Clonally derived CTLs can lyse only those cells that bear the same combination of antigen and class I MHC molecules originally recognized by the originally stimulated CTL from which the clone was generated. Death of the target cell can be induced via cell membrane injury through the action of perforins secreted by the CTL or the induction of target cell apoptosis by binding of target cell receptors by ligands on the surface of CTLs (e.g., Fas/FasL), by cytokines (e.g., TNF-a) secreted by the CTL, or by the release from CTLs of granzymes that can enter the target cells through the membrane pores caused by perforin.

DTH is an *in vivo* response by inflammatory T_H1 (or T_{dh}) cells (Fig. 1.11). Individuals presensitized against a particular antigen, then later challenged intradermally with a small amount of the same antigen, display local inflammatory responses 24 to 72 hours later at the site of challenge. Perhaps the best known example is a positive

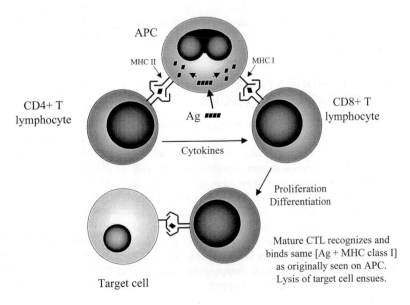

■ FIGURE 1.10 Cytotoxic T lymphocytes.

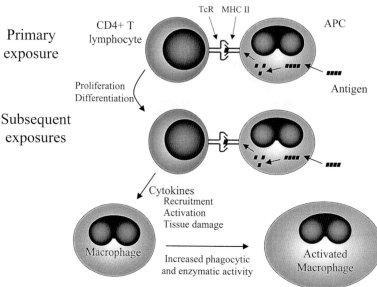

■ **FIGURE 1.11** Delayed-type hypersensitivity.

tuberculin skin test (Mantoux test). The response is mediated by $CD4^+$ T_H1 cells, previously sensitized against a particular combination of antigen and class II MHC molecules. On subsequent exposure to the same combination of antigen and class II MHC molecules, the T_H1 cells respond by secreting a series of cytokines (Table 1.3) that attract macrophages to the site and activate them. The activated macrophages exhibit increased size and activity, enabling them to destroy and phagocytize the antigenic stimulus. However, because macrophages are not antigen-specific, they can also destroy normal cells and tissues in the local area, causing *innocent bystander destruction.*

Contact dermatitis is an example of a normally protective T-cell–mediated immune response that becomes harmful under certain circumstances. Contact dermatitis is a DTH response, usually caused by the presence of small, chemically reactive antigens (e.g., heavy metals or, as in the case of poison ivy, plant lipids such as catechol) that bind to self proteins (e.g., class II MHC molecules) on the skin and produce neoantigens.

■ THE IMMUNE SYSTEM: A DOUBLE-EDGED SWORD

The immune system evolved to protect the body from a variety of external (infectious agents or harmful molecules) and internal (malignant cells) threats. In this regard, the immune system provides the body with a means for minimizing or preventing disease. This is most clearly illustrated by individuals who have defects in immune function (immunodeficiency disease) resulting from genetic, developmental, infective, or therapeutic causes. Because of its destructive potential, however, the immune system is also capable of causing disease when confronted with inappropriate antigenic stimulation or loss of regulatory control.

Transplantation

Transplantation involves the ability to replace damaged or diseased body parts by transplanting organs from one individual to another. Unfortunately, the immune system is exquisitely adept at recognizing nonself and rejecting transplanted organs from donors differing genetically from the recipient. The genetically encoded molecules that trigger the rejection response are termed *histocompatibility antigens* and are divided into two primary categories: major (encoded by class I and II MHC genes) and minor (scores, possibly hundreds, of antigens encoded by widely diverse genes scattered across the chromosomes). Because a genetically perfect match between host and donor in humans exists only between identical twins, transplantation surgeons are forced to minimize or eliminate the recipient immune response against the transplanted organ. Some of these responses can be minimized by using the closest possible genetic match between donor and recipient by tissue typing, but in humans, this is possible only for the HLA system. The alternative is the use of drugs to reduce immune responsiveness. Ideally, only the ability of the immune system to react to the antigens on the transplanted organ would be diminished (i.e., induction of antigen-specific immunologic tolerance), leaving the rest of the immune system intact. However, we currently must rely on drugs that depress the immune system in a relatively nonspecific fashion, thus leaving the patient susceptible to potentially fatal opportunistic infections. Recently, some agents (i.e., cyclosporine and FK506) have been found to diminish immune responses in a somewhat more specific fashion, but their long-term use may have secondary adverse effects on organs.

Bone marrow transplantation represents a special case in which the graft itself comprises immunocompetent tissue and the host is usually either immunodeficient or immunosuppressed. Thus, there is the possibility of the graft mounting an immune response against foreign host cells and tissues, leading to graft-versus-host disease.

Autoimmunity

Autoimmune diseases involve the development of antibody or cell-mediated immune responses directed against self antigens (54). In many autoimmune diseases, an individual's risk is affected by his or her HLA genes (55). There are several possible scenarios under which such undesirable responses might be initiated.

Autoimmune responses may arise when antigens that have been normally sequestered from the immune system (e.g., in immunologically privileged sites) are exposed as a result of trauma. Having never been detected previously by the immune system as it developed its sense of self versus nonself, such antigens are now seen as foreign. Secondly, immune responses against determinants on infectious agents may generate clones of lymphocytes with receptors capable of cross-reacting with self antigens (cross-reactive antigens). A classic example is rheumatic fever, which results from immune responses against streptococcal antigens that are cross-reactive with molecules found on cardiac tissue. Thirdly, some autoimmune responses, especially those that tend to develop in later life, may result from senescence of inhibitory mechanisms, such as suppressor and regulatory T lymphocytes, that keep autoimmune responses under control. For example, the onset of systemic lupus erythematosus is associated with aging and an accompanying decline in suppressor T-cell function. Finally, the interaction of self molecules with small reactive chemicals (e.g., haptens) or with infectious agents may produce alterations in self molecules (altered antigens or neoantigens), resulting in their detection as non-self. These are no longer truly self antigens, but the responses against them mimic autoimmune responses and may be mistaken for such in the absence of awareness of the chemical modifications.

Immune Complex Diseases

The humoral immune response is generally efficient in eliminating antigen–antibody complexes through the phagocytic cells of the reticuloendothelial system. There are, however, situations in which antigen–antibody complexes (involving IgG and IgM antibodies) reach such high concentrations that they leave solution and bind to cell surfaces or matrix and accumulate in tissues that are often unrelated to the source of the antigen. This may lead to systemic or localized inflammation as the complexes bind and activate serum complement components, attract phagocytic cells, and induce the release of proteolytic enzymes and other mediators of inflammation (56). Attempts to clear depositions of antigen–antibody complexes may lead to levels of inflammation intense enough to damage the tissues and organs involved. Such situations most often arise as a secondary effect of situations in which there is a persistence of antigen (e.g., chronic infection, cancer, autoimmunity, or frequent repeated administration of an external reagent), leading to continual stimulation of the immune system and production of high levels of antibodies against the persisting antigen. Among the most commonly damaged sites are the kidneys where the glomeruli tend to entrap and accumulate deposited complexes (glomerulonephritis), the synovial joint membranes (rheumatoid arthritis), the skin (vasculitis), and the endothelial walls of blood vessels (arteritis).

Allergies and Anaphylaxis (Immediate Hypersensitivity)

Allergies and anaphylaxis represent antigen-specific immunologic reactions involving IgE antibodies bound (by their Fc domain) to receptors on the surface of the membranes of mast cells and basophils (49, 50). When antigen is bound, resulting in cross-linking of the IgE molecules, human mast cells are stimulated to degranulate and release histamine, leukotrienes, kinins, platelet-activating factors, and other mediators of immediate hypersensitivity (49–50). The result is the rapid onset of an inflammatory response. Immediate hypersensitivity may develop against a wide array of environmental substances and may be localized (e.g., itching, tearing) or systemic (e.g., involving the circulatory system). The latter may be life-threatening if severe.

■ TOLERANCE

In many cases, it is desirable to diminish or eliminate immune responses, thus inducing tolerance to some particular antigen. For example, autoimmune responses, asthmatic and allergic responses, and the host responses against transplanted tissues or organs all represent situations in which such tolerance would be desirable. There are two approaches: nonspecific and specific.

Immunosuppression is the elimination of all immune responses, regardless of the specificity of those responses. This may occur naturally, as in the case of individuals who are deficient in immune function for genetic reasons (e.g., severe combined immunodeficiency disease) or as the result of infection (e.g., acquired immunodeficiency syndrome). Alternatively, it may be intentionally imposed by the application of radiation, drugs, or other therapeutic reagents (e.g., antilymphocyte sera). Such procedures, however, impose a new set of risks because their nonspecificity leaves the patient (or experimental animal) open to infections by opportunistic pathogens. Attempts to diminish these consequences involve the development of reagents with narrower effects, including drugs such as cyclosporine and FK506, or the application of antibodies specific for only particular subsets of lymphocytes. Immunologic tolerance is the *specific* acquired inability of individuals to respond to a specific immunogenic determinant toward which they would otherwise normally respond. Tolerance is more desirable than immunosuppression because it eliminates or inactivates only those lymphocytes involved in the responses of concern, leaving the remainder of the immune system intact to deal with opportunistic infections.

The natural induction of tolerance during the development of the immune system prevents immune responses against self antigens (*self tolerance*), thus preventing autoimmunity. Experimentally, tolerance can be induced in immunocompetent adult animals by manipulating a variety of factors, including age, the physical nature and dose of antigen, and the route of administration (57–60). Tolerance may be induced in both T and B lymphocytes, although tolerance of T cells generally requires lower doses of antigen and is effective for a longer period of time. In addition, because B lymphocytes require T-cell help, the induction of tolerance in T cells often also diminishes corresponding antibody responses.

The means by which specific tolerance is induced and maintained involves three general mechanisms, all of which probably occur in various situations. *Clonal deletion* or abortion is the actual elimination of those clones of lymphocytes that encounter the specific antigen under particular conditions. *Clonal anergy* is the functional inactivation of those clones of lymphocytes that encounter the specific antigen in a tolerogenic form, which may be reversible. *Antigen-specific suppression* relies on the presence of cells that inhibit the antigen-specific induction or expression of immune responses by other T or B lymphocytes. It is known that T_H1 cells (promoting cellular and inflammatory responses) and T_H2 cells (promoting antibody responses) directed against the same antigen may inhibit one another through the cytokines they secrete. Thus, a response against a given antigen may be dominated by cellular responses in one case and by antibody responses in another. And, for example, attempts to alleviate cellular inflammatory responses directed against a given antigen may involve the promotion of antibody responses against the same antigen. Recently, the importance of certain types of regulatory cells such as the $CD4^+CD25^+FoxP3^+$ T_{reg} cells in inducing and maintaining tolerance has created considerable interest, not only in dissecting the normal process, but suggesting clues for ways to manipulate the system to induce tolerance where it is absent but needed (44). For example, the association of autoimmune disorders with advancing age is often attributed to age-related declines in suppressor T cells.

The immune system is an amazing biologic system. Precise interactions must occur, in appropriate sequences and quantities, between a bewildering array of cells and molecules. Moreover, these highly specific cells and molecules must find one another, after patrolling throughout the entire body, in order to coordinate their activities. It is so complex that it seems incredible at times that it works at all. We still have far to go in learning how to reliably correct and alleviate the occasions when it malfunctions with potentially harmful consequences.

■ REFERENCES

1. Menendez AS, Finlay BB. Defensins in the immunology of bacterial infections. *Curr Opin Immunol.* 2007;19:385–391.
2. Janeway CA Jr, Medzhitov R. Innate immune recognition. *Annu Rev Immunol.* 2002;20:197.
3. Murphy K, Travers P, Walport M. *Janeway's Immunobiology.* 7th ed. New York: Garland Science, 2008.
4. Jinnushi M, Vanneman M, Munshi N, et al. MHC Class I chain-related protein A antibodies and shedding are associated with the progression of multiple myeloma. *Proc Natl Acad Sciences.* 2008;105:1285–1290.
5. Abbas A, Lichtman AH, Pilaj S. *Cellular and Molecular Immunology,* 6th ed. Philadelphia: Elsevier Health Sciences, 2007.
6. Takeda K, Kaisho T, Akira S. Toll-like receptors. *Annu Rev Immunol.* 2003;21:335–376.
7. Lauzon NM, Mian F, Ashkar AA. Toll-like receptors, natural killer cells and innate immunity. *Adv Exp Med Biol.* 2007;598:1–11.
8. Ravetch J, Aderem A. Phagocytic cells. *Immunol Rev.* 2007;219:5–7.
9. Cresswell P. Antigen processing and presentation. *Immunol Rev.* 2005;207:5–7.
10. Gasser S, Raulet DH. Activation and self-tolerance of natural killer cells. *Immunol Rev.* 2006;214:130–142.
11. Lanier LL. NK cell recognition. *Annu Rev Immunol.* 2005;23:225–274.
12. Gros P, Milder FJ, Jansson BJ. Complement driven by conformational changes. *Nat Rev Immunol.* 2008;8:48–58.
13. Berzofsky JA, Berkhower IJ. Immunogenicity and antigen structure. In: Paul WE, ed. *Fundamental Immunology,* 5th ed. Philadelphia: Lippincott Williams and Wilkins, 2003.
14. Brandtzaeg P. Induction of secretory immunity and memory at mucosal surfaces. *Vaccine* 2007;25:5467–5484.
15. Jung D, Giallourakis C, Mostoslavsky R, et al. Mechanism and control of V(D)J recombination at the immunoglobulin heavy chain locus. *Annu Rev Immunol.* 2006;24:451–470.
16. Spicuglia S, Franchini DM, Ferrier M. Regulation of V(D)J recombination. *Curr Opin Immunol.* 2006;18:158–163.
17. Edry M, Mohamed D. Class switch recombination: a friend and a foe. *Clin Immunol.* 2007;123:244–251.
18. Benedict CL, Gilfillian S, Thai TH, et al. Terminal deoxynucleotidyl transferase and repertoire development. *Immunol Rev.* 2000;175:150–157.
19. Di Noia JM, Neuberger MS. Molecular mechanisms of antibody somatic hypermutation. *Annu Rev Biochem.* 2007;76:1–22.
20. Krogsgaard M, Davis MM. How T cells see antigen. *Nat Immunol.* 2005;6:239–245.
21. Xiong N, Raulet DH. Development and selection of $\gamma\delta$ T cells. *Immunol Rev.* 2007;215:15–31.
22. Kuhns MS, Davis MM, Garcia KC. Deconstructing the form and function of the TCR/CD3 complex. *Immunity.* 2006;24:133–139.
23. Mazza C, Malisson B. What guides MHC-restricted TCR recognition? *Semin Immunol.* 2007;19:225–235.
24. Rudolph MG, Stanfield RL, Wilson, IA. How TCRs bind MHCs, peptides, and co-receptors. *Annu Rev Immunol.* 2006;24:419–466.
25. Williams A, Peh CA, Elliott T. The cell biology of MHC class I antigen presentation. *Tissue Antigens* 2002;59:3–17.
26. Holling TM, Schooten E, van Den Elsen PJ. Function and regulation of MHC class II molecules in T-lymphocytes: of mice and men. *Hum Immunol.* 2004;65:282–290.
27. Lai L, Alaverdi N, Maltais L, et al. Mouse cell surface antigens: nomenclature and immunophenotyping. *J Immunol.* 1998;160:3861–3868.

28. Kumanovics A, Takada T, Lindahl KF. Genomic organization of the mammalian MHC. *Annu. Rev. Immunol.* 2003;21:629–657.

29. Shao L, Kamalu O, Mayer L. Non-classical MHC class I molecules on intestinal epithelial cells: mediators of mucosal crosstalk. *Immunol Rev.* 2005;206:160–176.

30. Pestka S, Krause CD, Walter MR. Interferons, interferon-like cytokines, and their receptors. *Immunol Rev.* 2004;202:8–32.

31. Wan YY, Flavell RA. The roles for cytokines in the generation and maintenance of regulatory T cells. *Immunol Rev.* 2006;212:114–130.

32. Rot A, van Adrian UH. Chemokines in innate and adaptive host defense: basic chemokinese grammar for immune cells. *Annu Rev Immunol.* 2004;22:891–928.

33. Sharpe AH, Freeman GJ. The B7-CD28 superfamily. *Nat Rev Immunol.* 2002;2:116–126.

34. Sansom DM, Walker LS. The role of CD28 and cytotoxic T-lymphocyte antigen-4 (CTLA-4) in regulatory T-cell biology. *Immunol Rev.* 2006;212:131–148.

35. Xu Y, Song G. the role of CD40-CD154 interaction in cell immunoregulation. *J Biomed. Sci.* 2004;11:426–438.

36. Sela M, Pecht I. The nature of the antigen. *Adv Protein Chem.* 1996;49:289–328.

37. Vestweber D. Adhesion and signaling molecules controlling the transmigration of leukocytes through endothelium. *Immunol Rev.* 2007;218:178–196.

38. Lefrancois L. Development, trafficking, and function of memory T-cell subsets. *Immunol Rev.* 2006;211:93–103.

39. Rothenberg EV, Taghon T. Antigen-specific memory B cell development. *Annu Rev Immunol.* 2005;23:487–513.

40. Kalia V, Sarkar S, Gourley TS, et al. Differentiation of memory B and T cells. *Curr Opin Immunol.* 2006;18:255–264.

41. Romagnani S. Regulation of the T cell response. *Clin. Exp. Allergy.* 2006;36:1357–1366.

42. Wong P, Pamer EG. CD8 T cell responses to infectious pathogens. *Annu Rev Immunol.* 2003;21:29–70.

43. Raupach B, Kaufmann SH. Immune responses to intracellular bacteria. *Curr Opin Immunol.* 2001;13:417–428.

44. Sakaguchi S, Ono M, Setoguchi R, et al. Foxp3+CD25+CD4+ natural regulatory T cells in dominant self-tolerance and autoimmune disease. *Immunol Rev.* 2006;212:8–27.

45. Bendelac A, Savage PB, Teyton L. The biology of NKT cells. *Ann. Rev. Immunol.* 2007;25:297–336.

46. Van Kaer L. NKT cells: T lymphocytes with innate effector functions. *Curr Opin Immunol.* 2007;19:354–364.

47. Kronenberg M, Havran WL. Frontline T cells: γδ T cells and intraepithelial lymphocytes. *Immunol Rev.* 2007;215:5–7.

48. Sulica A, Morel P, Metes D, et al. Ig-binding receptors on human NK cells as effector and regulating surface molecules. *Int Rev Immunol.* 2001;20:371–414.

49. Robbie-Ryan M, Brown M. The role of mast cells in allergy and autoimmunity. *Curr Opin Immunol.* 2002;14:728–733.

50. Gould HJ, Sutton BK, Beavil AJ, et al. The biology of IgE and the basis of allergic disease. *Annu Rev Immunol.* 2003;21:579–628.

51. Dombrowicz D, Capron M. Eosinophils, allergy and parasites. *Curr Opin Immunol.* 2004;26:25–34.

52. Starr TK, Jameson SC, Hogquist KA. Positive and negative selection of T cells. *Ann Rev Immunol.* 2002;21:139–176.

53. Ollila J, Vihinen M. B cells. *Int J Biochem Cell Biol.* 2005;37:518–523.

54. Diamond B. Autoimmunity. *Immunol Rev.* 2005;204:5–8.

55. McDevitt HO. Discovering the role of the major histocompatibility complex in the immune response. *Annu Rev Immunol.* 2000;18:1–17.

56. Jancar S, Sanchez Crespo M. Immune complex-mediated tissue injury: a multistep paradigm. *Trends Immunol.* 2005;26:48–55.

57. Faria AM, Weiner HL. Oral tolerance. *Immunol Rev.* 2005;206:232–259.

58. Gallegos AM, Bevan MJ. Central tolerance: good but imperfect. *Immunol Rev.* 2006;209:290–296.

59. Kyewski B, Klein L. A central role for central tolerance. *Annu Rev Immunol.* 2006;24:571–605.

60. Romagnani S. Immunological tolerance and autoimmunity. *Intern Emerg Med.* 2006;1:187–196.

CHAPTER 2

Immunology of IgE-mediated and Other Hypersensitivity Responses

C. RAYMOND ZEISS

■ HISTORICAL REVIEW OF IgE-MEDIATED HYPERSENSITIVITY

In 1902, Richet and Portier described the development of anaphylaxis in dogs given sea anemone toxin; subsequently, anaphylaxis was described in humans after the injection of horse serum to achieve passive immunization against tetanus and diphtheria. In 1906, Clemens von Pirquet correctly predicted that immunity and hypersensitivity reactions would depend on the interaction between a foreign substance and the immune system, and that immunity and hypersensitivity would have similar underlying immunologic mechanisms (1).

The search for the factor responsible for immediate hypersensitivity reactions became a subject of intense investigation over several years. The transfer of allergy to horse dander by transfusion was reported by Ramirez in 1919 (2). In 1921, Prausnitz and Küstner (3) described the transfer of immediate hypersensitivity (to fish protein) by serum to the skin of a normal individual. This test for the serum factor responsible for immediate hypersensitivity reactions was termed the *Prausnitz-Küstner test*. Variations of this test remained the standard for measuring skin sensitizing antibody over the next 50 years.

In 1925, Coca and Grove (4) extensively studied the skin-sensitizing factor from sera of patients with ragweed hay fever. They called skin-sensitizing antibody *atopic reagin* because of its association with hereditary conditions and because of their uncertainty as to the nature of the antibody involved. Thereafter, this factor was called *atopic reagin*, *reaginic antibody*, or *skin-sensitizing antibody*. This antibody clearly had unusual properties and could not be measured readily by standard immunologic methods. Major research efforts from the 1920s through the 1960s defined its physical and chemical properties and measured its presence in allergic individuals (5,6).

In 1967, the Ishizakas discovered that skin-sensitizing antibody belonged to a unique class of immunoglobulin, which they called immunoglobulin E (IgE). In elegant studies using immunologic techniques, they clearly demonstrated that reagin-rich serum fractions from a patient with ragweed hay fever belonged to a unique class of immunoglobulin (7). Shortly thereafter, the Swedish researchers Johansson and Bennich discovered a new myeloma protein, termed *IgND*, which had no antigenic relation to the other immunoglobulin classes. In 1969, cooperative studies between these workers and Ishizakas confirmed that the proteins were identical and that a new class of immunoglobulin, IgE, had been discovered (8,9).

■ PHYSIOLOGY OF IgE

IgE Structure and Receptors

The immunochemical properties of IgE are shown in Table 2.1 in contrast to those of the other immunoglobulin classes. IgE is a glycoprotein that has a molecular weight of 190,000 with a sedimentation coefficient of 8S. Like all immunoglobulins, IgE has a four-chain structure with two light chains and two heavy chains. The heavy chains contain five domains (one variable and four constant regions) that carry unique, antigenic specificities termed the *epsilon* (ε) *determinants* (Fig. 2.1A). These unique antigenic structures determine the class specificity of this protein. Digestion with papain yields the Fc fragment, which contains the epsilon antigenic determinants and two Fab fragments. The Fab fragments contain the antigen-combining sites. The tertiary structure of the Fc fragment is responsible for the protein's ability to bind to the FcεRI receptors on mast cells and basophils (10).

The FcεR1 receptor is the high-affinity receptor for IgE found on mast cells, basophils, eosinophils, and human skin Langerhans cells (11). Cross-linking of high-affinity receptor-bound IgE by allergen results in the release of mediators from mast cells and basophils. Molecular biologic techniques have been used to clone the gene encoding the ε chain of human IgE (ND) and

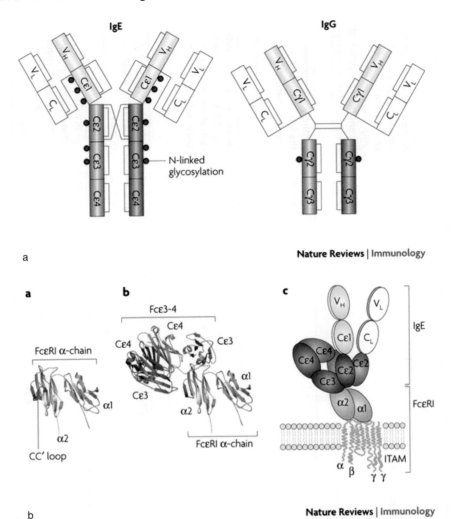

■ **FIGURE 2.1 A:** The domain structure of IgE and IgG. Schematic representations of the polypeptide and domain structures of human IgE and IgG1 showing the intra and inter-domain disulphide bridges, and sites of N-linked glycosylation. (From Gould HJ, and Sutton BJ. IgE in allergy and asthma today. *Nature Reviews Immunol* 2008; 8: 205–215.) **B:** The structures of the FcεRI α chain and its complex with IgE. (A) The structure of the extracellular domains of the FcεRI α chain taken from the crystal structure of the Fcε3-4-FcεRI α chain complex. (B) The structure of the high affinity complex between Fcε3-4 and the extracellular domains of the FcεRI α chain, showing the extensive interaction surface and engagement of both Cε3 domains. (C) Representation of the entire IgE molecule bound to the extracellular domains of the FcεRI α chain. The β and γ chains of the FcεRI, with their immunoreceptor tyrosine based activation motifs (ITAMS) are depicted (15).

to determine the site on IgE that binds to its receptor (12). Studies have localized this site to the Cε3 heavy chain domains (13). The high-affinity receptor for IgE is composed of an α chain, a β chain, and two γ chains, and it is the α chain that binds IgE (Fig. 2.1B). The crystal structure of the α chain has been determined, giving insights into the interaction of IgE with its receptor at the molecular level (14,15). The β and γ chains are involved in signal transduction when the receptors are aggregated by the cross-linking of IgE, resulting in mediator release (16). The IgE receptor on dendritic and other antigen-presenting cells is expressed in a heterotrimeric form α,γ,γ and is called FcεRII or CD23

(17,18). The capture of IgE allergen complexes by the dendritic cell IgE receptor is a highly efficient mechanism for allergen presentation to T cells (17).

Studies have delineated the central role that IgE molecules in the circulation play in determining the number of FcεRI receptors on mast cells and basophils (19,20) and consequently the release of mediators from these cells. After infusion of anti-IgE monoclonal antibody in allergic subjects, there is a significant reduction in serum levels of free IgE, with a dramatic fall in basophil FcεRI number and mediator release; of note, the total serum IgE is not reduced. The availability of anti-IgE monoclonal antibodies for the treatment of allergic

TABLE 2.1 IMMUNOGLOBULIN ISOTYPES

ISOTYPE	NO. OF C$_H$ DOMAINS	APPROXIMATE SIZE (KD)	ADDITIONAL COMPONENTS	PERCENTAGE OF SERUM IMMUNOGLOBULIN	APPROXIMATE HALF-LIFE (D)	FUNCTIONS
IgA						
Monomer[a]	3	160,000	J chain	13–19	6	Provides antibodies for external body fluids, including mucus, saliva, and tears; effective at neutralizing infectious agents, agglutination, and (when bound to antigen) activation of the alternative complement pathway
Dimer[b]	3	385,000	Secretory piece	0.3		
IgD						
Monomer[a,b]	3	180,000		<1	3	Found almost entirely in membrane-bound form; the function is unknown, but may be related to maturational stages
IgE						
Monomer[a,b]	4	190,000		<0.001	3	IgE is bound to mast cell surfaces; subsequent binding of antigen stimulates mast cell degranulation, leading to immediate hypersensitivity responses (allergy)
IgG						
Monomer[a,b]	3	145,000–170,000		72–80	20	Found in four subclasses: IgG1, IgG2, IgG3, and IgG4; prevalent isotype in secondary responses
IgM						
Monomer[a]	4	—	—	—	5–10	Prevalent isotype in primary responses; effective at agglutination and activation of classic complement pathway
Pentamer[b]	4	970,000	J chain	6–8	—	

C$_H$, constant heavy chain.
[a] Membrane-bound form.
[b] Secreted form.

subjects has led to a wealth of information on the complex physiology of lowering free IgE levels in serum (17). The monoclonal anti-IgE antibody, omalizumab, binds circulating IgE at the same site in the Cε3 domain as the FcεRI receptor. It therefore binds free IgE and not FcεRI receptor-bound IgE on mast cells and basophils, which would lead to mediator release (17). A low-affinity FcεRII receptor (CD23) has been localized to B lymphocytes, monocytes, macrophages, platelets, eosinophils, and epithelial cells (15, 21). The receptor has an A form found only on B lymphocytes and a B form found on all cells expressing CD23. The molecular structure of CD23 has been delineated in detail; its binding site for IgE has three domains and in this trimeric form has a binding affinity for the IgE Cε3 region approaching that of the FceR1 receptor (15). The expression of this receptor is markedly up-regulated on all cell types by interleukin-4 (IL-4) and IL-13. Binding of IgE to this receptor places IgE at the center of activation of many important effector cells and adds an additional receptor on the B cell whereby IgE can present allergen to T cells (15,21). The role of CD23 in regulation of the IgE response is complex, having both positive and inhibitory effects (15,21).

Sites of IgE Production, Turnover, and Tissue Localization

With the advent of a highly specific reagent for detecting IgE antibody against the Fc portion of IgE (anti-IgE), the sites of production of this immunoglobulin could be examined by fluorescent-labeled anti-IgE. It was found that lymphoid tissue of the tonsils, adenoids, and the bronchial and peritoneal areas contained IgE-forming plasma cells. IgE-forming plasma cells also were found in the respiratory and intestinal mucosa (22). This distribution is similar to that of IgA. However, unlike IgA, IgE is not associated with a secretory piece, although IgE is found in respiratory and intestinal secretions. The traffic of IgE molecules from areas of production to the tissues and the circulation has not been established. Areas of production in the respiratory and intestinal mucosa are associated with the presence of tissue mast cells (23). There has been renewed interest in the local mucosal production of IgE by IgE+ B cells. In grass- and ragweed-sensitive individuals there is clear evidence of marked local production of specific IgE after allergen challenge using elegant techniques to track gene activation (class switch recombination) involved in IgE production by B cells (24). It is speculated that most IgE production occurs in mucosal tissue sites (15,24)

With the development of techniques to measure total IgE in the blood and the availability of purified IgE protein, investigators were able to study the metabolic properties of this immunoglobulin in normal individuals (25). The mean total circulating IgE pool was found to be 3.3 μg/kg of body weight, in contrast to the total circulating IgG pool of about 500,000 μg/kg of body weight. IgE has an intravascular half-life of only 2.3 days. The rate of IgE production was found to be 2.3 μg/kg/day.

It had been known for several years that the half-life of reaginic antibody in human skin as determined by passive transfer studies was about 14 days. This was reconfirmed with studies that investigated the disappearance of radiolabeled IgE in human skin. The half-life in the skin was reported to be between 8 days and 14 days (7). The basophil and mast cell-bound IgE pool needs to be investigated thoroughly, but it has been estimated that only 1% of the total IgE is cell-bound. Direct quantification of specific IgE in the blood, in contrast to specific IgE on the basophil surface, indicates that for every IgE molecule on the basophil, there are 100 to 4,000 molecules in circulation (26).

IgE Synthesis

Major advances in the understanding of IgE synthesis have resulted from human and animal studies (27–33). Tada (27) studied the production of IgE antibody in rats and found that IgE antibody production is regulated by cooperation between T lymphocytes (T cells) and B lymphocytes (B cells). The T cells provide the helper function, and the B cells are the producers of IgE antibody.

In human systems, it became clear that IgE production from B cells required T-cell signals that were unique to the IgE system (28). In 1986, Coffman and Carty (29) defined the essential role of IL-4 in the production of IgE. The pathway to IgE production is complex, requiring not only IL-4 and IL-13 but also T- and B-cell contact, major histocompatibility complex (MHC) restriction, adhesion molecules, expression of FcεRII (CD23) receptors, CD40 and CD40 ligand interaction, and the terminal action of IL-5 and IL-6 (30).

IL-4 acts on precursor B lymphocytes and is involved in the class switch recombination to ε heavy chain production (28). Class switch recombination is a complex process that results in class switching to IgE generating in the process switch circles and circle transcripts that signify ongoing or recent B-cell switch recombination (15,24). IL-4 and IL-13 are not sufficient to complete the switch to functional ε messenger RNA, and several second signals have been described that result in productive messenger RNA transcripts (31,32). In the absence of those signals, sterile transcripts result. A key physiologic second signal is provided by CD4+ helper T-cell contact. This contact signal is provided by CD40 ligand on activated T cells, which interacts with the CD40 receptor on IL-4–primed B cells and completes isotype switching to IgE (30). Several studies indicate that IgE synthesis is critically dependent on the IL-4 receptor α chain and nuclear factors such as NF-κB and Stat6 (33). Another cytokine, interferon-γ (IFN-γ), suppresses IgE production, acting at the same point as IL-4 (30). This complex set of interactions is shown in Fig. 2.2.

During the secondary IgE response to allergen, allergen-specific B lymphocytes capture allergen by surface IgE, internalize and degrade it, and present it to T cells as peptides complexed to class II MHC molecules. This leads to T-cell–B-cell interaction, mutual exchange of cytokine and cell contact signals, and enhanced allergen-specific IgE production.

■ ROLE OF IgE IN HEALTH AND DISEASE

IgE in Health

The fetus is capable of producing IgE by 11 weeks gestation. Johansson and Foucard (34) measured total IgE in sera from children and adults. They found that cord serum contained 13 to 202 ng/mL and that the concentration of IgE in the cord serum did not correlate with

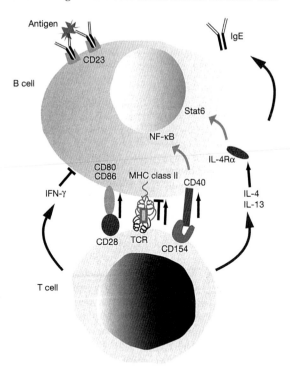

■ **FIGURE 2.2** The molecular control of the IgE response. Interleukin-4 (IL-4) and IL-13 are the most important cytokine inducers of IgE production acting at the IL-4 receptor α chain and through nuclear factor, Stat6. Interferon-γ (IFN-γ) is the most important inhibitor of IgE synthesis. CD154, the T-cell ligand for CD40 on the B cell, promotes IgE transcription through nuclear factor, NF-κB. Antigen presented to the T-cell receptor (TCR) by class II major histocompatibility complex molecules on the B cell initiates this complex process. (Adapted from Cory DB, Kheradmand F. Induction and regulation of the IgE response. *Nature* 1999;402s: 18–23, with permission.)

the serum IgE concentration of the mother, which confirmed that IgE does not cross the placenta. In children, IgE levels increase steadily and peak between 10 and 15 years of age. Johansson and Foucard illustrate well the selection of population groups for determining the normal level of serum IgE. Studies of healthy Swedish and Ethiopian children showed a marked difference in mean IgE levels: Swedish children had a mean of 160 ng/mL, and Ethiopian children had a mean of 860 ng/mL (35). Barbee and coworkers (36) studied the IgE levels in atopic and nonatopic people 6 to 75 years of age in Tucson, AZ. IgE levels peaked in those aged 6 to 14 years and gradually declined with advancing age; male subjects had higher levels of IgE than female subjects (Fig. 2.3).

Several roles for the possible beneficial effect of IgE antibody have been postulated. The presence of IgE antibody on mast cells in the tissues that contain heparin and histamine points to a role for IgE in controlling the microcirculation, and a role for the mast cell as a "sentinel" or first line of defense against microorganisms has been advanced. The hypothesis is that IgE antibody specific for bacterial or viral antigens could have a part in localizing high concentrations of protective antibody at the site of tissue invasion (37,38).

The role of IgE antibody has been studied extensively in an experimental infection of rats with the parasite *Nippostrongylus brasiliensis*. IgE antibody on the surface of mast cells in the gut may be responsible for triggering histamine release and helping the animal to reduce the worm burden (39). In experimental *Schistosoma mansoni* infection in the rat, IgE is produced at high levels to schistosome antigens. IgE complexed to these antigens has a role in antibody-dependent cell-mediated cytotoxicity, whereas eosinophils, macrophages, and platelets are effector cells that damage the parasite (40). IgE and IgE immune complexes are bound to these effector cells by the IgE FcεRII receptor, which has a high affinity for IgE immune complexes. Effector cells triggered by FcεRII receptor aggregation result in release of oxygen metabolites, lysosomal enzymes, leukotrienes, and platelet-activating factor. These observations in animals have relevance to human populations, where the IgE inflammatory cascade may protect against helminth infections (40).

IgE in Disease

The Atopic State and the T_H2 Paradigm

Extensive evidence has accumulated that may define the underlying immunologic basis for the atopic phenotype, that is, individuals with allergic asthma, allergic rhinitis, and atopic eczema (30). The atopic condition can be viewed as a T_H2 lymphocyte-driven response to allergens of complex genetic and environmental origins (41). The current view is that the immature T_H2 neonatal response

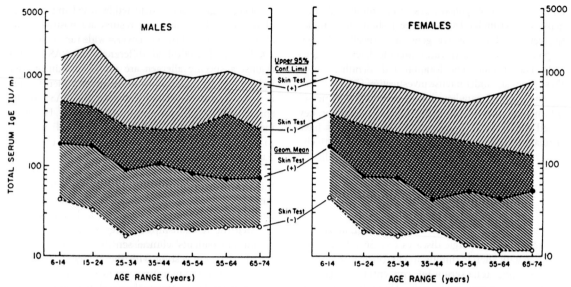

■ FIGURE 2.3 Serum IgE as function of age and sex among whites in the United States. Geometric means and upper 95% confidence intervals are plotted against age for males and females with positive and negative results from skin tests. Double cross-hatched area represents overlap of total IgE levels between the two groups of subjects. Age-related declines in serum IgE are significant in all groups. (From Knauer KA, Adkinson NF. Clinical significance of IgE. In: Middleton E, Reed CE, Ellis EJ, eds. *Allergy principles and practice*. St. Louis: CV Mosby, 1983, with permission.)

is modified by environmental microbial exposure early in postnatal life, is modulated to a more mature and balanced T_H1 dominant pattern in normal individuals, and the T_H2 pattern persists in atopic individuals. The reasons for this persistence of the T_H2 pattern of response in atopic individuals is complex and may be related to their early response to environmental microbial exposure, the "hygiene hypothesis" (42). This interface with environmental microbial exposure has led to the investigation of the important role of the innate immune system, Toll-like receptors, and barrier epithelium in the genesis and pathogenesis of allergic disease (43,44).

Historically, the reciprocal action of IL-4 and IFN-γ on IgE production led to several studies on the T-cell origin of these cytokines. Mosmann and Coffman (45) described two distinct types of helper T cells in murine systems and defined them as T_H1 or T_H2 cells by the pattern of cytokine secretion. T_H1 cells produced IL-2, IFN-γ, and IL-12. T_H2 cells produced IL-4, IL-5, IL-6, and IL-10.

A significant body of evidence has further defined the role of T_H2 cells in the human atopic state related to IL-4 production, IgE synthesis, and the maturation and recruitment of eosinophils by IL-5 and the maturation of IgE B cells by IL-5 and IL-6 (30,41). T cells having the T_H2 cytokine profile have been cloned from individuals with a variety of atopic diseases (30), have been identified in the airway of atopic asthmatic patients, and have been implicated as fundamental to persistent airway inflammation in asthma (46,47).

Once a T_H2 response is established, there is down-regulation of T_H1 cells by the cytokines IL-4 and IL-10.

T_H1 cells are capable of down-regulating T_H2 cytokine secretion through the reciprocal action of IFN-γ on T_H2 cells, a physiologic control that is abrogated by the predominant T_H2 cell response in the atopic individual (48) (Fig. 2.4).

The expression of the atopic state is dependent on genes that control the T_H2 response, total IgE production,

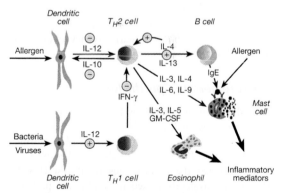

■ FIGURE 2.4 The T_H2 cell paradigm in allergic disease. The interaction of allergen, dendritic cell, and cytokine environment causes naïve CD4$^+$ T cells to differentiate to the T_H2 phenotype with the capacity for enhanced secretion of cytokines that drive and maintain the allergic inflammatory response. The established T_H2 response down-regulates the influence of T_H1 cells and the inhibitory effect of interferon-γ (IFN-γ), by the action of cytokines IL-10 and IL-4. These cytokine pathways are under complex genetic control that defines the atopic phenotype. (Adapted from Holgate ST. The epidemic of allergy and asthma. *Nature* 1999;402s:2–4, with permission.)

and specific IgE responsiveness to environmental allergens. High serum IgE levels have been shown to be under the control of a recessive gene, and specific allergen responses are associated with human leukocyte antigens (49). The chromosomal location and identification of these genes are under intense investigation (50,51).

The T_H1/T_H2 paradigm has been modified by newer information that includes the role of two other key T-cell populations, Tregs and T_H17 cells, that have regulatory and proinflamatory actions, respectively, each of which can shift the balance toward the allergic phenotype (52).

Measurement of Total IgE

Several early studies evaluated the role of IgE in patients with a variety of allergic diseases (34–36). Adults and children with allergic rhinitis and extrinsic asthma tend to have higher total serum IgE concentrations as compared to nonatopic individuals. About half of atopic patients have total IgE concentrations that are two standard deviations above the mean of a normal control group. Significant overlap of total serum IgE concentrations in normal subjects and in patients with allergic asthma and hay fever has been demonstrated (Fig. 2.3). Therefore, the total serum IgE concentration is neither a specific nor sensitive diagnostic test for the presence of atopic disorders.

Total serum IgE has been found to be markedly elevated in some patients with atopic dermatitis (AD), and the serum IgE concentration correlates with the severity of the AD and with the presence of allergic rhinitis, asthma, or both. Patients with AD without severe skin disease or accompanying asthma or hay fever may have normal IgE concentrations (53). Total IgE concentrations have been found to be markedly elevated in allergic bronchopulmonary aspergillosis.

Measurement of Specific IgE

Since the discovery of IgE in 1967, it is possible not only to measure total IgE in the serum but also to measure IgE antibody against complex as well as purified allergens. One of the first methods described by Wide et al. (54) was the radioallergosorbent test (RAST). Allergen is covalently linked to solid-phase particles, and these solid-phase particles are incubated with the patient's serum, which may contain IgE antibody specific for that allergen. After a period of incubation, the specific IgE present binds firmly to the solid phase. The solid phase is then washed extensively, and the last reagent added is radiolabeled anti-IgE antibody. The bound radiolabeled anti-IgE reflects amounts of specific IgE bound to the allergen. The results are usually given in RAST units or in units in which a standard serum containing significant amounts of IgE specific for a particular allergen is used as a reference.

Specific IgE antibody detected by RAST in the serum of patients whose skin test results are positive to an allergen has been shown to cover a wide range. Between 100-fold and 1,000-fold differences in RAST levels against a specific allergen are found in skin-reactive individuals. In studies of large groups of patients, there is a significant correlation between the RAST result, specific IgE level, and skin test reactivity. However, individuals with the same level of specific IgE antibody to ragweed allergen may vary 100-fold in their skin reactivity to that allergen (55).

The RAST concept has been extended to the use of fluorescent- and enzyme-labeled anti-IgE, which obviates the need for radiolabeled materials. Although RAST and other specific IgE measurement technologies have clarified the relationships between specific IgE in the serum and patients' clinical sensitivity, these tests do not replace skin testing with the allergens in clinical practice because skin testing is more sensitive.

It is possible to estimate the absolute quantity of specific IgE antibody per milliliter of serum against complex and purified allergens (56,57). Using one of these *in vitro* methods to measure IgE antibody against ragweed allergens, Gleich et al. (56) defined the natural rise and fall of ragweed-specific IgE over a 1-year period. In this population of ragweed-sensitive individuals, the IgE antibody specific for ragweed allergens varied from 10 to 1,000 ng/mL. A marked rise of specific IgE level occurred after the pollen season, with a peak in October followed by a gradual decrease. Specific IgE level reached a low point just before the next ragweed season in August (Fig. 2.5). It is also possible to measure basophil-bound, total, and specific IgE against ragweed antigen E, now called *Amb a1*. There are between 100,000 and 500,000 molecules of total IgE per basophil (58) and between 2500 and 50,000 molecules of specific IgE per basophil (26).

■ OTHER HYPERSENSITIVITY RESPONSES

All immunologically mediated hypersensitivity responses had been classified into four types by Gell and Coombs in 1964. This classification has been a foundation for an understanding of the immunopathogenesis of clinical hypersensitivity syndromes (59). This schema depends on the location and class of antibody that interacts with antigen resulting in effector cell activation and tissue injury.

In type I, or immediate, hypersensitivity, allergen interacts with IgE antibody on the surface of mast cells and basophils, resulting in the cross-linking of IgE, FcεRI receptor apposition, and mediator release from these cells. Only a few allergen molecules, interacting with cell-bound IgE, lead to the release of many mediator molecules, resulting in a major biologic amplifica-

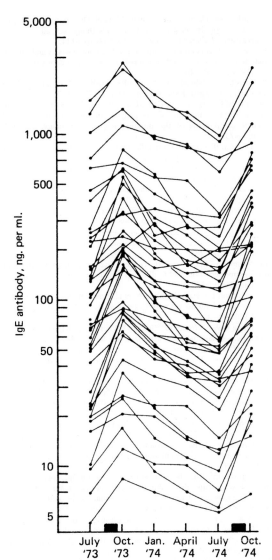

■ FIGURE 2.5 Levels and changes of IgE antibodies to ragweed allergens in 40 untreated allergy patients. The ragweed pollination season is indicated by the *black bar* on the abscissa. (From Gleich GJ, Jacob GL, Unginger JW, et al. Measurement of the absolute levels of IgE antibodies in patients with ragweed hay fever. *J Allergy Clin Immunol* 1977;60:188, with permission.)

tion of the allergen–IgE antibody reaction. Clinical examples include anaphylaxis, allergic rhinitis, and allergic asthma.

In type II, or cytotoxic, injury, IgG or IgM antibody is directed against antigens on the individual's own tissue. Binding of antibody to the cell surface results in complement activation, which signals white blood cell influx and tissue injury. In addition, cytotoxic killer lymphocytes, with Fc receptors for IgG, can bind to the tissue-bound IgG, resulting in antibody-dependent cellular cytotoxicity. Clinical examples include lung and kidney damage in Goodpasture syndrome, acute graft

rejection, hemolytic disease of the newborn, and certain bullous skin diseases.

In type III, or immune complex, disease, IgG and IgM antigen–antibody complexes of a critical size are not cleared from the circulation and fix in small capillaries throughout the body. These complexes activate the complement system, which leads to the influx of inflammatory white blood cells, resulting in tissue damage. Clinical examples include serum sickness (after foreign proteins or drugs), lupus erythematosus, and glomerulonephritis after common infections.

In type IV, or delayed-type, hypersensitivity, the T-cell antigen receptor on T_H1 lymphocytes binds to tissue antigens, resulting in clonal expansion of the lymphocyte population and T-cell activation with the release of inflammatory lymphokines. Clinical examples include contact dermatitis (e.g., poison ivy) and tuberculin hypersensitivity in tuberculosis and leprosy.

The classic Gell and Coombs classification has been adapted by Janeway et al. (60). Subsequently, Kay further expanded the adaptation (61). Type II reactions have been divided into two different subtypes. Type IIa reactions are characterized by cytolytic reactions produced by antibodies causing immune-mediated hemolytic anemia, whereas type IIb reactions are characterized by cell-stimulating reactions produced by thyroid-stimulating antibody in patients with Graves disease or antibodies to the high-affinity mast cell receptor in chronic idiopathic urticaria. The latter antibodies cause mast cell activation.

Type IV reactions are divided into four subtypes. Type IVa_1 reactions are mediated by $CD4^+$ T_H1 cells causing classic delayed-type hypersensitivity reactions, such as allergic contact dermatitis or tuberculin reactions. Type IVa_2 reactions are mediated by $CD4^+$ T_H2 cells resulting in cell-mediated eosinophilic hypersensitivity as occurs in asthma. Type IVb_1 reactions are mediated by cytotoxic $CD8^+$ cells that mediate graft rejection and Stevens-Johnson syndrome. Type IVb_2 reactions are mediated by $CD8^+$ lymphocytes that can produce IL-5, resulting in cell-mediated eosinophilic hypersensitivity, usually in association with viral mucosal infection.

■ REFERENCES

1. Von Pirquet C. Allergie. *Münch Med Wochenschr.* 1906; 53:1457.
2. Ramirez MA. Horse asthma following blood transfusion: Report of a case. *JAMA.* 1919;73:984.
3. Prausnitz C, Küstner H. Studien über ueberempfindlichkeit. *Centralbl Bakteriol.* 1921;86:160.
4. Coca AF, Grove EF. Studies in hypersensitiveness. XIII. A study of atopic reagins. *J Immunol.* 1925;10:444.
5. Stanworth DR. Reaginic antibodies. *Adv Immunol.* 1963;3:181.
6. Sehon AH, Gyenes L. Antibodies in atopic patients and antibodies developed during treatment. In: Samter M, ed. *Immunological Diseases.* 2nd ed. Boston: Little, Brown; 1971:785.
7. Ishizaka K, Ishizaka T. Immunology of IgE mediated hypersensitivity. In: Middleton E, Reed CE, Ellis EJ, eds. *Allergy Principles and Practice.* 2nd ed. St. Louis: CV Mosby, 1983:52.
8. Bennich H, Ishizaka K, Ishizaka T, et al. Comparative antigenic study of E globulin and myeloma IgND. *J Immunol.* 1969;102:826.
9. Johansson SGO. The discovery of immunoglobulin E. *Asthma Allergy Proceedings.* 2006;27: S3–S6.

10. Bennich H, Johansson SGO. Structure and function of human immunoglobulin E. *Adv Immunol.* 1971;13:1–55.

11. Wang B, Reiger A, Kigus O, et al. Epidermal Langerhans cells from normal human skin bind monomeric IgE via FcεR1. *J Exp Med.* 1992;175:1353.

12. Kenten JH, Molgaard HV, Hougton M, et al. Cloning and sequence determination of the gene for the human ε chain expressed in a myeloma cell line. *Proc Natl Acad Sci USA.* 1982;79:6661–6665.

13. Henry AJ, Cook JP, McDonnell JM, et al. Participation of the N-terminal region of Cepsilon3 in the binding of human IgE to its high affinity receptor FcεR1. *Biochemistry.* 1997;36:15568–15578.

14. Garman SC, Kinet JP, Jardetzky TS. Crystal structure of the human high-affinity IgE receptor. *Cell.* 1998;95:951–961.

15. Gould HJ, Sutton BJ. IgE in allergy and asthma today. *Nature Reviews Immunol.* 2008;8:205–215.

16. Turner H, Kinet JP. Signaling through the high-affinity IgE receptor FcεR1. *Nature.* 1999;402s:24–30.

17. Owen CE. Immunoglobulin E: role in asthma and allergic disease: lessons learned from the clinic. *Pharmacol Theraputics.* 2007;113:121–133.

18. Prussin C, Metcalfe DD. IgE, mast cells, basophils, and eosinophils. *J Allergy Clin Immunol.* 2006;117:S450–456.

19. Saini SS, MacGlashan DW, Sterbinsky SA, et al. Down-regulation of human basophil IgE and FC epsilon R1 alpha surface densities and mediator release by anti-IgE-infusions is reversible in vitro and in vivo. *J Immunol.* 1999;162:5624–5630.

20. Yamaguchi M, Lantz CS, Oettgen HC, et al. IgE enhances mouse mast cell Fc(epsilon)R1 expression in vitro and in vivo: evidence for a novel amplification mechanism in IgE-dependent reactions. *J Exp Med.* 1997;184:663–672.

21. Delespesse G, Sarfati M, Wu CY, et al. The low-affinity receptor for IgE. *Immunol Rev.* 1992;125:77–97.

22. Tada T, Ishizaka K. Distribution of gamma E-forming cells in lymphoid tissues of the human and monkey. *J Immunol.* 1970;104:377.

23. Callerame ML, Condemi JJ, Bohrod MG, et al. Immunologic reactions of bronchial tissues in asthma. *N. Engl J Med.* 1971;284:459–464.

24. Gould HJ, Takhar P, Harris HE, et al. Germinal-center reactions in allergic inflamation. *Trends in Immunol.* 2006;27:446–452.

25. Waldmann TA, Iio A, Ogawa M, et al. The metabolism of IgE: studies in normal individuals and in a patient with IgE myeloma. *J Immunol.* 1976;117:1139–44.

26. Zeiss CR, Pruzansky JJ, Levitz D, et al. The quantitation of IgE antibody specific for ragweed antigen E on the basophil surface in patients with ragweed pollenosis. *Immunology.* 1978;35:237–246.

27. Tada T. Regulation of reaginic antibody formation in animals. *Prog Allergy.* 1975;19:122–194.

28. Lebman DA, Coffman RL. Interleukin-4 causes isotype switching to IgE in T cell-stimulated clonal B cell cultures. *J Exp Med.* 1988;168:853–862.

29. Coffman RL, Carty J. A T-cell activity that enhances polyclonal IgE production and its inhibition by interferon-γ. *J Immunol.* 1986;136:949–954.

30. Leung DY. Mechanisms of the human allergic response: clinical implications. *Pediatr Clin North Am.* 1994;41:727–743.

31. Maggi E, Romagnani S. Role of T-cells and T-cell derived cytokines in the pathogenesis of allergic diseases. *Ann N Y Acad Sci.* 1994;725:2.

32. Gauchat JF, Lebman DA, Coffman RL, et al. Structure and expression of germline ε transcripts in human B cells induced by interleukin-4 to switch to IgE production. *J Exp Med.* 1990;172:463–473.

33. Cory DB, Kheradmand F. Induction and regulation of the IgE response. *Nature.* 1999;402s:18–23.

34. Johansson SGO, Foucard T. IgE in immunity and disease. In: Middleton E, Reed CE, Ellis EJ, eds. *Allergy Principles and Practice.* 1st ed. St Louis: CV Mosby, 1978:551.

35. Johansson SGO, Mellbin T, Vahlquist G. Immunoglobulin levels in Ethiopian preschool children with special reference to high concentrations of immunoglobulin E (IgND). *Lancet.* 1968;1:1118–1121.

36. Barbee RA, Halonen M, Lebowitz M, et al. Distribution of IgE in a community population sample: correlation with age, sex, allergen skin test reactivity. *J Allergy Clin Immunol.* 1981;68:106–111.

37. Lewis RA, Austen KF. Mediation of local homeostasis and inflammation by leukotrienes and other mast-cell dependent compounds. *Nature.* 1981;293:103–108.

38. Steinberg P, Ishizaka K, Norman PS. Possible role of IgE-mediated reaction in immunity. *J Allergy Clin Immunol.* 1974;54:359.

39. Dineen JK, Ogilvie BM, Kelly JD. Expulsion of *Nippostrongylus brasiliensis* from the intestine of rats: collaboration between humoral and cellular components of the immune response. *Immunology.* 1973;24:467–475.

40. Dessaint JP, Capron A. IgE inflammatory cells: the cellular network in allergy. *Int Arch Allergy Appl Immunol.* 1989;90:28–31.

41. Romagnani S. The role of lymphocytes in allergic disease. *J Allergy Clin Immunol* 2000;105:399–408.

42. Strachan DP. Family size, infection, and atopy: the first decade of the "hygiene hypothesis" *Thorax.* 2000;55:S2–S10.

43. Prescott SL. Allergy takes its Toll: The role of Toll like receptors in allergy pathogenesis. *WAO Journal.* 2008;1:4–-8.

44. Schleimer RP, Kato A, Kern R, et al. Epithelium: At the interface of innate and adaptive immune responses. *J Allergy Clin Immunol.* 2007;120:1279–1284.

45. Mosmann TR, Coffman RL. Th1 and Th2 cells: different patterns of lymphokine secretion lead to different functional properties. *Annu Rev Immunol.* 1989;7:145–146.

46. Robinson DS, Hamid Q, Ying S, et al. Predominant Th2-like bronchoalveolar T-lymphocyte population in atopic asthma. *N Engl J Med.* 1992;326:298–304.

47. Busse WW, Coffman RL, Gelfand EW, et al. Mechanisms of persistent airway inflammation in asthma: a role for T cells and T-cell products. *Am J Respir Crit Care Med.* 1995;152:388–393.

48. Holgate ST. The epidemic of allergy and asthma. *Nature.* 1999;402s:2–4.

49. Marsh DG, Huang S-K. Molecular genetics of human immune responsiveness pollen allergens. *Clin Exp Allergy.* 1991;21:168.

50. Cookson W. The alliance of genes and the environment in asthma and allergy. *Nature.* 1999;402s:5–11.

51. Vercilli D. Discovering susceptibility genes for asthma and allergy. *Nat Rev Immunol.* 2008;8:161–238.

52. Orihara K, Nahae S, Pawankar R, et al. Role of regulatory and proinflamatory T-cell populations in allergic disease. *WAO Journal.* 2008;1:9–14.

53. Johnson EE, Irons JJ, Patterson R, et al. Serum IgE concentrations in atopic dermatitis:relationship to severity of disease and presence of atopic respiratory disease. *J Allergy Clin Immunol.* 1974:54:94–99.

54. Wide L, Bennich H, Johansson SGO. Diagnosis of allergy by an *in vitro* test for allergenic antibodies. *Lancet.* 1967;2:1105–1107.

55. Norman P. Correlations of RAST and in vivo and in vitro assays. In: Evans R III, ed. *Advances in Diagnosis of Allergy: RAST.* Miami: Symposia Specialists;1975:45.

56. Gleich GJ, Jacobs GL, Yunginger JW, et al. Measurement of the absolute levels of IgE antibodies in patients with ragweed hay fever: effect of immunotherapy on seasonal changes and relationship to IgG antibodies. *J Allergy Clin Immunol.* 1977;60:188–198.

57. Zeiss CR, Pruzansky JJ, Patterson R, et al. A solid phase radioimmunoassay for the quantitation of human reaginic antibody against ragweed antigens. *J Immunol.* 1973;110:414–421.

58. Conroy MC, Adkinson NF, Lichtenstein LM. Measurement of IgE on human basophils: relation to serum IgE and anti-IgE induced histamine release. *J Immunol.* 1977;118:1317–1321.

59. Roitt I. Hypersensitivity. In: *Essential Immunology.* 8th ed. London: Blackwell Science; 1994:313.

60. Janeway C, Travers P, eds. *Immunobiology.* 2nd ed. London: Garland Press; 1995.

61. Kay AB. Concepts of allergy and hypersensitivity in allergy and allergic diseases. In: Kay AB, ed. *Allergy and Allergic Diseases.* Vol. 1. Oxford, UK: Blackwell Science; 1997;23–35.

CHAPTER 3

Biochemical Mediators of Allergic Reactions

CHHAVI GANDHI AND STEPHEN I. WASSERMAN

The cells and mediators involved in diseases of immediate-type hypersensitivity have been well described. The biologically active molecules responsible have been identified, and a thorough biochemical and structural elucidation of diverse lipid mediators has been accomplished. The activity of mediator-generating cells and their diverse products has been assigned a central role in both immunoglobulin E (IgE)-mediated acute and prolonged inflammatory events. More recently, a broadened understanding of the previously implicated mediators and newer agents has occurred both in human and animal model studies. This chapter places in perspective the mediator-generating cells, the mediators themselves and these newer concepts of their roles in pathobiologic and homeostatic events.

■ MEDIATOR-GENERATING CELLS

Mast cells and basophilic polymorphonuclear leukocytes (basophils) constitute the two cell types on which the high affinity FcεRI is expressed (1). Mast cells are most closely related to mononuclear leukocytes (2) and are richly distributed in the deeper region of the central nervous system, the upper and lower respiratory epithelium, the bronchial lumen, the gastrointestinal mucosa and submuscosa, bone marrow, and skin (3). They are especially prominent in bone, dense connective tissue adjacent to blood vessels (particularly small arterioles and venules)- and peripheral nerves. In the skin, lungs, and gastrointestinal tract, mast cell concentrations approximate 10,000 to 20,000 cells/mm³. (They develop from CD34+ bone marrow precursors through the action of stem cell factor (kit-ligand SCF), which binds to a specific receptor (c-kit, CD117) (4). Precursor cells exit the marrow and terminally differentiate in tissues under a variety of local influences, such as interleukin-3 (IL-3), IL-4, IL-6, IL-9, IL-10, and factors from fibroblasts (5).

Mast cells are large (10 to 15 mm in diameter) and possess a ruffled membrane, numerous membrane-bound granules (0.5 to 0.7 mm in diameter), mitochondria, a mononuclear nucleus, and scant rough endoplasmic reticulum. Ultrastructurally, human mast cell granules display whorl and scroll patterns. Mast cells are heterogeneous, and both connective tissue (MC_{TC}) and mucosal types (MC_T) have been recognized. MC_{TC} dominate in the skin and can be distinguished from the mucosal type by expressing CD-88 (C5aR) on their cell surface. They are also found in lesser quantities in the gastrointestinal system, bronchial smooth muscle, and glandular region of the lungs. In the asthmatic lung, elevated levels of MC_{TC} are found in the smooth muscle (6). This mast cell type expresses tryptase, chymase, cathepsin-G-like protease, and carboxypeptidase A in the granules. Mucosal-type mast cells (MC_T) predominate in the lamina propria of the gastrointestinal tract as well as the peripheral airways, alveolar septa, and epithelium of the lung. MC_T cells predominantly express tryptase (7) (Table 3.1). Recently, a c-kit mutant mouse has been developed using the W-*sash* mouse (Kit $^{W-sh/}$ $^{W-sh}$) producing an experimental mast cell-deficient mice model that, unlike prior c-kit knockout models, can successfully reproduce (8), has no other leukocyte deficiencies, and should thus be helpful in further describing the mast cell's role in inflammation.

Basophils, most closely related to eosinophils, are circulating leukocytes whose presence in tissue is unusual except in disease states. They originate in the bone marrow and constitute 0.1% to 2.0% of the peripheral blood leukocytes. Basophils possess a polylobed nucleus and differ from mast cells in their tinctorial properties, their relatively smooth cell surface, and their granule morphologic makeup, which is larger and less structured than that of the mast cell. Their growth is responsive, not to SCF, but rather to IL-3, and granulocyte-macrophage colony-stimulating factor (GM-CSF) (9).

Other mediator-generating cells include platelets, which express FcεRI and release serotonin, RANTES, platelet-activating factor (PAF), histamine, and platelet

TABLE 3.1   HUMAN MAST CELL SUBTYPES

FEATURE	MC_{TC} CELL	MC_T CELL
Structural features		
Grating/Lattice granule	++	−
Scroll granules	Poor	Rich
Tissue distribution		
Skin	++	−
Intestinal submucosa	++	+
Intestinal mucosa	+	++
Alveolar wall	−	++
Bronchi	+	++
Nasal mucosa	++	++
Conjunctiva	++	+
Mediator Synthesized		
Histamine	+++	+++
Chymase	++	−
Tryptase	++	++
Carboxypeptidase	++	−
Cathepsin G	++	−
LTC_4	++	++
PGD_2	++	++
TNF-α	++	++
IL-4, IL-5, IL-6, IL-13	++	++

Adapted from Krishnaswamy G, Chi DS. The Human Mast Cell: An Overview. *Methods in Molecular Biology* 2006;315:16 Table 1. ©Humana Press Inc.

factor 4, as well as cytokines and chemokines. Their role has been imputed from mouse studies of anaphylactoid shock in mast cell-deficient animals. Eosinophils have been suggested to play both a proinflammatory role, through release of granule-associated proteins, and an anti-inflammatory role, through the metabolism of vasoactive mediators (Table 3.1) (9).

■ ACTIVATION OF MAST CELLS AND BASOPHILS

Mast cells and basophils possess numerous high-affinity intramembranous receptors (FcεRI) for the Fc portion of IgE. The number of such receptors is up-regulated and their stability enhanced by exposure of the mast cell or basophil to increased amounts of IgE (10). Aggregation of two or more of these FcεRI receptors with antigen cross-linking of receptor-bound IgE molecules leads to receptor activation and complex signal transduction leading to the release of mediators from mast cells and basophils (11). Pre-formed mediators from mast cell cytoplasmic granules are released immediately and include histamine, neutral proteases, a small proportion of total cytokines, and proteoglycans. Unstored mediator synthesis is initiated in minutes and includes the production of lipid membrane-derived arachidonic acid, prostaglandins (PGD_2), PAF, and leukotrienes (LTB_4 and LTC_4). Chemokine and cytokine products are unstored and are produced within hours of the initial stimulus; their release can continue for days (12). Mast cell responsiveness may be heightened by exposure to SCF or other cytokines, whereas basophils are primed to respond by GM-CSF, IL-1, IL-3, and IL-5. Other important secreatagogues include a family of histamine-releasing factors and complement fragments C3a and C5a, the latter of which have not shown to be necessary to mount an anaphylactic episode. (The coagulation cascade and kallikrein-kinin contact system have also been implicated to be involved because of the reported decreases in fibrinogen, factor V and VIII, and factor XIIa-c1 inhibitor complexes, and the high-molecular weight kininogen and kallikrein-C1 that have been seen [13]).

The FcεRI receptor is composed of one extracellular subunit, α, which binds to IgE, and two intracellular subunits, β and γ, which are associated with enzymes and are essential in the subsequent signal transduction on the activation of mast cells and basophils. FcεRI receptor bridging is followed by phosphorylation of the immunoreceptor tyrosine-based activation motifs (ITAM) of the β and γ subunits, which acts as a scaffold to allow the binding of additional signaling molecules, the most important of which is the protein tyrosine kinase Syk. Syk binds, via the γ subunit of the receptor, becomes phosphorylated, and leads to the phosphorylation of several downstream proteins, directly and indirectly (11). The net result of this signaling is an increase in intracellular calcium, protein kinase C translocation, G protein activation, and cyclic adenosine monophosphate generation. At the same time, membrane phospholipids are metabolized to generate monoacylglycerols, diacylglycerols, and phosphorylated inositol species, which facilitate protein kinase C function and liberate Ca^{2+} from intracellular sites. While these biochemical events are underway, adenosine triphosphate (ATP) is catabolized and adenosine is liberated which further activates a mast cell adenosine receptor to enhance granule release. Finally, the cell gains control over mediator release, the process stops, and the cell regranulates (14).

Although initiated at the time of IgE and antigen activation, the generation of cytokines is expressed over a time frame of hours to days. Both mast cells and basophils are important sources of a variety of inflammatory cytokines, as described later. After the initiating event of allergen binding, cytokine synthesis proceeds through activation of such signaling pathways as the STAT and NF-κB-regulated processes, with gene transcription evident within hours and protein secretion occurring subsequently (15).

Recent work has added further complexity to mast cell and basophil activation and has suggested pathways for their regulation. Mast cells possess a receptor for IgG, FcγRII, which can modulate mediator release; these cells also respond to endotoxin through engagement of a Toll-like receptor complex. The presence of these additional modulatory pathways suggests that mast cell and basophil mediators participate in inflammatory conditions in which IgE may not be present. Murine models suggest further mechanisms in the activation and signaling of mast cells and basophils. Zinc has been implicated in inducing FCεRI-dependent mast cell degranulation, cytokine production (IL-6 and TNF-α), NF-κB activation, and possibly protein kinase C plasma membrane translocation (16). Sensory skin nerves may augment mast cell-derived inflammation by releasing neuropeptides such as substance P and calcitonin gene-related peptide in this setting, with less mast cell-driven inflammation being seen in denervated skin (17). A protein of the regulator of G-protein signaling (RGS) family, RGS13, has been shown to halt normal signal transduction downstream of FcεRI by blocking PIP3 phosphorylation from occurring in mast cells, suggesting it may have a role in their homeostasis (18). A human Ig fusion protein, Fcγ-Fcε (GE2 protein), has been shown to inhibit FcεRI signaling by cross-linking FcεRI with FcγRIIb, a negative regulatory molecule (19). Its role in the basal regulation mast cell and basophil activity has not been fully evaluated.

■ MEDIATORS

Whatever their final metabolic interrelationships, the early biochemical processes lead to the generation of a heterogenous group of molecules termed *mediators*. Some mediators are preformed and are stored in the granules of the cell; others are generated only after cell activation and originate in the cytosol or membrane. Mediators are classified in this chapter by their proposed actions (Tables 3.2 and 3.3), although some mediators subserve several functions.

Spasmogenic Mediators

Histamine, generated by decarboxylation of histidine, was the first mast cell mediator to be identified, and it is the sole preformed mediator in this functional class. It is bound to the proteoglycans of mast cell and basophil granules (5 and 1 mg/10^6 cells, respectively) (20). Histamine circulates at concentrations of about 300 pg/mL with a circadian maximum in the early morning hours. (Histamine excretion exceeds 10 mg/24 hours; a small fraction is excreted as the native molecule and the remainder as imidazole acetic acid or methyl histamine.) Histamine interacts with specific H_1, H_2, H_3, and newly discovered H_4 receptors (20). The H_4 receptor has low homology with the other histamine receptors but shares the most with the H_3 receptor with 35% amino acid homology; antihistamines specific for the H_1 and H_2 receptors do not bind to the H_4 receptor (20).

All of the histamine receptors are G-protein coupled receptors. H_1 receptors utilize G_q proteins, leading to phopholipase C activation, inositol phosphate production, and, eventually, calcium mobilization (20). H_2 receptors use $G\alpha_s$ proteins, causing an increase in cyclic AMP. H_3 receptors use $G\alpha_{i/o}$, causing inhibition of cAMP, increasing calcium mobilization, and activating MAP kinases and ion channels. H_4 receptors seem to work through pertussis-toxin sensitive $G\alpha_{i/o}$ proteins, which signal through increases in intracellular calcium; however, other pathways have been described (21).

H_1 receptors predominate in the skin and smooth muscle; H_2 receptors are the most prevalent in the skin, lungs, stomach, and on a variety of leukocytes; H_3 receptors predominate in the brain; H_4 receptors appear to be present on mast cells, basophils, eosinophils (22), dendritic cells, CD4$^+$ effector T cells (at low levels)

TABLE 3.2 MAST CELL VASOACTIVE AND SPASMOGENIC MEDIATORS

MEDIATOR	OTHER ACTIONS
Histamine	Alters cell migration Generates prostaglandins Increases mucus production Activates suppressor T lymphocytes
Platelet-activating factor	Activates platelets Attracts and activates eosinophils
Prostaglandin D_2	Prevents platelet aggregation Alters cell migration
Sulfidopeptide leukotrienes (C_4, D_4, E_4)	Generates prostaglandins
Adenosine	Prevents platelet aggregation Enhances mediator release Inhibits neutrophil superoxide production

(23), and may be present on neutrophils and monocytes (46) as well as on lung parenchymal cells (24). The biologic response to histamine reflects the ratio of these receptors in a given tissue. Increased levels of histamine have been reported in the blood or urine of patients with physical urticaria, anaphylaxis, systemic mastocytosis, and antigen-induced rhinitis and asthma (25). H_1 histamine effects include the contraction of bronchial and gut musculature, vascular permeability, pulmonary vasoconstriction, and nasal mucus production (26). By its H_2 pathway, histamine dilates respiratory musculature, enhances airway mucus production, inhibits basophils and skin (but not lung) mast cell degranulation, and activates suppressor T lymphocytes.

Both H_1 and H_2 actions are required for the full expression of pruritus, cutaneous vasodilation, and cardiac irritability (20). The H_3 actions of histamine suppress central nervous system histamine synthesis. The H_4 actions of histamine include eosinophil chemotaxis, cell shape change, and up-regulation of adhesion molecules, the induction of mast cell chemotaxis toward a histamine gradient (22,23) and an increase in cytokine production from dendritic and T cells (24,27). Studies using the H_4 receptor antagonist JNJ 7777120 help support these findings (28), and H_4 KO mice suggest the H_4 receptor has a role in allergic airway inflammation through activation of CD4$^+$ T cells (29). It is also possible that this receptor is an important factor in pruritus.

TABLE 3.3 MAST CELL MEDIATORS AFFECTING CELL MIGRATION

MEDIATOR	CELL TARGET
High molecular weight NCF	Neutrophils
ECF-A	Eosinophils
ECF oligopeptides	Eosinophils (secondary mononuclear)
T-lymphocyte chemotactic factors	T cells
Histamine	Nonselective
PGD_2	Eosinophils and neutrophils
Leukotriene B_4	Neutrophils
Leukotriene E_4	Eosinophils
PAF	Eosinophils and neutrophils
Lymphocyte chemokinetic factor	T and B cells

NCF, neutrophil chemotactic factor; ECF-A, eosinophil chemotactic factor of anaphylaxis; PGD_2, prostaglandin D_2; PAF, platelet-activating factor.

Platelet-activating Factor

Platelet-activating factor is a lipid identified structurally as 1-alkyl-2acetyl-sn-glyceryl-3-phoporylcholine (30). It is a metabolic product of phospholipase A2 and acetyltransferase and works through G-protein coupled receptors. PAF is primarily secreted by mast cells, monocytes, macrophages, and eosinophils (31). Functional receptors are found on platelets, monocytes, neutrophils, and eosinophils; degradation of PAF occurs by the action of acetyl hydrolase to remove acetate from the sn-2 position (30,31).

PAF causes aggregation of human platelets, wheal-and-flare permeability responses, eosinophil chemotaxis, smooth muscle contraction, and increased vascular permeability (30). PAF has the ability to induce histamine release from basophils and mast cells, cause eosinophils and neutrophils to degranulate, and increase LTC_4 formation by eosinophils (31). PAF also contracts pulmonary and gut musculature, induces vasoconstriction, and is a potent hypotensive agent. Effects mediated by PAF also include pulmonary artery hypertension, pulmonary edema, an increase in total pulmonary resistance, and a decrease in dynamic compliance. In addition, PAF is capable of inducing a prolonged increase in nonspecific bronchial hyperreactivity *in vivo*). Recently, the relative activity of PAF and acetylhydrolase has been directly and inversely linked to severity of anaphylaxis (but definitive strategies employing this information to target treatment or to stratify patients at risk for anaphylaxis remain to be elucidated) (32).

Nitric Oxide

Nitric oxide (NO) is a radical derived from L-arginine by NO synthase (NOS), on histamine binding to H_1 receptors, involved in smooth muscle relaxation, hypotension, and shock related to anaphylaxis. NO activates guanylate cyclase leading to vasodilation and the production of cyclic guanosine monophosphate. Three types of synthases have been discovered, including inducible NOS (i-NOS), neuronal NOS (n-NOS), and endothelial NOS (e-NOS). e-NOS (found on cardiac myocytes, hippocampal neurons, renal epithelial cells, and blood platelets) and n-NOS are constitutively expressed and produce low levels of NO through calcium-dependent pathways (33), whereas i-NOS is induced robustly in a calcium-independent fashion and has been traditionally assigned the role of causing the vascular responses seen in anaphylaxis. Newer discoveries have recognized the constant expression of e-NOS and variable expression of n-NOS on mast cells (34) with further suggestions that e-NOS (and not i-NOS) is the primary vasodilator working potentially through PI_3 and Akt kinases (35).

Oxidative Products of Arachidonic Acid

Arachadonic acid is a C20:4 fatty acid component of mast cell membrane phospholipids, from which it may be liberated by the action of phospholipase A_2 or by the concerted action of phospholipase C and diacylglycerol lipase. At least 20 potential end products may be generated from arachidonic acid by the two major enzymes, 5-lipoxygenase and cyclooxygenase, which regulate its fate.

Cyclooxygenase Products

Prostagladin (PG) D_2 is the predominant cyclooxygenase product generated by human mast cells, whereas human basophils do not generate this molecule. The production of PGD_2 from PGH_2 is glutathione dependent and is blocked by nonsteroidal anti-inflammatory drugs and dapsone. It is a potent vasoactive and smooth muscle reactive compound that causes vasodilation when injected into human skin, induces gut and pulmonary muscle contraction, and, *in vitro*, inhibits platelet aggregation (36). PGD_2 is thought to be responsible for flushing and hypotension in some patients with mastocytosis and to be an important mediator of allergic asthma. PGD_2 is further metabolized to PGJ_2, a natural ligand for peroxisome proliferators-activated receptor-γ, a nuclear receptor important in diabetes and atherosclerosis, and possibly in the inflammatory response.

Immediate IgE antigen-activated PGD_2 production is dependent on the constitutive expression of cyclooxygenase 1. Later and more prolonged PGD_2 synthesis occurs after antigen challenge of sensitized cells that are stimulated with SCF and IL-10 (36).

Lipooxygenase Products

Human mast cells generate 5-lipoxygenase products of arachidonic acid, starting with an unstable intermediate, 5-HPETE (which may be reduced to the monohydroxy fatty acid 5-HETE), or, through leukotrienes synthetase, LTC_4 by addition of glutathione through the action of LTC_4 synthase (LTC_4S). This enzyme and its activating factor, FLAP, resides on the outer surface of the nuclear membrane. The initial product of this pathway is LTC_4, from which LTD_4 may be generated by the removal of the terminal glutamine, and LTE_4 by the further removal of glycine. LTC_4, LTD_4, and LTE_4 collectively are termed the *cysteinyl leukotrienes*. A polymorphism in the LTC_4 synthase gene is thought to alter the amount of this mediator generated during biologic reactions. The newly discovered crystal structure of LTC_4S demonstrates that the glutathione residue resides in a U-shaped conformation within an interface of adjacent monomers from a trimer formed by four transmembrane α-helices providing a unique binding site for the precursor molecule LTA_4 (37). The biologic activity of the sulfidopeptide leukotrienes occurs by its binding to two specific receptors termed *Cys LTR_I* and *LTR_{II}*. Both receptors have been implicated in the development of microvascular leakage with suspected heterogeneous distribution in the microvasculature of different tissues (38). In particular, murine studies indicate that CysLT's from mast cells and monocytes/macrophages preferentially utilize $CysLTR_I$ (38), while transgenic animal model of human $CysLTR_{II}$ suggests $CysLTR_{II}$ has a contributory role in the vascular changes seen in models of passive cutaneous anaphylaxis (39). Recently evidence has been presented suggesting the presence of a third receptor for cysteinyl leukotrienes.

Degradation of leukotrienes is rapid and is accomplished by various oxygen metabolites. Clinically useful inhibitors of both 5-lipoxygenase and $CysLTR_I$ are available and demonstrate efficacy in clinical asthma (40). No clinically available inhibitor of $CysLTR_{II}$ or for the putative $CysLTR_{III}$ has been assessed *in vivo*, and the contribution of these receptors to the physiologic manifestations of LTC_4, LTD_4, or LTE_4 in human disease remains speculative.

Leukotrienes are potent and possess a broad spectrum of biologic activity (41). They induce wheal-and-flare responses that are long-lived and are accompanied historically by endothelial activation and dermal edema. In the airway, they enhance mucus production and cause bronchoconstriction, especially by affecting peripheral units. Experimentally, there is a decreased presence of T_H2-dependent pulmonary inflammation (eosinophil and goblet cell count, amount of mucus, and degree of mast cell infiltration) after antigen challenge in murine models lacking LTC_4S (42). In humans, LTD_4 is most active, LTC_4 is intermediate, and LTE_4 is the least potent. LTE_4 has been implicated as an inducer of nonspecific bronchial hyperreactivity. It has been suggested that the LTD_4 augments airway remodeling (43), possibly by stimulating matrix metalloproteinase release or activity. All depress cardiac muscle performance and diminish coronary flow rates. Suggestions have also been made that they contribute to venoconstriction in the liver during anaphylaxis (44). LTC_4 and LTD_4 have been recovered from nasal washings and bronchial lavage fluids of patients with allergic rhinitis or asthma, whereas LTE_4 has been recovered from the urine.

More recently, the development of 5-oxo-ETE through the alternative pathway for 5-HPETE metabolism has been delineated. 5-HPETE gives rise to 5-HETE through peroxidases and subsequently to 5-oxo-ETEs (eicosatetraenoic acids) by 5-hydroxyeicosanoid dehydrogenase (5-HEDH). 5-oxo-ETE is an extremely potent eosinophil chemoattractant, which supercedes PAF in this manner. It is also involved in eosinophilic intracellular calcium mobilization, actin polymerization, neutro-

philic chemotaxis, and at high levels (*in vitro*) airway smooth muscle contraction (45).

LTB_4 is the alternative product of LTA_4 via LTA_4 hydrolase, primarily formed in neutrophils and monocytes. Is a chemotactic agent of many cells, including neutrophils and eosinophils, is implicated in the trafficking of $CD4^+$ and $CD8^+$ cells into the airway on antigen challenge (46), and theorized to contribute to the late phase of anaphylaxis and to protracted reactions (14).

Phospholipase

Phospholipases are enzymes that convert phospholipids into fatty acids and lipophilic substances. There are four major classes (A–D) that catalyze different reactions in phospholipase breakdown, some of which have been implicated in mechanisms of mast cell and basophil reactions in anaphylaxis. Cytosolic phospholipase A_2 has direct effects in producing arachidonic acid from phospholipid membranes, leading to the formation of prostaglandins and leukotrienes. Exogenous phospholipase A_2 (honeybee venom secretory phospholipase A_2) can directly activate human basophils *in vivo* to induce leukotriene production (47). Phospholipase C has many different isoforms; it has been suggested that one of them, phospholipase $C\gamma_2$ ($PLC\gamma_2$), may be expressed in mast cells and monocytes/macrophages and may play a role in increasing intracellular calcium levels following FcεRI cross-linking of mast cells (48). Phospholipase D (PLD) has two isoforms, PDL_1 and PLD_2, which are actively involved in the signaling process of mast cells (49), but their exact function and mechanisms are still unclear. PLD can be activated (50) and cultured in mast cells (51) and, interfering with the presence of substrates for PLD, has led to suppression of mast cell degranulation (52)

Adenosine

The nucleoside adenosine generated from the breakdown of ATP is released from mast cells on IgE-mediated activation (53). In humans, circulating blood levels of adenosine are 0.3 µg/mL and are increased after hypoxia or antigen-induced bronchospasm. Adenosine is a potent vasodilator, inhibits platelet aggregation, and causes bronchospasm on inhalation by asthmatics. Adenosine, acting through a cell surface receptor, probably the A2b and A3 subtypes (53), enhances mast cell mediator release *in vitro* and potentiates antigen-induced local wheal-and–flare responses *in vivo*. Adenosine binding to its receptor is inhibited by methylxanthines.

Osteopontin

Osteopontin (OPN) is an extracellular matrix glycoprotein involved in bone metabolism but is also found in many cell types in the immune system and is being linked with multiple inflammatory and immune processes, including wound healing, dystrophic calcification, coronary atherosclerosis, tumor cell metastasis, and with the pathogenesis of diseases such as multiple sclerosis and rheumatoid arthritis (54). Recent discoveries have elucidated mast cell secretion of biologically active OPN and have suggested it has a role in augmenting mast cell degranulation by FcεRI aggregation and promoting mast cell migration (55). OPN has been found in the asthmatic lung and the secreted form has been implicated to have an opposing role in the development and containment of T_{H2} responses through plasmacytoid dendritic cells (56). Future studies are needed to further decipher its exact role in the allergic response.

Chemotactic Mediators

Several chemotactic molecules have been characterized by activities generated during IgE-dependent allergic responses. Most remain incompletely characterized. Chemokines, a family of cytokines, have chemoattractant activity for leukocytes and fibroblasts. In the C-X-C or α chemokines, the cysteines are separated by one amino acid, whereas the cysteines are adjacent in the C-C or β chemokines. Most α chemokines attract neutrophils, whereas β chemokines attract T cells and monocytes (some also attract basophils and eosinophils). The C-X-C chemokines that attract neutrophils include GRO-α, GRO-β, IL-8, NAP-2, and PF-4. The C-C chemokines that attract eosinophils include eotaxin, MIP-1α, MCP-2, MCP-3, and RANTES. IL-8, MIP-1α, and RANTES are also cell chemoattractants for both mast cells and basophils.

Eosinophil Chemotactic Factors

Historically, PAF was thought to be the most potent and selective eosinophil-directed agent (32) which induced skin or bronchial eosinophilia. More recently, 5-oxo-ETE has been found to be up to 30 times more potent in eosinophilic chemotaxis than LTB_4 or any CysLTs and nearly three times more potent than PAF (45). Other, less active eosinophil-directed mast cell products include the tetrapeptides Val or ala-gly-ser-glu (eosinophil chemotactic factor of anaphylaxis (ECF-A) and others, having a molecular weight of 1,000 to 3,000. The latter ones have been found in the blood of humans after induction of physical urticaria or allergic asthma. ECF-A is capable of inducing PAF production by eosinophils (45).

Mediators with Enzymatic Properties

Tryptase is the major protein found in human mast cells and its expression by peripheral blood cells is predominantly by the mast cell with <1% of its expression from the basophil. Although it was previously questioned, basophil cells secreting mast-cell tryptase have been characterized as their own entity, disputing previously reported hybrid lineages or mast-cell lineages as the source. Tryptase is a neutral serine protease that is stored in secretory granules as an active tetramer with a molecular weight of 134kD (57). There are two tryptase genes α and β. α-Protryptase is secreted constitutively from mast cells as an inactive proenzyme and is the major form of tryptase found in the circulation of normal subjects. β-Tryptase is stored in the secretory granules of mast cells and its activation involves two proteolytic steps. The first is an autocatalytic intermolecular cleavage of the molecule at an acidic pH and in the presence of heparin or dextran sulfate. The second involves the removal of the remaining precursor dipeptide by dipeptidyl peptidase I (58). Tryptase constitutes nearly 25% of mast call-granular protein and is released during IgE-dependent reactions. It is capable of cleaving kininogen to yield bradykinin, and can diminish clotting activity, and generate and degrade complement components such as C3a and a variety of other peptides. The proteolytic activities of tryptase work best in low pH environments, and β-tryptase is often released into acidic tissues such as areas of poor inflammation and poor vascularity. Although the exact mechanism for its regulation is not known, β-tryptase can be slowly and incompletely dissociated from heparin proteoglycan by basic proteins such as antithrombin III (57). Tryptase is not inhibited by plasma antiproteases and thus its activity may be persistent. β-Tryptase released during mast cell degranulation has been suggested to cleave IgE possibly acting as a natural mechanism for controlling allergic inflammation (59).

The ratio of α and β subtype assays have become useful markers in discerning between systemic mastocytosis and anaphylaxis in which α-tryptase is primarily released in the former and β-tryptase in the later. A ratio of total tryptase (α protryptase+ β tryptase) to mature (total β-tryptase) of less than 10 suggests the diagnosis of anaphylaxis whereas systemic mastocytosis is suggested if this ratio is greater than 20 (57).

A chymotryptic protease termed *chymase* is present in a subclass of human mast cells, particularly those in the skin and on serosal surfaces, and has thus been used as a marker to identify connective tissue mast cells. It cleaves angiotensinogen to yield angiotensin, activates IL-1, and is a mucus secretagogue. Other enzymes found in mast cells include carboxypeptidase, which converts angiotensin I to angiotensin II and cleaves bradykinin, and substance P and acid hydrolases (12).

Structural Proteoglycans

The structural proteoglycans include heparin, various chondroitin sulfates, and cytokines.

Heparin

Heparin is a highly sulfated proteoglycan that is contained in amounts of 5 pg/10^6 cells in human mast cell granules (60) and is released on immunologic activation. Human heparin is an anticoagulant proteoglycans and a complement inhibitor, and it modulates tryptase activity. Human heparin also may be important in angiogenesis by binding angiogenic growth factors and preventing their degradation, and it is essential for the proper packaging of proteases and histamine within the mast cell granule.

Chondroitin Sulfates

Human basophils contain about 3 pg to 4 pg of chondroitin 4 and 6 sulfates, which lack anticoagulant activity and bind less histamine than heparin. Human lung mast cells contain highly sulfated proteoglycans, chondroitin sulfates D and E, which account for the different staining characteristics of these mast cells. Chondroitin sulfate, along with heparin proteoglycans, helps to stabilize and regulate the secretion of granular proteases. Mouse models have suggested focal adhesion kinase (FAK), a nonreceptor protein kinase, increases the chondroitin/dermatan sulfate content of maturing mast cell granules, ensuring an intact microvillous cell surface (60).

Cytokines

Although cytokines traditionally have been viewed as products of monocytes-macrophages or lymphocytes, it has been well established that mast cells (61) generate many, including tumor necrosis factor-α (TNF-α), IL-1, IL-1ra, IL-3, IL-4, IL-5, IL-6, IL-9, IL-13, IL-16, and GM-CSF (62–64) in an NF-κB-dependent process (15). These molecules may be central to local regulation of mast cell growth and differentiation and may also provide new functions for mast cells in health and disease. Basophils are also a prominent source of IL-4 and IL-13 (61). These cytokines are categorized as those that cause inflammation (IL-1, IL-6, TNF-α); enhance IgE synthesis (IL-4, IL-13); stimulate eosinophil growth, survival, localization, and activation (IL-3, IL-5, GM-CSF); participate in airway remodeling (IL-9); and decrease inflammation (IL-1ra) (65).

■ MEDIATOR INTERACTIONS

The mediators generated and released after mast cell activation have been isolated, identified, and characterized as individual factors, whereas physiologic and pathologic events reflect their combined interactions. Given the number of mediators, the knowledge that may have yet to be purified (or even identified), and the lack of understanding of appropriate ratios of mediators generated or released in vivo, it is not surprising that there are no reliable data regarding these interactions in health or disease. The number and type of mast cell mediator interactions are potentially enormous, and their pathobiologic consequences are relevant to a variety of

homeostatic and disease processes. The best clues to the interaction of mediators are the known physiologic and pathologic manifestations of allergic diseases. It is hoped that the valuable tool of gene knockouts in mice will elucidate critical individual and interactive roles of these molecules (66).

■ THE ROLE OF THE MAST CELL AND ITS MEDIATORS IN TISSUE

The most compelling evidence for the role of mast cells and mediators in human tissue is derived from experiments in which IgE-dependent mast cell activation in skin is caused by specific antigen (or antibody to IgE). The participation of other immunoglobulin classes and immunologically activated cells, and thus of other inflammatory pathways, is excluded in such studies by using purified IgE to sensitize nonimmune individuals passively. Activation of cutaneous mast cells by antigen results initially in a pruritic wheal-and-flare reaction that begins in minutes and persists for 1 to 2 hours, followed in 6 to 12 hours by a large, poorly demarcated, erythematous, tender, and indurated lesion (66). Histologic analysis of the initial response shows mast cell degranulation, dermal edema, and endothelial cell activation. The late reaction is characterized by edema; by infiltration of the dermis by neutrophils, eosinophils, basophils, lymphocytes, and mononuclear leukocytes; and, in some instances, by hemorrhage, blood vessel wall damage, and fibrin deposition of sufficient severity to warrant the diagnosis of vasculitis. Similar studies of lung tissue responses, employing passive sensitization or mast cell-deficient subjects, have only been possible in mice. In humans, a similar dual-phase reaction is experienced by allergic patients who inhale antigen, but the participation of immunoglobulins other than IgE and of activating cells, other than mast cells cannot be excluded, therefore complicating assessment and preventing unambiguous assignment of any response to a particular immunologic pathway. Such challenges result in an immediate bronchospastic response followed by recovery, and, 6 to 24 hours later, by a recrudescence of asthmatic signs and symptoms (67). The mediators responsible for these pathophysiologic manifestations have not been delineated fully, but clues to their identity can be derived from knowledge of the effects of pharmacologic manipulation, by the identification of mediators in blood or tissue fluid obtained when the inflammatory response occurs, and by the known effects of isolated mediators.

Pharmacologic intervention suggests that the initial phase is mast cell-dependent in both skin and lung tissues. The initial response in skin may be inhibited by antihistamines, and in the lungs by cromolyn, aspirin, or antihistamines. In both tissues, corticosteroids effectively inhibit only the late response, reflecting its inflammatory nature. Histamine, TNF-α, tryptase, LTD$_4$, PGD$_2$, IL-5, and both neutrophil and eosinophil chemotactic activity are found soon after challenge. The late response is associated with leukocyte infiltration and cytokine release, but not with a unique profile of released mediators. The exact genesis of the early and late reactions is speculative. The concerted action of the spasmogenic mediators histamine, adenosine, PGD$_2$, leukotrienes, and PAF seems sufficient to account for all of the immediate pathophysiologic (anaphylactic) responses to antigen. This concept is supported by the knowledge that the early response occurs before a significant influx of circulating leukocytes.

However, mast cell mediators or mediators from antigen-reactive T lymphocytes, epithelial cells, or macrophages may induce such changes, either directly or indirectly. In response to mediators, vascular endothelium, fibroblast, and a variety of connective tissue and epithelial cells then could generate other inflammatory and vasoactive mediators. The late phases in lung and skin tissue are likely to represent the residue of the early response as well as the contribution of active enzymes, newly arrived plasma inflammatory cascades, various cytokines (particularly those inducing endothelial expression of adhesion molecules) (61), and the influx of activated circulating leukocytes. Of direct relevance to leukocyte recruitment are GM-CSF, IL-3, and especially IL-5, which promote eosinophil growth, differentiation, migration, adherence, and activation (68). The late inflammatory response is relevant to the progression of asthma in that patients experiencing the late responses have exacerbation of their nonspecific bronchial hyperreactivity, whereas this phenomenon does not occur after isolated early responses.

■ HOMEOSTATIC ROLE OF MAST CELLS

Mast cell mediators likely are important in maintaining normal tissue function and participate in the expression of innate immunity. Because mast cells are positioned near small blood vessels and at the host-environment interface, and are thus at crucial sites for regulating local nutrient delivery and for the entry of noxious materials, the potential regulatory role of mediators is obvious. They are likely to be especially important in the regulation of flow through small blood vessels, impulse generation in unmyelinated nerves, and smooth muscle and bone structural integrity and function. The ability to recruit and activate plasma proteins and cells may also provide preimmune defense against host invasion by infectious agents. Such a role is most apparent in parasitic infestation but is also likely in the case of other insults. Moreover, the recognition of mast cell heterogeneity implies that differences in mast cells relate to locally important biologic requirements.

Although the homeostatic and pathophysiologic role of mast cell mediators is understood imprecisely, the broadening understanding of their chemical nature and function provides a useful framework for addressing their role in health and disease.

■ REFERENCES

1. Williams CMM, Galli, SJ. The diverse potential effector and immunoregulatory roles of mast cells in allergic disease. *J Allergy Clin Immunol.* 2000;105:847–859.
2. Kirshenbaum AS, Goff JP, Semerc T, et al. Demonstration that human mast cells arise from a progenitor cell population that is CD 34+, cKit+ and expresses aminopeptidase N (CD13). *Blood.* 1999;94:2333–2342.
3. Church MK, Levi-Schaffer F. The human mast cell. *J Allergy Clin Immunol.* 1997;99:155–160.
4. Valent P, Bettelheim P. Cell surface structures on human basophils and mast cells. *Adv Immunol.* 1992;52:333–423.
5. DaSilva CA, Reber L, Frossard N. Stem cell factor expression, mast cells and inflammation in asthma. *Fundam Clin Pharmacol.* 2006; 20:21–39.
6. Oskeritzian CA, Zhao W, Min H, et al. Surface CD88 functionally distinguishes the MCTC from the MCT type of human lung mast cell. *J Allergy Clin Immunol.* 2005;115:1162–1168.
7. Brightling CE, Bradding P, Symon FA, et al. Mast-cell infiltration of airway smooth muscle in asthma. *N Engl J Med.* 2002;346:1699–1705.
8. Grimbaldeston MA, Chen C, Pilponsky AM, et al. Mast cell-deficient W-sash c-kit mutant kit$^{W-sh/W-sh}$ mice as a model for investigating mast cell biology in vivo. *Am J Pathol.* 2005;167:835–848.
9. Gessner A, Mohrs K, Mohrs M. Mast cells, basophils, and eosinophils acquire constitutive IL-4 and IL-13 transcripts during lineage differentiation that are sufficient for rapid cytokine production. *J Immunol.* 2005;174:1063–1072.
10. McGlashan D, Lichtenstein LM, McKenzie-White J, et al. Upregulation of FcεRI on human basophils by IgE antibody is mediated by interaction of IgE with FcεRI. *J Allergy Clin Immunol.* 1999;104: 492–498.
11. Siraganian, RP. Mast cell signal transduction from the high-affinity IgE receptor. *Curr Opin Immunol.* 2003;15:639–646. Review
12. Castells M. Mast cell mediators in allergic inflammation and mastocytosis. *Immunol Allergy Clin North Am.* 2006;26:465–485.
13. Krishnaswamy G, Ajitawi O, Chi DS. The human mast cell: an overview. *Methods Mol Bio.* 2006;315:13–34.
14. Dvorak AM, Morgan ES. Ribonuclease-gold ultrastructural localization of heparin in isolated human lung mast cells stimulated to undergo anaphylactic degranulation and recovery in vitro. *Clin Exp Allergy.* 1999;29:1118–1128.
15. Kelly-Welch AE, Hanson EM, Boothby MR, et al. Interleukin-4 and interleukin-13 signaling connections map. *Science.* 2003;300:1527–1528.
16. Kabu K, Yamasaki S, Kamimura D, et al. Zinc is required for FCεRI-mediated mast cell activation. *J Immunol.* 2006;177:1296–1305.
17. Siebenhaar, F, Magerl M, Peters EM, et al. Mast cell-driven skin inflammation is impaired in the absence of sensory nerves. *J Allergy Clin Immunol.* 2008;121:955–961. Epub 2007; Dec 22.
18. Bansal G, Xie Z, Rao S, et al. Suppression of immunoglobulin E-mediated allergic responses by regulator of G protein signaling 13. *Nat Immunol.* 2008;11:73–80.
19. Mertschung E, Bafetti L, Hess H, et al. A mouse Fcgamma-Fcepsilon protein that inhibits mast cells through activation of FcgammaRIIB, SH2 domain-containing inositol phosphatase 1, and SH2 domain-containing protein tyrosine phosphatases. *J Allergy Clin Immunol.* 2008;121:441–447.
20. Huang JF, Thurmond RL. The new biology of histamine receptors. *Curr Allergy Asthma Rep.* 2008;8:21–27.
21. Thurmond RL, Gelfand EW, Dunford PJ. The role of histamine H$_1$ and H$_4$ receptors in allergic inflammation: the search for new antihistamines. *Nat Rev Drug Discov.* 2008;7:41–53.
22. Hofstra CL, Desai PJ, Thurmond RL, et al. Hitsamine H$_4$ receptor mediates chemotaxis and calcium mobilization of mast cells. *J Pharmacol Exp Ther.* 2003;305:1212–1221.
23. Ling P, Ngo K, Nguyen S, et al. Histamine H$_4$ receptor mediates eosinophil chemotaxis with cell shape change and adhesion molecule upregulation. *Br J Pharmacol.* 2004;142:161–171.

24. Gantner F, Sakai K, Tusche MW, et al. Histamine H4 and H2 receptors control histamine-induced interleukin-16 from human CD8+ T cell. *J Pharmacol Exp Ther.* 2002;303:300–307.

25. Lin RY, Schwartz LB, Curr A, et al. Histamine and tryptase levels in patients with acute allergic reactions: an emergency department-based study. *J Allergy Clin Immunol.* 2000;106:65.

26. Roumestan C, Henriquet C, Gougat C, et al. Histamine H1-receptor antagonists inhibit nuclear factor kappaB and activator protein-1 activities via H1-recptor-dependent and –independent mechanisms. *Clin Exp Allergy.* 2008;38:947–956.

27. Gutzmer R, Diestel C, Mommert S, et al. Histamine H4 receptor stimulation suppresses IL-12p70 production and mediates chemotaxis in human monocytes-derived dendritic cells. *J Immunol.* 2005;174:5224–5232.

28. Thurmond RL, Desai PJ, Dunford PJ, et al. A potent and selective histamine H4 receptor antagonist with anti-inflammatory properties. *J Pharmacol Exp Ther.* 2004;309:404–413.

29. Dunford PJ, O'Donnell N, Riley JP, et al. The histamine H4 receptor mediates allergic airway inflammation by regulating the activation of CD4+ T cells. *J Immunol.* 2006;176:7062–7070.

30. Kasperska-Zajac A, Brzoza Z, Rogala B. Platelet activating factor as a mediator and therapeutic approach in bronchial asthma. *Inflammation.* 2008;31:112–120. Epub 2008 Jan 12.

31. Finkelman FD, Rothenberg ME, Brandt EB, et al. Molecular mechanisms of anaphylaxis: lessons from studies with murine models. *J Allergy Clin Immunol* 2005;115:449–457.

32. Vadas P, Gold M, Perelman B, et al. Platelet-activating factor, PAF acetylhydrolase and severe anaphylaxis. *N Engl J Med.* 2008;358:28–35.

33. Dudzinski DM, Igarashi J, Greif D, et al. The regulation and pharmacology of endothelial nitric oxide synthase. *Annu Rev Pharmacol Toxicol.* 2006;46:235–276.

34. Gilchrist M, McCauley SD, Befus AD. Expression, localization, and regulation of NOS in human mast cell lines effects on leukotriene production. *Blood.* 2004;104:462–469.

35. Cauewels A, Janssen B, Buys E, et al. Anaphylactic shock depends on PI3K and eNOS-derived NO. *J Clin Invest.* 2006;116:2241–2251.

36. Nagai H. Prostaglandin as a target molecule for pharmacotherapy of allergic inflammatory disease. *Allergol Int.* 2008;57:187–196. Epub 2008 Jun 1)

37. Ago H, Kanaoka Y, Irikura D, et al. Crystal structure of a human membrane protein involved in cysteinyl leukotriene biosynthesis. *Nature.* 2007;448:609–612.

38. Austen KF. Additional functions for the cysteinyl leukotrienes recognized through studies of inflammatory processes in null strains. *Prostaglandins Other Lipid Mediat.* 2007;83:182–187.

39. Hui Y, Cheng Y, Smalera I, et al. Directed vascular expression of human cysteinyl leukotriene 2 receptor modulates endothelial permeability and systemic blood pressure. *Circulation.* 2004;110:3360–3366.

40. Sorkness CA. Leukotriene receptor antagonists in the treatment of asthma. *Pharmacotherapy.* 2001;21:345–375.

41. Peters-Golden M, Henderson WR Jr. Leukotrienes. *N Engl J Med.* 2007;357:1841–1854.

42. Kim DC, Hsu FI, Barrett NA, et al. Cysteinyl leukotrienes regulate T_H2 cell-dependent pulmonary inflammation. *J Immunol.* 2006;176: 4440–4448.

43. Parettieri RA, Tan EM, Ciocca V, et al. Effects of LTD 4 on human airway smooth muscle cell proliferation, matrix expression, and contraction in vitro: differential sensitivity to cysteinyl leukotriene receptor antagonists. *Am J Respir Cell Mol Biol.* 1998;19:453–461.

44. Cui S, Shibamoto T, Takano H, et al. Leukotrienes and cyclooxygenase products mediate anaphylactic venoconstriction in ovalbumin sensitized rat livers. *Eur J Pharmacol.* 2007;576:99–106.

45. Powell WS, Rokach J. Biochemistry, biology and chemistry of the 5-lipoxygenase product 5-oxo-ETE. *Prog Lipid Res.* 2005;44:154–183.

46. Tager AM, Bromley SK, Medoff BD, et al. Leukotriene B4 receptor BLT1 mediates early effector T cell recruitment. *Nat Immunol.* 2003;4:982–990.

47. Mustafa FB, Ng FSP, Nguyen TH, et al. Honeybee venom secretory phospholipase A2 induces leukotriene production but not histamine release from human basophils. *Clin Exp Immunol.* 2008;151:94–100.

48. Wen R, Jou S, Chen Y, et al. Phospholipase Cγ2 is essential for specific functions of FcεR and FcγR. *J Immunol.* 2002;169:6743–6752.

49. Lee JH, Kim YM, Kim NW, et al. Phospholipase D2 acts as an essential adaptor protein the activation of Syk in antigen-stimulated mast cells. *Blood.* 2006;108:956–964.

50. Dinh TT, Kennerly DA. Assessment of receptor-dependent activation of phosphatidylcholine hydrolysis by both phospholipase D and phospholipase C. *Cell Regul* 1991;2:299–309.

51. Chahdi A, Choi WS, Kim YM, et al. Serine threonin kinases synergistically regulate phospholipase D1 and 2 and secretion of in RBL-2H3 mast cells. *Mol Immunol.* 2002:38:1269–1276.

52. Lee JH, Kim YM, Kim NW, et al. Phospholipase D2 acts as an essential adaptor protein in the activation of Syk in antigen-stimulated mast cells. *Blood.* 2006;108:956–964.

53. Brown RA, Spina D, Page CP. Adenosine receptors and asthma. *Br J Pharmacol.* 2008;153:S446–556.

54. Xu G, Nie H, Li N, et al. Role of osteopontin in amplification and perpetuation of rheumatoid arthritis. *J Clin Invest.* 2005;115:1060–1067.

55. Nagasaka A, Matsue H, Matsushima H, et al. Osteopontin is produced by mast cells and affects IgE-mediated degranulation and migration of mast cells. *Eur J Immunol.* 2008;38:489–499.

56. Xanthou G, Alissafi T, Semitekolou M, et al. Osteopontin has a crucial role in allergic airway disease through regulation of dendritic cell subsets. *Nat Med.* 2007;13:570–578.

57. Shakoory B, Fitzgerald SM, Lee SA, et al. The role of human mast cell-derived cytokines in eosinophil biology. *J Interferon Cytokine Res.* 2004;24:271–281.

58. Schwartz LB. Diagnostic value of tryptase in anaphylaxis and mastocytosis. *Immunol Allergy Clin North Am.* 2006;26:451–463. Review.

59. Rauter M, Krauth MT, Westritschnig K, et al. Mast cell-derived proteases control allergic inflammation through cleavage of IgE. *J Allergy Clin Immunol.* 2008;121:197–202.

60. Stevens RL, Adachi R. Protease-proteoglycan complexes of mouse and human mast cells and importance of their beta-tryptase-heparin complexes in inflammation and innate immunity. *Immunol Rev.* 2007; 217:155–167.

61. Kobayashi H, Ishizaka T, Okoyama Y. Human mast cells and basophils as sources of cytokines. *Clin Exp Allergy.* 2000;30:1205–1212.

62. Barata LT, Ying S, Meng O, et al. IL-4 and IL-5 positive T lymphocytes, eosinophils and mast cells in allergen induced late phase cutaneous reactions in atopic subjects. *J Allergy Clin Immunol.* 1998;101:222–230.

63. Toru H, Pawanhar R, Ra C, et al. Human mast cells produce IL-13 by high affinity IgE receptor cross-linking: enhanced IL-13 production by IL-4 primed mast cells. *J Allergy Clin Immunol.* 1998;102:491.

64. Wilson SJ, Shute JK, Holgate ST, et al. Localization of IL-4 but not IL-5 to human mast cell secretory granules by immunoelectron microscopy. *Clin Exp Allergy.* 2000;30:493–500.

65. Anthony RM, Rutitzky LI, Urban JF Jr, et al. Protective immune mechanisms in helminth infections. *Nat Rev Immunol.* 2007;7:975–987.

66. Nieuwenhuizen N, Herbert DR, Lopata AL, et al. CD4+ T cell-specific deletion of IL-4 receptor α prevents ovalbumin-induced anaphylaxis by an IFN-γ-dependent mechanism. *J Immunol.* 2007;179:2758–2765.

67. Gauvreau GM, Evans MY. Allergen inhalation challenge: a human model of asthma exacerbation. *Contrib Microbiol.* 2007;14:21–32.

68. Resnick MB, Weller PF. Mechanisms of eosinophil recruitment. *Am J Respir Cell Mol Biol.* 1993;8:349.

CHAPTER 4

Evaluation and Management of Immune Deficiency in Allergy Practice

MELVIN BERGER

There is considerable overlap between the manifestations of allergy and respiratory infection (i.e., rhinorrhea, sneezing, coughing, wheezing), and allergy may be a predisposing factor in sinusitis, otitis, and other respiratory infections. Therefore, the allergist must frequently evaluate patients with symptoms that have been attributed to recurrent infections and in which the competence of the patient's immune system has been or should be questioned. Because half or more of all patients with primary immune defects have antibody deficiencies (1,2) and most of them have problems with recurrent sinopulmonary infections, this is not an uncommon condition for which allergist-immunologists are consulted. Recent surveys suggest that the population prevalence of diagnosed primary immune deficiencies in the United States is at least 1 in 1,200, and many additional cases are undiagnosed (3). The intent of this chapter is to provide a practical approach to the diagnosis and management of such patients, not a comprehensive review of immune deficiency disorders or their molecular bases. Readers who wish a more in-depth analysis of immune deficiency disorders should consult comprehensive texts such as those edited by Ochs et al. (4) or Stiehm et al. (5).

■ INDICATIONS FOR AN IMMUNOLOGIC WORKUP

Although many immune-deficient patients present with a clear history of distinct episodes of severe infection, the allergist is frequently called on to see patients with less severe, nonspecific symptoms such as nasal stuffiness, chronic and recurrent rhinorrhea, or cough, which may be due to infection, allergy, or other factors. The first step in sorting out such complaints is to try to distinguish whether the symptoms are, in fact, due to

infection. Inciting factors, such as seasonality, and clearly identifiable triggers may suggest allergic etiologies; but changes in the weather and changes in seasons are frequently accompanied by changes in exposure to infectious diseases, especially among school-aged children.

A history of exposure to other people with similar symptoms; and details such as the presence or absence of fever, description of excessive secretions (clear and watery versus thick and purulent), and the response to antibiotics, may help to distinguish between infectious and noninfectious etiologies. After an estimate of the real incidence of infection is obtained, this can be compared with benchmarks such as the "10 Warning Signs of Immune Deficiency" (Fig. 4.1). The incidence of infection should be compared with the incidence for that age group in the community, but the exposure history should also be considered. For example, a 40-year-old who lives alone and sits at a computer all day would be expected to have a different degree of exposure to infectious agents than a kindergarten teacher, day care worker, or pediatric office nurse. College students moving from home to the dormitory for the first time and military recruits often have sharp increases in infectious disease exposure. Similarly, a first-born baby at home often has a very different degree of exposure than a similar-aged child in day care or with many siblings. Generally, the frequency of respiratory infection among school-aged children in the United States is about six to eight upper respiratory infections per year, but as many as one a month while school is in session is not unusual. About half of these may be primary bacterial infections or secondary bacterial sequelae, such as otitis media, sinusitis, pneumonia, or bronchitis.

Patients with clear histories of more than 10 distinct episodes of infection per year, more than two documented episodes of pneumonia per year, or more than

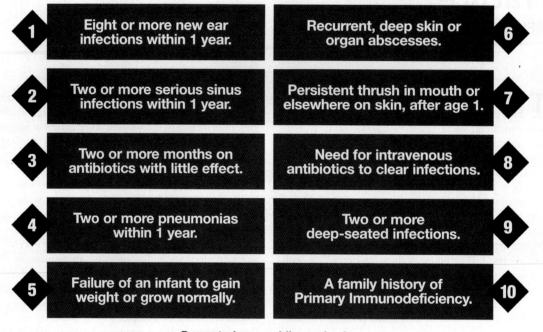

The 10 Warning Signs®
OF
Primary Immunodeficiency

Primary Immunodeficiency causes children and adults to have infections that come back frequently or are unusually hard to cure. In America alone, up to 1/2 million people suffer from one or more of the 80 known Primary Immunodeficiency diseases. If you or a child are affected by more than one of the following conditions, speak to your doctor about the possible presence of Primary Immunodeficiency.

1 Eight or more new ear infections within 1 year.

6 Recurrent, deep skin or organ abscesses.

2 Two or more serious sinus infections within 1 year.

7 Persistent thrush in mouth or elsewhere on skin, after age 1.

3 Two or more months on antibiotics with little effect.

8 Need for intravenous antibiotics to clear infections.

4 Two or more pneumonias within 1 year.

9 Two or more deep-seated infections.

5 Failure of an infant to gain weight or grow normally.

10 A family history of Primary Immunodeficiency.

Presented as a public service by:

 National Institute of Child Health and Human Development (NICHD)

 National Institute of Allergy and Infectious Disease (NIAID)

 National Cancer Institute (NCI)

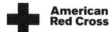
The Jeffrey Modell Foundation

American Red Cross

Aventis Behring
•
Baxter Healthcare Corporation
•
Bayer Corporation
•
Novartis Pharmaceuticals Corporation

For information or referrals contact The Jeffrey Modell Foundation: 1-800-JEFF-844 • www.jmfworld.com
These warning signs were developed by The Jeffrey Modell Foundation Medical Advisory Board • © 2000 The Jeffrey Modell Foundation

■ **FIGURE 4.1** The 10 warning signs of primary immune deficiency. (Presented as a public service by The Jeffrey Modell Foundation and American Red Cross. These warnings signs were developed by The Jeffrey Modell Foundation Medical Advisory Board.)

one life-threatening infection should be evaluated for possible immune deficiency or other underlying abnormalities. However, the specialist must be careful in interpreting the history from the patient or parent. Frequently, antibiotics are given when the patient does not have clear evidence for bacterial infection, then a failure to respond leads to the conclusion that "antibiotics do not work." This may, in turn, lead to the suggestion that there is something "wrong" with the patient's immune system. Frequent upper respiratory symptoms may represent individual viral upper respiratory infections. On the other hand, there may be prolonged symptoms from chronic infections such as sinusitis that have not been adequately treated despite multiple short courses of oral antibiotics. Patients who present with the complaint of "constant colds" may actually have allergic rhinitis. Densities on chest radiograph may represent atelectasis due to asthma rather than true infiltrates, and should not necessarily be taken as indicating recurrent pneumonia unless there is documentation of concomitant fever, elevated white blood cell count, or positive sputum Gram stain or culture.

Patients with unusually severe infections, such as those requiring parenteral antibiotics, prolonged or multiple courses of antibiotics for a single infection, or surgical intervention such as incision and drainage of abscesses or removal of seriously infected tissue (e.g., a segment of lung or infected bone), should probably also undergo at least screening (see later) to exclude immune deficiency. Patients with unusual or opportunistic infections, or with unusual responses, such as prostration or excessive fever to seemingly common organisms, should also be evaluated for immune deficiency.

Although many patients with primary immune deficiencies present with recurrent and chronic respiratory infections (2,5–7), gastrointestinal disorders are also common in these patients (8,9). The combination of recurrent respiratory infections with recurrent gastrointestinal symptoms may prompt immunologic screening even when the involvement of either organ system itself is not severe. Infection with *Giardia lamblia* (7,8) and bacterial overgrowth in the small intestine are not infrequent in patients with antibody deficiencies. These problems may present with symptoms such as cramps or diarrhea after eating, leading to suspicion of food allergy despite the absence of other manifestations of IgE-mediated reactions. In some immune-deficient patients, there may be organized lymphonodular hyperplasia in the intestine or infiltration of the submucosa with scattered aggregates of lymphocytes (7). Patients with gastrointestinal workups or biopsy results not typical for recognized patterns of inflammatory bowel disease should also undergo evaluation for immune deficiencies.

The presence of nonimmunologic findings on physical examination may also provide indications for evaluation to exclude immune deficiency (Table 4.1). Failure to thrive and/or leveling out of the growth curve in children, and unexplained weight loss in adults may indicate malabsorption due to intestinal infection or cumulative morbidity of other infections. The importance of recording accurate measurements of weight and height in children at every visit cannot be overemphasized. Eczema and thrombocytopenia may suggest

Wiskott-Aldrich syndrome (10). Facial, cardiac, or skeletal features are often suggestive of a recognizable pattern of malformation such as that seen in DiGeorge syndrome, short-limbed dwarfism, or cartilage-hair hypoplasia (11,12). Characteristic abnormalities of dentition have been described in NF-κB essential modulator (NEMO) deficiency and hyper IgE (Job) syndrome (13–15). The latter is also often accompanied by facial and skeletal abnormalities and a unique form of eczematoid dermatitis (14,15). Rib flaring and prominent costochondral junctions are skeletal abnormalities that may be present in severe combined immune deficiency (SCID) due to adenosine deaminase (ADA) deficiency (16). Alopecia and/or endocrinopathies occur with increased frequency in chronic mucocutaneous candidiasis due to mutations in the AIRE gene (17). Nystagmus, clumsiness, and other neurologic abnormalities may occur before observable telangiectasias and can suggest the diagnosis of ataxia-telangiectasia (18). Neurologic disorders are also common in purine nucleoside phosphorylase deficiency (19). Although delayed separation of the umbilical cord stump is widely recognized as an indicator of leukocyte adherence protein deficiency, in fact, there is a wide variation in the time at which the stump separates, and this should not be overemphasized in an otherwise well infant (20). Of course, patients with positive screening tests for human immunodeficiency virus (HIV) would also be candidates for immunologic evaluation.

Several immune deficiencies are clearly hereditary. For many, the patterns of inheritance and the precise molecular defects have been defined (21,22) (Table 4.2). Family members suspected of having these disorders, perhaps because an older sibling has already been diagnosed, should undergo assessment of their immune status. When available, tests for the specific molecular lesion should be included so that treatment aimed at correcting or compensating for the basic defect can be instituted early enough to prevent or minimize endorgan damage. Prenatal diagnosis and screening for the carrier state is now available for many of these disorders and can be used both in counseling and in ensuring that prompt and appropriate therapy is offered to affected newborns. It is important to realize, however, that a negative family history does not rule out a disease that is usually considered hereditary. For example, analysis of a large group of patients with confirmed mutations in Bruton tyrosine kinase revealed that 73% of the cases were sporadic, indicating a new mutation on the x-chromosome in that particular patient (6).

■ DOCUMENTING THE HISTORY OF INFECTION

A major goal in questioning the patient and reviewing the medical records is to develop a firm impression of

TABLE 4.1   PHYSICAL FINDINGS NOT DUE TO INFECTIOUS DISEASE ASSOCIATED WITH SELECTED IMMUNE DEFICIENCY SYNDROMES

I. Facial and Dental Abnormalities	
Broad nasal bridge, increased interalar distance	Hyper-IgE syndrome
Hypognathism; low, cupped ears	DiGeorge syndrome
Peg teeth	NEMO deficiency
Failure to lose primary teeth	Hyper-IgE syndrome
II. Other Skeletal Abnormalities	
Metaphysial chrondrodysplasia (short-limbed dwarfism)	Cartilage-hair hypoplasia
Cupped (dysplastic) costochondral junctions, abnormalities of apophyses of iliac bones and vertebrae	Adenosine deaminase deficiency
Multiple fractures	Hyper-IgE syndrome
III. Cardiac Defects	
Conotruncal (great vessel) defects	DiGeorge syndrome
Single chamber, anomalous pulmonary veins	Asplenia
IV. Thymic Abnormalities	
Hypoplasia or aplasia	DiGeorge syndrome
	Severe combined immune deficiency
Thymoma	Hypogammaglobulinemia (Good syndrome)
V. Central Nervous System Abnormalities	
Spasticity, retardation	Purine nucleoside phosphorylase deficiency
Ataxia (cerebellar), nystagmus, developmental delay	Ataxia telangiectasia
VI. Cutaneous Abnormalities	
Eczematoid rashes	Hyper-IgE syndrome
	Wiskott-Aldrich syndrome
Fine, sparse hair	Cartilage-hair hypoplasia
Poor wound healing, thin scars	Leukocyte adherence deficiency
Cutaneous and ocular telangiectasias	Ataxia telangiectasia
Oculocutaneous albinism	Chédiak-Higashi syndrome
Alopecia	Chronic mucocutaneous candidiasis
VII. Endocrine Defects	
Hypoparathyroidism/hypocalcemia	DiGeorge syndrome
Multiple (autoimmune) endocrinopathies	Chronic mucocutaneous candidiasis

the types of infections that the patient has suffered, so that subsequent laboratory tests can be targeted to specifically analyze those components of the immune system whose defects would most likely explain the patient's symptoms. This will be best served by keeping in mind general patterns of infection that might be caused by defects in specific immunologic defense mechanisms. Thus, infections with encapsulated extracellular bacterial pathogens, particularly of the respiratory tract, are suggestive of defects in antibody production (23), which

constitute the majority of all immune deficiencies (1). Noninvasive mucosal infections may particularly suggest isolated IgA deficiency (24). Infections with opportunistic pathogens, including protozoans and fungi, and severe or recurrent episodes of chickenpox or herpetic lesions, may suggest problems in cell-mediated immunity (4–7). Failure to clear bacteria promptly from the blood stream, resulting in bacteremia/sepsis, or hematogenously disseminated infections such as osteomyelitis, may be seen in deficiencies of C3 or early-acting

TABLE 4.2   MAJOR INHERITED IMMUNE DEFICIENCIES

DISORDER	DEFECTIVE GENE OR LOCUS
I. X-Linked	
Primarily B-cell Defect or Deficiency	
Bruton (X-linked) agammaglobulinemia	Bruton tyrosine kinase (BTK)
X-linked Hyper-IgM syndrome	CD40 ligand (gp39, CD154)
Wiskott-Aldrich syndrome	Wiskott-Aldrich syndrome protein (WASP)
Severe Combined Immune Deficiency	
X-linked severe combined immune deficiency	Cytokine receptor common chain (γ c chain)
Phagocyte Defects	
Chronic granulomatous disease (about 65%)	Gp91 phox component of cytochrome b245
Severe glucose-6-phosphatase deficiency	G-6-PD
Properdin deficiency	Properdin
II. Autosomal Recessive	
Primarily B-cell Defect or Deficiency	
Immunoglobulin heavy chain deletion	Indicated gene on chromosome 14
κ-Light chain deletion	22p11
Autosomal agammaglobulinemia	?
Common variable immune deficiency	TACI, ICOS, CD19 (together <10% of cases)
Ataxia telangiectasia	*ATM*, 11q22.3
Hyper IgM	Activation-induced cytidine deaminase
	Uracil-N-glycolase (UNG)
Primarily T-Cell Deficiency	
DiGeorge syndrome	22q11 microdeletion
Zeta chain associated protein deficiency (ZAP-70 def)	2q12
Severe Combined Immune Deficiency	
Adenosine deaminase deficiency	20q13
Janus kinase 3 (Jak 3) deficiency	19p13
Purine nucleoside phosphorylase deficiency	14q13.1
Natural Killer Cell Defect	
NEMO	NF-κB essential modifier
Phagocyte Defects	
Chronic granulomatous disease (35%)	Gp47phox or p22phox components of neutrophil oxidase
Leukocyte adherence deficiency type I	CD18 common β chain of leukocyte integrins
Leukocyte adherence deficiency type II	Sialyl-Lewis X (ligand for E-selectin)
Other complement component defects	Various autosomes

components of the complement system (25), but may also indicate asplenia or poor reticuloendothelial system function, as in sickle cell disease. Recurrent or disseminated neisserial infections may suggest deficiency of the later-acting complement components that form the membrane attack complex (25). Abscesses and infections with unusual bacteria or fungi may suggest neutropenia or defects in neutrophil function (6,7,26–28). Enteroviral meningoencephalitis may suggest X-linked agammaglobulinemia (29). On the other hand, it should be remembered that normal babies have increased susceptibility to infections usually controlled by T cells and γ-interferon (30), so that isolation of some organisms otherwise considered "opportunistic" should not always be cause for alarm.

The number and types of infections and their individual and cumulative morbidity should be assessed. It is necessary to carefully exclude other causes of nonspecific symptoms; for example, is sniffling or congestion due to recurrent upper respiratory infection, allergy, or other types of rhinitis? In contrast, documentable sinusitis is a frequent complication of primary immune deficiency (31). If cough is a major complaint, it is important to determine whether this is due to sputum production versus irritation, or other causes. Could it represent cough-equivalent asthma? If failure to thrive and cough are both present, could the patient have cystic fibrosis? Celiac or other forms of inflammatory bowel disease may mimic hypogammaglobulinemia in children with poor weight gain who also have frequent upper respiratory infections, which by themselves would not be considered significant.

Isolation and identification of responsible organisms is clearly the gold standard for rigorous diagnosis of infection. Documentation of fever, white blood count with differential, and sensitive but nonspecific measures such as the erythrocyte sedimentation rate and C-reactive protein can help distinguish between recurrent/chronic sinusitis and headaches due to other causes. These tests can also help with the differential diagnosis of recurrent cough or other chest symptoms. The importance of culture and examination of smears of nasal secretions for bacteria and neutrophils versus eosinophils cannot be overemphasized in distinguishing infectious from allergic and other noninfectious etiologies, particularly in small children. In some cases, the most appropriate step in the workup is to send the patient back to the primary care physician with instructions to have appropriate cultures and the readily available laboratory tests listed above performed every time an infection is suspected or the symptoms recur. Similar steps may also help in identifying adults with recurrent headaches erroneously attributed to chronic/recurrent sinusitis. Sometimes, culture results point to the diagnosis, as in the case of *Pseudomonas aeruginosa* suggesting cystic fibrosis, or invasive aspergillosis suggesting neutropenia or chronic granulomatous disease (CGD) (28). Chronic or recurrent *Cryptosporidium parvum* infection may suggest the X-linked hyper IgM syndrome (CD40 ligand deficiency) (32,33), and, of course, *Streptococcus pneumoniae* or *Haemophilus influenzae* suggest antibody deficiency (1,5–7,23).

Clues to the severity and overall morbidity resulting from infection may be obtained by asking whether hospitalization or intravenous antibiotics have been required to treat infections or whether oral antibiotics have generally been sufficient. The response to therapy should be evaluated carefully. Continued high fever or other symptoms suggesting a lack of response of

culture-confirmed bacterial infection to antibiotics is more likely indicative of a significant immune deficiency than is the frequently seen pattern in which the fever and symptoms resolve promptly when antibiotic therapy is started (e.g., for otitis media) only to recur again shortly after the prescribed course of therapy is concluded. The latter may actually represent a distinct new infection. This pattern is quite commonly seen in children in day care and in adults with frequent exposure to small children. Similarly, it is also important to distinguish inadequate or inappropriate therapy (i.e., antibiotics for viral URIs) from failure to respond, and it is important to differentiate chronic infections from recurrent episodes. Absence from school or work should be quantitated if possible, and any long-term sequelae or disability should be documented. The family history should include questions about siblings and preceding generations. Family trees with premature deaths of male infants should raise suspicion of X-linked immune deficiencies (Table 4.2). However, the absence of such a family history does not rule out X-linked disorders, which may have a high spontaneous mutation rate (6,22). Questions should also be asked about the family history of asthma and allergy as well as other genetic diseases that may present with recurrent infection such as cystic fibrosis. In evaluating a child, it may be important to determine whether the parents have died prematurely or have known risk factors for HIV infection.

The age at onset of infections of unusual frequency or severity may yield important insights into possible underlying immune deficiencies. It must be kept in mind that term newborns have IgG levels equivalent to those of their mothers, from whom most of their IgG has been transferred across the placenta (34). Thus, babies who have problems with infections during the first few months of life may have T-cell or phagocyte problems but are less likely to have agammaglobulinemia or other isolated problems in antibody production. In contrast, disorders of antibody production are more likely to present after the age of 6 months. The history of exposure must be carefully considered in evaluating this issue because the frequency of common types of infections often increases after a child's exposure to infectious agents increases on starting day care or preschool, particularly if there are no siblings in the home. Although patients with severe antibody deficiency such as that seen in Bruton agammaglobulinemia classically present between 6 months and 2 years of age (6,29), that diagnosis as well as the diagnosis of hyper-IgM syndromes is often delayed until later in childhood (6,29,31,32). Common variable immunodeficiency disease (CVID) may present at any age (35–37). That diagnosis is frequently delayed by 8 to 10 years from the onset of increased morbidity due to infection. Diagnosis of CVID in older children and young adults may represent an early-onset deficiency that has not been previously recognized or a newly acquired problem. Just as some infants may have delayed development of the full range of immune responses (38), it seems likely that some adults may undergo premature senescence of immune responsiveness (39) and may present with recurrent bacterial infections and/or activation of latent infections (i.e., shingles, tuberculosis) in their 40s or 50s, as opposed to their 60s or 70s.

THE PHYSICAL EXAMINATION IN CASES OF SUSPECTED IMMUNE DEFICIENCY

The physical examination often provides important evidence for or against immune deficiency and may also allow the physician to assess critically the cumulative morbidity due to infection. Most importantly, the presence or absence of lymphoid tissue should be carefully documented. The absence of visible tonsils in patients who have not had them surgically removed and the absence of palpable cervical or inguinal lymph nodes should promote a strong suspicion of a significant antibody deficiency because the bulk of these tissues is composed of B-lymphocytes involved in antibody synthesis. Conversely, the presence of palpable lymph nodes and easily visible tonsils essentially excludes Bruton agammaglobulinemia and may suggest the absence of SCID, but does not help one way or the other with the diagnosis of CVID or X-linked hyper-IgM syndrome. The presence of cervical or peripheral adenopathy, splenomegaly, or hepatomegaly may suggest CVID, HIV, CGD, or other abnormalities. Many anatomic findings are associated with immune defects in recognizable malformation syndromes (Table 4.1); characteristic rashes may suggest Wiskott-Aldrich (10) or hyper-IgE (Job) syndromes (14,15); clumsiness, nystagmus and ocular telangiectases may suggest ataxia-telangiectasia (18); and craniofacial abnormailities may suggest DiGeorge syndrome in patients who do not have major cardiac defects (12). Secondary effects, such as failure to thrive, weight loss, and short stature, may suggest significant morbidity due to chronic or recurrent infection. Scars from incision and drainage of abscesses or from drainage or surgical reduction of enlarged lymph nodes may indicate significant morbidity from neutrophil defects (27,28).

Autoimmune phenomena (40,41) and rheumatic complaints (40–42), including infectious or chronic arthritis, are common in patients with CVID and other primary immune deficiencies and may suggest evaluation for immune deficiency, even if the number or severity of acute infections has not been excessive.

Careful assessment of the tympanic membranes, paranasal sinuses, and chest is extremely important in evaluating patients suspected of having antibody deficiency syndromes. The quantity and characteristics of secretions should be documented and it should determined whether observed abnormalities are acute or chronic. In this regard, high-resolution (thin-slice) computed tomography (CT) scans of the chest and formal pulmonary function testing may be very helpful, because observation of bronchiectasis, areas of "ground-glass" density in the lung parenchyma, and/or hilar adenopathy may suggest the presence of subclinical chronic disease, which could be associated with antibody deficiency and/or CVID (43,44). Clubbing of the digits may also provide an important indication of chronic lung disease.

GENERAL LABORATORY SCREENING TESTS

Guidelines for the diagnosis and management of immunodeficiency and handy algorithims are available from the Joint Council on Allergy, Asthma, and Immunology (45), the Immune Deficiency Foundation (1), and the Jeffrey Modell Foundation (http://www.info4PI.org). These can help prioritize screening tests that might be ordered and interpreted by the primary physician and define situations in which referral to the specialist becomes appropriate. Often, the primary care physician can already have these results in hand when the specialist is called to determine if referral is appropriate.

A review of laboratory tests already obtained by the primary care physician may yield important clues to the presence of an immune deficiency disorder and may save steps in the evaluation of patients by suggesting which of the more specialized tests are most likely to be informative. The complete blood count (CBC) and differential is a critical first step. It is important to remember that lymphocyte counts in newborns should be higher than in older children and adults, and that age-appropriate norms should be used (46,47). Neutropenia may be a primary abnormality, or may accompany X-linked agammaglobulinemia (6,26). General blood chemistry panels will show low total protein but normal albumin in agammaglobulinemia. A low uric acid level may be indicative of ADA deficiency or purine nucleoside phosphorylase deficiency (16,48); while a low serum calcium level may suggest DiGeorge syndrome.

In addition to assessing the airways and lung parenchyma, the chest radiograph should be reviewed for the absence or presence of a thymus in infants and for the possibility of a thymoma, which may be associated with hypogammaglobulinemia in adults (49). Hyperinflation with patches of atelectasis, suggestive of asthma, might suggest that additional details of the past history should be carefully reviewed in patients referred because of cough or recurrent pneumonia. Particularly in small children, densities actually due to atelectasis may be misinterpreted as infiltrates suggestive of pneumonia. The presence of old scars and active disease should be documented. Hilar adenopathy may be seen in cellular and humoral immune defects. Abnormalities of the ribs resembling rickets can be seen in ADA deficiency (16); abnormalities of the great vessels may suggest asplenia (50) or DiGeorge syndrome (12,51) or may steer the workup away from immune deficiency and toward Kartagener syndrome (situs inversus and ciliary dysmotility).

■ IMMUNOLOGIC SCREENING TESTS

Initial laboratory tests, which may indicate that a patient has an immune deficiency, can be done in most regional laboratories and community hospitals, with results available in a few days. These should include measurement of the major immunoglobulins and consideration of IgG subclasses. In older adults, serum protein electrophoresis should be considered because patients with monoclonal gammopathy, multiple myeloma, or chronic lymphocytic leukemia (CLL) may have antibody deficiency co-existing with a normal total level of the class of immunoglobulin that includes the paraprotein. Interpreting serum concentrations of IgG and its subclasses is often less than straightforward (37,42). First of all, age-specific norms must be used, because of the marked changes in values during the first 2 years of life. Although some laboratories may report IgG concentrations as low as 200 mg/dL as "normal" in 3-month-old to 6-month-old infants, concentrations of less than 400 mg/dL frequently fail to provide sufficient protective antibody levels (52). Second, even within a given age group, most laboratories report a normal range whose upper limit may be two or more times its lower limit. It should be remembered that the total serum IgG concentration represents the sum of hundreds of separately regulated responses, rather than a single variable whose physiology requires reasonably tight control, like that of an electrolyte or the blood glucose. Concentrations of IgG, and particularly its subclasses, vary not only among individuals of the same age who have different exposure histories but also in a single individual at different times. Thus, before any conclusions are reached about the diagnosis of IgG subclass deficiency, the tests should be repeated several weeks apart, and analysis of specific antibody titers should also be considered in pediatric patients and should be performed in adults (see discussion later in this chapter). In 2-month-old to 8-month-old babies, the results of any single measurement may be less important than the trend observed in two or more measurements at monthly intervals (38).

In judging the adequacy of the IgG concentration in a given individual, the history of exposure and the frequency of documented infections must be considered. Thus, normal individuals with frequent exposure to pathogens and those whose host defenses are compromised by conditions that do not affect lymphocyte responses, such as cystic fibrosis and chronic granulomatous disease, often have elevated total serum IgG concentrations. This may be considered a physiologic adaptation or the response of a normal immune system to increased or persistent antigen stimulation. IgG concentrations toward the lower limit of normal in patients with comparably increased frequency of or morbidity due to infection (but without underlying nonimmunologic defects) may thus actually indicate relative deficiency in specific antibodies and should be evaluated further, as explained below.

In addition to those conditions in which paraproteins may conceal true antibody deficiencies within normal total IgG levels, several diseases may be associated with nonspecific polyclonal B-cell activation that may cause the total IgG and/or IgM level to be within the normal range or even elevated, while specific antibodies may actually be deficient. This is not unusual in systemic lupus erythematosus, Epstein-Barr virus infection, and HIV infection (53,54). Finding low or absent serum IgA together with low-normal or borderline levels of one or more IgG subclasses, particularly subclass 2, should also raise suspicion of more severe defects in specific antibody production than would be suggested by the total IgG concentration per se, and such patients should also be investigated further (55). Elevated serum IgE and IgA concentrations may be found co-existing with deficiency of antibodies to polysaccharides in Wiskott-Aldrich syndrome, and extremely high IgE levels may suggest, but are not by themselves diagnostic of, hyper-IgE (Job) syndrome.

Quantitation of lymphocyte subtypes by flow cytometry is now widely available and should be included as a screening test in all patients in whom cellular immune deficiency is suspected (56,57). A CBC with differential should always accompany lymphocyte surface marker analysis so that the absolute number of any given type of cell per cubic millimeter of blood can be calculated. As with immunoglobulin determinations, age-specific norms should be used (46). This is extremely important since normal newborns and infants should have higher T-cell counts than older children or adults, and T-lymphopenia suggests SCID (46,47). The physician should be careful about the specific test that is ordered because, in the era of widespread treatment of HIV, many laboratories offer a standard "lymphocyte surface marker panel," which includes only CD3, CD4, and CD8 T cells. Because antibody deficiency due to decreased B-cell number or function is the most common type of immune deficiency overall, a complete analysis, including enumeration of B cells and natural killer (NK), cells should be performed. In addition, because patients with chronic CLL may present with antibody deficiency, the ratio of lymphocytes expressing κ and λ light chains should also be determined. Analysis of T-cell subsets, B cells, and NK cells frequently provides important clues to the actual molecular defect in many cases of SCID (see below). The exact defect can often be confirmed by analysis of intracellular signaling molecules, which can now also be accomplished using flow cytometry (56,57). Disorders due to mutations in lymphocyte surface molecules such as CD40-ligand (CD154) deficiency in X-linked hyper-IgM syndrome, and Fas (CD95) deficiency in the autoimmune lymphoproliferative syndrome (ALPS), are readily diagnosable by flow cytometry, as are several disorders of neutrophil surface molecule expression. Defects in the neutrophil microbicidal oxidase pathway (i.e., in chronic granulomatous disease) can also be detected by flow cytometry, using dyes such as dihydrorhodamine, which are taken up by the cells and whose fluorescence changes when the cells produce H_2O_2 (58).

More rare deficiencies involving other arms of the immune system can also be identified and characterized at this level of testing. In patients suspected of defects in T-cell–mediated immunity, the overall functional activity of T cells is best assessed by determining the patient's ability to mount cutaneous delayed hypersensitivity reactions to recall antigens such as candida, mumps, or tetanus toxoid (58). Obviously, delayed hypersensitivity skin tests have little meaning in children younger than 2 years of age, who may not be adequately immunized. Patients who have infections suggestive of defects in T-cell–mediated immunity should also undergo HIV screening.

The CBC will give an indication of the number of phagocytes. Assessing their function can often be done by flow cytometry but may require more specialized laboratory capabilities (58,59). Complement screening should include measurement of the serum C3 concentration and the total hemolytic activity (CH_{50}) because the former may be seriously reduced without affecting the latter. The CH_{50} is the best overall screening test for complement defects and is zero in cases of late component defects, such as those that predispose to recurrent or disseminated Neisserial infections (25). However, serum for this test must be handled carefully or partially reduced values will be measured, and repeat testing is often required. In patients with a history of bacteremia, sepsis, or hematogenously spread infection, a careful review of the peripheral blood smear, looking for Howell-Jolly bodies in the erythocytes, and/or special microscopic examination for pits in their membranes (60), may suggest anatomic or functional asplenia or severely impaired reticuloendothelial system function.

■ DETAILED IMMUNOLOGIC LABORATORY EVALUATION

Although frank hypogammaglobulinemia, neutropenia, and complete deficiency of a component of the classic complement pathway can be detected by the screening laboratory tests described previously, more detailed testing is necessary to detect more subtle immune deficiencies. This level of testing is also frequently necessary to characterize severe defects more completely.

Because of the possibility that clinically significant antibody deficiency may be present even when the total serum concentrations of the major immunoglobulin classes and IgG subclasses are normal, specific antibody production should be assessed in all cases in which the clinical presentation suggests recurrent bacterial infections, particularly of the respiratory tract. This may not be necessary if the major immunoglobulin classes themselves are absent or severely depressed. Specific antibody titers should be measured against polysaccharide as well as protein antigens (61–63). Although measurement of isohemagglutinins, (antibodies to the A, B, or both blood group substances in patients of other blood groups) may be used to screen for the ability to produce antibodies against polysaccharides, the availability of measurement of antibodies against specific bacterial antigens has decreased dependence on those assays.

If specific pathogens have been isolated and identified (e.g., from effusions at the time of insertion of tympanostomy tubes, endoscopic drainage of paranasal sinuses, or expectorated or induced sputum samples), antibodies against those specific organisms could also be measured. In addition, antibodies against common immunizing agents should be measured. We usually request measurement of antibodies against tetanus and diphtheria toxins and several pneumococcal polysaccharides as well as *H. influenzae* type B polysaccharide (61–63). Testing for these and additional antibody titers are available in many commercial laboratories and are sometimes referred to as a *humoral immunity panel*.

An advantage of using these particular antigens is that they are contained in readily available, well-tested vaccines, which often have already been given or will be clinically indicated for the patients in question, so that exposure to the antigen is definite. Obtaining titers before, as well as 4 to 8 weeks after, immunization allows comparison of the response to each antigen. The absence of a threefold rise in titer after immunization and/or failure to achieve protective levels indicates that the patient is unable to mount specific antibody responses. This may be seen either with protein or polysaccharide antigens and may indicate a failure to process properly or recognize an entire class of antigens., This may occur in what has been termed *specific polysaccharide antibody deficiency*; or the failure to respond to certain particular antigens may be considered a "lacunar" defect. Deficient vaccine responses may also be seen with "normal" Ig levels in patients with polyclonal B-cell activation or lymphoma (see above).

In some rare cases, patients already receiving immunoglobulin infusions may require assessment of their own specific antibody production, which may be difficult because antibodies against many common antigens will have been acquired passively. In many cases, the immunoglobulin therapy can be stopped for a few months so that the patients can be immunized and their own antibody production measured while they are being reassessed clinically. If this is not possible, special test antigens, such as keyhole limpet hemocyanin and the bacteriophage øX174, can be obtained from specialized centers (64). Because most individuals and plasma donors have not been commonly exposed to these antigens, commercial immunoglobulin preparations do not contain antibodies against them, and they can be used to assess *de novo* specific antibody formation.

Specific T-cell function is most commonly tested by measuring the incorporation of ^{3}H-thymidine into the newly formed DNA of rapidly proliferating lymphocytes after cultures of peripheral blood mononuclear cells are stimulated *in vitro* (65). Lectins, proteins that bind common polysaccharides on the surface of human cells, are frequently used as the stimuli. Because these proteins stimulate most human lymphocytes, regardless of prior antigen sensitization, they are called *mitogens*, and tests using them should be referred to as *lymphocyte mitogen proliferation assays*. Plant-derived lectins typically used for mitogen proliferation assays include concanavalin A, phytohemagglutinin, and pokeweed mitogen. Incorporation of ^{3}H-thymidine, a low-molecular-weight precursor, into high-molecular-weight cellular DNA in newly proliferating lymphocytes serves as the basis for the measurements, and the results may be expressed as the amount incorporated (in counts per minute) or as the ratio of incorporation in parallel cultures of mitogen-stimulated versus unstimulated lymphocytes, also referred to as the *stimulation index*. Mitogen stimulation tests are useful even in newborns who have not received any immunizations. These tests may be particularly informative about lymphocyte function and immune competence in babies with partial T-cell deficiency, such as in DiGeorge syndrome (66). Disadvantages of these tests include the requirements for several milliliters of blood, which may be prohibitive for small newborns; time constraints that may be imposed by the laboratory to facilitate isolation of the mononuclear cells during normal working hours; and the fact that the cells must be cultured for several days (usually 48 hours to 72 hours) before they are "pulsed" with ^{3}H-thymidine to assess its incorporation.

To surmount these difficulties, many laboratories are now using flow cytometry assays based on the appearance on the lymphocyte plasma membrane of early activation markers such as CD69 (67). Mixed lymphocyte cultures, in which a patient's T cells are stimulated by a relative or other potential donor's lymphocytes that have been irradiated to prevent them from proliferating (and vice versa), are also used to test T-cell competence and to determine histocompatability in cases in which bone marrow transplantation is contemplated. Staphylococcal enterotoxins are also often employed as stimuli in proliferation assays because they function as "superantigens," which stimulate broad families of T cells by binding to parts of their T-cell receptors other than the antigen-binding site. The response to these superantigens is thus also independent of prior antigen sensitization. T-cell proliferative responses to recall antigens may also be assessed using similar techniques. However, because fewer T cells respond to any given antigen than to the more broadly reacting mitogens discussed above, these tests commonly involve 4- to 5-day incubation periods before the ^{3}H-thymidine incorporation is determined. The Cowen strain of *Staphylococcus aureus* may be used as a T-cell–independent stimulus for B-cell proliferation.

Obviously, antigen responses can only be expected if it is documented that the patient has been exposed to the antigen in question. Thus, antigen stimulation tests are usually not useful in early infancy. However, if an older child is known to have received his or her scheduled immunizations, or if candidal infection has been obvious, the response to soluble candida preparations and vaccine antigens such as tetanus toxoid may be useful. Patients with normal responses to mitogens who fail to respond to candida may be considered to have chronic mucocutaneous candidiasis rather than a more pervasive T-cell defect. In patients with opportunistic infections suggestive of AIDS or positive screening tests for HIV, confirmatory tests, such as Western blot, and quantitation of p24 antigen or viral load should be performed. Absolute CD4 number, T-cell function, and viral load should also be assessed as part of the detailed evaluation (68).

Detailed laboratory analysis in patients suspected of phagocyte disorders should include assessment of neutrophil chemotaxis and the oxidative respiratory burst that accompanies phagocytosis (69,70). Chemotaxis is assessed by measuring the migration of polymorphonuclear leukocytes through agar gels or across filters. The oxidative burst can be assessed by the nitroblue tetrazolium test, in which a soluble yellow dye is reduced to an easily visible insoluble blue intracellular precipitate (71). Flow cytometric assays in which oxidized products are detected by fluorescence may also be employed (58,69). If the CH_{50} was abnormal on screening, the actual deficient component can be identified by functional testing in reference laboratories. These laboratories can also screen for abnormalities of the alternative and lectin pathways, which may be indicated in patients who have recurrent bacterial infections or bacteremia and sepsis despite normal results in tests for antibodies and the classic complement pathway.

■ MOLECULAR GENETIC DIAGNOSIS AND OTHER ADVANCED TESTING

Advanced testing to pinpoint the molecular lesion in cases of confirmed immune deficiency is usually performed at a university or research center laboratory by a specialized immunologist. However, an additional level of definition is now possible in many hospital and commercial laboratories and may aid the practitioner in providing prognostic and genetic counseling information for patients and their families. The pattern of X-chromosome inactivation (22,72,73) can be used to determine whether female family members are carriers of Bruton agammaglobulinemia, Wiskott-Aldrich syndrome, neutrophil defects, and other, but not all, X-linked disorders (72,73). Furthermore, practitioners should recognize that defining the molecular defect is important in the management of immune-deficient patients because several forms of specific therapy are already available and new modalities are being developed at a rapid rate. Patients with SCID should be classified as completely as possible with flow cytometry, which may be highly suggestive of the exact molecular lesion and may have important prognostic implications (56,57,74). Identification of lymphopenia in babies using age-specific norms for the CBC and differential should prompt complete evaluation of lymphocyte subsets as quickly as possible (46,47). In particular, relative preservation of B cells in SCID patients with very low T- and NK-cell counts may suggest deficiency of the important signaling kinase Jak 3 (75) or the common γ cytokine receptor chain (76). The latter is a component of multiple receptors necessary for lymphocyte development and is the site of mutations in most cases of X-linked SCID. These disorders may be cured by hematopoietic stem cell transplantation (HSCT)) and have been successfully treated by gene therapy, increasing the importance of prompt recognition of this specific defect (78,79). B, T and NK cells may be present in equal numbers in forms of autosomal recessive SCID not due to ADA deficiency (74,79). Relatively selective deficiency of CD8 cells is characteristic of deficiency of Zap 70, a protein kinase important in signaling from the T-cell receptor. The most likely defect can then be confirmed in specialized research laboratories using assays for the specific protein (by Western blot or flow cytometry) or gene that is suspect. Fluorescence *in situ* hybridization (FISH) (80) can be used to confirm the chromosome abnormality in patients suspected of having DiGeorge or velocardiofacial syndrome, compound anomaly syndromes that may be associated with partial T-cell deficiencies and are due to microdeletions in chromosome 22q11.2 (12,51).

Advances in technology have made detection of defects in gene transcription readily detectable by real-time PCR, and greatly facilitated identification of specific mutations by microarray or actual DNA sequencing. Definitive DNA tests for known mutations are becoming increasingly available in commercial laboratories, and the scope of such molecular testing is increasing rapidly.

Babies with SCID, their parents, and siblings should promptly undergo human leukocyte antigen typing to begin to evaluate the possibility of HSCT, which may be accompanied by minimal morbidity if performed before serious infection is established, and is curative in many cases (74). This is best accomplished in the first month of life, before there has been end-organ damage and/or chronic infection. If there is no potential donor who matches at all loci, transplantation of T-cell–depleted marrow from a donor with a mismatch at one or more loci might be considered, but is performed only at certain research centers. There may be mild or delayed presentations of SCID due to enzyme deficiencies such as purine nucleoside phosphorylase deficiency or ADA deficiency. Making the correct diagnosis as early as possible is especially important in the latter because enzyme replacement with bovine ADA conjugated with polyethylene glycol (Adagen) is readily available and often results in marked amelioration of the immune defect. This can serve as a bridge until stem cell transplantation is performed or as long-term replacement if the patient does not have a matched donor (81). In cases of T-cell deficiency with impaired mitogen responses, anticoagulated whole blood should be sent to a research center with expertise in these assays (48,81). Gene therapy has been used with some success in ADA deficiency and in deficiency of the common γ chain of the T-cell cytokine receptor (77,78). Therefore, in cases of apparent SCID in which B cells are present (74,79), early definition of the exact defect, which may often be determined by flow cytometry, is important.

■ EARLY MANAGEMENT OF CELLULAR AND SEVERE COMBINED IMMUNE DEFICIENCY

Infants with significant defects in T-cell number or function and those with SCID are not only at great risk for infection with opportunistic pathogens but also may suffer from severe or overwhelming infection with attenuated live viruses used for immunization. They may present with rashes and eosinophilia due to disregulated oligoclonal autologous T cells or graft-versus-host disease (GVHD) from maternal or transfused leukocytes, as in Omenn syndrome and other severe defects (82). Some states in the United States have already started neonatal screening for SCID based on correlates of lymphopenia (83). For these reasons, special precautions must be initiated as soon as this type of immune defect is suspected, while the immunologic workup is proceeding and plans for referral and definitive treatment are being formulated. First, any blood products that are given must be irradiated to prevent transfusion of viable lymphocytes that could cause GVHD. Second, live virus vaccines must be avoided.

With current recommendations in the United States abandoning the use of the live attenuated oral polio vaccine and replacing it with inactivated vaccine only, polio is less of a risk. However, immunization with

Bacille-Calmette-Guérin vaccine is practiced in many other countries and may lead to fatal infection. Live measles-mumps-rubella and varicella vaccines should also be avoided. Prophylaxis with varicella-zoster immune globulin should be given if infants with T-cell defects or SCID are exposed to children with chickenpox. Trimethoprim-sulfamethoxazole or other appropriate regimens should be should be used for prophylaxis against *P. carinii* pneumonia (84), and prolonged courses of nystatin and/or systemic antifungals may be necessary to control candida. The use of passive immunization against respiratory syncytial virus (Synagis®) and intravenous or subcutaneous immune globulin should be considered, particularly in low-birth-weight infants and in those older than 6 months of age. This may be required for more than a year, even in children who have received HSCT, because functional B-cell engraftment is often delayed and/or incomplete.

■ MANAGEMENT OF ANTIBODY DEFICIENCY SYNDROMES

Because half or more of all primary immune deficiencies involve defects in antibody production, management of these patients is a common part of allergy-immunology practice. Patients with X-linked agammaglobulinemia, hyper-IgM syndromes, and other severe immunoglobulin deficiencies clearly require immunoglobulin replacement (see below). On the other hand, decisions about IgG supplementation in patients with less severe deficiencies often require close observation, subjective evaluation, and clinical judgement, in addition to laboratory data. A useful scheme is presented in Table 4.3. In deciding which form of therapy may be most appropriate for any given patient, the practitioner must consider not only the underlying diagnosis but also the exposure history, the cumulative morbidity and future risk for end-organ damage from infection, and the risks and adverse effects of the various therapeutic options. The number of days lost from school or work due to infection, as well as the number of days which might be required for IgG infusions at a hospital or infusion center must be considered, along with other interferences with the patient's lifestyle. Formal pulmonary function tests and CT scans may indicate progressive yet subclinical chronic lung disease which may mandate chronic treatment, despite a lack of acute pneumonias. The absence of symptomatic complaints of chronic lung disease may represent accommodation and/or denial by the patient (43,44,85). Often, antibody-deficient patients who present with repeated acute infections also have systemic morbidity, about which they may or may not complain. This may include fatigue, lack of stamina, poor weight gain (in infants), and musculoskeletal/rheumatic symptoms that have been attributed to other causes or ignored. Because these symptoms often improve with appropriate management of chronic infection and immunoglobulin replacement, they must be carefully evaluated in the review of systems and weighed in considering the options for therapy. Patients with a history of inflammatory bowel disease, recurrent problems with *Clostridium difficile,* and/or drug allergies may have decreased tolerance for antibiotics, which can limit the alternatives to IgG therapy. Patients diagnosed with chronic obstructive pulmonary disease and those with asthma triggered by infection may actually have underlying antibody deficiencies. If so, the patient may experience a marked amelioration of lower airway symptoms if infection is prevented with IgG supplementation and/or the astute use of antibiotics (86).

A hierarchy of treatments may be employed across the range of severities of antibody deficiency, or sequentially in any given patient. Some patients, particularly small children, with partial antibody deficiency who have not had significant permanent end-organ damage may be managed by limiting their exposure to infectious agents (e.g., by removing them from day care or preschool) and being sure that they have received all appropriate vaccines, including conjugated polysaccharide vaccines and annual immunization against influenza. Measurement of specific antibody titers after administration of these vaccines may provide reassurance for parents and referring physicians and may suggest that additional therapy is not indicated. In some cases of partial antibody deficiency, immunization, prompt and rigorous treatment of likely bacterial infections such as sinusitis and bronchitis, with verification that these are continued until the infection has been completely resolved, may provide satisfactory control of infection. Freedom from chronic or progressive symptoms should be assessed by frequent clinical follow-up. In other cases, prolonged courses of oral antibiotics and/or parenteral treatment may be required. The

---

TABLE 4.3   WHEN IS IGG REPLACEMENT/SUPPLEMENTATION INDICATED?

- IgG <200 mg/dL: All patients.
- IgG 200 mg/dL to 500 mg/dL: If specific antibody deficiency documented and frequent infections.
- IgG >500 mg/dL: If specific antibody deficiency identified and severe/recurrent infections, and/or intolerance or failure of antibiotics.

After presentation by Dr. Anders Fasth, European Society for Immune Deficiency, Budapest, 2006.

next step would be the use of prophylactic antibiotics. Many patients attain satisfactory freedom from infection by a once-daily dose of trimethoprim-sulfamethoxazole* (e.g., half of the total daily dose that would be used for otitis media). Other oral antibiotics, such as ampicillin or a cephalosporin, may also be used, especially in patients who are allergic to sulfonamides, but these may be associated with a higher risk for resistant bacteria. Patients who develop diarrhea or other excessive gastrointestinal side effects, oral thrush, or vaginal candidiasis may be poor candidates for this approach. Because of the possible development of antibiotic resistance, when patients on prophylactic antibiotics develop infections likely to be of bacterial origin, a full course of different agent should be used for treatment, then the prophylactic regimen may be resumed.

In patients with severe antibody deficiency, in those for which antibiotic therapy is problematic, and in those in whom prophylaxis has not been satisfactory, immunoglobulin replacement therapy is indicated (1,45,87,88). This can be be conveniently done by the intravenous or subcutaneous routes (45,88,89). Intramuscular injections of immune serum globulin are rarely used in the current era, except as occasional prophylaxis for travelers.

Currently available immunoglobulin preparations are made from the pooled plasma of thousands of donors and contain a broad spectrum of molecularly intact specific IgG antibodies of all four subclasses, with little or no IgM or IgE. The content of albumin and IgA varies. Most preparations contain stabilizers such as the sugars maltose or dextrose, and/or amino acids such as glycine or proline. Because IgG is a blood product, the possibility of transmission of blood-borne viruses must be considered. The risk for viral transmission is minimized by careful screening and selection of donors, by the processes used to purify the IgG (usually a modification of the Cohn-Oncley cold alcohol precipitation procedure), and by specific viral inactivation steps (88,90–93). These may include treatment with solvent-detergent, fatty acids, and/or fatty alcohols to inactivate enveloped viruses (90–92). Pasteurization (91), and/or low pH incubation denature capsid proteins in nonenveloped viruses (92). Most products also undergo nanofiltration. Several recent, comprehensive reviews of IgG therapy are available (87,88).

Because the average half-life of IgG in the circulation is about 21 days, intravenous infusions are usually given every 3 to 4 weeks (45,87,88). Alternatively, subcutaneous infusions can be given at home once a week or even more often (88,89). Regardless of the route of administration, the dose should be individualized to control infections and other symptoms, but usually falls

in a range of 300 mg/kg/month to 800 mg/kg/month. The higher doses are often used in patients with chronic lung and/or sinus infection (45,87,88,94,95). Serum IgG concentrations determined at the trough, just before the next infusion, can be used to provide an index and to assist decisions about the adequacy of dose and treatment interval but should not by themselves be used as an end point (45,87,88). This is particularly important in patients with CVID, IgG subclass deficiency, or selective antibody deficiencies, such as those who are unable to respond to polysaccharide antigens. These patients often require full replacement doses to remain free from infection despite having pretreatment serum IgG levels on the border of or within the normal range.

Antibody-deficient patients with active acute or chronic infection may experience severe systemic symptoms, including shaking chills and spiking fevers, and inflammatory reactions at the site of infection (e.g., the sinuses or airways) when they first receive IV infusions of IgG (88,96). It may therefore be preferable to defer initiation of treatment until a satisfactory course of antibiotics is given in such patients. IV infusions are generally initiated at the rate of 0.5 mg/kg/min to 1 mg/kg/min (0.01 mL/kg/min to 0.02 mL/kg/min of 5% solution) and increased in a stepwise manner at 15- to 30-minute intervals, as tolerated, until a maximum rate of 4 mg/kg/min to 6 mg/kg/min is achieved. Occasional patients may tolerate rates as fast as 8 mg/kg/min to 10 mg/kg/min. Most stable patients can thus complete their infusions within 2 to 3 hours. A minority of patients may experience adverse reactions during IV infusions, which may consist of headache, backache, flushing, chills, and mild nausea (96). In severe cases, there may be dyspnea, a sense of anxiety, and chest pain. These are usually not true anaphylactic reactions, are not mediated by IgE, and are frequently associated with increased rather than decreased blood pressure. Such reactions can usually be treated by decreasing the rate of infusion and/or by administration of diphenhydramine, acetaminophen, or aspirin. Patients who demonstrate consistent patterns of reactions can be kept at slower rates for subsequent infusions or pretreated with the previously mentioned drugs. In rare cases, pretreatment with corticosteroids (e.g., 0.5 mg/kg to 1 mg/kg of prednisone or intravenous methylprednisolone) may be necessary. True anaphylaxis is extremely uncommon but has been reported in a very small number of patients with IgA deficiency who have IgE antibodies against IgA (97). Because this is so rare, IgA deficiency should not be regarded as a contraindication against IVIG therapy in patients who also have significant deficiency of IgG antibodies, but slow starting rates and caution should be used with such patients. Rarely, aseptic meningitis, thrombotic events, and acute renal failure have been associated with IVIG, generally when high doses (>1,000 mg/kg) are used for anti-inflammatory or immunomodulatory effects (96). These

---

*Note that this would not provide satisfactory prophylaxis against *P. carinii* infection for patients with T-cell deficiencies. Recommendations for that situation may be found in reference 84.

are rare in patients receiving conventional doses as replacement therapy for immune deficiencies. Late adverse reactions may include headache, which may have features of migraine including nausea and fever, and may occur up to 48 hours after the infusion. These generally respond to acetaminophen, aspirin, or other nonsteroidal anti-inflammatory drugs. Occasionally, antiemetics, serotonin receptor antagonists, or other anti-migraine preparations may be required. Patients with recurrent febrile reactions should be carefully evaluated for the presence of chronic infection, which should be treated with appropriate antibiotics. In many cases, the IVIG infusions are sufficiently benign to be safely given in the home by a home care nurse, parent, or spouse (98). We usually establish the safety, maximally tolerated rate, and need for premedication in our clinic before allowing the patient to go to home care. IVIG is not irritating to the veins, and conventional preparations are not viscous or difficult to administer; hence, in-dwelling venous access devices such as a MediPort should not be required. If a patient is particularly sensitive to the pain of having the IV started, advance application of a local anesthetic, such as lidocaine/prilocaine (EMLA), which is available as a cream or presaturated disk, may be helpful.

Subcutaneous IgG treatment is remarkably free from systemic adverse effects and most patients can easily learn to administer the IgG at home (87–89,99). Usually, one-quarter of the previous monthly IVIG dose is given weekly, but with this route, individual treatment regimens can be very flexible. Frequently, two or three subcutaneous sites are used simultaneously for each infusion with a small portable pump and a tubing set that branches into one to three individual needles. For most adults, 25-gauge to 27-gauge needles, 9-mm to 11-mm in length, are satisfactory and the infusions are completed in ≤2 hours. The incidence of local adverse effects, most often resembling a single large hive, may be quite high, especially when this route is first employed (99). These reactions usually resolve within hours and become less frequent when subcutaneous treatment is continued. The subcutaneous route may be particularly preferable for patients in whom establishing venous access is difficult, those who have significant adverse effects from IV infusions, and those who live at a distance from an IV infusion facility and/or desire flexibility in scheduling their infusions to fit into their schedules of work, school, and other activities. Formal quality-of-life studies have shown that the ability to infuse at home, whether SC or IV, is appreciated by most patients and results in less overall intrusion of their disease into their lives (100,101).

Although prevention of acute, severe bacterial infections is the major goal of antibody replacement therapy, freedom from the symptoms of chronic infections and/or bronchiectasis can often be achieved, and many patients report amelioration of other symptoms such as arthralgia or arthritis when appropriate replacement has been achieved. The pulmonary status, chest CT scan results, or both in all patients with significant antibody deficiencies should be carefully documented at the beginning of therapy and followed at regular intervals, even if they become asymptomatic, because some patients may have progressive subclinical lung disease even when they do not complain of chronic symptoms or acute exacerbations (43,44).

In some infants with normal lymphoid tissues and B-cell numbers in whom IgG supplementation is started because of problems with bacterial or viral infections, the antibody deficiency may represent a maturational delay in the full range of antibody responses rather than a fixed and permanent defect (38). This is most likely to involve delayed development of T-independent antibody responses, such as those to bacterial capsular polysaccharides. After these patients have had a satisfactory interval with a normal or decreased incidence of infections, the IgG infusions should be stopped, and the patient's own antibody production should be reassessed. We find it best to try such interruptions of therapy during the summer months, when the exposure to droplet-spread respiratory infection is reduced. Serum concentrations of the major immunoglobulin classes and subclasses and specific antibody titers can be redetermined after 2 to 3 months off therapy to allow sufficient catabolism of the therapeutic IgG so that the infant's own production can be assessed. In our experience, children whose IgG levels or specific antibody responses are not satisfactory by 5 years of age are not likely to improve in subsequent years, and this exercise is rarely productive above that age.

In summary, immune deficiencies include a range of disorders spanning a spectrum from SCID and X-linked agammaglobulinemia to subtle specific antibody defects. The former may be relatively straightforward to detect in early infancy, but a high index of suspicion is necessary. Common variable immunodeficiency disease and specific antibody deficiencies may present with symptoms of recurrent or chronic respiratory or gastrointestinal infections at any age, but the diagnosis is often delayed because it has not been considered. Recognition of the possibility that immune deficiency may be responsible for a patient's problems is the first step in determining whether an immunologic evaluation is appropriate. The pattern of infections and the associated historical and physical features may provide important clues to the underlying diagnosis and should be kept in mind as a progression through screening and specialized and definitive laboratory tests is pursued. Therapeutic efforts aimed at minimizing the morbidity from infection or correcting the underlying problem will be suggested by the specific diagnosis and should be individualized. Because subclinical chronic infection that can lead to long-term pulmonary damage may be present (43,44) and because there is an increased incidence of malignancy in patients with primary immune deficiencies (36), close follow-up is necessary. With rapid advances in our understanding of the molecular pathogenesis of these disorders, additional specific therapies lie just over the horizon.

■ REFERENCES

1. Buckley R, ed. *Diagnostic and Clinical Care Guidelines for Primary Immmunodeficiency Diseases.* Towson, MD: Immune Deficiency Foundation; 2006. Available at: http://www.primaryimmune.org/pubs. Accessed 3/1/08.

2. Geha RS, Notarangelo LD, Casanova JL, et al. Primary immunodeficiency diseases: an update from the International Union of Immunological Societies Primary Immunodeficiency Diseases Classification Committee. *J Allergy Clin Immunol.* 2007;120:776–794.

3. Boyle JM, Buckley RH. Population prevalence of diagnosed primary immunodeficiency diseases in the United States. *J Clin Immunol.* 2007;27:497–502.

4. Ochs HD, Smith CIE, Puck JM, eds. *Primary Immunodeficiency Diseases: A Molecular and Genetic Approach.* 2nd ed. New York: Oxford University Press, 2006.

5. Stiehm ER, Ochs H, Winkelstein J, et al., eds. *Immunologic Disorders in Infants and Children.* 5th ed. Philadelphia: WB Saunders, 2004.

6. Conley ME, Howard V. Clinical findings leading to the diagnosis of X-linked agammaglobulinemia. *J Pediatr.* 2002;141:566–571.

7. Stiehm ER, Chin TW, Haas A, et al. Infectious complications of the primary immunodeficiencies. *Clin Immunol Immunopathol.* 1986;40:69–86.

8. Washington K, Stenzel TT, Buckley RH, et al. Gastrointestinal pathology in patients with common variable immunodeficiency and X-linked agammaglobulinemia. *Am J Surg Pathol.* 1996;20:1240–1252.

9. Ochs HD, Ament ME, Davis SD. Giardiasis with maladsorption in x-linked agammaglobulinemia. *N Engl J Med.* 1972;287:341–342.

10. Notarangelo LD, Miao CH, Ochs HD. Wiskott-Aldrich syndrome. *Curr Hematol.* 2008;15:30–36.

11. Ming JE, Stiehm ER, Graham JM Jr. Syndromes associated with immunodeficiency. *Adv Pediatr.* 1999;46:271–351.

12. Jones KL, ed. *Smith's Recognizable Patterns of Human Malformation.* 6th ed. Philadelphia: WB Saunders, 2005.

13. Uzel G. The range of defects associated with nuclear factor kappa B essential modulator. *Curr Opinion Allergy Clin Immunol.* 2005:5:513–518.

14. Grimbacher B, Holland SM, Gallin JI, et al. Hyper-IgE syndrome with recurrent infections: an autosomal dominant multisystem disorder. *N Engl J Med.* 1999;340:692–702.

15. Holland SM, DeLeo FR, Elloumi HZ, et al. STAT3 mutations in the hyper- IgE syndrome. *N Engl J Med.* 2007;357:1608–1619.

16. Cedarbaum SD, Kautila I, Rimoin DL, et al. The chondro-osseous dysplasia of adenosine deaminase deficiency with severe combined immune deficiency. *J Pediatr.* 1976;89:737–742.

17. Ahonen P, Myllamiemi S, Sipela I, et al. Clinical variation of autoimmune polyendocrinopathy candidiasis-ectodermal dystrophy (ADECED) in a series of 68 patients. *N Engl J Med.* 1990;322:1829–1836.

18. Becker-Catania SG, Gatti RA. Ataxia-telangiectasia. *Adv Exp Med Biol.* 2001;495:191–198.

19. Markert ML. Purine nucleoside phosphorylase deficiency. *Immunodefic Rev.* 1991;3:45–81.

20. Novak AH, Mueller B, Ochs H. Umbilical cord separation in the normal newborn. *Am J Dis Child.* 1988;142:220–223.

21. Jones AM, Gaspar HB. Immunogenetics: changing the face of immunodeficiency. *J Clin Pathol.* 2000;53:60–65.

22. Ochs HD, Notarangelo LD. X-linked immunodeficiencies. *Curr Allergy Asthma Rep.* 2004; 4:339–348.

23. Holland SM, Gallin JI. Evaluation of the patient with recurrent bacterial infections. *Annu Rev Med.* 1998;49:185–199.

24. Schaeffer FM, Monteiro RC, Volanakis JE, et al. IgA deficiency. *Immunodefic Rev.* 1991;3:15–44.

25. Figueroa JE, Densen P. Infectious diseases associated with complement deficiencies. *Clin Microbiol Rev.* 1991;4:359–395.

26. Cham B, Bonilla MA, Winkelstein J. Neutropenia associated with primary immunodeficiency syndromes. *Semin Hematol.* 2002; 39:107–112.

27. Malech HL, Hickstein DD. Genetics, biology and clinical management of myeloid cell primary immune deficiencies: chronic granulomatous disease and leukocyte adhesion deficiency. *Curr Opin Hematol.* 2007;14:29–36.

28. Winkelstein JA, Marino MC, Johnston RB Jr, et al. Chronic granulomatous disease: report on a national registry of 368 patients. *Medicine.* 2000;79:155–169.

29. Winkelstein JA, Marino MC, Lederman HM, et al. X-linked agammaglobulinemia: report on a United States registry of 201 patients. *Medicine.* 2006; 85:193–202.

30. Wilson CB, Penix L, Weaver WM, et al. Ontogeny of T lymphocyte function in the neonate. *Am J Reprod Immunol.* 1992;28:132–135.

31. Wise MT, Hagaman DD. An immunological approach to chronic and recurrent sinusitis. *Curr Opin Otolaryngol Head Neck Surg.* 2007;15:10–7.

32. Durandy A, Peron S, Fischer A. Hyper-IgM syndromes. *Curr. Opin. Rheumatol.* 2006;18:369–376.

33. Etzioni A, Ochs HD. The hyper IgM syndrome—an evolving story. *Pediatr Res.* 2004;56:519–525.

34. Einhorn MS, Granoff DM, Nahm MH, et al. Concentrations of antibodies in paired material and infant sera: relationship to IgG subclass. *J Pediatr.* 1987;111:783–788.

35. Azar AE, Ballas ZK. Evaluation of the adult with suspected immunodeficiency. *Am J Med.* 2007;120:764–768.

36. Cunningham-Rundles C. Clinical and immunologic analyses of 103 patients with common variable immunodeficiency. *J Clin Immunol.* 1989;9:22–33.

37. Cunningham-Rundles C, Knight AK. Common variable immune deficiency: reviews, continued puzzles, and a new registry. *Immunol Res.* 2007;38:78–86.

38. Whelan MA, Hwan WH, Beausoleil J, et al. Infants presenting with recurrent infections and low immunoglobulins: characteristics and analysis of normalization. *J Clin Immunol.* 2006:26:7–11.

39. Hakim FT, Gress RE. Immunosenescence: deficits in adaptive immunity in the elderly. *Tissue Antigens.* 2007;70:179–189.

40. Conley ME, Park CL, Douglas SD. Childhood common variable immunodeficiency with autoimmune disease. *J Pediatr.* 1986;108:915–922.

41. Iyer M, Gorevic PD. Reactive arthropathy and autoimmunity in non-HIV-associated immunodeficiency. *Curr Opin Rheumatol.* 1993;5:475–482.

42. Knight AK, Cunningham-Rundles C. Inflammatory and autoimmune complications of common variable immune deficiency. *Autoimmun Rev.* 2006;5:156–159.

43. Thickett KM, Kumararatne DS, Banerjee AK, et al. Common variable immune deficiency: respiratory manifestations, pulmonary function and high-resolution CT scan findings. *Quarterly J Med.* 2002;95:655–662.

44. Kainulainen L, Varpula M, Liippo K, et al. Pulmonary abnormalities in patients with primary hypogammaglobulinemia. *J Allergy Clin Immunol.* 1999;104:1031–1036.

45. Bonilla FA, Bernstein IL, Khan DA, et al. Practice parameter for the diagnosis and management of primary immunodeficiency. *Ann Allergy Asthma Immunol.* 2005;94 (Suppl 1):S1–63.

46. Shearer WT, Rosenblatt HM, Gelman RS, et al. Lymphocyte subsets in healthy children from birth through 18 years of age: the Pediatric AIDS Clinical Trials Group P1009 study. *J Allergy Clin Immunol.* 2003;112:973–980.

47. Lindegren ML, Kobrynski L, Rasmussen SA, et al. Applying public health strategies to primary immunodeficiency diseases: a potential approach to genetic disorders. *MMWR Recomm Rep.* 2004;53(RR-1):1–29.

48. Hershfield MS, Kurtzberg J, Aiyar VN, et al. Abnormalities in S-adenosylhomocysteine hydrolysis, ATP catabolism, and lymphoid differentiation in adenosine deaminase deficiency. *Ann N Y Acad Sci.* 1985;451:78–86.

49. Gary G, Gutowski WTI. Thymoma: a clinicopathologic study of 54 cases. *Am J Surg Pathol.* 1979;3:235–249.

50. Phoon CK, Neill CA. Asplenia syndrome: insight into embryology through an analysis of cardiac and extracardiac anomalies. *Am J Cardiol.* 1994;73:581–587.

51. Hong R. The DiGeorge anomaly (catch 22, DiGeorge/velocardiofacial syndrome). *Semin Hematol.* 1998;35:282–290.

52. Thórarinsdóttir HK, Lúdvíksson BR, Víkingsdóttir T, et al. Childhood levels of immunoglobulins and mannan-binding lectin in relation to infections and allergy. *Scand J Immunol.* 2005;61:466–474.

53. Shirai A, Consentino M, Leitman-Klinman SF, et al. Human immunodeficiency virus infection induces both polyclonal and virus-specific B-cell activation. *J Clin Invest.* 1992;89:561–564.

54. Granholm NA, Cavallo T. Autoimmunity, polyclonal B cell activation and infection. *Lupus.* 1992;1:63–74.

55. Oxelius V, Laurell A, Lindquist B, et al. IgG subclasses in selective IgA deficiency: importance of IgG2-IgA deficiency. *N Engl J Med*. 1981;304:1476–1478.

56. Fleisher TA. Evaluation of suspected immunodeficiency. *Adv Exp Med Biol*. 2007;601:291–300.

57. O'Gorman MR. Role of flow cytometry in the diagnosis and monitoring of primary immunodeficiency disease. *Clin Lab Med*. 2007;27:591–626.

58. Vowells SJ, Sekhsaria S, Malech HL, et al. Flow cytometric analysis of the granulocyte respiratory burst: a comparison study of fluorescent probes. *J Immunol Methods*. 1995;178:89–97.

59. McCormick T, Shearer WT. Delayed-type hypersensitivity skin testing. In: Detrick B, Hamilton RG, Folds JD, eds. *Manual of Molecular and Clinical Laboratory Immunology*. 7th ed. Washington, DC: ASM Press, 2006:234–240.

60. Corazza GR, Tarozzi C, Vaira D, et al. Return of splenic function after splenectomy: how much tissue is needed? *Br Med J. (Clin Res Ed.)*. 1984;289:861–864.

61. Agarwal S, Cunningham-Rundles C. Assessment and clinical interpretation of reduced IgG values. *Ann Allergy Asthma Immunol*. 2007;99:281–283.

62. Chouksey AK, Berger M. Assessment of protein antibody response in patients with suspected immune deficiency. *Ann Allergy Asthma Immunol*. 2008;100:166–168.

63. Paris K, Sorensen RU. Assessment and clinical interpretation of polysaccharide antibody responses. *Ann Allergy Asthma Immunol*. 2007;99:462–464.

64. Wedgwood RJ, Ochs HD, Davis SD. The recognition and classification of immunodeficiency diseases with bacteriophage ΦX174. *Birth Defects Orig Artic Ser*. 1975;11:331–338.

65. Currier JR. T-lymphocyte activation and cell signaling. In: Detrick B, Hamilton RG, Folds JD, eds. *Manual of Molecular and Clinical Laboratory Immunology*. 7th ed. Washington, DC: ASM Press, 2006: 315–327.

66. Bastian J, Law S, Vogler L, et al. Prediction of persistent immunodeficiency in the Di George anomaly. *J Pediatr*. 1989;115:391–396.

67. Perfetto SP, Mickey TE, Blair PJ, et al. Measurement of CD69 induction in the assessment of immune function in asymptomatic HIV-infected individuals. *Cytometry*. 1997;30:1–9.

68. Branson BM, Handsfield HH, Lampe MA. CDC Revised recommendations for HIV testing of adults, adolescents, and pregnant women in health-care settings. *MMWR Recomm Rep*. 2006 Sep 22;55(RR-14):1–17.

69. Holland, SM. Neutropenia and neutrophil defects. Chap 103. In: Detrick B, Hamilton RG, Folds JD, eds. *Manual of Molecular and Clinical Laboratory Immunology*. 7th ed. Washington, DC: ASM Press, 2006:924–932.

70. Nauseef WM. The NADPH-dependent oxidase of phagocytes. *Proc Assoc Am Physicians*. 1999;111:373–382.

71. Ochs HD, Igo RP. The NBT slide test: a simple method for detecting chronic granulomatous disease and female carriers. *J Pediatr*. 1973;83:77–82.

72. Puck JM, Willard HF. X-inactivation in females with x-linked disease. *N Engl J Med*. 1998;338:325–328.

73. Allen RC, Nachtman RG, Rosenblatt HM, et al. Application of carrier testing to genetic counseling for x-linked agammaglobulinemia. *Am J Hum Genet*. 1994;54:25–35.

74. Buckley RH. Molecular defects in human severe combined immunodeficiency and approaches to immune reconstitution. *Annu Rev Immunol*. 2004;22:625–655.

75. O'Shea JJ, Husa M, Li D, et al. Jak3 and the pathogenesis of severe combined immunodeficiency. *Mol Immunol*. 2004;41:727–737.

76. Kovanen PE, Leonard WJ. Cytokines and immunodeficiency diseases: critical roles of the gamma(c)-dependent cytokines interleukins 2, 4, 7, 9, 15, and 21, and their signaling pathways. *Immunol Rev*. 2004; 202:67–83.

77. Gaspar HB, Thrasher AJ. Gene therapy for severe combined immunodeficiencies. *Expert Opin Biol Ther*. 2005;5:1175–1182.

78. Puck, J, Malech HL. Gene therapy for immune disorders: good news tempered by bad news. *J Allergy Clin Immunol*. 2006;117:865–869.

79. Roifman C. Approach to the diagnosis of severe combined immune deficiency. In: Detrick B, Hamilton RG, Folds JD, eds. *Manual*

of Molecular and Clinical Laboratory Immunology. 7th ed. Washington, DC: ASM Press, 2006:895–900.

80. Thomas JA, Graham JM Jr. Chromosome 22q11 deletion syndromes: an update and review for the primary pediatrician. *Clin Pediatr (Phila)*. 1997;36:253–266.

81. Booth C, Hershfield M, Notarangelo L, et al Management options for adenosine deaminase deficiency. *Clin Immunol*. 2007;123(2): 139–147.

82. Villa A, Sobacchi C, Notarangelo LD, et al. V(D)J recombination defects in lymphocytes due to RAG mutations: severe immunodeficiency with a spectrum of clinical presentations. *Blood*. 2001;97:81–88.

83. Puck JM. SCID Newborn Screening Working Group. Population-based newborn screening for severe combined immunodeficiency: steps toward implementation. *J Allergy Clin Immunol*. 2007; 120:760–768.

84. Report of the Committee for Infectious Diseases. Recommendations for *Pneumocystis carinii* pneumonia prophylaxis. In: Georges P, ed. *American Academy of Pediatrics Red Book*. Elk Grove Village, IL: Amercan Academy of Pediatrics;1997:423.

85. Watts WJ, Watts MB, Dai W, et al. Respiratory dysfunction in patients with common variable hypogammaglobulinemia. *Am Rev Respir Dis*. 1986;134:699–703.

86. Schwartz HJ, Hostoffer RW, McFadden ER Jr, et al. The response to intravenous immunoglobulin replacement therapy in patients with asthma with specific antibody deficiency. *Allergy Asthma Proc*. 2006;27:53–58.

87. Orange JS, Hossny EM, Weiler CR, et al. Use of intravenous immunoglobulin in human disease: a review of evidence by members of the Primary Immunodeficiency Committee of the American Academy of Allergy, Asthma and Immunology. *J Allergy Clin Immunol*. 2006;117(4 Suppl):S525–S553. Erratum in: *J Allergy Clin Immunol*. 2006;117:1483.

88. Berger M. Advances in immunoglobulin replacement therapy. *Immunol Allergy Clin N Amer*. 2008;28:413–437.

89. Berger M. Subcutaneous immunoglobulin replacement in primary immunodeficiencies. *Clin Immunol*. 2004;112:1–7.

90. Biesert L. Virus validation studies of immunoglobulin preparations. *Clin Exp Rheumatol*. 1996;104:547–552.

91. Chandra S, Cavanaugh JE, Lin CM, et al. Virus reduction in the preparation of intravenous immune globulin: in vitro experiments. *Transfusion*. 1999;39:249–257.

92. Bos OJ, Sunye DG, Nieuweboer CE, et al. Virus validation of pH 4-treated human immunoglobulin products produced by the Cohn fractionation process. *Biologicals*. 1998;26:267–276.

93. Korneyeva M, Hotta J, Lebing W, et al. Enveloped virus inactivation by caprylate: a robust alternative to solvent-detergent treatment in plasma derived intermediates. *Biologicals*. 2002;30:153–162.

94. Roifman CM, Levison H, Gelfand EW. High-dose versus low-dose intravenous immunoglobulin in hypogammaglobulinaemia and chronic lung disease. *Lancet*. 1987;1:1075–1077.

95. Eijkhout HW, van Der Meer JW, Kallenberg CG. The effect of two different dosages of intravenous immunoglobulin on the incidence of recurrent infections in patients with primary hypogammaglobulinemia. A randomized, double-blind, multicenter crossover trial. *Ann Intern Med*. 2001;135:165–174.

96. Pierce LR, Jain N. Risks associated with the use of intravenous immunoglobulin. *Transfusion Med Rev*. 2003;17:241–254.

97. Burks AW, Sampson HA, Buckley RH. Anaphylactic reactions after gamma globulin administration in patients with hypogammaglobulinemia. *N Engl J Med*. 1986;314:560–564.

98. Sorensen RU, Kallick MD, Berger M. Home treatment of antibody deficiency syndromes with intravenous immunoglobulin. *J Allergy Clin Immunol*. 1987;80:810–815.

99. Ochs HD, Gupta S, Kiessling P, et al. Safety and efficacy of self-administered subcutaneous immunoglobulin in patients with primary immunodeficiency diseases. *J Clin Immunol*. 2006;26:265–274.

100. Gardulf A, Nicolay U. Replacement IgG therapy and self-therapy at home improve the health-related quality of life in patients with primary antibody deficiencies. *Curr Opin Allergy Clin Immunol*.; 6: 434–442.

101. Nicolay U, Kiessling P, Berger M, et al. Health-related quality of life and treatment satisfaction in North American patients with primary immunodeficiency diseases receiving subcutaneous IgG self-infusions at home. *J Clin Immunol*. 2006;26:65–72.

CHAPTER 5

Evaluation of Eosinophilia

ROBERT M. ZEMBLE AND ANDREA J. APTER

Eosinophilia is defined in this chapter as the presence of excess numbers of eosinophils in the blood or tissues. The upper limit of normal number of eosinophils in the circulation has been variably described as approximately 400 cells/µL (1–3). Eosinophilia is associated with allergic, infectious, neoplastic, or idiopathic disorders. This chapter focuses on the diagnosis and management of disease characterized by eosinophilia.

■ EOSINOPHILS IN THE BLOOD

Wharton Jones is believed to have been the first scientist to recognize the eosinophil in unstained preparations of peripheral blood in 1876. Paul Ehrlich gave the cell the name *eosinophil* in 1879 because of the intense staining of its granules with acidic aniline dyes like eosin. The staining procedures he developed allowed the cell to be recognized and studied (4).

The eosinophil count can be estimated by multiplying the percentage of eosinophils from the differential white blood cell count by the total number of white blood cells. Normally, 1% to 5% of blood leukocytes are eosinophils (2,5). A manual differential should be obtained if eosinophilia is suspected. Various conditions may influence the eosinophil count. In patients with leukopenia, the percentages of eosinophils may be increased, but not their absolute number. This has been called *pseudoeosinophilia* (5). The number of eosinophils in the blood has a diurnal variation, being highest at night and falling in the morning when endogenous glucocorticoid levels increase (5). Exogenous glucocorticoids, endogenous glucocorticoid production, stress, and some bacterial and viral infections may suppress eosinophil counts (5,6). Thus, a condition promoting eosinophilia could be masked if it occurred in the presence of such events.

■ EOSINOPHILS IN THE TISSUES

Eosinophils are present in only small numbers in the circulation; they are primarily tissue-dwelling cells, with more than a hundred times as many present in the tissues as compared with the circulation (5). Eosinophils are generated in the bone marrow and reside in the hematopoietic and lymphatic organs such as the bone marrow, spleen, lymph nodes, and thymus (2). However, they are most prevalent in tissues with mucosal epithelial cells, primarily the gastrointestinal and also the respiratory and lower genitourinary tracts (4). In disease, they can accumulate in any tissue, particularly in the tissues interfacing with the environment, such as the respiratory (e.g., asthma, nasal polyps, and allergic and nonallergic rhinitis with eosinophilia), dermatologic (eosinophilic cellulitis or fasciitis), gastrointestinal (eosinophilia-associated gastrointestinal disorders), and lower genitourinary systems (eosinophilic cystitis), suggesting a role in host defense or tissue immunoregulation (7).

The peripheral blood half-life of eosinophils is as short as 8 hours to as long as 18 hours (8), but eosinophils survive for weeks within tissues (5). Thus, blood eosinophil numbers do not necessarily reflect the extent of eosinophil involvement in affected tissues in various diseases. Prolonged eosinophilia, such as in the hypereosinophilic syndrome (HES), has been associated with organ damage, particularly cardiovascular, but also cutaneous, neurologic, pulmonary, splenic, hepatic, ocular, and gastrointestinal (9).

Routine eosin staining of eosinophils may underestimate eosinophil numbers. Immunofluorescent stains with monoclonal antibodies directed against the cationic proteins from the granules or fluorescent staining techniques based on granule autofluorescense are used to detect eosinophils in tissues. Degranulation, cytolysis, apoptosis, and necrosis alter the morphology of the eosinophil and its granules and, thus, staining properties (5).

Morphology and Development of Eosinophils

To better understand the diagnosis and management of conditions characterized by eosinophilia, we present a brief synopsis of the morphology, development, and recruitment into tissue of the eosinophil. *Fig. 5.1* illustrates some of these concepts. Eosinophils are bone marrow-derived granulocyte leukocytes arising from $CD34^+$ hematopoietic progenitor cells (10). They are distinguished by their bilobed nuclei and large acidophilic cytoplasmic granules (15). The cytokines granulocyte-macrophage colony-stimulating factor (GM-CSF), interleukin-3 (IL-3), and IL-5 are associated with promoting their growth and differentiation in the bone marrow (10). Of these, the actions of IL-5 are most specific for eosinophils, potently and specifically stimulating eosinophil production in the marrow. IL-5 stimulates eosinophil precursors to synthesize granule proteins (5), and mediates eosinophil expansion, priming, recruitment, and tissue survival (10). Despite the importance of IL-5 in eosinophilia, it is not required for eosinophil growth and differentiation under homeostatic conditions, and IL-5 gene-depleted mice produce mature eosinophils, although not in large numbers (11, 12).

IL-5 and eotaxins promote the migration of eosinophils and progenitor cells through the bone marrow sinus endothelium and their release into the circulation (13). Eotaxins are chemoattractant cytokines (chemokines) that promote eosinophil recruitment to tissues via chemoattractant cytokine receptor 3 (CCR3), which is expressed predominantly on eosinophils (10). Eosinophils exit the circulation and migrate to mucosal surfaces, including the lung, gut, and lower genitourinary tract (5,10). This migration is mediated by adhesion molecules on endothelial and eosinophil surfaces. Through binding of P-selectin glycoprotein ligand 1 (PSGL-1) on eosinophils with P-selectin on endothelial cells, tethering, rolling, and margination of eosinophils occurs. The eosinophil then adheres to the endothelial wall by the binding of the β_1 integrin very late antigen-4 (VLA-4) on eosinophils to the vascular cell adhesion molecule-1 (VCAM-1) (5,10). The β_2 integrin, lymphocyte function-associated antigen-1 (LFA-1), which binds to intercellular adhesion molecule-1 (ICAM-1), is also important in eosinophil migration (12). With the binding of integrins and their ligands, the rolling stops, the eosinophil adheres more firmly to the endothelium and then migrates out of the vascular compartment. The migration of eosinophils into the tissues is controlled by chemoattractants. These include platelet-activating factor (PAF), complement components (C3a and C5a), leukotrienes, lipoxygenase-derived products, and chemokines. The most important group of chemokines is the eotaxins and their chemoattractive effect is augmented by IL-5. Other chemokines have also been classified as eosinophil chemoattractants. These include RANTES (chemoattractant cytokine ligand 5 [CCL5]) and macrophage inflammatory protein 1α (CCL3), but their chemoattractive properties are not specific for eosinophils. Once eosinophils migrate into inflamed tissue, they are activated by many stimuli, including receptors for immunoglobulin A (IgA) and IgG, and cytokines, including IL-3, IL-5, and GM-CSF. IL-3,

IL-5, GM-CSF, and eotaxin prolong survival of eosinophils and inhibit eosinophil apoptosis (5,10,12, 13).

In tissue, eosinophils modulate immune responses using a variety of mechanisms, including antigen presentation, cytokine release, and secretion of cytotoxic granule cationic proteins (14). After engagement of their receptors by cytokines, immunoglobulins, and complement, eosinophils can release an assortment of cytokines (IL-2, IL-4, IL-5, IL-10, IL-12, IL-13, IL-16, IL-18, TGF-α, and TGF-β), chemokines (RANTES and eotaxin-1), and lipid mediators (PAF and leukotriene C4) (14). These factors can then cause inflammation through upregulating adhesion, altering cellular trafficking, and regulating vascular permeability, mucus secretion, and smooth muscle contraction (14,15). Although eosinophils originally were considered to be effector cells participating in host defense against parasites, it is now recognized that eosinophils may also play a role in both innate and acquired immunity. They may act as initial responders to cell death and tissue damage, participate in remodeling and repair processes, and play these roles in immune responses that do not involve parasite or IgE-mediated responses (7).

Mature eosinophils can produce their end effector toxic and inflammatory effects by the release of mediators stored in their specific granules. The crystalloid core of these granules is composed of cationic major basic protein (MBP); the matrix contains eosinophil cationic protein, eosinophil-derived neurotoxin, and eosinophil peroxidase. These proteins produce hydrogen peroxide. In addition, eosinophil peroxidase generates halide acids (15). Eosinophil cationic protein can disrupt membranes by causing pore formation that facilitates the entry of other toxic molecules. It also can suppress T-cell proliferation and immunoglobulin synthesis, induce mast cell degranulation, and stimulate airway mucus secretion by fibroblasts (15). In the respiratory epithelium, activated eosinophil granule products can impair cilia beating and increase vascular permeability. MBP increases smooth muscle reactivity by acting on the epithelium and by antagonizing M2 muscarinic receptor function (16). Eosinophil granule proteins trigger degranulation of mast cells and basophils and amplify the inflammatory cascade by promoting release of chemoattractants such as eotaxin, RANTES, and PAF.

■ DIFFERENTIAL DIAGNOSIS OF EOSINOPHILIA

Eosinophilia can result from either cytokine-mediated increased differentiation and survival of eosinophils or mutation-mediated clonal expansion of eosinophils. The most common cause of eosinophilia results from an increased generation of IL-5 producing T cells regardless of the initial trigger. Eosinophilia has been classified into primary and secondary causes (3). Primary causes include clonal eosinophilia resulting from a hematologic malignancy or idiopathic eosinophilia, which is a diagnosis of exclusion. Secondary eosinophilia includes atopic, infectious, drug-induced, vasculitic, tissue-associated inflammatory, and malignant conditions in which the eosinophils are not part of the neoplastic condition (3). Table 5.1 displays the differential diagnosis of eosinophilia in blood and tissues. It is beyond the scope of this chapter to discuss all causes of eosinophilia in detail, but Table 5.1 contains references for each. These references include the original description of disease, a review of the clinical presentation, or an update on the possible immunopathogenic mechanisms involved. Below is a review of some of the causes of eosinophilic infiltration of blood and tissues most pertinent to the allergist-immunologist and not covered in other chapters. Topics include helminthic infections, drugs, HES, Churg-Strauss syndrome (CSS), and tissue-specific eosinophilic conditions of the lung, gut, and lower genitourinary tract.

Infections and Eosinophilia: Helminthic Diseases

In developing countries, helminthic diseases are the most common cause of eosinophilia, whereas in developed countries, atopic diseases are most common. Infections with bacteria and most viruses are generally associated with eosinopenia. However, respiratory syncytial virus has been shown to stimulate endothelial cells to produce eosinophil chemoattractants and activate eosinophils (17). These findings may explain in part how viral infections trigger asthma exacerbations.

Parasitic, particularly helminthic, infections are associated with eosinophilia. Helminths generate TH_2 responses leading to IL-4 and IL-5 production (18,19). Although IL-5 may be sufficient to cause helminth-mediated eosinophilia in most cases, helminthic infection also results in endothelial expression of eotaxin and RANTES, which promote eosinophil recruitment to tissues (19). However, the precise function of eosinophils in parasitic function in vivo is not certain. Although eosinophils have been shown to be potent effectors in killing parasites in vitro and to aggregate and degranulate in the vicinity of damaged parasites in vivo (15), in vivo data in animal models do not strongly support a requisite role for eosinophils in helminth immunity (19).

Helminthic diseases causing significant eosinophilia include strongyloidiasis, ascariasis, hookworm infection (ankylostomiasis), schistosomiasis, trichinosis, filariasis (caused by Wucheria bancrofti or Brugia species), gnathostomiasis, Toxocara canis infection causing visceral larva migrans, cysticercosis, and echinococcosis. Other helminths associated with eosinophilia include Mesocestoides corti, Hymenolepis diminuta, Angiostrongylus species, Anisakis species, Baylisascaris species, Enterobius vermicularis, Heligmosomoides polygyrus, Litomosoides species, Nippostrongylus species, Onchocerca species, Trichuris species, and Fasciola species (2,20). With the exception of Isospora belli and Dientamoeba fragilis, protozoan infections generally have not been recognized to elicit eosinophilia. Giardia does not cause eosinophilia. Eosinophilia has also been seen in Plasmodium falciparum infection (20), and recently infection with Babesia species has been suggested as a cause of eosinophilia (21). In parasitic infections associated with eosinophilia, the level of peripheral blood eosinophilia may be modest or even nonexistent if the infection is well contained in tissues such as in an echinococcal cyst. The levels of peripheral eosinophilia may fluctuate as these cysts leak or adult filaria migrate. Blood eosinophil levels tend to parallel the extent of tissue involvement and may be very marked as, for example, in disseminated Strongyloides species infection.

It is particularly important to diagnose Strongyloides species infection, which sometimes may be dormant and unrecognized in a patient for years. Potentially fatal dissemination of this helminth can occur if the patient becomes immunosuppressed or receives corticosteroids, which is the treatment for many other eosinophilic conditions (22).

Serial stool examinations with appropriate serologic tests are the initial diagnostic tests for parasites that infect the gastrointestinal tract. However, this test is not sensitive for strongyloidiasis as only small numbers of larvae are shed in the stool (20). The CDC offers a blood test with a sensitivity and negative predictive value of greater than 95% (20,23).

Eosinophilia may also be seen in primary and disseminated coccidioidomycosis (5). While eosinophilia may also be seen in HIV infected patients, it is often due to secondary causes, such as adrenal insufficiency rather than direct induction by HIV. It is also present in human T-lymphotropic virus-1 (HTLV-1) and HTLV-II infected patients (5).

Drug Reactions Associated with Eosinophilia

Table 5.2 displays drugs most commonly associated with eosinophilia of blood and tissues as an adverse reaction. Among the drugs most frequently reported are nitrofurantoin, minocycline, and nonsteroidal anti-inflammatory agents (NSAIDs). Although numerous drugs have been cited, in many cases these citations are based on case reports, as is evident from those provided in Table 5.2, making the associations difficult to interpret. When information is based on case reports, it is not clear how often eosinophilia occurs in all of the patients who take the drug. Furthermore, it is possible that a case report can describe a true association between the drug and eosinophilia, or temporally associated but causally unrelated events, such as an

TABLE 5.1   DISEASES MOST FREQUENTLY ASSOCIATED WITH EOSINOPHILIA OF BLOOD OR TISSUES

DISEASE	REFERENCE(S)
Infectious	
Parasitic infections (helminths)	(20,79)
Fungal (aspergillosis, coccidiomycosis)	(80,81)
Retroviral (e.g., human immunodeficiency virus)	(82)
Chronic tuberculosis	(83)
Pneumocystis carinii infection	(84)
Respiratory	
Asthma	(85,86) See Chapter 21
Allergic rhinitis	(87) See Chapter 9
Nonallergic rhinitis with eosinophilia syndrome	(88) See Chapter 19
Nasal polyposis	(89) See Chapter 19
Chronic rhinosinusitis	(90) See Chapter 19
Allergic bronchopulmonary aspergillosis	See Chapter 24
Allergic fungal sinusitis	(91) See Chapter 19
Acute eosinophilic pneumonia (drugs, parasites, other)	See text
Chronic eosinophilic pneumonia	See text
Eosinophilic granuloma (histiocytosis X)	(92)
Dermatologic	
Atopic dermatitis	(93) See Chapter 15
Eosinophilic panniculitis	(94)
Eosinophilic cellulitis (Wells syndrome)	(95)
Eosinophilic fasciitis (Shulman syndrome)	(96)
Angioedema and chronic urticaria	(97) See Chapter 13
Eosinophilic folliculitis	(98)
Vasculitic	
Churg-Strauss syndrome (CSS)	See text
Eosinophilic vasculitis	(99)
Hematologic and neoplastic	
Hypereosinophilic syndrome (HES)	See text
Leukemia	(3, 100)
Lymphoma (Hodgkin, non-Hodgkin)	(101)
Sézary syndrome	(102)
Solid tumors (e.g., cervical tumors; large cell carcinoma of the lung; squamous cell carcinoma of skin, penis, vagina; adenocarcinoma of gastrointestinal tract; transitional cell bladder carcinoma; breast)	(2, 103)
Mastocytosis	(104)
Gastrointestinal	
Eosinophilic gastrointestinal disorders	See text and Chapters 14 and 34
Inflammatory bowel disease	(105)
Cardiac (see HES)	

(continued)

TABLE 5.1   DISEASES MOST FREQUENTLY ASSOCIATED WITH EOSINOPHILIA OF BLOOD OR TISSUES (*CONTINUED*)

DISEASE	REFERENCE(S)
Urologic	
Eosinophilic cystitis	See text
Immunologic	
Omenn syndrome	(106)
Hyper-IgE syndrome	(107)
Transplant rejection	(108)
Endocrine	
Hypoadrenalism	(109, 110)

occurrence of eosinophilia and a concurrent but unrelated exposure. For example, inhaled beclomethasone and cromolyn, prescribed for asthma, a disease associated with eosinophilia, have both been associated with eosinophilia in case reports (24,25). Asthma and associated eosinophilia may wax and wane as part of the disease course and this may be incidental to whether a drug is taken. In contrast, doses of systemic steroids for asthma may have been reduced when inhaled steroids were added, resulting in an increase in peripheral blood eosinophilia. Thus, the true association may be between the extent of eosinophilia and the underlying asthma, and not the drug used for treatment. Indeed, the suggested association between leukotriene antagonists and eosinophilia in asthma patients appears to result from unmasking of underlying CSS rather than a direct association between leukotriene antagonists and eosinophilia (26).

When taking a history for possible therapeutic agents associated with eosinophilia, inquiry about the use of agents used in complementary and alternative medicine and over-the-counter preparations should be made. For example, contaminated L-tryptophan and rapeseed oil were associated with the eosinophilia-myalgia syndrome (27,28). Patients should also be asked about the use of illicit drugs because cocaine and heroin use have been associated with eosinophilia. The mechanisms by which a drug might cause eosinophilia have not been fully elucidated; however, presumably it results from an increase in eosinophil growth factors such as IL-5. Investigators have associated *in situ* drug-induced eosinophilia with IL-5 production by infiltrating CD4 T-cells. Drug-induced eosinophilia usually resolves with discontinuation of the offending agent (1,3,28).

Hypereosinophilic Syndromes

Recently, diseases characterized by significant peripheral blood or tissue eosinophilia without identifiable precipitants were classified as hypereosinophilic syndromes by the Hypereosinophilic Syndromes Working Group (50). Included were the syndromes characterized by hypereosinophilia: HES; platelet-derived growth factor receptor α (PDGFRA)-associated HES; lymphocyte variant HES; familial hypereosinophilia; as well as CSS and EGID. The Working Group sponsored by the National Institutes of Health, a pharmaceutical company, and a nonprofit advocacy organization for those living with eosinophilic gastrointestinal disorders, aimed to promote research to identify markers of disease progression and new therapeutics for these diseases (29).

Hypereosinophilic Syndrome

HES was described in 1968 by Hardy and Anderson (30). It was a diagnosis of exclusion, characterized by eosinophilia and damage to heart, lungs, skin, or other organs infiltrated with eosinophils (31). In 1975, Chusid and colleagues (32) proposed diagnostic criteria on which the diagnosis is based today: (a) blood eosinophilia greater than 1,500/μL persisting for at least 6 months; (b) exclusion of diseases associated with eosinophilia, such as parasitic infections, HIV, allergic diseases, drug hypersensitivity, or malignancy; and (c) evidence of organ involvement. In addition, diseases generally restricted to one organ system (e.g., EGID, eosinophilic pneumonias, and eosinophilic cystitis) were excluded in this first description of HES. Although eosinophilia should be documented on more than one occasion, a delay in treatment for the 6 months required in Chusid's criteria could be detrimental to a patient's health (33) and a patient can be considered to have HES if he or she appears to have a chronic and unremitting clinical course (9).

HES is more common in men, with a male-to-female ratio of 9:1 (5). It usually presents between the ages of 20 and 50 years and is rare in childhood. Presenting symptoms are often insidious and may be respiratory, cardiac, neurologic, or constitutional (such as low-grade fever or fatigue). Patients may also present with myalgias, angioedema, or skin rashes. Eosinophilia may be detected coincidentally during routine blood testing (9,34). Sweating, pruritus, abdominal discomfort, flushing, or alcohol intolerance may be seen. Weight loss is unusual, and patients do not have increased infections or anergy.

In HES, total leukocyte counts are usually less than 25,000/μL, with 30% to 70% of the total leukocyte count being eosinophils; some patients may develop very high white blood cell counts (>90,000/μL), which is associated with a poor prognosis (31). Examination of the bone marrow reveals increased numbers of eosin-ophils, often 30% to 60% of marrow cells. There are increased numbers of early forms compared with nor-mal bone marrow, but blast forms are not usually pres-ent (31). When blast forms are present in the blood or make up more than 10% of the eosinophils in the mar-row, the diagnosis is eosinophilic leukemia. In addition to eosinophilia, neutrophilia is common in HES. Ane-mia and basophilia have been described. The clinical spectrum of hematologic findings ranges from very mild abnormalities to signs and symptoms typical of a myeloproliferative disease, such as abnormal leukocyte alkaline phosphatase levels, anemia, splenomegaly (in 43% of HES patients), cytogenetic abnormalities, and myelodysplasia. Cardiac manifestations are common in HES and are present in about 58% of patients (31) (*Table 5.3*). Cardiac damage is thought to progress through three stages: acute necrosis, the development of endocardial thrombi, and endocardial fibrosis (31,34). The first acute stage is frequently clinically silent, although on histologic examination, damage to the endocardium including necrosis and eosinophilic infil-tration of myocardium with eosinophil degranulation products and microabscesses are present. It is hypothe-sized that treatment in the first stage with corticosteroids will prevent progression to the other nonreversible stages (31). The second stage is characterized by thrombi in either ventricle and occasionally in the atrium. In the third stage, fibrosis may lead to entrapment of the chor-dae tendineae and resultant mitral or tricuspid valve insufficiency or a restrictive cardiomyopathy. Clinically, patients may present with dyspnea, chest pain, or con-gestive heart failure. Murmurs of mitral regurgitation can be heard. Because the heart is the most common site of organ involvement and because the first stage may be clinically silent, an electrocardiogram and echocardio-gram must be obtained if HES is under consideration. Serial echocardiograms should be used to monitor cardiac involvement in patients in whom HES is a diag-nostic possibility and in those with established disease. Cardiac MRI may prove to be a more reliable test for the rapid noninvasive diagnosis of myocardial complications of hypereosinophilic syndrome (35).

The most common cutaneous findings are erythro-derma, urticarial plaques, angioedema, pruritic papules, and nodules (31,34). A less common manifestation is mucosal ulcerations that can be difficult to treat and are found most often in the myeloproliferative variant (34). Patients who have urticaria or angioedema as skin man-ifestations tend to have a better prognosis; they are more likely to have no cardiac or neurologic manifesta-tions (531,34). Biopsy specimens of the papular and nodular lesions are characterized by perivascular infil-trates of eosinophils, neutrophils, and mononuclear cells without evidence of vasculitis (31).

Neurologic involvement occurs in about half of cases and has three forms: thromboembolic disease resulting from thrombotic cardiac disease, primary cen-tral nervous system dysfunction, and peripheral neu-ropathy (31,36). Clinically, patients who present with thromboembolic events have had strokes or transient ischemic attacks. Visual symptoms, occurring in 23% of patients, are also attributed to microemboli or possibly local thrombi. The most frequent visual abnormality is blurred vision. Central nervous system dysfunction is manifested as gait disturbances, behavioral changes, memory loss, or upper motor neuron signs such as increased muscle tone. Peripheral neuropathy may be expressed as mononeuritis multiplex with symmetric or asymmetric sensory deficits or painful paresthesias, or as motor neuropathies.

About half of HES patients have respiratory findings, with the most frequent being a nonproductive cough (31). Pulmonary involvement is believed to result from infiltration of lung tissue by eosinophils or originate from primary cardiac events such as congestive heart failure or emboli originating from right ventricular thrombi. Interestingly, asthma does not occur more fre-quently in HES than in the general population, and its presence raises the suspicion for CSS (9,31).

Diarrhea is the most frequent sign of gastrointestinal tract involvement. Eosinophilic gastritis, enterocolitis, colitis, pancreatitis, hepatitis, and the Budd-Chiari syn-drome all have been described in HES (31). Rheumato-logic symptoms include arthralgias, joint effusions, arthritis, Raynaud phenomenon, and digital necrosis.

The Emerging Immunologic Findings Surrounding HES

According to the Hypereosinophilic Syndromes Work-ing Group (Figure 5.2) (29), HES syndrome is now grouped into a myeloproliferative variant (M-HES) and a lymphocytic variant (L-HES), although most patients fall into an undefined subtype (19). A small group of patients are considered to have familial form.

The M-HES classification was motivated by clonal abnormalities observed in some patients (37). Subse-quently, Gleich et al. found that imatinib was effective in several patients with HES (38). Since imatinib is a

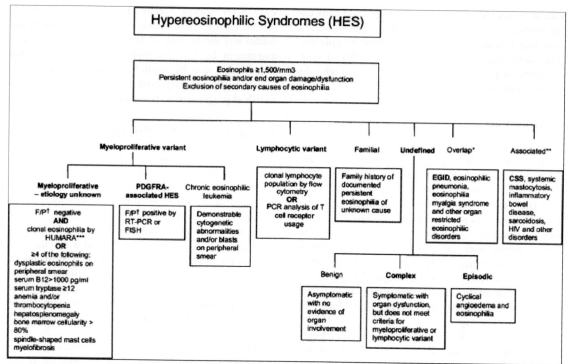

■ FIGURE 5.2 Classification of HESs. Specific syndromes discussed by Hypereosinophilic Syndromes Working group during the International Eosinophil Society in 2005 are indicated in bold. *Incomplete criteria, apparent restriction to specific tissues-organs. **Peripheral eosinophilia $\geq$1500/mm³ in association with a defined diagnosis. †Presence of the *FIP1L1/PDGFRA* mutation. ***Clonality analysis based on the digestion of genomic DNA with methylation-sensitive restriction enzymes followed by PCR amplification of the CAG repeat at the human androgen receptor gene (*HUMARA*) locus at the X chromosome. *FISH,* Fluorescence *in situ* hybridization. Reproduced with permission from Klion, A.D., et al. *Approaches to the treatment of hypereosinophilic syndromes: a workshop summary report.* J Allergy Clin Immunol, 2006. **117**(6): p. 1292–1302.

tyrosine-kinase inhibitor with activity against several oncogenes including PDGFR, Coon et al. searched and in 2003, discovered a deletion on chromosome 4q12 that leads to fusion of the FIP1-like 1 (FIP1L1) and PDGFRA genes. The fusion product produces a protein with significant constitutive tyrosine kinase activity (9,39). Thus, these discoveries demonstrated clonal expansion of eosinophils in some patients and the relationship of HES to myeloproliferative disease.

L-HES-variant patients are thought to have an abnormal T-cell population driving the recruitment of eosinophils with the clonal lymphocyte population identified by flow cytometry or reverse transcriptase polymerase chain reaction for the T-cell receptor. For example, clonal expansions of abnormal T cells (CD3⁻CD4⁺CD8⁻ and CD3⁺CD4⁻CD8⁻) have been described (40). In addition, overproduction of IL-5 has been observed in almost all reports in which IL-5 has been measured in HES patients who have not already received corticosteroids (40).

Studies suggest that 11% to 17% of HES patients have the FIPL1-PDGFRA M-HES variant and 27% to 31% have L-HES, but definite frequencies of the subtypes have not been established and the above numbers were subject to referral biases (9,41). According to the

workshop summary report, patients may be classified with the M-HES variant if they are FIP1L1/PDGRA-positive, demonstrate cytogenetic abnormalities or blasts on peripheral smear (technically chronic eosinophilic leukemia), or have four or more of the characteristics displayed in Figure 5.2 (29).

Patients with M-HES are predominantly male and have more frequent cardiac involvement (9). L-HES affects males and females equally. The most common T-cell subpopulation is CD3⁻CD4⁺ with rare reports of CD3⁺CD4⁻CD8⁻ expression, with an increased activated (CD25 or HLA-DR⁺) memory (CD45RO⁺) pattern with a high expression of CD5 and loss of CD7 or CD27 in many cases (9). Elevated IgE is common, but it is also found in M-HES patients. Nearly all L-HES patients have cutaneous involvement, typically with a lymphocytic inflammatory pattern (9).

The familial form of HES is very rare and has a benign course that my be related to a lack of eosinophil activation (9,41). The overlap category is designed to capture eosinophilia that is restricted to specific tissues (29). The associated category captures patients with peripheral eosinophilia greater than 1500/mm³ that is associated with a defined diagnosis (29). The undefined category consists of benign cases that are asymptomatic with no evidence of end-organ damage (and thus do not technically meet criteria for HES); episodic cases including patients with Gleich syndrome of episodic angioedema and eosinophilia; and the complex subtype consisting of patients with organ dysfunction who do not meet criteria for M-HES or L-HES (50).

Treatment of HES

An algorithm for the treatment of hypereosinophilic syndromes (*Fig. 5.3*) was proposed by Klion (33). Imatinib is the first-line treatment for all FIP1L1/PDGFRA-positive patients and also has been reported successful in M-HES patients lacking the FIP1L1/PDGFRA mutation (33,39,42). As acute eosinophilic myocarditis has been reported following the initiation of imatinib in three patients with HES, a screening troponin is obtained before therapy and corticosteroid therapy initiated if it is elevated (33,42,43). Young males are advised to store sperm before initiation of imatinib (33,44). Imatinib resistance has been reported in FIP1L1/PDGFRA positive patients with a T6741 mutation in PDGFRA and alternative tyrosine kinase inhibitors such as dasatinib, nilotinib, and sorafenib could be considered, but their side effect profile is less favorable than imatinib (33,39). Nonmyeloablative bone marrow transplantation has also been used in patients with HES and is the only potentially curative therapy but is associated with significant morbidity and even mortality (45).

Corticosteroids remain the first-line treatment for most patients without the FIP1L1/PDGFRA mutation if there is evidence of organ damage. The initial dose is usually 1 mg/kg or at least 40 mg of prednisone equivalent daily with a very slow taper while monitoring eosinophil level (29). Prognostic factors indicative of a prolonged response to corticosteroid therapy include episodic angioedema, positive response to a corticosteroid challenge, elevated serum IgE, and the lack of hepatosplenomegaly (29,31).

Various cytoxic therapies have been used for corticosteroid refractory HES. Hydroxyurea and IFN-α have been used singly and together for synergy (29). Vincristine can lower eosinophil counts rapidly in patients with extremely high levels (>100,000/mm³). A recent randomized, double-blind, placebo-controlled trial of mepolizumab, an anti-IL5 antibody, showed a reduction in the prednisone dose required by steroid-dependent patients who lacked the FIP1L1-PDGRFRA fusion gene (46). Alemtuzamab, an anti-CD52 antibody, has been used with limited experience in HES patients (47).

In patients with L-HES, corticosteroids are first-line therapy. Therapies that target eosinophils or eosinophil precursors (hydroxyurea, imatinib) are less effective second-line therapies as clonal T cells are the primary cause of the eosinophilia (33). IFN-α has been shown to inhibit *in vitro* proliferation and IL-5 production from clonal T cells, but also to prolong survival of

CD3⁻/CD4⁺ clonal T cells (33). Therefore, it should not be used as monotherapy without corticosteroids. Additional monitoring of therapy in L-HES includes assessment for lymphadenopathy and lymphocytosis every 3 to 4 months, quantification of aberrant T cells semiannually and karyotyping annually for monitoring of risk of progression to lymphoma (55,80).

Churg-Strauss Syndrome

The major vasculitis associated with eosinophilia is CSS, which was originally called *allergic angiitis* and *granulomatosis* in 1951 (49,50). The syndrome is characterized by a necrotizing vasculitis in patients with asthma and eosinophilia. The diagnostic criteria generally followed are formulated by the American College of Rheumatology, yielding a sensitivity of 85% and a specificity of 99.7% (51). For a diagnosis of CSS, four of the following six criteria must be satisfied: asthma, peripheral eosinophilia (>10%), mononeuropathy or polyneuropathy, nonfixed pulmonary infiltrates, paranasal sinus abnormality, and biopsy containing a blood vessel with extravascular eosinophils (49,50).

Estimates of the frequency of CSS is about 5 cases per 1,000,000 patient-years with an estimate of 1.8 cases in patients without asthma and 64.4 cases per 1,000,000 patient-years in asthmatics (52,53). However, the true incidence of CSS is likely unknown because it is relatively rare and therefore not readily recognized. In addition, some cases initially treated as asthma, the prodrome of CSS, may be controlled by corticosteroid therapy and any progression to vasculitis may not be recognized until steroids are tapered (26).

The mean age at diagnosis is 48 years, with new cases reported in both pediatric and geriatric age groups (54,55). Men are affected slightly more frequently than women (9). There are three distinct clinical phases in most CSS patients: asthma; tissue eosinophilia; and vasculitis (52). Typically, asthma or rhinitis precedes the development of the other manifestations by a mean of 8.9 ± 10.9 years and may present as new "allergies" in a patient without an allergic family history (5,10,50). This vasculitic phase is often accompanied by constitutional symptoms, such as fever, malaise, and weight loss, and typically begins years after asthma is diagnosed but sometimes occurs within months of the diagnosis of asthma.

The distribution of organ involvement is enumerated in *Table 5.4*. Virtually all patients have pulmonary involvement as asthma or pulmonary infiltrates that are fleeting and nonspecific (52). Chest x-ray abnormalities include bilateral patchy consolidations in a nonsegmental distribution (52,56). Bilateral ground-glass opacities and peripheral airspace consolidation are typical CT findings (55,56). Allergic rhinitis occurs in about 75% of patients and is frequently the initial symptom. Recurrent sinusitis, nasal polyps, and nasal obstruction may also be seen (52). Mononeuritis multiplex is the most common form of neurologic involvement (55). Skin lesions are common and include palpable purpura, nodules, pustules, urticaria, and livedo (52). Skin biopsy shows leukocytoclastic vasculitis. Clinically, cardiac manifestations include congestive heart failure, eosinophilic endomyocarditis, coronary vasculitis, valvular heart disease, pericarditis, pericardial effusions, and dysrhythmias (52). In one review, only about one-third of patients had clinical cardiac disease, but almost two-thirds were found to have findings at autopsy, including fibrosis, myocarditis, pericarditis, and eosinophilic granulomas in the pericardium (55). The most common gastrointestinal symptoms are abdominal pain, nausea, vomiting, diarrhea, and hematochezia. Ulcers and bowel perforation have been reported infrequently. Proteinuria is the most common manifestation of renal disease associated with CSS. Renal disease in CSS is less severe than in other related vasculitides, such as polyarteritis nodosa and Wegener granulomatosis; renal failure is rare (55). Renal biopsy has shown pauci-immune focal segmental glomerulonephritis with necrosis or crescent formation (55). Myalgias and arthralgias are the most common musculoskeletal symptoms; however, true arthritis is rare (56).

Laboratory studies are most notable for fluctuating peripheral blood eosinophilia, with peaks ranging from 20% to 90% of the differential white blood cell count. Perinuclear antineutrophil cytoplasmic antibodies directed against myeloperoxidase occur in 50% to 70% of patients. The erythrocyte sedimentation rate is frequently elevated, with a mean of 52.7 ± 32.6 in one series of patients (55). Anemia is often present (52). Biopsy of involved tissues is characterized by necrotizing vasculitis of the small arteries and veins, eosinophils, and extravascular granulomas.

The pathogenesis of CSS is unknown, but it likely derives from autoimmune mechanisms involving endothelial cells and leukocytes (57). Although ANCA has been detected in approximately half of CSS patients, its role in the pathogenesis of the disease is not established (55). CSS has been associated with various asthma therapies, including leukotriene inhibitors and inhaled corticosteroids; however, there has been no causal link and rather it seems that the syndrome is either coincidental or that the medications facilitate systemic steroid withdrawal, thus unmasking the syndrome (55). A recent multivariable analysis controlling for the use of oral corticosteroids, inhaled corticosteroids, and number of categories of asthma drugs dispensed supported the thinking that the use of leukotriene modifiers was not associated with the development of CSS (58). CSS has now also been reported in patients following the usage of the humanized anti-IgE omalizumab (59).

Without treatment, the prognosis is poor, with 50% dying within 3 months of the onset of vasculitis (52). Currently, long-term outcomes showed overall remission rates ranging from 81% to 92% with relapse in 26% to 28% of patients in remission. However, the overall mortality in treated patients who relapsed was only 3.1% (52,60). The patients at risk for a poor outcome are those with myocardial involvement (vasculitis, cardiomyopathy, or congestive heart failure), severe gastrointestinal symptoms (intestinal bleeding, perforation, pancreatitis, or requiring laparotomy), proteinuria greater than 1 g/day, or a short duration of asthma before the presentation of the vasculitic phase (52). In patients without systemic involvement or indicators of poor prognosis, therapy consists of corticosteroids alone with prednisone 1 mg/kg for 1 month or until there is no evidence of disease. The prednisone is tapered over the course of a year if no disease activity recurs (52). If there is systemic involvement or indicators of poor prognosis, cyclophosphamide is given either orally (2 mg/kg/day) or via intravenous pulses (0.6 mg/m^2 monthly) concurrently with the steroids (52). Other attempted treatment regimens have included IVIG, cyclosporine, interferon-α, mycophenolate mofetil, and azathioprine (29).

Eosinophilic Pneumonias

The eosinophilic pneumonias are a group of disorders characterized by blood or tissue eosinophilia and pulmonary infiltrates. In 1952, Reeder and Goodrich introduced the term *pulmonary infiltrates with eosinophilia* (PIE) for diseases with peripheral blood eosinophilia and pulmonary infiltrates (61). In 1969, Liebow and Carrington broadened the diseases that had been included in the PIE group by defining *eosinophilic pneumonias* as pulmonary diseases characterized by eosinophilic infiltrates with or without peripheral blood eosinophilia (62). Pulmonary eosinophilic syndromes are currently characterized by an increased number of eosinophils in peripheral blood, lung tissue, sputum, bronchoalveolar lavage (BAL) fluid, or any combination of the above.

Eosinophilic pneumonias can be thought of as primary or secondary, in which eosinophilia is attributed to a specific cause such as drug reaction, infection, malignancy, or other pulmonary conditions such as asthma (55). *Table 5.5* lists the pulmonary eosinophilic syndromes. Reviews of the topic (49,55) provide further details and descriptions of disorders for which space does not allow inclusion here. Drug-induced pulmonary eosinophilia was discussed previously and in Table 5.2. CSS (previously discussed) and HES with pulmonary eosinophilia are the only primary eosinophilic pneumonias with extrapulmonary involvement. Allergic bronchopulmonary aspergillosis is discussed in Chapter 24.

Four eosinophilic pneumonias were not discussed earlier: tropical pulmonary eosinophilia, Löffler syndrome, chronic eosinophilic pneumonia, and acute eosinophilic pneumonia. Tropical pulmonary eosinophilia is thought to be a hypersensitivity response to filarial parasites, *Wuchereria bancrofti* and *Brugia malayi*. It is characterized by paroxysmal cough, dyspnea, and wheezing predominantly at night with marked peripheral eosinophilia and diffuse reticulonodular infiltrates on chest radiographs (63). Diagnostic criteria include appropriate exposure history such as a mosquito bite after travel to an endemic area of filariasis, a history of paroxysmal nocturnal cough and breathlessness, pulmonary infiltrates, leukocytosis, eosinophilia >3000 cells/mm^3, increased serum IgE, serum antifilarial antibodies (IgE and/or IgG), and a clinical response to diethylcarbamazine citrate (63). Treatment is typically 3 weeks of oral diethylcarbamazine citrate, which can be obtained from the Centers for Disease Control and Prevention under an Investigational New Drug protocol (63).

Löffler syndrome, or simple pulmonary eosinophilia, is characterized by fleeting migratory infiltrates, peripheral blood eosinophilia, low-grade fever, dry cough, and dyspnea (49). There is no age predominance. Most patients with Löffler syndrome have either a parasitic infection or drug reaction, although no cause can be found in about one-third of cases (64). The condition resolves spontaneously within 4 weeks.

Chronic eosinophilic pneumonia (CEP) has an insidious onset. Its symptoms include cough, dyspnea, malaise, fever, and weight loss. The cough is initially nonproductive, but may become productive. Wheezing occurs in half the cases with respiratory failure being extremely rare; women are affected twice as often as men (65). Although CEP may affect every age group, patients are generally at least 30 years of age; many have a history of atopy and more than one-third have a history of asthma (65). There has been an association in some patients with prior radiation for breast cancer (66). The course is chronic, with symptoms usually present for at least a month before diagnosis with a mean duration of 20 weeks (65). Blood eosinophilia is present in about 90% of patients, but its absence does not exclude the diagnosis (67). Of the cell counts from bronchoaveolar lavage, more than 25% of the cells are eosinophils. The classic chest radiograph reveals progressive peripheral dense infiltrates, which resemble a "photographic negative of pulmonary edema" (67). However, this finding occurs in less than half of patients. Other radiographic findings may include nodular infiltrates, atelectasis, unilateral or bilateral involvement, cavitation, and pleural effusion. High-resolution computed tomography scans of the chest may identify peripheral infiltrates not evident on the radiograph and may also reveal mediastinal adenopathy. Pulmonary function tests may reveal a restrictive, normal, or obstructive pattern (49,65). The diffusion capacity is frequently reduced. Biopsy is not necessary for diagnosis of CEP, but histopathologic examination reveals a predominantly eosinophilic infiltrate involving the alveoli and interstitium. Interstitial fibrosis, bronchiolitis, and bronchiolitis obliterans can be present, and occasionally eosinophilic microabscesses and noncaseating granulomas are observed. Necrosis is rare. Symptoms and pulmonary infiltrates resolve rapidly with initiation of corticosteroids, usually 0.5–1 mg/kg of prednisone. The duration of treatment has ranged from 6 weeks to 1 year, but shorter courses are favored because relapses are exceedingly responsive to reinstitution of steroids (65). Although the prognosis is excellent, up to one-half of patients experience relapses (49,65,67).

Acute eosinophilic pneumonia (AEP) is a febrile illness characterized by hypoxemia and respiratory failure with profound eosinophilia on bronchoalveolar lavage fluid. Patients commonly present with rapid onset of cough, tachypnea, and dyspnea of less than 7 days duration; however, the largest published case series reported patients with a duration of symptoms of up to a month before presentation. Chest pain and myalgias are also present in 73% and 50% of patients, respectively (68). There is no gender difference in prevalence in contrast to the female predominance of chronic eosinophilic pneumonia. AEP is a diagnosis of exclusion; hypersensitivity reactions, reactions to medications and toxins, and infectious etiologies must be ruled out.

Various inhalational exposures have been associated with AEP, including World Trade Center dust, indoor renovation work, gasoline tank cleaning, tear gas, firework smoke, cave exploration, woodpile moving, plant repotting, and, most frequently, new-onset smoking (68,69). In a case series of AEP in deployed U.S. military personnel, all patients were smokers and 14 of 18 had recently began smoking compared with controls in whom 48/72 were smokers and only 2/72 were new-onset smokers (70). In a retrospective case series in France, 6 of 8 patients who were smokers had begun within 3 months of disease onset, and several patients in Japan were described with AEP developing soon after beginning smoking (71).

Early radiographic findings of AEP show reticular markings with Kerley B-lines and small pleural effusions. Subsequent findings include mixed reticular and alveolar infiltrates with progression to dense alveolar infiltrates; CT scan findings are consistent with diffuse interstitial infiltrates, patchy alveolar infiltrates, or diffuse ground-glass infiltrates (68).

Eosinophils generally exceed 25% of the cells in the bronchoalveolar lavage; patients generally do not present with peripheral blood eosinophilia, but most develop peripheral blood eosinophilia during the hospitalization (68). Thymus and activation-regulated chemokine (TARC/CCL17) has been suggested as a possible peripheral blood marker to help differentiate AEP from other acute lung injuries as its level is elevated in the acute phase before peripheral eosinophilia is present (72). Biopsy in not necessary for diagnosis, but histopathology is characterized by marked infiltration of eosinophils in the interstitium and alveolar spaces with common findings including diffuse alveolar damage with hyaline membranes, fibroblast proliferation, and inflammatory cells (68). Pulmonary function testing can be notable for a restrictive defect with reduced diffusion capacity (55).

The treatment is respiratory support and high-dose corticosteroids. Recommended regimens have consisted of methylprednisolone 125 mg every 6 hours until respiratory failure resolves, then a total corticosteroid course of 2- to 12-weeks, duration (68). There have been reports of some patients recovering without corticosteroids (70), but they are currently recommended for all patients. Most patients recover without long-term complications, and relapse is extremely rare.

Eosinophil-Associated Gastrointestinal Disorders

The eosinophil-associated gastrointestinal disorders (EGID) include eosinophilic esophagitis, eosinophilic gastritis, eosinophilic gastroenteritis, and eosinophilic enteritis. They are characterized by eosinophilic inflammation of the GI tract in the absence of known causes for eosinophilia and are reviewed in more detail in Chapters 14 and 34. Under homeostatic conditions, eosinophils typically are present throughout the GI tract with the exception of the esophagus (73). Eosinophils may accumulate in abnormal numbers in the GI tract in numerous disorders including IgE-mediated food allergy, inflammatory bowel disease, gastroesophageal reflux, HES syndrome, and eosinophilia resulting from secondary causes such as drug reactions, parasitic infections, and malignancy (73).

Over the past decade, eosinophilic esophagitis (EE) has increased in recognition, particularly in Westernized, developed countries in a similar manner as other atopic diseases (1,3). Prevalence in children in outpatient settings has been reported to range from 8.9 to 43 per 100,000, but is increasing with the intense interest in this disease (74). EE is also increasingly recognized in adults. Among those with esophageal food impaction, EE frequency estimates range from 11% to 54% (73,74). EE occurs more often in males and has a possible familial pattern with approximately 8% of pediatric patients having at least one sibling or parent with eosinophilic esophagitis (73). Recently a single-nucleotide polymorphism in the gene encoding for eotaxin-3 was shown to be associated with disease susceptibility (73).

Recently, the First International Gastrointestinal Eosinophil Research Symposium (FIGERS) presented consensus recommendations for diagnostic criteria for EE (75). It was defined as a clinicopathologic disease with clinical symptoms of food impaction and dysphagia in adults and GERD symptoms or feeding intolerance in children, with esophageal biopsy showing

evidence of at least 15 eosinophils/hpf. The diagnosis requires the exclusion of GERD or other similar diseases by either failure of high-dose proton pump inhibitor therapy or presence of a normal distal esophageal pH (75). Other histologic features associated with EE include eosinophil microabscesses, superficial layering of eosinophils, and basal zone hyperplasia; the gross appearance of the esophagus can be normal or abnormalities, can include longitudinal furrowing, friability, edema, longitudinal shearing, exudates, granularity, narrowing, or strictures (75).

The FIGERS consensus report summarized skin prick testing (SPT) results in the pediatric population with about two-thirds of children having positive skin tests to at least one food allergen, with the most common allergens being peanuts, eggs, soy, cow milk, wheat, beans, and rye. Atopy patch testing has been used successfully to direct food elimination diets but is not yet a standardized procedure (73). Eosinophilic colitis is often manifested as allergic colitis of infancy (dietary protein-induced proctocolitis of infancy syndrome) and is the most common cause of bloody stools in the first year of life (73). There is a bimodal distribution of eosinophilic colitis patients, either presenting in infancy or adolescence and early adulthood. Diarrhea is the classic symptom, but other symptoms include abdominal pain, weight loss, and anorexia. Histology shows aggregates of eosinophils in the lamina propria, crypt epithelium, and muscularis mucosa. Treatment is withdrawal of the offending protein trigger in allergic colitis of infancy and anti-inflammatory agents including aminosalicylates and glucocorticoids in older patients (73).

Eosinophilic Cystitis

Eosinophilic cystitis is a rare disease characterized by urinary frequency (present in 67%), hematuria (68%), suprapubic pain (49%), and urinary retention (10%) (76). It is distributed equally between males and females, but in childhood, males are more commonly affected. Peripheral eosinophilia is present in 43% of patients; cystoscopy reveals hyperemic mucosa with areas of elevation and nodularity (76). Biopsy is characterized by eosinophilic infiltrate, mucosal edema, and muscle necrosis. This inflammatory pattern may progress to chronic inflammation and fibrosis of the bladder mucosa and muscularis. No underlying etiology has been associated with 29% of patients, other cases have been associated with transitional cell carcinoma of the bladder, intravesical chemotherapy, various medications, allergic respiratory disease, bladder outlet obstruction, autoimmune disorders, nonurological parasitic disorders, and eosinophilic enteritis (77). Recommended treatment has varied between primarily conservative treatment and radical transurethral resection of the lesions in the bladder with a combination of corticosteroids and antihistamines depending on assessment of the underlying cause (76).

■ EVALUATION OF THE PATIENT WITH EOSINOPHILIA

In the approach to the evaluation of a patient with eosinophilia, (see Figure 5.4) the most important factor is

the history, with careful attention to travel and dietary history. Medications including over-the-counter and complementary medicine preparations must be considered and any nonessential medications discontinued. A history consistent with atopy should be sought, with the caveat that atopy causes only a modest increase in peripheral eosinophil count (<15%). Possible family history of diseases associated with eosinophila should

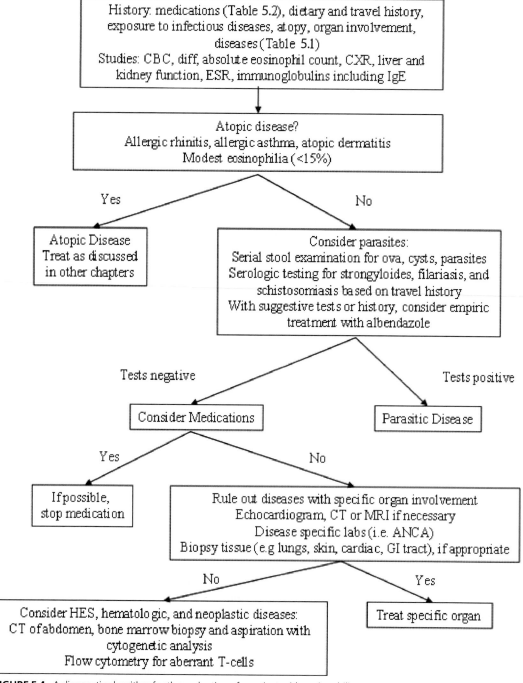

■ **FIGURE 5.4** A diagnostic algorithm for the evaluation of a patient with eosinophilia.

be elicited. If parasitic disease remains a consideration, multiple examinations of the stool and appropriate serologic tests based on travel history should be ordered. Physical exam with particular attention to skin, lymphadenopathy, organomegaly, and possible masses should be performed (78). Laboratory tests to assess hematologic and organ function should be performed including complete blood count, liver function tests, renal function tests, urinalysis, inflammatory markers, and immunoglobulins (78). Evidence of tissue infiltration should be sought. An echocardiogram and chest radiograph should be obtained. If the etiology remains unclear or the degree of eosinophilia is substantial, further examination for lymphoproliferative disease and HES should be pursued. Additional tests necessary would include screening for autoantibodies, CT examination of the abdomen, tissue or specimen analyses, bone marrow examination with cytogenetics, testing for FIP1L1/PDGFRA, and assessment for lymphocyte clonality (33). Patients with persistent eosinophilia without a clear etiology should be monitored with physical examination, echocardiography for evidence of cardiac damage, including thrombi and endomyocardial fibrosis, and assessment of pulmonary function or CT imaging based on clinical manifestations of individual patients (33).

■ ACKNOWLEDGMENTS

This chapter was adapted from: Irani C and Apter AJ: Evaluation of Eosinophilia. In Grammer LC and Greenberger PA, editors: *Patterson's Allergic Disease*, ed. 6, Philadelphia, 2002, Lippincott Williams and Wilkins, Chapter 33 pp 683–701.

■ REFERENCES

1. Holland SMG, Gallin JI. Disorders of granulocytes and monocytes. In: Kasper DLB, Braunwald E, Fauci A, et al., eds. *Harrison's Principles of Internal Medicine*. New York: McGraw-Hill, Medical Pub. Division; 2005:v, xxvii, 2, 128, 2607, 128 p. 349–356).
2. Simon D, Simon HU. Eosinophilic disorders. *J Allergy Clin Immunol.* 2007;119(6):1291–3000; quiz 1301–1302.
3. Tefferi A. Blood eosinophilia: a new paradigm in disease classification, diagnosis, and treatment. *Mayo Clin Proc.* 2005;80(1):75–83.
4. Wardlaw AJM, Moqbel RM, Kay AB. Eosinophils and the allergic inflammatory response. In: Kay AB, ed. *Allergy and Allergic Diseases*. Malden, MA: Blackwell Science; 1997:171–188.
5. Weller PF. Eosinophilia and eosinophil-related disorders. In: Adkinson NB, Yunginger JW, Holgate ST, et al., eds. *Middleton's Allergy: Principles & Practice*. Philadelphia: Mosby; 2003:1105–1126.
6. Malathi A, Parulkar VG. Evaluation of anxiety status in medical students prior to examination stress. *Indian J Physiol Pharmacol.* 1992;36(2):121–122.
7. Jacobsen EA, Taranova AG, Lee NA, et al. Eosinophils: singularly destructive effector cells or purveyors of immunoregulation? *J Allergy Clin Immunol.* 2007;119(6):1313–1320.
8. Prussin C, Metcalfe DD. 5. IgE, mast cells, basophils, and eosinophils. *J Allergy Clin Immunol.* 2006;117(2 Suppl Mini-Primer):S450–S456.
9. Sheikh J, Weller PF. Clinical overview of hypereosinophilic syndromes. *Immunol Allergy Clin North Am.* 2007;27(3):333–355.
10. Weller PF. Human eosinophils. *J Allergy Clin Immunol.* 1997;100(3):283–287.
11. Kopf M, Brombacher F, Hodgkin PD, et al. IL-5-deficient mice have a developmental defect in CD5+ B-1 cells and lack eosinophilia

but have normal antibody and cytotoxic T cell responses. *Immunity.* 1996;4(1):15–24.
12. Watt AP, Schock BC, Ennis M. Neutrophils and eosinophils: clinical implications of their appearance, presence and disappearance in asthma and COPD. *Curr Drug Targets Inflamm Allergy.* 2005;4(4): 415–423.
13. Collins PD, Mareau S, Griffiths-Johnson DA, et al. Cooperation between interleukin-5 and the chemokine eotaxin to induce eosinophil accumulation in vivo. *J Exp Med.* 1995;182(4):1169–1174.
14. Hogan SP. Recent advances in eosinophil biology. *Int Arch Allergy Immunol.* 2007;143(Suppl 1):3–14.
15. Rothenberg ME, Hogan SP. The eosinophil. *Annu Rev Immunol.* 2006;24:147–174.
16. Jacoby DB, Gleich GJ, Fryer AD. Human eosinophil major basic protein is an endogenous allosteric antagonist at the inhibitory muscarinic M2 receptor. *J Clin Invest.* 1993;91(4):1314–1318.
17. Harrison AM, Bonville CA, Rosenberg HF, et al. Respiratory syncytial virus-induced chemokine expression in the lower airways: eosinophil recruitment and degranulation. *Am J Respir Crit Care Med.* 1999;159(6):1918–1924.
18. Anthony RM, Rutitzky LI, Urban JF, et al. Protective immune mechanisms in helminth infection. *Nat Rev Immunol.* 2007;7(12):975–987.
19. Klion AD, Nutman TB. The role of eosinophils in host defense against helminth parasites. *J Allergy Clin Immunol.* 2004;113(1):30–37.
20. Page KR, Zenilman J. Eosinophilia in a patient from South America. *JAMA.* 2008;299(4):437–444.
21. Schaller JL, Burkland GA, Langhoff PJ. Are various *Babesia* species a missed cause for hypereosinophilia? A follow-up on the first reported case of imatinib mesylate for idiopathic hypereosinophilia. *Med Gen Med.* 2007;9(1):38.
22. Genta RM, Miles P, Fields K. Opportunistic Strongyloides stercoralis infection in lymphoma patients. Report of a case and review of the literature. *Cancer.* 1989;63(7):1407–1411.
39. Loutfy MR, Wilson M, Keystone JS, et al. Serology and eosinophil count in the diagnosis and management of strongyloidiasis in a nonendemic area. *Am J Trop Med Hyg.* 2002;66(6):749–752.
23. Schermoly MJ, Hinthorn DR. Eosinophilia in coccidioidomycosis. *Arch Intern Med.* 1988;148(4):895–896.
24. Lobel H, Machtey I, Eldror MY. Pulmonary infiltrates with eosinophilia in an asthmatic patient treated with disodium cromoglycate. *Lancet.* 1972;2(7785):1032.
25. Mollura JL, Bernstein R, Fine SR, et al. Pulmonary eosinophilia in a patient receiving beclomethasone dipropionate aerosol. *Ann Allergy.* 1979;42(5):326–329.
26. Wechsler ME, Finn D, Gunawardena D, et al. Churg-Strauss syndrome in patients receiving montelukast as treatment for asthma. *Chest.* 2000;117(3):708–713.
27. Sternberg EM. Pathogenesis of L-tryptophan eosinophilia myalgia syndrome. *Adv Exp Med Biol.* 1996;398:325–330.
28. Mikami C, Ochiai K, Umemiya K, et al. Eosinophil activation and in situ interleukin-5 production by mononuclear cells in skin lesions of patients with drug hypersensitivity. *J Dermatol.* 1999;26(10):633–639.
29. Klion AD, Bochner BS, Gleich GJ, et al. Approaches to the treatment of hypereosinophilic syndromes: a workshop summary report. *J Allergy Clin Immunol.* 2006;117(6):1292–1302.
30. Hardy WR, Anderson RE. The hypereosinophilic syndromes. *Ann Intern Med.* 1968;68(6):1220–1229.
31. Weller PF, Bubley GJ. The idiopathic hypereosinophilic syndrome. *Blood.* 1994;83(10):2759–2779.
32. Chusid MJ, Dale DC, West BC, et al. The hypereosinophilic syndrome: analysis of fourteen cases with review of the literature. *Medicine* (Baltimore). 1975;54(1):1–27.
33. Klion AD. Approach to the therapy of hypereosinophilic syndromes. *Immunol Allergy Clin North Am.* 2007;27(3):551–560.
34. Leiferman KM, Gleich GJ. Hypereosinophilic syndrome: case presentation and update. *J Allergy Clin Immunol.* 2004;113(1):50–58.
35. Plastiras SC, Economopoulos N, Kelekis NL, et al. Magnetic resonance imaging of the heart in a patient with hypereosinophilic syndrome. *Am J Med.* 2006;119(2): 130–132.
36. Moore PM, Harley JB, Fauci AS. Neurologic dysfunction in the idiopathic hypereosinophilic syndrome. *Ann Intern Med.* 1985;102(1): 109–114.
37. Chang HW, Leong KH, Koh DR, et al. Clonality of isolated eosinophils in the hypereosinophilic syndrome. *Blood.* 1999;93(5):1651–1657.
38. Gleich GJ, Leiferman KM, Pardanani A, et al. Treatment of hypereosinophilic syndrome with imatinib mesilate. *Lancet.* 2002;359(9317): 1577–1578.

39. Cools J, DeAngelo DJ, Gotlib J, et al. A tyrosine kinase created by fusion of the PDGFRA and FIP1L1 genes as a therapeutic target of imatinib in idiopathic hypereosinophilic syndrome. N Engl J Med. 2003;348(13):1201–1214.

40. Brugnoni D, Airo P, Rossi G, et al. A case of hypereosinophilic syndrome is associated with the expansion of a CD3−CD4+ T-cell population able to secrete large amounts of interleukin-5. Blood. 1996;87(4): 1416–1422.

41. Roche-Lestienne C, Lepers S, Soenen-Cornu V, et al. Molecular characterization of the idiopathic hypereosinophilic syndrome (HES) in 35 French patients with normal conventional cytogenetics. Leukemia. 2005;19(5): 792–798.

42. Pardanani A, Brockman SR, Paternoster SF, et al. FIP1L1-PDGFRA fusion: prevalence and clinicopathologic correlates in 89 consecutive patients with moderate to severe eosinophilia. Blood. 2004;104(10):3038–3045.

43. Pitini V, Arrigo C, Azzarello D, et al. Serum concentration of cardiac Troponin T in patients with hypereosinophilic syndrome treated with imatinib is predictive of adverse outcomes. Blood. 2003;102(9):3456–3457.

44. Seshadri T, Seymour JF, McArthur GA. Oligospermia in a patient receiving imatinib therapy for the hypereosinophilic syndrome. N Engl J Med. 2004;351(20):2134–2135.

45. Ueno NT, Anagnostopoulos A, Rondon G, et al. Successful nonmyeloablative allogeneic transplantation for treatment of idiopathic hypereosinophilic syndrome. Br J Haematol. 2002;119(1):131–134.

46. Rothenberg ME, Klion AD, Roufosse FE, et al. Treatment of patients with the hypereosinophilic syndrome with mepolizumab. N Engl J Med. 2008;358(12): 1215–1228.

47. Simon HU, Cools J. Novel approaches to therapy of hypereosinophilic syndromes. Immunol Allergy Clin North Am. 2007;27(3): 519–527.

48. Roufosse F, Cogan E, Goldman M. Recent advances in pathogenesis and management of hypereosinophilic syndromes. Allergy. 2004;59(7):673–689.

49. Allen JN, Davis WB. Eosinophilic lung diseases. Am J Respir Crit Care Med. 1994;150(5 Pt 1):1423–1438.

50. Churg J, Strauss L. Allergic granulomatosis, allergic angiitis, and periarteritis nodosa. Am J Pathol. 1951;27(2):277–301.

51. Masi AT, Hunder GG, Lie JT, et al. The American College of Rheumatology 1990 criteria for the classification of Churg-Strauss syndrome (allergic granulomatosis and angiitis). Arthritis Rheum. 1990;33(8):1094–1100.

52. Noth I, Strek ME, Leff AR. Churg-Strauss syndrome. Lancet. 2003;361(9357):587–594.

53. Watts RA, Lane SE, Bentham G, et al. Epidemiology of systemic vasculitis: a ten-year study in the United Kingdom. Arthritis Rheum. 2000; 43(2):414–419.

54. Boyer D, Vargas SO, Slattery D, et al. Churg-Strauss syndrome in children: a clinical and pathologic review. Pediatrics. 2006; 118(3):e914–e920.

55. Wechsler ME. Pulmonary eosinophilic syndromes. Immunol Allergy Clin North Am. 2007;27(3):477–492.

56. Choi YH, Im JG, Han BK, et al. Thoracic manifestation of Churg-Strauss syndrome: radiologic and clinical findings. Chest. 2000;117(1):117–124.

57. Weller PF, Plaunt M, Taggart V, et al. The relationship of asthma therapy and Churg-Strauss syndrome: NIH workshop summary report. J Allergy Clin Immunol. 2001;108(2):175–183.

58. Harrold LR, Patterson MK, Andrade SE, et al. Asthma drug use and the development of Churg-Strauss syndrome (CSS). Pharmacoepidemiol Drug Saf. 2007; 16(6):620–626.

59. Ruppert AM, Averous G, Stanciu D, et al. Development of Churg-Strauss syndrome with controlled asthma during omalizumab treatment. J Allergy Clin Immunol. 2008;121(1):253–254.

60. Solans R, Bosch JA, Perez-Bocanegra C, et al. Churg-Strauss syndrome: outcome and long-term follow-up of 32 patients. Rheumatology (Oxford). 2001;40(7):763–771.

61. Reeder WH, Goodrich BE. Pulmonary infiltration with eosinophilia (PIE syndrome). Ann Intern Med. 1952;36(5):1217–1240.

62. Liebow AA, Carrington CB. The eosinophilic pneumonias. Medicine (Baltimore). 1969;48(4):251–285.

63. Vijayan VK. Tropical pulmonary eosinophilia: pathogenesis, diagnosis and management. Curr Opin Pulm Med. 2007;13(5):428–433.

64. Alberts WM. Eosinophilic interstitial lung disease. Curr Opin Pulm Med. 2004;10(5):419–424.

65. Marchand E, Cordier JF. Idiopathic chronic eosinophilic pneumonia. Semin Respir Crit Care Med. 2006. 27(2):134–141.

66. Cottin V, Frognier R, Monnot H, et al. Chronic eosinophilic pneumonia after radiation therapy for breast cancer. Eur Respir J. 2004;23(1):9–13.

67. Jederlinic PJ, Sicilian L, Gaensler EA. Chronic eosinophilic pneumonia. A report of 19 cases and a review of the literature. Medicine (Baltimore). 1988;67(3):154–162.

68. Allen J. Acute eosinophilic pneumonia. Semin Respir Crit Care Med. 2006; 27(2):142–147.

69. Pope-Harman AL, Davis WB, Allen ED, et al. Acute eosinophilic pneumonia. A summary of 15 cases and review of the literature. Medicine (Baltimore). 1996;75(6):334–342.

70. Shorr AF, Scoville SL, Cersovsky SB, et al. Acute eosinophilic pneumonia among US Military personnel deployed in or near Iraq. JAMA. 2004;292(24):2997–3005.

71. Nakajima M, Manabe T, Niki Y, et al. Cigarette smoke-induced acute eosinophilic pneumonia. Radiology. 1998;207(3):829–831.

72. Miyazaki E, Nureki S, Ono E, et al. Circulating thymus- and activation-regulated chemokine/CCL17 is a useful biomarker for discriminating acute eosinophilic pneumonia from other causes of acute lung injury. Chest. 2007;131(6):1726–1734.

73. Zuo L, Rothenberg ME. Gastrointestinal eosinophilia. Immunol Allergy Clin North Am. 2007;27(3):443–455.

74. Chehade M, Sampson HA. Epidemiology and etiology of eosinophilic esophagitis. Gastrointest Endosc Clin North Am. 2008;18(1):33–44;viii.

75. Furuta GT, Liacouras CA, Collins MH, et al. Eosinophilic esophagitis in children and adults: a systematic review and consensus recommendations for diagnosis and treatment. Gastroenterology. 2007; 133(4):1342–1363.

76. van den Ouden D. Diagnosis and management of eosinophilic cystitis: a pooled analysis of 135 cases. Eur Urol. 2000;37(4):386–394.

77. Itano NM, Malek RS. Eosinophilic cystitis in adults. J Urol. 2001;165(3):805–807.

78. Nutman TB. Evaluation and differential diagnosis of marked, persistent eosinophilia. Immunol Allergy Clin North Am. 2007;27(3):529–549.

79. Wolfe MS. Eosinophilia in the returning traveler. Med Clin North Am. 1999;83(4):1019–1032, vii.

80. Lombard CM, Tazelaar HD, Krasne DL, Pulmonary eosinophilia in coccidioidal infections. Chest. 1987;91(5):734–736.

81. Warren WP, Rose B. Hypersensitivity bronchopulmonary aspergillosis. Dis Chest. 1969;55(5):415–421.

82. Skiest DJ, Keiser P. Clinical significance of eosinophilia in HIV-infected individuals. Am J Med. 1997;102(5):449–453.

83. Riantawan P, Bangpattanasiri K, Chaowalit P, et al. Etiology and clinical implications of eosinophilic pleural effusions. Southeast Asian J Trop Med Public Health. 1998;29(3):655–659.

84. Fleury-Feith J, Van Nhieu JT, Picard C, et al. Bronchoalveolar lavage eosinophilia associated with Pneumocystis carinii pneumonitis in AIDS patients. Comparative study with non-AIDS patients. Chest. 1989;95(6):1198–1201.

85. Matsumoto K, Tamari M, Saito H. Involvement of eosinophils in the onset of asthma. J Allergy Clin Immunol. 2008;121(1):26–27.

86. Expert Panel Report 3 (EPR-3): Guidelines for the Diagnosis and Management of Asthma—Summary Report 2007. J Allergy Clin Immunol. 2007;120(5 Suppl):S94–138.

87. Bahls C. In the clinic. Allergic rhinitis. Ann Intern Med. 2007;146(7):ITC4-1-ITC4-16.

88. Ellis AK, Keith PK. Nonallergic rhinitis with eosinophilia syndrome and related disorders. Clin Allergy Immunol. 2007;19:87–100.

89. Hamilos DL, Leung DY, Huston DP, et al. GM-CSF, IL-5 and RANTES immunoreactivity and mRNA expression in chronic hyperplastic sinusitis with nasal polyposis (NP). Clin Exp Allergy. 1998;28(9):1145–1152.

90. Meltzer EO, Hamilos DL, Hadley JA, et al. Rhinosinusitis: establishing definitions for clinical research and patient care. J Allergy Clin Immunol. 2004;114(6 Suppl):155–212.

91. Ponikau JU, Sherris DA, Kern EB, et al. The diagnosis and incidence of allergic fungal sinusitis. Mayo Clin Proc. 1999;74(9):877–884.

92. Sundar KM, Gosselin MV, Chung HL, et al. Pulmonary Langerhans cell histiocytosis: emerging concepts in pathobiology, radiology, and clinical evolution of disease. Chest. 2003;123(5):1673–1683.

93. Akdis CA, Akdis M, Bieber T, et al. Diagnosis and treatment of atopic dermatitis in children and adults: European Academy of Allergology and Clinical Immunology/American Academy of Allergy, Asthma and Immunology/PRACTALL Consensus Report. J Allergy Clin Immunol. 2006;118(1):152–169.

94. Adame J, Cohen PR. Eosinophilic panniculitis: diagnostic considerations and evaluation. *J Am Acad Dermatol.* 1996;34(2 Pt 1):229–234.

95. Caputo R, Marzano AV, Vezzoli P, et al. Wells syndrome in adults and children: a report of 19 cases. *Arch Dermatol.* 2006;142(9):1157–1161.

96. Bischoff L, Derk CT. Eosinophilic fasciitis: demographics, disease pattern and response to treatment: report of 12 cases and review of the literature. *Int J Dermatol.* 2008;47(1):29–35.

97. Matsuda M, Fushimi T, Nakamura A, et al. Nonepisodic angioedema with eosinophilia: a report of two cases and a review of the literature. *Clin Rheumatol.* 2006;25(3):422–425.

98. Sufyan W, Tan KB, Wong ST, et al. Eosinophilic pustular folliculitis. *Arch Pathol Lab Med.* 2007;131(10):1598–1601.

99. Chen KR, Su WP, Pittelkow MR, et al. Eosinophilic vasculitis in connective tissue disease. *J Am Acad Dermatol.* 1996;35(2 Pt 1):173–182.

100. Maric I, Robyn J, Metcalfe DD, et al. KIT D816V-associated systemic mastocytosis with eosinophilia and FIP1L1/PDGFRA-associated chronic eosinophilic leukemia are distinct entities. *J Allergy Clin Immunol.* 2007;120(3):680–687.

101. Utsunomiya A, Ishida T, Inagaki A, et al. Clinical significance of a blood eosinophilia in adult T-cell leukemia/lymphoma: a blood eosinophilia is a significant unfavorable prognostic factor. *Leuk Res.* 2007;31(7):915–920.

102. Tancrede-Bohin E, Ionescu MA, de La Salmoniere P, et al. Prognostic value of blood eosinophilia in primary cutaneous T-cell lymphomas. *Arch Dermatol.* 2004;140(9):1057–1061.

103. Saliba WR, Dharan M, Bisharat N, et al. Eosinophilic pancreatic infiltration as a manifestation of lung carcinoma. *Am J Med Sci.* 2006;331(5):274–276.

104. Bohm A, Fodinger M, Wimazal F, et al. Eosinophilia in systemic mastocytosis: clinical and molecular correlates and prognostic significance. *J Allergy Clin Immunol.* 2007;120(1):192–199.

105. Al-Haddad S, Riddell RH. The role of eosinophils in inflammatory bowel disease. *Gut.* 2005;54(12):1674–1675.

106. Wada T, Takei K, Kudo M, et al. Characterization of immune function and analysis of RAG gene mutations in Omenn syndrome and related disorders. *Clin Exp Immunol.* 2000;119(1):148–155.

107. Kishi Y, Sugawara Y, Tamura S, et al. Histologic eosinophilia as an aid to diagnose acute cellular rejection after living donor liver transplantation. *Clin Transplant.* 2007;21(2):214–218.

109. Beishuizen A, Vermes I, Hylkema BS, et al. Relative eosinophilia and functional adrenal insufficiency in critically ill patients. *Lancet.* 1999;353(9165):1675–1676.

110. Thorn GW, Prunty FTG, Hills AG. A test for adrenal cortical insufficiency. *JAMA.* 1948;137:105–109.

111. Lanham JG, Elkon KB, Pusey CD, et al. Systemic vasculitis with asthma and eosinophilia: a clinical approach to the Churg-Strauss syndrome. *Medicine* (Baltimore). 1984;63(2):65–81.

112. Saxon A, Beall GN, Rohr AS, et al. Immediate hypersensitivity reactions to beta-lactam antibiotics. *Ann Intern Med.* 1987;107(2):204–215.

113. Poe RH, Condemi JJ, Weinstein SS, et al. Adult respiratory distress syndrome related to ampicillin sensitivity. *Chest.* 1980;77(3):449–451.

114. Hawkins EP, Berry PL, Silva FG. Acute tubulointerstitial nephritis in children: clinical, morphologic, and lectin studies. A report of the Southwest Pediatric Nephrology Study Group. *Am J Kidney Dis.* 1989;14(6):466–471.

115. Tsakiri A, Balslev I, Klarskov P. Eosinophilic cystitis induced by penicillin. *Int Urol Nephrol.* 2004;36(2):159–161.

116. Fiegenberg DS, Weiss H, Kirshman H. Migratory pneumonia with eosinophilia associated with sulfonamide administration. *Arch Intern Med.* 1967;120(1):85–89.

117. Sitbon O, Bidel N, Dussopt C, et al. Minocycline pneumonitis and eosinophilia. A report on eight patients. *Arch Intern Med.* 1994;154(14):1633–1640.

118. MacNeil M, Haase DA, Tremaine R, et al. Fever, lymphadenopathy, eosinophilia, lymphocytosis, hepatitis, and dermatitis: a severe adverse reaction to minocycline. *J Am Acad Dermatol.* 1997;36(2 Pt 2):347–350.

119. Ho D, Tashkin DP, Bein ME, et al. Pulmonary infiltrates with eosinophilia associated with tetracycline. *Chest.* 1979;76(1):33–36.

120. Tsuruta D, Someda Y, Sowa J, et al. Drug hypersensitivity syndrome caused by minocycline. *J Cutan Med Surg.* 2006;10(3):131–135.

121. Wai AO, Lo AM, Abdo A, et al. Vancomycin-induced acute interstitial nephritis. *Ann Pharmacother.* 1998;32(11):1160–1164.

122. Zuliani E, Zwahlen H, Gilliet F, et al. Vancomycin-induced hypersensitivity reaction with acute renal failure: resolution following cyclosporine treatment. *Clin Nephrol.* 2005;64(2):155–158.

123. Rastogi S, Atkinson JL, McCarthy JT. Allergic nephropathy associated with ciprofloxacin. *Mayo Clin Proc.* 1990;65(7):987–989.

124. Wong PC, Yew WW, Wong CF, et al. Ethambutol-induced pulmonary infiltrates with eosinophilia and skin involvement. *Eur Respir J.* 1995;8(5):866–868.

125. Takami A, Nakao S, Asakura H, et al. Pneumonitis and eosinophilia induced by ethambutol. *J Allergy Clin Immunol.* 1997;100(5):712–713.

126. Davidson AC, Bateman C, Shovlin C, et al. Pulmonary toxicity of malaria prophylaxis. *BMJ.* 1988;297(6658):1240–1241.

127. Lor E, Liu YQ. Didanosine-associated eosinophilia with acute thrombocytopenia. *Ann Pharmacother.* 1993;27(1):23–25.

128. Hogan MB, Piktel D, Landreth KS. IL-5 production by bone marrow stromal cells: implications for eosinophilia associated with asthma. *J Allergy Clin Immunol.* 2000;106(2):329–336.

129. Taskinen E, Tukiainen P, Sovijarvi AR. Nitrofurantoin-induced alterations in pulmonary tissue. A report on five patients with acute or subacute reactions. *Acta Pathol Microbiol Scand (A).* 1977;85(5):713–720.

130. Santos RP, Ramilo O, Barton T. Nevirapine-associated rash with eosinophilia and systemic symptoms in a child with human immunodeficiency virus infection. *Pediatr Infect Dis J.* 2007;26(11):1053–1056.

131. Knudtson E, Para M, Boswell H, et al. Drug rash with eosinophilia and systemic symptoms syndrome and renal toxicity with a nevirapine-containing regimen in a pregnant patient with human immunodeficiency virus. *Obstet Gynecol.* 2003;101(5 Pt 2):1094–1097.

132. Davis CM, Shearer WT. Diagnosis and management of HIV drug hypersensitivity. *J Allergy Clin Immunol.* 2008;121(4):826–832 e5.

133. Santos RP, Awa E, Anbar RD. Inhaled tobramycin solution-associated recurrent eosinophilia and severe persistent bronchospasm in a patient with cystic fibrosis: a case report. *BMC Pediatr.* 2007;7:11.

134. Gaffey CM, Chun B, Harvey JC, et al. Phenytoin-induced systemic granulomatous vasculitis. *Arch Pathol Lab Med.* 1986;110(2):131–135.

135. Mahatma M, Haponik EF, Nelson S, et al. Phenytoin-induced acute respiratory failure with pulmonary eosinophilia. *Am J Med.* 1989;87(1):93–94.

136. Cullinan SA, Bower GC. Acute pulmonary hypersensitivity to carbamazepine. *Chest.* 1975;68(4):580–581.

137. Mizoguchi S, Setoyama M, Higashi Y, et al. Eosinophilic pustular folliculitis induced by carbamazepine. *J Am Acad Dermatol.* 1998;38(4):641–643.

138. Gonzalez FJ, Carvajal MJ, del Pozo V, et al. Erythema multiforme to phenobarbital: involvement of eosinophils and T cells expressing the skin homing receptor. *J Allergy Clin Immunol.* 1997;100(1):135–137.

139. Conilleau V, Dompmartin A, Verneuil L, et al. Hypersensitivity syndrome due to 2 anticonvulsant drugs. *Contact Dermatitis.* 1999;41(3):141–144.

140. Mahoney JM, Bachtel MD. Pleural effusion associated with chronic dantrolene administration. *Ann Pharmacother.* 1994;28(5):587–589.

141. Pot C, Oppliger R, Castillo V, et al. Apomorphine-induced eosinophilic panniculitis and hypereosinophilia in Parkinson disease. *Neurology.* 2005;64(2):392–393.

142. Jeandel PY, Traissac T, Rainfray M, et al. Drug hypersensitivity syndrome with lamotrigine two cases in elderly. *Presse Med.* 2005;34(7):516–518.

143. Szczeklik A, Sladek K, Dworski R, et al. Bronchial aspirin challenge causes specific eicosanoid response in aspirin-sensitive asthmatics. *Am J Respir Crit Care Med.* 1996;154(6 Pt 1):1608–1614.

144. Buscaglia AJ, Cowden FE, Brill H. Pulmonary infiltrates associated with naproxen. *JAMA.* 1984;251(1):65–66.

145. Goodwin SD, Glenny RW. Nonsteroidal anti-inflammatory drug-associated pulmonary infiltrates with eosinophilia. Review of the literature and Food and Drug Administration Adverse Drug Reaction reports. *Arch Intern Med.* 1992;152(7):1521–1524.

146. Rich MW, Thomas RA. A case of eosinophilic pneumonia and vasculitis induced by diflunisal. *Chest.* 1997;111(6):1767–1769.

147. Bruyn GA, Velthuysen E, Joosten P, et al. Pancytopenia related eosinophilia in rheumatoid arthritis: a specific methotrexate phenomenon? *J Rheumatol.* 1995;22(7):1373–1376.

148. Mok CC, Lau CS, Wong RW. Toxicities of dapsone in the treatment of cutaneous manifestations of rheumatic diseases. *J Rheumatol.* 1998;25(6):1246–1247.

149. Tomioka R, King TE Jr. Gold-induced pulmonary disease: clinical features, outcome, and differentiation from rheumatoid lung disease. *Am J Respir Crit Care Med.* 1997;155(3):1011–1020.

150. Davis P, Hughes GR. Significance of eosinophilia during gold therapy. *Arthritis Rheum.* 1974;17(6):964–968.

151. Michel F, Navellou JC, Ferraud D, et al. DRESS syndrome in a patient on sulfasalazine for rheumatoid arthritis. *Joint Bone Spine.* 2005;72(1):82–85.

152. Fam AG, Lewtas J, Stein J, et al. Desensitization to allopurinol in patients with gout and cutaneous reactions. *Am J Med.* 1992;93(3):299–302.

153. Raptis L, Pappas G, Katsanou A, et al. Diltiazem-induced eosinophilic pleural effusion. *Pharmacotherapy.* 2007;27(4):600–602.

154. Steinman TI, Silva P. Acute renal failure, skin rash, and eosinophilia associated with captopril therapy. *Am J Med.* 1983;75(1): 154–156.

155. Schatz PL, Mesologites D, Hyun J, et al. Captopril-induced hypersensitivity lung disease. An immune-complex-mediated phenomenon. *Chest.* 1989;95(3):685–687.

156. Serratrice J, Pellissier JF, Champsaur P, et al. Fasciitis with eosinophilia: a possible causal role of angiotensin-converting enzyme inhibitor. *Rev Neurol* (Paris). 2007;163(2):241–243.

157. Higa K, Hirata K, Dan K. Mexiletine-induced severe skin eruption, fever, eosinophilia, atypical lymphocytosis, and liver dysfunction. *Pain.* 1997;73(1):97–99.

158. Hall D, Link K. Eosinophilia associated with Coumadin. *N Engl J Med.* 1981;304(12):732–733.

159. Volpi A, Ferrario GM, Giordano F, et al. Acute renal failure due to hypersensitivity interstitial nephritis induced by warfarin sodium. *Nephron.* 1989;52(2):196.

160. d'Adamo G, et al. Omeprazole-induced acute interstitial nephritis. *Ren Fail.* 1997;19(1):171–175.

161. Tishler M, Abramov AL. Cimetidine-induced eosinophilia. *Drug Intell Clin Pharm.* 1985;19(5):377–378.

162. Kendell KR, Day JD, Hruban RH, et al. Intimate association of eosinophils to collagen bundles in eosinophilic myocarditis and ranitidine-induced hypersensitivity myocarditis. *Arch Pathol Lab Med.* 1995;119(12):1154–1160.

163. Andreu V, Bataller R, Caballeria J, et al. Acute eosinophilic pneumonia associated with ranitidine. *J Clin Gastroenterol.* 1996;23(2):160–162.

164. Tanigawa K, Sugiyama K, Matsuyama H, et al. Mesalazine-induced eosinophilic pneumonia. *Respiration.* 1999;66(1):69–72.

165. Makino H, Haramoto T, Sasaki T, et al. Massive eosinophilic infiltration in a patient with the nephrotic syndrome and drug-induced interstitial nephritis. *Am J Kidney Dis.* 1995;26(1):62–67.

166. Cutler NR, Anderson DJ. Proven asymptomatic eosinophilia with imipramine. *Am J Psychiatry.* 1977;134(11):1296–1297.

167. Panuska JR, King TR, Korenblat PE, et al. Hypersensitivity reaction to desipramine. *J Allergy Clin Immunol.* 1987;80(1):18–23.

168. Fleisch MC, Blauer F, Gubler JG, et al. Eosinophilic pneumonia and respiratory failure associated with venlafaxine treatment. *Eur Respir J.* 2000;15(1):205–208.

169. Raz A, Bergman R, Eilam O, et al. A case report of olanzapine-induced hypersensitivity syndrome. *Am J Med Sci.* 2001;321(2):156–158.

170. Salerno SM, Strong JS, Roth BJ, et al. Eosinophilic pneumonia and respiratory failure associated with a trazodone overdose. *Am J Respir Crit Care Med.* 1995;152(6 Pt 1):2170–2172.

171. Banov MD, Tohen M, Friedberg J. High risk of eosinophilia in women treated with clozapine. *J Clin Psychiatry.* 1993;54(12):466–469.

172. White DA, Kris MG, Stover DE. Bronchoalveolar lavage cell populations in bleomycin lung toxicity. *Thorax.* 1987;42(7):551–552.

173. Weiss RB, Donehower RC, Wiernik PH, et al. Hypersensitivity reactions from taxol. *J Clin Oncol.* 1990;8(7):1263–1268.

174. Rutella S, Sica S, Rumi C, et al. Hypereosinophilia during 2-chlorodeoxyadenosine treatment for hairy cell leukaemia. *Br J Haematol.* 1996;92(2):426–428.

175. Aglietta M, Sanavio F, Stacchini A, et al. Interleukin-3 in vivo: kinetic of response of target cells. *Blood.* 1993;82(7):2054–2061.

176. Rodgers S, Rees RC, Hancock BW. Changes in the phenotypic characteristics of eosinophils from patients receiving recombinant human interleukin-2 (rhIL-2) therapy. *Br J Haematol.* 1994;86(4):746–753.

177. Donhuijsen K, Haedicke C, Hattenberger S, et al. Granulocyte-macrophage colony-stimulating factor-related eosinophilia and Loeffler's endocarditis. *Blood.* 1992;79(10):2798.

178. Le Nouail P, Viseux V, Chaby G, et al. Drug reaction with eosinophilia and systemic symptoms (DRESS) following imatinib therapy. *Ann Dermatol Venereo.* 2006;133(8–9 Pt 1):686–688.

179. Wong PW, Macris N, DiFabrizio L, et al. Eosinophilic lung disease induced by bicalutamide: a case report and review of the medical literature. *Chest.* 1998;113(2):548–550.

180. Jennings CA, Deveikis J, Azumi N, et al. Eosinophilic pneumonia associated with reaction to radiographic contrast medium. *South Med J.* 1991;84(1):92–95.

181. Nadeem S, Nasir N, Israel RH. Loffler's syndrome secondary to crack cocaine. *Chest.* 1994;105(5):1599–1600.

182. Bond GR. Hepatitis, rash and eosinophilia following trichloroethylene exposure: a case report and speculation on mechanistic similarity to halothane induced hepatitis. *J Toxicol Clin Toxicol.* 1996;34(4):461–466.

183. Hertzman PA, Blevins WL, Mayer J, et al. The eosinophilia-myalgia syndrome: status of 205 patients and results of treatment 2 years after onset. *Ann Intern Med.* 1995;122(11):851–855.

184. Norgard N, Wall GC. Possible drug rash with eosinophilia and systemic symptoms syndrome after exposure to epoetin alfa. *Am J Health Syst Pharm.* 2005;62(23):2524–2526.

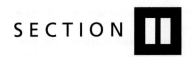
Pathogenic and Environmental Aspects in Allergy and Asthma

CHAPTER 6

Allergens and Other Factors Important in Atopic Disease

G. DANIEL BROOKS AND ROBERT K. BUSH

An allergen is an antigen that produces a clinical allergic reaction. In atopic diseases, allergens are antigens that elicit an immunoglobulin E (IgE) antibody response. Sensitivity to an allergen can be demonstrated by a wheal-and-flare reaction to that antigen in a skin test, or by *in vitro* immunoassays such as the radioallergosorbent test (RAST), or enzyme-linked immunosorbent assay (ELISA), which measures antigen-specific IgE in serum. Other methods, usually restricted to research laboratories, also may be used to demonstrate the presence of specific IgE antibodies. These include crossed radioimmunoelectrophoresis (CRIE), immunoblotting technique, and leukocyte histamine release assay. When assessing the contribution of a particular antigen to an observed symptom, the nature of the immune response must be clarified. The clinician must differentiate the allergic (or atopic) response from the irritant response. The immediate Type I IgE-mediated allergic response is distinctly different from the Type 1Va pathophysiologic mechanism mediating the delayed hypersensitivity reactions, which result from contact antigens, such as poison ivy or nickel.

Allergens most commonly associated with atopic disorders are inhalants or foods, reflecting the most common entry sites into the body. Drugs, biologic products, insect venoms, and certain chemicals also may induce an immediate-type reaction. In practice, however, most atopic reactions involve pollens, fungal spores, house dust mites, animal epithelial materials, and other substances that impinge directly on the respiratory mucosa. They cross-link IgE antibodies attached to mast cells or basophils, initiating a series of intracellular process that result in mediator release and allergic symptoms. This chapter is confined to the exploration of these naturally occurring inhalant substances; other kinds of allergens are discussed elsewhere in this text. Aeroallergens are airborne proteins that can cause respiratory or conjunctival allergy. It is common for a single airborne particle, such as a mold spore or a pollen grain, to contain multiple allergens.

■ AEROALLERGENS

Certain aeroallergens, such as animal danders, may be localized to individual homes. Others may be associated with occupational exposures, as is the case in bakers who inhale flour. Some sources of airborne allergens are narrowly confined geographically, such as the mayfly and the caddis fly, whose scales and body parts are a cause of respiratory allergy in the eastern Great Lakes area in the late summer. In addition, endemic asthma has been reported in the vicinity of factories where castor beans are processed.

Several methods can be used to determine whether a protein is an allergen. The most clinically related method is an allergen challenge. In a conjunctival or nasal challenge, the extract is introduced directly to the affected mucosa to look for typical allergy symptoms. In a bronchoprovocation challenge, the allergen is inhaled and pulmonary function is deemed significantly different if there is a 20 % decline in FEV1. These methods are generally too impractical to perform in an office setting. Most often a skin test is performed to determine whether an extract can elicit the typical wheal-and-flare response. Finally, tests to estimate allergen-specific IgE can be performed with patient sera. Although most tests are performed with crude extracts, specific IgE tests can be performed on serum to examine individual allergenic proteins within an extract. From a practical standpoint, it is the presence of specific IgE to a protein in the sera of clinically allergic patients that defines it as an allergen.

The chemical nature of certain allergens has been studied intensively, although the precise composition of many other allergens remains undefined. For an increasing number of allergens, the complementary DNA (cDNA) sequence has been derived. For others, the physiochemical characteristics or the amino acid sequence is known. Still other allergens are known only as complex mixtures of proteins and polypeptides with varying amounts of carbohydrate. Details of the chemistry of known allergens are described under their appropriate headings.

The methods of purifying and characterizing allergens include biochemical, immunologic, and biologic techniques. The methods of purification involve techniques such as chromatography, immunoprecipitation, and molecular biology. All of these purification techniques rely on sensitive and specific assay techniques for the allergen as reviewed below.

Allergen Nomenclature

To be recognized as an allergen by the International Union of Immunological Societies (IUIS), a protein must have evidence of allergenicity in at least five individuals and 5% of the population studied (1). Allergens to a specific source such as ragweed pollen or cat dander, can be classified as either major or minor allergens. Major allergens are those that result in IgE greater than 50% of the population sensitized to the source. Minor allergens are those that result in specific IgE in less than 50% of those individuals sensitized to the specific source, be it a pollen or dust mite. Sometimes authors refer to allergens that result in specific IgE in about 50% of the sensitized population as intermediate allergens.

The nomenclature for individual allergen proteins has been established by the IUIS: the first three letters of the genus, followed by the first letter of the species and an Arabic numeral. For example, the primary allergen in cat (*Felis domesticus*) is Fel d 1. Prior to the adoption of this nomenclature system, grass allergens, ragweed allergens, cockroach allergens, and dust mite allergens all had separate naming systems, that are now only of historical interest. The numbering given to the allergen is often adjusted to account for proteins in separate species that are either cross-reactive or structurally similar. The nomenclature of the German cockroach (*Blatella germanica*) and the American cockroach (*Periplaneta americana*) allergens illustrates this principle well (Table 6.1). Notice that *Bla g 6* and *Per a 6* are both members of the

TABLE 6.1 COCKROACH ALLERGENS

GERMAN COCKROACH	BIOCHEMICAL NAME	AMERICAN COCKROACH	BIOCHEMICAL NAME
Bla g 1		*Per a 1*	
Bla g 2	Aspartic protease		
		Per a 3	Arthropod hemocyanin
Bla g 4	Calycin		
Bla g 5	Glutathione S transferase		
Bla g 6	Troponin C	*Per a 6*	Troponin C
Bla g 7	Tropomyosin	*Per a 7*	Tropomyosin

Troponin C family of molecules. *Bla g 1* and *Per a 1* have similar attributes, though they do not have an identified function. There has not yet been an allergen identified in the American cockroach that is similar to *Bla g 2*, so there is no *Per a 2*. As allergenic proteins are matched by number, they often must be assigned new names, which can lead to confusion when reading even relatively recent journal articles. An updated list of all established allergens with reference to obsolete names is maintained by the IUIS (1).

Isoallergens are proteins within a species that have similar immunologic properties and/or molecular structures, but differ in some way such as isoelectric point, carbohydrate content, or amino acid composition. For example, the ragweed allergen *Amb a 1* has four isoallergenic variants based on biochemical studies and cDNA analyses (1). The *Amb a 1* isoallergen sequences all have the same first 25 proteins, but vary in the rest of their structure.

Sampling Methods for Airborne Allergens

Patients commonly seek out daily reports of pollen or mold spore levels from the newspaper, television, or Internet. They often use these levels to correlate and predict their allergy symptoms. It is important to understand that all of the current methods for reporting these levels involve averaging pollen levels from the day before. Thus the levels may be helpful in correlating previous symptoms but are of limited use in correlating current symptoms or predicting future symptoms. There are commercial companies that claim to have computer models that predict pollen counts. However, there are no publications that have prospectively determined the value of computer models in predicting pollen counts (2,3).

Aerobiological sampling attempts to identify and quantify the allergenic particles in the ambient atmosphere, both outdoors and indoors. Commonly, an adhesive substance is applied to a microscope slide or other transparent surface, and the pollens and spores that stick to the surface are microscopically enumerated. Devices of varying complexity have been used to reduce the most common sampling errors relating to particle size, wind velocity, and rain. Fungi also may be sampled by culture techniques. Although many laboratories use various immunoassays to identify and quantify airborne allergens, the microscopic examination of captured particles remains the method of choice. Two types of sampling devices are most commonly used: impaction and suction. Gravitational samplers were used historically, but are rarely used today because they provide qualitative data not quantitative.

Impaction Samplers

Impaction samplers are the most common outdoor allergen samplers. Rotating arm impaction samplers have two vertical, adhesive-coated collecting arms mounted on a crossbar, which is rotated by a vertical motor shaft. Small particles, particularly pollen grains, are prone to blowing in the wind in a way that interferes with gravitational settling. They become more likely to impact on an adhesive surface. The sampler rotates up to several thousand revolutions per minute to overcome the effects of wind. However, at this speed turbulence may "push" the pollen away and decrease sampling. For this reason the sampling surface is small (1 to a few millimeters) to get the highest rate of impaction. Small surface areas, however, are rapidly overloaded, causing a decrease in the efficiency of capture. These samplers usually are run intermittently (20 to 60 seconds every 10 minutes) to reduce overloading. In some models, the impacting arms are retracted or otherwise protected while not in use. The Rotorod sampler (Fig. 6.1) is a commercially available impaction sampler and has been shown to be over 90% efficient at capturing pollen particles of approximately 20 μm diameter. It is much less efficient at capturing smaller particles, especially those <5 μm diameter.

Suction Samplers

Suction samplers employ a vacuum pump to draw the air sample into the device. Although suitable for pollens, they are more commonly used to measure smaller particles such as mold spores. Disorientation with wind direction and velocity skews the sampling efficiencies of particles of different sizes. For example, if the wind

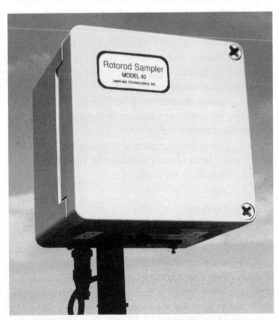

■ **FIGURE 6.1** Rotating impaction sampler: Rotorod sampler model 40 (Sampling Technologies, Minnetonka, MN). (Courtesy of Medical Media Service, Wm. Middleton Memorial Veteran's Hospital, Madison, WI.)

velocity is less than that generated by the sampler, smaller particles are collected in greater concentrations than exist in the ambient air. The reverse is true for greater wind velocities. The Hirst spore trap is an inertial suction sampler with a clock mechanism that moves a coated slide at a set rate along an intake orifice. This enables discrimination of diurnal variations. A wind vane orients the device to the direction of the wind. The Burkard spore trap collects particles on an adhesive-coated drum that takes 1 week to make a full revolution around an intake orifice. Both of these spore traps are designed to measure nonviable material. Spore traps are the most flexible devices for sampling particles over a wide range of sizes.

The Anderson sampler is another suction device, but it is unique in its adaptability for enumerating viable fungal spores. Air passes through a series of sieve-like plates (either two or six), each containing 400 holes. Although the air moves from plate to plate, the diameter of the holes decreases. The larger particles are retained by the upper plates and the smaller ones by successive lower plates. A Petri dish containing growth medium is placed beneath each sieve plate, and the spores that pass through the holes fall onto the agar and form colonies. This method has value for identifying fungi whose spore morphologic features do not permit microscopic identification. In general, however, nonviable volumetric collection techniques more accurately reflect the actual spore prevalence than do volumetric culture methods. The volume of air sampled is easy to calculate for suction devices because the vacuum pumps may be calibrated. In the case of rotation impaction samplers, there are formulas that depend on the surface area of the exposed bar of slide, the rate of revolution, and the exposure time. After the adherent particles are stained and counted, their numbers can be expressed as particles per cubic meter of air. Gravitational samplers cannot be quantified volumetrically.

The location of samplers is important. Ground level is usually unsatisfactory because of liability, tampering, and similar considerations. Rooftops are used most frequently. The apparatus should be placed at least 6 m (20 ft) away from obstructions and 90 cm (3 ft) higher than the parapet on the roof.

Fungal Culture

Fungi also may be studied by culture techniques. This is often necessary because many spores are not morphologically distinct enough for microscopic identification. In such cases, characteristics of the fungal colonies are required. Most commonly, Petri dishes with appropriate nutrient agar are exposed to the air at a sampling station for 5 to 30 minutes. The plates are incubated at room temperature for about 5 days, and then inspected grossly and microscopically for the numbers and types of colonies present. Cotton-blue is a satisfactory stain for fungal morphologic identification. Potato-dextrose agar supports growth of most allergenic fungi, and rose bengal may be added to retard bacterial growth and limit the spread of fungal colonies. Specialized media such as Czapek agar may be used to look for particular organisms (e.g., *Aspergillus* or *Penicillium*).

The chief disadvantage of the culture plate method is a gross underestimation of the spore count. This may be offset by using a suction device such as the Anderson or Burkard sampler. A microconidium containing many spores still grows only one colony. There may be mutual inhibition or massive overgrowth of a single colony such as *Rhizopus nigricans*. Other disadvantages are short sampling times, as well as the fact that some fungi (rusts and smuts) do not grow on ordinary nutrient media. Furthermore, avoiding massive spore contamination of the laboratory is difficult without precautions such as an isolation chamber and ventilation hood.

Immunologic Methods

Numerous immunologic methods of identifying and quantifying airborne allergens have been developed. In general, these methods require more sophisticated instruments and thus are unlikely to replace the physical pollen count. The immunologic assays do not depend on the morphologic features of the material sampled, but on the ability of eluates of this material collected on filters to interact in immunoassays with human IgE or IgG or with mouse monoclonal antibodies (4,5). Studies at the Mayo Clinic have used a high-volume air sampler that retains 95% of particles larger than 0.3 μm on a fiberglass filter. The antigens, of unknown composition, are eluted from the filter sheet by descending chromatography. The eluate is dialyzed, lyophilized, and reconstituted as needed. This material is analyzed by RAST inhibition for specific allergenic activity or, in the case of antigens that may be involved in hypersensitivity pneumonitis, by interaction with IgG antibodies. The method is extremely sensitive. An eluate equivalent to 0.1 mg of pollen produced 40% to 50% inhibition in the short ragweed RAST. An equivalent amount of 24 μg of short ragweed pollen produced over 40% inhibition in the *Amb a 1* RAST (6). The allergens identified using this method have correlated with morphologic studies of pollen and fungal spores using traditional methods and with patient symptom scores. The eluates also have produced positive results on prick skin tests in sensitive human subjects (7). These techniques demonstrate that with short ragweed, different-sized particles from ragweed plant debris can act as a source of allergen in the air before and after the ragweed pollen season. Unexpectedly, appreciable ragweed allergenic activity has been associated with particles less than 1 μm in diameter (8).

Use of low-volume air samples that do not disturb the air and development of a sensitive two-site monoclonal antibody immunoassay for the major cat allergen (*Fel d 1*) have made accurate measurements of airborne cat allergen possible (5). These studies confirm that a high proportion of *Fel d 1* is carried on particles smaller than 2.5 μm. During house cleaning, the amount of the small allergen-containing particles in the air approached that produced by a nebulizer for bronchial provocation (40 ng/m^3). The results indicate that significant airborne *Fel d 1* is associated with small particles that remain airborne for long periods. This is in contrast to prior studies with house dust mites (9) in which the major house dust mite allergen *Der p 1* was collected on large particles with diameters greater than 10 μm. Little of this allergen remained airborne when the room was undisturbed.

Many pollen grains may be difficult to distinguish morphologically by normal light microscopic study. Immunochemical methods may permit such distinctions. Grass pollen grains collected from a Burkard trap were blotted onto nitrocellulose; then, by using specific antisera to Bermuda grass, a second antibody with a fluorescent label, and a fluorescent microscope study, Bermuda grass pollen grains could be distinguished from grass pollens of other species (10). These newer methods show promise because they measure allergenic materials that react with human IgE. Currently, immunochemical assays to quantify the major house dust mite allergens *Der p 1* and *Der f 1* and the major cat allergen *Fel d 1* in settled dust samples are commercially available. Further studies with these techniques may lead to a better understanding of exposure–symptom relationships.

■ STANDARDIZATION OF ALLERGENIC EXTRACTS

The need to standardize allergenic extracts has been recognized for many years. Variability in antigen composition and concentration is a major problem in both allergy testing and allergen immunotherapy. Without standardization of extracts, there is no accurate system of quality control. The clinician often is forced to alter immunotherapy schedules with each new vial of extract because of lot-to-lot variability. Each allergen extract supplier uses its own assays and rarely compares specific antigen concentrations with competitors. The result of this disparity is that the clinician must bring more art than science to the field of allergen immunotherapy. Fortunately, this is changing, with the requirement for standardization of ragweed pollen, house dust mite, cat dander, and grass pollen extracts. The development of purified and even cloned allergens that can be expressed in bacteria or yeast hosts have allowed the production of vast quantities of allergen extract with little or no variance between batches (11). With investigators, clinicians, and government agencies that license extracts demanding improved standardization, it is expected that

more progress in this area of allergy will be made in the near future.

Quantification of Allergens

The traditional method of preparing and labeling allergens for clinical use is to extract a known weight of defatted pollen or other allergenic particle in a specified volume of fluid. For example, 1 g in 100 mL of fluid would yield a 1% (1:100) solution. This weight per volume (w/v) system still is one of the most commonly used in clinical practice. This solution can be concentrated or diluted as needed.

Another system of measurement, used by some extract manufacturers, is the protein-nitrogen unit (PNU). The basis of the PNU system is the fact that most allergenic moieties of pollens are proteins, and that the ratio of protein to dry weight of pollen varies from plant to plant. In this method, nitrogen is precipitated by phosphotungstic acid and measured by the micro-Kjeldahl technique. One PNU is 0.01 μg of protein nitrogen.

Both of these methods are used for nonstandardized inhalant and food allergens; clinicians generally must communicate in terms of these measurements. Unfortunately, neither the w/p nor the PNU truly measures allergenic activity, because not all measured proteins and extractable components in the solution are allergenic. In addition, many complex allergens are destroyed during the harsh extraction procedure. Such problems have been circumvented through the use of biologic assays of "functional" allergen reactivity. Currently, ragweed pollen, grass pollen, house dust mite, and cat allergen extracts are standardized, and their activity is expressed in allergen units or biologic allergenic units. Other allergen extracts may be added to this list in the future. It is essential for anyone devising immunotherapy regimens to have an appreciation for the biologic assays of allergenicity, which are described later.

■ CHARACTERIZATION OF ALLERGENS

While any methods are available to characterize an allergen, many of these, such as the determination of protein content, molecular weight, and isoelectric point, are not unique to the study of allergenic compounds. These are simply methods of describing any protein. Several categories of tests, however, are restricted to studying molecules responsible for IgE-mediated symptoms.

Radioallergosorbent Test

The RAST is described elsewhere in this text. Although primarily used in the quantification of antigen-specific IgE, the test may be adapted to determine antigen concentrations. To measure potency, the unknown allergen is immobilized onto solid-phase supports (cellulose disks or beads) and reacted with a known quantity of antigen-specific IgE in a standard test system. For comparison, the extracts are compared with a reference standard, which should be carefully chosen. The quantity of extract required to obtain a specified degree of reactivity is determined. The greater the binding of IgE to the antigen, the greater the allergenicity.

RAST Inhibition Assay

The most widely used assay for *in vitro* potency of allergenic extract is the RAST inhibition method. This test is a variation of the direct RAST. Serum from an allergic individual (containing IgE) is first mixed with the soluble unknown allergen. Next, a standard amount of the solid-phase (immobilized) allergen is added. The more potent the fluid phase allergen, the less IgE is free to bind to the solid-phase allergen. The technique and its statistical analysis have been standardized. RAST inhibition usually is the key technique to assess total allergenic activity of an extract and is used by manufacturers to calibrate new batches by comparison with the in-house reference preparation. Some have raised concern regarding the continued use of RAST inhibition as a standard technique. The arguments concern the fact that the choice of antigen for the solid-phase reaction is variable and may influence results. In addition, the finite supply of allergenic reference sera limits reproducibility: without identical reference sera and immobilized allergen, comparisons are impossible. Further development of monoclonally derived IgE and recombinant allergens may help with these concerns.

Assessment of Allergenicity

Biochemical methods for analyzing allergens, such as protein composition and concentration, are practical but tell nothing about the allergenicity of the extract. Immunologic reactivity with IgE antibodies as assessed *in vitro* and *in vivo* provides this information. Preparations of inhalant allergens contain more than one antigen. Of the several antigens in a mixture, usually one or more dominate in both frequency and intensity of skin reactions in sensitive persons. It is inferred from this that these antigens are the most important clinically. Not all persons allergic to a certain pollen allergen react to the same antigens from that pollen allergen extract, however. The antigens of tree, grass, and weed pollens are immunologically distinct, and this agrees with the clinical and skin test data. As more allergens are isolated and purified, correlations between immunogenicity and biochemical structure have emerged.

There are two methods of determining the allergenicity of an individual protein. One method is to look at how many people make an IgE response against a certain allergen. A major allergen has been defined as one that binds IgE in 50% or more of sensitized patients

(12). A second method of determining the allergenicity of a protein is to determine how much of the IgE is bound to that protein. For example, in experiments involving the major cat allergen, *Fel d 1*, it has been reported that 90% of the IgE antibodies against cat are reacting against *Fel d 1* (1).

Theories of Allergenicity

What characteristics determine whether a particle or a protein can become an important allergen? For a particle to be clinically significant as an aeroallergen, it must be buoyant, present in significant numbers, and allergenic. In general, the insect-pollinated plants do not produce appreciable amounts of airborne pollen, as opposed to wind-pollinated plants, which, by necessity, produce particles that travel for miles. However, being present in high concentrations is not enough. For example, pine pollen is abundant in certain regions and is buoyant, but because it does not readily elicit IgE antibodies, it is not a significant aeroallergen. The characteristics of allergenic particles have been examined and theories relating to their allergenicity are described below.

Structural Properties of Aeroallergens

Some protein structures do seem to be more likely to be associated with allergenicity. One factor that may be important is the simultaneous exposure of multiple allergenic epitopes on a single structure to promote cross-linking of IgE. The major birch allergen, *Bet v 1*, has been compared to a naturally occurring, nonallergenic protein with significant sequence homology using three-dimensional computer modeling. The nonallergenic protein appears to have fewer epitopes on the exposed surface of the molecule and is more likely to be a monomer than *Bet v 1* (13). Computer models that predict allergenicity suggest that the presence of multiple allergenic motifs on a protein makes it more likely to be allergenic (14). There is also evidence from computer modeling of known allergen sequences that a number of diverse allergens have a common structural motif, a groove inside an alpha-beta motif, which is also found in some toxins and defensins (15).

Do specific carbohydrate determinants promote allergenicity? Serum from allergic patients often has IgE that interacts with cross-reacting carbohydrate determinants. Many of these cross-reacting carbohydrate determinants are present in a wide variety of proteins and across very different species. There may be some *in vivo* effects of these epitopes on an immunologic level. However, cross-reacting carbohydrate epitopes often appear to be a source of positive serologic results without clinical significance (16). Carbohydrates have recently been identified in IgE-mediated reactions, and further investigations are underway.

It has been hypothesized that proteins might be more allergenic because of their structural similarity to invasive organisms. Helminths are classically associated with high IgE levels and intuitively might be associated with allergy, but studies in animal models and human populations suggest that helminthic infection is generally protective against the development of allergies (17). An exception, the fish parasite Anisakis, is associated with allergenic symptoms during infection and has been reported as an occupational respiratory allergen in fish-processing factories (18).

Chemical Properties of Allergens and Immune Interactions

It has been known for some time that the major house dust mite allergen, Der p 1, has structural similarity to cysteine protease enzymes (19). The enzymatic activity of this allergen may have a role in the development of atopic sensitization and asthma. A series of experiments have been done in which mice are sensitized using enzymatically active or inactive Der p 1. In the presence of the active enzyme, the mice create more total IgE and Der p 1-specific IgE (20). Active Der p 1 also has been used as an adjuvant to increase production of ovalbumin-specific IgE (21). A third experiment involved nasal sensitization with either active or inactive Der p 1. The active enzyme group had increased cellular inflammatory cells in the lungs and increased total IgE levels (22). Thus, the enzymatic activity appears to contribute to the allergenicity of the molecule.

Several mechanisms have been proposed to explain the relation between enzymatic function and the development of sensitization. Enzymatically active Der p 1 can disrupt tight junction between respiratory epithelia in cell cultures (23). This has been proposed as a mechanism by which the allergen can be delivered through the epithelium to the immune cells. Other dust mite allergens, Der p 3, 6, and 9, have been categorized as serine proteases. These allergens can also disrupt the tight junctions in respiratory epithelium (24).

Several immunologic mechanisms have also been proposed to explain the apparent allergenic effects of dust mite enzymes. The enzymatic activity of Der p 1 has been shown to cleave the low-affinity IgE FcR CD23 from human B cells, which may augment IgE synthesis. (25,26). It has also been shown that dendritic cells incubated with enzymatically active Der p 1 generate less IL-12, which would favor T_H2 cell responses (27).

The role of allergenic enzymes in activating protease activated receptors (PARs) has also been investigated. It appears that serine proteases, but not cysteine proteases are involved in the activation of protease activated receptors. The major mold allergen from penicillium, Pen c 13, is also a serine protease. Incubation of a respiratory epithelial cell line with Pen c 13 induces IL-8 release through a pathway that is dependent on

activation of both PAR-1 and PAR-2 (28,29). Several other major mold allergens have been shown to increase IL-8 and IL-6 secretion in epithelial cell lines. Crude cockroach extracts also activate PAR-2 and stimulate IL-8 production in respiratory epithelial cell lines (30,31). Cysteine proteases, such as Der p 1, can activate respiratory epithelial cells to secrete IL-8, but the mechanism does not involve PAR-2 (32).

Properties of Pollen Grains

It is important to remember that pollen grains are complex structures designed to deliver plant reproductive material. They have many chemicals and proteins that are presented to the respiratory mucosa at the same time as the most allergenic proteins. The biochemical properties of these pollen grains also contribute to their allergenicity. It has been shown that birch, grass, and ragweed pollens contain both serine proteases and cysteine proteases and that these proteases can also disrupt epithelial tight junctions (33). Type 1 grass pollen allergens appear to migrate into the stratum corneum skin via the hair follicles as soon as 15 minutes. This has been proposed as a mechanism of sensitization in atopic dermatitis (34).

Pollen extracts also appear to have direct effects on the immune system. In cell culture, birch pollen extracts have been found to direct dendritic cells toward a more T_H2 type of antigen presentation and to recruit more T_H2 cells for antigen presentation (35).

Effects of Particle Size

Aeroallergen particle size is an important element of allergic disease. Airborne pollens are in the range of 20 μm to 60 μm in diameter; mold spores usually vary between 3 μm and 30 μm in diameter or longest dimension; house dust mite particles are 1 μm to 10 μm. Protective mechanisms in the nasal mucosa and upper tracheobronchial passages remove most of the larger particles, so only those 3 μm or smaller are thought to reach the alveoli of the lungs. Hence, the conjunctivae and upper respiratory passages receive the largest dose of airborne allergens. Despite this conventional wisdom, examination of tracheobronchial aspirates and surgical lung specimens has revealed whole pollen grains in the lower respiratory tract (36). These are considerations in the pathogenesis of allergic rhinitis and bronchial asthma as well as the effects of chemical and particulate atmospheric pollutants.

The development of asthma after pollen exposure is enigmatic because pollen grains are thought to be deposited in the upper airways as a result of their large particle size. Experimental evidence suggests that rhinitis, but not asthma, is caused by inhalation of whole pollen in amounts encountered naturally (37). Asthma caused by bronchoprovocation with solutions of pollen extracts is easily achieved in the laboratory, however. Pollen asthma may be caused by the inhalation of pollen debris that is small enough to access the bronchial tree.

Ragweed asthma supports this hypothesis. The major ragweed allergen, *Amb a 1*, has been found in ambient air, even in the absence of whole pollen (7). Extracts of materials collected on an 8-μm filter that excludes ragweed pollen grains still appear to contain ragweed allergen based on skin testing and ragweed-IgG inhibition (38).

In Melbourne and London, severe outbreaks of asthma have been reported during some thunderstorms. This phenomenon has been referred to as thunderstorm asthma. People who had asthma exacerbations during a thunderstorm were more likely to be sensitive to grass pollen (39). Grass pollen is generally considered to be too large to access the smaller airways of the lungs. However, exposure of grass pollen grains to water creates rupture into smaller, respirable-size starch granules with intact allergens (40). These starch granules have been found to increase 50-fold during a rainstorm and thunderstorm asthma patients are more likely to be sensitive to the starch granules than other asthma patients (39,41). There is evidence for a similar effect of *Alternaria* spores. Thunderstorm asthma patients were more likely to be sensitive to *Alternaria*, and counts of broken *Alternaria* spores correlate with hospital admissions during a thunderstorm (42).

■ POLLEN ALLERGENS

Pollen grains are living male gametophytes of higher plants (gymnosperms and angiosperms). Each grain has an internal limiting cellulose membrane, the intine, and a two-layered external covering, the exine, composed of a durable substance called sporopollenin. Sporopollenin is primarily a high molecular weight polymer of fatty acids.

Morphologic studies of pollens using the scanning electron microscope disclose an intricate infrastructure. The morphologic structure varies in relation to size, number of furrows, form and location of pores, thickness of the exine, and other features of the cell wall (spines, reticulations, an operculum in grass pollens, and air sacs [bladders] in certain conifers). Ragweed pollen is about 20 μm in diameter, tree pollens vary from 20 μm to 60 μm, and grass pollens, which are all morphologically similar, are usually 30 μm to 40 μm. The identification of pollens important in allergic disease is not difficult and is certainly within the capabilities of the physician with no special expertise in botany (43,44).

Some plants produce prodigious amounts of pollen. A single ragweed plant may expel 1 million pollen grains in a single day. Trees, especially conifers, may release so much pollen that it is visible as a cloud and may be scooped up by the handful after settling. The seasonal onset of pollination of certain plants (e.g.,

ragweed) is determined by the duration of light received daily. Pollination occurs earlier in the northern latitudes and demonstrates little year-to-year variation in terms of date. In the belt from the central Atlantic to the north-central states, August 15 is a highly predictable date for the onset of ragweed pollination. Most ragweed pollen is released between 6:00 AM and 8:00 AM, and release is enhanced by high temperature and humidity. Extended dry spells in early summer inhibit flower development, reduce ragweed pollen production, and thus result in lower counts in August and September.

Most brightly colored flowering plants are of little clinical importance in inhalant allergy because their pollen generally is carried by insects (entomophilous plants) rather than the wind (anemophilous plants). Entomophilous plants have relatively scant, heavy, and sticky pollen. Roses and goldenrod are examples of plants that often are erroneously thought to cause pollinosis because of the time they bloom. Nevertheless, in isolated cases, the pollens of most entomophilous plants can sensitize and then cause symptoms if exposure is sufficient. Of the pollens of anemophilous plants, ragweed has a long range, having been detected 400 miles out at sea. The range of tree pollens is much shorter. Thus, an individual living in the center of a city is more likely to be affected by weed and grass pollens than by trees. Local weed eradication programs, more often legislated than accomplished, are futile in light of the forgoing information. Air conditioners significantly reduce indoor particle recovery because windows are shut when they operate and they largely exclude outdoor air.

■ CLASSIFICATION OF ALLERGENIC PLANTS

The botanical considerations and taxonomic scheme given here are not exhaustive (43,44). Individual plants, their common and botanical names, geographic distributions, and relative importance in allergy are considered elsewhere in this book.

Anatomy

Seed-bearing plants produce their reproductive structures in cones or flowers. Gymnosperms ("naked seeds"; class Gymnospermae) are trees and shrubs that bear their seeds in cones. Pines, firs, junipers, spruces, yews, hemlocks, savins, cedars, larches, cypresses, retinisporas, and ginkgoes are gymnosperms. Angiosperms produce seeds enclosed in the female reproductive structures of the flower. Angiosperms may be monocotyledons, whose seeds contain one "seed leaf" (cotyledon), or dicotyledons, with two seed leaves. Leaves of monocotyledons have parallel veins, whereas leaves of dicotyledons have branching veins. Grasses are monocotyledons; most other allergenic plants are dicotyledons.

The flower has four fundamental parts:

1. *Pistils* (one or more) are the female portion of the plant and consist of an ovary at the base, a style projecting upward, and a stigma, the sticky portion to which pollen grains adhere.
2. *Stamens*, which are the male portions of the plant, are variable in number and consist of anthers borne on filaments. Pollen grains are produced in the anthers.
3. *Petals*, the colored parts of the flower, vary from three to many in number.
4. *Sepals*, the protective portion of the flower bud, are usually green and three to six in number.

The phylogenetically primitive flower had numerous separate parts, as typified by the magnolia. Fusion of flower parts and reduction of their number is a characteristic of phylogenetic advancement. As a group, dicotyledons are more primitive than monocotyledons.

A "perfect" flower contains both male and female organs; an "imperfect" flower contains only stamens or only pistils. Monoecious ("one house") plants bear both stamens and pistils; the individual flowers may be perfect or imperfect. Dioecious ("two houses") plants have imperfect flowers, and all flowers on a particular plant are the same type (male and female). Ragweed is a monoecious plant with perfect flowers; corn is a monoecious plant with imperfect flowers; willows are dioecious plants. Like the flowering plants, gymnosperms may be either monoecious (pines) or dioecious (cypresses and ginkgoes).

Taxonomy

Plants are classified in a hierarchical system. The principal ranks, their endings, and some examples are as follows:

Class (-ae): Angiospermae, Gymnospermae
Subclass (-ae): Monocotyledonae, Dicotyledonae
Order (-ales): Coniferales, Salicales
Suborder (-ineae)
Family (-aceae): Asteraceae, Poaceae
Subfamily (-oideae)
Tribe (-eae)
Genus (no characteristic ending; italicized): *Acer*
Species (genus name plus "specific epithet"): *Acer rubrum*

Trees: Gymnosperms

Trees may be gymnosperms or angiosperms. The gymnosperms include two orders, the Coniferales (conifers) and the Ginkgoales. Neither is of particular importance in allergy, but because of the prevalence of conifers and the incidence of their pollens in surveys, some comments are in order.

Conifers grow mainly in temperate climates. They have needle-shaped leaves. The following three families are germane to this discussion.

Pinaceae (Pines, Spruces, Firs, and Hemlocks)

Pines are monoecious evergreens whose leaves are arranged in bundles of two to five and are enclosed at the base by a sheath (all other members of the Pinaceae family bear leaves singly, not in bundles). The pollen grains of pines are 45 μm to 65 μm in diameter and have two bladders (Fig. 6.2). This pollen occasionally has been implicated in allergy. Spruces produce pollen grains morphologically similar to pine pollen but much larger, ranging from 70 μm to 90 μm exclusive of the bladders. Hemlock pollen grains may have bladders, depending on the species. The firs produce even larger pollen grains, ranging from 80 μm to 100 μm, not including the two bladders.

Cupressiaceae (Junipers, Cypresses, Cedars, and Savins)

Most of these trees are dioecious and produce large quantities of round pollen grains 20 μm to 30 μm in diameter with a thick intine (internal membrane). The mountain cedar is an important cause of allergic rhinitis in certain parts of Texas and has proliferated where the ecosystem has been disturbed by overgrazing of the grasslands.

Taxodiaceae (Bald Cypress and Redwood)

The bald cypress may be a minor cause of allergic rhinitis in Florida.

Trees: Angiosperms

Most allergenic trees are in this group. The more important orders and families are listed here with relevant notations. Other trees have been implicated in pollen allergy, but most of the pollinosis in the United States can be attributed to those mentioned here.

Order Salicales, Family Salicaceae (Willows and Poplars)

Willows are mainly insect pollinated and are not generally considered allergenic (Fig. 6.2). Poplars, however, are wind pollinated, and some (e.g., species of *Populus*) are of considerable allergenic importance. Poplar pollen grains are spherical, 27 μm to 34 μm in diameter, and characterized by a thick intine (Fig. 6.2). The genus *Populus* includes poplars, aspens, and cottonwoods. Their seeds are borne on buoyant cotton-like tufts that may fill the air in June like a localized snowstorm. Patients often attribute their symptoms to this "cottonwood," but the true cause usually is grass pollens.

Order Betulales, Family Betulaceae (Birches)

Betula species are widely distributed in North America and produce abundant pollen that is highly allergenic.

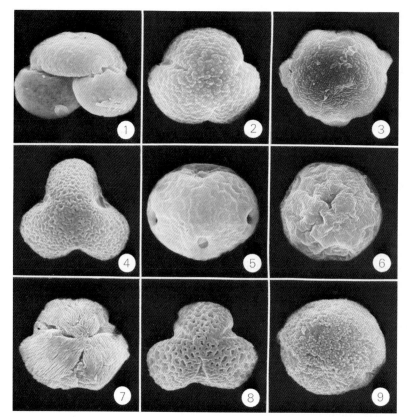

■ **FIGURE 6.2** Scanning electron photomicrographs of early spring airborne hay fever–producing pollen grains: *1*, pine (*Pinus*); *2*, oak (*Quercus*); *3*, birch (*Betula*); *4*, sycamore (*Platanus*); *5*, elm (*Ulmus*); *6*, hackberry (*Celtis*); *7*, maple (*Acer*); *8*, willow (*Salix*); *9*, poplar (*Populus*). (Courtesy of Professor James W. Walker.)

The pollen grains are 20 μm to 30 μm and flattened, generally with three pores, although some species have as many as seven (Figs. 6.2 and 6.3). The pistillate catkins may persist into winter, discharging small winged seeds.

Order Fagales, Family Fagaceae (Beeches, Oaks, Chestnuts, and Chinquapins)

Five genera of Fagaceae are found in North America, of which only the beeches (*Fagus*) and oaks (*Quercus*) are wind pollinated and of allergenic importance. The pollens of these two genera are morphologically similar but not identical. They are 40 μm in diameter, with an irregular exine (outer covering) and three tapering furrows (Figs. 6.2 and 6.4). Both produce abundant pollen; oaks in particular cause a great deal of tree pollinosis in areas where they are numerous.

Order Urticales, Family Ulmaceae (Elms and Hackberries)

About 20 species of elms are in the Northern Hemisphere, mainly distributed east of the Rocky Mountains. They produce large amounts of allergenic pollen and continue to be a major cause of tree pollinosis despite the almost total elimination of the American elm by Dutch elm disease. Elm pollen is 35 μm to 40 μm in diameter with five pores and a thick, rippled exine (Fig. 6.2). Hackberries are unimportant for this discussion.

Order Juglandales, Family Juglandaceae (Walnuts)

Walnut trees (*Juglans*) are not important causes of allergy, but their pollen often is found on pollen slides. The pollen grains are 35 μm to 40 μm in diameter, with about 12 pores predominantly localized in one area and a smooth exine (Fig. 6.5).

The Hickories (Carya)

These trees produce large amounts of highly allergenic pollen. Pecan trees in particular are important in the etiology of allergic rhinitis where they grow or are cultivated. The pollen grains are 40 μm to 50 μm in diameter and usually contain three germinal pores.

Order Myricales, Family Myricaceae (Bayberries)

Bayberries produce windborne pollen closely resembling the pollen of the *Betulaceae*. The wax myrtles are thought to cause pollinosis in some areas.

Order Urticales, Family Moraceae (Mulberries)

Certain members of the genus *Morus* may be highly allergic. The pollen grains are small for tree pollens, about 20 μm in diameter, and contain two or three germinal pores arranged with no geometric pattern (neither polar nor meridial).

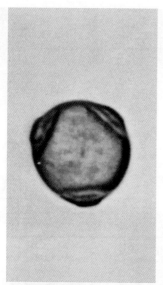

■ **FIGURE 6.3**   Birch (*Betula nigra*). Average diameter is 24.5 μm. Pollen grains have three pores and a smooth exine. (Courtesy of Center Laboratories, Port Washington, NY.)

Order Hamamelidales, Family Platanaceae (Sycamores)

These are sometimes called "plane trees." The grains of their plentiful pollen are oblate (flattened at the poles), about 20 μm in diameter, and without pores. There are three or four furrows on the thin, granular exine (Fig. 6.2). Regionally, sycamores may be of allergenic significance.

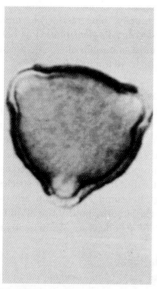

■ **FIGURE 6.4**   Oak (*Quercus* species). Average diameter is 32 μm. Pollens of the various species are similar, with three long furrows and a convex, bulging, granular exine. (Courtesy of Center Laboratories, Port Washington, NY.)

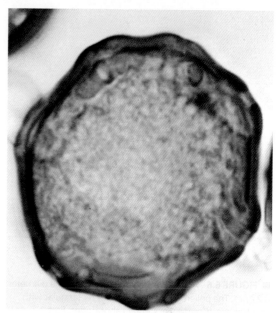

■ **FIGURE 6.5**   Walnut (*Juglans nigra*). Average diameter is 36 μm. Grains have multiple pores surrounded by thick collars arranged in a nonequatorial band. (Courtesy of William P. Solomon, M.D., University of Michigan, Ann Arbor.)

Order Rutales, Family Simaroubaceae (Ailanthus)

Only the tree of heaven (*Ailanthus altissima*) is of allergenic importance regionally. Its pollen grains have a diameter of about 25 μm and are characterized by three germinal furrows and three germinal pores.

Order Malvales, Family Malvaceae (Lindens)

One genus, *Tilia* (the linden or basswood tree), is of allergenic importance, although it is insect pollinated. The pollen grains are distinct, 28 μm to 36 μm, with germ pores sunk in furrows in a thick, reticulate exine.

Order Sapindales, Family Aceraceae (Maples)

There are more than 100 species of maple, many of which are important in allergy. Maple pollen grains have three furrows but no pores (Fig. 6.2). Box elder, a species of *Acer*, is particularly important because of its wide distribution, its prevalence, and the amount of pollen it sheds.

Order Oleales, Family Oleaceae (Ashes)

This family contains about 65 species, many of which are prominent among the allergenic trees. Pollen grains have a diameter of 20 μm to 25 μm, are somewhat flattened, and usually have four furrows (Fig. 6.6). The exine is coarsely reticulate.

Grasses (Poaceae)

Grasses are monocotyledons of the family Poaceae (or Gramineae). The flowers usually are perfect (Figs. 6.7 and 6.8). Pollen grains of most allergenic grasses are

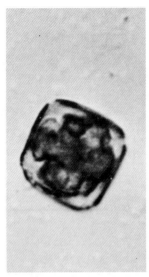

■ **FIGURE 6.6** Ash (*Fraxinus americana*). Average diameter is 27 μm. The pollen grains are square or rectangular with four furrows. (Courtesy of Center Laboratories, Port Washington, NY.)

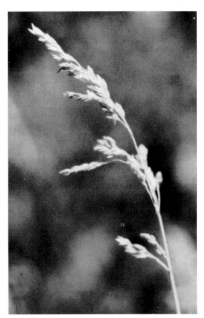

■ **FIGURE 6.8** June grass or bluegrass (*Poa pratensis*). Morphologic features of the flowering head. (Courtesy of Arnold A. Gutman, M.D., Associated Allergists Ltd., Chicago, IL.)

20 μm to 25 μm in diameter, with one germinal pore or furrow and a thick intine (Fig. 6.9). Some grasses are self-pollinated and therefore noncontributory to allergies. The others are wind-pollinated, but of the more than 1,000 species in North America, only a few are significant in producing allergic symptoms. Those few, however, are important in terms of the numbers of patients affected and the high degree of morbidity produced. Most of the allergenic grasses are cultivated and therefore are prevalent where people live.

The grass family contains several subfamilies and tribes of varying importance to allergists. The most important are listed here.

Subfamily Festucoideae, Tribe Festuceae

The tribe Festuceae contains meadow fescue (*Festuca elatior*), Kentucky bluegrass (*Poa pratensis*), and orchard grass (*Dactylis glomerata*) (Fig. 6.9), which are among the most important allergenic grasses. The pollens are 30 μm to 40 μm in diameter.

Tribe Argostideae

The Argostideae tribe includes timothy (*Phleum pratense*) (Fig. 6.8) and redtop (*Agrostis alba*), two particularly significant grasses in terms of the amount of pollen shed, their allergenicity, and the intensity of symptoms produced. Both are cultivated as forage, and timothy is used to make hay. Other species of *Agrostis* immunologically similar to redtop are used for golf course greens. Timothy pollens are 30 μm to 35 μm in diameter. Redtop pollens are 25 μm to 30 μm.

Tribe Phalarideae

Sweet vernal grass (*Anthoxanthum odoratum*) is an important cause of allergic rhinitis in areas where it is indigenous. In the total picture of grass allergy, however, it is not as important as the species previously mentioned. The pollen grains are 38 μm to 45 μm in diameter.

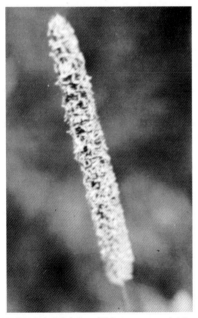

■ **FIGURE 6.7** Timothy grass (*Phleum pratense*). Morphologic features of the flowering head. (Courtesy of Arnold A. Gutman, M.D., Associated Allergists Ltd., Chicago, IL.)

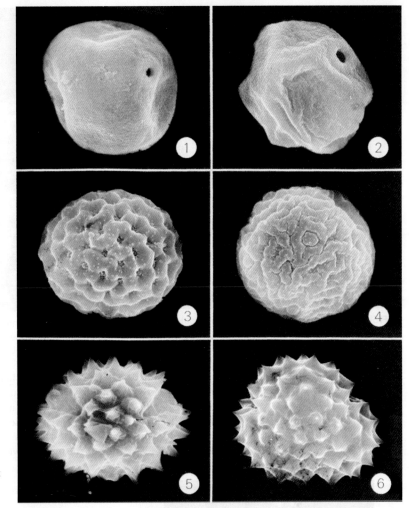

■ **FIGURE 6.9** Early and late summer airborne hay fever–producing pollen grains: *1*, timothy (*Phleum*); *2*, orchard grass (*Dactylis*); *3*, lambs quarter's (*Chenopodium*); *4*, plantain (*Plantago*); *5*, goldenrod (*Solidago*); *6*, ragweed (*Ambrosia*). (Courtesy of Professor James W. Walker.)

Tribes Triticaceae (Wheat and Wheat Grasses), Aveneae (Oats), and Zizaneae (Wild Rice)

The Triticaceae, Aveneae, and Zizaneae tribes are of only minor or local importance in allergy because they are self-pollinating or produce pollen that is not abundant or readily airborne.

Subfamily Eragrostoideae, Tribe Chlorideae

Bermuda grass (*Cynodon dactylon*) is abundant in all the southern states. It is cultivated for decorative and forage purposes. It sheds pollen almost year round and is a major cause of pollen allergy. The pollen grains are 35 μm in diameter.

Weeds

A weed is a plant that grows where people do not intend it to grow. Thus, a rose could be considered a weed if it is growing in a wheat field. What are commonly called weeds are small annual plants that grow without cultivation and have no agricultural or ornamental value.

All are angiosperms and most are dicotyledons. Those of interest to allergists are wind pollinated, and thus tend to have relatively inconspicuous flowers.

Family Asteraceae (Compositae)

The composite family is perhaps the most important allergenic weed group. Sometimes called the sunflower family, it is characterized by multiple tiny flowers arranged on a common receptacle and usually surrounded by a ring of colorful bracts. There are many tribes within this family; only those of allergenic or general interest are mentioned.

Tribe Heliantheae includes sunflower, dahlia, zinnia, and black-eyed Susan. The flowers cause pollinosis mainly among those who handle them.

Tribe Ambrosieae, or the ragweed tribe, is the most important cause of allergic rhinitis and pollen asthma in North America. Other common weeds in this tribe are the cocklebur and marsh elder. *Ambrosia trifida*, giant ragweed, may grow to a height of 4.5 m (15 ft) (Fig. 6.10). The leaves are broad with three to five

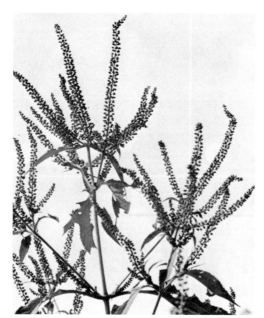

■ **FIGURE 6.10** Giant ragweed (*Ambrosia trifida*). Arrangement of staminate heads. (Courtesy of Arnold A. Gutman, M.D., Associated Allergists Ltd., Chicago, IL.)

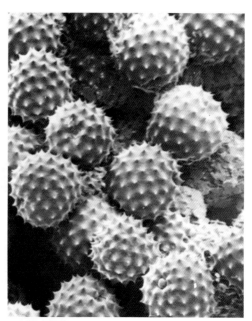

■ **FIGURE 6.12** Scanning electron photomicrograph of ragweed pollen. Notice the pore on the pollen grain (*lower right*). (Courtesy of D. Lim, M.D., and J.I. Tennenbaum, M.D.)

lobes. The staminate heads are borne on long terminal spikes, and the pistillate heads are borne in clusters at the base of the staminate spikes. The pollen grains, 16 μm to 19 μm in diameter, are slightly smaller than those of *Ambrosia artemisiifolia*, short ragweed. Short ragweed grows to a height of 120 cm (4 ft) (Fig. 6.11).

Its leaves are more slender and usually have two pinnae on each side of a central axis. Pollen grains range from 17.5 μm to 19.2 μm in diameter and are almost indistinguishable from those of giant ragweed (Figs. 6.9, 6.12, and 6.13). There is no practical reason, however, for distinguishing between the two. *Ambrosia bidentia*,

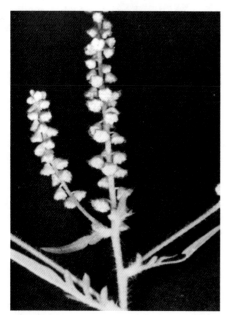

■ **FIGURE 6.11** Short ragweed (*Ambrosia artemisiifolia*). Close-up of staminate head. The anthers are full of pollen just before anthesis. (Courtesy of Arnold A. Gutman, M.D., Associated Allergists Ltd., Chicago, IL.)

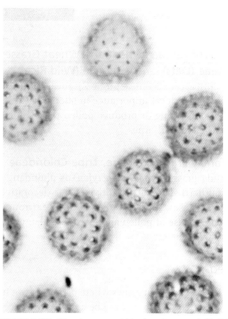

■ **FIGURE 6.13** Short ragweed (*Ambrosia artemisiifolia*). Average diameter is 20 μm. Pollen grains have spicules on the surface. (Courtesy of Schering Corporation, Kenilworth, NJ.)

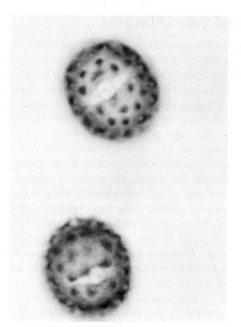

■ **FIGURE 6.14** Burweed marsh elder (*Cyclachaerna xanthifolia*). Average diameter is 19.3 μm. Three pores are centered in furrows, distinguishing it from ragweed. (Courtesy of Schering Corporation, Kenilworth, NJ.)

southern ragweed, is an annual that grows from 30 cm to 90 cm (1 ft to 3 ft) tall. The pollen grains are 20 μm to 21 μm in diameter and resemble those of giant ragweed. *Ambrosia psilostachya*, western ragweed, grows to a height of 30 μm to 120 μm (1 ft to 4 ft). It has the largest pollen grains of all the ragweeds, ranging from 22 μm to 25 μm in diameter. *Franseria acanthicarpa*, false ragweed, is found mainly in the South and Southwest, where it may cause allergic symptoms. *Franseria tenuifolia*, slender ragweed, is another allergenic species of this tribe.

Xanthium (cocklebur) is morphologically distinct from the ragweeds, but its pollen grains are similar. Most species of *Xanthium* produce scanty pollen and are relatively unimportant causes of allergic rhinitis. Many patients with ragweed sensitivity also give strong skin test reactions to the cockleburs; this is probably a cross-reaction.

Cyclachaerna xanthifolia, burweed marsh elder, is antigenically distinct from ragweed, and the pollen grains are morphologically different from those of ragweed (Fig. 6.14).

Tribe Anthemideae, or the mayweed tribe, is important to allergy because it contains chrysanthemums. Pyrethrum is an insecticide made from flowers of these plants, and inhalation of this substance may cause allergic symptoms in ragweed-sensitive persons as well as in those who have been sensitized to the pyrethrum itself. The genus *Artemisia* includes the sagebrushes, mugworts, and wormwoods and is one of the most important groups of allergenic weeds. *Artemisia*

vulgaris is the common mugwort, found mainly on the east coast and in the Midwest in the United States. It is indigenous to Europe and Asia. The pollen grains, like those of other *Artemisia* species, are oblately spheroidal, 17 μm to 28 μm in diameter with three furrows and central pores, a thick exine, and essentially no spines. Other similar species are found on the West Coast and in the Southeast, Great Plains, and Rocky Mountains. *Artemisia tridentata* is common sagebrush, the most important allergenic plant of this tribe. It is most prevalent in the Great Plains and the Northwest, where overgrazing of grassland has increased its presence.

Polygonaceae (Buckwheat Family)

The docks, comprising the genus *Rumex*, are the only allergenic members of the buckwheat family. *Rumex acetosella* (sheep sorrel), *Rumex crispus* (curly dock), and *Rumex obtusifolius* (bitter dock) are the most important species. In the whole spectrum of pollen allergy, however, the docks are of minor significance.

Amaranthaceae (Pigweed and Waterhemp Family)

The best known of the amaranths are *Amaranthus retroflexus* (red-root pigweed), *Amaranthus palmeri* (carelessweed), and *Amaranthus spinosus* (spring amaranth). They are prolific pollen producers and should be considered in the etiology of "hay fever" in the areas where they abound. Western waterhemp (*Amaranthus tamariscinus*), a potent allergen, is most prevalent in the Midwest.

Chenopodiaceae (Goosefoot Family)

The genus *Chenopodium*, "goosefoot," is best represented by *Chenopodium album* (lamb's quarters) (Fig. 6.9). Each plant produces a relatively small amount of pollen, but in some areas the abundance of plants assures a profusion of pollen in the air. *Salsola pestifer*, Russian thistle, and *Kochia scoparia*, burning bush, are other Chenopodiaceae whose allergenic presence is more significant than that of lamb's quarters. Russian thistle also is known as tumbleweed because in the fall the top of the plant separates from its roots and is rolled along the ground by the wind. Burning bush may be recognized easily by the thin wing-like projections along its stems and, in the fall, by the fire engine red color of its leaves. It is often cultivated as an ornamental plant. Indigenous to Europe and Asia, these two weeds first became established in the prairie states but have migrated eastward, and are now important in the pathogenesis of pollinosis. *Atriplex* is the genus of the salt bushes, wingscale, and shadscale. These are of some allergenic significance in the Far West and Southwest.

Two crops numbered among the Chenopodiaceae are the sugar beet (*Beta vulgaris*) and spinach (*Spinacea oleracea*). The former has been implicated in allergy where it is cultivated.

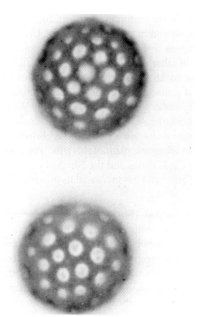

■ FIGURE 6.15 Pigweed (*Amaranthus retroflexus*). Average diameter is 25 µm. The "golf ball" appearance of these grains is characteristic of the chenopod-amaranth group. (Courtesy of Schering Corporation, Kenilworth, NJ.)

Pollens of the Amaranthaceae and Chenopodiaceae are so morphologically similar that they are generally described as chenopodamaranth when found in pollen surveys. Although subtle differences exist, it is generally fruitless and impractical to attempt to identify them more precisely. They have the appearance of golf balls, which makes them unique and easy to identify (Fig. 6.15). Multiple pores give this peculiar surface appearance. The grains are 20 µm to 25 µm in diameter and spheroidal.

Plantaginaceae (Plantain Family)
English plantain (*Plantago lanceolata*) is the only member of this family that is important for allergy. It sheds pollen mainly in May and June, corresponding to the time when grasses pollinate. The pollen grains may be distinguished by their multiple pores (numbering 7 to 14) and variable size (25 µm to 40 µm) (Fig. 6.9). English plantain may be a potent cause of allergic rhinitis, which may be confused with grass pollinosis.

Urticaceae (Nettle Family)
Spreading pellitory (*Parietaria judaica*) and pellitory of the wall (*Parietaria officinalis*) have both been implicated in allergic disease. It is the leading cause of pollen sensitization in southern Europe, and is often referred to as the asthma weed in Australia. It is native to the Mediterranean, but also found in coastal areas of the United Kingdom, Australia, and North America. *Parietaria* species have a very long pollen season with peaks in the spring and fall. *Parietaria judaica* has a small, triporate pollen.

Weed Pollen Allergens

King and Norman (45,46) were pioneers in the purification and analysis of allergens. *Amb a 1* (antigen E) and *Amb a 2* (antigen K), were purified by gel filtration and ion exchange chromatography. These two major ragweed allergens plus eight intermediate or minor allergens have been isolated. *Amb a 1* is mainly found in the intine of the pollen grain (47). Roughly 6% of the protein in ragweed extract is *Amb a 1*. There is no correlation between protein-nitrogen content in six commercial preparations and quantitative studies of ragweed (48). However, *Amb a 1* can be quantified in allergenic extracts to determine potency using RAST inhibition. The U.S. Food and Drug Administration requires *Amb a 1* content to be labeled for ragweed allergen extracts. *Amb a 1* consists of two fragments that are easily dissociated, though they are resistant to enzymatic degradation. The amount of *Amb a 1* produced by an individual ragweed plant appears to be determined genetically. There is considerable variation in the amount extractable by standard methods from pollen from plants grown under identical conditions (59 µg/mL to 468 µg/mL) (49).

Amb a 2 constitutes about 3% of extractable ragweed pollen protein. Approximately 90% to 95% of ragweed-sensitive subjects show skin reactivity to this antigen. *Amb a 2* may cross-react slightly with *Amb a 1*, a finding reinforced by a 68% sequence homology at a DNA level (50).

Since the isolation of *Amb a 1* and 2, additional minor allergens have been identified. In contrast to *Amb a 1*, these low-molecular-weight fractions are rapidly extractable (<10 minutes) from pollen and have basic isoelectric points (51). *Amb a 3* has a relatively high carbohydrate content, making it similar to certain grass pollen antigens. It consists of a single peptide chain of 102 amino acids. Two variants of *Amb a 3* differing by a single amino acid residue have been described; however, this difference does not alter the allergenic specificity (52). This gene has not been cloned. Individuals who are allergic to *Amb a 3* have elevated IgE levels and are more likely to have the HLA-A2 and HLA-B12 phenotype (53).

Amb a 5 consists of a single polypeptide chain whose 45 amino acids have been sequenced. The two isoallergenic forms differ at the second position by the substitution of leucine for valine in about 25% of samples. The frequency of positive skin test results to these antigens in ragweed-sensitive subjects demonstrates that approximately 90% to 95% react to *Amb a 1* and *Amb a 2*, 20% to 25% react to *Amb a 3* and *Amb a 6*, and about 10% to *Amb a 5*. A small fraction (10%) of ragweed-sensitive patients is more sensitive to *Amb a 3* and 5 than to *Amb a 1*. *Amb a 6* and *Amb a 7* show sequence homology to other plant proteins involved in lipid metabolism and electron transport, respectively.

The remaining weed allergens are summarized in Table 6.2. Giant ragweed (*A trifida*), *Amb t 5*, has been

TABLE 6.2   WEED ALLERGENS

COMMON NAME	TAXONOMIC NAME	PURIFIED/CLONED ALLERGENS
Short ragweed	*Ambrosia artemisiifolia*	*Amb a 1–3, 5–10*
Giant ragweed	*Ambrosia trifida*	*Amb t 5*
Western ragweed	*Ambrosia psilostachya*	*Amb p 5*
Russian thistle	*Salsola kali*	*Sal k 1–2*
Mugwort	*Artemisia vulgaris*	*Art v 1–6*
Coccharia (Pellitory)	*Parietaria judaica, officinalis*	*Par j 1–4, Par o 1*
Pigweed	*Chenopodium album*	*Chen a 1–3*

identified (54). Other allergens that cause allergic rhinitis have been purified from additional weeds. These include *Sal p 1* from *S pestifer* (Russian thistle) (55), *Par j 1* and *Par j 2* from *Parietaria judaica* pollen (Coccharia) (56,57), and *Par o 1* from *Parietaria officionalis* (58). The cDNA for *Par j 1* and *Par o 1* also have been described (59,60). *Art v 1* and *Art v 2* from *A vulgaris* (mugwort) also have been purified (61). Mugwort has shown significant cross-reactivity with ragweed, including *Art v1* and profilin (62).

Grass Pollen Allergens

Grass pollen sensitivity is a significant problem worldwide. Important temperate grass species involved in allergic reactions are *Lolium perenne* (ryegrass), *Phleum pratense* (timothy), *Poa pratensis* (June grass, Kentucky bluegrass), *Festuca pratensis* (meadow fescue), *Dactylis glomerata* (cocksfoot, orchard grass), *Agrotis tenuis* (redtop), and *Anthoxanthum odoratum* (sweet vernal). Subtropical grasses that are involved in allergy include *Sorghum halepense* (Johnson grass), and *Cynodon dactylon* (Bermuda grass). Grass allergens are generally remarkable for the high degree of cross-reactivity between species. Due to this cross-reactivity, the allergens were once referred to in groups I to IX that were present in most species studied. Now, however, the grasses are named according to standard allergen nomenclature (1).

Lol p 1 (ryegrass) and *Phl p 1* (timothy) are located in the outer wall and cytoplasm of the pollen grains, but can also be found in starch granules (63). As discussed earlier, these granules release on contact with water and are small (3 µm diameter) enough to reach the lower airways. These allergens are referred to as the beta expansions and have been characterized as cell wall loosening agents (64). There is some debate whether these allergens have protealytic activity. The group 1 allergens have significant cross-reactivity based on IgE RAST inhibition, crossed immunoelectrophoresis (CIE), monoclonal antibody mapping, and amino acid sequence homology (65–68). Other studied group I members include *Poa p 1* (Kentucky bluegrass), *Cyn d 1* (Bermuda), *Dac g 1* (orchard), and *Sor h 1* (Johnson). These allergens are present in 90% to 95% of grass pollen–allergic patients by skin testing. Groups 2 and 3 cause reactions in 60% and 70% of patients (69).

Group 2 allergens include *Lol p 2*, a ryegrass allergen, which has been cloned and is present in about 45% of rye-grass allergic patients (70). *Lol p 3* and *Dac g 3* have both been cloned and have 84% identity, but the predicted secondary structures suggest they may not be cross-reactive (71). Only 20% of grass-pollen sensitive patients react to the group 4 allergen, which appears to have a significant cross-reactivity with *Amb a 1* (71). *Phl p 5* is present in excess of 95% of patients, but its functions are still not certain (1). The cDNA of *Cyn d 7* also has been cloned and has two calcium binding sites. Depletion of calcium causes a loss of IgE reactivity (72). Profilin, a compound involved in actin polymerization, has been identified as an allergen in tree pollens (73). It is allergenic and also has been found to be a minor allergen in the grass allergens and is currently classified in *Phl p 12* and *Cyn d 12* (1).

The cDNA cloning of multiple grass allergens has some potential diagnostic applications. A strategy to take advantage of the extensive cross-reactivity between species using recombinant allergens has been studied. A mixture of *Phl p 1*, *Phl p 2*, *Phl p 5*, and *Bet v 2* (birch profilin) accounted for 59% of grass-specific IgE (74). A study of purified *Lol p 1* and *Lol p 5* versus recombinant *Phl p 1* and *Phl p 5* was performed on RAST-positive patients. The *Lol p* extracts reacted with 80% of the IgE, whereas the recombinant *Phl p* reacted with 57% of the IgE (75).

One of the most innovative applications of DNA technology has been the development of ryegrass plants with down regulation of the *Lol p 5* gene. This transgenic ryegrass pollen maintained its fertility, but had a significant decrease in its IgE-binding capacity compared with normal pollen. This creates the possibility of genetic engineering of less allergenic grasses (76).

TABLE 6.3   TREE ALLERGENS

COMMON NAME	TAXONOMIC NAME	PURIFIED/CLONED ALLERGENS
Birch	*Betula verrucosa*	*Bet v 1–4, 6-7*
Alder	*Alnus glutinosa*	*Aln g 1,4*
Hazel	*Corylus avellana*	*Cor a 1–2, 8–11*
White oak	*Quercus alba*	*Que a 1*
Olive	*Olea europaea*	*Ole e 1–10*
Sugi	*Cryptomeria japonica*	*Cry j 1, 2*
Mountain cedar	*Juniperus ashei*	*Jun a 1–3*

Tree Pollen Allergens

There seems to be a higher degree of specificity to skin testing with individual tree pollen extracts compared with grass pollens because pollens of individual tree species may contain unique allergens. Despite this observation, several amino acid homologies and antigenic cross-reactivities have been noted. Most tree pollen characterization has been done using birch (*Betula verrucosa*), alder (*Alnus glutinosa*), hazel (*Corylus avellana*), white oak (*Quercus alba*), olive (*Olea europaea*), and Sugi (*Cryptomeria japonica*) allergens. Common tree allergens are listed in Table 6.3.

A major birch-pollen allergen, *Bet v 1*, has been isolated by a combination chromatographic technique. Both the amino acid sequence as well as a cDNA clone coding for the *Bet v 1* antigen have been described (77). *Bet v 1* is the birch tree allergen that cross-reacts with a low-molecular-weight apple allergen, a discovery that helps to explain the association between birch sensitivity and oral apple sensitivity (78). Further investigations by the same workers extend this cross-reactivity to include pear, celery, carrot, and potato allergens. Most of the 20 patients tested had birch-specific serum IgE (anti–*Bet v 1* and anti–*Bet v 2*) that cross-reacted to these fruits and vegetables. *Bet v 2* has been cloned and identified as profilin, a compound responsible for actin polymerization in eukaryotes. There is approximately 33% amino acid homology between the human and birch profilin molecules (73).

Bet v 3 and *Bet v 4* have both been cloned and further described as calcium-binding molecules (79,80). Recombinant *Bet v 5* appears to have sequence homology with isoflavone reductase, but the biochemical function remains unknown (81). *Bet v 7* is the most recent to be cloned. It reacts with IgE from 20% of birch allergic patients and has been identified as a cyclophilin (82).

Cryptomeria japonica, the national tree of Japan, is a significant source of allergenic pollen. For a long time, this tree was incorrectly called Japanese cedar, though it is a member of the cypress family. It is distinct from Japanese cypress and is now simply called by its Japanese name, Sugi. *Cry j 1* was initially separated by a combination of chromatographic techniques. Four subfractions were found to be antigenically and allergenically identical (83). There is some amino acid homology between *Cry j 1* and *Amb a 1* and 2, but the significance of this is unclear. A second Sugi allergen, *Cry j 2*, also has been described (84). Allergens from mountain cedar (*Juniperus ashei*) are important in the United States. The major allergen, *Jun a 1*, has a 96% homology with *Cry j 1* and some homology with Japanese cypress (*Chamaecyparis obtusa*) (85). Olive tree pollen is an important allergen in the Mediterranean and California. *Ole e 1* through *Ole e 10* have all been described (86).

■ ROLE OF FUNGAL ALLERGENS

The first description of fungal allergy came in 1726, when Sir John Floyer noted asthma in patients who had just visited a wine cellar. More recently, inhalation challenge studies have suggested a role for fungal sensitivity (87). A prospective cohort suggests that fungal sensitization is a significant risk factor for developing asthma later in life (88). Atmospheric fungal spore counts frequently are 1,000-fold greater than pollen counts (89), and exposure to indoor spores can occur throughout the year (90). Most fungal extracts used clinically are extracts of spore and mycelial material. They also may be derived from culture filtrates.

Estimating the extent to which a sensitive person's symptoms can be attributed to fungal allergy is a major clinical problem because exposure to fungus is continuous, often without definite seasonal end points. This is in contrast to pollens, which have distinct seasons, and to animal dander, for which a definitive history of exposure usually can be obtained. Such a history is sometimes possible for fungal exposure (e.g., raking leaves, or being in a barn with moldy hay), but these exposures are not common for many patients. Some species do show distinctive seasons; nevertheless, during any season, and especially during winter, the number and types of spores a patient inhales on a given day are purely conjectural.

In the natural environment, people are exposed to more than 100 species of airborne or dust-bound microfungi. The variety of fungi is extreme, and dominant types have not been established directly in most areas. The spores produced by fungi vary enormously in size, which makes collection difficult. In addition, more than half of the outdoor fungus burden (Ascomycetes and Basidiomycetes) have spores that have not been studied or are practically unobtainable. Moreover, both microscopic evaluation of atmospheric spores and culturing to assess viability are necessary to fully understand the allergenic potential of these organisms. Fungal spores are currently counted to estimate the burden of allergen, but it is likely that fungal fragments also play a significant role in allergic disease. Fragments of fungi are in much higher concentration than spores and a recent study demonstrated that 25% of hyphal fragments contained allergenic epitopes (91).

Fungi are members of the phylum Thallophyta, plants that lack definite leaf, stem, and root structures. They are separated from the algae in that they do not contain chlorophyll and therefore are saprophytic or parasitic. Almost all allergenic fungi are saprophytes. The mode of spore formation, particularly the sexual spore, is the basis for taxonomic classification of fungi. Many fungi have two names because the sexual and asexual stages initially were described separately. Many fungi produce morphologically different sexual and asexual spores that may become airborne. Thus, describing symptom–exposure relationships becomes difficult. The Deuteromycetes ("fungi imperfecti") are an artificial grouping of asexual fungal stages that includes many fungi of allergenic importance (*Aspergillus*, *Penicillium*, and *Alternaria*). These fungi were considered "imperfect," but are now known to be asexual stages (form genera or form species of Ascomycetes). These fungi reproduce asexually by the differentiation of specialized hyphae called conidiophores, which bear the conidia or asexual spore-forming organs. The various species of these fungi are differentiated morphologically by the conidia. Other classes of fungi also can reproduce asexually by means of conidia. Hyphae are filamentous strands that constitute the fundamental anatomic units of fungi. Yeasts are unicellular and do not form hyphae. The mycelium is a mass of hyphae, and the undifferentiated body of a fungus is called a thallus. One taxonomic scheme follows, with annotations of interest to allergists.

■ CLASSES OF ALLERGENIC FUNGI

Oomycetes

This class of fungi is of little allergenic importance, but *Phytophthoria infestans* has been reported to be associated with occupational allergy.

Zygomycetes

The sexual forms of Zygomycetes are characterized by thick-walled spinous zygospores; the asexual forms are characterized by sporangia. Spores of this group generally are not prominent in the air, but can be found in abundance in damp basements and around composting vegetation. The order Mucorales includes the allergenic species *Rhizopus nigricans* and *Mucor racemosus*. *Rhizopus nigricans* is the black bread mold whose hyphae are colorless but whose sporangia (visible to the naked eye) are black.

Ascomycetes

The Ascomycetes are the "sac fungi." Their spores are produced in spore sacs called asci. Concentrations of ascospores reaching thousands of particles per cubic meter occur in many areas and are especially numerous during periods of high humidity. Two significant allergenic Ascomycetes are *Saccharomyces cerevisiae*, a yeast, and *Chaetomium indicum*. The former, known as baker's yeast, is seen most commonly in its asexual budding form, but under certain culture conditions it forms hyphae and asci. Skin sensitivity to conidia of a powdery mildew, *Microsphaera alni*, has been reported, but the clinical significance of this is unknown.

The conidial forms of several Ascomycetes may represent the sexual form genera of imperfect fungi. For example, *Leptosphaeria* species are prominent and represent asexual stages of *Alternaria*.

Basidiomycetes

Two major subgroups occur within the class Basidiomycetes. The subclass Homobasidiomycetidae comprises mushrooms, bracket fungi, and puffballs. The spores of these organisms constitute a significant portion of the spores found in the air during nocturnal periods and wet weather. These abundant spores are confirmed to be allergenic (92–95) and can provoke bronchoconstriction in sensitive asthmatic subjects (96). Numerous species, including *Pleurotus ostreatus*, *Cantharellus cibarius*, *Clavata cyanthiformis*, *Geaster saccatum*, *Pisolithus tinctorius*, *Scleroderma aerolatum*, *Ganoderma lucidum*, *Psilocybe cubensis*, *Agaricus*, *Armillaria*, and *Hypholoma* species, and *Merulisus lacrymans* ("dry rot") have been identified as allergens.

The Heterobasidiomycetidae include the rusts (Uredinales), smuts (Ustilaginales), and jelly fungi. The Ustilaginales and Uredinales are plant parasites of enormous agricultural importance and may cause allergy where cereal grains are grown or in the vicinity of granaries. Rust spores are encountered primarily by agricultural workers, whereas smut spores can be identified in urban areas surrounded by areas of extensive cultivation. Among the important allergenic species are *Ustilago*, *Urocystis*, and *Tilletia* species.

Deuteromycetes (Fungi Imperfecti)

Asexual spores (conidia) rather than sexual spores characterize the reproductive mechanism of Deuteromycetes and are the basis for subclassification into the following orders.

Sphaeropsidales

The conidiospores are grouped in spherical or flask-shaped structures called pycnidia. The genus *Phoma* is the only common allergenic fungus in this order. It frequently yields positive skin test results in patients sensitive to *Alternaria*.

Melanoconoiales

The order Melanoconoiales is not of allergenic importance.

Moniliales

The conidiophores are spread over the entire colony. Moniliales is by far the largest and most diverse order of the Deuteromycetes and contains most of the recognized and suspected fungus allergens. Three families account for most of the fungi that cause allergy in humans: Moniliaceae, Dematiaceae, and Tuberculariaceae.

The Moniliaceae are characterized by colorless or light-colored hyphae and conidia; the colonies are usually white, green, or yellow. The genera *Aspergillus* (Fig. 6.16), *Penicillium* (Fig. 6.17), *Botrytis, Monilia,* and *Trichoderma* are "moniliaceous molds" associated with allergic disease.

The family Dematiaceae, one of the most important from the standpoint of allergy, is characterized by the production of dark pigment in the conidia and often in the mycelia. It contains the genera *Alternaria* (Fig. 6.18), *Cladosporium (Hormodendrum)* (Fig. 6.19), *Helminthosporium* (Fig. 6.20), *Stemphyllium* (Fig. 6.21), *Nigrosporia, Curvularia,* and *Aureobasidium (Pullularia)*. The last is morphologically similar to the yeasts, and is sometimes classified with them and called the "black" yeast. This group often is described as the "dematiaceous molds." The Tuberculariaceae produce a sporodochium, a round mass of conidiospores containing macroconidia

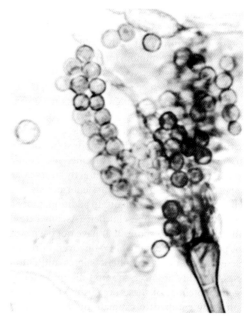

■ FIGURE 6.16 *Aspergillus* species. Average spore diameter is 4 μm. The spores are borne in chains and have connecting collars. (Courtesy of Bayer Allergy Products [formerly Hollister-Stier Labs], Spokane, WA.)

and microconidia in a slimy substrate. The genera *Fusarium* (Fig. 6.22) and *Epicoccum* (Fig. 6.23) are important allergenic fungi in this family.

The family Cryptococcaceae contains the true yeasts, which do not produce hyphae under known

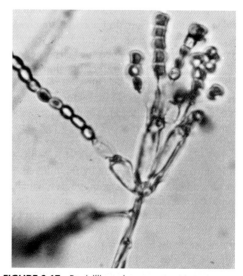

■ FIGURE 6.17 *Penicillium chrysogenum.* Average spore diameter is 2.5 μm. The spores appear in unbranched chains on phialides, the terminal portions of the conidiophores. The phialides and chains of spores resemble a brush. (Courtesy of Bayer Allergy Products [formerly Hollister-Stier Labs], Spokane, WA.)

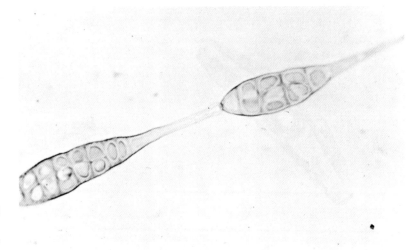

■ **FIGURE 6.18** *Alternaria alternata*. Average spore size is 12 × 33 μm. Spores are snowshoe shaped and contain transverse and longitudinal septae with pores. (Courtesy of Schering Corporation, Kenilworth, NJ.)

cultural or natural circumstances. Allergenic genera within this family include *Rhodotorula* and *Sporobolomyces*.

This classification and list of genera are not exhaustive, but do represent most of the important allergenic fungi found in environmental surveys. The fungi listed here are a framework on which an individual allergist can build or make deletions, depending on the region or clinical judgment. Most fungal sensitivity is specific for genus, although species and strain differences have been reported. Where more than one species occurs for a genus, allergenic extracts usually are mixed together, as in *Aspergillus* mixture or *Penicillium* mixture. It should be remembered that extracts prepared from fungi are extremely variable in allergenic content and composition.

Certain data concerning the prevalence and ecology of fungi make the list less formidable in practice. With the exception of the Pacific Northwest, *Alternaria* and *Cladosporium* (*Hormodendrum*) are the most numerous genera encountered in most surveys of outdoor air. These fungi are "field fungi" and thrive best on plants in the field and decaying plant parts in the soil. They require a relatively high moisture content (22% to 25%) in their substrate. They are mainly seasonal, from spring to late fall, and diminish markedly with the first hard frost. Their spores generally disappear from air samples during the winter months when snow cover is present. *Helminthosporium* and *Fusarium* are the other common field fungi. These and certain other fungi propagate in the soil, and their spores are released in large numbers when the soil is tilled.

Aspergillus and *Penicillium*, conversely, sometimes are called "storage fungi" because they are common causes of rot in stored grain, fruits, and vegetables. *Aspergillus* in particular thrives on a substrate with low moisture content (12% to 16%). These are the two fungi most commonly cultured from houses, especially from basements, crawl spaces, and bedding. *Penicillium* is the green mildew often seen on articles stored in basements. *Rhizopus* causes black moldy bread and proliferates in vegetable bins in homes, especially on onions.

The foremost allergenic fungi, based not only on their incidence in atmospheric surveys, but on allergenic skin test reactivity, are *Alternaria*, *Aspergillus*, *Cladosporium*, and *Penicillium*. Most patients allergic to fungi typically react on skin testing to one or more of these allergens. Many patients also react to other fungi, however, and some to fungi other than these four.

The designations "field" and "storage" fungi or "indoor" and "outdoor" fungi are not precise because exceptions are common in environmental surveys.

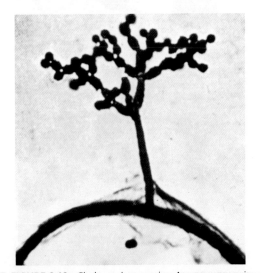

■ **FIGURE 6.19** *Cladosporium* species. Average spore size is 4 × 16 μm. Spores occur in chains and have small attaching collars at one end. The first spore buds off from the conidiophore, then the spore itself buds to form a secondary spore. (Courtesy of Bayer Allergy Products [formerly Hollister-Stier Labs], Spokane, WA.)

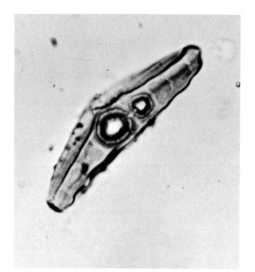

■ **FIGURE 6.20** *Helminthosporium* species. Average spore size is 15 × 75 mm. The spores, which occur in the ends of the conidiophores, are large, brownish, and have transverse septae. (Courtesy of Schering Corporation, Kenilworth, NJ.)

Moreover, indoor colonization from molds varies with the season, particularly in homes that are not air conditioned (97). During the warmer months, *Alternaria* and *Cladosporium* spores are commonly found indoors, having gained entry into the home through open windows.

In contrast to field and storage fungi, yeasts require a high sugar content in their substrates, which limits their habitat. Certain leaves, pasture grasses, and flowers exude a sugary fluid that is a carbon source for

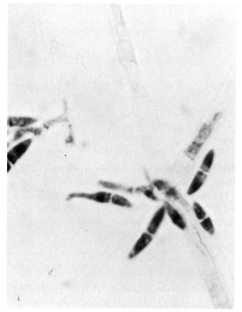

■ **FIGURE 6.22** *Fusarium vasinfectum*. Average spore size is 4 × 50 μm. The most prevalent spore type is the macrospore, which is sickle shaped and colorless, and contains transverse septae and a point of attachment at one end. (Courtesy of Bayer Allergy Products [formerly Hollister-Stier Labs], Spokane, WA.)

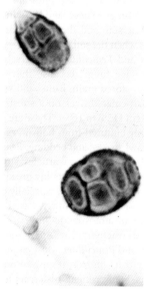

■ **FIGURE 6.21** *Stemphyllium* species. The spores superficially resemble those of *Alternaria* but lack the "tail" appendage. Also, they are borne singly rather than in chains. (Courtesy of Schering Corporation, Kenilworth, NJ.).

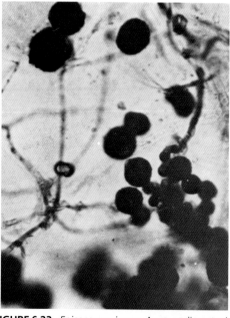

■ **FIGURE 6.23** *Epicoccum nigrum*. Average diameter is 20 μm. Large spores are borne singly on the ends of conidiophores. They are yellowish brown and rough, and develop transverse septae when old. (Courtesy of Bayer Allergy Products [formerly Hollister-Stier Labs], Spokane, WA.)

the nonfermentative yeasts such as *Aureobasidium* (*Pullularia*) and *Rhodotorula*. Hundreds of millions of yeast colonies may be obtained per gram of leaf tissue. Berries and fruit also are commonly colonized. The soil is not a good habitat for yeasts unless it is in the vicinity of fruit trees. Yeasts are often cultured indoors, however.

The relationship of weather to spore dissemination is clinically important, because the symptoms of patients with respiratory allergy are often worse in damp or rainy weather. This has been attributed by some to an increase in the fungal spore count. Absolute fungal spore counts decrease during and after a rainstorm because some spores, like pollen grains, are washed out or made less buoyant. Most of the common allergenic fungi, such as *Aspergillus* and *Cladosporium*, are of the dry spore type, with the spores being released by the wind during dry periods. Alternatively, some so-called "wet weather spores," including certain yeasts such as *Aureobasidium*, *Trichoderma*, and *Phoma* and biologically dispersed ascospores, increase. Although these spores are loosened during wet periods and are dispersed by rain droplets, it is unlikely that they are responsible for the mass symptoms that occur during inclement weather. High spore counts are found in clouds and mist, and it is reasonable to attribute some of the symptoms encountered during long periods of high humidity to fungal allergy. Recall that other allergens, such as the house dust mite, also propagate in conditions of high humidity. Snow cover obliterates the outdoor fungal spore count, but the conditions subsequent to thawing predispose to fungal growth and propagation.

The relationship of house plants to indoor fungal exposure has been studied. Contrary to common belief, indoor plantings are associated with only a slight increase in the numbers of spores from such genera as *Cladosporium*, *Penicillium*, *Alternaria*, and *Epicoccum*. Greenhouses do show an increased number of spores, particularly when plants are agitated by watering or fanning (98).

■ FUNGAL ALLERGENS

Alternaria is an important allergenic fungus that has strong associations with asthma. The major allergenic fraction, *Alt a 1*, has been cloned (99,100), but its biologic function remains unknown. About 90% of *Alternaria*-allergic individuals have IgE to this protein. The *Alt a 1* allergen is rich in carbohydrates, and glycosylation of proteins may be important for allergenic activity (101). Interestingly, the fungus *Stemphyllium* shares at least 10 antigens with *Alternaria* and an allergen immunochemically identical to *Alt a 1* (102). Commercial *Alternaria* extracts contain widely varying amounts of *Alt a 1*, and improved methods of standardization are needed (103).

Alt a 2 also has been cloned, but its function remains unknown (104). *Alt a 5*, a P_2 ribosomal protein, *Alt a 7*,

a YCP4 yeast protein, *Alt a 8*, a mannitol dehydrogenase, and *Alt a 10*, an alcohol dehydrogenase, have all been cloned and sequenced (105,106). *Alt a 2* is a major allergen, recognized by 60% of *Alternaria*-sensitive patients' IgE and *Alt a 8* is present in about 40%, whereas the other three are minor allergens with less than 10% (104,105). Enolase has been obtained from both *Alternaria* (*Alt a 6*) and *Cladosporium* (*Cla h 6*). This is a highly conserved protein among fungi. About 50% of patients reactive to *Alternaria* or *Cladosporium* have IgE to enolase. There is also evidence of further cross-reactivity with *Saccharomyces* and *Candida* (107).

Cladosporium species are among the most abundant airborne spores in the world. Two major allergens have been isolated from *Cladosporium herbarum*: *Cla h 1* and *Cla h 2* (108). *Cla h 1* was isolated by chromatographic and isoelectric focusing techniques. *Cla h 2* is a glycoprotein that is reactive in a smaller percentage of patients than *Cla h 1*. Neither allergen is cross-reactive, as determined by passive transfer skin testing. Two cDNA clones of the minor allergens from *C. herbarum* have been isolated in addition to enolase. *Cla h 5* is a ribosomal P_2 protein found with RNA in the cytosol (109). Heat shock protein (hsp) 70 also has been cloned (110). *Cla h 8* is a mannitol dehydrogenase that is a major allergen (111).

In contrast to *Cladosporium* and *Alternaria* extracts, which are traditionally prepared by extracting mycelia and spores, *Aspergillus fumigatus* extracts generally are prepared from culture filtrate material. Freshly isolated spores from *A. fumigatus* have nearly undetectable levels of the major allergen *Asp f 1*, but begin to produce it within 6 hours of germination. *A. fumigatus* and other *Aspergillus* species have been studied with particular reference to allergenic bronchopulmonary aspergillosis. This disorder is characterized by the presence of both IgE and IgG antibodies to the offending fungal antigens. Analysis by CRIE has demonstrated some components that bind IgE avidly but bind IgG poorly, whereas other components precipitate strongly (bind IgG) but react poorly with IgE (112). When the strains used in the extract were investigated individually, they varied in their quantities of the four most important allergens. Other studies demonstrated that disrupted spore antigens did not cross-react with either mycelial or culture filtrate allergen (113). Common allergens occur within the *fumigatus* and *niger* groups, which are allergenically distinct from the *versicolor*, *nidulans*, and *glaucus* groups (89).

Asp f 1 has been cloned and identified as a cytotoxin, mitogillin, which is excreted from the fungus only during growth (114,115). Approximately 50% of *Aspergillus*-sensitive patients react to *Asp f 1* (116). *Asp f 3* is a peroxisomal membrane protein, and *Asp f 5* is a metalloprotease. A combination of *Asp f 1*, *Asp f 3*, and *Asp f 5* has a sensitivity of 97% for diagnosing *Aspergillus* sensitivity (117).

Diagnostic testing for allergic bronchopulmonary aspergillosis (ABPA) may be greatly simplified in the future using recombinant *Aspergillus* allergens. *Asp f 2*, *Asp f 4*, and *Asp f 6* have all been cloned and are associated with ABPA (117,118). *Asp f 3* and *Asp f 5* are secreted proteins that are recognized by patients with *Aspergillus* sensitivity with or without ABPA, but *Asp f 4* and *Asp f 6* are nonsecreted proteins that are only recognized by patients with ABPA (117). A combination of *Asp f 4* and *Asp f 6* yielded positive skin test results in 11 of 12 ABPA patients, but in 0 of 12 patients sensitized to *Aspergillus* without ABPA. Serologic IgE determinations using ImmunoCAPs and a PharmacaciaCAP system with *Asp f 4* and *Asp f 6* also correlated well with ABPA (119).

Sensitivity to spores of the Basidiomycetes can also cause allergic disease. Several species have been shown to be allergenic, and extracts from these species show multiple antigens and allergens (92). Up to 20% of asthmatic individuals demonstrate positive skin test results to Basidiomycetes species (93). Only two basidiomycete allergens have been well characterized. *Cop c 1* from *Coprinus comatus* has been cloned, but only 25% of basidiomycete-allergic patients respond (120). *Psi c 2* from *Psilocybe cubensis* mycelia was also cloned and shows some homology with *Schizosaccharomyces pombe* cyclophilin (121).

Candida albicans is the most frequently isolated fungal pathogen in humans; however, its role in allergic disease is relatively minimal. Candida sensitivity is associated with eczema related to infection with the human immunodeficiency virus (122). Candida has two major allergens, an alcohol dehydrogenase, and an enolase (123), which cross-reacts as noted before (124). *Candida* also secretes an acid protease, which produces IgE antibodies in 37% of *Candida*-allergic patients (125).

■ DUST MITES

Mites are small (0.33-mm long), eight-legged animals that are easily identified microscopically using a low-power lens. They are a subclass of arachnids that constitute several orders of Acarina, and dust mites are members of the family Pyroglyphidae. The primary dust mites found inside homes in North America and Europe are *Dermatophagoides farinae* and *Dermatophagoides pteronyssinus*. Other house dust mite species are *Dermatophagoides microceras*, *Euroglyphus maynei*, and the tropical *Blomia tropicalis*. Dust mites feed off shed human skin and other high protein debris in their environment. They obtain water from the ambient water in the air.

In North America, dust mites appear to grow more rapidly in the summer months. The major factors governing mite reproduction are temperature, and particularly humidity. When the relative humidity is greater

than 60% at 21°C (70°F) dust mites tend to grow (126). If the relative humidity falls below 40% to 50% for more than 11 days, adult dust mites are unable to survive at temperatures above 25°C (77°F), because increased transpiration of water leads to dehydration (127). The larval form (protonymph) of *Dermatophagoides farinae*, however, is resistant to dessication and may account for the resurgence of dust mites after the winter heating season.

Regional patterns have been observed in dust mite species distribution. High altitudes are associated with low number of dust mites, presumably due to the reduced humidity (128). Areas with a long dry season favor growth of *Dermatophagoides farina*, but humid areas favor *Dermatophagoides pteronyssinus*. *Euroglyphus maynei* will sometimes be the predominant species under damp conditions. *Blomia tropicalis* is important in the southeastern United States (e.g., Florida) as well as in Central and South America.

Dust mites typically are found in the greatest numbers in mattress dust, but can certainly be found anywhere in the house that people routinely traffic, including rugs, bedding, and furniture. Housekeeping or the presence of household pets does not necessarily influence the mite load. The primary methods recommended to reduce dust mites include mattress covers, pillow covers, and frequent washing of bedding. Whether dust mite control measures have a significant clinical effect on asthma remains a point of controversy (129,130).

Both the mite body and the feces contain allergen, though the major allergens are found in feces extracts. A high percentage of dust mite–sensitive patients have positive skin tests to both *Dermatophagoides farinae* and *Dermatophagoides pteronyssinus*. Studies show that many allergens cross-react between the two species although some are unique (131).

Group 1 dust mite allergens include *Der p 1*, *Der f 1*, *Der m 1*, and *Eur m 1*. These allergens have 80% to 85% homology between the mite species, with moderate levels of antigenic cross-reactivity measured by IgE antibodies. Studies of *Der p 1* suggest that it is responsible for 75% of the IgE binding in mite feces (132). Using sequence data, the group I allergens have been identified as members of the cysteine protease family and the possible importance of this function is addressed earlier in the chapter (19). The group 2 allergens include *Der p 2* and *Der f 2*. Both allergens have been cloned and reveal over 85% sequence homology (133). Their structure is similar to an LPS binding protein involved in activation of toll-like receptor 4, but the function appears to be unrelated (134).

Der p 3 and *Der f 3*, are found primarily in fecal material from the house dust mites. *Der p 3* has been cloned (135), and enzymatic studies have demonstrated serine protease activities consistent with trypsin (136). *Der p 6*, *Der f 6*, and *Der p 9* have been described as serine proteases with activity similar to chymotrypsin (137–139). *Der p 4* and *Eur m 4* have been cloned and identified as alpha-amylases (140).

There are other species of mites that are pests in areas of stored grain and can cause allergy, particularly in farm workers. Species include *Acarus siro, Tyrophagus putresentiae, Lepidoglyphus (Glycyphagus) domesticus,* and *Lepidoglyphus destructor.* Spider mites (*Paronychus ulmi* and *Tetranychus urticae*) have been implicated in occupational allergy among apple farmers, and citrus red mite (*Panonychus citri*) among citrus farmers (141,142).

■ EPITHELIAL AND OTHER ANIMAL ALLERGENS

Animal allergens can be found in many types of tissues: hair, feathers, saliva, urine, and dander. *Dander* is the word for desquamated animal epithelium, which is shed constantly. People often believe that a short-haired or hairless animal is not allergenic, which is not the case.

The most severe symptoms tend to be in people allergic to cats. It is unknown whether this is due to the strength of the allergic reaction, the quantities in the air, or the size of the airborne particles. The major allergen, *Fel d 1*, is present in 80% of cat-sensitive individuals and has traditionally been thought to be the primary antigen responsible for allergic disease. *Fel d 1* is produced primarily in cat saliva, but is also found in the sebaceous glands of the skin (143). The *Fel d 1* molecule has some sequence homology with uteroglobin (144). Crystal structures of recombinant *Fel d 1* also have a significant resemblance to uteroglobin, which is cytokine-like molecule with anti-inflammatory and immunomodulatory properties (145). Recently, two additional major allergens have been identified using molecular techniques. *Fel d 3* (cystatin) has been identified, and appears to be a cysteine protease based on molecular modeling (146,147). *Fel d 4* has been suggested as a major allergen, and 47% of patients having a significantly higher IgE titer against *Fel d 4* than against *Fel d 1*. *Fel d 4* is a lipocalin that has sequence homology with other known animal allergens (148).

Cats have significant individual variation in the production of *Fel d 1*, with male cats generally producing greater amounts of allergen than females. The variability of *Fel d 3* and *Fel d 4* have not been studied. These factors may explain why some patients are more allergic to certain cats than to others.

A company claims to have a genetically engineered cat that is less allergenic, but very expensive. They state that they have used naturally occurring genetic divergences in the structure of *Fel d 1* to create a cat with a less allergenic *Fel d 1*. No peer-reviewed evaluation of the allergenicity of these cats can be found in a literature search or on the company website at the time of writing though the company claims a 95% success rate (149).

Air sampling in rooms occupied by cats show abundant cell fragments smaller than 5 μm. Particles this size are able to reach small bronchioles. The quantity of *Fel d 1* allergen detected in room air is similar to the quantity required to cause a 20% decrease in forced expiratory volume in 1 second (FEV$_1$) on pulmonary function in conventional bronchoprovocation testing (approximately 0.09 μg/mL) (150). The small particle size may also explain why cat allergen can remain airborne in undisturbed conditions for extended periods. Further studies have indicated that it takes up to 24 weeks after removing a cat from inside the home to get back to the baseline quantity of *Fel d 1* found in a home with no cat (151).

Dog allergens can be found in dander, saliva, urine, and serum. Three allergens have been described, *Can f 1, Can f 2,* and albumin. The allergens *Can f 1* and *Can f 2* are lipocalins with dimeric structures (152). *Can f 1* accounts for slightly more than 50% of dog allergic patients, and about one-third of patients react to *Can f 2* or albumin. Sera from albumin-sensitive patients has a high cross-reactivity with cat and other animal albumins (153). There is also evidence of a dog allergen that cross-reacts in 25% of *Fel d 1* allergic patients (154). Dander from all breeds is allergenic, including poodle, but differences between breeds occur in the number and quantity of antigens (155). Individual patients vary in their skin test results to different dog breeds, but in one study these variations did not correlate with the patient perception of specific breed allergy (156).

Many patients who are sensitive to animals, are also sensitive to other perennial allergens, which complicates the determination of which allergen is responsible for their symptoms. Patients often have difficulty accepting that a pet is causing their symptoms, even with a positive skin test. Cat allergen can persist in the environment for 6 months after a pet is removed. For this reason, moving a pet from the house is not a good indicator. It is necessary for the patient to be removed to another environment to determine the role of the animal.

Horse allergy can cause severe symptoms, similar to the symptoms seen with cat allergy, though it typically is easier to manage because the horses do not live in the house. Some antigens are common to horse dander and serum, creating the potential for a serious problem in patients when horse serum (such as an antivenom) may be urgently needed. Two horse allergens have been identified so far. *Equ c 1* and *Equ c 2* have been cloned and both described as members of the lipocalin family (157,158). Allergy to cows, goats, and sheep usually is primarily found in farmers.

Mouse and rat allergy are significant problems for laboratory workers and for people living in the inner city (159,160). In most mouse-sensitive subjects, a major urinary protein, *Mus m 1*, is a significant allergen.

It is also a lipocalin and has sequence homology with *Can f 2* (161). The two predominant rat urinary allergens are *Rat n 1* and *Rat n 2*. In one study, rat sebaceous glands were not found to be the source of allergenic secretions (162), but other studies have reported a high-molecular-weight protein (over 200 kDa), which was believed to originate from rat sebaceous glands (163). *Rat n 2* has been definitively demonstrated in the liver, lacrimal, and salivary glands (164).

Several occupational issues exist for laboratory workers. Feeding and cleaning rats produce the highest airborne concentrations of the prealbumin protein *Rat n 1* (165). Using ventilated cages and negative air pressure appears to reduce exposure to mouse allergens (166). Many companies prefer to screen patients for atopy prior to employment. There is some controversy over the predictive value of atopy in determining whether someone will develop occupational animal allergy (167,168).

■ INSECTS

Cockroach infestation is greater in the inner cities and in southern climates, though it can occur in northern climates as well. Cockroach allergens have been shown to be a cause of allergic asthma using RASTs and bronchoprovocation studies.

The two most common indoor species of cockroaches are *Blattella germanica* (German cockroach) and *Periplaneta americana* (American cockroach). Immunoelectrophoretic studies of roach allergens suggest that most allergens are present in the whole-body and cast-skin fractions, with feces and egg casings less allergenic. *Per a 1* and *Bla g 1* are cross-reactive and have sequence homology with a mosquito digestive protein (169). Cockroaches that eat less food secrete less of this allergen (170). *Bla g 2* shows sequence homology to an aspartic protease but shows weak activity (171). Cockroaches secrete more of this allergen when exposed to sublethal concentrations of boric acid (172). *Per a 3* has been defined and may have some cross-reactivity with a German cockroach allergen (173). *Bla g 4* is a lipocalin (174). *Bla g 5* is a glutathione-S-transferase (175). In addition, a tropomyosin has been identified as an allergen from *Periplanta americana*, with sequence homology to dust mite and shrimp tropomyosins (176).

Moth allergy has been found in considerable frequency in some studies. In Minnesota, the moth *Pseudaletia unipuncta* (Haworth) appears to be a significant outdoor allergen with outdoor levels similar to pollens. The allergen peaked in June and again in August to September. Of patients with other positive skin tests, 45% reacted to whole body extract of the moth (177). In Japan, 50% of asthmatics have sensitivity to the silkworm moth (*Bombyx mori*) (178). Finished silk products generally are not allergenic, but quilts that are stuffed with silk may contribute to asthma and rhinitis.

Asian lady beetle infestation of homes appears to be an allergen in multiple regions of the United States (179). Mayfly, house fly, and caddis fly sensitization has been reported in significant numbers (180). In the Sudan, the "green nimmiti midge" has been associated with seasonal allergies, apparently a reaction to the hemoglobin molecule (181). Some insects are used as food or bait and can cause allergy for the people using them. Crickets used for frog food, chironomid larvae used for fish food, or mealworms (*Tenebrio molitor*) used as fishing bait or reptile food have all been demonstrated to be significant allergens for some hobbyists (182–184).

■ AIR POLLUTANTS AND CHEMICALS

Many patients report that their asthma or rhinitis is made worse by airborne pollution, second hand smoke, chemical irritant or strong fragrances. Air pollution appears to have an impact on asthma and rhinitis. Multiple epidemiologic studies have demonstrated a correlation between levels of common outdoor air pollutants and hospital admissions or emergency room visits (185,186). However, these epidemiologic studies are limited by confounding factors, including air temperature and levels of other outdoor aeroallergens. For this reason, experiments also have been performed under controlled conditions involving short exposures to individual pollutants.

Ozone is generated by the action of ultraviolet light on precursor pollutants from such sources as automobiles and power plants. Ozone causes decreased FEV_1 and forced vital capacity as well as increases in bronchial hyperresponsiveness in both asthmatics and nonasthmatics at concentrations as low as the National Ambient Air Quality Standard of 0.12 ppm (185). A few bronchoprovocation studies have suggested that ozone increases the respiratory response to allergen (187,188). Ozone is a highly reactive oxygen intermediate and people with a genetic defect in glutathione reduction appear to be more susceptible to its effects (189). Nitrogen oxides from car emissions also may play a role, although the evidence in controlled exposures is less convincing than for ozone (190).

Diesel exhaust particles (DEPs) also have been implicated in allergic disease. When they are given in combination with an allergen, they promote both allergen-specific IgE production and a T_H2 cytokine profile (191). One study attempted to sensitize atopic individuals to keyhole limpet hemocyanin, a protein isolated from a marine mollusk, with no known cross-reactive antibodies in humans. Exposure to this allergen with DEPs generated a specific IgE response, whereas exposure to the allergen alone did not (192).

Sulfur dioxide is a product of soft coal burned for industrial use that correlates with respiratory and conjunctival symptoms. Metabisulfites, sulfiting agents used as preservatives agents, may also be a respiratory irritant (193). Carbon monoxide impairs oxygen transport, which is only likely to be important for the individual with low respiratory reserve.

Formaldehyde is released into the air from particle board, foam insulation, furnishings, tobacco smoke, and gas stoves. Symptoms are often most prominent for people in mobile homes, where large amounts of particle board have been used in a relatively small enclosed space. Symptoms may start after exposure to as low as 1 ppm in some individuals and is still thought to be irritative, not allergenic.

The term *sick building syndrome* is used to describe symptoms that happen to multiple people in the same building during a similar time frame. Buildings with this problem tend to have less air exchange with the outdoors and less efficient filtrations systems. Conjunctival and respiratory tract symptoms are most common, but are often accompanied by nonspecific complaints such as headache, fatigue, and inability to concentrate. Mechanisms are usually not allergic and determination of specific irritants is very difficult in a clinical setting. Formaldehyde and second-hand smoke are among the most common associations. Sometimes contamination of the ventilation system with mold can generate allergic reactions or even hypersensitivity pneumonitis. A psychogenic cause of the sick building symptoms should be considered, but not assumed. Symptoms usually improve when the ventilation problems are corrected.

■ REFERENCES

1. Allergen Nomenclature. International Union of Immunological Societies. http://www.allergen.org/Allergen.aspx.
2. Castellano-Mendez M, Aira MJ, Iglesias I, et al. Artificial neural networks as a useful tool to predict the risk level of Betula pollen in the air. *Int J Biometeorol.* 2005;49:310–316.
3. Sanchez Mesa JA, Galan C, Hervas C. The use of discriminant analysis and neural networks to forecast the severity of the Poaceae pollen season in a region with a typical Mediterranean climate. *Int J Biometeorol.* 2005;49:355–362.
4. Reed CE. Measurement of airborne antigens. *J Allergy Clin Immunol.* 1982;70:38–40.
5. Luczynska CM, Li Y, Chapman MD, et al. Airborne concentrations and particle size distribution of allergen derived from domestic cats (Felis domesticus). Measurements using cascade impactor, liquid impinger, and a two-site monoclonal antibody assay for Fel d I. *Am Rev Respir Dis.* 1990;141:361–367.
6. Agarwal MK, Yuninger JW, Swanson MC, et al. An immunochemical method to measure atmospheric allergens. *J Allergy Clin Immunol.* 1981;68:194–200.
7. Agarwal MK, Swanson MC, Reed CE, et al. Immunochemical quantitation of airborne short ragweed, Alternaria, antigen E, and Alt-I allergens: a two-year prospective study. *J Allergy Clin Immunol.* 1983;72:40–45.
8. Agarwal MK, Swanson MC, Reed CE, et al. Airborne ragweed allergens: association with various particle sizes and short ragweed plant parts. *J Allergy Clin Immunol.* 1984;74:687–693.
9. Platts-Mills TA, Heymann PW, Longbottom JL, et al. Airborne allergens associated with asthma: particle sizes carrying dust mite and rat allergens measured with a cascade impactor. *J Allergy Clin Immunol.* 1986;77:850–857.
10. Schumacher MJ, Griffith RD, O'Rourke MK. Recognition of pollen and other particulate aeroantigens by immunoblot microscopy. *J Allergy Clin Immunol.* 1988;82:608–616.
11. Bush RK, Kagen SL. Guidelines for the preparation and characterization of high molecular weight allergens used for the diagnosis of occupational lung disease. Report of the Subcommittee on Preparation and Characterization of High Molecular Weight Allergens. *J Allergy Clin Immunol.* 1989;84:814–819.
12. Lowenstein H. Quantitative immunoelectrophoretic methods as a tool for the analysis and isolation of allergens. *Prog Allergy.* 1978;25:1–62.
13. Ghosh D, Gupta-Bhattacharya S. Structural insight into protein T1, the non-allergenic member of the Bet v 1 allergen family-An in silico analysis. *Mol Immunol.* 2008;45:456–462.
14. Kong W, Tan TS, Tham L, et al. Improved prediction of allergenicity by combination of multiple sequence motifs. *In Silico Biol.* 2007;7:77–86.
15. Furmonaviciene R, Shakib F. The molecular basis of allergenicity: comparative analysis of the three dimensional structures of diverse allergens reveals a common structural motif. *Mol Pathol.* 2001;54:155–159.
16. Malandain H. IgE-reactive carbohydrate epitopes—classification, cross-reactivity, and clinical impact. *Allerg Immunol* (Paris). 2005; 37:122–128.
17. Maizels RM. Infections and allergy—helminths, hygiene and host immune regulation. *Curr Opin Immunol.* 2005;17:656–661.
18. Nieuwenhuizen N, Lopata AL, Jeebhay MF, et al. Exposure to the fish parasite Anisakis causes allergic airway hyperreactivity and dermatitis. *J Allergy Clin Immunol.* 2006;117:1098–1105.
19. Chua KY, Stewart GA, Thomas WR, et al. Sequence analysis of cDNA coding for a major house dust mite allergen, Der p 1. Homology with cysteine proteases. *J Exp Med.* 1988;167:175–182.
20. Gough L, Schulz O, Sewell HF, et al. The cysteine protease activity of the major dust mite allergen Der p 1 selectively enhances the immunoglobulin E antibody response. *J Exp Med.* 1999;190:1897–1902.
21. Gough L, Sewell HF, Shakib F. The proteolytic activity of the major dust mite allergen Der p 1 enhances the IgE antibody response to a bystander antigen. *Clin Exp Allergy.* 2001;31:1594–1598.
22. Gough L, Campbell E, Bayley D, et al. Proteolytic activity of the house dust mite allergen Der p 1 enhances allergenicity in a mouse inhalation model. *Clin Exp Allergy.* 2003;33:1159–1163.
23. Wan H, Winton HL, Soeller C, et al. Der p 1 facilitates transepithelial allergen delivery by disruption of tight junctions. *J Clin Invest.* 1999;104:123–133.
24. Wan H, Winton HL, Soeller C, et al. The transmembrane protein occludin of epithelial tight junctions is a functional target for serine peptidases from faecal pellets of Dermatophagoides pteronyssinus. *Clin Exp Allergy.* 2001;31:279–294.
25. Hewitt CR, Brown AP, Hart BJ, et al. A major house dust mite allergen disrupts the immunoglobulin E network by selectively cleaving CD23: innate protection by antiproteases. *J Exp Med.* 1995;182:1537–1544.
26. Schulz O, Laing P, Sewell HF, et al. Der p I, a major allergen of the house dust mite, proteolytically cleaves the low-affinity receptor for human IgE (CD23). *Eur J Immunol.* 1995;25:3191–3194.
27. Ghaemmaghami AM, Gough L, Sewell HF, et al. The proteolytic activity of the major dust mite allergen Der p 1 conditions dendritic cells to produce less interleukin-12: allergen-induced Th2 bias determined at the dendritic cell level. *Clin Exp Allergy.* 2002;32:1468–1475.
28. Chiu LL, Perng DW, Yu CH, et al. Mold allergen, pen C 13, induces IL-8 expression in human airway epithelial cells by activating protease-activated receptor 1 and 2. *J Immunol.* 2007;178:5237–5244.
29. Kauffman HF, Tomee JF, van de Riet MA, et al. Protease-dependent activation of epithelial cells by fungal allergens leads to morphologic changes and cytokine production. *J Allergy Clin Immunol.* 2000;105:1185–1193.
30. Page K, Strunk VS, Hershenson MB. Cockroach proteases increase IL-8 expression in human bronchial epithelial cells via activation of protease-activated receptor (PAR)-2 and extracellular-signal-regulated kinase. *J Allergy Clin Immunol.* 2003;112:1112–1118.
31. Hong JH, Lee SI, Kim KE, et al. German cockroach extract activates protease-activated receptor 2 in human airway epithelial cells. *J Allergy Clin Immunol.* 2004;113:315–319.
32. Adam E, Hansen KK, Astudillo FO, et al. The house dust mite allergen Der p 1, unlike Der p 3, stimulates the expression of interleukin-8 in human airway epithelial cells via a proteinase-activated receptor-2-independent mechanism. *J Biol Chem.* 2006;281:6910–6923.
33. Runswick S, Mitchell T, Davies P, et al. Pollen proteolytic enzymes degrade tight junctions. *Respirology.* 2007;12:834–842.

34. Jacobi U, Engel K, Patzelt A, et al. Penetration of pollen proteins into the skin. *Skin Pharmacol Physiol.* 2007;20:297–304.

35. Traidl-Hoffmann C, Mariani V, Hochrein H, et al. Pollen-associated phytoprostanes inhibit dendritic cell interleukin-12 production and augment T helper type 2 cell polarization. *J Exp Med.* 2005;201:627–636.

36. Michel FB, Marty JP, Quet L, et al. Penetration of inhaled pollen into the respiratory tract. *Am Rev Respir Dis.* 1977;115:609–616.

37. Busse WW, Reed CE, Hoehne JH. Where is the allergic reaction in ragweed asthma? *J Allergy Clin Immunol.* 1972;50:289–293.

38. Solomon WR, Burge HA, Muilenberg ML. Allergen carriage by atmospheric aerosol. I. Ragweed pollen determinants in smaller micronic fractions. *J Allergy Clin Immunol.* 1983;72:443–447.

39. Bellomo R, Gigliotti P, Treloar A, et al. Two consecutive thunderstorm associated epidemics of asthma in the city of Melbourne. The possible role of rye grass pollen. *Med J Aust.* 1992;156:834–837.

40. Schappi GF, Taylor PE, Pain MC, et al. Concentrations of major grass group 5 allergens in pollen grains and atmospheric particles: implications for hay fever and allergic asthma sufferers sensitized to grass pollen allergens. *Clin Exp Allergy.* 1999;29:633–641.

41. Suphioglu C. Thunderstorm asthma due to grass pollen. *Int Arch Allergy Immunol.* 1998;116:253–260.

42. Pulimood TB, Corden JM, Bryden C, et al. Epidemic asthma and the role of the fungal mold Alternaria alternata. *J Allergy Clin Immunol.* 2007;120:610–617.

43. Lewis WR, Vinay P, Zenger VE. *Airborne and allergenic pollen of North America.* Baltimore: The Johns Hopkins University Press, 1983.

44. Smith EG. *Sampling and identifying allergenic pollens and molds.* San Antonio: Blewstone, 1986.

45. King TP, Norman PS. Standardized extracts, weeds. *Clin Rev Allergy.* 1986;4:425–433.

46. King TP, Norman PS, Lichtenstein LM. Studies on ragweed pollen allergens. V. *Ann Allergy.* 1967;25:541–553.

47. Marsh DG, Berlin L, Bruce CA, et al. Rapidly released allergens from short ragweed pollen. I. Kinetics of release of known allergens in relation to biologic activity. *J Allergy Clin Immunol.* 1981;67:206–216.

48. Baer H, Godfrey H, Maloney CJ, et al. The potency and antigen E content of commercially prepared ragweed extracts. *J Allergy.* 1970;45:347–354.

49. Lee YS, Dickinson DB, Schlager D, et al. Antigen E content of pollen from individual plants of short ragweed (Ambrosia artemisiifolia). *J Allergy Clin Immunol.* 1979;63:336–339.

50. Rogers BL, Morgenstern JP, Griffith IJ, et al. Complete sequence of the allergen Amb alpha II. Recombinant expression and reactivity with T cells from ragweed allergic patients. *J Immunol.* 1991;147:2547–2552.

51. Hussain R, Norman PS, Marsh DG. Rapidly released allergens from short ragweed pollen. II. Identification and partial purification. *J Allergy Clin Immunol.* 1981;67:217–222.

52. Goodfriend L, Roebber M, Lundkvist U, et al. Two variants of ragweed allergen Ra3. *J Allergy Clin Immunol.* 1981;67:299–304.

53. Marsh DG, Hsu SH, Hussain R, et al. Genetics of human immune response to allergens. *J Allergy Clin Immunol.* 1980;65:322–332.

54. Roebber M, Klapper DG, Goodfriend L, et al. Immunochemical and genetic studies of Amb.t. V (Ra5G), an Ra5 homologue from giant ragweed pollen. *J Immunol.* 1985;134:3062–3069.

55. Shafiee A, Yuninger JW, Gleich GJ. Isolation and characterization of Russian thistle (Salsola pestifer) pollen allergens. *J Allergy Clin Immunol.* 1981;67:472–481.

56. Cocchiara R, Locorotondo G, Parlato A, et al. Purification of Parj I, a major allergen from Parietaria, judaica pollen. *Int Arch Allergy Appl Immunol.* 1989;90:84–90.

57. Costa MA, Duro G, Izzo V, et al. The IgE-binding epitopes of rParj 2, a major allergen of Parietaria judaica pollen, are heterogeneously recognized among allergic subjects. *Allergy.* 2000;55:246–250.

58. Coscia MR, Ruffilli A, Oreste U. Basic isoforms of Par o 1, the major allergen of Parietaria officinalis pollen. *Allergy.* 1995;50:899–904.

59. Duro G, Colombo P, Assunta CM, et al. Isolation and characterization of two cDNA clones coding for isoforms of the Parietaria judaica major allergen Par j 1.0101. *Int Arch Allergy Immunol.* 1997;112:348–355.

60. Menna T, Cassese G, Di Modugno F, et al. Characterization of a dodecapeptide containing a dominant epitope of Par j 1 and Par o 1, the major allergens of P. judaica and P. officinalis pollen. *Allergy.* 1999;54:1048–1057.

61. Nilsen BM, Grimsoen A, Paulsen BS. Identification and characterization of important allergens from mugwort pollen by IEF, SDS-PAGE and immunoblotting. *Mol Immunol.* 1991;28:733–742.

62. Hirschwehr R, Heppner C, Spitzauer S, et al. Identification of common allergenic structures in mugwort and ragweed pollen. *J Allergy Clin Immunol.* 1998;101:196–206.

63. Staff IA, Taylor PE, Smith P, et al. Cellular localization of water soluble, allergenic proteins in rye-grass (Lolium perenne) pollen using monoclonal and specific IgE antibodies with immunogold probes. *Histochem J.* 1990;22:276–290.

64. Cosgrove DJ, Bedinger P, Durachko DM. Group I allergens of grass pollen as cell wall-loosening agents. *Proc Natl Acad Sci USA.* 1997;94:6559–6564.

65. Van Ree R, Driessen MN, Van Leeuwen WA, et al. Variability of crossreactivity of IgE antibodies to group I and V allergens in eight grass pollen species. *Clin Exp Allergy.* 1992;22:611–617.

66. Matthiesen F, Lowenstein H. Group V allergens in grass pollens. II. Investigation of group V allergens in pollens from 10 grasses. *Clin Exp Allergy.* 1991;21:309–320.

67. Mourad W, Mecheri S, Peltre G, et al. Study of the epitope structure of purified Dac G I and Lol p I, the major allergens of Dactylis glomerata and Lolium perenne pollens, using monoclonal antibodies. *J Immunol.* 1988;141:3486–3491.

68. Petersen A, Schramm G, Bufe A, et al. Structural investigations of the major allergen Phl p I on the complementary DNA and protein level. *J Allergy Clin Immunol.* 1995;95:987–994.

69. Ford SA, Baldo BA. A re-examination of ryegrass (Lolium perenne) pollen allergens. *Int Arch Allergy Appl Immunol.* 1986;81:193–203.

70. Tamborini E, Brandazza A, De Lalla C, et al. Recombinant allergen Lol p II: expression, purification and characterization. *Mol Immunol.* 1995;32:505–513.

71. Guerin-Marchand C, Senechal H, Bouin AP, et al. Cloning, sequencing and immunological characterization of Dac g 3, a major allergen from Dactylis glomerata pollen. *Mol Immunol.* 1996;33:797–806.

72. Suphioglu C, Ferreira F, Knox RB. Molecular cloning and immunological characterisation of Cyn d 7, a novel calcium-binding allergen from Bermuda grass pollen. *FEBS Lett.* 1997;402:167–172.

73. Valenta R, Duchene M, Ebner C, et al. Profilins constitute a novel family of functional plant pan-allergens. *J Exp Med.* 1992;175:377–385.

74. Niederberger V, Laffer S, Froschl R, et al. IgE antibodies to recombinant pollen allergens (Phl p 1, Phl p 2, Phl p 5, and Bet v 2) account for a high percentage of grass pollen-specific IgE. *J Allergy Clin Immunol.* 1998;101:258–264.

75. Van Ree R, Van Leeuwen WA, Aalberse RC. How far can we simplify in vitro diagnostics for grass pollen allergy?: A study with 17 whole pollen extracts and purified natural and recombinant major allergens. *J Allergy Clin Immunol.* 1998;102:184–190.

76. Bhalla PL, Swoboda I, Singh MB. Antisense-mediated silencing of a gene encoding a major ryegrass pollen allergen. *Proc Natl Acad Sci USA.* 1999;96:11676–11680.

77. Breiteneder H, Pettenburger K, Bito A, et al. The gene coding for the major birch pollen allergen Betv1, is highly homologous to a pea disease resistance response gene. *EMBO J.* 1989;8:1935–1938.

78. Valenta R, Duchene M, Vrtala S, et al. Recombinant allergens for immunoblot diagnosis of tree-pollen allergy. *J Allergy Clin Immunol.* 1991;88:889–894.

79. Ferreira F, Engel E, Briza P, et al. Characterization of recombinant Bet v 4, a birch pollen allergen with two EF-hand calcium-binding domains. *Int Arch Allergy Immunol.* 1999;118:304–305.

80. Seiberler S, Scheiner O, Kraft D, et al. Characterization of a birch pollen allergen, Bet v III, representing a novel class of Ca2+ binding proteins: specific expression in mature pollen and dependence of patients' IgE binding on protein-bound Ca2+. *EMBO J.* 1994;13:3481–3486.

81. Karamloo F, Schmitz N, Scheurer S, et al. Molecular cloning and characterization of a birch pollen minor allergen, Bet v 5, belonging to a family of isoflavone reductase-related proteins. *J Allergy Clin Immunol.* 1999;104:991–999.

82. Cadot P, Diaz JF, Proost P, et al. Purification and characterization of an 18-kd allergen of birch (Betula verrucosa) pollen: identification as a cyclophilin. *J Allergy Clin Immunol.* 2000;105:286–291.

83. Yasueda H, Yui Y, Shimizu T et al. Isolation and partial characterization of the major allergen from Japanese cedar (Cryptomeria japonica) pollen. *J Allergy Clin Immunol.* 1983;71:77–86.

84. Sakaguchi M, Inouye S, Taniai M, et al. Identification of the second major allergen of Japanese cedar pollen. *Allergy.* 1990;45:309–312.

85. Midoro-Horiuti T, Goldblum RM, Kurosky A, et al. Molecular cloning of the mountain cedar (Juniperus ashei) pollen major allergen, Jun a 1. *J Allergy Clin Immunol.* 1999;104:613–617.

86. Tejera ML, Villalba M, Batanero E, et al. Identification, isolation, and characterization of Ole e 7, a new allergen of olive tree pollen. *J Allergy Clin Immunol.* 1999;104:797–802.

87. Licorish K, Novey HS, Kozak P, et al. Role of Alternaria and Penicillium spores in the pathogenesis of asthma. *J Allergy Clin Immunol.* 1985;76:819–825.

88. Halonen M, Stern DA, Wright AL, et al. Alternaria as a major allergen for asthma in children raised in a desert environment. *Am J Respir Crit Care Med.* 1997;155:1356–1361.

89. Bush RK, Yunginger JW. Standardization of fungal allergens. *Clin Rev Allergy.* 1987;5:3–21.

90. Solomon WR. Assessing fungus prevalence in domestic interiors. *J Allergy Clin Immunol.* 1975;56:235–242.

91. Green BJ, Tovey ER, Sercombe JK, et al. Airborne fungal fragments and allergenicity. *Med Mycol.* 2006;44 Suppl 1:S245–S255.

92. Koivikko A, Savolainen J. Mushroom allergy. *Allergy.* 1988;43:1–10.

93. Lehrer SB, Lopez M, Butcher BT, et al. Basidiomycete mycelia and spore-allergen extracts: skin test reactivity in adults with symptoms of respiratory allergy. *J Allergy Clin Immunol.* 1986;78:478–485.

94. Ibanez MD, Horner WE, Liengswangwong V, et al. Identification and analysis of basidiospore allergens from puffballs. *J Allergy Clin Immunol.* 1988;82:787–795.

95. Weissman DN, Halmepuro L, Salvaggio JE, et al. Antigenic/allergenic analysis of basidiomycete cap, mycelia, and spore extracts. *Int Arch Allergy Appl Immunol.* 1987;84:56–61.

96. Lopez M, Voigtlander JR, Lehrer SB, et al. Bronchoprovocation studies in basidiospore–sensitive allergic subjects with asthma. *J Allergy Clin Immunol.* 1989;84:242–246.

97. Hirsch DJ, Hirsch SR, Kalbfleisch JH. Effect of central air conditioning and meteorologic factors on indoor spore counts. *J Allergy Clin Immunol.* 1978;62:22–26.

98. Burge HA, Solomon WR, Muilenberg ML. Evaluation of indoor plantings as allergen exposure sources. *J Allergy Clin Immunol.* 1982;70:101–108.

99. Barnes CS, Pacheco F, Landuyt J, et al. Production of a recombinant protein from Alternaria containing the reported N-terminal of the Alt a1 allergen. *Adv Exp Med Biol.* 1996;409:197–203.

100. De Vouge MW, Thaker AJ, Curran IH, et al. Isolation and expression of a cDNA clone encoding an Alternaria alternata Alt a 1 subunit. *Int Arch Allergy Immunol.* 1996;111:385–395.

101. Horner WE, Helbling A, Salvaggio JE, et al. Fungal allergens. *Clin Microbiol Rev.* 1995;8:161–179.

102. Agarwal MK, Jones RT, Yunginger JW. Shared allergenic and antigenic determinants in Alternaria and Stemphylium extracts. *J Allergy Clin Immunol.* 1982;70:437–444.

103. Helm RM, Squillace DL, Aukrust L, et al. Production of an international reference standard alternaria extract. I. Testing of candidate extracts. *Int Arch Allergy Appl Immunol.* 1987;82:178–189.

104. Bush RK, Sanchez H, Geisler D. Molecular cloning of a major Alternaria alternata allergen, rAlt a 2. *J Allergy Clin Immunol.* 1999;104:665–671.

105. Achatz G, Oberkofler H, Lechenauer E, et al. Molecular cloning of major and minor allergens of Alternaria alternata and Cladosporium herbarum. *Mol Immunol.* 1995;32:213–227.

106. Schneider PB, Denk U, Breitenbach M, et al. Alternaria alternata NADP-dependent mannitol dehydrogenase is an important fungal allergen. *Clin Exp Allergy.* 2006;36:1513–1524.

107. Breitenbach M, Simon B, Probst G, et al. Enolases are highly conserved fungal allergens. *Int Arch Allergy Immunol.* 1997;113:114–117.

108. Aukrust L, Borch SM. Partial purification and characterization of two Cladosporium herbarum allergens. *Int Arch Allergy Appl Immunol.* 1979;60:68–79.

109. Zhang L, Muradia G, Curran IH, et al. A cDNA clone coding for a novel allergen, Cla h III, of Cladosporium herbarum identified as a ribosomal P2 protein. *J Immunol.* 1995;154:710–717.

110. Zhang L, Muradia G, De Vouge MW, et al. An allergenic polypeptide representing a variable region of hsp 70 cloned from a cDNA library of Cladosporium herbarum. *Clin Exp Allergy.* 1996;26:88–95.

111. Simon-Nobbe B, Denk U, Schneider PB, et al. NADP-dependent mannitol dehydrogenase, a major allergen of Cladosporium herbarum. *J Biol Chem.* 2006;281:16354–16360.

112. Longbottom JL. Aspergillus fumigatus antigens: the Pepys' years. *Clin Exp Allergy.* 1997;27 Suppl 1:6–8.

113. Kauffman HF, van der HS, Beaumont F, et al. The allergenic and antigenic properties of spore extracts of Aspergillus fumigatus: a comparative study of spore extracts with mycelium and culture filtrate extracts. *J Allergy Clin Immunol.* 1984;73:567–573.

114. Moser M, Crameri R, Menz G, et al. Cloning and expression of recombinant Aspergillus fumigatus allergen I/a (rAsp f I/a) with IgE binding and type I skin test activity. *J Immunol.* 1992;149:454–460.

115. Arruda LK, Mann BJ, Chapman MD. Selective expression of a major allergen and cytotoxin, Asp f I, in Aspergillus fumigatus. Implications for the immunopathogenesis of Aspergillus-related diseases. *J Immunol.* 1992;149:3354–3359.

116. Moser M, Crameri R, Brust E, et al. Diagnostic value of recombinant Aspergillus fumigatus allergen I/a for skin testing and serology. *J Allergy Clin Immunol.* 1994;93:1–11.

117. Crameri R. Recombinant Aspergillus fumigatus allergens: from the nucleotide sequences to clinical applications. *Int Arch Allergy Immunol.* 1998;115:99–114.

118. Banerjee B, Kurup VP, Phadnis S, et al. Molecular cloning and expression of a recombinant Aspergillus fumigatus protein Asp f II with significant immunoglobulin E reactivity in allergic bronchopulmonary aspergillosis. *J Lab Clin Med.* 1996;127:253–262.

119. Hemmann S, Menz G, Ismail C, et al. Skin test reactivity to 2 recombinant Aspergillus fumigatus allergens in A fumigatus-sensitized asthmatic subjects allows diagnostic separation of allergic bronchopulmonary aspergillosis from fungal sensitization. *J Allergy Clin Immunol.* 1999;104:601–607.

120. Brander KA, Borbely P, Crameri R, et al. IgE-binding proliferative responses and skin test reactivity to Cop c 1, the first recombinant allergen from the basidiomycete Coprinus comatus. *J Allergy Clin Immunol.* 1999;104:630–636.

121. Horner WE, Reese G, Lehrer SB. Identification of the allergen Psi c 2 from the basidiomycete Psilocybe cubensis as a fungal cyclophilin. *Int Arch Allergy Immunol.* 1995;107:298–300.

122. Nissen D, Nolte H, Permin H, et al. Evaluation of IgE-sensitization to fungi in HIV-positive patients with eczematous skin reactions. *Ann Allergy Asthma Immunol.* 1999;83:153–159.

123. Shen HD, Choo KB, Lee HH, et al. The 40-kilodalton allergen of Candida albicans is an alcohol dehydrogenase: molecular cloning and immunological analysis using monoclonal antibodies. *Clin Exp Allergy.* 1991;21:675–681.

124. Breitenbach M, Simon B, Probst G, et al. Enolases are highly conserved fungal allergens. *Int Arch Allergy Immunol.* 1997;113:114–117.

125. Akiyama K, Shida T, Yasueda H, et al. Allergenicity of acid protease secreted by Candida albicans. *Allergy.* 1996;51:887–892.

126. Platts-Mills TA, Chapman MD. Dust mites: immunology, allergic disease, and environmental control. *J Allergy Clin Immunol.* 1987;80:755–775.

127. Arlian LG, Bernstein IL, Gallagher JS. The prevalence of house dust mites, Dermatophagoides spp, and associated environmental conditions in homes in Ohio. *J Allergy Clin Immunol.* 1982;69:527–532.

128. Vervloet D, Penaud A, Razzouk H, et al. Altitude and house dust mites. *J Allergy Clin Immunol.* 1982;69:290–296.

129. Gotzsche PC, Hammarquist C, Burr M. House dust mite control measures in the management of asthma: meta-analysis. *BMJ.* 1998;317:1105–1110.

130. Platts-Mills TA, Chapman MD, Wheatly LM. Control of house dust mite in managing asthma. Conclusions of meta-analysis are wrong. *BMJ.* 1999;318:870–871.

131. Arlian LG, Bernstein IL, Vyszenski-Moher DL, et al. Investigations of culture medium-free house dust mites. IV. Cross antigenicity and allergenicity between the house dust mites, Dermatophagoides farinae and D. pteronyssinus. *J Allergy Clin Immunol.* 1987;79:467–476.

132. Tovey ER, Chapman MD, Platts-Mills TA. Mite faeces are a major source of house dust allergens. *Nature.* 1981;289:592–593.

133. Heymann PW, Chapman MD, Aalberse RC, et al. Antigenic and structural analysis of group II allergens (Der f II and Der p II) from house dust mites (Dermatophagoides spp). *J Allergy Clin Immunol.* 1989;83:1055–1067.

134. Keber MM, Gradisar H, Jerala R. MD-2 and Der p 2—a tale of two cousins or distant relatives? *J Endotoxin Res.* 2005;11:186–192.

135. Smith WA, Chua KY, Kuo MC, et al. Cloning and sequencing of the Dermatophagoides pteronyssinus group III allergen, Der p III. *Clin Exp Allergy.* 1994;24:220–228.

136. Stewart GA, Ward LD, Simpson RJ, et al. The group III allergen from the house dust mite Dermatophagoides pteronyssinus is a trypsin-like enzyme. *Immunology.* 1992;75:29–35.

137. Yasueda H, Mita H, Akiyama K, et al. Allergens from Dermatophagoides mites with chymotryptic activity. *Clin Exp Allergy.* 1993;23:384–390.

138. Kawamoto S, Mizuguchi Y, Morimoto K, et al. Cloning and expression of Der f 6, a serine protease allergen from the house dust mite, Dermatophagoides farinae. *Biochim Biophys Acta.* 1999; 1454:201–207.

139. King C, Simpson RJ, Moritz RL, et al. The isolation and characterization of a novel collagenolytic serine protease allergen (Der p 9) from the dust mite Dermatophagoides pteronyssinus. *J Allergy Clin Immunol.* 1996;98:739–747.

140. Mills KL, Hart BJ, Lynch NR, et al. Molecular characterization of the group 4 house dust mite allergen from Dermatophagoides pteronyssinus and its amylase homologue from Euroglyphus maynei. *Int Arch Allergy Immunol.* 1999;120:100–107.

141. Kim YK, Lee MH, Jee YK, et al. Spider mite allergy in apple-cultivating farmers: European red mite (Panonychus ulmi) and two-spotted spider mite (Tetranychus urticae) may be important allergens in the development of work-related asthma and rhinitis symptoms. *J Allergy Clin Immunol.* 1999;104:1285–1292.

142. Kim YK, Son JW, Kim HY, et al. Citrus red mite (Panonychus citri) is the most common sensitizing allergen of asthma and rhinitis in citrus farmers. *Clin Exp Allergy.* 1999;29:1102–1109.

143. Bartholome K, Kissler W, Baer H, et al. Where does cat allergen 1 come from? *J Allergy Clin Immunol.* 1985;76:503–506.

144. Morgenstern JP, Griffith IJ, Brauer AW, et al. Amino acid sequence of Fel d 1, the major allergen of the domestic cat: protein sequence analysis and cDNA cloning. *Proc Natl Acad Sci USA.* 1991; 88:9690–9694.

145. Kaiser L, Gronlund H, Sandalova T, et al. The crystal structure of the major cat allergen Fel d 1, a member of the secretoglobin family. *J Biol Chem.* 2003;278:37730–37735.

146. Ichikawa K, Vailes LD, Pomes A, et al. Identification of a novel cat allergen–cystatin. *Int Arch Allergy Immunol.* 2001;124:55–56.

147. Ichikawa K, Vailes LD, Pomes A, et al. Molecular cloning, expression and modelling of cat allergen, cystatin (Fel d 3), a cysteine protease inhibitor. *Clin Exp Allergy.* 2001;31:1279–1286.

148. Smith W, Butler AJ, Hazell LA, et al. Fel d 4, a cat lipocalin allergen. *Clin Exp Allergy.* 2004;34:1732–1738.

149. Allerca. http://www.allerca.com.

150. Van MT Jr, Marsh DG, Adkinson NF Jr, et al. Dose of cat (Felis domesticus) allergen 1 (Fel d 1) that induces asthma. *J Allergy Clin Immunol.* 1986;78:62–75.

151. Wood RA, Chapman MD, Adkinson NF Jr, et al. The effect of cat removal on allergen content in household-dust samples. *J Allergy Clin Immunol.* 1989;83:730–734.

152. Kamata Y, Miyanomae A, Nakayama E, et al. Characterization of dog allergens Can f 1 and Can f 2. 2. A comparison of Can f 1 with Can f 2 regarding their biochemical and immunological properties. *Int Arch Allergy Immunol.* 2007;142:301–308.

153. Spitzauer S, Pandjaitan B, Soregi G, et al. IgE cross-reactivities against albumins in patients allergic to animals. *J Allergy Clin Immunol.* 1995;96:951–959.

154. Reininger R, Varga EM, Zach M, et al. Detection of an allergen in dog dander that cross-reacts with the major cat allergen, Fel d 1. *Clin Exp Allergy.* 2007;37:116–124.

155. Moore BS, Hyde JS. Breed-specific dog hypersensitivity in humans. *J Allergy Clin Immunol.* 1980;66:198–203.

156. Lindgren S, Belin L, Dreborg S, et al. Breed-specific dog-dandruff allergens. *J Allergy Clin Immunol.* 1988;82:196–204.

157. Gregoire C, Tavares GA, Lorenzo HK, et al. Crystallization and preliminary crystallographic analysis of the major horse allergen Equ c 1. *Acta Crystallogr D Biol Crystallogr.* 1999;55:880–882.

158. Bulone V, Krogstad-Johnsen T, Smestad-Paulsen B. Separation of horse dander allergen proteins by two-dimensional electrophoresis—molecular characterisation and identification of Equ c 2.0101 and Equ c 2.0102 as lipocalin proteins. *Eur J Biochem.* 1998;253:202–211.

159. Phipatanakul W, Eggleston PA, Wright EC, et al. Mouse allergen. I. The prevalence of mouse allergen in inner-city homes. The National Cooperative Inner-City Asthma Study. *J Allergy Clin Immunol.* 2000;106:1070–1074.

160. Perry T, Matsui E, Merriman B, et al. The prevalence of rat allergen in inner-city homes and its relationship to sensitization and asthma morbidity. *J Allergy Clin Immunol.* 2003;112:346–352.

161. Konieczny A, Morgenstern JP, Bizinkauskas CB, et al. The major dog allergens, Can f 1 and Can f 2, are salivary lipocalin proteins: cloning and immunological characterization of the recombinant forms. *Immunology.* 1997;92:577–586.

162. Walls AF, Longbottom JL. Comparison of rat fur, urine, saliva, and other rat allergen extracts by skin testing, RAST, and RAST inhibition. *J Allergy Clin Immunol.* 1985;75:242–251.

163. Longbottom JL, Austwick PK. Allergy to rats: quantitative immunoelectrophoretic studies of rat dust as a source of inhalant allergen. *J Allergy Clin Immunol.* 1987;80:243–251.

164. Laperche Y, Lynch KR, Dolan KP, et al. Tissue-specific control of alpha 2u globulin gene expression: constitutive synthesis in the submaxillary gland. *Cell.* 1983;32:453–460.

165. Eggleston PA, Newill CA, Ansari AA, et al. Task-related variation in airborne concentrations of laboratory animal allergens: studies with Rat n I. *J Allergy Clin Immunol.* 1989;84:347–352.

166. Schweitzer IB, Smith E, Harrison DJ, et al. Reducing exposure to laboratory animal allergens. *Comp Med.* 2003;53:487–492.

167. Platts-Mills TA, Longbottom J, Edwards J, et al. Occupational asthma and rhinitis related to laboratory rats: serum IgG and IgE antibodies to the rat urinary allergen. *J Allergy Clin Immunol.* 1987;79: 505–515.

168. Slovak AJ, Hill RN. Does atopy have any predictive value for laboratory animal allergy? A comparison of different concepts of atopy. *Br J Ind Med.* 1987;44:129–132.

169. Melen E, Pomes A, Vailes LD et al. Molecular cloning of Per a 1 and definition of the cross-reactive Group 1 cockroach allergens. *J Allergy Clin Immunol.* 1999;103:859–864.

170. Gore JC, Schal C. Expression, production and excretion of Bla g 1, a major human allergen, in relation to food intake in the German cockroach, Blattella germanica. *Med Vet Entomol.* 2005;19:127–134.

171. Wunschmann S, Gustchina A, Chapman MD, et al. Cockroach allergen Bla g 2: an unusual aspartic proteinase. *J Allergy Clin Immunol.* 2005;116:140–145.

172. Zhang YC, Perzanowski MS, Chew GL. Sub-lethal exposure of cockroaches to boric acid pesticide contributes to increased Bla g 2 excretion. *Allergy.* 2005;60:965–968.

173. Wu CH, Wang NM, Lee MF, et al. Cloning of the American cockroach Cr-PII allergens: evidence for the existence of cross-reactive allergens between species. *J Allergy Clin Immunol.* 1998;101:832–840.

174. Arruda LK, Vailes LD, Hayden ML, et al. Cloning of cockroach allergen, Bla g 4, identifies ligand binding proteins (or calycins) as a cause of IgE antibody responses. *J Biol Chem.* 1995;270:31196–31201.

175. Arruda LK, Vailes LD, Platts-Mills TA, et al. Induction of IgE antibody responses by glutathione S-transferase from the German cockroach (Blattella germanica). *J Biol Chem.* 1997;272:20907–20912.

176. Santos AB, Chapman MD, Aalberse RC, et al. Cockroach allergens and asthma in Brazil: identification of tropomyosin as a major allergen with potential cross-reactivity with mite and shrimp allergens. *J Allergy Clin Immunol.* 1999;104:329–337.

177. Wynn SR, Swanson MC, Reed CE, et al. Immunochemical quantitation, size distribution, and cross-reactivity of lepidoptera (moth) aeroallergens in southeastern Minnesota. *J Allergy Clin Immunol.* 1988;82:47–54.

178. Kino T, Oshima S. Allergy to insects in Japan. II. The reaginic sensitivity to silkworm moth in patients with bronchial asthma. *J Allergy Clin Immunol.* 1979;64:131–138.

179. Albright DD, Jordan-Wagner D, Napoli DC, et al. Multicolored Asian lady beetle hypersensitivity: a case series and allergist survey. *Ann Allergy Asthma Immunol.* 2006;97:521–527.

180. Smith TS, Hogan MB, Welch JE, et al. Modern prevalence of insect sensitization in rural asthma and allergic rhinitis patients. *Allergy Asthma Proc.* 2005;26:356–360.

181. Baur X, Dewair M, Fruhmann G, et al. Hypersensitivity to chironomids (non-biting midges): localization of the antigenic determinants within certain polypeptide sequences of hemoglobins (erythrocruorins) of Chironomus thummi thummi (Diptera). *J Allergy Clin Immunol.* 1982;69:66–76.

182. Mazur G, Baur X, Modrow S, et al. A common epitope on major allergens from non-biting midges (Chironomidae). *Mol Immunol.* 1988;25:1005–1010.

183. Bagenstose AH III, Mathews KP, Homburger HA, et al. Inhalant allergy due to crickets. *J Allergy Clin Immunol.* 1980;65:71–74.

184. Bernstein DI, Gallagher JS, Bernstein IL. Mealworm asthma: clinical and immunologic studies. *J Allergy Clin Immunol.* 1983;72: 475–480.

185. Health effects of outdoor air pollution. Committee of the Environmental and Occupational Health Assembly of the American Thoracic Society. *Am J Respir Crit Care Med.* 1996;153:3–50.

186. Koenig JQ. Air pollution and asthma. *J Allergy Clin Immunol.* 1999;104:717–722.

187. Jorres R, Nowak D, Magnussen H. The effect of ozone exposure on allergen responsiveness in subjects with asthma or rhinitis. *Am J Respir Crit Care Med.* 1996;153:56–64.

188. Kehrl HR, Peden DB, Ball B, et al. Increased specific airway reactivity of persons with mild allergic asthma after 7.6 hours of exposure to 0.16 ppm ozone. *J Allergy Clin Immunol.* 1999;104:1198–1204.

189. David GL, Romieu I, Sienra-Monge JJ, et al. Nicotinamide adenine dinucleotide (phosphate) reduced:quinone oxidoreductase and glutathione S-transferase M1 polymorphisms and childhood asthma. *Am J Respir Crit Care Med.* 2003;168:1199–1204.

190. Health effects of outdoor air pollution. Part 2. Committee of the Environmental and Occupational Health Assembly of the American Thoracic Society. *Am J Respir Crit Care Med.* 1996;153:477–498.

191. Casillas AM, Hiura T, Li N, et al. Enhancement of allergic inflammation by diesel exhaust particles: permissive role of reactive oxygen species. *Ann Allergy Asthma Immunol.* 1999;83:624–629.

192. Diaz-Sanchez D, Garcia MP, Wang M, et al. Nasal challenge with diesel exhaust particles can induce sensitization to a neoallergen in the human mucosa. *J Allergy Clin Immunol.* 1999;104:1183–1188.

193. Yang WH, Purchase EC, Rivington RN. Positive skin tests and Prausnitz-Kustner reactions in metabisulfite-sensitive subjects. *J Allergy Clin Immunol.* 1986;78:443–449.

CHAPTER 7

Airborne Pollen Prevalence in the United States

WILLIAM R. SOLOMON

The dramatic seasonal appearance of windborne pollens, and resulting symptoms, are events familiar to physicians and lay persons alike. By knowing where and when symptoms occur annually, the informed allergist can focus on probable offenders with some confidence. Therefore, appreciating patterns of pollen prevalence confers an important advantage in providing informed patient care.

Despite this imperative, the growth of dependable prevalence information has been slow and remains incomplete. Only recently have data generated from volumetric sampling been widely based and a network of accredited North American reporting stations established. Clearly, the allergist arriving in an unfamiliar area needs to obtain or, more often, generate the information on which he or she will rely. Many difficulties attend the interpretation of traditional data as well as compilations such as this chapter presents. First, of course, is the bias of older, "gravity" data to preferentially recover larger bioaerosols in, at best, semi-quantitative fashion. In addition, much "conventional wisdom" (and practice) reflects observations of source plants and "land use" or skin test surveys rather than aerometric data. However, even the best available analysis can tell us only the genus or affinity group of origin for many pollen types (e.g., most oaks and grasses), leaving inferences of source species to field surveys; considering this, gaps in the species listed below are inevitable. Where allergen extract suppliers provide information, an obvious conflict of interest potential, favoring overly numerous "important" candidates for testing and treatment, must be resisted. Finally, it must be recalled that pollen-exposure levels sufficient to evoke threshold symptoms are largely unknown; exposure-induced sensitivity without disease is, thus, possible and, perhaps, widespread.

Much of the appeal of North America's landscape arises from its climatic, and resulting floristic, diversity. This variety provides inherent challenge for the allergist, especially so because plant growth and land use rarely conform to political boundaries. Even regional groupings, as attempted here, must be qualified for marked internal climatic differences due especially to effects of mountain ranges and upwind bodies of water.

Although published pollen data are often treated as "revealed truth," there is little to justify such optimism. Local plantings of crops such as sugar beets, pecans, or dates may affect circumscribed populations. By contrast, long-distance transport, (e.g., of mountain cedar pollen from west Texas), is documented and may be more common and/or extensive than suspected. Because bioaerosols smaller than intact grains may carry pollen allergens, their potential for more extended travel without detection is obvious. Land-use practices may modify pollen exposure patterns indirectly as well as by directly providing source species. Midwestern ragweeds, for example, selectively colonize cultivated fields and the margins of winter-salted roads and are overgrown rapidly when such disturbance is removed. Changes in pollen prevalence over several decades also are referable to effects as diverse as street tree planting, reforestation (planned or as natural succession), and range extension by opportunistic species (e.g., mugwort recently in northeastern states). The last of these effects deserves special attention in a setting of climate change as well as mounting international travel and commerce. A trend toward earlier annual appearance of spring tree pollens, for example, is now evident.

Variable similarities among pollen of some related taxa are well-described. Efforts to prioritize clinical impact of pollen types reflect also a growing economic imperative to avoid "duplication" among allergens employed for diagnosis and treatment. Unfortunately, a firm factual basis for such strategy cannot be easily assumed. Shared, largely vegetative, structural components such as profilins are known as one basis for similarities among pollen of quite disparate taxa. However, these are seldom principal allergens. Among botanically related species, pollen allergen similarities often are assumed for purposes of expediency, despite limited proof.

TABLE 7.1   NORTH AMERICAN WINDBORNE POLLEN SOURCES AND THEIR GENERIC (LATIN) NAMES

FAMILIAR NAME	*LATIN GENUS*	FAMILIAR NAME	*LATIN GENUS*
Alder	*Alnus*	Mugwort	*Artemisia*
Amaranth	*Amaranthus*	Mulberry	*Morus*
Ash	*Fraxinus*	Oak	*Quercus*
Aspen	*Populus*	Pecan	*Carya*
Beech	*Fagus*	Pigweed	*Amaranthus*
Birch	*Betula*	Plantain	*Plantago*
Butternut	*Juglans*	Ragweed	*Ambrosia*
Dock	*Rumex*	Red cedar	*Juniperus*
Elm	*Ulmus*	Sage	*Artemisia*
Hickory	*Carya*	Sorrel	*Rumex*
Juniper	*Juniperus*	Sweet gum	*Liquidambar*
Maple	*Acer*	Sycamore	*Platanus*
Marsh elder	*Iva*	Walnut	*Juglans*
Mesquite	*Prosopis*	Willow	*Salix*
Mountain cedar	*Juniperus*		

Recently promulgated guidelines for immunotherapy have variably reflected these concerns in a search for minimally adequate allergen panels. The Betulaceae offer perhaps the best-documented example of shared pollen components among genera with major allergens of prominent birch, alder, and hazelnut species essentially interchangeable immunochemically. Comparable similarities, if they exist, remain to be documented for many anemophilous families—even within genera. Pollen allergen sharing among members of the oak-beech-chestnut group, within the ash and olive family, among some ragweeds, in the chenopod and the related amaranth groups, and within individual tribes of related grasses are well described. Similarities among *Artemisia* species pollen and within the Cupressaceae (junipers, etc.) also are documented. However, since emissions of related taxa usually are microscopically indistinguishable, field surveys and known patterns of allergen content remain key in choosing materials for clinical use.

Despite the aforementioned reservations, this chapter attempts to list clinically significant pollen on a state-by-state basis with their botanical names and approximate periods of peak prevalence. Where reference to two or more species of a single genus is intended, *spp.* is used after the generic term; *sp.* designates an uncertain species of a stated genus. Relative importance is implied by a three-level scale: + + +, generally quite important; + +, of secondary importance; +, occasionally or locally worth considering. Among the last of these, those chosen versus those excluded require, ultimately, an arbitrary decision, however refined by facts. Finally, cardinal directions, abbreviated as N, S, E, W, and L (for local occurrence) should pose no problem. Pollen sources for each state or group are listed in the order: trees, grasses, weeds (i.e., broad-leaved, nonwoody plants, or "forbs") (Tables 7.1 and 7.2).

For many prominent genera, the first letter of the Latin epithet only may be given to conserve space; Table 7.1 should allay any resulting uncertainty. Table 7.2 lists the geographic units considered.

TABLE 7.2   U.S. REGIONS AND COMPONENT DIVISIONS CONSIDERED IN THIS CHAPTER

The Northeast

Connecticut and New York
Delaware and New Jersey
Massachusetts and Rhode Island
Pennsylvania, Maryland, District of Columbia, and West Virginia
Maine, New Hampshire, and Vermont

(continued)

TABLE 7.2   U.S. REGIONS AND COMPONENT DIVISIONS CONSIDERED IN THIS CHAPTER (CONTINUED)

The Southeast

Kentucky and Tennessee
North Carolina and Virginia
Georgia, South Carolina, Alabama, and Mississippi
Arkansas and Louisiana
Florida

The Midwest

Illinois and Indiana
Ohio and Michigan
Iowa and Missouri
Minnesota and Wisconsin

The Great Plains

North and South Dakota
Kansas and Nebraska
Oklahoma and Texas
Colorado, Wyoming, and Montana

The Southwest

Arizona and New Mexico
Nevada and Utah
California

The Pacific Northwest

Idaho, Oregon, and Washington

The Noncontiguous United States

Alaska
Hawaii
Puerto Rico
U.S. Virgin Islands

THE NORTHEAST*

POLLEN TYPE	GENUS AND SPECIES	IMPACT	PREVALENCE
Connecticut and New York			
Trees			
Juniper, yew	*Juniperus spp., Taxus spp.*	+	Mar–Apr
Alder	*Alnus spp.*	+(L)	Mar–Apr
Elm, white	*U. americana*	++	Apr
Birch, gray, red, etc.	*Betula spp.*	+	Apr
Cottonwood	*P. deltoides*	++	Apr
Maple, sugar, red	*A. saccharum, rubrum*	+	Apr–May
Ash, white	*F. americana*	+	Apr–May
Oak, white, red	*Q. alba, rubra*	+++	Apr–May
Hickory	*C. ovata, Carya spp.*	+	May
Beech	*F. grandifolia*	++(L)	May
Hackberry (SE)	*C. occidentalis*	+(L)	May–June
Mulberry, red, black (L)	*M. rubrum, nigra*	+	May
Grasses			

(continued)

TABLE 7.2 U.S. REGIONS AND COMPONENT DIVISIONS CONSIDERED IN THIS CHAPTER (*CONTINUED*)

POLLEN TYPE	GENUS AND SPECIES	IMPACT	PREVALENCE
June/blue	*Poa pratensis*	+++	May–July
Orchard	*Dactylis glomerata*	+++	May–July
Timothy	*Phleum pratense*	+++	June–July
Red top	*Agrostis alba*	+	May–July
Rye	*Lolium spp.*	+	June–July
Sweet vernal	*Anthoxanthum odoratum*	++	May–July
Weeds			
Sorrel; dock	*R. acetosella, Rumex spp.*	+	May–June
Ragweed, short	*A. artemisiifolia*	+++	Aug–Sep
Ragweed, giant	*A. trifida*	+	
Plantain, English	*P. lanceolata*	+	June–Sep
Lambs quarters	*Chenopodium album*	+	Aug–Sep
Pigweed, amaranths	*Amaranthus spp.*	+	Aug–Sep
Mugwort	*Artemisia vulgaris*	+(L)	Aug–Sep

Sweet fern (*Myrica asplenifolia*) and bayberry (*M. caroliniana*) of sandy soils are modest local factors in pollinosis.

Delaware and New Jersey			
Trees			
Red cedar	*J. virginiana*	+	Mar–Apr
Alder	*Alnus spp.*	+ (L)	Mar–Apr
Elm, white	*U. americana*	++	Apr
Birch, gray, red, etc.	*B. alba, nigra, Betula spp.*	+	Apr
Cottonwood	*P. deltoides*	+	Apr
Red maple	*A. rubrum*	+	Apr
Ash, white	*F. americana*	++	Apr–May
Sycamore, eastern, hybrids	*Platanus spp.*	+	Apr–May
Oak, white, red, etc.	*Quercus spp.*	+++	Apr–May
Beech	*F. grandifolia*	+ (N)	May
Walnut, black	*J. nigra*	+ (L)	May
Hickory	*Carya spp.*	+	May
Sweet gum	*L. styraciflua*	+ (S)	May
Mulberry	*Morus spp.*	+ (L)	May

Grasses

Strongly similar to Connecticut and New York. In addition, Bermuda grass occurs in more southern areas. Others, including fescue (*Festuca elatior, Festuca spp.*) are marginal, local sources; velvet grass (*Holcus lanatus*), Johnson grass (*Sorghum halepense*), and others may evoke symptoms locally.

Weeds

Closely similar to Connecticut and New York. In addition, yellow dock (*Rumex crispus*) may contribute in June, but mugwort is less prominent.

Massachusetts and Rhode Island

Trees

(continued)

TABLE 7.2   U.S. REGIONS AND COMPONENT DIVISIONS CONSIDERED IN THIS CHAPTER (CONTINUED)

POLLEN TYPE	GENUS AND SPECIES	IMPACT	PREVALENCE
Red cedar	*J. virginiana*	+	Mar–Apr
Elm, white	*U. americana*	+	Apr
Poplar, aspen(s)	*Populus spp.*	+	Apr
Willow, black	*S. nigra*	+	Apr–June
Ash, white	*F. americana*	+	Apr–May
Birch, yellow	*B. alleghaniensis, papyrifera,*	+++	Apr–May
Paper, gray	*populifolia*	+	
Maple, sugar	*A. saccharum*	++	Apr–May
Oak, white, red	*Q. alba, rubra*	+++	May
Beech	*F. grandifolia*	+	May
Mulberry, red, black (L)	*M. rubra, nigra*	+(L)	May
Hemlock	*Tsuga canadensis*	+(W)	May

Grasses

Strongly similar to Connecticut and New York.

Weeds

Strongly similar to Connecticut and New York. Mugwort (*A. vulgaris*) is found increasingly in the east and merits clinical concern.

Pennsylvania, Maryland, District of Columbia, and West Virginia

Trees

Elm, white	*U. americana*	+	Mar–Apr
Birch, yellow	*B. alleghaniensis*	++	Apr
Maple, red	*A. rubrum*	+	Apr
Cottonwood, aspen	*Populus spp.*	+	Apr
Ash, white	*F. americana*	++	Apr
Sycamore	*Platanus spp.*	+	Apr–May
Oak, white, red, etc.	*Quercus spp.*	+++	Apr–May
Hickory	*Carya spp.*	+	Apr–May
Walnut, butternut	*Juglans spp.*	+(L)	Apr–May
Sweet gum	*L. styraciflua*	+	Apr–May
Mulberry, red, black (L)	*M. rubra, nigra*	+	May

Grasses

June (blue), orchard, timothy, and rye grasses produce abundant late May to late July pollen. Bermuda grass appears also in Maryland, District of Columbia, and West Virginia.

Weeds

Strongly similar to Connecticut and New York.

Maine, New Hampshire, and Vermont

Trees

Elm, white	*U. americana*	+	Apr
Ash, white	*F. americana*	+	May
Birch, yellow, paper, etc.	*B. lutea, papyrifera, Betula spp.*	++	Apr–May

(continued)

TABLE 7.2   U.S. REGIONS AND COMPONENT DIVISIONS CONSIDERED IN THIS CHAPTER (*CONTINUED*)

POLLEN TYPE	GENUS AND SPECIES	IMPACT	PREVALENCE
Aspen, cottonwood, poplar	*P. tremuloides, grandidentata, deltoides, balsamifera (N)*	++	Apr–May
Oak, red, white	*Q. rubra, alba*	++	May
Maple, sugar	*A. saccharum*	++	May
Beech	*F. grandifolia*	+	May
Hickory	*Carya spp.*	+(S)	May
Grasses			
Strongly similar to Connecticut and New York; May–July period shortens to the north.			
Weeds			
Sorrel, docks	*Rumex spp.*	+	May–June
Ragweed, short	*A. artemisiifolia*	+++	Aug–Sep
Lambs quarters	*Chenopodium album*	+	July–Sep
Pigweed, redroot	*A. retroflexus*	+	July–Sep
Plantain, English	*P. lanceolata*	+	June–Aug
Mugwort	*A. vulgaris*	+(SE)	Aug

*As the area longest intensively colonized by Europeans, the paradigm of a brief, hectic spring tree pollen season, grass pollen from late May to July, and the ragweed debacle in late summer originated here. Despite their size, metropolitan areas receive ample pollen from upwind sources and occasionally from intraurban planting of ash, oak, and sycamore. Traditional havens from ragweed exposure in northern states today offer minimal protection, at best. Rye grass–related northern grass species predominate, with Bermuda grass appearing only in the southernmost tier.

THE SOUTHEAST*

POLLEN TYPE	GENUS AND SPECIES	IMPACT	PREVALENCE
Kentucky and Tennessee			
Trees			
Elm, white, slippery, etc.	*U. americana, rubra, Ulmus spp.*	+	Feb–Mar
Red cedar	*J. virginiana*	+(W)	Feb–Mar
Ash, white, green	*F. americana, pennsylvanica*	++	Mar–May
Red maple	*A. rubrum*	+	Feb–Mar
Oak, red, white, other	*Quercus spp.*	+++	Mar–Apr
Hornbeam, American	*Carpinus caroliniana*	+(L)	Mar–Apr
Birch, sweet, yellow	*B. lenta, alleghaniensis*	+(L)	Mar–Apr
Sweet gum	*L. styraciflua*	+	Apr
Cottonwood	*P. deltoides*	++	Mar–Apr
Hickory, pecan	*Carya spp.*	+++	Apr–May
Sycamore	*P. occidentalis*	+	Apr–May
Mulberry, red	*M. rubra*	+	Apr–May
Walnut, butternut	*Juglans spp.*	+	Apr–May
Grasses			
June (blue)	*Poa pratensis*	+++	Apr–Sep

(continued)

TABLE 7.2   U.S. REGIONS AND COMPONENT DIVISIONS CONSIDERED IN THIS CHAPTER (*CONTINUED*)

POLLEN TYPE	GENUS AND SPECIES	IMPACT	PREVALENCE
Timothy	*Phleum pratense*	+++	May–July
Orchard	*Dactyis glomerata*	++	May–June
Bermuda	*Cynodon dactylon*	+++	May–Sep
Red top	*Agrostis alba*	+	May–July
Johnson	*Sorghum halepense*	+	June–Sep
Weeds			
Sorrel, dock	*Rumex spp.*	+	Apr–June
Plantain, English	*P. lanceolata*	+	May–Aug
Amaranths, pigweed	*Amaranthus spp.*	+	July–Sep
Burning bush	*Kochia scoparia*	+	July–Sep
Ragweed, short, giant	*A. artemisiifolia, trifida*	+++	Aug–Sep
Burweed marsh elder	*I. xanthifolia*	+(W)	Aug–Sep
North Carolina and Virginia			
Trees			
Alder, hazel	*A. serrulata*	+	Feb–Mar
Elm, white, slippery	*U. americana, rubra*	+	Feb–Apr
Maple, red	*A. rubrum*	++	Feb–Apr
Ash, white, green	*F. americana, pennsylvanica*	+	Feb–Apr
Oak, red, white, live[a]	*Quercus spp.*	+++	Mar–May
Sycamore	*P. occidentalis*	+	Apr–May
Hickory; pecan	*Carya spp.*	+++	Apr–May
Willow, black, etc.	*Salix nigra, Salix spp.*	+	Apr–May
Sweet gum	*L. styraciflua*	+	Apr–May
Hackberry	*C. laevigata*	+(S)	Apr–May
Bayberry	*Myrica spp.*	+(L)	Apr–May
Grasses			
Strongly similar to Kentucky and Tennessee, although Bermuda grass is an incrementally dominant offender.			
Weeds			
Strongly similar to Kentucky and Tennessee.			
Georgia, South Carolina, Alabama, and Mississippi			
Trees			
Red cedar	*J. virginiana*	+	Jan–Feb
Cottonwood	*P. deltoides*	+	Feb–Mar
Elm, white, slippery	*U. americana, rubra*	+	Feb–Mar
Maple, red	*A. rubrum*	+++	Mar–Apr
Birch, river	*B. nigra*	+	Mar–Apr
Mulberry	*Morus spp.*	+	Mar–Apr
Ash, white, green, etc.	*Fraxinus spp.*	+	Apr
Oak, red, white, live	*Quercus spp.*	+++	Feb–Mar
Hickory, pecan	*Carya spp.*	+++	Apr–May
Sweet gum	*L. styraciflua*	+	Mar–Apr

(continued)

TABLE 7.2 U.S. REGIONS AND COMPONENT DIVISIONS CONSIDERED IN THIS CHAPTER (*CONTINUED*)

POLLEN TYPE	GENUS AND SPECIES	IMPACT	PREVALENCE
Bayberry	*Myrica spp.*	+(E)	Apr–May
Sugar (hack) berry	*C. laevigata*	++(L)	Apr–May
Grasses			
Bermuda	*Cynodon dactylon*	+++	May–Oct
June (blue)	*Poa pratensis*	++	Apr–July
Johnson	*Sorghum halepense*	++	May–Oct
Rye	*Lolium spp.*	+	May–July
Weeds			
Sorrel, dock	*Rumex spp.*	+ (N)	Apr–June
Ragweed, short, giant	*A. artemisiifolia, trifida*	+++	Aug–Oct
Pigweed, amaranths	*Amaranthus spp.*	+	May–Sep
Plantain, English	*P. lanceolata*	+	Apr–Oct
Nettle	*Urtica spp.*	+	July–Oct
Marsh elder, rough	*I. ciliata*	+(W)	July–Oct
Arkansas and Louisiana			
Trees			
Juniper; cedar	*Juniperus spp.*	+++	Jan–Mar
Elm	*Ulmus spp.*	+	Jan–Mar
Sugar (hack) berry	*C. laevigata*	++	Mar–May
Oak, white, red	*Quercus spp.*	+++	Mar–Apr
Oak, live	*Q. virginiana*	++(S)	Mar–Apr
Mulberry, red	*M. rubra*	+	Mar–Apr
Hickory, pecan	*Carya spp.*	+++	Apr–May
River birch	*B. nigra*	+	Mar–Apr
Sweet gum	*L. styraciflua*	+	Apr–May
Grasses			
Bermuda	*Cynodon dactylon*	+++	Apr–Nov
June (blue)	*Poa spp.*	++	Apr–Nov
Johnson	*Sorghum halepense*	+	Apr–Nov
Rye	*Lolium spp.*	+	May–Nov
Weeds			
Ragweed, giant, short,	*A. trifida, artemisiifolia*	+++	Aug–Oct
Marsh elder, rough	*I. ciliata*	+++	Aug–Oct
Western water hemp	*Acnida tamarascina*	++	July–Sep
Russian thistle	*Salsola pestifer*	+	June–Sep
Pigweed, amaranths	*Amaranthus spp.*	+	June–Sep

*Warmer average temperatures provide a long growing season with early appearance of common tree pollens. In certain areas, some airborne grass pollen occurs in every month; Bermuda grass is the principal source. In the south and east especially, multiple oaks contribute, including several evergreen species, e.g., live, willow and laurel oaks at lower elevations. Vast areas of yellow, long-leaf, short-leaf and loblolly pines produce copiously, although human effects remain uncertain. Throughout the Southeast the imported paper mulberry (*Broussonetia papyrifera*) has local importance.

[a]Live is used here as a surrogate for several evergreen oaks, including also laurel and willow.

(continued)

TABLE 7.2 U.S. REGIONS AND COMPONENT DIVISIONS CONSIDERED IN THIS CHAPTER (CONTINUED)

FLORIDA

POLLEN TYPE	GENUS AND SPECIES	IMPACT	PREVALENCE
Trees			
Alder	A. serrulata	+(N)	Dec–Feb
Juniper, cedar	Juniperus, cupressus spp.	+	Jan–Mar
Bald cypress	Taxodium distichum	+	Jan–Apr
Australian pine	Casuarina spp.	++	Feb–Apr/Oct–Dec
Oak, post (N), Southern	Q. stellata, falcata, virginiana,	+++	Feb–Apr
Oak red (N), live, laurel	laurifolia	+	Feb–Mar
Box elder	Acer negundo	+(N)	
Mulberry, red, white	Morus spp.	++(L)	Mar–Apr
Sweet gum	L. styraciflua	+(L)	Feb–Mar
Maple, red	A. rubrum	++(N)	Jan–Feb
Elm, white, etc.	U. americana, Ulmus spp.	+(N)	Jan–Mar
Hickory, pecan	Carya is., Carya spp.	++(N)	Sep–Nov
Palm, sabal, date,	Palmaceae	?+(L)	Mar–Sep
Canary, etc.			
Grasses			
Bermuda	Cynodon dactylon	+++	Mar–Nov
Johnson	Sorghum halepense	+	Apr–Aug
Bahia	Paspalum notatum	+	Apr–Oct
June (blue)	Poa spp.	+	Apr–Aug
Weeds			
Sorrel; dock	Rumex spp.	+	May–Aug
Ragweed, short, giant (N)	A. artemisiifolia, trifida	++	May–Nov
Groundsel tree (shrub)	Baccharis spp.	+(E)	July–Sep
Nettle group	Urtica spp.	?+	Jan–July
Pigweed; amaranths	Amaranthus spp.	+	Mar–Nov

*The peninsula of Florida extends almost 600 miles into warm seas and supports a subtropical flora at its tip. Elsewhere, wind-pollinated species resemble those of Georgia and Alabama, even to major pine formations on sandy soil. A few introduced types (e.g., casuarina, eucalypts, palms) merit at least local concern and may yet be recognized as significant.

THE MIDWEST*

POLLEN TYPE	GENUS/SPECIES	IMPACT	PREVALENCE
Illinois and Indiana			
Trees			
Red cedar	J. virginiana	+	Feb–Mar
Cottonwood	P. deltoides	+	Mar–Apr
Elm, white, slippery, etc.	U. americana, rubra, Ulmus spp.	++	Feb–Apr
Box elder	Acer negundo	++	Mar–Apr
Ash, white, green, etc.	Fraxinus spp.	++	Apr–May
Oak, red, white, bur	Quercus rubra, alba, macrocarpa	+++	Apr–May

(continued)

TABLE 7.2   U.S. REGIONS AND COMPONENT DIVISIONS CONSIDERED IN THIS CHAPTER (*CONTINUED*)

POLLEN TYPE	GENUS/SPECIES	IMPACT	PREVALENCE
Hickory, pecan	*Carya spp.*	++(SW)	Apr–May
Mulberry, red	*M. rubra*	++(L)	Apr–May
Birch, river, etc.	*Betula spp.*	+	Apr–May
Walnut, black	*J. nigra*	+	Apr–May
Sycamore	*Platanus spp.*	+(S.L.)	Apr–May
Grasses			
June (blue)	*Poa spp.*	+++	Apr–July
Orchard	*Dactylis glomerata*	+++	May–July
Timothy	*Phleum pratense*	++	May–July
Red top	*Agrostis alba*	+	May–July
Bermuda	*Cynodon dactylon*	+++(S)	May–Aug
Johnson	*Sorghum halepense*	+(S)	May–Aug
Rye	*Lolium spp.*	+	May–Aug
Weeds			
Ragweed, short, giant	*Ambrosia spp.*	+++	Aug–Sep
Burweed marsh elder	*Iva xanthifolia*	++(S)	Aug–Sep
Burning bush[a]	*Kochia scoparia*	++	July–Oct
Russian thistle[a]	*Salsola pestifer*	+++	July–Oct
Plantain, English	*P. lanceolata*	+	May–Oct
Pigweed, amaranths	*Amaranthus spp.*	+	July–Oct
Ohio and Michigan			
Trees			
Red cedar	*J. virginiana*	+	Feb–Mar
Elm, white, etc.	*U. americana, Ulmus spp.*	++	Mar–Apr
Cottonwood, aspen (N)	*Populus spp.*	+	Mar–Apr
Box elder	*Acer negundo*	+++	Apr–May
Birch, river, gray, etc.	*Betula spp.*	+	Apr–May
Ash, white, green, etc.	*Fraxinus spp.*	+++	Apr–May
Oak, red, white, bur, etc.	*Quercus spp.*	++	Apr–May
Hickory	*Carya spp.*	+	Apr–May
Sycamore	*Platanus spp.*	+(L)	Apr–May
Walnut, butternut	*Juglans spp.*	+	Apr–May
Mulberry, red	*M. rubra*	+++(L)	Apr–May
Grasses			
Orchard grass	*Dactylis glomerata*	+++	May–June
June (blue)	*Poa pratensis*	+++	May–June
Timothy	*Phleum pratense*	+++	June–July
Red top	*Agrostis alba*	+	May–June
Bermuda	*Cynodon dactylon*	+++(S)	May–July
Johnson	*Sorghum halepense*	+(S)	May–July
Rye	*Lolium spp.*	+	June–July

(continued)

TABLE 7.2   U.S. REGIONS AND COMPONENT DIVISIONS CONSIDERED IN THIS CHAPTER (*CONTINUED*)

POLLEN TYPE	GENUS/SPECIES	IMPACT	PREVALENCE
Weeds[b]			
Ragweed, short, giant	*A. artemisiifolia, trifida*	+++	Aug–Sep
Burning Bush[a]	*Kochia scoparia*	++(L)	Aug–Sep
Pigweed; amaranths	*Amaranthus spp.*		
Plantain, English	*P. lanceolata*	+	May–Sep
Iowa and Missouri			
Trees			
Red cedar	*J. virginiana*	+	Feb–Apr
Oak, white, red, bur, etc.	*Quercus spp.*	+++	Mar–Apr
Elm, white, slippery, etc.	*Ulmus spp.*	++	Feb–Apr
Cottonwood, eastern, swamp (SE)	*P. deltoides, heterophylla*	+	Mar–Apr
Red maple	*A. rubrum*	+(SE)	Mar–Apr
Box elder	*Acer negundo*	++(N)	Mar–Apr
Willow, black, etc.	*Salix nigra, Salix spp.*	+	Mar–Apr
Ash, green, white, etc.	*Fraxinus spp.*	+(S)	Apr–May
Oak, white, red, bur, etc.	*Quercus spp.*	+++	Mar–May
Mulberry, red	*M. rubra*	++(L)	Apr–May
Hickory, pecan	*Carya spp.*	++	Apr–May
Sycamore, eastern	*P. occidentalis*	+	Apr–May
Butternut (E), black walnut	*J. cinerea, nigra*	+(L)	Apr–May
Grasses			
Both Bermuda and the rye-related, more northern species flower April–July (Aug).			
Weeds			
Strongly similar to Illinois and Indiana with the addition of rough marsh elder (S) and hemp (*Cannabis sativa*) in extreme NW Iowa as ++ factors as well Palmer amaranth (++) in western Missouri.			
Minnesota and Wisconsin			
Trees			
Juniper, red cedar (S)	*Juniperus spp.*	++	Apr–May
Cottonwood, aspen	*Populus spp.*	+	Apr
Maple, red, sugar, black, box elder	*Acer spp.*	++	Apr–May
Birch, yellow, paper, etc.	*Betula spp.*	++	Apr–May
Ash, white, green, etc.	*Fraxinus spp.*	++	Apr–May
Oak, red, bur, pin, white, etc.	*Quercus spp.*	+++	Apr–May
Mulberry, red	*M. rubrum* (S)	++(L)	May
Hickory	*Carya spp.*	+	May
Walnut black	*J. nigra* (S)	+	May
Grasses			
June (blue)	*Poa pratensis*	+++	June–July
Orchard	*Dactylis glomerata*	+++	May–June

(continued)

TABLE 7.2 U.S. REGIONS AND COMPONENT DIVISIONS CONSIDERED IN THIS CHAPTER (*CONTINUED*)

POLLEN TYPE	GENUS/SPECIES	IMPACT	PREVALENCE
Timothy	*Phleum pratense*	+++	June–July
Red top	*Agrostis alba*	+	June–July
Rye	*Lolium spp.*	++	June–Aug
Weeds			
Ragweed, short, giant	*A. artemisiifolia, trifida*	+++	Aug–Sep
Burweed marsh elder	*Iva xanthifolia*	+++(W)	July–Sep
Russian thistle[a]	*Salsola kali*	++(W)	July–Sep
Amaranths	*Amaranthus spp.*	+	July–Sep
Plantain, English	*P. lanceolata*	+	June–Aug
Hemp	*Cannabis sativa*	++(L)	July–Sep

*This broad, largely agricultural area forms the transition between the Great Plains and the (traditional) eastern forest domain. To the west, woodlands are increasingly confined to river bottoms. Bermuda becomes a principal grass pollen below central Ohio, Indiana, and Illinois, whereas the more northern types (i.e., orchard, timothy, june, red top, and rye) predominate around, and west of, the Great Lakes. Sorrel and dock pollen is a variable but usually modest spring factor throughout. Nettle (-like) pollen is surprisingly abundant (July–August) in many areas, but sources such as wood nettle (*Laportea canadensis*) and a native parietaria (*P. pennsylvanica*) also may contribute.

[a]Additional chenopod sources are negligible by comparison

[b]Sorrel, dock and nettle; see introductory note.

*THE GREAT PLAINS**

POLLEN TYPE	GENUS/SPECIES	IMPACT	PREVALENCE
North Dakota and South Dakota			
Trees			
Juniper, red cedar	*Juniperus spp.*	+	Mar–May
Cottonwood, aspen	*Populus spp.*	++	Mar–Apr
Elm, white, Siberian, etc.	*Ulmus spp.*	+++	Mar–Apr Aug–Oct
Ash, white, green, etc.	*Fraxinus spp.*	++(S)	Apr–May
Box elder	*Acer negundo*	++	Apr–May
Birch, paper, yellow, etc.	*Betula spp.*	+	Apr–May
Ash, white, green, etc.	*Fraxinus spp.*	+	Apr–May
Oak, bur, white (E), etc.	*Quercus spp.*	+++	Apr–May
Mulberry, red	*M. rubra*	++	May
Grasses			
June (blue)	*Poa pratensis*	+++	May–July
Timothy	*Phleum pratense*	++	June–July
Orchard (E)	*Dactylis glomerata*	+	May–July
Brome (chess)	*Bromus spp.*	+	May–July
Wheatgrass, crested, western, etc.	*Agropyron spp.*	+	June–July

(continued)

TABLE 7.2   U.S. REGIONS AND COMPONENT DIVISIONS CONSIDERED IN THIS CHAPTER (*CONTINUED*)

POLLEN TYPE	GENUS/SPECIES	IMPACT	PREVALENCE
Weeds			
Ragweed, short, giant, perennial, etc.	*Ambrosia spp.*	+++	Aug–Sep
Burning bush	*Kochia scoparia*	+++*	July–Sep
Russian thistle	*Salsola kali*	+++*	July–Sep
Western water hemp	*Acnida tamarascina*	++	July–Sep
Pigweed, amaranths	*Amaranthus spp.*	+	July–Sep
Nettle	*Urtica spp.*	+?	July–Aug
Hemp	*Cannabis sativa*	++(E)	July–Aug
Kansas and Nebraska			
Trees			
Red cedar, juniper	*Juniperus spp.*	++	Feb–Apr
Elm, white	*U. americana*	+	Feb–Mar
Box elder	*Acer negundo*	+	Mar–Apr
Cottonwood	*P. deltoides*	+	Mar–Apr
Oak, white, bur, post (E), etc.	*Quercus spp.*	++	Apr–May
Ash, green	*F. pennsylvanica*	+(E)	Apr–May
Mulberry, red	*M. rubra*	++(SE)	Apr–May
Grasses			
Strongly similar to North and South Dakota.			
Weeds			
Strongly similar to North and South Dakota; Palmer amaranth is a factor in eastern Kansas.			
Oklahoma and Texas			
Trees			
Mountain cedar, Juniper	*Juniperus ashei, Juniperus spp.*	+++	Dec–Mar
Elm, white, slippery, etc.	*Ulmus spp.*	+++	Jan–Apr
Cottonwood	*P. deltoides*	+ (E)	Mar–Apr
Ash, green, white, etc.	*Fraxinus spp.*	++ (S.E.)	Feb–Mar
Sugarberry; hackberry	*Celtis spp.*	++	Feb–Apr
Box elder	*Acer negundo*	+(E)	Mar–Apr
Oak, bur, post, live (E), etc.	*Quercus spp.*	+++	Feb–May
Mulberry, red	*M. rubra*	++	Mar–Apr
Willow, black	*S. nigra*	++	Mar–June
Hickory, pecan	*Carya spp.*	+(L)	Apr–May
Osage orange	*Maclura pomifera*	++(E)	Apr–June
Mesquite	*P. glandulosa*	+(W)	Mar–May
Elm, cedar	*U. crassifolia*	+++	Aug–Oct
Grasses			

(continued)

TABLE 7.2   U.S. REGIONS AND COMPONENT DIVISIONS CONSIDERED IN THIS CHAPTER (*CONTINUED*)

POLLEN TYPE	GENUS/SPECIES	IMPACT	PREVALENCE
June (blue)	*Poa pratensis*	++	Apr–Aug
Orchard	*Dactylis glomerata*	+	May–July
Bermuda	*Cynodon dactylon*	+++	May–July
Rye	*Lolium spp.*	+	June–Aug
Johnson	*Sorghum halepense*	+	May–Sep
Weeds			
Ragweed, short, giant, perennial, southern (E)	*Ambrosia spp.*	+++	Aug–Oct
Marsh elder, burweed (N), rough (E)	*Iva spp.*	++	June–Sep
Burning bush[a]	*Kochia scoparia*	++	June–Sep
Russian thistle[a]	*Salsola kali*	++	June–Sep
Water hemp, western[a]	*Acnida tamariscina*	++(N)	June–Sep
"Scales"[a]	*Atriplex spp.*	++(W)	June–Sep
Colorado, Wyoming, and Montana			
Trees			
Juniper, common, Utah (S), one-seeded (S), rocky mountain, etc.	*Juniperus spp.*	+++	Feb–May
Elm	*Ulmus spp.*	++	Feb–Apr
Cottonwood, eastern (E), black (NW), fremont, narrowleaf, etc; aspen, quaking (W)	*Populus spp.*	+	Mar–June
Maple, rocky mountain, etc., box elder	*Acer spp.*	+	Apr–May
Willow, pacific, peach leaf, etc.	*Salix spp.*	+	Mar–May
Alder, mountain, etc.	*Alnus spp.*	+	Mar–Apr
Oak, gambel's	*Q. gambelii*	++	Apr–June
Grasses			
June (blue)	*Poa spp.*	++	June–Aug
Brome	*Bromus spp.*	+	May–July
Fescue	*Festuca spp.*	+	June–Aug
The contribution of these and other grass genera to the modest total levels recorded, including *Koeleria*, Agropyron, Buchlöe, Bouteloua, etc., remain speculative.			
Weeds			
Russian thistle[b]	*Salsola kali*	+++	June–Oct
Burning bush[b]	*Kochia scoparia*	+++	June–Oct
Scales[b]	*Atriplex spp.*	+++	June–Oct
Sages	*Artemisia spp.*	++	July–Oct
Ragweeds[c]	*Ambrosia spp.*	++	July–Sep
Burweed marsh elder	*Iva xanthifolia*	+	July–Sep

(continued)

TABLE 7.2   U.S. REGIONS AND COMPONENT DIVISIONS CONSIDERED IN THIS CHAPTER (*CONTINUED*)

POLLEN TYPE	GENUS/SPECIES	IMPACT	PREVALENCE
Sorrel, dock (L)	*Rumex spp.*	+(N)	May–July

*This region was previously the domain of long (east) and short (west) grass prairies; however, little original cover remains, and grass pollen levels are moderate, at best. Grass pollen sources also are numerous and difficult to assign rank. Most woodland is limited to river courses and related wetlands, except in the extreme Northwest (Rocky Mountains) and South (Texas).

[a]Additional chenopods and amaranths appear to make small contributions, by comparison. Moderate levels of partly wind-pollinated composites such as *Parthenium hysterophorus* occur, but health impact remains unclear.

[b]Pollen production of types listed far exceeds that of other chenopods and amaranths.

[c]Prominently including the bur ("false") ragweeds previously designated *Franseria* (now *Ambrosia*).

THE SOUTHWEST*

POLLEN TYPE	GENUS AND SPECIES	IMPACT	PREVALENCE
Arizona and New Mexico			
Trees			
Mountain cedar	*J. ashei*	+++(SE)	Dec–Feb
Ash, velvet, etc.	*Fraxinus spp.*	++(L)	Jan–Apr
Juniper, other cedar	*Juniperus spp.*	+++	Mar–May
Elm	*Ulmus spp.*	+++	Feb–May
Cottonwood, fremont, etc., aspen, quaking (W)	*Populus fremontii, Populus spp.*	+	Feb–May
Mulberry, white	*Morus alba*	++	Apr–June
Olive	*Olea europaea*	+++(L)	Apr–June
Box elder	*Acer negundo*	+(N, L)	Apr–May
Oak, gambel's, etc.	*Quercus gambelii, Quercus spp.*	++(L)	Apr–June
Mesquite	*Prosopis spp.*	+	Apr–June
Grasses			
Bermuda	*Cynodon dactylon*	++	Apr–Sep
Johnson	*Sorghum halepense*	+(L)	Apr–Aug
June (blue)	*Poa spp.*	+(L)	Apr–July
The relative contributions of other types must still be defined.			
Weeds			
Ragweed, canyon, rabbit bush, burroweed	*A. ambrosioides, deltoidea, dumosa*	+++	Mar–May
Russian thistle[a]	*Salsola kali*	++	June–Sep
Burning bush	*Kochia scoparia*	+(N)	June–Sep
Scales	*Atriplex spp.*	++	June–Sep
Sage	*Artemisia spp.*	++(L)	June–Oct
Ragweeds, short, slender, etc.	*Ambrosia spp.*	+	July–Sep
Sugar beet	*Beta vulgaris*	+(L)	Apr–June
Nevada and Utah			
Trees			

(continued)

TABLE 7.2   U.S. REGIONS AND COMPONENT DIVISIONS CONSIDERED IN THIS CHAPTER (*CONTINUED*)

POLLEN TYPE	GENUS AND SPECIES	IMPACT	PREVALENCE
Elm	*Ulmus spp.*	+(L)	Feb–Mar
Juniper, cedar	*Juniperus spp., Cupressus spp.*	++	Feb–May
Box elder	*Acer negundo*	+(L)	Apr–May
Cottonwood, aspen	*Populus spp.*	+(L)	Apr–May
Ash, velvet, etc.	*Fraxinus spp.*	+++(L)	Apr–May
Mulberry	*Morus spp.*	+(L)	Apr–May
Mesquite	*Prosopis spp.*	+(L)	Apr–June
Grasses			
See Arizona and New Mexico listing and note.			
Weeds			
Sage	*Artemisia spp.*	+++	Aug–Sep
Ragweed, annual bur, etc.	*A. acanthacarpa, Ambrosia spp.*	+	Aug–Sep
Russian thistle[b]	*Salsola pestifer*	+++	July–Sep
Scales	*Atriplex spp.*	+++	July–Sep

*This group of states is best known for flat arid terrain and a limited variety of potent "hay fever plants." However, substantial mountains are found here, and multipurpose irrigation is increasingly extensive, creating broad "islands" of pollen exposure with a background that is neither simple nor fully described.

[a]Contribution by congeners is probably small.

[b]Additional chenopods (and amaranths), including burning bush, carelessweeds, greasewood, etc., are also variable contributors to exposure.

THE PACIFIC NORTHWEST*

POLLEN TYPE	GENUS AND SPECIES	IMPACT	PREVALENCE
Idaho, Oregon, and Washington			
Trees			
Alder, red, white	*A. rubra, rhombifolia*	+++	Feb–May
Cedar, juniper[a]	*Cupressaceae*	+++	Jan–May
Cottonwood, black, etc., aspen	*Populus spp.*	++	Feb–Apr
Birch, paper, etc.	*Betula spp.*	+++(NW)	Feb–Apr
Willow, pacific, Sitka, etc.	*Salix spp.*	+(L)	Feb–Apr
Elm	*Ulmus spp.*	+(L)	Feb–Mar
Box elder	*Acer negundo*	+++	Mar–Apr
Ash, Oregon, etc.	*Fraxinus spp.*	+	Mar–Apr
Oak, Oregon white, California, black, etc.	*Q. garryana, kelloggii, Quercus spp.*	+(L)	Apr–May
Walnut, English, etc.	*Juglans regia, Juglans spp.*	++(L)	Apr–May
Grasses			
June (blue)	*Poa pratensis, Poa spp.*	+++	May–Aug
Timothy	*Phleum pratense*	+	June–Aug

(continued)

TABLE 7.2   U.S. REGIONS AND COMPONENT DIVISIONS CONSIDERED IN THIS CHAPTER (*CONTINUED*)

POLLEN TYPE	GENUS AND SPECIES	IMPACT	PREVALENCE
Rye, perennial, etc.	*Lolium spp.*	+(L)	June–Aug
Brome	*Bromus spp.*	+(E)	May–Sep
Red top	*Agrostis alba*	+(L)	June–Sep
Weeds			
Nettle and related types	Urticaceae[b]	+	May–July
Sorrel, dock	*Rumex spp.*	+	May–July
	Salsola kali	++(E)	July–Sep
Pigweed, amaranths	*Amaranthus spp*	+	July–Sep
Sage	*Artemisia spp.*	+++(EL)	July–Sep
Additional chenopods appear to contribute little, by comparison			

*The north–south course of the Cascades Mountain Range is the arbiter of moisture here, with well-watered western slopes, a dryer region downwind, and, ultimately, high desert to the east. Regional features include red alder as a preeminent tree pollen source, a grass flora recalling the Northeast and heightened grass pollen levels in the Willamette valley of Oregon where seed is produced commercially. Idaho presents a mountainous spine with a patchwork of dry and moist, agricultural lowlands.

[a]May include other sources, among them incense cedar (*Calocedrus decurrens*), Douglas fir (*Pseudotsuga menziesii*), etc.; hence, the family is listed.

[b]Contributions of types other than nettle (*Urtica spp.*) are uncertain; hence the family name is used here.

CALIFORNIA*

POLLEN TYPE	GENUS AND SPECIES	IMPACT	PREVALENCE
Trees			
Alder, red, white, etc.	*A. rubra, rhombifolia, Alnus spp.*	+(W)	Jan–Feb
Cedar; juniper	*Cupressus spp., Juniperus spp.*	++	Jan–Apr
Cottonwood, Fremont	*Populus fremontii*	++	Feb–Apr
Oak, black, interior live, coast live (W), etc.	*Q. Kelloggii, wislizenii, agrifolia, Quercus spp.*	+++	Jan–May
Ash, velvet (S) Oregon, etc.	*F. velutina, latifolia, Fraxinus spp.*	++	Jan–Apr
Acacia (S)	*Acacia spp.*	+(L)	Feb–Oct
Sycamore, California	*P. racemosa*	+	Feb–Apr
Mulberry, white, etc.	*Morus alba, morus spp.*	+++	Mar–May
Australian pine (Casuarina)	*Casuarina spp.*	+	Mar–May
Walnut, English, etc.	*J. regia, Juglans spp.*	+	
Olive (S)	*Olea europaea*	+++(L)	Apr–June
Castor bean[a]	*Ricinus communis*	+(L)	Apr–July
Elm, Siberian, etc.	*Ulmus pumila spp.*	+++(L)	Aug–Oct
Grasses			
Bermuda	*Cynodon dactylon*	+++	Apr–Oct

(continued)

TABLE 7.2 U.S. REGIONS AND COMPONENT DIVISIONS CONSIDERED IN THIS CHAPTER (*CONTINUED*)

POLLEN TYPE	GENUS AND SPECIES	IMPACT	PREVALENCE
Rye	*Lolium spp.*	+(N)	May–Aug
Brome	*Bromus spp.*	+	Apr–Sep
Fescue	*Festuca spp.*	+	May–Sep
Johnson	*Sorghum halepense*	+(S)	May–Sep
June (blue)	*Poa spp.*	+	Apr–Sep
Diverse additional species are noted and may contribute.			
Weeds			
Sage	Artemisia spp.	+++(S)	June–Oct
Russian thistle[b]	*Salsola kali*	+++(L)	June–Sep
Scale[b]	*Atriplex spp.*	++(E)	June–Sep
Ragweed (L)	*Ambrosia spp.*	++(E, L)	July–Sep
Pigweed, amaranth	*Amaranthus spp.*	+	July–Sep
Nettle	Urticaceae	?+(L)	Apr–Sep
Burning bush[b]	*Kochia scoparia*	++(S)	Mar–July

*The diversity of life zones that California presents argues for separate treatment as well as care in discriminating the many circumscribed pollen sources. A complex oak flora is prominent and (northern) conifer pollens of uncertain significance abound. Bermuda is the dominant grass offender, with many more minor sources recognized. To the south, seasonal rains determine pollen output, both varying between extremes. Clinical reactivity to eucalypts, bottle brush, maples, and mesquite probably is uncommon, although skin test reactivity is documented.

[a]Additional shrubby species, including pepper-tree (*Schinus spp.*), chamise (*Adenostoma*), and blue blossom or California lilac (*Ceanothus spp.*) produce appreciable windborne pollen of uncertain significance clinically.

[b]Pollen output by other chenopods is comparatively minor.

THE NONCONTIGUOUS UNITED STATES

Alaska

A somewhat limited wind-pollinated flora, sources with pollen output limited, at best, and a short growing season serve to allow relief for many "stateside" sufferers. Throughout the state, birch (*B. papyrifera*) pollen is paramount, and grasses and sedges are secondary sources, with Sitka and mountain alders (*A. sinuata and A. tenuifolia*) locally significant. Quaking aspen, balsam poplar, and black cottonwood are factors in moist areas, where brief pollination by several scrubby willows also is recognized. Primarily in the south, limited shedding by docks, chenopods, amaranth, and sages is recognized, but probably none have clinical impact, and ragweeds are absent.

Hawaii

With its unfailing pleasant temperatures and high humidity, Hawaii provides perennially favorable conditions for much plant growth. However, like many other tropical sites, abundant, wind-pollinated species are distinctly limited. Bermuda grass pollen is present potentially at all times, but other sources including sugar cane (*Sorghum vulgare var.*), Johnson grass (*Sorghum halepense*), panic grasses (*Panicum spp.*), and pennisetum appear minimal. Sufficient weed pollen to elicit symptoms also must be rare, indeed. When grouped, mesquite (*Prosopis spp.*), casuarina (*Casuarina spp.*), and several palms (Palmaceae) have been implicated as occasional offenders.

■ BIBLIOGRAPHY

1. Anderson JH. Allergenic airborne pollens and spores in Anchorage, Alaska. *Ann Allergy.* 1985;54:390–399.

2. Anderson EF, Dorsett CS, Fleming EO. Airborne pollens of Walla Walla, Washington. *Ann Allergy.* 1978;41:232–235.

3. Beggs PJ: Impacts of climate change on aeroallergens: past and future. *Clin Exper Allergy.* 2004; 34:1507–1513.

4. Bucholtz GA, Hensel AE III, Lockey RF, et al. Australian pine (*Casuarina equistifolia*) pollen as an aeroallergen. *Ann Allergy.* 1987;59:52–56.

5. Bucholtz GA, Lockey RF, Serbousek D. Bald cypress tree (*Taxodium distichum*) pollen, an allergen. *Ann Allergy.* 1985;55:805–810.

6. Bucholtz GA, Lockey RF, Wunderlin RP, et al. A three year aerobiologic pollen survey of the Tampa Bay area, Florida. *Ann Allergy.* 1991;67:534–543.

7. Buck P, Levetin E. Airborne pollens and mold spores in a subalpine environment. *Ann Allergy*. 1985;55:794–801.

8. Durham OC, LaFalla H. A study of the air-borne allergens of the Virgin Islands National Park and adjacent parts of St. John Islands. *J. Allergy*. 1961;32:27–29.

9. Ellis MH, Gallup J. Aeroallergens of Southern California. *Immunol Allergy Clin N Am*. 1989;9:365–380.

10. Fitter AH, Fitter RS: Rapid changes in flowering time in British plants. *Science*. 2002; 296(5573):1689–1691.

11. Freeman GL. Pine pollen allergy in northern Arizona. *Ann Allergy*. 1993;70:491–494.

12. Gergen PJ, Turkeltaub PC, Kovar MG. The prevalence of allergic skin test reactivity to eight common aeroallergens in the US population: results from the second National Health and Nutritional Examination Survey. *J Allergy Clin Immunol*. 1987;80:669–679.

13. Girsh L. Ragweed pollen in the United States: utilization of graphic maps. *Ann Allergy*. 1982;49:23–28.

14. Jelks ML. Aeroallergens of Florida. *Immunol Allergy Clin N Am*. 1989;9:381–397.

15. Leavengood DC, Renard RL, Martin BG, et al. Cross allergenicity among grasses determined by tissue threshold changes. *J Allergy Clin Immunol*. 1986;76:789–794.

16. Levetin E, Buck P. Evidence of mountain cedar pollen in Tulsa, Oklahoma. *Ann Allergy*. 1986;56:295–299.

17. Lewis WH, Dixit AB, Wedner HJ. Asteraceae aeropollen of the western United States Gulf Coast. *Ann Allergy*. 1991;67:37–46.

18. Lewis WH, Imber WE. Allergy epidemiology in the St. Louis Missouri area. II. Grasses. *Ann Allergy*. 1975;35:42–50.

19. Lewis WH, Imber WE. Allergy epidemiology in the St. Louis Missouri area. III. Trees. *Ann Allergy*. 1975;35:113–119.

20. Lewis WH, Imber WE. Allergy epidemiology in the St. Louis Missouri area. IV. Weeds. *Ann Allergy*.1975;35:180–187.

21. Mansfield LE, Harris NS, Rael E, et al. Regional individual allergen based miniscreen to predict IgE-mediated airborne allergy. *Ann Allergy*. 1988;61:259–261.

22. McLean AC, Parker L, von Reis J, et al. Airborne pollen and fungal spore sampling on the central California coast: the San Luis Obispo pollen project. *Ann Allergy*. 1991;67:441–449.

23. Newark FM. The hayfever plants of Colorado. *Ann Allergy*. 1978;40:18–24.

24. Phillips JW, Bucholtz GA, Fernandez-Caldas E, et al. Bahia grass pollen, a significant aeroallergen: evidence for the lack of clinical cross-reactivity with timothy grass pollen. *Ann Allergy*. 1989;63: 503–507.

25. Prince HE, Meyers GH. Hayfever from the southern wax myrtle (*Myrica cerifera*): a case report. *Ann Allergy*. 1977;38:252–254.

26. Reid MJ, Moss RB, Hsu Y-P, et al. Seasonal asthma in northern California: Allergic causes and efficacy of immunotherapy. *J. Allergy Clin Immunol*. 1986;78:590–600.

27. Reiss NM, Kostic SR. Pollen season severity and meteorologic parameters in central New Jersey. *J Allergy Clin Immunol*. 1976;57: 609–614.

28. Roth A, Shira J. Allergy in Hawaii. *Ann Allergy*. 1966;24:73–78.

29. Samter M, Durham OC. *Regional Allergy of the United States, Canada, Mexico, and Cuba*. Springfield, IL: Charles C Thomas, 1955.

30. Seggev JS, Cruz-Perez P, Naylor MH, et al. Outdoor aeroallergens in the Las Vegas valley. *Ann Allergy*. 1997;78:145. (Abstract)

31. Silvers WS, Ledoux RA, Dolen WK, et al. Aerobiology of the Colorado Rockies: pollen count comparisons between Vail and Denver, Colorado. *Ann Allergy*. 1992;69:421–426.

32. Sneller MR, Hayes HD, Pinnas JL. Pollen changes during five decades of urbanization in Tucson, Arizona. *Ann Allergy*. 1993;71:519–524.

33. Solomon WR. Volumetric studies of aerollergen prevalence. I. Pollens of weedy forbs at a midwestern station. *J Allergy*. 1976;57: 318–327.

34. *Statistical Report of the Pollen and Mold Committee*. Milwaukee, WI: American Academy of Allergy, Asthma & Immunology 1978–1999.

35. Street DH, Hamburger RN. Atmospheric pollen and spore sampling in San Diego, California. I. Meterological correlations and potential clinical relevance. *Ann Allergy*. 1976;37:32–40.

36. Valenta R, Steinberger P, Duchene M, et al. Immunological and structural similarities among allergens: prerequisite for a specific and component-based therapy of allergy. *Immunology and Cell Biology*. 1996;74:187–194.

37. Vaughan WT, Black JH. *Practice of Allergy*. 3rd ed. St Louis: CV Mosby, 1954.

38. Weber R. Cross reactivity among pollens. *Ann Allergy*. 1981;46:208–215.

39. Wodehouse RP. Hayfever plants. Waltham, MA: Chronica Botanica, 1945.

40. Yoo T-J, Spitz E, McGerrity JL. Conifer pollen allergy: studies of immunogenicity and cross antigenicity of conifer pollens in rabbits and man. *Ann Allergy*. 1975;34:87–93.

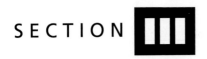

SECTION III

Principles of Evaluation and Treatment

CHAPTER 8

Diagnosis of Immediate Hypersensitivity

ANJU T. PETERS AND JENNIFER S. KIM

Immediate hypersensitivity is defined as the presence of immunoglobulin E (IgE) antibodies in response to an allergen. It is one of the explanations for conjunctivitis, rhinitis, and asthma. In addition, it may be responsible for some cases of anaphylaxis, urticaria, angioedema, atopic dermatitis, and drug reactions. Many other causative explanations are possible for each of these conditions. Consequently, when a patient has been troubled enough with one of these conditions to consult a physician, it is necessary to perform a complete medical evaluation.

First, it must be determined if the symptoms are allergic in origin or if they have another cause. If the symptoms are considered to be allergic in origin, a more specific diagnostic evaluation must be completed to identify the allergen responsible for producing symptoms. In addition, various other factors must be evaluated. The degree of sensitivity to an allergen may vary among patients, as may the degree of exposure to a particular allergen. Many patients are sensitized to multiple allergens, and the cumulative effects of exposure to several antigens may produce severe or persistent symptoms. The influence of nonimmunologic

phenomena also must be evaluated. Infections, inhaled irritants, fatigue, and emotional problems can be significant factors in varying degrees. Considering the large number of variables, it is not surprising that the most important portion of any clinical evaluation is the expertly taken history.

■ PATIENT HISTORY

Many techniques have been used in obtaining a history, including the use of forms by the patient or the interviewer (Fig. 8.1). These may be convenient, but they can only facilitate and not replace the careful inquiries of a skilled historian. In some cases, the salient points can be obtained with relative ease, but generally a complete history is attainable only after considerable time and energy has been invested.

The history provides most of the information necessary for diagnosis. Diagnostic testing may be indicated to confirm or refute the suspected diagnosis. It is the clinician's responsibility to select allergens appropriately and to be cognizant of potential adverse effects, particularly in patients suspected to be highly sensitized.

Allergy Survey Sheet

Name_____Age_____Sex_____Date_____

I. **Chief complaint:**
II. **Present illness:**
III. **Collateral allergic symptoms:**

Eyes:	Pruritus_____	Burning _____	Lacrimation _____
	Swelling _____	Infection_____	Discharge_____
Ears:	Pruritus _____	Fullness _____	Popping _____
	Frequent infections _____		
Nose:	Sneezing _____	Rhinorrhea _____	Obstruction _____
	Pruritus _____	Mouth breathing _____	
	Purulent discharge _____		
Throat:	Soreness _____	Postnasal discharge _____	
	Palatal	Mucus in the morning _____	
	pruritus _____		
Chest:	Cough _____	Pain _____	Wheezing _____
	Sputum _____	Dyspnea_____	
	Color _____	Rest _____	
	Amount _____	Exertion_____	
Skin:	Dermatitis_____	Eczema_____	Urticaria _____

IV. **Family allergies:**
V. **Previous allergic treatment or testing:**
Prior skin test:
Drugs:

Antihistamines	Improved _____	Unimproved _____
Bronchodilators	Improved _____	Unimproved _____
Nose drops	Improved _____	Unimproved _____
Immunotherapy	Improved _____	Unimproved _____
Duration _____		
Antigens _____		
Reactions_____		
Antibiotics	Improved _____	Unimproved _____
Steroids	Improved _____	Unimproved _____

VI. **Physical agents and habits:**

		Bothered by:
Tobacco for _____years	Alcohol _____	Air cond. _____
Cigarettes _____ packs/day	Heat _____	Muggy
Cigars _____per day	Cold _____	weather _____
Pipe _____per day	Perfumes_____	Weather _____
Never smoked _____	Paints_____	changes _____
Bothered by smoke _____	Insecticides _____	Hair spray _____
Illicit drugs_____	Cosmetics _____	Newspapers_____

Time and circumstances of 1st episode:
Prior health:
Course of illness over decades: progressing _____ regressing_____

Time of year   Exact dates
       Perennial _____
       Seasonal _____
       Seasonally exacerbated _____
Monthly variations (menses, occupation): _____
Time of week (weekends vs weekdays):_____
Time of day or night: _____
After insect stings: _____

■ **FIGURE 8.1** *(Continued)*

■ HISTORY TO ESTABLISH PRESENCE OF IMMEDIATE HYPERSENSITIVITY

The history is taken in the same way as any medical history. The patient is asked to state the major complaint and to describe the symptoms. During the history, the presence or absence of symptoms of nonallergic conditions must be determined. Particular attention should be focused on which organs are affected. Characteristic details of the allergic history should be specifically noted.

1. *Are there other symptoms in addition to the presenting complaint that may be allergic in origin?* In patients complaining of upper or lower airway disease, the presence of sneezing, rhinorrhea, nasal congestion, anosmia, ear fullness, palatal pruritus, ocular

VII.   Where symptoms occur:

Living where at onset: _____

Living where since onset: _____

Effect of vacation or major geographic change: _____

Symptoms better indoors or outdoors: _____

Effect of school or work: _____

Effect of staying elsewhere nearby: _____

Effect of hospitalization: _____

Effect of specific environments: _____

Do symptoms occur around: _____

old leaves _____ hay _____ lakeside _____ barns _____

summer homes _____ damp basement _____ dry attic _____

lawn mowing _____ animals _____ other _____

Do symptoms occur after eating:

melons _____

bananas _____ fish _____ nuts _____ citrus fruits _____

other foods (list) _____

Home: city _____ rural _____ house _____ age _____

apartment _____ basement _____ damp _____ dry _____

heating system _____

pets (how long) _____ dog _____ cat _____ other _____

Bedroom:	Type	Age	**Living Room:**	Type	Age
Pillow	____	____	Rug	____	____
Mattress	____	____	Matting	____	____
Blankets	____	____	Furniture	____	____
Quilts	____	____			
Furniture	____	____			

Anywhere in home symptoms are worse: _____

VIII.   What does patient think makes symptoms worse: _____

IX.   Under what circumstances is he or she free of symptoms:

_____

X.   Summary and additional comments:

■ **FIGURE 8.1** Diagnosis of immediate hypersensitivity.

irritation, intermittent hearing loss, wheezing, dyspnea, or cough should be determined. Several allergic symptoms frequently exist simultaneously even if the patient does not associate them with a common cause. If several of these symptoms are present, it is more likely that they all have an allergic origin. Conversely, a symptom in a single organ system, such as isolated nasal obstruction, is less likely to be allergic.

2. *Are symptoms bilateral?* Unilateral symptoms, whether they are ocular, nasal, or pulmonary, suggest the presence of nonallergic conditions, often anatomic in nature.

3. *Is there a family history of atopic disease?* Most allergic patients have a positive family history (1,2). Specifically ask about allergic diseases in parents, grandparents, siblings, aunts, uncles, cousins, and children.

4. *How has the patient responded to previous treatment?* Information about response to previous therapy is useful. A good response to antihistamines increases the likelihood that the symptoms have an allergic origin. Response to a bronchodilator or anti-inflammatory therapy, either systemically or by inhalation, may give valuable information regarding the presence of reversible airway obstruction. A good response to previously administered immunotherapy would strongly implicate an allergic problem.

5. *Are symptoms continuous or intermittent?* Allergic symptoms are often intermittent. Moreover, intermittent exacerbations can occur for patients in whom symptoms appear to be continuous.

6. *Are there specific triggers?* A careful historian can often narrow the list of suspected allergens responsible for the symptoms of allergic diseases. This facilitates selection of further diagnostic tests and minimizes the number of tests performed. Specifically, a detailed survey of the patient's home, work, or school environment may identify potential triggers. Moreover, a list of medications, both prescription and over-the-counter, should be elicited and their potential role as a causative factor considered. For example, oral contraceptives, certain antihypertensives, and phosphodieserase type 5 inhibitors can cause rhinitis (3). Most cardioselective beta blockers are safe in asthmatics, but β-adrenergic blockers rarely can be responsible for wheezing and dyspnea (4–6). Angiotensin-converting enzyme (ACE) inhibitors can produce a severe persistent cough or angioedema (7,8). Chronic use of topical decongestants in the nose or eyes may lead to chronic nasal congestion or ocular irritation respectively (9,10). Awareness of these reactions can prevent unnecessary and expensive allergic evaluations. History is especially important in selecting appropriate food extracts for testing because of the

low specificity of *in vivo* and *in vitro* specific IgE testing (11).

7. *Did the time course suggest an allergic reaction?* Most anaphylactic reactions occur within minutes to hours of exposure to the allergen. For example, IgE-mediated reactions to oral antigens (i.e., food, medication) typically occur within 2 hours of exposure to a particular agent.

The evaluation should address the severity of the illness. Symptom severity helps to determine the extent of the diagnostic evaluation and the intensity of therapy. Whether the symptoms are nasal, ocular, pulmonary, or dermatologic, it is necessary to judge the subjective degree of discomfort they cause. Health care providers must also take into account the patient's perceptions and expectations. Perceived severity may relate closely to its effect on spouses or parents, for example. The assessment of severity also includes more objective measures, such as frequency: the number of days that symptoms occur, number of hours that they persist, number of days lost from or being unproductive at work or school, and the number of days hospitalized. Certainly, special consideration should be given to life-threatening events.

■ CHARACTERISTICS OF ALLERGENS

See Table 8.1 for a review of the important aeroallergens. Some general characteristics of the antigens responsible for allergic illnesses must be appreciated before an adequate clinical history can be obtained or interpreted. Although foods may be contributing factors in cases of infantile eczema, acute urticaria/angioedema, or anaphylaxis, they are rarely responsible for triggering chronic respiratory symptoms. Patients with concomitant food allergy and asthma are more likely to exhibit acute respiratory symptoms on exposure to the offending food antigen. However, asthmatics without a clear history of an acute reaction after ingestion of a particular food are not likely to have food allergy. The allergens most important in asthma and rhinitis are airborne environmental allergens. Several different groups of these aeroallergens are of major clinical significance, including pollen, molds, house dust mites, cockroach, and animal dander.

Pollen

The grains of pollen from plants are among the most important antigens that cause clinical symptoms. Most plants produce pollen that is rich in protein and therefore potentially antigenic. Whether a specific pollen regularly causes symptoms depends on several factors. The pollens that routinely cause illness usually fulfill four criteria: (1) the pollen grains are produced in large quantities by a plant that is prevalent locally; (2) they depend primarily on the wind for dispersal; (3) they are 2 μm to 60 μm in diameter; and (4) they are antigenic.

TABLE 8.1   SYMPTOMS CHARACTERISTICALLY PRODUCED BY COMMON AEROALLERGENS

ANTIGENS	SYMPTOMS
Pollens	Seasonal symptoms or seasonal exacerbation of symptoms
Mold spores	Perennial symptoms in warm climates Seasonal exacerbations in some moderate climates Reduced symptoms when living or vacationing in dry climates Symptoms that decrease with snow Sudden increase in symptoms if exposed to basements, moldy hay or leaves, barns or silos, dairies, breweries, food storage areas, buildings with contaminated air conditioning systems, rotting wood, or any location that might have high humidity Rarely may have exacerbation after ingesting mold products
House dust mites	Characteristically perennial symptoms Exacerbations when making beds, cleaning or dusting the home Occasional exacerbations when entering older homes with older furnishings
Animal danders	Perennial symptoms Marked improvement in symptoms when leaving home for several days or weeks, if animal lives in the home Sudden exacerbations of symptoms after a new pet has been introduced to the home Sudden increase in symptoms when visiting a home where animals live Less frequently, sudden increase in symptoms when playing with an animal Worsening of symptoms at work and clearing of symptoms on weekends or vacations if exposure is occupational

Many plants produce pollen grains that are large, thick, and waxy. Under natural conditions, transfer of pollen between flowering plants is accomplished chiefly by insects. The pollen is not widely dispersed in the air and therefore rarely clinically significant. In contrast, pollen grains that are small, light, widely dispersed by the wind, and highly antigenic cause significant allergic symptoms. In the United States, many trees, grasses, and weeds produce large quantities of highly antigenic, wind-borne pollen. The seasonal occurrence of tree, grass, and weed pollens varies with the geographic location, as discussed in Chapter 7. Even though many factors may alter the total amount of pollen produced in any year, the season of pollination of a plant remains remarkably constant in any one area from year to year. This is because pollen release is determined by length of day, which is consistent from year to year. The treating physician must know which pollens abound in the patient's primary geographical area and the seasons of pollination.

Fungi and Molds

Many thousands of different fungi exist. The role of molds in many conditions is speculative, but some species have been definitely implicated in exacerbating symptoms in mold allergic individuals (12,13). Because fungi can colonize almost every possible habitat and reproduce spores prolifically, the air is seldom free of spores. Consequently, they are important in some patients with perennial symptoms. However, seasonal or local influences can greatly alter the number of airborne spores.

Periods of warm weather with relatively high humidity allow optimal growth of molds. If this period is followed by hot, dry, windy weather, the spores often become airborne in large concentrations. "Thunderstorm asthma" has been associated with increases in mold spores. A frost may produce a large amount of dying vegetation, but the decreased temperature may reduce the growth rate of fungi. In contrast, spring and fall provide the relative warmth, humidity, and adequate substrate necessary for the growth of fungi.

High local concentrations of mold spores are encountered frequently. Deep shade may produce high humidity because of water condensing on cool surfaces. High humidity may occur in areas of water seepage such as basements, refrigerator drip trays, or garbage pails. Food storage areas, dairies, breweries, air conditioning systems, piles of fallen leaves or rotting wood, and barns or silos containing hay or other grains may provide nutrients as well as a high humidity, and therefore may have high concentrations of mold spores.

Indoor Allergens

The indoor environment contains multiple potential allergens, including fungi, dust mites, and pet dander; their role as indoor antigens has been definitely established (14–16). *Dermatophagoides* species are recognized as the major source of antigen in house dust (17). Carpeting, bedding, upholstered furniture, and draperies are the main sanctuaries of dust mites in a home. They are discussed in Chapter 10. In tropical climates, storage mites such as *Lepidoglyphus destructor* and *Blomia tropicalis* are important indoor allergens (18,19). Dust mite–sensitive patients may have perennial symptoms, although these may be somewhat improved outdoors with less humidity or during summer months. They may have a history of sneezing, lacrimation, rhinorrhea, or mild asthma whenever the house is cleaned or the beds are made. In many dust mite–sensitive patients, the history is not so obvious, and the presence of perennial symptoms is the only suggestive feature.

In the inner city, cockroaches are an important allergen. Exposure and IgE sensitivity to cockroach is associated with increased asthma morbidity especially in inner city children (20,21). Both mite and cockroach allergen are airborne in rooms with activity. In the absence of activity, airborne levels decline rapidly.

Proteins from sebaceous, salivary, or perianal glands, and urinary proteins of animals can act as potent allergens (22–24). When warm-blooded pets live inside a home, these products can reach high concentrations and completely permeate the furniture, bedding, rugs, and air. The small particle size and aerodynamic characteristics of pet allergens make them easily airborne especially with minimal disturbance of the environment (25). A short-haired pet does not eliminate this hazard since skin and fur are reservoirs and not the source of the allergens. Although cats and dogs are involved most frequently, many other animals such as hamsters, guinea pigs, rabbits, or mice are occasionally responsible (26–28). Certain occupational groups such as laboratory workers, veterinarians, ranchers, farmers, or pet shop owners may be exposed to an unusual variety of animal dander (29,30).

A patient with clinical sensitivity to a household pet may have a history similar to that of dust mite–sensitive patients with perennial symptoms. In addition, they may have symptomatic improvement when leaving home. Symptoms may persist outside the home because allergen is often carried on clothing, however, and patients may use this as inappropriate evidence that animals that they do not wish to eliminate from the environment are not a cause of their problem. Many patients may relate a history of wheal and erythema at a skin site that was in contact with the animal. If a physician does not inquire about the presence of a pet, the patient's symptoms may be completely misinterpreted and improper therapy may be prescribed.

Other Allergens

IgE-mediated food reactions may be responsible for anaphylaxis or urticarial reactions. These are discussed further in Chapter 14. Similarly, certain drugs or venom stings may be responsible for immediate hypersensitivity reactions and are discussed in Chapters 17 and 12, respectively.

■ NONIMMUNOLOGIC FACTORS

Certain nonimmunologic factors so frequently aggravate allergic conditions that they should always be evaluated. Primary irritants such as tobacco smoke, paint fumes, hair spray, perfumes, cleaning agents, or other strong odors or more generalized air pollution may precipitate flares of allergic respiratory conditions (31). In addition, infections, especially viral, weather changes, exercise, and stress can worsen airway allergic diseases (32).

■ PHYSICAL EXAMINATION

Every patient should have a complete physical examination. Particular attention must be directed to sites affected by common allergic diseases: eyes, nose, oropharynx, ears, chest, and skin.

Conjunctivitis

Physical findings of allergic conjunctivitis are hyperemia and edema of the conjunctiva. Occasionally, a pronounced chemosis occurs associated with clear, watery discharge. Periorbital edema may be present, and, rarely, a bluish discoloration or "allergic shiner" around the eyes may occur.

Rhinitis

The examination of the nose requires good exposure and adequate light. In a patient with allergic rhinitis, the inferior turbinates usually appear to be swollen and actually may meet the nasal septum. They may have a uniform bluish or pearly gray discoloration, but more frequently there may be adjacent areas where the membrane is red, giving a mottled appearance. Polyps may or may not be seen within the nose. The skin of the nose, and particularly of the upper lip, may show irritation and excoriation produced by the nasal discharge and continuous nose wiping. In patients with nasal allergic disease, the ears should be examined for evidence of acute or chronic otitis media, either serous or infectious in nature. Nasal secretions also may be observed draining into the posterior pharynx. "Cobblestoning" of retropharyngeal lymphoid tissue may be observed.

Asthma

Physical findings in asthmatic patients are highly variable, not only between patients but also in the same patient at different times. When the asthmatic patient is not having an acute exacerbation, there may be no demonstrable abnormalities on auscultation even when evidence of reversible airway obstruction can be demonstrated with pulmonary function studies. In many instances, asthma is persistent, and wheezes may be heard even while the patient is feeling subjectively well. In some cases, wheezes will not be heard during normal respiration but can be heard if the patient exhales forcefully.

During an acute attack of asthma, the patient is often tachycardic and tachypneic. The patient appears to be in respiratory distress and usually uses the accessory muscles of respiration. Mechanically, these muscles are more effective if the patient stands or sits and leans slightly forward. Intercostal, subcostal, and supraclavicular retraction, as well as flaring of the alae nasi, may be present with inspiratory effort. On auscultation, musical wheezes may be heard during both inspiration and expiration, and the expiratory phase of respiration may be prolonged. These auscultory findings tend to be present uniformly throughout the lungs in uncomplicated asthma exacerbation. Asymmetry of auscultory findings might be caused by concomitant disease such as pneumonia, or by a complication of the asthma itself, such as occlusion of a large bronchus with a mucous plug. In severely ill patients, extreme bronchial plugging and loss of effective mechanical ventilation may be associated with disappearance of the wheezing and decrease in audible breath sounds. In critically ill patients, once alveolar ventilation has decreased significantly, they may have distant breath sounds along with hypoxemia and cyanosis.

Atopic Dermatitis

The findings on physical examination of a patient with atopic dermatitis vary widely. Individual lesions feature initial erythema followed by a fine papular eruption. The papules may coalesce to form ill-defined plaques, or they may progress to papulovesicles that may rupture to produce oozing and crusting. These lesions uniformly are markedly pruritic. Chronic lesions are characterized by lichenification. The skin appears thickened, coarse, and xerotic. There may be moderate scaling and alteration in pigmentation.

The distribution of the lesions varies with the age of the patient. In an infant 4 to 6 months of age, the initial lesions commonly occur on the cheeks, scalp, ears, and the neck. Older children typically have lesions in flexural areas specifically the antecubital and popliteal fossae. Adults may have localized involvement such as on the hands or generalized disease. Secondary bacterial infection is frequently present. Further details are described in Chapter 15.

Anaphylaxis, Urticaria, or Angioedema

During an anaphylactic episode, vital signs need to be closely monitored. Tachycardia and tachypnea are often present. Most anaphylaxis is accompanied by skin manifestations varying from flushing to urticaria and/or angioedema (33). Upper or lower airway involvement may be present with tongue/laryngeal edema or wheezing respectively. Severe laryngeal edema or bronchospasm may result in respiratory arrest; hypotension or cardiac arrest may occur with cardiovascular collapse.

Urticaria is suggested by erythematous lesions that blanch under pressure and resolve typically within hours without sequelae, such as bruising or discoloration. Angioedema involves subcutaneous swelling especially of the lips, eyelids, tongue, or genitals. IgE-mediated angioedema typically resolves in 24 to 48 hours without sequelae. Angioedema that is bradykinin-mediated may require 3 to 5 days to resolve.

■ OTHER EXAMINATIONS

Abnormalities of red cells or of the sedimentation rate are not associated with atopic disease. If such abnormalities are present, other illnesses or complications should be suspected. The differential white blood cell count is usually normal, with the frequent exception of eosinophilia that may range from 3% to 12%, especially in patients who have both atopic dermatitis and asthma. Higher eosinophil counts are not ordinarily seen in atopic diseases. The evaluation of eosinophilia is reviewed in Chapter 33.

Extensive laboratory evaluation for urticaria and angioedema is generally not required and is not cost effective. Laboratory evaluation and further work up including skin biopsy is suggested by the history. See Chapter 13 for further details.

Chest radiographs may be necessary to rule out concomitant disease or complications of asthma. Chest radiographs in patients with asthma may reveal hyperinflation or bronchial cuffing; however, most often they are normal (34). The utility of chest radiographs prior to admission for acute asthma exacerbations is controversial but radiographs are often recommended since they have been reported to reveal clinically significant abnormalities in 15% to 34% of patients (35–37). A screening sinus computed tomography (CT) scan without contrast material may be required in the evaluation of upper airways of patients with chronic or recurrent sinus infections. Conventional radiographs of the sinuses provide limited information and have high false-positive and false-negative rates (38).

Sputum Gram stain and culture, rhinoscopy, bronchoscopy, bronchial lavage, and electrocardiograms, as well as CT and magnetic resonance imaging (MRI) of the chest aid in the diagnosis of some patients. All or some of these procedures may be necessary to establish the correct diagnosis. Gross and microscopic findings in nasal secretions and in sputum have been described in allergic patients. These changes include eosinophils, Curschmann spirals, Charcot-Leyden crystals, and Creola bodies. Although these are interesting findings, their presence or absence may not be of diagnostic value.

Fractional exhaled nitric oxide (FeNO) is elevated in asthmatics and decreases after corticosteroid therapy and is a noninvasive measure of airway inflammation (39–41). FeNO has potential utility in managing asthma in terms of monitoring disease severity and adjusting anti-inflammatory therapy and is currently being utilized in research protocols as well as some clinical practices (42).

■ EVALUATION OF RESPIRATORY FUNCTION

Quantitative tests of ventilation can be of great value. They may yield some insight into the type and severity of the functional defect and, more importantly, may provide an objective means for assessing changes that may occur with time or may be induced by treatment. These tests are detailed in Chapter 32. It must be remembered that single sets of values describe conditions at designated points in time, and conditions such as asthma have rapid pathophysiologic changes. A flow–volume loop may demonstrate extrathoracic obstruction such as vocal cord dysfunction that may mimic asthma symptoms. Guidelines recommend spirometry both for diagnosis and periodic monitoring (43). More extensive pulmonary function testing in a specialized pulmonary function laboratory may be necessary if the office spirometry is indeterminate or shows severe abnormalities.

Provocation Tests

Although nasal or bronchial challenges with specific antigens to confirm immediate sensitivity are rarely performed in routine practice, they are nevertheless important tools in research studies. Nonspecific bronchial reactivity may be assessed with methacholine or histamine and is occasionally used to refute the diagnosis of asthma. Because positive methacholine challenges occur in patients with a variety of disorders, including allergic rhinitis, upper respiratory infections, chronic obstructive airway diseases, sarcoidosis, and in smokers, the utility of confirming a diagnosis is limited (44).

Food challenges may be necessary in the diagnosis of food allergy and open challenges are performed on a regular basis in clinical practice. Double-blind placebo-controlled food challenges are the gold standard in the diagnosis of food allergy and may occasionally be required. Provocation testing should be performed in a medically supervised setting with emergency equipment and treatment readily available. Details can be found in Chapter 14.

Skin Tests

Skin tests are the corroborative diagnostic test of choice for many allergic diseases. Used in the evaluation of conjunctivitis, rhinitis, asthma, and anaphylaxis, skin tests confirm or exclude allergic factors, such as airborne allergens, reactions to foods, certain drugs, and venom.

Pathogenesis of Skin Testing

Immediate response elicited by skin testing peaks in 15 to 20 minutes and involves production of the wheal-and-flare reaction characteristic of atopic sensitization. Mast cell degranulation and subsequent release of histamine and other mediators is responsible for the immediate reaction (45). The wheal and erythema reaction can be reproduced by introduction of histamine into the skin.

Skin Testing Techniques

Currently, two methods of skin testing are widely used: prick/puncture/epicutaneous tests and intradermal tests. Both are easy to perform, fairly reproducible, reliable, and relatively safe. The tests should be read in 15 to 20 minutes.

Prick/Puncture/Epicutaneous Test

Prick tests are more specific than intradermal tests in corroborating allergic disease (46,47). These tests can be performed with a minimum of equipment and are the most convenient and precise method of eliciting the presence of IgE antibodies. A drop of allergen extract is placed on the skin surface and a needle is gently penetrated into the epidermis through the drop. The epidermis is then gently raised without causing any bleeding. If appropriate antigen concentrations are used, there is relatively little risk of anaphylaxis, although large local skin reactions may occur occasionally.

Intradermal Test

If the skin-prick test result is negative, an intradermal test may be performed by injecting the allergen into the dermis. The skin is held tense and the needle is inserted almost parallel to its surface, just far enough to cover the beveled portion. Allergen extract (0.01 mL to 0.02 mL) is injected using a 26-gauge needle to form a small bleb. There is a small risk of a systemic reaction with intradermal testing. Therefore, dilute concentrations of the antigen are used. If the skin-prick test is positive, the intradermal test is not needed and should be avoided. Intradermal tests are more sensitive but less specific compared to prick tests. Some studies have questioned the clinical utility of intradermal testing if prick tests are negative (46,48,49). Intradermal testing to food allergens is avoided due to the high false-positive rate and the risk of systemic reactions. (50).

Grading of Skin Tests

Currently no standardized system exists for recording and interpreting skin test results. Many systems for grading positive reactions have been devised. A simple semi-quantitative system that measures wheal and erythema is shown in Table 8.2 (51). In general, a wheal size of 3 mm or greater than the negative control suggests the presence of allergen specific IgE antibody (52).

The tests rely on the skills of the tester. Both positive and negative controls must be performed for the proper interpretation of the test results. Histamine is the preferred agent for positive control. Saline or extract diluent may be used for the negative control. Because large reactions at adjacent test sites might coalesce, the test sites should be at least 2 cm apart (53). In cases of dermographism, there may be reactivity at the control site. This should be noted when the results of the tests are recorded. Interpretation of the tests is then more difficult. Tests that do not clearly have a greater reaction (of at least 3 mm) than the negative control should be considered indeterminate.

Variables Affecting Skin Testing

Site of Testing

The skin tests may be performed on the back or on the volar surface of the forearm. The back is more reactive than the forearm (53), but the clinical significance of the greater reactivity of the back is considered to be minimal. Skin testing on the forearm, however, enables

TABLE 8.2	GRADING SYSTEM FOR SKIN TESTING
GRADE	SKIN APPEARANCE
0	No reaction or a reaction no different than negative control
1+	Erythema less than 21 mm and larger than negative control No wheal formation
2+	Erythema larger than 21 mm and larger than negative control Wheal formation of less than 3 mm
3+	Erythema and wheal formation of 3 mm or greater without pseudopod
4+	Erythema and wheal formation of 3 mm or greater with pseudopod formation

Adapted from Doan T, Zeiss CR. Skin testing in allergy. *Allergy Proc* 1993;14:110–111; with permission.

the patient to witness the positive skin test results which may assist in patient education.

Age

Although all ages can be skin tested, skin reactivity has been demonstrated to be reduced in infants (<12 to 18 months of age) and the elderly (54,55).

Gender

There is no significant difference in skin test reactivity between males and females (55).

Medications

Antihistamines reduce skin reactivity to histamine and allergens and thus should be withheld for a period of time corresponding to three half-lives of the drug (56). Histamine (H_2) antagonists also may blunt dermal reactivity, although this is usually not clinically significant (57,58). Other medications, such as tricyclic antidepressants and chlorpromazine, can block skin test reactivity for extended periods of time and may need to be avoided for up to 2 weeks before testing (59).

Short courses of oral corticosteroids do not affect skin reactivity (60). Long-term systemic corticosteroid therapy may affect mast cell response; however, it does not appear to affect skin testing with airborne allergens (61,62). Topical corticosteroid preparations may inhibit skin reactivity and should not be applied at the site of testing for at least 1 week before testing (63). Leukotriene antagonists may affect skin tests, but this is usually not clinically significant. One study showed that montelukast given for 5 days suppressed the itching and flare response from skin prick tests but not the wheal size (64). β-agonists, theophylline, decongestants, cromolyn, and inhaled or nasal corticosteroids have no effect on skin reactivity.

Immunotherapy

Individuals who have previously received allergen immunotherapy can have diminished skin reactivity to allergens when repeat testing is performed (65–67). The diminution is less than 10-fold on end-point titration and therefore rarely clinically relevant.

Circadian Rhythm and Seasonal Variation

There are conflicting data whether cutaneous reactivity changes during the day (68,69). Testing during certain times of the year also may influence skin reactivity (70,71). These variations, however, are of no clinical significance.

Extracts

Skin testing should be performed with clinically relevant and potent allergens. Currently a number of standardized allergenic extracts are available and should be used when possible. Standardized extracts increase skin test reproducibility, decrease false positives, and facilitate cross-comparison among extracts from different physicians (72). Factors that decrease stability of extracts include extended periods of storage, temperatures above 40°F or below 33°F, and presence of proteases. Refrigeration of extracts and addition of glycerin diminishes loss of potency (73). Food extracts often lose potency over time and may be less stable. Prick testing with fresh plant food may be advisable if a food extract skin test is negative and there is suspicion for food allergy. Currently many recombinant allergen extracts are being investigated for skin testing. However these have not been approved for clinical practice (74,75)

Late Phase Response

Occasionally delayed reactions characterized by erythema and induration will occur at the site of skin tests. They become apparent 1 hour to 2 hours after application, peak at 6 hours to 12 hours, and usually disappear after 24 hours to 48 hours (76). In contrast to the immediate reactions, they are inhibited by conventional doses of corticosteroids but not by antihistamines (77,78). It is uncertain if the presence of a cutaneous late phase response (LPR) to an antigen will predict occurrence of LPR in the nose or lung of the same patient. Some investigators believe there is a correlation and others do not (79–83).

Adverse Reactions from Skin Testing

Large local reactions at the site of testing are the most common adverse reaction from skin testing. These usually resolve with cold compresses and antihistamines. Systemic reactions are rare but have been reported particularly with intradermal testing. They usually occur within 20 minutes of testing (84–86). Emergency treatment should be available during testing, and patients should be kept under observation for at least 20 minutes after testing. Patients with unstable asthma are at a greater risk of an adverse reaction from skin testing and should not be tested until their asthma is stabilized.

Interpretation of Skin Tests

A positive skin test result demonstrates only the presence of specific IgE antibody or sensitization. A positive result does not necessarily indicate that a person has an allergic disease; sensitization may not correspond with a clinically significant reaction to a specific antigen.

Both false-positive and false-negative skin test results may occur, due to improper technique. False-positive results may also result from dermatographism or from "irritant" reactions. For intradermal skin tests, injection of an excessive volume (>0.05mL) can cause mechanical irritation of the skin, resulting in false-positive results. False-negative skin tests may be caused by outdated extracts or decreased skin reactivity due to disease or age.

TABLE 8.3   INTERPRETATION OF SKIN TESTS

IF:	AND:	THEN:
History suggests sensitivity,	skin tests are positive,	strong possibility that antigen is responsible.
History does not suggest sensitivity,	skin test results are positive,	may want to observe patient during time of high natural exposure.
History suggests sensitivity,	skin tests are negative,	1. Review medications the patient has taken: antihistamines, antidepressants 2. Review other reasons for false-negative tests such as poor quality of testing materials or poor technique or assess for other conditions that cause similar symptoms 3. Observe patient during a period of high natural exposure 4. Perform provocative challenge (rarely)

Test Interpretations of Inhalant Allergens

Table 8.3 provides a guide for the interpretation of skin tests to aeroallergens. Population studies have demonstrated that asymptomatic individuals may have positive allergy results (87–90). Clinical history should guide the selection of aeroallergens to which skin prick tests are performed. Geographical location and antigen cross-reactivity should also be considered. Satisfactory information can usually be obtained with a relatively small number of tests that are carefully chosen. Positive skin tests with a corresponding history of clinical reactivity may strongly incriminate an antigen. Conversely, negative skin tests (to aeroallergens) with a negative history exclude the antigens as being clinically significant.

Interpretation of skin tests that do not correlate with the clinical history or physical findings is less straightforward. If there is no history suggesting sensitivity to an aeroallergen, and the skin test result is positive, the patient can be interviewed and examined during a period of maximal exposure to the antigen (i.e., peak pollen season). At that time, if there are no symptoms or physical findings of allergic disease, the positive skin test finding may be ignored based on the lack of clinical relevance. Positive results may also precede the onset of clinical symptoms (88,89). A study of college students (89) demonstrated that asymptomatic students who were skin test positive were more than twice as likely to develop allergic rhinitis 23 years later than asymptomatic students who were skin test negative. Having positive skin tests was found to be a significant risk factor for developing asthma as well.

Test Interpretations of Foods

In general, properly performed skin prick tests to food allergens have a high negative predictive value (>95%) (91,92), but the positive predictive value is much lower at 30% to 65% (91–95). Therefore, a positive test indicates sensitization that may or may not be symptomatic. As with aeroallergens, a response of a 3-mm wheal or greater (associated with a flare) indicates the presence of specific IgE in the setting of a negative saline response. Larger wheal sizes (>8 mm to 10 mm) indicate an even greater likelihood of clinical reactivity with ingestion (95). Intradermal testing is contraindicated for food allergens due to its high false-positive rate and risk of systemic reactions.

Occasionally, patients with a history highly suggestive for allergic disease may have negative skin test results for the suspected antigens. In these cases, the history and physical exam should be revisited, and the possibility of false-negative skin test results must be excluded.

Skin testing for Hymenoptera venoms, latex allergy, and drug hypersensitivity is discussed in Chapters 12 and 17.

■ *IN VITRO* MEASUREMENT OF IgE ANTIBODIES

Total Serum IgE

Total serum IgE is generally elevated in atopic individuals, especially patients with atopic dermatitis. However, concentrations fluctuate widely around a mean of 125 IU/mL (300 ng/mL) among atopic and nonatopic individuals (96–99). Generally, measuring total IgE is not of diagnostic significance and rarely provides useful information (100,101).

Total serum IgE determinations are indicated in patients suspected of having allergic bronchopulmonary allergic aspergillosis, both in the diagnosis and monitoring of the course of the disease (102). IgE concentrations are also necessary in the evaluation of certain immunodeficiencies such as hyper-IgE (or Job) syndrome.

Specific IgE (sIgE)

In vitro procedures detect allergen specific (sIgE) antibodies in the patient's serum. High quality *in vitro* tests are comparable to skin tests in diagnostic value, especially for demonstration of aeroallergen and food sensitivity (103–108). Although skin testing is the diagnostic test of choice for IgE-mediated disease, *in vitro* testing may be indicated in specific circumstances:

1. Because there are no medications that interfere with *in vitro* testing, this modality may be useful in patients who are unable to withhold medications with antihistamine properties.
2. In patients with a history of extreme sensitivity to allergens, use of *in vitro* tests would avoid uncomfortable local reactions potentially associated with skin testing. Moreover, there is no risk of anaphylaxis with *in vitro* testing.
3. In patients who demonstrate dermatographism or have skin lesions affecting testing sites (i.e., forearm or back), *in vitro* testing may be preferable over skin testing.

"RAST" or the radioallergosorbent test is the colloquial term that refers to an antiquated *in vitro* method of measuring sIgE. Although this is no longer the method used in most laboratories, the name has stuck. The most predictive and most useful method of measuring sIgE is the Phadia CAP system (Uppsala, Sweden), a fluoroenzyme-immunoassay (FEIA) that has been approved for use by the U.S. Food and Drug Administration. This is a quantitative test with a reportable range of 0.1 kU$_A$/L to 100 kU$_A$/L. This assay, also referred to as ImmunoCAP, has been used in prior studies (108–111) to define diagnostic points for certain foods (112). These data curves have been generated for some of the more common food allergens, including egg, milk, peanut, and fish (108). It is important to note that higher sIgE levels do not correlate with severity of reactions but rather they indicate an increased probability of a food-induced reaction. Therefore, the 95% predictive values are helpful in determining which patients are at higher risk of developing a reaction with ingestion and in whom oral challenges may not be advisable. On the other hand, there are limitations to this assay as patients (up to 20%, depending on the food) may react to a food despite very low or undetectable levels of food sIgE as demonstrated by oral challenges (108). Simply establishing the presence of sIgE against allergens (sensitization), whether measured *in vivo* or *in vitro*, does not automatically designate disease or clinical relevance in a given patient. Among children who have elevated sIgE to food as measured by ImmunoCAP, Perry et al. (114) demonstrated that those without a clear history of a food reaction were more likely to be tolerant to the food in double-blind placebo-controlled food challenges. Therefore, sensitization may be symptomatic (as in food allergy) or asymptomatic (as in food tolerance).

In contrast to foods, diagnostic values for *in vitro* tests have not yet been firmly established for aeroallergens. As a rule, test results must correlate with allergic signs and symptoms to a specific antigen to have any meaning. Consequently, the history and physical examination carefully performed by the physician remain the fundamental investigative procedure for the diagnosis of allergic disease.

■ REFERENCES

1. Mrinho S, Simpson A, Lowe L, et al. Rhinoconjunctivitis in 5-year-old children: a population-based birth cohort study. *Allergy.* 2007;62(4):385–393.
2. Grasi M, Bugiani M, de Marco R. Investigating indicators and determinants of asthma in young adults. *European J Epidemiol.* 2006;21(11):831–842.
3. Ramey JT, Bailen E, Lockey RF. Rhinitis medicamentosa. *J Investig Allergol Clin Immunol.* 2006;16 (3):148–155.
4. Hanania NA, Singh S, El-Wali R, et al. The safety and effects of the beta-blocker, nadolol, in mild asthma: an open-label pilot study. *Pulm Pharmacol Therap.* 2008;21(1):134–141.
5. Brooks TW, Creekmore FM, Young DC, et al. Rates of hospitalizations and emergency department visits in patients with asthma and chronic obstructive pulmonary disease taking beta-blockers. *Pharmacotherapy.* 2007;27(5):684–690.
6. Zaid G, Beall GN. Bronchial response to beta-adrenergic blockade. *N Engl J Med.* 1966;275:580–584.
7. Tumanan-Mendoza BA, Dans AL, Villacin LL, et al. Dechallenge and rechallenge method showed different incidences of cough among four ACE-Is. *J Clin Epidemiol.* 2007;20(6):547–553.
8. Grant NN, Deeb ZE, Chia SH. Clinical experience with angiotensin-converting enzyme inhibitor-induced angioedema. *Otolaryngol Head Neck Surg.* 2007;137(6):931–935.
9. Graf P. Rhinitis medicamentosa: a review of causes and treatment. *Treat Respir Med.* 2005;4(1):21–29.
10. Spector SL, Raizman MB. Conjunctivitis medicamentosa. *J Allergy Clin Immunol.* 1994;94(1):134–136.
11. Food Allergy: A practice parameter. *Ann Allergy Asthma Immunol.* 2006;96:S1–S68.
12. Pulimood TB, Corden JM, Bryden C, et al. Epidemic asthma and the role of the fungal mold Alternaria alternata. *J Allergy Clin Immunol.* 2007;120(3):610–617.
13. O'Hollaren MT, Yunginger JW, Offord KP, et al. Exposure to an aeroallergen as a possible precipitating factor in respiratory arrest in young patients with asthma. *New Engl J Med.* 1991;325(3):206–208.
14. Sears MR, Greene JM, Willan AR, et al. A longitudinal, population-based, cohort study of childhood asthma followed into adulthood. *N Engl J Med.* 2003;349:1414–1422.
15. Chinn S, Heinrich J, Anto JM, et al. Bronchial responsiveness in atopic adults increases with exposure to cat allergen. *Am J Respir Crit Care.* 2007;176(1):20–26.
16. Salo PM, Arbes SJ Jr, Crockett PW, et al. Exposure to multiple indoor allergens in US homes and its relationship to asthma. *J Allergy Clin Immunol.* 2008;121(3):678–684.
17. Platts-Mills TAE, Chapman MD. Dust mites: immunology, allergic diseases, and environmental control. *J Allergy Clin Immunol.* 1987;80:755–775.
18. Valdivieso R, Iraola V, Estupinan M, et al. Sensitization and exposure to house dust and storage mites in high-altitude areas of Ecuador. *Ann Allergy Asthma Immunol.* 2006;97(4):532–538.
19. Korsgaard J, Harving H. House-dust mites and summer cottages. *Allergy.* 2005;60(9):1200–103.
20. Rosentreich D, Eggleston P, Kattan M, et al. The role of cockroach allergy and exposure to cockroach allergen in causing morbidity among inner-city children with asthma. *N Engl J Med.* 1997;336:1356–1363.
21. Gruchalla RS, Pongracic J, Plaut M, et al. Inner city asthma study: relationships among sensitivity, allergen exposure, and asthma morbidity. *J Allergy Clin Immunol.* 2005;115(3):478–485.
22. Mata P, Charpin P, Charpin C, et al. Fel d 1 allergen: skin or saliva? *Ann Allergy.* 1992;69:321–322.

23. Dornelas de Andrade A, Birnbaum J, Magalon C, et al. Fel d 1 levels in cat anal glands. *Clin Exp Allergy.* 1996;26:178–180.

24. Siraganian RP, Sandberg AL. Characterization of mouse allergens. *J Allergy Clin Immunol.* 1979;63(6):435–442.

25. Liccardi G, D'Amato G, Russo M, et al. Focus on cat allergen (Fel d 1): immunological and aerodynamic characteristics, modality of airway sensitization and avoidance strategies. *Int Arch Allergy Immunol.* 2003;132(1):1–12.

26. Fahlbusch B, Rudeschko O, Szilagyi U, et al. Purification and partial characterization of the major allergen, Cav p 1, from guinea pig Cavia porcellus. *Allergy.* 2002;57(5):417–422.

27. Choi JH, Kim HM, Park HS. Allergic asthma and rhinitis caused by household rabbit exposure: identification of serum-specific IgE and its allergens. *J Korean Med Sci.* 2007;22(5):820–824.

28. Niitsuma T, Tsuji A, Nukaga M, et al. Thirty cases of bronchial asthma associated with exposure to pet hamsters. *J Investig Allergol Clin Immunol.* 2004;14(3):221–224.

29. Krakowiak A, Wiszniewska M, Krawczyk P, et al. Risk factors associated with airway allergic diseases from exposure to laboratory animal allergens among veterinarians. *Int Arch Occup Environ Health.* 2007;80(6):465–475.

30. Ruoppi P, Loistinen T, Susitaival P, et al. Frequency of allergic rhinitis to laboratory animals in university employees as confirmed by chamber challenges. *Allergy.* 2004;59(3):295–301.

31. Bernstein JA, Alexis N, Bacchus H, et al. The health effects of nonindustrial indoor air pollution. *J Allergy Clin Immunol.* 2008; 121(3):585–591.

32. Green RM, Custovic A, Sanderson G, et al. Synergism between allergens and viruses and risk of hospital admission with asthma: case-control study. *BMJ.* 2002;324:763–769.

33. Webb LM, Lieberman P. Anaphylaxis: a review of 601 cases. *Ann Allergy Asthma Immunol.* 2006;97(1):39–43.

34. Findley LJ, Sahn SA. The value of chest roentgenograms in acute asthma in adults. *Chest.* 1981;80:535–536.

35. Brooks LJ, Cloutier MM, Afshani E. Significance of roentgenographic abnormalities in children hospitalized for asthma. *Chest.* 1982;82:315–318.

36. Pickup CM, Nee PA, Randall PE. Radiographic features in 1016 adults admitted to hospital with acute asthma. *J Accid Emerg Med.* 1994;11(4):234–237.

37. White CS, Cole RP, Lubetsky HW, et al. Acute asthma. Admission chest radiography in hospitalized patients. *Chest.* 1991;100(1):14–16.

38. Mafee MF, Tran BH, Chapa AR. Imaging of rhinosinusitis and its complications: plain film, CT, and MRI. *Clin Rev Allergy Immunol.* 2006;30(3):165–186.

39. Kharitonov SA, Yates DH, Robbins R, et al. Increased nitric oxide in exhaled air of asthmatic patients. *Lancet.* 1994;343:133–135.

40. Yates D, Kharitonov S, Robbins R, et al. Effect of a nitric oxide synthase inhibitor and a glucocorticoid on exhaled nitric oxide. *Am J Respir Crit Care Med.* 1995;152:892–896.

41. Strunk R, Szefler S, Phillips BR, et al. Relationship of exhaled nitric oxide to clinical and inflammatory markers of persistent asthma in children. *J Allergy Clin Immunol.* 2003;112:883–892.

42. Smith AD, Cowan JO, Brassett KP, et al. Use of exhaled nitric oxide measurements to guide treatment in chronic asthma. *N Engl J Med.* 2005;352:2163–2173.

43. Expert Panel Report 3: *Guidelines for the Diagnosis and Management of Asthma.* Bethesda, MD:National Heart, Lung, and Blood Institute, 2007.

44. Guidelines for methacholine and exercise challenge testing—1999. *Am J Respir Crit Care Med.* 2000;161:309–329.

45. Friedman MM, Kaliner M. Ultrastructural changes in human skin mast cells during antigen-induced degranulation in vivo. *J Allergy Clin Immunol.* 1988;82: 988–1005.

46. Nelson HS, Oppenheimer J, Buchmeier A, et al. An assessment of the role of intradermal skin testing in the diagnosis of clinically relevant allergy to timothy grass. *J Allergy Clin Immunol.* 1996;97:1193–1201.

47. Idrajana T, Spieksma FTM, Vorrhorst R. Comparative study of the intracutaneous, scratch, and prick tests in allergy. *Ann Allergy.* 1997;29:639–660.

48. Wood RA, Phipatanakul W, Hamilton RG, et al. A comparison of skin prick tests, intradermal skin tests, and RASTS in the diagnosis of cat allergy. *J Allergy Clin Immunol.* 1999;103:773–779.

49. Schwindt PG, Hutcheson CS, Leu SY, et al. Role of intradermal skin tests in the evaluation of clinically relevant respiratory allergy assessed using patient history and nasal challenges. *Ann Allergy Asthma Immunol.* 2005;94:627–633.

50. Bock SA, Lee WY, Remigio L, et al. Appraisal of skin tests with food extracts for diagnosis of food hypersensitivity. *Clin Allergy.* 1978;8:559–564.

51. Doan T, Zeiss CR. Skin testing in allergy. *Allergy Proc.* 1993;14:110–111.

52. Practice parameters for allergy diagnostic testing. *Ann Allergy Asthma Immunol.* 1995;75:543–625.

53. Nelson HS, Knoetzer J, Bucher B. Effect of distance between sites and region of the body on results of skin prick tests. *J Allergy Clin Immunol.* 1996;97: 596–601.

54. Menardo JL, Bousquet J, Rodiere M, et al. Skin test reactivity in infancy. *J Allergy Clin Immunol.* 1985;75;646–651.

55. Skassa-Brociek W, Manderscheid JC, Michel FB, et al. Skin test reactivity to histamine from infancy to old age. *J Allergy Clin Immunol.* 1987;80;711–716.

56. van Steelkelenburg J, Clement PA, Beel MH. Comparison of five new antihistamines (H1-receptor antagonists) in patients with allergic rhinitis using nasal provocation studies and skin tests. *Allergy.* 2002;57(4):346–350.

57. Harvey RP, Schocket AL. The effect of H_1 and H_2 blockage on cutaneous histamine response in man. *J Allergy Clin Immunol.* 1980;65:136–139.

58. Kupczyk M, Kuprys I, Bochenska-Marciniak M, et al. Ranitidine (150 mg daily) inhibits wheal, flare, and itching reactions in skin-prick tests. *Allergy & Asthma Proceedings.* 2007;28(6):711–715.

59. Rao KS, Menon PK, Hilman BC, et al. Duration of the suppressive effect of tricyclic antidepressants on histamine-induced wheal-and-flare reactions in human skin. *J Allergy Clin Immunol.* 1988;82:752–757.

60. Slott RJ, Zweiman B. A controlled study of the effects of corticosteroids on immediate skin test reactivity. *J Allergy Clin Immunol.* 1974;54:229–235.

61. Olson R, Karpink MH, Shelanki S, et al. Skin reactivity to codeine and histamine during prolonged corticosteroid therapy. *J Allergy Clin Immunol.* 1990;86:153–159.

62. Des Roches A, Paradis L, Bougeard YH, et al. Long-term oral corticosteroid therapy does not alter the results of immediate-type allergy skin prick tests. *J Allergy Clin Immunol.* 1996;98(3):522–527.

63. Pipkorn U, Hammarlund A, Enerbäck L. Prolonged treatment with topical glucocorticoids results in an inhibition of the allergen-induced weal-and-flare response and a reduction in skin mast cell numbers and histamine content. *Clin Exp Allergy.* 1989;19(1):19–25.

64. Kupczyk M, Kuprys I, Gorski P, et al. The effect of montelukast (10 mg daily) and loratadine (10 mg daily) on wheal, flare, and itching reactions in skin prick tests. *Pulm Pharmacol Therap.* 2007;20(1):85–89.

65. Varney VA, Tabbah K, Mavroleon G, et al. Usefulness of specific immunotherapy in patients with severe perennial allergic rhinitis induced by house dust mite: a double-blind, randomized, placebo-controlled trial. *Clin Exp Allergy.* 2003;33(8):1076–1082.

66. Eng PA, Reinhold M, Gnehm HM. Long-term efficacy of preseasonal grass pollen immunotherapy in children. *Allergy.* 2002;57(4): 306–312.

67. Graft DF, Schuberth KC, Kagey-Sobotka A, et al. The development of negative skin tests in children treated with venom immunotherapy. *J Allergy Clin Immunol.* 1984;73:61–68.

68. Paquet F, Boulet LP, Bedard G, et al. Influence of time of administration on allergic skin prick tests response. *Ann Allergy.* 1991; 67:163–166.

69. Seery JP, James SM, Ind PW, et al. Circadian rhythm of cutaneous hypersensitivity reactions in nocturnal asthma. *Ann Allergy Asthma Immunol.* 1998;30:329–330.

70. Haahtela T, Jokela H. Influence of the pollen season on immediate skin test reactivity to common allergens. *Allergy.* 1980;35:15–21.

71. Nahm DH, Park HS, Kang SS, et al. Seasonal variation of skin reactivity and specific IgE antibody to house dust mite. *Ann Allergy Asthma Immunol.* 1997;78:589–593.

72. American Academy of Allergy, Asthma, and Immunology Position Paper. The use of standardized allergen extracts. *J Allergy Clin Immunol.* 1999;99:583–586.

73. Plunkett G. Stability of allergen extracts used in skin testing and immunotherapy. *Curr Opin Otolaryngol Head Neck Surg.* 2008;16: 285–291.

74. Champman MD, Smith AM, Vailes LD, et al. Recombinant allergens for diagnosis and therapy of allergic disease. *J Allergy Clin Immunol.* 2000;106:419–418.

75. Astier C, Morisset M, Roitel O, et al. Predictive value of skin prick tests using recombinant allergens for diagnosis of peanut allergy. *J Allergy Clin Immunol.* 2006;118:250–256.

76. Reshef A, Kagey-Sobotka A, Adkinson N Jr, et al. The pattern and kinetics in human skin of erythema and mediators during the acute and late-phase response (LPR). *J Allergy Clin Immunol.* 1989;84: 678–687.

77. Umemoto L, Poothullil J, Dolovich J, et al. Factors which influence late cutaneous allergic responses. *J Allergy Clin Immunol.* 1976;58:60–68.

78. Poothullil J, Umemoto L, Dolovich J, et al. Inhibition by prednisone of late cutaneous allergic response induced by antiserum to human IgE. *J Allergy Clin Immunol.* 1976;57:164–167.

79. Atkins PC, Martin GL, Yost R, Zweiman B. Late onset reactions in humans: correlation between skin and bronchial reactivity. *Ann Allergy.* 1988;60:27–30.

80. Price KF, Hey EN, Soothill JF. Antigen provocation to the skin, nose, and lung in children with asthma: immediate and dual hypersensitivity reactions. *Clin Exp Immunol.* 1982;47:587–594.

81. Warner JO. Significance of late reactions after bronchial challenge with house dust mite. *Arch Dis Child.* 1976; 51:905–911.

82. Boulet LP, Robert RS, Dolovich JE, et al. Prediction of late asthmatic responses to inhaled allergen. *Clin Allergy.* 1984;14:379–385.

83. Taylor G, Shivalkor PR. Arthus-type reactivity in the nasal airways and skin in pollen sensitive subjects. *Clin Allergy.* 1971;1:407–414.

84. Valyasevi MA, Maddox DE, Li JT. Systemic reactions to allergy skin tests. *Ann Allergy Asthma Immunol.* 1999;83:132–136.

85. Lockey RF, Benedict LM, Turkeltaub PC, et al. Fatalities from immunotherapy (IT) and skin testing (ST). *J Allergy Clin Immunol.* 1987;79:660–677.

86. Codreanu F, Moneret-Vautrin DA, Morriset M, et al. The risks of systemic reactions to skin prick-tests using food allergens. CICBAA data and literature review. *Eur Ann Allergy Clin Immunol.* 2006;38(2): 52–54.

87. Droste JH, Kerkhof M, de Monchy JGR, et al. Association of skin test reactivity, specific IgE, total IgE, and eosinophils with nasal symptoms in a community based population study. *J Allergy Clin Immunol.* 1996;97(4):922–932.

88. Hagy GW, Settipane GA. Prognosis of positive allergy skin tests in asymptomatic population. A three year followup of college students. *J Allergy Clin Immunol.* 1971;48(4):200–212.

89. Settipane RJ, Hagy GW, Settipane GA. Long-term risk factors for developing asthma and allergic rhinitis: a 23-year follow-up study of college students. *Allergy Proc.* 1994;15(1):21–25.

90. Pastorello EA, Incorvaia C, Ortolani C, et al. Studies on the relationship between the level of specific IgE antibodies and the clinical expression of allergy: I. Definition of levels distinguishing patients with symptomatic from patients with asymptomatic allergy to common aeroallergens. *J Allergy Clin Immunol.* 1995;96(5Pt1):580–587.

91. Bock SA, Buckley J, Holst A, et al. Proper use of skin tests with food extracts in diagnosis of food hypersensitivity. *Clin Allergy.* 1977;7(4):375–383.

92. Sampson HA, Albergo R. Comparison of results of skin tests, RAST, and double-blind, placebo-controlled food challenges in children with atopic dermatitis. *J Allergy Clin Immunol.* 1984;74(1):26–33.

93. Sampson HA, Scanlon SM. Natural history of food hypersensitivity in children with atopic dermatitis. *J Pediatr.* 1989;115(1):23–27.

94. Burks AW, James JM, Hiegel A, et al. Atopic dermatitis and food hypersensitivity reactions. *J Pediatr.* 1998;132(1):132–136.

95. Hill DJ, Hosking CS, Reyes-Bonito LV. Reducing the need for food allergen challenges in young children: a comparison of in vitro with in vivo tests. *Clin Exp Allergy.* 2001;31(7):1031–1035.

96. Klink M, Cline MG, Halonen M, et al. Problems in defining normal limits for serum IgE. *J Allergy Clin Immunol.* 1990;85(2):440–444.

97. Sunyer J, Anto JM, Castellsague J, et al. Total serum IgE is associated with asthma independently of specific IgE levels. *Eur Respir J.* 1996;9(9):1880–1884.

98. Luoma R, Koivikko A, Viander M. Development of asthma, allergic rhinitis and atopic dermatitis by the age of five years. *Allergy.* 1983;38(5):339–346.

99. Peat JK, Toelle BG, Dermand J, et al. Serum IgE levels, atopy, and asthma in young adults: results from a longitudinal cohort study. *Allergy.* 1996;51(11):804–810.

100. Ezeamuzie CI, Ali-Ali AF, Al-Dowaisan A, et al. Reference values of total serum IgE and their significance in the diagnosis of allergy among the young adult Kuwaiti population. *Clin Exp Allergy.* 1999;29(3):375–381.

101. Wittig HJ, Belloit J, De Fillippi L, et al. Age-related serum immunoglobulin E levels in healthy subjects and in patients with allergic disease. *J Allergy Clin Immunol.* 1980;66(4):305–313.

102. Roberts ML, Greenberger PA. Serologic analysis of allergic bronchopulmonary aspergillosis. In: Patterson R, Greenberger PA, eds. *Allergic Bronchopulmonary Aspergillosis.* Providence, RI: Oceanside Publications, 1995:11–15.

103. Anonymous. The use of in vitro tests for IgE antibody in the specific diagnosis of IgE-mediated disorders and in the formulation of allergen immunotherapy. *J Allergy Clin Immunol.* 1992;90(2):263–267.

104. Plebani M, Borghesan F, Faggian D. Clinical efficiency of in vitro and in vivo tests for allergic diseases. *Ann Allergy Asthma Immunol.* 1995;74(1):23–28.

105. Williams PB, Dolen WK, Koepke JW, et al. Comparison of skin testing and three in vitro assays for specific IgE in the clinical evaluation of immediate hypersensitivity. *Ann Allergy.* 1992;68(1):35–42.

106. Kam KL, Hsieh KH. Comparison of three in vitro assays for serum IgE with skin testing in asthmatic children. *Ann Allergy.* 1994;73(4): 329–336.

107. Kelso JM, Sodhi N, Gosselm VA, et al. Diagnostic performance characteristics of the standard Phadebas RAST, modified RAST, and Pharmacia CAP system versus skin testing. *Ann Allergy.* 1991; 67(5):511–514.

108. Nepper-Christensen S, Backer V, DuBuske LM, Nolte H. In vitro diagnostic evaluation of patients with inhalant allergies: summary of probability outcomes comparing results of CLA- and CAP-specific immunoglobulin E test systems. *Allergy Asthma Proc.* 2003;24(4):253–2258.

109. Sampson HA. Utility of food-specific IgE concentrations in predicting symptomatic food allergy. *J Allergy Clin Immunol.* 2001; 107(5):891–896.

110. Boyano MT, Garcia-Ara C, Diaz-Pena JM, et al. Validity of specific IgE antibodies in children with egg allergy. *Clin Exp Allergy.* 2001; 31(9):1464–1469.

111. Garcia-Ara C, Boyano-Martinez T, Diaz-Pena JM, et al. Specific IgE levels in the diagnosis of immediate hypersensitivity to cows' milk protein in the infant. *J Allergy Clin Immunol.* 2001;107(1):185–190.

112. Clark AT, Ewan PW. Interpretation of tests for nut allergy in one thousand patients, in relation to allergy or tolerance. *Clin Exp Allergy.* 2003;33(8):1041–1045.

113. Sampson HA. Update on food allergy. *J Allergy Clin Immunol.* 2004;113(5):805–819.

114. Perry TT, Matsui EC, Conover-Walker MK, Wood RA. The relationship of allergen-specific IgE levels and oral food challenge outcome. *J Allergy Clin Immunol.* 2004;114(1):144–149.

CHAPTER 9

Physiologic and Biologic Evaluation of Allergic Lung Diseases

RAVI KALHAN AND JANE E. DEMATTE

Allergic and immunologic lung disease can be assessed through a variety of physiologic and biologic measurements. Physiologic measurements include comprehensive pulmonary function testing, such as forced spirometry, measurement of lung volumes, and determination of diffusing capacity. Peak expiratory flow measurement is easy to obtain and may serve as a useful surrogate for complete spirometric evaluation. Bronchoprovocation testing represents a combined physiologic–biologic approach to assessing airway hyperreactivity, and fraction of expired nitric oxide is a biologic test that correlates with the amount of eosinophilic inflammation in the airways. Finally, bronchoalveolar lavage fluid provides a window into the biologic make-up of lung inflammatory cells and can be used in the diagnosis of hypersensitivity pneumonitis and eosinophilic pneumonia.

■ SPIROMETRY

Essential Components of Forced Spirometry

Forced spirometry is an important component of pulmonary function testing and the key component of the physiologic assessment of obstructive airways diseases. The American Thoracic Society (ATS)/European Respiratory Society (ERS) task force on the Standardization of Lung Function Testing assert several indications for spirometry including diagnosis and monitoring of diseases that affect lung function and determining prognosis or response to therapeutic interventions in those diseases (1). A forced spirometry contains the following components:

- The *forced vital capacity (FVC)* is the maximum amount of air exhaled with a maximal forced effort from total lung capacity (TLC).

- The *forced expiratory volume in 1 second (FEV_1)* is the maximal volume of air exhaled in the first second of the FVC maneuver.
- The *mean forced expiratory flow between 25% and 75% of the FVC ($FEF_{25-75\%}$)*, also termed the *maximum mid-expiratory flow* (MMEF), provides a measurement of expiratory flow during the middle phase of the FVC maneuver and provides a measure of small airways obstruction albeit an inconsistent and nonspecific one in individual patients (1,2).

With worsening obstructive airways disease, airflow at low lung volumes can become very slow, and it may be difficult for older patients, or those with severe airflow obstruction, to sustain a complete FVC maneuver. Some experts have therefore advocated the use of the *forced expiratory volume in 6 second (FEV_6)*, the volume of air exhaled in the first 6 seconds of the FVC maneuver, as a substitute for FVC (3,4). The *FEV_1/FVC ratio (or FEV_1/FEV_6 ratio)* can be calculated from the above data and, when low, serves as one of the defining features of obstructive airways disease. A *flow-volume loop* is also constructed as a part of forced spirometry and when analyzed visually can reinforce the presence of airflow obstruction, provide an early indication of airflow obstruction when the FEV_1/FVC ratio is not yet reduced, and provide information regarding extrathoracic (upper airway) obstruction.

The *peak expiratory flow (PEF)* is the maximum expiratory flow achieved from a forced expiration starting, without hesitation, from TLC. *Reversibility testing* can be obtained as a part of forced spirometry by repeat testing after administration of a bronchodilator. Patients are considered to have reversible airflow obstruction when, following the administration of a bronchodilator, the FEV_1 and/or FVC increases by more than 12% *and* 200 mL in a single testing session. Repeat spirometry should be performed 10 minutes to 15 minutes after administration of a short-acting beta-agonist or 30 minutes after administration of a short-acting anticholinergic (2). Increases of less than 8% in FEV_1 or FVC are likely related to normal variability of the test and do not represent significant responses to a bronchodilator (5).

The FVC maneuver has three phases: maximal inspiration to TLC from relaxed breathing, a forced exhalation, and continued complete exhalation until the end of the test. Because false reductions in FEV_1 and PEF have been observed when the maximal inspiration is slow or there is a prolonged pause at TLC (6), the initial inspiration should be fast and pauses at TLC minimized. For an accurate FVC maneuver, specific criteria for the end of the test are essential. The volume-time

curve should show no change in volume for 1 second or greater, and the patient should have tried to exhale for 3 seconds or longer if younger than 10 years old or 6 seconds or longer if 10 years or older (7). In summary, an adequate FVC maneuver must have a maximum inspiration, a rapid start followed by a smooth continuous exhalation, and maximal effort until the volume-time curve reaches a plateau. Idealized flow-volume loops and volume-time curves are shown in Fig. 9.1.

Spirometry in Asthma

The Expert Panel Report 3 of the National Asthma Education and Prevention Program (NAEPP) of the

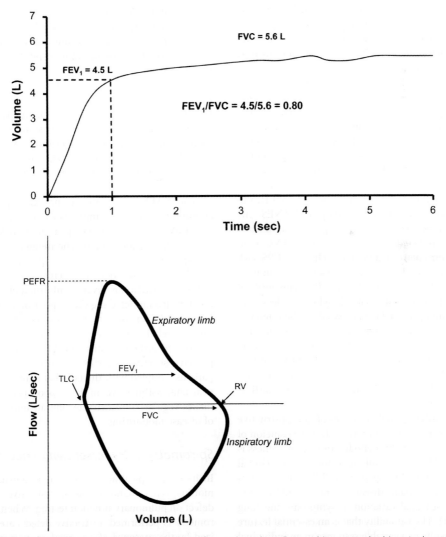

■ **FIGURE 9.1** Stereotypical volume-time curve (top) and flow-volume loop (bottom) in a normal subject. In the volume-time curve, approximately 80% of volume is expired in the first second resulting in a normal FEV_1/FVC ratio of 0.80. The quality of the maneuver is documented by a volume-plateau at the termination of the test after 6 seconds. After inspiration to total lung capacity (TLC), the expiratory limb of the flow-volume loop has a sharp increase in peak expiratory flow rate (PEFR) and then a smooth deceleration in flow over the entire expiration until complete at residual volume (RV).

National Heart, Lung, and Blood Institute recommends the use of forced spirometry in asthma at the following four time periods (3):

1. When the diagnosis of asthma is being considered
2. At the time of initial assessment
3. After treatment is initiated and symptoms have stabilized to document attainment of normal or near-normal airway function
4. At least every year to 2 years to assess the maintenance of airway function

While clinical symptoms are important factors in diagnosing asthma, symptoms often do not correlate well with lung function in either adults or children (8–11) creating a well-documented disconnect between severity of asthma symptoms and severity of airflow obstruction (12). The NAEPP further recommends that forced spirometry should be followed over the patient's lifetime to detect the possible rate in decline in lung function over time (3).

Airway obstruction that is spontaneously reversible or reversible with medical intervention on forced spirometry is a principle clinical feature of asthma (3). The ATS/ERS task force defines an obstructive ventilatory defect as occurring when there is a disproportionate reduction of *maximum airflow* relative to *maximum volume* (i.e., FVC) that can be displaced from the lung (2). Obstructive defects are identified on spirometry by a reduction in the FEV_1/FVC ratio. The National Health and Nutrition Examination survey (NHANES III) derived reference equations (13) provide ethnically appropriate predicted values for the FEV_1/FVC ratio and other spirometric parameters. The ATS/ERS task force suggests that obstruction is present when an individual's FEV_1/FVC ratio is below the fifth percentile of the predicted value or alternatively when it is less than the lower limit of normal (LLN) based on the reference equations (2). While in small airways obstruction the $FEF_{25-75\%}$ can be reduced as well, and often this occurs earlier in disease than a decrease in the FEV_1, abnormalities in MMEF are not specific for small airways disease and should not be used to identify airflow obstruction (2).

After identifying the presence of an obstructive defect in patients in whom there is clinical suspicion of asthma, assessment of bronchodilator responsiveness is appropriate. The Global Initiative for Asthma Global Strategy for Asthma Management and Prevention notes that asthma is a variable disease characterized by daily, monthly, or seasonal variation in symptoms and lung function (14). The variability that is an essential feature of asthma results in a variable response in an individual patient to bronchodilator testing. An individual patient is unlikely to exhibit bronchodilator responsiveness every time he or she is tested, particularly if the disease is well-controlled (14). Repeated testing at different times, therefore, is important to confirm the diagnosis of asthma as well as assess asthma control (3,14).

After an FEV_1/FVC ratio less than the LLN is detected by spirometry, the ATS/ERS task force recommends that the severity of airflow obstruction be assessed by the magnitude of reduction in the FEV_1.

- Mild obstruction—FEV_1 >70% predicted, but below LLN
- Moderate obstruction—FEV_1 60% to 69% predicted
- Moderately severe obstruction—FEV_1 50% to 59% predicted
- Severe obstruction—FEV_1 35% to 49% predicted
- Very severe obstruction—FEV_1 < 35% predicted

Obstructive ventilatory defects are visually detected by a delayed plateau on the volume-time curve as well as "scooping," "coving," or upward concavity to the shape of the expiratory limb of a flow-volume curve (Fig. 9.2). The inspiratory limb of the flow-volume loop is normal in asthma. If the inspiratory limb is flattened, extrathoracic causes of airflow obstruction should be considered. Vocal cord dysfunction (VCD) can clinically mimic asthma and has been reported to be concomitant with asthma in many patients (15). When asthma symptoms persist despite therapy, a flattening of the inspiratory limb of the flow-loop, termed *variable extrathoracic obstruction,* can prove useful in raising suspicion of VCD as an etiology of persistent symptoms.

The NAEPP recommends periodic spirometry in addition to assessing symptoms (3) as individuals with low FEV_1 represent a group at high risk for acute asthma exacerbations (16). The frequency of performing spirometry in an individual patient depends on whether he or she does not perceive symptoms until airflow obstruction is severe. Unfortunately, there is no good means for detecting these "poor perceivers" (3). It has been documented that in asthma patients, there is little correlation between FEV_1 and self-perception of severity of airflow obstruction (17). This inability to perceive severity of airflow obstruction among some patients, coupled with the fact that many patients with near-fatal asthma are in fact "poor perceivers" (18) makes regular spirometry testing an important aspect of disease monitoring.

Spirometry in Hypersensivity Pneumonitis

In its stereotypical acute form, hypersensitivity pneumonitis (HP) manifests as a restrictive ventilatory defect on pulmonary function testing. When forced spirometry is performed, restrictive defects are characterized by the presence of a normal or increased (>85%) FEV_1/FVC ratio and a diminished FVC (2). In the setting of restrictive lung disease, the flow-volume loop is often narrowed and the expiratory limb has a convex upward shape (2). This spirometric pattern

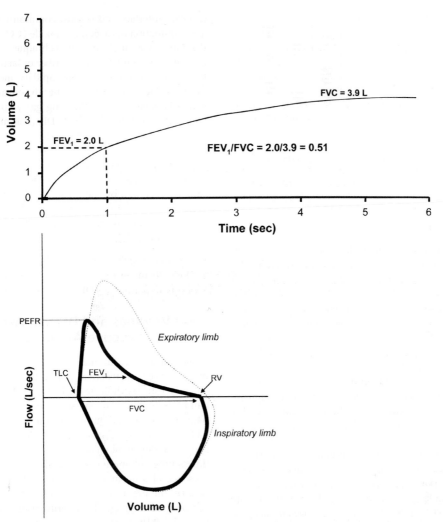

■ **FIGURE 9.2** Volume-time curve (top) and flow-volume loop (bottom) in obstructive airways disease such as asthma. On the volume time curve, note that only approximately 50% of volume is expired in the first second resulting in a decreased FEV_1/FVC ratio of 0.51. In addition, the plateau of expired volume is delayed and not achieved until later in the expiratory compared with the example in Figure 9.1, but a plateau is still achieved at 6 seconds indicating a test of adequate quality. The flow-volume loop shows a decreased PEFR compared to normal (dashed curve) and the expiratory curve demonstrates the characteristic concave upward (or "scooped") appearance reflecting decreased expiratory flow throughout the maneuver.

lacks specificity for restrictive lung disease and can be associated with poor patient effort on the forced spirometry. A low FVC, therefore, cannot be deemed diagnostic for a restrictive ventilatory defect and measurement of lung volumes and diffusing capacity is required. A diminished FVC carries a positive predictive value for an actual restrictive ventilatory defect of only 41% (19). The negative predictive value for an FVC in excluding a restrictive defect, however, is 97.5% (19). Therefore, forced spirometry may serve as a useful screening tool to exclude restrictive lung diseases such as acute HP; the spirometry of subacute and chronic HP is generally a mixed obstructive and restrictive pattern (Chapter 23).

■ **FULL PULMONARY FUNCTION TESTING**

Essential Components of Full Pulmonary Function Testing

Full pulmonary function tests (PFTs) comprise measurement of absolute lung volumes and diffusing capacity in addition to forced spirometry. Absolute lung volumes include: *Residual Volume (RV)*, the volume of gas that remains in the lung after a complete expiration; *Functional Residual Capacity (FRC)*, the volume of gas remaining in the lung after exhaling a normal tidal breath; and *Total Lung Capacity (TLC)*, the maximal

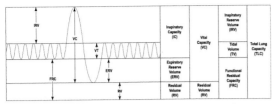

■ **FIGURE 9.3** Residual Volume (RV): the volume of gas that remains in the lung after a complete expiration; Functional Residual Capacity (FRC): the volume of gas remaining in the lung after exhaling a normal tidal breath; Total Lung Capacity (TLC): the maximal amount of gas in the lung after maximal inspiration; Inspiratory Capacity (IC): the difference between TLC and FRC; Expiratory Reserve Volume (ERV): the difference between FRC and RV.

amount of gas in the lung after maximal inspiration (Fig. 9.3). Lung volumes are typically measured by plethysmographic, helium gas dilution or nitrogen washout methods. Body plethsymography is considered the optimal method as both ventilated and nonventilated lung volumes are measured. A discussion of the methodology used to measure lung volumes is beyond the scope of this chapter but was recently published by the ATS/ERS task force (20).

Measurement of lung volumes is required for the definitive diagnosis of a restrictive ventilatory impairment, defined as a reduction of the TLC below the fifth percentile of the predicted value (2). While reductions in vital capacity (VC) are sometimes interpreted as indicating restriction, VC is poorly predictive of an associated reduction in TLC (19, 21). A restrictive pattern on PFTs suggests the presence of parenchymal lung disease wherein there is concentric reduction in all volumes, the TLC, FRC, RV, and VC. Measurement of lung volumes is also required to establish a mixed obstructive and restrictive impairment. Severity of the impairment is based on the degree of reduction in the TLC as set forth by the ATS in 1991 (22).

- Mild restriction—TLC >70% predicted <LLN
- Moderate restriction—TLC 60% to 69% predicted
- Moderately severe restriction—TLC 50% to 59% predicted
- Severe restriction—TLC 34% to 49% predicted
- Very severe restriction—TLC <34% predicted

A significant drawback to lung volume testing is the lack of robust reference standards. The studies from which lung volume reference values were derived are obsolete, lack standardized and detailed description of measurement technique, included asymptomatic smokers, had small sample sizes, and were Caucasian-based and cannot be directly applied to other ethnic groups (23). Lung volumes should be adjusted for ethnicity when race based reference values are not available (2,24).

The *Diffusing Capacity (DL$_{CO}$)* measures the capacity of the lung to exchange gas across the alveolar capillary interface and is most commonly measured by a determination of carbon monoxide (CO) uptake from the lung in a single breath technique. The diffusing capacity is dependent on a number of factors including the thickness of the alveolar capillary membrane, the intact surface area between the alveoli and capillary, which is dependent on the lung gas volume and thoracic blood volume at which DL$_{CO}$ is measured, the matching of ventilation and perfusion, and the hemoglobin concentration available for CO binding (25). Thus, many factors have the ability to alter the measured DL$_{CO}$. The technique to measure the DL$_{CO}$ was recently reviewed by the ATS/ERS task force (25). Severity of the diffusing impairment is based on the extent of the reduction in the DL$_{CO}$ as set forth by the ATS/ERS task force (2).

- Mild impairment—DL$_{CO}$ > 60% predicted <LLN
- Moderate impairment—DL$_{CO}$ 40% to 60 % predicted
- Severe impairment—DL$_{CO}$ <40 % predicted

Lung Volumes and DL$_{CO}$ in Asthma and Other Obstructive Airway Diseases

Lung volume measurements are essential to discriminate between obstructive and restrictive impairment when spirometry indicates reductions in both the FEV$_1$ and FVC. In moderate and severe obstruction, air trapping and hyperinflation may lead to a reduction in the FVC and a deceptively normal FEV$_1$/FVC ratio. The diagnosis of obstruction can be overlooked in this setting unless lung volume measurements are performed. The presence of a normal or increased TLC or RV would confirm the presence of airflow obstruction. The FEV$_1$ can be used to gauge the severity of disease; however, the FEV$_1$/FVC ratio is not useful in this setting. Increases in the TLC and RV indicate the presence of gas trapping, loss of elastic recoil, and hyperinflation in severe obstruction and emphysema and can be important indicators of disease severity (26,27).

The DL$_{CO}$ is useful in discriminating among forms of obstructive lung diseases. In patients with a concomitant history of asthma and tobacco abuse, the DL$_{CO}$ is the best means by which to distinguish between asthma, and chronic obstructive pulmonary disease/emphysema. In asthma, DL$_{CO}$ should be normal or elevated (28), whereas the DL$_{CO}$ will be reduced in the presence of emphysema (29).

Pulmonary Function Testing in Restrictive Lung Diseases

Hypersensitivity Pneumonitis

PFTs alone are rarely helpful in establishing a diagnosis of, or in classifying HP; however, they are useful in quantifying the extent of disease and monitoring response to exposure avoidance and/or treatment. The prevailing pattern of impairment in acute HP is restriction; although in subacute or chronic HP, obstructive and mixed patterns are common (30–33). A restrictive pattern correlates with ground-glass infiltrates and reticulation on chest computed tomography (CT). Obstructive patterns, which include decreased FEV_1, decreased MMEF, and air trapping, correlate with areas of decreased attenuation and bronchiolitis on chest CT (33,34). In chronic HP, emphysematous changes are also seen on chest CT scans and correspond with obstructive patterns on PFTs (31). Patients with HP related to farmers lung demonstrate airflow obstruction and gas trapping after acute exposure to antigen and airway hyperreactivity to methacholine (35). Regardless of the pattern of impairment, the DL_{CO} is often reduced (30,31) in HP. In early, acute forms of the disease, an isolated reduction in DL_{CO} may be the only abnormality detected (31). PFTs may be normal in early, mild disease (36).

In patients with acute or subacute HP, the PFT abnormalities are reversible with removal from exposure and/or treatment. In subacute disease, abnormalities may be intermittent corresponding to exposure, but may become chronically progressive. In chronic HP, the impairment in pulmonary function is irreversible (31,33,37,38).

Idiopathic Eosinophilic Pneumonia

PFT data in eosinophilic pneumonia (EP) are limited but most studies describe abnormalities in the majority of patients. The pattern of impairment on presentation may be either obstructive or restrictive, mixed patterns are rarely seen (39–42). Idiopathic chronic eosinophilic pneumonia (ICEP) is often associated with underlying asthma and although obstruction is more common in those with a history of asthma, it was also seen in those without this preexisting diagnosis. The presence of obstructive impairment is consistent with extension of eosinophilic inflammation to the distal airways (40). Abnormalities in DL_{CO} are also found in the majority of patients (40,43). In ICEP, pulmonary function test normalized rapidly with treatment; however, long-term follow-up demonstrated an obstructive impairment in a high percentage of patients, some of whom had fixed disease (39,40). Those with underlying asthma often experienced worsening of symptoms (44).

Idiopathic acute eosinophilic pneumonia (IAEP) is also associated with abnormal PFTs, most often with small airway disease as evidenced by reduced mid and low lung volume flows, but mild restrictive impairment is also reported. DL_{CO} is reduced in nearly all patients and hypoxemia is common at presentation (45,46). PFTs return to normal with treatment in most patients (45–47); however, residual restriction has been reported (46).

■ PEAK EXPIRATORY FLOW RATE

Handheld peak flow meters serve as a convenient tool for monitoring lung function in asthma. They are not, however, diagnostic tools for the presence of airflow obstruction, and it is recommended that patients who monitor peak expiratory flow rates (PEFR) have yearly correlation with FEV_1 performed to check the accuracy of the peak flow meter (3,48). PEFR is dependent on patient effort and an adequate inspiration to TLC before initiating the maneuver. After inhaling to TLC, the patient should deliver a maximal expiratory blow without any hesitation and with the neck in a neutral position. Hesitation before the forced blow, neck flexion, spitting, and coughing diminish the accuracy of the PEFR measurement (1). When PEFR monitoring is used in clinical practice, initial teaching followed by regular evaluations of the patient's technique are appropriate. The NAEPP report recommends consideration of long-term home peak flow monitoring when patients

- Have moderate or severe persistent asthma
- Have a history of severe asthma exacerbations
- Are "poor perceivers" of airflow obstruction
- Prefer this method of monitoring asthma.

PEFR, when placed in the context of a patient's "personal best" PEFR, can be used to diagnose, understand the severity of, and evaluate the rate of resolution of an asthma exacerbation. Results of the utility of PEFR monitoring have been inconsistent in clinical studies and the decision to use this modality of monitoring should be made on a case-by-case basis (1,49).

■ BRONCHOPROVOCATION TESTING

Although methacholine is the most common agent used in bronchoprovocation testing, challenge testing may be performed with a variety of stimuli including cold air, histamine, or exercise. Bronchoprovocation testing is indicated when asthma is suspected clinically, but spirometry is normal (3). When performing bronchoprovocation testing, clinicians should remain mindful that a positive methacholine bronchoprovocation test is diagnostic for the presence of bronchial hyperresponsiveness (BHR) which may be present in a variety of conditions (chronic obstructive pulmonary disease, allergic rhinitis, and congestive heart failure among others) including asthma (50). In a typical methacholine bronchoprovocation test, dilute concentrations of methacholine are given via a dosimeter and nebulizer system and serial spirometric measurements made. In the recommended methacholine dosing protocol, increasing concentrations of methacholine are delivered serially and after each inhalation an FEV_1 is measured within 90 seconds. The test is terminated when the FEV_1 declines by 20%, a dose termed the *provocative concentration* 20% (PC_{20}) to methacholine. The test is deemed negative if the FEV_1 has not declined by more than 20% after the highest dose of methacholine (16 mg/mL) is delivered (50). The ATS suggests the following interpretation of methacholine bronchoprovocation testing (50):

- PC_{20} >16 mg/mL—Normal bronchial responsiveness
- PC_{20} 4 mg/mL to 16 mg/mL—Borderline BHR
- PC_{20} 1 mg/mL to 4 mg/mL—Mild BHR (positive test)
- PC_{20} <1.0 mg/mL—Moderate to severe BHR

Because BHR is not specific to asthma, bronchoprovocation testing may have more utility in excluding asthma than in actually confirming a diagnosis (3).

■ FRACTION OF EXHALED NITRIC OXIDE

Nitric oxide (FE_{NO}) is a noninvasive marker of eosinophilic airway inflammation (51–53) with potential utility in monitoring asthma (3). FE_{NO} is elevated in asthma patients never treated with steroids (54,55) and decreases following treatment with inhaled steroids (52). The magnitude of FE_{NO} may be a useful predictor of steroid responsiveness (56). A commercially available system which provides instantaneous FE_{NO} measurement has been approved by the U.S. Food and Drug Administration for monitoring asthma (57).

Because of its correlation with eosinophilic airways inflammation and potential predictive power of FE_{NO} in determining steroid responsiveness, recent studies have attempted to use FE_{NO} to guide therapy with inhaled corticosteroids and determine asthma control. The results of studies using FE_{NO} to guide therapy have been inconsistent (58,59). Two studies have indicated that FE_{NO}, may be helpful as a marker of asthma control (60,61) with the test having particular utility in patients treated with low doses of inhaled corticosteroids (61). Several issues remain before FE_{NO} becomes routine clinical practice including a better understanding of normal and abnormal cut-point values and a determination of the minimally important clinical difference (MICD) for a FE_{NO} reduction.

■ ANALYSIS OF BRONCHOALVEOLAR LAVAGE FLUID CELLS

Analysis of bronchoalveolar lavage fluid (BALF) provides important, and often diagnostic, information in allergic lung diseases. In health, macrophages predominate in BALF constituting 89% of cells in nonsmokers. Lymphocytes account for 9%; most are T-cells with a CD4:CD8 ratio averaging 1.9 (+/−1). Neutrophils make up 1% of BALF cells (62,63).

BALF in Hypersensitivity Pneumonitis

In contrast to healthy subjects, BALF in patients with HP demonstrates a lymphocytic alveolitis (64). The percentage of lymphocytes is higher in subacute disease as compared to chronic disease (in one study, 53% versus 38% respectively). Furthermore, lymphocytes are more abundant in patients without radiographic evidence of fibrosis, 59% compared with 20% in those with fibrosis (65). Neutrophils are also present in a higher percentage (31,32) and may be the predominant cell in early acute HP (66). BALF lymphocytosis is more sensitive for the diagnosis of early and/or mild HP wherein both high resolution chest CT and PFTs may be normal (36). A lymphoctye percentage of <30% in the BALF makes the diagnosis of HP less likely (32).

While the lymphocytes are predominantly T-cells, the prevalent T-cell phenotype is less clear. Numerous studies have demonstrated either an increase in CD8 cells with a CD4/CD8 ratio of <1 (38, 67) or an increase in CD4 cells with a ratio >1 (64). The observed variation may be due to time from antigen exposure until sampling. A predominant $CD8^+$ lymphoctyosis may be found in the acute stage of disease but shift to the predominant $CD4^+$ at quiescent stage after antigen avoidance (68–70). The type of antigen may also be important in determining the phenotypic response (71). A marked predominance of $CD4^+$ cells is seen in mycobacterium avian complex associated HP with CD4/CD8 ratios ranging from 6 to 49 (30,72). Similarly, HP in pigeon breeder's lung is associated with an increased CD4/CD8 ratio whereas summer type HP is associated with a decreased CD4/CD8 ratio (71, 73).

BALF in Eosinophilic Pneumonia

BALF analysis is also useful in the diagnosis of eosinophilic lung disease. Measurement of eosinophils in the alveolar space has nearly replaced lung biopsy for diagnosis of eosinophilic pneumonia. Normally eosinophils account for <2% of cells in the BALF (63), counts between 2% and 25% are nonspecific and are found in diseases such as asthma or eosinophilic bronchitis; however, counts >25% are seen in IAEP and > 40% in ICEP (40,44,46).

In patients with IAEP, the eosinophils are atypical with few granules and greater than two nuclear lobes. Eosinophils decrease to <1% of BALF cells on post treatment analysis (46). While blood eosinophilia is uncommon at presentation of IAEP (45–47), it is common in ICEP. The combination of blood and BALF eosinophilia can provide a noninvasive diagnosis in the proper clinical setting. While ICEP is also associated with increased BALF lymphocytes, eosinophils are always more abundant than lymphocytes which is useful in distinguishing it from other diseases (39,40,47).

■ REFERENCES

1. Miller MR, Hankinson J, Brusasco V, et al. Standardisation of spirometry. *Eur Respir J*. 2005;26:319–338.

2. Pellegrino R, Viegi G, Brusasco V, et al. Interpretative strategies for lung function tests. *Eur Respir J*. 2005;26:948–968.

3. NHLBI National Asthma Education and Prevention Program. *Expert Panel Report 3: Guidelines for the Diagnosis and Management of Asthma*. Available at: http://www.nhlbi.nih.gov/guidelines/asthma/asthgdln.pdf 2007.

4. Swanney MP, Beckert LE, Frampton CM, et al. Validity of the American Thoracic Society and other spirometric algorithms using FVC and forced expiratory volume at 6 s for predicting a reduced total lung capacity. *Chest*. 2004;126:1861–1866.

5. Brand PL, Quanjer PH, Postma DS, et al. Interpretation of bronchodilator response in patients with obstructive airways disease. The Dutch Chronic Non-Specific Lung Disease (CNSLD) Study Group. *Thorax*. 1992;47:429–436.

6. D'Angelo E, Prandi E, Milic-Emili J. Dependence of maximal flow-volume curves on time course of preceding inspiration. *J Appl Physiol*. 1993;75:1155–1159.

7. Eigen H, Bieler H, Grant D, et al. Spirometric pulmonary function in healthy preschool children. *Am J Respir Crit Care Med*. 2001;163:619–623.

8. Shingo S, Zhang J, Reiss TF. Correlation of airway obstruction and patient-reported endpoints in clinical studies. *Eur Respir J*. 2001;17:220–224.

9. Stout JW, Visness CM, Enright P, et al. Classification of asthma severity in children: the contribution of pulmonary function testing. *Arch Pediatr Adolesc Med*. 2006;160:844–850.

10. Bacharier LB, Strunk RC, Mauger D, et al. Classifying asthma severity in children: mismatch between symptoms, medication use, and lung function. *Am J Respir Crit Care Med*. 2004;170:426–432.

11. Fuhlbrigge AL, Weiss ST, Kuntz KM, et al. Forced expiratory volume in 1 second percentage improves the classification of severity among children with asthma. *Pediatrics*. 2006;118:e347–355.

12. Stahl E. Correlation between objective measures of airway calibre and clinical symptoms in asthma: a systematic review of clinical studies. *Respir Med*. 2000;94:735–741.

13. Hankinson JL, Odencrantz JR, Fedan KB. Spirometric reference values from a sample of the general U.S. population. *Am J Respir Crit Care Med*. 1999;159:179–187.

14. Global Initiative for Asthma: Global Strategy for Asthma Prevention and Management. Available at: http://www.ginasthma.com 2007.

15. Mikita JA, Mikita CP. Vocal cord dysfunction. *Allergy Asthma Proc*. 2006;27:411–414.

16. Fuhlbrigge AL, Kitch BT, Paltiel AD, et al. FEV(1) is associated with risk of asthma attacks in a pediatric population. *J Allergy Clin Immunol*. 2001;107:61–67.

17. Teeter JG, Bleecker ER. Relationship between airway obstruction and respiratory symptoms in adult asthmatics. *Chest*. 1998;113:272–277.

18. Kikuchi Y, Okabe S, Tamura G, et al. Chemosensitivity and perception of dyspnea in patients with a history of near-fatal asthma. *N Engl J Med*. 1994;330:1329–1334.

19. Aaron SD, Dales RE, Cardinal P. How accurate is spirometry at predicting restrictive pulmonary impairment? *Chest*. 1999;115:869–873.

20. Wanger J, Clausen JL, Coates A, et al. Standardisation of the measurement of lung volumes. *Eur Respir J*. 2005;26:511–522.

21. Glady CA, Aaron SD, Lunau M, et al. A spirometry-based algorithm to direct lung function testing in the pulmonary function laboratory. *Chest*. 2003;123:1939–1946.

22. Lung function testing: selection of reference values and interpretative strategies. American Thoracic Society. *Am Rev Respir Dis.*. 1991;144:1202–1218.

23. Stocks J, Quanjer PH. Reference values for residual volume, functional residual capacity and total lung capacity. ATS Workshop on Lung Volume Measurements. Official Statement of the European Respiratory Society. *Eur Respir. J* 1995;8:492–506.

24. Harik-Khan RI, Fleg JL, Muller DC, et al. The effect of anthropometric and socioeconomic factors on the racial difference in lung function. *Am J Respir Crit Care Med*. 2001;164:1647–1654.

25. Macintyre N, Crapo RO, Viegi G, et al. Standardisation of the single-breath determination of carbon monoxide uptake in the lung. *Eur Respir J*. 2005;26:720–735.

26. Dykstra BJ, Scanlon PD, Kester MM, et al. Lung volumes in 4,774 patients with obstructive lung disease. *Chest*. 1999;115:68–74.

27. Pellegrino R, Brusasco V. On the causes of lung hyperinflation during bronchoconstriction. *Eur Respir J*. 1997;10:468–475.

28. Collard P, Njinou B, Nejadnik B, et al. Single breath diffusing capacity for carbon monoxide in stable asthma. *Chest*. 1994;105:1426–1429.

29. McLean A, Warren PM, Gillooly M, et al. Microscopic and macroscopic measurements of emphysema: relation to carbon monoxide gas transfer. *Thorax*. 1992;47:144–149.

30. Marras TK, Wallace RJ, Jr., Koth LL, et al. Hypersensitivity pneumonitis reaction to Mycobacterium avium in household water. *Chest*. 2005;127:664–671.

31. Remy-Jardin M, Remy J, Wallaert B, et al. Subacute and chronic bird breeder hypersensitivity pneumonitis: sequential evaluation with CT and correlation with lung function tests and bronchoalveolar lavage. *Radiology*. 1993;189:111–118.

32. Selman M. Hypersensitivity pneumonitis: a multifaceted deceiving disorder. *Clin Chest Med*. 2004;25:531–547, vi.

33. Hansell DM, Wells AU, Padley SP, et al. Hypersensitivity pneumonitis: correlation of individual CT patterns with functional abnormalities. *Radiology*. 1996;199:123–128.

34. Chung MH, Edinburgh KJ, Webb EM, et al. Mixed infiltrative and obstructive disease on high-resolution CT: differential diagnosis and functional correlates in a consecutive series. *J Thoracic Imaging*. 2001;16:69–75.

35. Lalancette M, Carrier G, Laviolette M, et al. Farmer's lung. Long-term outcome and lack of predictive value of bronchoalveolar lavage fibrosing factors. *Am Rev Respir Dis*. 1993;148:216–221.

36. Lynch DA, Rose CS, Way D, et al. Hypersensitivity pneumonitis: sensitivity of high-resolution CT in a population-based study. *Am J Roentgenol*. 1992;159:469–472.

37. Allen DH, Williams GV, Woolcock AJ. Bird breeder's hypersensitivity pneumonitis: progress studies of lung function after cessation of exposure to the provoking antigen. *Am Rev Respir Dis*. 1976;114:555–566.

38. Mohr LC. Hypersensitivity pneumonitis. *Curr Opin Pulm Med*. 2004;10:401–411.

39. Durieu J, Wallaert B, Tonnel AB. Long-term follow-up of pulmonary function in chronic eosinophilic pneumonia. Groupe d'Etude en Pathologie Interstitielle de la Societe de Pathologie Thoracique du Nord. *Eur Respir J*. 1997;10:286–291.

40. Marchand E, Reynaud-Gaubert M, Lauque D, et al. Idiopathic chronic eosinophilic pneumonia. A clinical and follow-up study of 62 cases. The Groupe d'Etudes et de Recherche sur les Maladies "Orphelines" Pulmonaires (GERM"O"P). *Medicine*. 1998;77:299–312.

41. Allen JN, Davis WB. Eosinophilic lung diseases. *Am J Respir Crit Care Med*. 1994;150:1423–1438.

42. Cottin V, Cordier JF. Eosinophilic pneumonias. *Allergy*. 2005;60:841–857.

43. Jederlinic PJ, Sicilian L, Gaensler EA. Chronic eosinophilic pneumonia. A report of 19 cases and a review of the literature. *Medicine*. 1988;67:154–162.

44. Marchand E, Etienne-Mastroianni B, Chanez P, et al. Idiopathic chronic eosinophilic pneumonia and asthma: how do they influence each other? *Eur Respir J*. 2003;22:8–13.

45. Ogawa H, Fujimura M, Matsuda T, et al. Transient wheeze. Eosinophilic bronchobronchiolitis in acute eosinophilic pneumonia. *Chest*. 1993;104:493–496.

46. Pope-Harman AL, Davis WB, Allen ED, et al. Acute eosinophilic pneumonia. A summary of 15 cases and review of the literature. *Medicine*. 1996;75:334–342.

47. Cottin V, Frognier R, Monnot H, et al. Chronic eosinophilic pneumonia after radiation therapy for breast cancer. *Eur Respir J*. 2004;23:9–13.

48. Miles JF, Bright P, Ayres JG, et al. The performance of Mini Wright peak flow meters after prolonged use. *Respir Med*. 1995;89:603–605.

49. Jain P, Kavuru MS, Emerman CL, et al. Utility of peak expiratory flow monitoring. *Chest*. 1998;114:861–876.

50. Crapo RO, Casaburi R, Coates AL, et al. Guidelines for methacholine and exercise challenge testing—1999. This official statement of the American Thoracic Society was adopted by the ATS Board of Directors, July 1999. *Am J Respir Crit Care Med*. 2000;161:309–329.

51. ATS/ERS Recommendations for Standardized Procedures for the Online and Offline Measurement of Exhaled Lower Respiratory Nitric Oxide and Nasal Nitric Oxide, 2005. *Am J Respir Crit Care Med*. 2005;171:912–930.

52. Kharitonov SA, Yates DH, Barnes PJ. Inhaled glucocorticoids decrease nitric oxide in exhaled air of asthmatic patients. *Am J Respir Crit Care Med*. 1996;153:454–457.

53. Mahut B, Delclaux C, Tillie-Leblond I, et al. Both inflammation and remodeling influence nitric oxide output in children with refractory asthma. *J Allergy Clin Immunol.* 2004;113:252–256.

54. Alving K, Weitzberg E, Lundberg JM. Increased amount of nitric oxide in exhaled air of asthmatics. *Eur Respir J.* 1993;6:1368–1370.

55. Kharitonov SA, Yates D, Robbins RA, et al. Increased nitric oxide in exhaled air of asthmatic patients. *Lancet.* 1994;343:133–135.

56. Smith AD, Cowan JO, Brassett KP, et al. Exhaled nitric oxide: a predictor of steroid response. *Am J Respir Crit Care Med.* 2005;172:453–459.

57. Silkoff PE, Carlson M, Bourke T, et al. The Aerocrine exhaled nitric oxide monitoring system NIOX is cleared by the US Food and Drug Administration for monitoring therapy in asthma. *J Allergy Clin Immunol.* 2004;114:1241–1256.

58. Smith AD, Cowan JO, Brassett KP, et al. Use of exhaled nitric oxide measurements to guide treatment in chronic asthma. *N Engl J Med.* 2005;352:2163–2173.

59. Shaw DE, Berry MA, Thomas M, et al. The use of exhaled nitric oxide to guide asthma management: a randomized controlled trial. *Am J Respir Crit Care Med.* 2007;176:231–237.

60. Jones SL, Kittelson J, Cowan JO, et al. The predictive value of exhaled nitric oxide measurements in assessing changes in asthma control. *Am J Respir Crit Care Med.* 2001;164:738–743.

61. Michils A, Baldassarre S, Van Muylem A. Exhaled nitric oxide and asthma control: a longitudinal study in unselected patients. *Eur Respir J.* 2008;31:539–546.

62. Ancochea J, Gonzalez A, Sanchez MJ, et al. Expression of lymphocyte activation surface antigens in bronchoalveolar lavage and peripheral blood cells from young healthy subjects. *Chest.* 1993;104:32–37.

63. Schwartz J, Weiss ST. Dietary factors and their relation to respiratory symptoms. The Second National Health and Nutrition Examination Survey. *Am J Epidemiol.* 1990;132:67–76.

64. Ratjen F, Costabel U, Griese M, et al. Bronchoalveolar lavage fluid findings in children with hypersensitivity pneumonitis. *Eur Respir J.* 2003;21:144–148.

65. Murayama J, Yoshizawa Y, Ohtsuka M, et al. Lung fibrosis in hypersensitivity pneumonitis. Association with CD4+ but not CD8+ cell dominant alveolitis and insidious onset. *Chest.* 1993;104:38–43.

66. Fournier E, Tonnel AB, Gosset P, et al. Early neutrophil alveolitis after antigen inhalation in hypersensitivity pneumonitis. *Chest.* 1985;88:563–566.

67. Semenzato G. Immunology of interstitial lung diseases: cellular events taking place in the lung of sarcoidosis, hypersensitivity pneumonitis and HIV infection. *Eur Respir J.* 1991;4:94–102.

68. Costabel U, Bross KJ, Marxen J, et al. T-lymphocytosis in bronchoalveolar lavage fluid of hypersensitivity pneumonitis. Changes in profile of T-cell subsets during the course of disease. *Chest.* 1984;85:514–522.

69. Yoshizawa Y, Ohtani Y, Hayakawa H, et al. Chronic hypersensitivity pneumonitis in Japan: a nationwide epidemiologic survey. *J Allergy Clin Immunol.* 1999;103:315–320.

70. Mornex JF, Cordier G, Pages J, et al. Activated lung lymphocytes in hypersensitivity pneumonitis. *J Allergy Clin Immunol.* 1984;74:719–727.

71. Ando M, Konishi K, Yoneda R, et al. Difference in the phenotypes of bronchoalveolar lavage lymphocytes in patients with summer-type hypersensitivity pneumonitis, farmer's lung, ventilation pneumonitis, and bird fancier's lung: report of a nationwide epidemiologic study in Japan. *J Allergy Clin Immunol.* 1991;87:1002–1009.

72. Aksamit TR. Hot tub lung: infection, inflammation, or both? *Semin Respir Infect.* 2003;18:33–39.

73. Suda T, Sato A, Ida M, et al. Hypersensitivity pneumonitis associated with home ultrasonic humidifiers. *Chest.* 1995;107:711–717.

Radiologic Evaluation of Allergic and Related Diseases of the Upper Airway

ACHILLES KARAGIANIS, MICHELLE NAIDICH, AND ERIC J. RUSSELL

■ ANATOMY

The complex anatomy, and the terminology used to describe the anatomy of the paranasal sinuses and nasal cavity, is best approached by first reviewing the normal drainage pattern of sinonasal secretions. Functional anatomy is intimately related to the pathophysiology of sinus inflammatory disease, and understanding it is critical to plan for functional endoscopic sinus surgery (FESS).

The anatomy of the sinuses can be viewed in two separate but interrelated groups: the sinuses themselves and their associated outflow tracts. There are paired frontal and maxillary sinuses, paired anterior and posterior ethmoid air cells, and a paired sphenoid sinus. Some radiologists consider the sphenoid sinus to be a single sinus subdivided by a sphenoid septum. There are three main outflow tracts for the paranasal sinuses: the ostiomeatal complex, the sphenoethmoidal recess, and the frontoethmoidal (frontal) recess (Fig. 10.1). The sinuses all eventually drain into the nasal cavity.

The nasal cavity is divided vertically by the nasal septum. The anterior portion of the septum is cartilaginous (quadrangular cartilage) and the osseous posterior portion is comprised of the vomer inferiorly and the perpendicular plate of the ethmoid bone superiorly. The nasal vestibule is a paired air passage at the level of the nasal ala. The pyriform aperture is the osseous opening to the nasal cavity. The nasal cavity communicates posteriorly with the nasopharynx via the nasal choanae (Fig. 10.2). The floor of the nasal cavity consists of the hard palate (anteriorly) and the soft palate (posteriorly) (1–3). There are typically three paired sets of inferiorly directed bony projections in the nasal cavity. These are termed the *superior, middle,* and *inferior turbinates* (Fig. 10.2).

The basal lamella is a thin osseous plate that arises from the middle turbinate and has several attachments. The vertical portion of the basal lamella attaches to the cribriform plate superiorly (*Fig. 10.3*), the middle and posterior portions attach to the lamina papyracea laterally, and the posterior margin attaches to the palatine bone (4). The significance of the basal lamella is that it anatomically separates the anterior ethmoids from the posterior ethmoids.

The ostiomeatal complex (OMC) comprises the primary functional drainage unit for the maxillary sinuses, the frontal sinuses, and the anterior ethmoid air cells. This region has several components including the natural maxillary sinus ostium (internal maxillary os), infundibulum, uncinate process, ethmoid bulla, hiatus semilunaris, and the middle meatus (Fig. 10.1) (5).

Mucus secretions, trapped dust particles, and inflammatory cells in the maxillary sinus are propelled centripetally by pseudostratified columnar ciliated epithelium (5,6). The cilia beat 250 to 300 times per minute in a synchronous manner (6), directed superomedially toward the natural ostium of the antrum (Fig. 10.4). Because of this phenomenon, FESS is most often performed to expand this ostium and the remainder of the OMC. Indeed, any surgery neglecting the natural ostium in the setting of an OMC obstruction will most often fail in adequately treating the patient. This was seen years ago in patients who received a Caldwell-Luc procedure (*Fig. 10.5*), in which a nasal antral window was created along the inferior aspect of the maxillary antrum; this did not address the OMC and was prone to failure. Extending superiorly from the maxillary sinus ostium is an aerated channel termed the *infundibulum,* which is bordered by the infero-medial orbital wall laterally and by the uncinate process medially. The

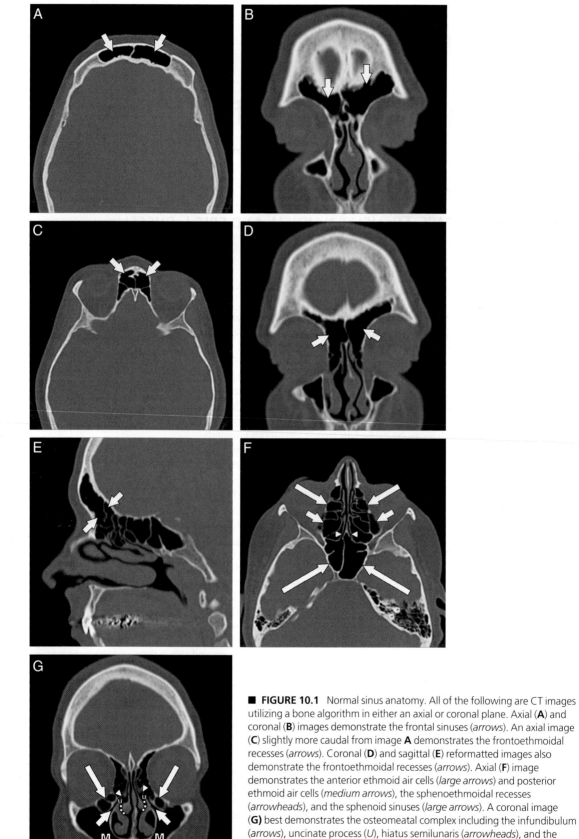

■ **FIGURE 10.1** Normal sinus anatomy. All of the following are CT images utilizing a bone algorithm in either an axial or coronal plane. Axial (**A**) and coronal (**B**) images demonstrate the frontal sinuses (*arrows*). An axial image (**C**) slightly more caudal from image **A** demonstrates the frontoethmoidal recesses (*arrows*). Coronal (**D**) and sagittal (**E**) reformatted images also demonstrate the frontoethmoidal recesses (*arrows*). Axial (**F**) image demonstrates the anterior ethmoid air cells (*large arrows*) and posterior ethmoid air cells (*medium arrows*), the sphenoethmoidal recesses (*arrowheads*), and the sphenoid sinuses (*large arrows*). A coronal image (**G**) best demonstrates the osteomeatal complex including the infundibulum (*arrows*), uncinate process (*U*), hiatus semilunaris (*arrowheads*), and the middle meatus (*dots*). Haller cells are present bilaterally (*medium arrows*). The maxillary sinuses (*M*) drain into the osteomeatal complexes.

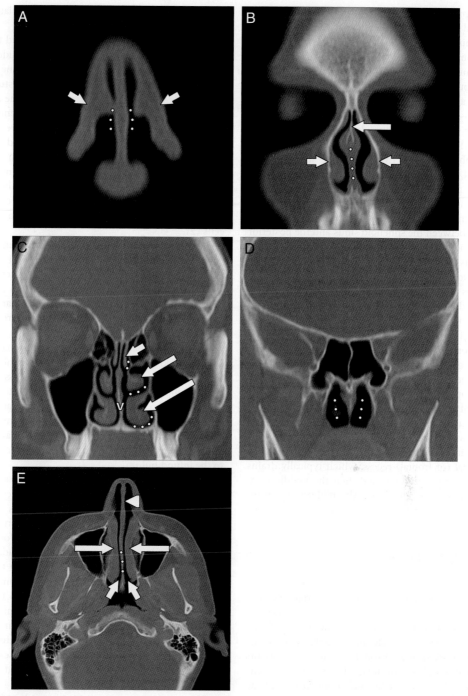

■ **FIGURE 10.2** Normal nasal cavity anatomy. All the following images are CT images utilizing a bone algorithm in either an axial or coronal plane. Coronal CT image (**A**) demonstrates the nasal ala (*arrows*) and the nasal vestibule (*dots*). Coronal CT image (**B**) slightly more posterior to **A** demonstrates the perpendicular plate of the ethmoid (*medium arrow*), the cartilaginous portion of the nasal septum (*dots*), and the piriform aperture (*small arrows*). Coronal CT image (**C**) slightly more posterior to **B** demonstrates the superior (*small arrow*), middle (*medium arrow*), and inferior (*large arrow*) turbinates as well as the vomer (*V*). The superior, middle, and inferior meati are located below their respective turbinates (*small dots*). Coronal CT image (**D**) slightly more posterior to **C** demonstrates the nasal choana (*dots*). Axial image (**E**) at the level of the inferior turbinates (*large arrows*) demonstrates the cartilaginous portion of the nasal septum (*arrowhead*), the vomer (*dots*), and the nasal choana (*medium arrows*).

uncinate process is a thin osseous plate that arises as a cephalad extension from the lateral wall of the nasal cavity behind the nasolacrimal fossa (Fig. 10.1). Secretions passing through the infundibulum reach the hiatus semilunaris, which is a region located below the ethmoid bulla (the largest antero-inferior ethmoid air cell) and above the uncinate process (4,5,7). This in turn opens into the middle meatus inferiorly. Secretions from the middle meatus drain into the nasal cavity, posteriorly through the nasal choanae, and into the nasopharynx (1,2). Eventually, the secretions are swallowed.

The superior meatus is the region lateral to the superior turbinate. It receives secretions from the posterior ethmoid cells and the sphenoid sinus. The outflow tract between the sphenoid sinus and the posterior ethmoids is termed the *sphenoethmoidal recess* (Fig. 10.2). This distinct functional unit is sometimes called the *posterior ostiomeatal complex*. The inferior meatus, which lies lateral to the inferior turbinate, does not serve as a drainage passageway for sinus secretions, but rather receives tears draining from the nasolacrimal sac and duct (1–3).

The frontal sinus outflow tract is a third functional unit and comprises the lower frontal sinus, the frontal ostium, and the frontoethmoidal recess (7). The frontal sinus outflow tract has an hourglass configuration on sagittal reformatted images. As the frontal sinus tapers inferiorly, it forms the frontal ostium, which is the narrowest portion of this hourglass configuration (7). Just inferior to the frontal ostium is the frontoethmoidal (or frontal) recess, which typically drains into the anterior ethmoids and then the middle meatus via anterior ethmoid ostia. Alternatively, the frontoethmoidal recess may directly drain into the middle meatus.

Anatomic Variants

Earwaker (8) analyzed the computerized tomography (CT) scans of 800 patients who were referred for evaluation prior to FESS. He found that only 57 of these 800 patients did not have anatomic variants. Of the described 52 types of anatomic variants, 93% of the patients had one or more variants. While these variants are frequently of no clinical significance, in some circumstances they may predispose to obstruction of the normal pathways of mucus drainage, or they may serve to increase the risk of complications associated with FESS. Consequently, familiarity with some of the more common variants is important.

Several variations in the anatomy of the nasal cavity can result in narrowing of the nasal cavity and obstruction to the drainage of the ipsilateral maxillary sinus and ethmoid air cells. For example, the nasal septum may be severely deviated toward one side (Fig. 10.6), narrowing the nasal cavity. Similarly, a bony nasal

septal spur, with or without nasal septal deviation, may compromise the OMC and nasal cavity.

A concha bullosa (Fig. 10.7) is an aerated turbinate head, most commonly associated with the middle turbinate, although aeration can also be seen in the superior and inferior turbinate heads (5). Various studies use different degrees of pneumatization to define a concha bullosa; consequently, the reported prevalence ranges from 4% to 80% (9). There is a strong relationship between the presence of a concha bullosa and contralateral nasal septal deviation although Stallman et al. (10) found no significant increase in paranasal sinus disease associated with a concha bullosa. Concha bullosa are lined by secretory mucoperiosteum and are therefore prone to the same sinus disease processes as other air cells (2).

Normally, middle turbinates are convex medially. A paradoxical middle turbinate (Fig. 10.4 and Fig. 10.8) refers to a middle turbinate that is convex laterally. This is a common variant and is most often an incidental finding. Rarely, the middle meatus may be narrowed by a paradoxical middle turbinate and this narrowing can predispose to sinus obstruction when associated with mucosal inflammation or edema. Occasionally, paradoxical middle turbinates may make surgical access to the OMC difficult (7). The uncinate process can have varying appearances. The orientation of the uncinate process may be vertical, horizontal (particularly in conjunction with a large ethmoid bulla) or anywhere in between (8,11). The uncinate process may also be pneumatized and expanded, resulting in compromise to the infundibulum.

A deviated nasal septum and an associated osseous spur often contact and deform the adjacent turbinates. Since the nose and paranasal sinuses are innervated by the first and second divisions of the trigeminal nerve (12), the potential exists for "contact point" headaches. These contact point headaches are referred headaches from stimulation of the trigeminal nerve and can significantly improve following surgical removal of the spur and a septoplasty (13,14). However, the presence or severity of a contact point between a septal deviation/spur and a turbinate is not a primary indication for surgery (13). Careful history, physical exam, and other potential causes for the patient's headaches should be considered prior to surgery.

Many common variants arise from the ethmoid air cells and extend into the adjacent sinuses or outflow tracts. These are collectively termed *extramural ethmoid air cells* (7). One of the more common variants is the Haller cell (Fig. 10.1 and Fig. 10.9). The Haller cell is an air cell that lies within the superomedial maxillary antrum and along the inferior medial margin of the orbit (Fig. 10.4). A large Haller cell may narrow the maxillary sinus ostium or the infundibulum, depending on its specific position along the sinus margin. Agger nasi cells (*Fig. 10.10*) are extremely common and are the most anterior ethmoidal air cells, located just ventral to the nasolacrimal canal. These cells are in, or adjacent to, the lacrimal bones and may anatomically narrow the frontoethmoidal recess (7). Agger nasi cells are important surgical landmarks for the position of the frontoethmoidal recess. A frontal bulla (*Fig. 10.11*) is an ethmoid air cell that extends along the back wall of the frontoethmoidal recess into the frontal sinus, occasionally resulting in obstruction of the frontal sinus and/or frontoethmoidal recess (15). Onodi cells (Fig. 10.12) are posterior ethmoid air cells that share a common wall with the optic canal and typically lie above the sphenoid sinus. The significance of the Onodi cell relative to surgery is discussed below.

Complications of Functional Endoscopic Sinus Sugery—Anatomic Considerations

The anatomy of the nasal cavity and ethmoid labyrinth is extremely complex and variable. Endoscopy provides a two-dimensional view of three-dimensional anatomy. Conventional cross sectional imaging, and more recently intraoperative framed and frameless stereotactic guided imaging techniques, can help avoid complications from endoscopic sinus surgery.

When surgical complications do occur, CT and magnetic resonance imaging (MRI) are essential for evaluation. A common site prone to complications is the lamina papyracea (the medial orbital wall), which

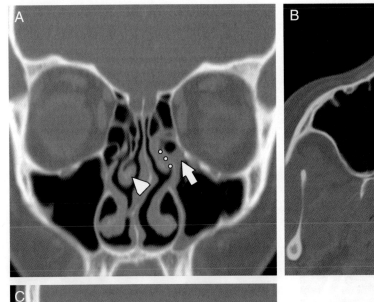

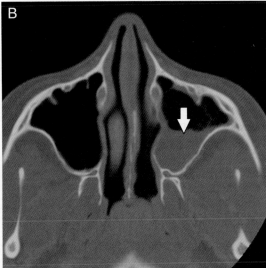

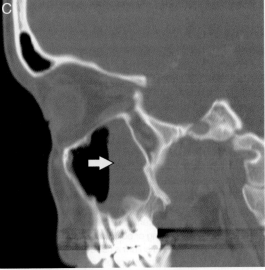

■ **FIGURE 10.4** Opacified osteomeatal complex. Coronal reformatted CT image (**A**) demonstrates opacification of the left infundibulum (*arrow*) and left middle meatus (dots). A paradoxical right middle turbinate is incidentally noted (*arrowhead*). Axial (**B**) and sagittal reformatted (**C**) CT images in the same patient demonstrate a moderate sized air fluid level layering dependently in the left maxillary sinus (*arrow*).

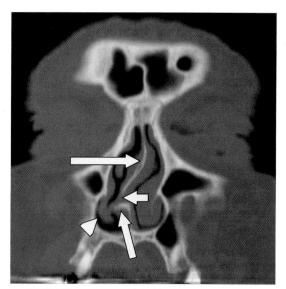

■ **FIGURE 10.6** Nasoseptal deviation. Coronal reformatted CT image with a bone algorithm demonstrates marked deviation of the nasal septum with the vomer deviated to the right (*small arrow*) and the perpendicular plate of the ethmoid (*large arrow*) deviated to the left. A superimposed spur (*medium arrow*) is associated with deformity of the right inferior turbinate (*arrowhead*).

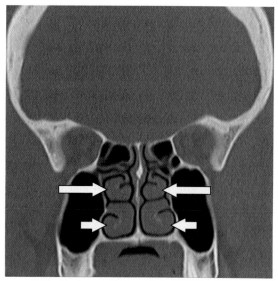

■ **FIGURE 10.8** Paradoxical middle turbinates. Coronal reformatted CT image demonstrates bilateral paradoxical middle turbinates (*medium arrows*). The heads of these middle turbinates curve inward rather than outward as opposed to the inferior turbinates (*small arrows*).

may be breached during ethmoid surgery. The surgeon should be aware of any preexisting lamina papyracea deformities to avoid inadvertent breach of the orbit.

Variations in the degree of pneumatization of the sphenoid sinus can also result in surgical mishap. The

internal carotid artery runs lateral to the sphenoid sinus wall, and if medially positioned, may bulge into the sphenoid sinus lumen, with the possibility of injury during sinus surgery; this may lead to serious hemorrhage or pseudoaneurysm formation (**Fig. 10.13**).

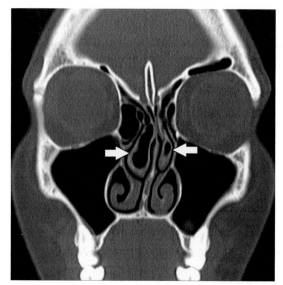

■ **FIGURE 10.7** Concha bullosa. Coronal reformatted CT image with a bone algorithm through the mid nasal cavity demonstrates bilateral concha bullosa involving the middle turbinates, right larger than left (*arrows*).

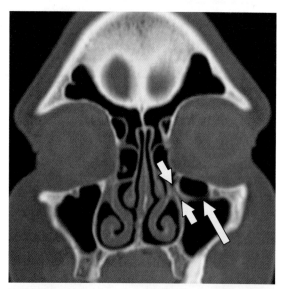

■ **FIGURE 10.9** Haller cell. Coronal CT image demonstrates a moderate-sized Haller cell (*medium arrow*) that forms the lateral margin of the left infundibulum (*small arrows*). Haller cells can result in narrowing or obstruction of an infundibulum. In this case, the left infundibulum is narrowed by the Haller cell and opacified due to superimposed mucosal thickening.

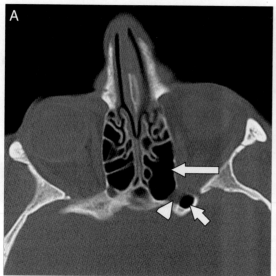 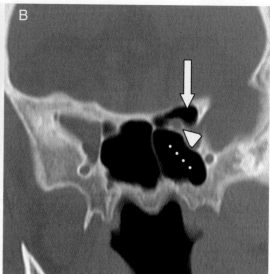

■ **FIGURE 10.12** Onodi cell. Axial (**A**) and coronal (**B**) CT images with a bone algorithm demonstrate a posterior most left ethmoid air cell (Onodi cell) (*medium arrow*) forming a margin with the left optic canal (*arrowhead*). The Onodi cell extends into and pneumatizes the left anterior clinoid process (*small arrow*). The typical location for an Onodi cell is superior to the sphenoid sinus (*dots*), as the coronal image demonstrates.

Pneumatization of the sphenoid sinus can extend into the anterior clinoid processes. The anterior clinoid processes (and the optic struts) normally form the lateral wall of the optic canal. Clinoid pneumatization can therefore expose the optic nerve to surgical damage during sphenoid sinus surgery. Oftentimes the sphenoid septum attaches to one of the carotid canals. If this is present, the potential exists for a fracture to the carotid canal on resection of the sphenoid septum. As discussed above, Onodi cells (Fig. 10.12) are posterior ethmoid air cells that share a common wall with the optic canal. If a surgeon is unaware of the presence of an Onodi cell, the surgeon could inadvertently breach the optic canal and damage the optic nerve. The presence and exact location of an Onodi cell can only be defined prior to surgery with cross sectional imaging, ideally with CT.

The roof of the ethmoid sinus is formed by the frontal bone (16). An asymmetric low-lying ethmoid roof increases the chances of inadvertent breech by the unsuspecting surgeon and may result in herniation of the brain and/or meninges. The cribriform plate lies at the midline between the roofs of the ethmoids. The cribriform plate contains a medial and a lateral lamella (*Fig. 10.3*). The lateral lamella is an extremely thin osseous structure and is a point of structural weakness in the anterior skull base (7,17). The anterior ethmoidal artery enters the intracranial compartment through the lateral lamella of the cribriform plate. If the lateral lamella is breached, the anterior ethmoidal artery may be damaged with risk of intracranial hemorrhage (2,5,8,18) or arteriovenous fistula formation. The

anterior ethmoidal artery also traverses within the orbit, lateral to a notch located along the superomedial margin of the orbit. This notch serves as a surgical landmark to the location of the anterior ethmoidal artery. The anterior ethmoidal artery exits the orbit via the anterior ethmoidal foramen (7). Occasionally, the anterior ethmoidal artery traverses within a small canal that crosses the ethmoid air cells as it ascends intracranially; if this small canal is surgically breached, the anterior ethmoidal artery can retract into the orbit resulting in uncontrolled intraorbital hemorrhage, increased intraorbital pressure, and possibly blindness from retinal artery occlusion (5). Operative injuries to the orbital walls, cribriform plate, and ethmoid roofs may be best seen on coronal CT (Fig. 10.14), but the resulting complications of cerebritis, meningitis, empyema, or abscess are best demonstrated on contrast-enhanced MR (18,19).

CSF leak is another known complication of FESS. The CSF leak in this population of patients is usually located in the region of the roof of ethmoids or cribriform plate. Patients may present with CSF rhinorrhea, recurrent meningitis, and meningoencephalocele. Symptoms may occur immediately or be delayed up to 2 years after the operative procedure (5,11). A radionuclide cisternogram can be performed to confirm the presence of a leak, but this test provides only limited anatomic information concerning the exact location of the leak. A noncontrast CT can be performed in the axial and coronal planes to localize a fracture and has been shown to demonstrate the site of a CSF fistula 71% of the time (20). A CT cisternogram is a procedure

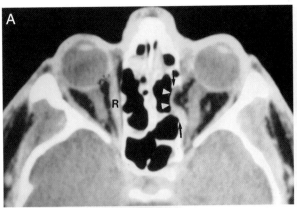

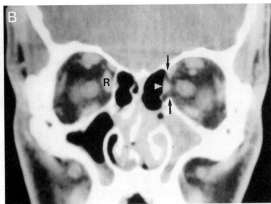

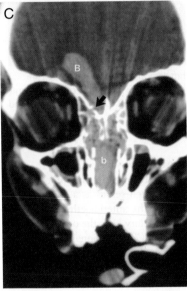

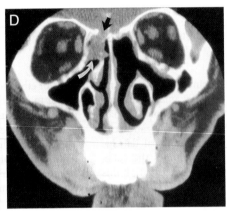

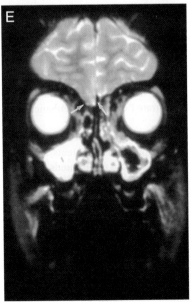

■ **FIGURE 10.14** Surgical complications. Axial (**A**) and coronal (**B**) computed tomography (CT) images from a patient who experienced left medial rectus palsy following sinus surgery. There has been inadvertent resection of the left medial orbital wall (*black arrows*). The left medial rectus muscle is seen herniating through the defect (*white arrowhead*) into the adjacent ethmoid air cell. The normal position of the medial rectus muscle is seen on the right (*R*). A coronal CT (**C**) from a different patient demonstrates an intracranial hemorrhage (*B*) as a result of injury to the fovea ethmoidalis (*black arrow*). Blood (*b*) is also filling the sinus and nasal cavities. A coronal CT (**D**) from another postoperative patient who suffered a similar injury shows abnormal soft tissue density (*curved white arrow*) adjacent to an apparent discontinuity of the bony fovea ethmoidalis and cribriform plate (*black arrow*). A coronal T2-weighted magnetic resonance image (**E**) illustrates this soft tissue density to be brain parenchyma herniating through the bone defect (*white arrows*). This is called a postoperative encephalocele.

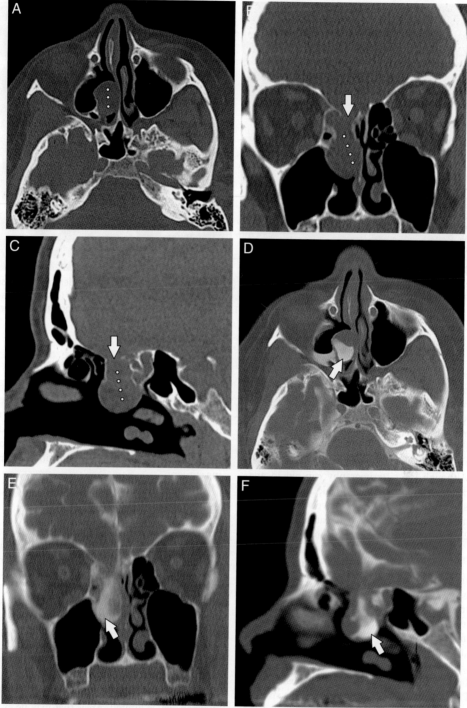

■ **FIGURE 10.15** Encephalocele. Axial (**A**), coronal reformatted (**B**), and sagittal reformatted (**C**) noncontrast CT images through the sinuses with a bone algorithm demonstrate a relatively large osseous defect involving the roof of the right ethmoid including the right lateral lamella (*arrow*, **B**). A nonspecific opacity is present in the posterior ethmoid suggestive of a cephalocele (*dots*). Axial (**D**), coronal reformatted (**E**), and sagittal reformatted (**F**) CT images through the sinuses with a bone algorithm following intrathecal administration of contrast demonstrate contrast extending into the lesion within the right posterior ethmoids. The partial opacification of the lesion with contrast (*arrow*) confirm that the lesion is partially CSF and partially brain tissue. This is consistent with an encephalocele.

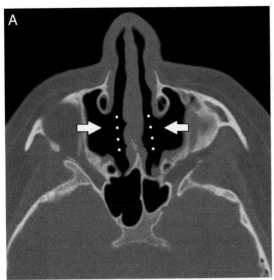 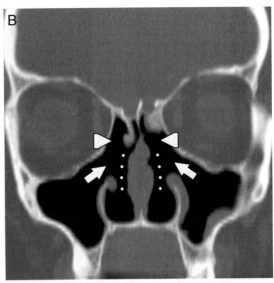

■ **FIGURE 10.17** Empty nose syndrome. Axial (**A**) and coronal (**B**) CT images with a bone algorithm demonstrate absent turbinates (*dots*), uncinectomies with antrostosmies (*small arrows*) and ethmoidectomies (*arrowheads*). This patient had symptoms of chronic sinusitis. Turbinates humidify inhaled air. The lack of the turbinates results in a congested sensation for the patient.

whereby contrast is placed into the subarachnoid space (via a lumbar puncture) and a CT is performed with direct coronal images (Fig. 10.15). The coronal images are ideally obtained with the patient placed prone and with the neck extended to promote leakage of contrast through the defect. The reported sensitivity of CT cisternography to detect CSF leaks (of all causes) is 36% to 81%. Although CT cisternography can aid in anatomical localization of the site of a leak, the sensitivity is diminished if the patient is not actively leaking CSF at the time of the exam (21). If a patient is leaking CSF, a β2-transferrin can be sent for laboratory analysis to verify that there is a CSF leak. Some authors advocate the use of MRI with or without intrathecal gadolinium contrast to localize the site of a CSF leak (20) (*Fig. 10.16*). T2-weighted images provide excellent contrast between the CSF and bone/air interface. Continuity of high T2 signal CSF from the intracranial subarachnoid space through an osseous defect into extracranial sites can sometimes be identified (22). However, a potential drawback to MRI cisternography is that the CSF and gadolinium may be obscured by fluid and enhancing mucosal thickening in the sinuses, respectively. Additionally, CT provides superior bone detail compared to MRI (21). Currently, most practitioners perform either a noncontrast CT with or without a β2-transferrin assay, or CT cisternography.

Empty nose syndrome (Fig. 10.17) refers to the sensation of nasal congestion that occurs from an atrophic rhinitis or following resection of the inferior turbinate, middle turbinate, or both (23). The function of the turbinates is to filtrate, warm, and humidify inhaled air.

Absence of the nasal turbinates due to surgery results in alteration of air flow and a deficient nasal sensation. However, the patient paradoxically experiences a congested nasal sensation despite a widely patent nasal cavity (23). The empty nose syndrome is considered rare (23), although this entity is likely directly proportional to the extent of the turbinate resection performed during surgery.

■ IMAGING TECHNIQUE

Full radiographic imaging of the sinuses is usually reserved for those patients with clinical signs and symptoms of rhinosinusitis who have failed standard medical treatment, such as patients with chronic rhinosinusitis, or who have recurrent episodes of rhinosinusitis and are potentially surgical candidates. Anatomic causes and underlying disease processes can be visualized, and the feasibility as well as the risk of surgery can be evaluated. Additionally, any patient with a suspected complication of rhinosinusitis or a presumed surgical complication should be imaged.

Standard radiography, while being fast and relatively inexpensive, is limited. Areas that may be evaluated by standard radiography include the lower third of the nasal cavity and the maxillary, frontal, and sphenoid sinuses as well as the posterior ethmoid air cells. The anterior ethmoid cells, the upper two-thirds of the nasal cavity, and the outflow tracts are often obscured by overlapping structures. Consequently, cross sectional imaging modalities, which eliminate the overlap of adjacent structures, are more definitive (2,18).

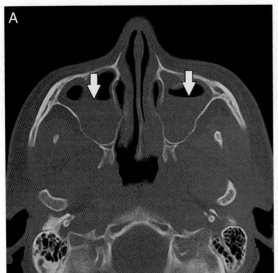
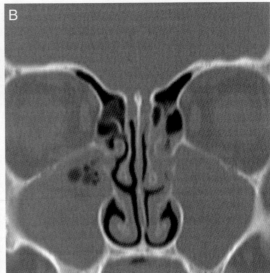

■ **FIGURE 10.18**   Acute sinusitis. Axial CT image with a bone algorithm (**A**) demonstrates air fluid levels (*arrows*) layering dependently in the maxillary sinuses. In the appropriate clinical setting, this is consistent with acute sinusitis. Coronal reformatted image with a bone algorithm (**B**) through the posterior aspect of the maxillary antra in the same patient gives the false impression that the maxillary antra are nearly completely opacified. The axial image reveals the true configuration of the fluid at the time of scanning as the patient lies supine during the image acquisition.

CT is the imaging modality of choice for routine evaluation of the sinuses. When performed for preoperative evaluation of fixed sinus obstructive disease, some clinicians recommend pre-imaging patient preparation consisting of a course of antibiotics to eliminate any acute or transient mucoperiosteal disease. This is followed by sympathomimetic spray just prior to the scan to minimize reversible congestion and mucus (1,18,24). In theory, this will allow for optimal delineation of the chronic nonreversible sinus disease which should be the target of operative intervention. This also serves to optimally evaluate the anatomy and to determine if there are any anatomic causes of obstruction resulting in sinus disease.

With the advent of helical CT scanning, several of the difficulties with patient positioning have been eliminated, and there are opportunities for reducing radiation dose and examination time. This technology allows for rapid acquisition of volumetric data that can be subsequently reformatted at narrow increments in any plane chosen, providing orthogonal reformatted images instead of a second set of direct images, further reducing the exam time and radiation dose. Consequently, the imaging time for the helical technique is faster than with the conventional methods.

Coronal and axial imaging is preferred prior to FESS (18,24). Coronal plane images optimally visualize the OMC and demonstrate anatomy that corresponds to the surgeon's orientation during endoscopy. With current CT scanners, axial imaging with coronal reformatted images can easily be performed. Images are obtained and displayed at both wide "bone" windows and narrow "soft

tissue" windows. One should remember that when viewing the coronal reformatted images, an air fluid level will not be seen. Since axial images are acquired when the patient is in the supine position, air fluid levels lie dependently along the back wall of the sinuses on axial images but not on the coronal reformatted images (Fig. 10.18).

An advantage of MRI over CT scans is the lack of ionizing radiation and improved soft tissue contrast. In addition, the extensive artifact from dental hardware that can occur with CT is usually less problematic than with MRI. It is clear that the bone detail necessary for evaluating the paranasal sinuses is superior on CT, while intraorbital and intracranial contents are better demonstrated on MR. Consequently, MRI is the technique of choice for evaluating the complications of rhinosinusitis, primary sinus neoplasms, the spread of neoplastic processes and postoperative complications. MRI is not the primary modality for evaluating simple inflammatory disease, which is the role of CT (25).

■ RHINOSINUSITIS (SINUSITIS)

Acute Rhinosinusitis

Rhinosinusitis is the preferred term for describing sinus inflammatory disease, since sinusitis is often preceded by rhinitis and rarely occurs without concomitant nasal inflammation (26). Acute rhinosinusitis often occurs following an upper respiratory tract infection. The respiratory infection causes mucoperiosteal congestion. At the level of the ostia, there is apposition of mucosal surfaces with obstruction of normal mucociliary clearance, resulting in retention of secretions and stasis. Transient ostial obstruction may lead to sterile fluid accumulation. This obstruction results in a decrease in oxygen tension and an increase in carbon dioxide tension in the sinus; in combination with stagnant fluid, this environment provides an excellent medium for bacterial growth (5, 27). Clinically, rhinosinusitis may be classified as acute, recurrent acute, subacute, and chronic (28). These clinical categories do not have well-defined imaging correlates. Bhattacharyya et al. (29) examined the relationship of patients' symptoms and CT findings in 221 subjects. These patients responded to a clinical questionnaire that assessed the severity of their symptoms prior to undergoing CT. Thirty-four percent of these patients had a normal CT scan. There was no significant correlation between the subset of patients with "positive" and "very positive" CT findings and the severity of their symptoms. Furthermore, the subgroup of patients reporting facial pain as their primary symptom had overall less impressive imaging findings than the patients without facial pain.

It has been noted that the mucoperiosteum lining the nasal turbinates, nasal septum, and ethmoid air cells demonstrates normal cyclic congestion (Fig. 10.19) over each 6-hour period (30). Consequently, mild 1 mm to 2 mm ethmoid air cell mucoperiosteal thickening may not represent an infectious process but rather transient congestion. It is not surprising that a prospective study performed by Rak et al. (31) showed that 69% of a group of patients undergoing brain MR for unrelated reasons demonstrated minimal (1 mm to 2 mm) ethmoid mucosal thickening. Sixty-three percent of these patients did not report any symptoms of rhinosinusitis. In fact, only when the mucosal thickening

was 4 mm or greater was there a significant correlation to the symptoms of rhinosinusitis.

The best imaging correlate for acute rhinosinusitis is the air-fluid level (Fig. 10.18), although fluid may accumulate without infection. Acute infection is a clinical diagnosis; imaging can support this impression (11). Consequently, sinus images may be interpreted descriptively, without necessarily drawing conclusions regarding the patient's clinical status.

The degree of mucoperiosteal thickening can be graded as mild (<5 mm), moderate (5 mm to 10 mm), and severe (>10 mm) (11). The location of mucoperiosteal thickening is also important. It is intuitive that a patient with a mild degree of thickening in the region of the infundibulum is more likely to suffer from obstructive sinusitis than a patient with moderate thickening involving the inferior aspect of the maxillary antrum.

Chronic Rhinosinusitis

Chronic rhinosinusitis (CRS) may be difficult to define on a single imaging study. CRS often demonstrates reactive bony sclerosis and thickening of the walls of the sinus (osteitis) (Fig. 10.20). This is the single best radiographic sign for CRS. Also, if there are a series of exams demonstrating persistent mucoperiosteal thickening in a symptomatic patient, the diagnosis of CRS is likely.

On CT scans, chronic inspissated secretions will appear as focal areas of higher attenuation, often with more peripheral low attenuation from edematous mucoperiosteum. This hyperdense appearance can also be seen with polyps, fungal colonization, and fungal sinusitis (Fig. 10.25) (18). The MRI appearance of the soft tissue contents within the sinus cavity is variable,

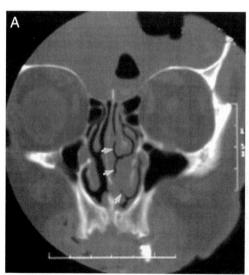
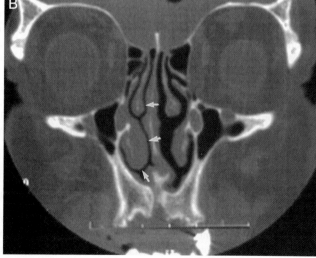

■ **FIGURE 10.19** Nasal cycle. Two coronal computed tomography images of the same patient shown in Fig. 29.6 obtained the same day. The first examination (**A**) was performed at 4 PM and the second study (**B**) at 7 PM. There is congestion of the nasal turbinates on the left initially. Later in the same day the congestion is on the right; this is the normal cyclic pattern of congestion of the turbinates (nasal cycle).

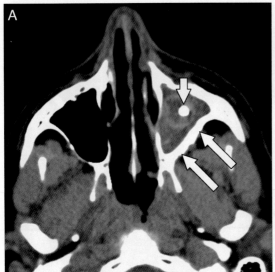 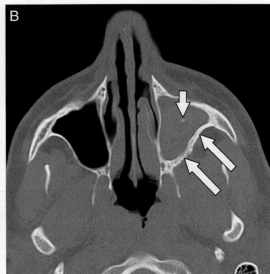

■ **FIGURE 10.20** Mycetoma. Axial CT in soft (**A**) and bone (**B**) windows demonstrates a completely opacified left maxillary sinus with a small focus of mineralization within the center of the opacity (*arrow*). Thickened and sclerotic maxillary sinus walls (*medium arrows*) are consistent with chronic sinusitis, in this case chronic sinusitis related to a mycetoma.

dependent on the proportion of water and protein contents within the secretions. Normal sinus secretions, predominantly glycomucoproteins, are comprised of 95% water and 5% solid materials. On MRI, the appearance of normal secretions reflects water content with isointense or hypointense signal on T1-weighted images and hyperintense signal on T2-weighted images. With chronic obstruction, there is continuous secretory activity and also resorption of water. Also, there are mucosal changes resulting in an increased number of glycomucoprotein producing goblet cells. As a result, the overall water content of the secretions is decreased and the protein concentration and viscosity is increased. Initially, these changes are reflected in shortening of the T1 relaxation time causing the secretions to become hyperintense on T1-weighted images. T2 relaxation time is not noticeably affected until the protein concentration is greater than 25%. At this protein concentration, there is cross-linking of the protein molecules, which increases the viscosity of the secretions. This diminishes macromolecular motion which further decreases the T2 relaxation time and results in decreased T2 signal intensity. Eventually, as the secretions become completely dessicated, there is elimination of free water resulting in marked hypointensity on both T1 and T2 sequences. The sinus may, as a result, appear as a signal "void" on T1 and T2 imaging. Consequently, a chronically obstructed sinus cavity may be falsely interpreted as aerated because the contents will be completely devoid of signal (32,33). A significant sinus infection, such as a fungal sinusitis, can have this appearance. Therefore, MRI is not the study of choice to evaluate inflammatory sinus disease.

Abnormalities Associated with Rhinosinusitis

Sinonasal Polyps and Retention Cysts

If there is obstruction of a solitary mucus gland duct and not the whole sinus cavity, a mucus retention cyst arises (Fig. 10.22). A mucus retention cyst is a homogeneous, dome shaped lesion, with a very thin wall that easily ruptures during surgery. It rarely fills the entire sinus cavity and does not cause sinus expansion. Serous retention cysts develop secondary to serous fluid accumulation beneath the submucosa (5). It is not possible to differentiate a serous retention cyst from a mucus retention cyst by imaging, although this has no clinical significance as both are benign and generally asymptomatic. On MRI, retention cysts demonstrate hyperintense signal on T2-weighted imaging due to their relatively high water content (34). Unlike malignancies, retention cysts demonstrate peripheral enhancement but never central or homogeneous enhancement on MRI.

Sinonasal polyps are also associated with CRS. Polyps develop as a result of mucoperiosteal hyperplasia, with abnormal accumulation of submucosal fluid. These lesions usually appear as abnormal rounded soft tissue masses, similar to retention cysts, and cannot be differentiated from retention cysts by CT, unless the lesion is clearly pedunculated (7). Additionally, polyps are generally not as hyperintense as retention cysts on T2-weighted MRI. Polyps are most commonly located in the nasal cavity (Fig. 10.25 and Fig. 10.23). Small, isolated polyps are of little clinical concern although if large or multiple, they may cause obstruction of a

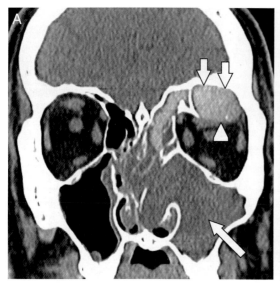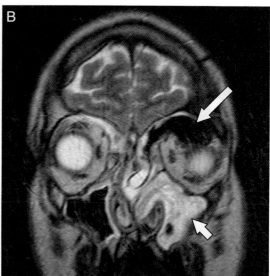

■ **FIGURE 10.21** Mucocele. Coronal CT image with a soft tissue algorithm (**A**) through the frontal and maxillary sinuses demonstrates completely opacified left frontal (*small arrows*) and left maxillary (*medium arrow*) sinuses associated with sinus expansion. The left frontal sinus demonstrates osseous dehiscence along its inferior wall resulting in extension of the mucocele into the superior left orbit (*arrowhead*). Notice the increased attenuation in the left frontal sinus. This is related to inspissated secretions and/or fungal colonization. Coronal T2-weighted MR image (**B**) demonstrates decreased signal in the left frontal sinus mucocele (*medium arrow*) due to the inspissation and/or fungal colonization. The increased signal in the left maxillary sinus mucocele (*small arrow*) reflects this mucocele's relatively higher water content.

drainage pathway or the nasal cavity. When a large solitary polyp arises in the maxillary antrum and extends through the infundibulum (or an accessory ostium) into

the middle meatus and subsequently into the choana, it is termed an *antrochoanal polyp* (Fig. 24). There is usually expansion of the infundibulum or accessory ostium. An antro-choanal polyp may protrude into the nasopharynx and mimic a mass originating in the nasopharynx. Surgery requires resecting not only the protruding portion of the polyp, but also the sinus component in order to prevent reccurrence (35).

Mucocele

A mucocele (Fig. 10.21 and Fig. 10.25) is an obstructed, expanded, and completely mucus-filled sinus that occurs with chronic sinus outlet obstruction (36). The accumulation of mucus under pressure results in sinus wall remodeling. In fact, it is the most common expansile lesion of the sinuses. Mucoceles are typically solitary, although multiple lesions may occur. Mucoceles most commonly occur in the frontal sinuses (60% to 65%) where they may remodel the orbit, resulting in proptosis. The ethmoid sinuses are the second most commonly involved area (20% to 25%) followed by the maxillary and rarely the sphenoid sinuses (37). Initially, a mucocele may be indistinguishable from a completely opacified sinus due to acute sinusitis. However, with time, there is expansion of the sinus cavity and bony remodeling. Focal lytic changes may also occur, resulting in wall dehiscence. Sinus contents may bulge through osseous defects into adjacent regions, and these destructive osseous changes may mimic sinus malignancy on CT.

■ **FIGURE 10.22** Retention cyst. Coronal reformatted CT image with a bone algorithm demonstrates a small dome shaped structure (*medium arrow*) along the floor of the left maxillary antrum, consistent with a small retention cyst. This could also represent a small sinus polyp, although there is no clinical relevance in distinguishing between these entities. A concha bullosa (*small arrow*) involving the right middle turbinate is also seen.

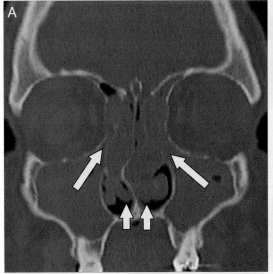

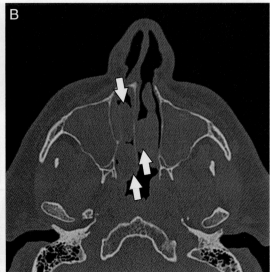

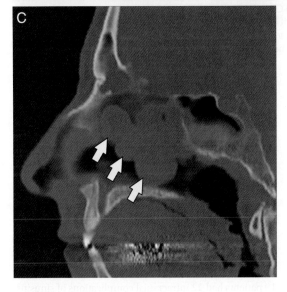

■ **FIGURE 10.23** Sinonasal polyposis. Coronal reformatted CT image (**A**) with a bone algorithm demonstrates multiple polypoid opacities (*small arrows*) in the nasal cavity that are not clearly delineated as they are closely apposed to the adjacent turbinates. Notice that the osteomeatal complexes are opacified bilaterally (*medium arrows*). Axial (**B**) and sagittal reformatted (**C**) CT images also demonstrate the multiple polypoid opacities (*small arrows*).

Although a mucocele may resemble a neoplasm on CT, differentiating a mucocele from a malignancy should be fairly straightforward by MRI. The MRI appearance of a mucocele depends on the relative water and protein concentration of its contents. Generally, the T1 and T2 patterns will suggest the presence of proteinaceous fluid typical of mucoceles. The more the water content, the more T2 hyperintense the mucocele will be on MRI. With the intravenous administration of gadolinium, an MRI contrast agent, a mucocele typically demonstrates thin, regular peripheral enhancement of the mucoperiosteal lining, while a sinus neoplasm rarely demonstrates peripheral enhancement and much more commonly solidly enhances (38,39). The lack of central enhancement with mucoceles following gadolinium administration aids in differentiating a sinus tumor from a mucocele. However, if a mucocele becomes superinfected (termed a *mucopyocele*), differentiation from a malignancy is more difficult.

Silent Sinus Syndrome

Silent sinus syndrome (Fig. 10.26) is a progressive and gradual disorder whereby a hypoventilated maxillary sinus becomes atelectatic resulting in ipsilateral enophthalmos (posterior positioning of the globe in the orbit) and hypoglobus (caudal positioning of the globe compared to the contralateral globe) (40). Silent sinus syndrome occurs in the setting of chronic OMC obstruction. Since the maxillary sinus walls are fairly malleable, when there is chronic OMC obstruction, negative pressure in the maxillary sinus results in inward retraction of the maxillary sinus walls (40). This inward retraction of the maxillary sinus walls is termed an *atelectatic maxillary sinus*. Since the floor of the orbit shares a common wall with the roof of the maxillary sinus, the floor of the orbit becomes depressed in the setting of an atelectatic maxillary

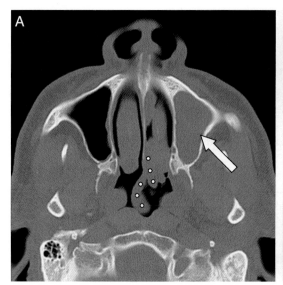
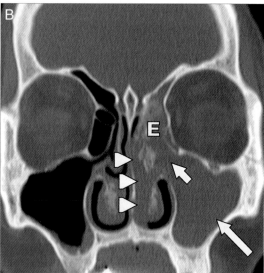

■ **FIGURE 10.24**   Antrochoanal polyp. Axial (**A**) and coronal (**B**) CT images with a bone alogorithm demonstrate complete opacification of the left maxillary antrum (*medium arrow*). The left infundibulum is widened (*small arrow*, **B**) and the polypoid opacity extends medial to the left middle and inferior turbinates (*arrowheads*). Contiguous polypoid opacity is present extending through the left choana into the nasopharynx (*dots*). The left ethmoids air cells (*E*) are opacified as well, either due to fluid or additional polyps.

sinus, thereby increasing the overall volume of the orbit (41). The orbital contents subsequently sag into the depressed orbital floor, resulting in enophthalmos and hypoglobus. When enophthalmos and/or hypoglobus are present, the constellation of findings is termed *silent sinus syndrome* as the enophthalmos and hypoglobus are generally painless. Visual acuity is typically unaffected in silent sinus syndrome (41). Atelectasis of the infundibulum occurs when the uncinate process becomes laterally positioned and immediately apposed to the inferomedial orbital wall, effectively obstructing the osteomeatal complex. This often results in concomitant enlargement of the ipsilateral middle meatus. An atelectatic infundibulum likely precedes and almost always coexists with an atelectatic maxillary sinus.

Odontogenic Sinusitis

Odontogenic sinusitis (*Fig. 10.27*) is thought to account for up to 10% to 12% of cases of maxillary sinusitis (42). The most common causes of odontogenic sinusitis include dental abscesses and periodontal disease that perforate the maxillary antral floor, intra-antral foreign bodies related to dental procedures, and maxillary antral perforation from a dental extraction (42). The patient may experience dental pain, headache, and anterior maxillary tenderness with odontogenic sinusitis (42). The treatment requires management of the odontogenic abnormality as well as the sinusitis, which generally includes both medical and dental surgical intervention (42).

Intracranial Complications of Rhinosinusitis

The incidence of intracranial complications from sinusitis has markedly decreased in the past decades, due to improved management of these cases and imaging guidance for treatment planning. There are a range of complications that may occur (*Fig. 10.28* and *Fig 10.29*) including meningitis, epidural abscess, subdural empyema, brain abscess, cortical venous thrombosis, and dural venous sinus thrombosis (18,43). Gallagher et al. (44) performed a chart review during a 5-year period of all patients admitted to their institution with one of the above diagnoses. They identified 176 cases of which 15 patients had 22 intracranial complications of sinusitis. The incidence of complications among this group was as follows: epidural abscess—23%, subdural empyema—18%, meningitis—18%, cerebral abscess—14%, superior sagittal sinus thrombosis—9%, cavernous sinus thrombosis—9%, and osteomyelitis—9%. Intracranial spread of infection can be secondary to direct communication with the intracranial contents via anatomic pathways. These pathways may arise from congenital or traumatic dehiscences, bone erosion, or through normal foramina such as those seen in the cribriform plate. Additionally, the diploic spaces of the sinus walls have draining veins that connect to intracranial veins and draining venous sinuses. These routes may permit the spread of infection without obvious bone destruction. Such spread may also give rise to orbital complications (*Fig. 10.30*) including preseptal cellulitis, postseptal cellulitis, and subperiosteal orbital abscess from spread of infection via valveless ethmoidal veins (43).

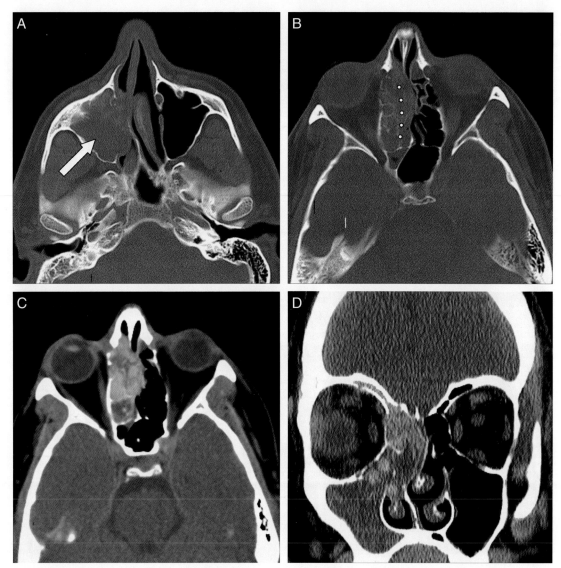

■ **FIGURE 10.25**   Allergic fungal sinusitis. Axial CT images with a bone algorithm through the level of the maxillary sinuses (**A**) and ethmoid air cells (**B**) demonstrate complete opacification of the right maxillary antrum (*arrow*) and ethmoid air cells (*dots*) associated with sinus expansion. Axial (**C**) and coronal CT reformatted (**D**) images with a soft tissue algorithm demonstrate increased attenuation in the involved sinuses consistent with fungal colonization. Allergic fungal sinusitis in a different patient (**E** through **H**). Coronal reformatted image with a bone algorithm (**E**) demonstrates marked expansion of the ethmoid air cells (*medium arrows*) and the visualized frontal sinuses (*small arrows*) with complete opacification of the paranasal sinuses and nasal cavity. The nasal cavity opacification is likely due to confluent polyposis. Axial CT image with a soft tissue algorithm (**F**) demonstrates marked expansion of the left frontal sinus, representing mucocele formation, with an imperceptible inner table of the left frontal sinus (*small arrows*). The increased attenuation in the right frontal sinus (*medium arrows*, **F**) is consistent with fungal colonization. Axial T1 noncontrast (**G**) and coronal T2 (**H**) MR images also demonstrate the markedly expanded left frontal sinus (*small arrow*) with imaging characteristics consistent with a mucocele. Compression of the left orbital soft tissues is present (*medium arrow*).

Association of Allergy, Rhinosinusitis and Polyposis

The exact relationship between allergy and sinusitis has not been determined. It is thought that in response to an inhaled allergen, an IgE-mediated (type 1 hypersen-sitivity) response occurs within the nasal mucosa. Nasal mucosal edema results in obstruction of the sinus ostia, decreased ciliary action, and increased mucus production with subsequent sinusitis. One study demonstrated that those patients with CT findings of extensive sinus disease had more markers of allergy. Specifically, this

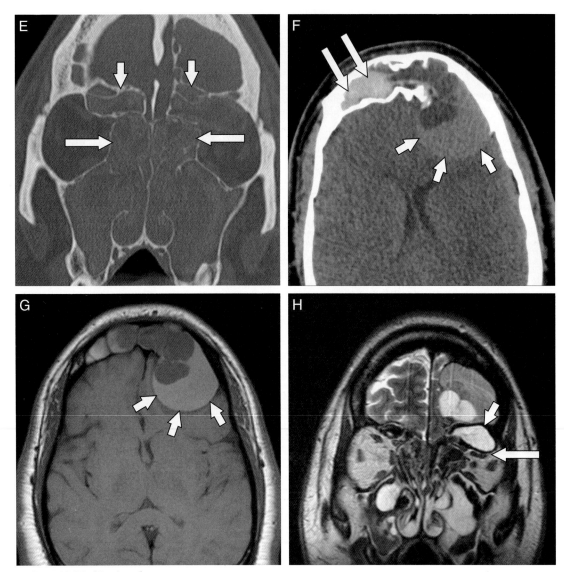

■ **FIGURE 10.25** *(Continued)*

group had a much higher prevalence of IgE antibodies to common inhalant allergens than the group of patients with limited sinus disease (45).

Sinonasal polyposis is the term used to describe extensive polyp disease (Fig. 10.23). As with sinusitis, there is debate concerning the relationship of nasal polyps (NP) with allergy. It is likely multifactorial although allergy is a suspected factor (46). The triad of aspirin intolerance, NP, and asthma is well-documented, supporting an allergic component to the development of sinonasal polyposis (47). Additionally, studies have shown that elevated mucosal IgE levels and eosinophilic inflammation are present in NP biopsy specimens from asthmatic patients (48,49). It is reported that 3% to 70% of patients with NP develop asthma, while 4% to 32% of asthmatic patients have NP (46).

Regardless of the etiologic factors, the imaging appearance of polyposis can be quite dramatic (*Fig. 10.16*). Rounded masses are seen filling the nasal cavities (unilateral or bilateral), often extending into and filling the adjacent sinuses. The involved ostia and outflow tracts are typically enlarged. The lateral walls of the ethmoid sinus often bulge laterally. The osseous sinus walls may be thinned and at times appear eroded making the possibility of a malignant mass a differential consideration. On CT, sinonasal polyposis is generally low in attenuation, although high attenuation can sometimes be seen surrounding the polyps. On MRI, the appearance of sinonasal polyposis will depend on the relative free water and protein concentration. Following the administration of contrast, the polypoid mucosa does not enhance homogenously (as one

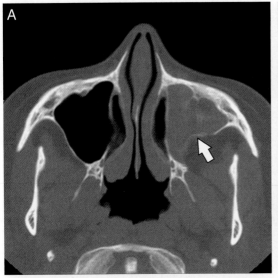

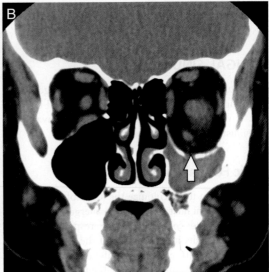

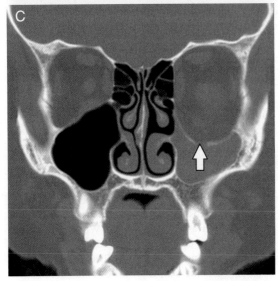

■ **FIGURE 10.26** Silent sinus syndrome. Axial CT image with a bone algorithm (**A**) demonstrates a completely opacified left maxillary antrum with a ventrally bowed posterolateral maxillary wall (*arrow*) and a smaller size compared to the right maxillary antrum. Coronal CT with soft tissue (**B**) and bone (**C**) algorithm images demonstates caudal bowing of the floor of the left orbit (*arrow*) toward the completely opacified small left maxillary antrum. An axial CT image with a soft tissue algorithm through the orbits (**D**) demonstrates subtle enophthalmos of the left globe (*L*) relative to the right (*R*).

would expect with malignancy) but rather only peripherally (18, 50).

■ GRANULOMATOUS DISEASES

Wegener Granulomatosis

Wegener granulomatosis (*Fig. 10.31*) is an idiopathic necrotizing granulomatous vasculitis that involves virtually any organ system, including the paranasal sinuses and in particular the nasal cavity (26,51). Common but nonspecific imaging findings with Wegener granulomatosis include nodular mucosal thickening, osseous destruction, osseous sclerosis, and nasal septal perforation. An orbital mass or extension of granulomatous disease from the paranasal sinuses into the orbit is

the most common extra-sinonasal head and neck lesion associated with Wegener granulomatosis (52).

Sarcoidosis

Sarcoidosis is a systemic granulomatous disease that is characterized by noncaseating granulomas and multinucleated giant cells (26). Sarcoidosis is most often indistinguishable from Wegener granulomatosis and may result in osseous destruction and nasal septal perforation (*Fig. 10.32*), although sarcoidosis generally does not result in bone destruction. Occasionally, nodules representing noncaseating granulomas can be seen along the nasal septum (26).

Advanced cases of Wegener granulomatosis and sarcoidosis can result in a so-called *saddle-nose* deformity, where the dominant abnormality is nasal bridge depression from cartilage and osseous destruction (*Fig. 10.31*).

■ FUNGAL SINUSITIS

Fungal sinusitis can be divided into four categories: allergic fungal sinusitis (AFS), mycetoma (fungal ball), chronic invasive fungal sinusitis, and acute invasive fungal sinusitis.

Allergic Fungal Sinusitis

AFS occurs when fungi colonize the sinus of an atopic immunocompetent host, and act as an allergen, eliciting both humoral and cellular immune responses. The inflammation results in obstruction of the sinus, stasis of secretions, and further fungal proliferation. The diagnostic criteria for AFS are as follows: the presence of allergic mucin (fungal hyphae and eosinophils); evidence of fungal specific IgE; the absence of fungal invasion of the submucosa, blood vessels, or bone; immunocompetency; and radiologic confirmation (53–54).

The CT findings of air-fluid levels associated with acute bacterial sinusitis are less common in fungal sinusitis; in fact, the absence of fluid levels can be suggestive of fungal disease. There is often complete opacification of the involved sinus. In a study performed by Mukherji et al. (54), it was noted that 96% of the patients had more than one sinus involved by the disease process. The sinuses involved with AFS disease, particularly the ethmoid air cells, are expanded and remodeled, occasionally with small osseous dehiscences. The bone resorption and remodeling is due to pressure from the expanding allergic mucin mass rather than invasion of fungi into the sinus mucosa or bone (55). The secretions in AFS may demonstrate areas of high CT attenuation. This is felt to be secondary to the presence of calcium, heavy metals (iron and manganese) and inspissated secretions (54,56). A similar appearance may occur with inspissated secretions in chronic bacterial sinusitis. However, one study (57) demonstrated that the calcifications seen in fungal sinusitis are more commonly central in location and more likely to be punctate in morphology. The calcifications in nonfungal sinusitis are more likely at the periphery of the sinus. Most cases of allergic fungal sinusitis are associated with nasal polyposis (55). In summary, allergic fungal sinusitis on CT is manifested as expansile disease with multiple sinus involvement and high density content, with or without calcifications (Fig. 10.21).

On MRI, the T1 signal of the secretions in allergic fungal sinusitis is isointense or hypointense. As a result of the presence of calcification and/or paramagnetic ions within the inspissated secretions, T2-weighted images show marked low signal and often a signal void (57).

Mycetoma

A mycetoma (or fungal ball) is also seen in immunocompetent nonatopic individuals; the fungus is in the secretions of the sinus without penetration of the mucosa (55). Mycetomas are tangled mats of hyphae that result in a low-grade chronic noninvasive fungal sinus disease. A mycetoma typically involves only one sinus, with the maxillary sinus being most commonly involved (58). Mycetomas generally cause sinus wall sclerosis (Fig. 10.20) and are usually asymptomatic or only minimally symptomatic. A mycetoma often contains calcification or a concretion within an opacified sinus. Osseous erosion usually does not occur. MRI demonstrates intermediate T1-weighted signal and hypointense T2-weighted signal. However, as is seen with other fungal sinus disease processes, the sinus can be completely hypointense on T1 and T2 without any MRI findings of sinus disease.

Chronic Invasive Fungal Sinusitis

Chronic invasive fungal sinusitis typically occurs in an immunocompetent individual. The fungus in this entity proliferates in the sinus cavity and penetrates the mucosa. Chronic invasive fungal sinusitis is extremely rare in the United States; most reports come from India or Sudan (7).

Acute Invasive Fungal Sinusitis

Acute invasive fungal sinusitis is a rapidly progressive disease seen in the immunocompromised host, with *Aspergillus*, *Rhizopus*, and *Mucor* being the most common offending organisms (55). There is usually soft tissue and vascular invasion with necrosis. While invasive fungal sinusitis may erode or destroy bone, often the bone is intact on imaging (*Fig. 10.33*). Silverman et al. (59) noted that in some cases there is loss of the normal periantral fat planes since invasive fungal sinusitis spreads outside the sinus lumen via perivascular channels. This occurs prior to bone destruction and may be an early sign of an invasive process. It is very important to inspect the premaxillary and retromaxillary fat in cases of significant maxillary sinus disease to exclude early extension by an invasive fungal sinusitis. Typically, invasive fungal sinusitis demonstrates an enhancing mass with or without bone erosion/destruction. The infection often extends beyond the sinus walls to involve the superficial soft tissues, orbit, or intracranial contents. Acute invasive fungal sinusitis is extremely aggressive and quickly spreads to adjacent structures. If untreated, invasive fungal sinusitis can be lethal.

■ SINONASAL TUMORS

Definitive radiologic diagnosis of sinonasal pathology is difficult as many processes demonstrate nearly identical imaging features. Imaging of sinonasal neoplasms is no exception, although some generalizations can be made. On MRI, tumors most often are intermediate to low in signal intensity on T2-weighted images. Hydrated secretions and hypertrophic mucosa (such as polyps or retention cysts) are generally more hyperintense on T2-weighted imaging. This assumes that the secretions are not inspissated. Neoplasms often demonstrate homogenous enhancement, while sinusitis, polyps, retention cysts, and mucoceles do not; this is a key finding. The problem with using bone destruction and extension to surrounding structures as a distinguishing feature is apparent, as this may be seen in aggressive non-neoplastic processes as well.

The most common benign sinonasal tumor is the osteoma (*Fig. 10.34*) (60). An osteoma is a well-defined, bone-forming tumor (52) covered by mucosa that is most commonly located in the frontal sinus (60) but can be seen in any sinus. An osteoma is generally an incidental finding and patients are asymptomatic, unless an osteoma results in obstruction, such as at the frontoethmoidal recess. A sinus osteoma rarely may also be associated with spontaneous pneumocephalus. If multiple osteomas are present, one should consider Gardener syndrome, which is an autosomal dominant condition of multiple osteomas, colorectal polyps, and soft tissue tumors (such as epidermal inclusion cysts and subcutaneous fibrous tumors) (60).

An inverted papilloma is an epithelial tumor that typically occurs in 50-year-olds to 70-year-olds, with a male to female ratio of 3:1 (60). This tumor is unusual in that the epithelium grows (inverts) into the underlying stroma, rather than initially growing exophytically. It is usually a unilateral mass that arises from the lateral nasal wall adjacent to the middle turbinate, and commonly extends into the maxillary sinus. An inverted papilloma is locally aggressive and commonly recurs following local resection. There is an association between inverted papilloma and squamous cell carcinoma; the numbers range from 2% to 56%. The malignancy may arise directly from the inverted papilloma or adjacent to the papilloma (synchronous tumors) (61,62). Squamous cell carcinoma may also arise following resection of an inverted papilloma (metachronous tumor), although metachronous tumors are much less common that synchronous tumors (60). An inverted papilloma is primarily soft tissue density on CT, and may have a lobulated surface with foci of calcification. The MRI appearance of an inverted papilloma nonspecific although one can see a "cerebriform" pattern on T2-weighted MR imaging characterized by curvilinear striations (*Fig. 10.35*) (52). At surgery, these lesions are often gritty in consistency, as opposed to polyps which are soft. Given the proclivity of an inverted papilloma for local destruction as well as its association with malignancy, surgery is part of the treatment paradigm (60).

A juvenile nasopharyngeal angiofibroma (JNA) is a benign vascular neoplasm that is unencapsulated (52). A JNA is generally thought to arise in the sphenopalatine foramen (60) and almost always involves the pterygopalatine fossa. This tumor usually presents in the second decade of life and occurs almost exclusively in males, often with epistaxis or nasal obstruction. Although a JNA is histologically benign, it is locally aggressive. It commonly widens and destroys the pterygopalatine fossa and erodes the pterygoid plates as it extends into the nasopharynx. The characteristic location, often with destruction or displacement of the posterolateral wall of the maxillary sinus, is one of the specific features that can be identified on CT (*Fig. 10.36*). In addition, the tumor is highly vascular and will show extensive vascular flow voids on MRI and high flow architecture on magnetic resonance angiography (63), computed tomographic angiography and conventional angiography. Tumor vascular supply often arises from the internal maxillary and ascending pharyngeal branches of the external carotid artery. When a JNA extends intracranially, small branches from the cavernous internal carotid artery may supply the tumor.

Malignancies of the nasal cavity and paranasal sinuses are rare. When they do occur they most often involve the maxillary sinus, followed by the ethmoid sinuses, and finally the nasal cavity. Eighty percent of all sinus malignancies are squamous cell carcinoma (*Fig. 10.37*) (11). CT findings include bone erosion and destruction with extension of the tumor beyond the sinus lumen or nasal cavity. MRI has a clear advantage over CT in evaluating sinus malignancies by helping differentiate tumor from post obstructive sinus disease. Malignancies generally homogeneously enhance on MRI and are often hypointense on T2-weighted imaging while postobstructive sinus disease will only peripherally enhance and is most commonly hyperintense on T2. MRI can also help delineate the extent of the tumor and any invasion into adjacent structures. CT is complementary to MRI by providing better bone detail.

Other sinonasal neoplasms that occur with variable frequency are esthesioneuroblastoma, sinonasal undifferentiated carcinoma (SNUC), osteosarcoma, non-Hodgkin lymphoma, minor salivary gland tumors, and melanoma, to name a few. Many of these tumors do not have specific imaging findings.

An esthesioneuroblastoma is a neural crest tumor that arises from the olfactory epithelium of the nasal cavity. There is a bimodal age distribution affecting teenagers and individuals in their sixth decade. These tumors are typically located at the level of the cribriform plate in the superior aspect of the nasal cavity. When these tumors extend intracranially, they may be associated apical cysts along their cephalad margin. Esthesioneuroblastomas are mostly hypointense on T2-weighted imaging due to their high cellularity (64).

SNUC (*Fig. 10.38*) is believed to be part of a spectrum that includes esthesioneuroblastoma (least malignant), neuroendocrine carcinomas, and small cell carcinoma (most malignant) (65); these tumors are roughly equivalent in prognosis with neuroendocrine carcinomas (65). SNUC tumors usually arise in the nasal cavity and ethmoid air cells and are locally advanced when diagnosed (5,66). These tumors also have a high nuclear to cytosplasmic ratio.

Adenoid cystic carcinomas (*Fig. 10.39*) account for up to 5% to 15% of all sinonasal malignant neoplasms and occur in minor salivary glands within the sinonasal cavities (5). These tumors are locally aggressive neoplasms and are classically known for their propensity for perineural spread. Hematogenous spread to lungs and bones is relatively common, but lymphatic involvement is not common (67).

Osteosarcoma (*Fig. 10.40*) is a malignant tumor that produces an osteoid matrix with many subtypes. This lesion may or may not be associated with a destructive pattern, and generally produces dense sclerotic bone, particularly when it occurs in the maxillary sinus.

Melanoma of the nasal and paranasal sinus mucosa has a unique MR appearance that may suggest the diagnosis. Melanotic tumors are hyperintense on T1-weighted images and hypointense on T2-weighted images (11). Patients with sinonasal melanoma present with advanced disease and most succumb to the disease within 3 years of diagnosis (68).

■ CONCLUSION

The intricate anatomy of the paranasal sinuses makes interpreting sinus examinations a challenge. Imaging examinations are designed not only to recognize acute disease processes, but also to identify any anatomic variations that may predispose to infection, which is best evaluated with CT. The anatomical guidance provided by cross sectional imaging helps map out a course of action for the surgeon and helps to identify potential areas at risk for complications. While sinusitis is essentially a clinical diagnosis, there are important imaging correlates. In addition, the complications from the natural progression of the primary disease process or from surgery are best diagnosed by imaging studies. The exact relationship of allergy to the various inflammatory disease processes affecting the sinus remains unclear. Inflammatory disease processes can have a similar appearance to the more aggressive fungal and malignant entities; therefore, close attention to the imaging findings, and clinical correlation, is required in order to differentiate these processes.

■ REFERENCES

1. Babbel RW, Harnsberger HR. A contemporary look at the imaging issues of sinusitis: sinonasal anatomy, physiology and computed tomography technique. *Semin Ultrasound CT MR.* 1991;12(6):526–540.

2. Zinreich J. Imaging of inflammatory sinus disease. *Otolaryngol Clin North Am.* 1993;26(4):535–547.

3. Davis WE, Templer J, Parsons DS. Anatomy of the paranasal sinuses. *Otolaryngol Clin North Am.* 1996;29(1):57–74.

4. Daniels DL, Mafee MF, Smith MM, et al. The frontal sinus drainage pathway and related structures. *AJNR Am J Neuroradiol.* 2003;24(8):1618–1627.

5. Rao VM, El-Noueam K. Sinonasal imaging anatomy and pathology. *Radiol Clin North Am.* 1998;36(5):921–939.

6. Kubal WS. Sinonasal anatomy. *Neuroimaging Clin N Am.* 1998; 8(1):143–156.

7. Zeifer B. Update on sinonasal imaging: anatomy and inflammatory disease. *Neuroimaging Clin N Am.* 1998;8(3):607–630.

8. Earwaker J. Anatomic variants in sinonasal CT. *Radiographics.* 1993;13:381–415.

9. Laine FJ, Smoker WRK. The ostiomeatal unit and endoscopic surgery: anatomy, variations, and imaging findings in inflammatory diseases. *AJR Am J Roentgenol.* 1992;159:849–857.

10. Stallman JS, Lobo JN, Som PM. The incidence of concha bullosa and its relationship to nasal septal deviation and paranasal sinus disease. *AJNR Am J Neuroradiol.* 2004;25(9):1613–1618.

11. Hudgins PA. Sinonasal imaging. *Neuroimaging Clin N Am.* 1996;6(2):319–331.

12. Seiden AM, Martin VT. Headache and the frontal sinus. *Otolaryngol Clin North Am.* 2001;34(1):227–241.

13. Parsons DS, Batra PS. Functional endoscopic sinus surgical outcomes for contact point headaches. *Laryngoscope.* 1998;108(5): 696–702.

14. Harley DH, Powitzky ES, Duncavage J. Clinical outcomes for the surgical treatment of sinonasal headache. *Otolaryngol Head Neck Surg.* 2003;129(3):217–221.

15. Lee WT, Kuhn FA, Citardi MJ. 3D computed tomographic analysis of frontal recess anatomy in patients without frontal sinusitis. *Otolaryngol Head Neck Surg.* 2004;131(3):164–673.

16. Stammberger HR, Kennedy DW. Paranasal sinuses:anatomic terminology and nomenclature. The Anatomic Terminology Group. *Ann Otol Rhinol Laryngol Suppl.* 1995;167:7–16.

17. Kainz J, Stammberger H. The roof of the anterior ethmoid: A place of least resistance in the skull base. *Am J Rhinol.* 1989;4:191.

18. Yousem DM. Imaging of sinonasal inflammatory disease. *Radiology.* 1993;188:303–314.

19. Hudgins PA, Browning DG, Gallups J, et al. Endoscopic paranasal sinus surgery: radiographic evaluation of severe complications. *Am J Neuroradiol.* 1992;14:1161–1167.

20. Arbeláez A, Medina E, Rodríguez M, et al. Intrathecal administration of gadopentetate dimeglumine for MR cisternography of nasoethmoidal CSF fistula. *AJR Am J Roentgenol.* 2007;188(6):W560–W564.

21. La Fata V, McLean N, Wise SK, et al. CSF leaks: correlation of high-resolution ct and multiplanar reformations with intraoperative endoscopic findings. *AJNR Am J Neuroradiol.* 2008;29(3):536–541. Epub 2007, Dec 13.

22. Stafford DB, Brennan P, Toland J, et al. Magnetic resonance imaging in the evaluation of cerebrospinal fluid fistula. *Clin Radiol.* 1996;51:837–841.

23. Houser SM. Empty nose syndrome associated with middle turbinate resection. *Otolaryngol Head Neck Surg.* 2006;135(6):972–973.

24. Nelson KL. CT of sinonasal inflammatory disease. *Imaging Decisions.* 1994:26–38.

25. Hahnel S, Ertl-Wagner B, Tasman A, et al. Relative value of MR imaging as compared with CT in the diagnosis of inflammatory paranasal sinus disease. *Radiology.* 1999; 210:171–176.

26. Eggesbø HB. Radiological imaging of inflammatory lesions in the nasal cavity and paranasal sinuses. *Eur Radiol.* 2006;16(4):872–88. Epub 2006, Jan 4.

27. Silberstein SD. Headaches due to nasal and paranasal sinus disease. *Neurol Clin.* 2004;22(1):1–19.

28. Shapiro G, Rachelefsky G. Introduction and definition of sinusitis. *J Allergy Clin Immunol.* 1992; 90(3):417–418.

29. Bhattacharyya T, Piccirillo J, Wippold FJ. Relationship between patient based descriptions of sinusitis and paranasal sinus computed tomographic findings. *Arch Otolaryngol Head Neck Surg.* 1997; 123(11):1189–1192.

30. Zinreich SJ, Kennedy DW, Kumar AJ, et al. MR imaging of the normal nasal cycle: comparison with sinus pathology. *J Comput Assist Tomogr.* 1988;12(6):1014–1019.

31. Rak KM, Newell JD, Yakes WF, et al . Paranasal sinuses on MR images of the brain: significance of mucosal thickening. *Am J Neuroradiol.* 1990;11:1211–1214.

32. Som PM, Dillon WP, Fullerton GD, et al. Chronically obstructed sinonasal secretions: observations on T1 and T2 shortening. *Radiology.* 1989;172:515–520.

33. Dillon WP, Som PM, Fullerton GD. Hypointense MR signal in chronically inspissated sinonasal secretions. *Radiology.* 1990;174: 73–78.

34. Som PM, Shugar JM. CT classification of ethmoid mucoceles. *J Comput Assist Tomogr.* 1980;4(2):199–203.

35. Weissman JL, Tabor EK, Curtin HD. Sphenochoanal polyps: evaluation with CT and MR imaging. *Radiology.* 1991;178:145–148.

36. Lim CC, Dillon WP, McDermott MW. Mucocele involving the anterior clinoid process: MR and CT findings. *AJNR Am J Neuroradiol.* 1999;20(2):287–290.

37. Weissman JL, Curtin HD, Eibling DE. Double mucocele of the paranasal sinuses. *Am J Neuroradiol.* 1994;15:1263–1264.

38. Lanziero CF, Shah M, Krauss D, et al. Use of Gadolinium-enhanced MR imaging for differentiating mucocele from neoplasms in the paranasal sinuses. *Radiology.* 1991;179;425–428.

39. VanTassel P, Lee Y, Jing B, et al. Mucoceles of the paranasal sinuses: MR imaging with CT correlation. *AJR,* 1989;153:407–412.

40. Annino DJ Jr, Goguen LA. Silent sinus syndrome. *Curr Opin Otolaryngol Head Neck Surg.* 2008;16(1):22–25.

41. Buono LM. The silent sinus syndrome: maxillary sinus atelectasis with enophthalmos and hypoglobus. *Curr Opin Ophthalmol.* 2004;15(6):486–489.

42. Brook I. Sinusitis of odontogenic origin. *Otolaryngol Head Neck Surg.* 2006;135(3):349–355.

43. Wegenmann M, Naclerio RM. Complications of sinusitis. *J Allergy Clin Immunol.* 1992;90(3):552–554.

44. Gallagher RM, Gross CW, Phillips CD. Suppurative intracranial complications of sinusitis. *Laryngoscope.* 1998;108(11 pt 1):1635–1642.

45. Phillips CD, Platts-Mills TAE. Chronic sinusitis: relationship between CT findings and clinical history of asthma, allergy, eosinophilia and infection. *AJR.* 1995;164:185–187.

46. Ceylan E, Gencer M, San I. Nasal polyps and the severity of asthma. *Respirology.* 2007;12(2):272–276.

47. Slavin RG. Nasal polyps and sinusitis. *JAMA.* 1997;278(22):1849–1854.

48. Bachert C, Patou J, Van Cauwenberge P. The role of sinus disease in asthma. *Curr Opin Allergy Clin Immunol.* 2006;6(1):29–36.

49. Penn R, Mikula S. The role of anti-IgE immunoglobulin therapy in nasal polyposis: a pilot study. *Am J Rhinol.* 2007;21(4):428–432.

50. Drutman J, Babbel RW, Harnsberger JR, et al. Sinonasal polyposis. *Semin Ultrasound CT MR.* 1991;12(6);561–574.

51. Lohrmann C, Uhl M, Warnatz K, et al. Sinonasal computed tomography in patients with Wegener granulomatosis. *J Comput Assist Tomogr.* 2006;30(1):122–125.

52. Harnsberger HR, Hudgins, PA, Wiggins RH, et al., eds. *Diagnostic Imaging: Head and Neck.* 1st ed. Salt Lake City: Amirsys; 2004; II:2–60.

53. Meltzer EO, Hamilos DL, Hadley JA, et al. Rhinosinusitis: developing guidance for clinical trials. *J Allergy Clin Immunol.* 2006;118:S17–S61.

54. Mukherji SK, Figueroa RE, Ginsberg LE, et al. Allergic fungal sinusitis: CT findings. *Radiology.* 1998;207:417–422.

55. Schubert MS. Allergic fungal sinusitis. *Clin Allergy Immunol.* 2007;20:263–271.

56. Zinreich SJ, Kennedy DW, Malat J, et al. Fungal sinusitis: diagnosis with CT and MR imaging. *Radiology,* 1988;169:439–444.

57. Yoon JH, Na DG, Byun HS, et al. Calcification in chronic maxillary sinusitis: comparison of CT findings with histopathologic results. *Am J Neuroradiol.* 1999;20:571–574.

58. Senocak D, Kaur A. What's in a fungus ball? Report of a case with submucosal invasion and tissue eosinophilia. *Ear Nose Throat J.* 2004;83(10):696–698.

59. Silverman CS, Mancuso AA. Periantral soft tissue infiltration and its relevance to early detection of invasive fungal sinusitis: CT and MR findings. *Am J Neuroradiol.* 1998;19:321–325.

60. Melroy CT, Senior BA. Benign sinonasal neoplasms: a focus on inverting papilloma. *Otolaryngol Clin North Am.* 2006;39(3):601–617.

61. Woodruff WW, Vrabec DP. Inverted papilloma of the nasal vault and paranasal sinuses: spectrum of CT findings. *AJR,* 1994;162:419–423.

62. Dammann F, Pereira P, Laniado M, et al. Inverted papilloma of the nasal cavity and the paranasal sinuses: using CT for primary diagnosis and follow-up. *AJR.* 1999;172:543–548.

63. Albery SM, Chaljub G, Cho NL, et al. MR imaging of nasal masses. *RadioGraphics,* 1995;15:1311–1327.

64. Li C, Yousem DM, Hayden RE, et al. Olfactory neuroblastoma: MR evaluation. *Am J Neuroradiol.* 1993;14:1167–1171.

65. Rosenthal DI, Barker JL Jr, El-Naggar AK, et al. Sinonasal malignancies with neuroendocrine differentiation: patterns of failure according to histologic phenotype. *Cancer.* 2004;101(11):2567–2573.

66. Mendenhall WM, Mendenhall CM, Riggs CE Jr, et al. Sinonasal undifferentiated carcinoma. *Am J Clin Oncol.* 2006;29(1):27–31.

67. Rhee CS, Won TB, Lee CH, et al. Adenoid cystic carcinoma of the sinonasal tract: treatment results. *Laryngoscope.* 2006; 116(6):982–986.

68. Ferraro RE, Schweinfurth JM, Highfill GR. Mucosal melanoma of the sinonasal tract. *Am J Otolaryngol.* 2002;23(5):321–323.

Radiologic Evaluation of Allergic and Related Diseases of the Lower Airway

THOMAS GRANT

The radiographic appearance of thoracic manifestations of systemic immunologic and allergic disorders comprises a variety of abnormalities that are influenced by the pathophysiologic characteristics of the underlying disease. These disorders include collagen vascular diseases and the systemic vasculitides. The clinician must also be familiar with the diseases in this category, a diverse group including Churg-Strauss syndrome (CSS), Wegener granulomatosis, asthma, allergic bronchopulmonary aspergillosis (ABPA), bronchocentric granulomatosis, hypersensitivity pneumonitis, eosinophilic lung disease, and drug induced lung injury.

Immunologic and allergic diseases of the lungs can manifest radiographically as diffuse or focal pulmonary parenchymal and airway abnormalities (1,2). In earlier stages of the disease, radiographs may be normal. Although chest radiographs are usually abnormal in advanced disease, characterization is frequently impossible. Thin section, or high resolution computed tomography (HRCT) has become the most important imaging technique to confirm the diagnosis.

■ COMPUTED TOMOGRAPHY

Recent developments using multi-detector CT (MDCT) change the way in which radiologists perform and interpret studies of the thorax (3,4). Current generation CT scanners with 16 or more detector rows can acquire isotropic volumetric data in a single breath hold. For example, MDCT scanners can cover the entire chest with a <1 mm collimation (section of thickness) in less than 20 seconds. MDCT not only generates traditional axial images but can acquire volumetric data sets to view the computer-generated information in multiple nonaxial planes if desired (4). The volumetric acquired data make CT ideal for detecting, characterizing, and distinguishing among diseases of the lungs, mediastinum, and pleura.

HRCT involves obtaining narrow (<2 mm) collimation, a small field of view, and a high spatial frequency reconstruction algorithm to obtain detailed images of the lungs. By using a very thin section, structural superimposition within the section of thickness is reduced, permitting optimal evaluation of lung detail. At our institution, the HRCT is typically performed with the patient in the supine position. Images are obtained in full inspiration from the apex to the diaphragm using 1.0 mm collimation. This is followed by a fewer number of inspiratory images obtained in a prone position. Expiratory images are obtained to look for air trapping. HRCT can detect lung disease at an early and potentially treatable stage. HRCT is also valuable in differentiating acute from chronic disease and optimizing the site for bronchoscopic or open lung biopsy (3–5). The HRCT findings of certain immunologic lung diseases are often so characteristic that a lung biopsy is not required (6,7).

The use of intravenous contrast is frequently unnecessary for chest CT examinations, particularly for evaluating pulmonary nodules or interstitial lung disease. However, intravenous contrast can help to distinguish lymph nodes from pulmonary vessels, characterize pleural disease, demonstrate vascular components of an arterial venous malformation, and detect pulmonary emboli.

Intravenous contrast should be avoided in patients with a creatinine level above 1.5 mg/dL, in patients with multiple myeloma, and in patients with suspected pheochromocytoma. Low osmotic contrast is now preferred because it has fewer side effects. Corticosteroid pretreatment supplemented with antihistamine, diminishes the risk of adverse reactions in patients with a previous anaphylactoid reactions to contrast material.

■ COMPUTED TOMOGRAPHY ANATOMY

The lung is composed of lobes, segments, subsegments, secondary lobules, and acini (8,9). Each level contains an airway, a pulmonary artery, and a supporting structure, the peribronchovascular interstitium. The airway is a branching series of 20 generations that leads to the alveoli.

The secondary pulmonary lobule is the smallest unit of lung structure marginated by connective tissue septa (10). These lobules measure 1 cm to 2.5 cm and are supplied by a small bronchial and pulmonary artery. The secondary lobule can be identified in both normal and abnormal lungs. There are distinct patterns of abnormality on HRCT that help to define acute and chronic infiltrative lung diseases (Tables 11.1 and 11.2).

Reticular opacities result from thickening of the pulmonary interstitium by fluid, fibrosis, or other materials. Pulmonary fibrosis on HRCT is characterized by honeycombing. In usual interstitial pneumonia honeycombing is most often observed peripherally at the lung bases (5,7). In chronic hypersensitivity pneumonitis the fibrosis is usually most severe in the mid or upper lung zones (11,12). Cysts or rounded air-containing nodules are present in a number of acute and chronic infiltrative diseases. Nodules in a centrilobular distribution that involve the secondary pulmonary lobule can be seen in subacute hypersensitivity pneumonitis,

pulmonary hemorrhage, cryptogenic organizing pneumonia, nonspecific interstitial pneumonia, and respiratory bronchiolitis-associated interstitial lung disease (13).

Ground-glass attenuation is characterized by the presence of hazy increased attenuation of lung without obscuration of the underlying bronchial or vascular anatomy. If the vessels are obscured, the term *consolidation* is used. Ground-glass attenuation can result from interstitial thickening, air space filling, or both. Although ground-glass attenuation is nonspecific, it usually indicates the presence of an active, potentially treatable disease.

■ RADIOLOGIC FINDINGS IN IMMUNOLOGIC LUNG DISEASE

Churg-Strauss Syndrome

CSS is a rare allergic necrotizing vasculitis of unknown etiology (15–17). The syndrome is most commonly seen in patients 30 years to 50 years of age and has no gender predilection. Patients are typically asthmatic and present with eosinophilia, fever, and multisystem vasculitis. Findings of chest radiography are often abnormal and most often consist of patchy nonsegmental areas of consolidation with no zonal predominance. The areas of consolidation may have peripheral distribution and are often transient. A pleural effusion is present in approximately 30% of patients, usually due

TABLE 11.1 COMMON COMPUTED TOMOGRAPHIC (CT) FEATURES OF IMMUNOLOGIC LUNG DISEASES

CT FINDING	ABPA	HYPERSENSITIVITY PNEUMONITIS (HP)	CHURG-STRAUSS SYNDROME	WEGENER GRANULO-MATOSIS	EOSINOPHILIC PNEUMONIA (EP)	ASTHMA
Ground-glass opacities		Acute		Present with cytotoxic drug treatment		
Consolidating/ air trappings			Consolidation		Consolidation	Air trappings
Irregular linear opacities		Chronic		Common		
Nodules	Centrilobular		0.5 cm to 3.0 cm in diameter	Common/ cavitation		
Distribution	Central	Mid and lower lung	Peripheral		Upper lobe peripheral in chronic EP	
Honeycombing fibrosis	Late stage (for ABPA)	Late stages chronic HP		Late	Chronic EP	
Bronchial abnormality	Bronchiectasis, mucoid impaction	Bronchiectasis in chronic HP	Wall thickening	Focal and diffuse narrowing		Bronchial wall thickening

ABPA, allergic bronchopulmonary aspergillosis.

TABLE 11.2   COMPUTED TOMOGRAPHIC (CT) APPEARANCE OF IMMUNOLOGIC/ EOSINOPHILIC LUNG DISEASE

DISEASE	CT APPEARANCE
Wegener granulomatosis	Multiple nodules or masses with or without cavitation, peripheral wedge-shaped areas of consolidation
Asthma	Air trapping on expiratory HRCT, bronchial wall thickening
Bronchocentric granulomatosis	Bronchiectasis, atelectasis, peripheral consolidation, ground-glass attenuation
Chronic eosinophilic pneumonia	Patchy unilateral or bilateral airspace consolidation, predominantly peripheral distribution, areas of ground-glass attenuation predominantly in the middle and upper lung zones
Acute eosinophilic pneumonia	Ground-glass attenuation, diffuse areas of ground-glass attenuation, defined nodules, smooth interlobular septal thickening
Churg-Strauss syndrome	Airspace consolidation, areas of ground-glass attenuation, peripheral predominance or random distribution, nodules, bronchial wall thickening or dilatation, interlobular septal thickening
ABPA	Bronchiectasis, mucous plugging, atelectasis, peripheral airspace consolidation or ground-glass attenuation
Simple pulmonary eosinophilia	Patchy unilateral or bilateral airspace consolidation, predominantly peripheral distribution, areas of ground-glass attenuation predominantly in the middle and upper lung zones, usually transient and migratory
Drug-induced eosinophilic pneumonia	Areas of ground-glass attenuation, airspace consolidation, nodules, irregular lines
Hypereosinophilic syndrome	Patchy areas of consolidation of nodules with or without pleural effusion

ABPA, allergic bronchopulmonary aspergillosis; HRCT, high resolution computed tomography

to cardiac involvement or eosinophilic pleuritis (15). Up to 25% of patients with CSS have few or no imaging abnormalities.

Recent reports on the HRCT findings of CSS have shown that they are nonspecific. Findings include ground-glass opacities, consolidation, small centrilobular nodules, interlobular septal thickening, and bronchial wall thickening (Fig. 11.1). The ground glass opacities and consolidation reflect the presence of chronic eosinophilic pneumonia (15).

Wegener Granulomatosis

Wegener granulomatosis (WG) is a systemic autoimmune disease characterized by a necrotizing granulomatous vasculitis of the upper and lower respiratory tracts and kidneys. The histologic features are a necrotizing vasculitis of small arteries and veins and granuloma formation. The clinical triad of classical WG is pulmonary disease, febrile sinusitis, and glomerulonephritis (2,18). A limited form of WG can be confined to the lungs. It is a disease that predominantly affects male patients. The imaging findings in most patients are multiple nodules or irregularly marginated masses

with no zonal predominance. The nodules or masses are usually multiple but can be solitary in approximately 25% of cases. Cavitation of the nodules occurs in approximately 50% of cases. The cavities usually have irregular, thick walls (2). After treatment, the

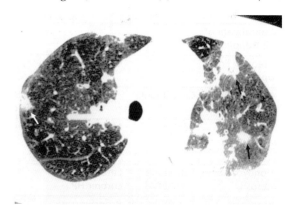

■ **FIGURE 11.1** Churg-Strauss syndrome. Computed tomography demonstrates irregular areas of consolidation (*arrows*) in this 57-year-old woman with previous episodes of eosinophilic pneumonia. An open lung biopsy revealed a necrotizing vasculitis.

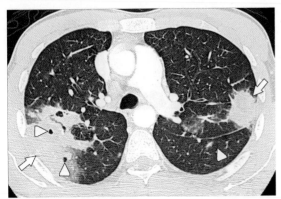

■ **FIGURE 11.2** Wegener granulomatosis in a 26-year-old man who presented with chronic cough, hemoptysis, and weight loss. Computed tomography demonstrates bilateral irregularly marginated masses (*arrows*) and small areas of cavitation (*arrowheads*).

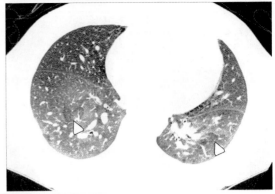

■ **FIGURE 11.3** Asthma in a 29-year-old man. Expiratory high resolution computed tomography demonstrates focal air trapping (*arrowheads*).

nodules or cavities may resolve completely or result in a scar. On CT, the nodules typically have irregular margins and often have a peribronchovascular distribution (Fig. 11.2). Peripheral, wedge-shaped areas of consolidation representing an infarct may be present.

A localized or diffuse area of air space consolidation may be present; these areas usually represent pulmonary hemorrhage. Involvement of the trachea or bronchial walls usually consists of mucosal or submucosal granulomatosis thickening. CT may show smooth nodular thickening of the tracheobronchial wall. If the thickening becomes severe, narrowing of the lumen and eventually calcification also may occur (1,2).

Asthma

HRCT findings of asthma have been assessed in several studies and include bronchial wall thickening, bronchial wall narrowing, and to a lesser extent bronchial wall dilatation (17). Air trapping and hyperinflation are common findings on HRCT. Emphysema is uncommon in the asthmatic nonsmoker. CT performed on expiration is helpful to determine the amount of air trapping (Fig. 11.3). Asthmatic patients with an FEV_1 of less than 60% of the predicted value had more bronchial wall thickening and a lower bronchial arterial diameter ratio than did patients with normal airflow or only mild airflow obstruction. The use of inspiratory and expiratory thin-section CT is of value in distinguishing asthmatic patients with normal to mild airflow obstruction from healthy subjects (19).

Allergic Bronchopulmonary Aspergillosis and Bronchocentric Granulomatosis

The primary radiographic presentation of ABPA on HRCT is severe bronchiectasis. The presence of bronchial dilatation, bronchial wall thickening, and

centrilobular nodules in an asthmatic patient should strongly suggest the diagnosis of an ABPA (20,21). The diagnosis is even more likely if the bronchial dilatation is moderate to severe, affects three or more lobes, and involves the central bronchi (Fig. 11.4). If bronchial dilatation is present in asthmatic patients without ABPA, it is most often mild and has an upper lobe distribution. Other findings include mucoid plugging involving the dilated ectatic bronchi. Several studies have concluded that HRCT is highly suggestive of ABPA when the classic findings are present (17,21).

Bronchocentric granulomatosis often occurs in patients with ABPA. It is characterized by a pattern of necrotizing granulomatous inflammation that destroys the walls of small bronchi and bronchioles (22).

Hypersensitivity Pneumonitis

Hypersensitivity pneumonitis (HP) is a diffuse granulomatous interstitial lung disease caused by inhalation of airborne organic particulate matter (12,23). Causative

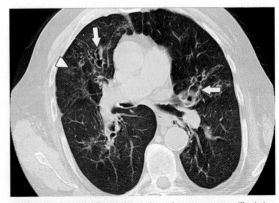

■ **FIGURE 11.4** Allergic bronchopulmonary aspergillosis in a 50-year-old man with asthma and eosinophilia. High resolution computed tomography demonstrates extensive bilateral central bronchiectasis (*arrows*) and peripheral centrilobular nodules (*arrowhead*).

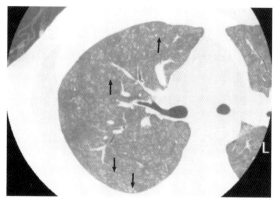

■ **FIGURE 11.5** Subacute hypersensitivity pneumonitis in a 30-year-old woman with acute dyspnea, hypoxemia, and chills after cleaning her attic. High resolution computed tomography shows numerous centrilobular nodules (*arrows*). The radiologic and clinical findings resolved 5 days after initiating corticosteroid therapy.

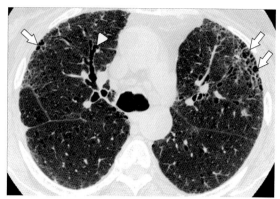

■ **FIGURE 11.6** Chronic hypersensitivity pneumonitis in a 52-year-old man with progressive dyspnea. Computed tomography shows traction bronchiectasis (*arrowhead*) and honeycombing (*arrows*).

factors are numerous and include bacteria, fungi, avian proteins, wood dusts, and chemicals. HP has been traditionally classified as manifesting in three phases: acute, subacute, and chronic. HRCT can be useful since patients with normal chest radiographs often have characteristic findings of centrilobular nodules and ground glass opacities. These findings are most common in the middle to lower lung fields (23,24).

Acute HP occurs after intense exposure to antigens. The radiographic manifestations have not been studied until recently. HRCT findings of acute HP are those of acute pulmonary edema and include diffuse ground glass opacities and thickening interlobular septa (23). The HRCT findings of subacute HP include diffuse or patchy ground glass opacities and small focal areas of decreased attenuation on expiratory images due to air trapping (23) (Fig. 11.5).

Chronic HP occurs after long-standing exposure to an offending antigen and can result in chronic pulmonary fibrosis. In chronic HP the HRCT findings include small nodules, irregular linear opacities, traction bronchiectasis, small areas of lobular lucency, and honeycombing that typically tend to spare the lung bases (11,23) (Fig. 11.6).

Eosinophilic Lung Disease

Eosinophilic lung disease of unknown cause includes simple pulmonary eosinophila (SPE), acute eosinophilic pneumonia, chronic eosinophic pneumonia, and idiopathic hypereosinphilic syndrome.

SPE, also known as Loeffler syndrome, is characterized by migratory pulmonary opacities, increased peripheral eosinophilia, little or no pulmonary symptoms, and spontaneous resolution within one month. The HRCT findings consist of ground-glass opacity and consolidation involving mainly the peripheral regions of the upper- and mid-lung zones (25,26) (Fig. 11.7).

Acute eosinophilc pneumonia (AEP) is an idiopathic disease, with a male predominance, in which acute upper respiratory failure is accompanied by markedly elevated levels of eosinophilia in fluid recovered from bronchoalveolar lavage (25,27). Peripheral blood eosinophilia is rarely present. Patients with AEP present with fever and acute respiratory failure (25). Pleural effusions are a common feature associated with AEP. The CT findings include patchy ground-glass opacities, interlobular septal thickening, and sometimes by pulmonary consolidation or nodules (Fig. 11.8). The radiographic differential diagnosis includes hydrostatic pulmonary edema, adult respiratory distress syndrome, and atypical viral or bacterial pneumonia.

Chronic eosinophilic pneumonia is an idiopathic condition histologically characterized by filling of the air spaces with eosinophils and macrophages and associated mild interstitial pneumonia. The patients are most often middle-aged and half of them have asthma. Patients usually present after several months of cough, low-grade fever, weight loss, and dyspnea (25,26,28).

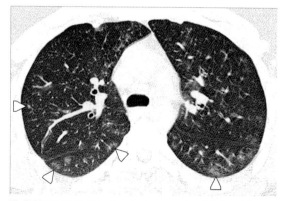

■ **FIGURE 11.7** Simple pulmonary eosinophila in a 19-year-old man with a cough and peripheral eosinophilia. HRCT shows peripheral small ground-glass opacities and centrilobular nodules in the upper lung zones (*arrowheads*).

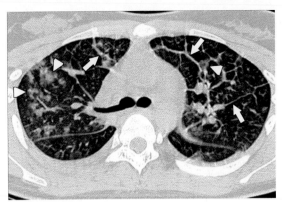

■ **FIGURE 11.8** Acute eosinophilc pneumonia in a 34-year-old woman with respiratory failure. The HRCT demonstrates thickening of the interlobular septum (*arrows*) and ground-glass opacities (*arrowheads*).

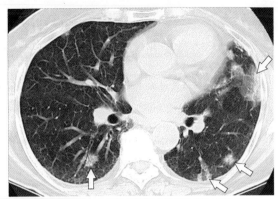

■ **FIGURE 11.10** Drug-induced lung disease in a 49-year-old woman on chemotherapy for lymphoma. There are lower lobe peripheral poorly defined ground opacities (*arrows*). The lung biopsy showed crytogenic organizing pneumonia.

On HRCT a peripheral distribution of consolidation is often present, even when it is not apparent on chest radiographs (Fig. 11.9). The combination of peripheral unilateral or bilateral patchy consolidation and peripheral blood eosinophilia is virtually diagnostic of chronic eosinophilic pneumonia (28).

Idiopathic hypereosinophilic syndrome (HES) is a rare and often fatal disorder characterized by elevated blood eosinophil levels (>1,500/μL) for more than 6 months. Cardiac involvement, including endocardial fibrosis and restrictive cardiomyopathy is one of the major complications of this entity. Pulmonary involvement occurs in up to 40% of patients, and typically presents on radiography as interstitial, nonlobar opacities (25,29,30). The heart and central nervous system are typically involved. The radiographic manifestations of HES while nonspecific, usually include diffuse pulmonary opacities related to severe cardiac failure.

Drug-induced Lung Disease

Pulmonary drug hypersensitivity is increasingly being diagnosed as a cause of acute and chronic lung disease (31–33). Numerous agents including cytotoxic and noncytotoxic drugs have the potential to cause pulmonary disturbances. The clinical and radiologic manifestation of these drugs generally reflects the underlying histopathologic processes. These manifestations include diffuse alveolar damage, cryptogenic organizing pneumonia (COP), eosinophilic pneumonia, and pulmonary hemorrhage (32,33).

Radiographic manifestation on CT includes diffuse areas of ground-glass opacity, diffuse areas of heterogeneous opacity, and, in the later stages, fibrosis, especially in a basilar distribution (Fig. 11.10). COP which is commonly caused by cytotoxic drugs, appears on radiographs as heterogeneous and homogenous peripheral opacities and on CT as poorly defined nodules and consolidation (32,33).

The prevalence of drug-induced pulmonary hypersensitivity or toxicity is increasing, and more than 100 drugs are now known to cause injury. Because of its progressive nature, early recognition is important. The diagnosis of pulmonary drug hypersensitivity should be considered in any patient with drug therapy who presents with new progressive respiratory complaints.

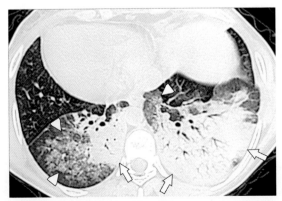

■ **FIGURE 11.9** Chronic eosinophilic pneumonia in a 60-year-old man. Transverse thin-section computed tomography demonstrates extensive areas of air space consolidation (*arrows*) and ground-glass attenuation (*arrowhead*) involving the periphery of the lungs.

■ **REFERENCES**

1. Mayberry JP, Primack SL, Muller NL. Thoracic manifestations of systemic autoimmune diseases: radiographic and high resolution CT findings. *Radiographics*. 2000;20:1623–1635.
2. Frazier AA, Roado-de-Christenson ML, Galvin JR. Pulmonary angiitis and granulomatosis: radiologic–pathologic correlation. *Radiographics*. 1998;18:687–710.
3. Beigelman-Aubry C, Hill C, Guibal A, et al. Multi-detector row CT and postprocessing techniques in the assessment of diffuse lung disease. *Radiographics*. 2005;25:1639–1652.
4. Gruden JF. Thoracic CT performance and interpretation in the multi-detector era. *J Thorac Imaging*. 2005;20(4),253–264.
5. Nishimura K, Izumi T, Kitaichi M, et al. The accuracy of high-resolution computed tomography in diffuse infiltrative lung disease. *Chest*. 1993;104:1149–1155.

6. Swensen SJ, Aughenbaugh GL, Myers JL. Diffuse lung disease: diagnostic accuracy of CT in patients undergoing surgical biopsy the lung. *Radiology.* 1997;205:229–234.

7. Itoh H, Murata K, Konishi J, et al. Diffuse lung disease: pathologic basis for the high-resolution computed tomography findings. *J Thorac Imaging.* 1993;8:176–188.

8. Kuhn C III. Normal anatomy and histology. In: Thurlbeck WM, Churg AM, eds. *Pathology of the Lung.* 2nd ed. New York: Thieme, 1995:1–36.

9. Miller WS. *The Lung.* 2nd ed. Springfield, IL: Charles C Thomas, 1950.

10. Heitzman ER, Markarian B, Berger I, et al. The secondary pulmonary lobule: a practical concept for interpretation of chest radiographs. *Radiology.* 1969;93:507–512.

11. Silva CI, Muller NL, Lynch DA, et al. Chronic hypersensitivity pneumonitis: differentiation from idiopathic pulmonary fibrosis and nonspecific interstitial pneumonia by using thin-section CT. *Radiology.* 2008;246:288–297.

12. Matar LD, McAdams HP, Sporn TA. Hypersensitivity pneumonitis. *AJR.* 2000;174:1061–1066.

13. Lynch DA, Travis WD, Muller NL, et al. Idiopathic interstitial pneumonias: CT features. *Radiology.* 2005; 236:10–21.

14. Silva CI, Muller NL, Fujimoto K, et al. Churg-Strauss Syndrome: high resolution CT and pathologic findings. *J Thorac Imaging.* 2005;20(2),74–80.

15. Hansell DM. Small-vessel diseases of the lung: CT-pathologic correlates. *Radiology.* 2002;225:639–653.

16. Silva CI, Colby TV, Mueller NL. Asthma and associated conditions: high-resolution CT and pathologic findings. *AJR.* 2004;183: 817–824.

17. Aderelo DR, Gamsu G, Lynch D. Thoracic manifestations of Wegener granulomatosis: diagnosis and course. *Radiology.* 1990;174: 703–709.

18. Newman RB, Lynch DA, Newman LS, et al. Quantitative computed tomography detects air trapping due to asthma. *Chest.* 1994;160: 105–109.

19. Park CS, Muller NL, Worthy SA, et al. Airway obstruction in a asthmatic and healthy individuals: inspiratory and expiratory thin-section CT findings. *Radiology.* 1997;203:361–367.

20. Allen JN, Davis BW. Eosinophic lung diseases. *Am J Respir Crit Care Med.* 1994;150:1423–1438.

21. Angus RM, Davies ML, Cowan MD, et al. Computed tomographic scanning of the lung in patients with allergic bronchopulmonary aspergillosis and in asthmatic patients with a positive skin test to *Aspergillus fumigatus. Thorax.* 1994;49:586–589.

22. Sulavik SB. Bronchocentric granulomatosis and allergic bronchopulmonary aspergillosis. *Clin Chest Med.* 1988;9:609–621.

23. Silva CI, Churg A, Mueller NL. Hypersensitivity pneumonitis: spectrum of high-resolution CT and pathologic findings. *AJR.* 2007; 188:334–344.

24. Hansell DM, Wells AU, Padley SP, et al. Hypersensitivity pneumonitis: correlation of individual CT patterns with functional abnormalities. *Radiology.* 1996;199:123–128.

25. Jeong YJ, Kun-II K, Seo IJ, et al. Eosinophilic lung diseases: a clinical, radiologic and pathologic overview. *Radiographics.* 2007;27: 617–637.

26. Takeshi J, Muller NL, Akira M, et al. Eosinophilic lung disease: diagnostic accuracy of thin-section CT in ill patients. *Radiology.* 2000;216:773–780.

27. King MA, Dope-Harman AJ, Allen JN, et al. Acute eosinophilic pneumonia: radiologic and clinical features. *Radiology.* 1997;203: 715–719.

28. Ebara H, Ikezoe J, Johkoh T, et al. Chronic eosinophilic pneumonia: evaluation of chest radiograms and CT features. *J Comput Assist Tomogr.* 1994;18:737–744.

29. Weller PF, Bubley GJ. The idiopathic hypereosinophilic syndrome. *Blood.* 1994;83:2759–2779.

30. Winn RE, Koller MH, Meyer JI. Pulmonary involvement in the hypereosinophilic syndrome. *Chest.* 1994;105:656–660.

31. Padley SP, Adler B, Hansell DM, et al. High resolution computed tomography of drug-induced lung disease. *Clin Radiol.* 1992;46: 232–236.

32. Epler GR, Colby TV, McLoud TC, et al. Bronchiolitis obliterans organizing pneumonia. *N Engl J Med.* 1985;312:152–158.

33. Souza CA, Muller NL, Johkoh T, et al. Drug induced eosinophilic pneumonia: high resolution CT findings in 14 patients. *AJR.* 2006; 186:368–373.

CHAPTER 12

Chronic Rhinosinusitis Role of Rhinoscopy and Surgery

RAKESH K. CHANDRA, DAVID B. CONLEY AND ROBERT C. KERN

■ INTRODUCTION AND HISTORICAL PERSPECTIVE

Chronic rhinosinusitis (CRS) affects an estimated 31 million people in the United States. Management of this disorder, which accounts for approximately 16 million patient visits per year, has changed dramatically in the past 50 years. This is due to new insights into the pathophysiology of sinusitis, advances in rhinoscopy (nasal endoscopy), improved radiographic imaging, and availability of antibiotics (1). Technical advances in endoscopic instrumentation have defined a new era in the office diagnosis and surgical management of sinusitis, permitting an unprecedented level of precision. Understanding the indications as well as the technical limitations of diagnostic and therapeutic rhinoscopy is now essential for practitioners who manage CRS.

Hirschman performed the first fiberoptic nasal examination using a modified cystoscope (2). Refinements in instrumentation after World War II allowed the development of smaller scopes that provided better illumination. In the early 1950s, investigators at Johns Hopkins University designed a series of endoscopes with relatively small-diameter, wide-field, high-contrast optics, and adequately bright illumination. At this time W. Messerklinger of Graz Austria began to use this technology for systematic nasal airway evaluation. He reported that primary inflammatory processes in the lateral nasal wall, particularly in the middle meatus, result in secondary disease in the maxillary and frontal sinuses (2). This region, which represents a common drainage site for the maxillary, frontal, and anterior ethmoid sinuses, is termed the *osteomeatal complex* (OMC). Messerklinger found that small anatomic variations or even minimal inflammatory activity in this area could result in significant disease of the adjacent sinuses as a result of impaired ventilation and drainage. With this observation, he used endoscopes to develop a surgical approach to relieve the obstruction in such a way that normal sinus physiology was preserved. Specifically, he demonstrated that even

limited surgical procedures directed toward the osteomeatal complex and the anterior ethmoid air cells could relieve obstruction of drainage from the frontal and maxillary sinuses. This philosophy was markedly different from the ablative sinus procedures advocated in the past, such as Caldwell-Luc, in that cilia and sinus mucosal function were preserved. Hence these procedures were termed *functional endoscopic sinus surgery* (FESS); Stammberger and Kennedy further refined these techniques in the 1980s.

■ ANATOMY AND PHYSIOLOGY OF THE SINONASAL TRACT

The frontal, maxillary, ethmoid, and sphenoid sinuses are formed early in development as evaginations of nasal respiratory mucosa into the facial bones. The ethmoid sinus develops into a labyrinth of 3 to 15 small air cells. In contrast, the other sinuses exist as a single bony cavity on each side of the facial skeleton. The ethmoid and maxillary sinuses are present at birth and can be imaged in infancy. The frontal sinuses develop anatomically by 12 months and can be evaluated radiographically at 4 to 6 years of age. Sphenoid sinuses begin to develop in children by the age of 3 years but cannot be imaged until they are 9 years or 10 years of age. The point at which mucosal outpouching occurs persists as the sinus ostium, through which the sinus drains (3).

Diagnostic rhinoscopy offers a wealth of information regarding the distribution of inflammatory foci within the sinonasal labyrinth and the associated anatomic variations that may impair physiologic sinus drainage. It is usually performed in an office setting with the aid of topical decongestants and topical anesthesia. It is essentially an extension of the physical examination that helps confirm the diagnosis, gain insight into the pathophysiologic factors at work, and guide medical or surgical therapy. The principles of diagnostic and therapeutic rhinoscopy are based on a firm understanding of

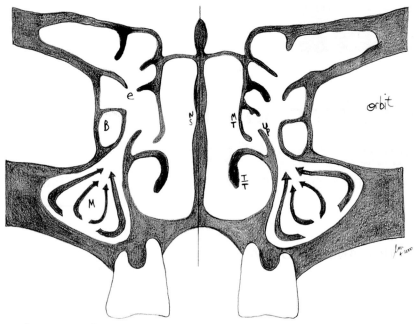

■ **FIGURE 12.1** A schematic view of sinonasal anatomy in the coronal plane. The maxillary sinus (*M*), ethmoid labyrinth (*e*) and bulla (*B*), uncinate process (*up*), nasal septum (*NS*), and middle (*MT*) and inferior (*IT*) turbinates are identified. The arrows demonstrate mucociliary clearance patterns in the maxillary sinuses. Cilia drive mucus toward the natural ostium.

the anatomy and physiology of the nose and sinuses (Fig. 12.1). The lateral nasal walls are each flanked by three turbinate bones, designated the superior, middle, and inferior turbinates. The region under each turbinate is known respectively as the superior, middle, and inferior meatus. The anatomy of the lateral nasal wall is of key importance for the understanding of sinonasal physiology and the principles of FESS, because the ostium of each sinus drains into an anatomically specific location. The frontal, maxillary, and anterior ethmoid sinuses drain on the lateral nasal wall in a region within the middle meatus, known as the OMC. This is an anatomically narrow space where even minimal mucosal disease can result in impairment of drainage from any of these sinuses.

The posterior ethmoid sinuses drain into the superior meatus but are often aerated via the middle meatus during FESS. The sphenoid sinus drains into a region known as the sphenoethmoidal recess, which lies at the junction of the sphenoid and ethmoid bones in the posterior superior nasal cavity. The nasolacrimal duct courses anteriorly to the maxillary sinus ostium and drains into the inferior meatus. The ethmoid bone is the most important component of the OMC and lateral nasal wall. It is a T-shaped structure, of which the horizontal portion forms the cribriform plate of the skull base. The vertical part forms most of the lateral nasal wall and consists of the superior and middle turbinates, as well as the ethmoid sinus labyrinth. Within the middle meatus, a sickle-shaped projection of the ethmoid bone, known as the uncinate process, forms a recess,

called the *infundibulum*, into which the maxillary sinus drains (4).

A collection of anterior ethmoid air cells forms a bulla, which is suspended from the remainder of the ethmoid bone, and hangs just superiorly to the opening of the infundibulum into the meatus. The drainage duct for the frontal sinus courses inferiorly such that its ostium lies posterior and often just medial to the anterior-most ethmoid air cell. Therefore, the main components of the OMC are the maxillary sinus ostium/infundibulum, the anterior ethmoid cells/bulla, and the frontal recess. The infundibulum and frontal recess exist as narrow clefts; thus, it is possible that minimal inflammation of the adjacent ethmoidal mucosa can result in secondary obstruction of the maxillary and frontal sinuses.

The paranasal sinuses are lined by pseudostratified-ciliated columnar epithelium, over which lays a thin blanket of mucus. The cilia beat in a predetermined direction such that the mucous layer is directed toward the natural ostium and into the appropriate meatus of the nasal airway. This is the process by which microbial organisms and debris are cleared from the sinuses (4). This principle of mucociliary flow is analogous to the "mucociliary elevator" described for the tracheobronchial tree. The maxillary ostium and infundibulum are located superior and medial to the maxillary sinus cavity itself. Therefore, mucociliary clearance in the maxillary sinus must overcome the tendency for mucus to pool in dependent areas of the sinus. Successful FESS entails enhancement of drainage via the natural ostium.

Antrostomies placed in dependent portions of the sinus are less effective because they interfere with normal sinus physiology.

PATHOPHYSIOLOGY OF CHRONIC RHINOSINUSITIS

The American Academy of Otolaryngology–Head and Neck Surgery Task Force on Rhinosinusitis (5) defines sinusitis as "inflammation of the mucosa of the nose and paranasal sinuses." *Rhinosinusitis*, rather than *sinusitis*, is the more appropriate term, because sinus inflammation is often preceded by rhinitis and rarely occurs without coexisting rhinitis. Primary inflammation of the nasal membranes, specifically in the region of the OMC, results in impaired sinus drainage and bacterial superinfection, resulting in further inflammation (Fig. 12.2). In most patients, a variety of host and environmental factors serve to precipitate initial inflammatory changes. Host factors include systemic processes such as allergic and immunologic conditions, various genetic disorders (e.g., immotile cilia syndrome and cystic fibrosis), and metabolic/endocrine disorders. Host variations in sinonasal anatomy also occur, predisposing some to ostial obstruction with even minimal degrees of mucosal inflammation. Neoplasms of the nose and maxilla and nasal polyps also may cause anatomic obstruction. Environmental factors play a vital role, including infectious agents, allergens, medications, trauma, and noxious fumes such as tobacco smoke (5). The pathophysiology of CRS can be influenced by sinonasal anatomy, infection, and allergic/immunologic disorders. Rhinoscopy can provide significant insight into the relative importance of these elements in each individual patient. The infectious, allergic, and immunologic elements of CRS are typically subjected to intense pharmacologic treatment. It should be noted that the specific immunologic factors that predispose a patient to CRS is an area of active investigation, and current evidence implicates many potential factors beyond IgE-mediated allergy. The disease process is better understood as a clinical syndrome caused by inflammatory etiologies, rather than as an infectious disease. Microorganisms, however, play a significant role in the progression and exacerbation of the condition.

Some of these underlying inflammatory factors may predispose the CRS patient to polyp growth, and prevailing thought suggests that polyp growth is associated with a $CD4^+$ T helper 2 (T_H2) cytokine profile (interleukins such as IL-4, IL-5, IL-13) and eosinophilic inflammation, while nonpolypoid CRS tends to exhibit a $CD4^+$ T_H1 cytokine profile and neutrophilic inflammation. This distinction may have significant therapeutic implications (6).

Anatomic Influences

Anatomic variations can contribute to the symptomatology in patients with CRS; these variations would include congenital, surgical, traumatic, or postinflammatory alterations in the normal structure. Common variations include septal deviations and spurs, and hypertrophic, pneumatized (concha bullosa), bent, or flattened turbinates. These entities create inherent anatomic narrowing of the bony channels through which mucus and air flow. When superimposed on inflammatory edema of the overlying mucosa, these factors may initiate the cascade of events resulting in symptoms of nasal airway obstruction, and possibly limitation of mucocilliary flow. Anatomic obstruction may also be precipitated or exacerbated by mass effect from inflammatory polyps, and occasionally, true neoplasms are encountered.

Accessory sinus ostia may result in recirculation of mucus with diminished net mucociliary clearance. These factors may, theoretically, induce progression to CRS, although the exact relationship between various anatomic factors and the development of CRS has been difficult to demonstrate statistically. Diagnostic nasal endoscopy is an important modality to elucidate which of these entities (or combination thereof) may be implicated in any individual patient with CRS. A sample of commonly encountered endoscopic findings is illustrated in Fig. 12.3. Although paranasal sinus imaging is beyond the scope of this chapter, it should be noted that computed tomography (CT) scan of the sinuses and nasal endoscopy are complimentary diagnostic modalities, as illustrated in Fig. 12.4.

Infection

Rhinosinusitis often is preceded by an acute viral illness such as the common cold (5). This leads to mucosal swelling, obstruction of sinus outflow, stasis of secretions, and subsequent bacterial colonization and infection. From the acute phase, four possible courses are possible. These include resolution, progression with

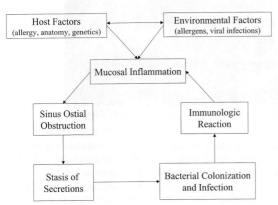

■ **FIGURE 12.2** Pathophysiology of chronic rhinosinusitis—the cycle of inflammation.

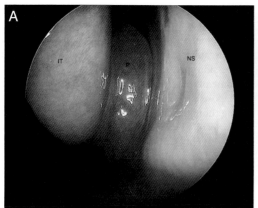 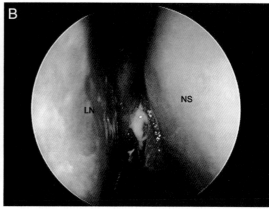

■ **FIGURE 12.3** Rhinoscopic diagnosis. (**A**) View into right side of nose revealing a nasal polyp (*P*) occupying the nasal airway between the inferior turbinate (*IT*) and nasal septum (*NS*). (**B**) View into right side of nose revealing polypoid change associated with pus in the middle meatus, which is the space between the middle turbinate (*MT*) and lateral nasal wall (*LN*) into which the frontal, maxillary, and anterior ethmoid sinuses drain. The nasal septum (*NS*) is also identified. A swab can be used for culture, as shown.

adverse sequelae such as orbital or intracranial infection, development of silent CRS, or the development of symptomatic CRS. In turn, CRS may undergo resolution, persistence, or the development of adverse seque-

lae, depending on the host and environmental variables at work (5). In the chronic persistent state, microbial colonization and infection lead to additional inflammation, further exacerbating the process.

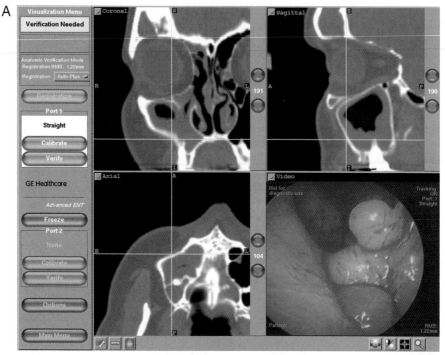

■ **FIGURE 12.4** Triplanar CT reconstructions with endoscopic view. For each figure, the axial, coronal, and saggital views are seen in the left lower, left upper, and right upper panels, respectively. Endoscopic correlation is seen in the right lower panel of each figure. (**A**) These images reveal opacification within the right maxillary sinus. Endoscopic visualization demonstrates this to be a neoplasm, rather than a fluid collection or mucosal thickening, which may have similar radiologic appearances. This particular neoplasm was an inverting papilloma, which is the most common benign neoplasm of the sinonasal tract, but may have malignant potential. (**B**) In this patient, although the endoscopic view clearly demonstrates a neoplasm (capillary hemangioma) pedicled to the head of the left middle turbinate, the CT images are relatively nondescript. Knowing that the pathology is present endoscopically, one is able to appreciate it on the saggital image (*crosshairs, right upper panel*).

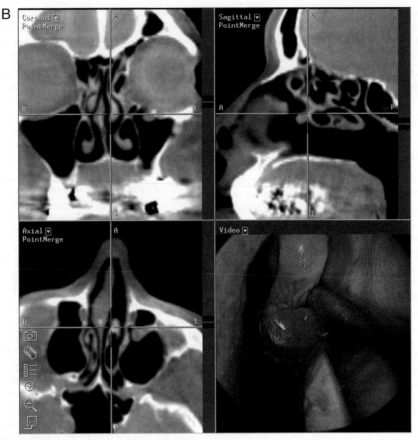

■ **FIGURE 12.4** *(Continued)*

With the development of symptomatic CRS, multiple bacteria usually are cultured, including anaerobes and β-lactamase–producing organisms (7,8). Some are apparently pathogens, whereas others are opportunistic, nonvirulent strains. Cultures obtained under rhinoscopic guidance or those obtained from tissue removed at surgery may help to guide appropriate antibiotic selection. Histopathologic studies of sinus mucosa taken from patients with CRS do not generally demonstrate bacterial tissue invasion. A pronounced inflammatory response with a dense lymphocytic infiltrate typically is seen, at least in part, as a response to the bacteria. The symptomatology associated with CRS is probably a result of this inflammatory reaction.

Allergic Rhinitis

The exact incidence of allergy in patients with CRS is unclear. It is reported that 38% to 67% of patients with CRS who require FESS have comorbid allergic rhinitis (9). This observation is true in children as well as adults. In susceptible individuals, provocation by airborne inhalant allergens triggers the release of mediators from mast cells that reside in the nasal mucosa.

Immunoglobulin E (IgE)-mediated inflammation may hypothetically lead to mucosal edema and osteomeatal obstruction, with secondary sinusitis. The early phase is primarily mediated by histamine and leukotrienes, whereas late-phase reactions result from cytokines and cellular responses. It should be noted that the prevalence of positive immediate skin testing is sometimes less than what would be expected intuitively, so that the overall impact of systemic IgE-mediated disease is still unclear. Nonallergic rhinitis, including vasomotor rhinitis, also can result in osteomeatal obstruction and secondary sinusitis.

Nasal Polyps

The exact etiology of nasal polyps (NPs) is unknown, and likely mutifactorial. NP growth is associated with high-grade chronic sinonasal inflammation in *susceptible* individuals. Degranulated eosinophils often are present (10); such eosinophils are known to secrete IL-5, IL-3, and granulocyte-macrophage colony-stimulating factor (GMC-SF), all of which are eosinophil growth factors. NPs also can be associated with specific disorders, such as aspirin-sensitive asthma and cystic fibrosis (CF).

The latter diagnosis should be excluded by chloride sweat test in any pediatric patient with NPs (2). The relationship of NPs to allergic rhinitis is uncertain (11). Because NPs observed on rhinoscopic examination may coexist with specific underlying disorders such as asthma, CF, or allergic fungal sinusitis (AFS), their detection may indicate the need for further evaluation of these conditions (12).

Immune Deficiency

Immune deficiencies should be considered in patients with CRS or recurrent sinusitis. Some individuals with recurrent, acute sinusitis or CRS may have a humoral immune deficiency. The most common is IgA deficiency, but IgG deficiency also may occur. Antibody defects predispose the patient to infection with encapsulated gram-positive and some gram-negative organisms. This is in contrast to T-cell deficiencies, which render the patient more susceptible to viral, fungal, and protozoal infections. Terminal complement component defects are associated with *Neisserial* infections. Thus, the particular type of immune deficiency dictates the nature of the infectious organisms (9). These observations are particularly important in this era of widespread acquired immunodeficiency in which sinusitis can be more atypical than in the general population. Subjects with HIV/AIDS can have CRS with normal to elevated total IgE concentration but absent immunity to *S. pneumonia*. Rhinoscopically directed cultures may be useful in the diagnosis and management of atypical infections.

Allergic Fungal Sinusitis

Allergic fungal sinusitis (AFS) is a pathologic entity distinct from invasive fungal sinusitis. The latter is a fulminant infectious process with tissue invasion; chronicity is rare. In AFS, however, chronic hypersensitivity to dematiaceous fungi is associated with nasal polyposis, obstruction, and multiple sinus involvement. Initially, the immunologic processes at work in AFS were thought to involve type I, type III, and/or type IVa_2 hypersensitivity, which are also observed in allergic bronchopulmonary aspergillosis (12). Recent studies, however, have suggested that AFS is predominantly mediated by eosinophils and that non-IgE-mediated mechanisms of T_H2 stimulation (especially IL-5 production) are most important. Furthermore, it has been speculated by some that the eosinophilic response to fungi, particularly Alternaria, may be responsible for CRS in general, while classic AFS merely reflects the end stage of the disease process (13). This view of a continuum is not held widely, however.

The hallmark rhinoscopic finding in classic AFS is thick, tenacious "peanut butter-like" inspissated mucus within one or more paranasal sinuses. Histologic examination of this "allergic mucin" reveals embedded eosinophils, Charcot-Leyden crystals (eosinophil breakdown products), and extramucosal fungal hyphae. Although bone destruction and expansion may occur, the disease most often follows a slow, progressive course and thus represents a unique form of CRS. In fact, classic AFS may occur in up to 7% of patients with CRS. The incidence of nasal polyposis in this disorder is high and, by some definitions, is required for diagnosis. NPs, in combination with allergic mucin, often lead to secondary osteomeatal obstruction. Fungal specific IgE can be detected by immediate skin testing or *in vitro* assay.

Superantigens

One area of active investigation involves the role of immunologic response to *Staphylococcus aureus* enterotoxins A and B in the pathophysiology of CRS. In addition to causing ciliostasis (14), these proteins, in susceptible patients, appear to have the ability to function as "superantigens," in that they are able to crosslink the class II major histocompatability complex of antigen presenting cells and the beta chain variable region of the T-cell receptor (6). This is reported to result in vigorous production of T_H2 cytokines, including IL-4, IL-5, IL-13, and eotaxin with concomitant NP formation. These data underscore the principle that although CRS is not primarily an infectious disease, microorganisms may have a significant role in the pathophysiology in susceptible individuals.

Innate Immunity

All of the aforementioned etiologic processes rely on susceptibility of the patient to infection, antigen exposure, and/or immunologic responsiveness. In this vein, recent studies also have examined the role of innate immune defenses of sinonasal epithelial cells in the development of CRS (15). It appears that airways epithelial cells themselves are immunologically active participants that are able to respond to microbial exposure. Notable innate defenses appear to involve Toll-like receptors, that mediate proinflammatory responses to microbes, and surfactant proteins.

Any combination of the previously discussed inflammatory and anatomic factors can result in the histopathologic picture of CRS, a proliferative process associated with fibrosis of the lamina propria and an inflammatory infiltrate of eosinophils, lymphocytes, and plasma cells. Chronic mucosal inflammation also may induce osteitic changes of the ethmoid bone (5). Although the precipitating and potentiating causes for CRS are multifactorial, the common outcome is a cycle by which ostial obstruction leads to stasis of secretions, microbial colonization, and further inflammatory changes and NP formation in susceptible individuals.

■ THE DIAGNOSIS OF CRS

Classification

Working definitions for CRSwNP, CRSsNP, AFS, and acute presumed bacterial rhinosinusitis (APBR) have been established by the Task Force on Rhinosinusitis sponsored by the American Academy of Otolaryngology–Head and Neck Surgery. This group also identified clinical factors that are associated with the diagnosis of rhinosinusitis. These are grouped into two categories: major factors and minor factors (Table 12.1) (5). The presence of two or more major factors or one major and two minor factors is considered a "strong history for sinusitis." Nasal purulence alone is considered diagnostic of sinusitis, and rhinoscopic examination clearly can document this physical sign. A stream of purulent mucus (Fig. 12.3B) may be apparent draining from beneath the middle turbinate, and endoscopically directed cultures of this drainage may be of particular value in guiding antibiotic therapy. The findings of polyps, polypoid changes, or mucosal inflammation are also suggestive of CRS. The current guidelines suggest that one or more of these physical manifestations of CRS should be present to satisfy the diagnosis. Endoscopy is thus critical in the evaluation of patients who meet the symptomatic criteria of CRS. This is often confirmed by CT scan that may reveal mucosal thickening, sinus opacification, and/or air fluid level.

Classification of sinusitis as acute (<4 weeks), subacute (4 to <12 weeks), recurrent acute, or chronic is dependent on temporal patterns (5). A diagnosis of CRS requires that signs and symptoms consistent with a "strong history for sinusitis" persist for longer than 12 weeks. Patients also may have acute exacerbations of CRS in which they experience worsening of the chronic baseline signs and symptoms or the development of new ones. These patients do not have complete resolution of symptoms between exacerbations, in contrast to those with recurrent acute sinusitis. Given the multifactorial nature of its etiology and the diversity of signs and symptoms, CRS can be considered a syndrome. Generally, CRS is the most common indication for FESS; the goal of surgery is to remove symptomatic anatomic obstruction that has failed to respond to aggressive medical therapy. The resulting improvement in sinus ventilation and drainage often promotes relief of inflammation and resolution of symptoms.

Rhinoscopic Diagnosis

Nasal endoscopy is an extension of the physical examination that offers significant insight into the pathologic factors at work in CRS. For centuries, the standard of diagnosis was visualization anteriorly using a nasal speculum and posteriorly using an angled mirror placed in the pharynx. Rhinoscopy using a rigid fiberoptic telescope, however, is considered more accurate and thorough, and can be performed at a reasonable cost. Several scopes are available to provide visualization with different angles of deflection (Fig. 12.5). The zero degree telescope, for example, gives a direct and magnified view of structures directly in front of the tip of the scope. In contrast, the 30°-scope evaluates structures located at a 30°-inclination from the long axis of the instrument in the direction of the bevel. Flexible endoscopy is preferable for patient comfort. Prior to the performance of endoscopy, the nose is topically decongested and anesthetized with a combination of phenylephrine or oxymetazoline (for decongestion), and lidocaine or pontocaine (for anesthesia). These are administered in aerosolized spray form. Decongestion temporarily shrinks the inflamed nasal mucosa, allowing the scope greater access to critical areas. The topical anesthesia improves patient comfort and compliance during the examination. Most endoscopists examine the key areas in a systematic sequence. Regardless of the order, attempts should be made to

TABLE 12.1 MAJOR AND MINOR FACTORS IN THE DIAGNOSIS OF RHINOSINUSITIS

MAJOR FACTORS	MINOR FACTORS
Facial pain/pressure	Headache
Facial congestion/fullness	Fever (all nonacute forms of sinusitis)
Nasal obstruction/blockage	Halitosis
Nasal discharge/purulence	Fatigue
Discolored post-nasal drip	Dental pain
Hyposmia/anosmia	Cough
Purulence in nasal cavity	Ear pain/pressure/fullness
Fever (acute sinusitis only)	

Adapted from Lanza DC, Kennedy DW. Adult rhinosinusitis defined. *Otolaryngol Head Neck Surg* 1997;117 (suppl):1–7; with permission.

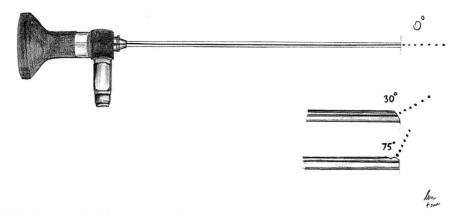

■ **FIGURE 12.5**   Representative rhinoscopes. Note the variation in angle of view between the 0°, 30°, and 75° tips.

visualize the following: nasal septum, inferior turbinate and meatus, middle turbinate and meatus, superior meatus, sphenoethmoidal recess, and the presence of accessory ostia.

In examining patients who have a history consistent with sinusitis, specific pathology that is not evident by a speculum examination may be detected by fiberoptic rhinoscopy. These include middle meatal polyps, pus, turbinate pathology, alterations in mucous viscosity, and synechiae (scar bands). In AFS, allergic mucin may be apparent in addition to NPs. Anatomic abnormalities of the septum, turbinates, or meatus are noted. These may contribute to the development of CRS by causing ostial obstruction. In the absence of symptoms and mucosal inflammatory changes, findings such as a deviated septum or a concha bullosa are considered incidental. In each particular case, the surgeon must assess the degree of pathology and the contribution of anatomic abnormalities to that pathology. Those factors that appear to affect sinus drainage can then be addressed.

An additional role of diagnostic rhinoscopy is to rule out the presence of benign or malignant neoplasms of the nose and paranasal sinuses. These pathologies can cause anatomic obstruction of sinus drainage and thus produce symptoms of CRS. Suspicious lesions observed rhinoscopically can be examined via biopsy with endoscopic guidance, often in the office setting. The differential diagnosis of sinonasal masses includes benign and malignant salivary gland tumors, inverting papilloma, and sinonasal carcinoma. These entities are relatively rare; their discussion is beyond the scope of this chapter. It is nonetheless important to note that rhinoscopic examination may reveal pathology that may not be suspected on the initial history and physical examination in a patient with symptoms of CRS.

Radiologic Diagnosis

Imaging has become a critical element in the diagnosis of sinusitis, the extent of inflammatory disease, and the evaluation of sinonasal anatomy. By the time FESS was introduced in the United States in 1984, CT had become the radiologic modality of choice for diagnosis of sinusitis. Prior to this, imaging studies for sinusitis were conventional radiography and polytomography. CT has continued to be the gold standard, and its advantages continue to grow. At many institutions the cost of a screening coronal sinus CT scan limited sinus series is comparable with that of a plain film sinus series and provides far more clarity of bony detail. With improved technology, CT is being performed more quickly and with lower radiation doses. Therefore, CT stands as a cost-effective, efficient, safe, and informative modality. CT is also being used with ever-increasing frequency for image-guided surgery. In this practice, CT data are digitized into a computer system that allows the surgeon to correlate endoscopic anatomic points with those on the digitized CT scan (Fig. 12.4) (16).

Magnetic resonance imaging (MRI) has become more widespread, accessible, and affordable during recent years. Its utility in sinonasal imaging, however, is limited secondary to its inability to display fine bony detail. MRI, nonetheless, is useful in the detection of disease extension into adjacent compartments such as the brain and orbit. Compared with CT, MRI may better distinguish neoplastic from inflammatory processes and may more accurately distinguish fungal disease from other inflammatory conditions (16).

Computed tomography accurately demonstrates mucosal thickening within the sinus cavities and deep in the OMC (16), the degree of bony thickening, and the presence of NPs, air-fluid levels, or sinus opacification (Fig. 12.4). The number and location of the involved sinuses also can be determined. In fact, several staging systems have been developed attempting to grade the severity of sinusitis based on these variables (17). The presence of bony anatomic variations that may contribute to the pathology of CRS also can be detected. The CT scan should be viewed as an adjunct to rhinoscopy rather than a replacement for this procedure. Most importantly, the CT scan confirms and documents osteomeatal obstruction. A patient with sinusitis symptoms despite aggressive medical therapy who has sinus outflow obstruction on a CT scan is a typical candidate for FESS.

■ FUNCTIONAL ENDOSCOPIC SINUS SURGERY

Indications

Initial treatment for CRS is medical. This may include any combination, depending on underlying causes, of topical steroid nasal sprays, oral steroids, antihistamines, decongestants, antibiotics, and nasal saline irrigations. Identification and avoidance of causative allergens are also indicated. Medical therapy usually should be the first-line treatment in uncomplicated cases, with course of a broad spectrum antibiotic, generally recommended for a minimum duration of 3 weeks. It should be noted that this recommendation is based on consensus opinion rather than controlled scientific evidence. Surgical indications include chronic or recurrent acute pansinusitis, frank nasal polyposis, mucocele, pending orbital or cranial complications, mycotic infections, debilitating headache, and olfactory dysfunction (18,19). The most common clinical setting for FESS is persistent sinusitis symptoms despite an extended course of comprehensive medical therapy coupled with a CT scan demonstrating osteomeatal obstruction. There are some data to suggest that FESS can reduce significantly both the number of infections requiring antibiotics and the severity of facial pain or headache in patients with recurrent acute sinusitis who have normal CT scans; this subset of patients is thought to have reversible nasal mucosal disease (20). Although FESS may have a role in the management of carefully selected symptomatic patients with normal CT scans, the exact indications for surgery in this patient population are unclear.

CF may be etiologic in children and adults with NPs, and this scenario is a strong indication for FESS (21). In cases of extensive polyp disease, surgery is not curative but does improve symptoms. These patients often require revision surgery and are committed to long-term topical or oral steroid therapy. Thus, surgery is considered palliative in these cases because it cannot address the underlying pathophysiologic process (18). Uncomplicated pediatric CRS that is refractory to medical management is only considered a relative indication for FESS. In these cases, adenoidectomy is first-line surgical therapy if the adenoid pad is enlarged (21).

Preoperative Imaging

The importance of preoperative CT scanning cannot be overstated. This is crucial prior to the performance of FESS, not only for diagnostic purposes, but to demonstrate the relationships between the paranasal sinuses and critical surrounding structures such as the brain, orbit, and carotid artery. The ethmoid sinus system forms the skull base, and the frontal, maxillary, and ethmoid sinuses surround the orbit (Fig. 12.1). Anatomic details vary from patient to patient and must be correlated with endoscopic data for the safe performance of FESS (16). It is important to remember, however, that the CT scan represents only one point in time, and thus does not always predict the extent of inflammatory disease that will be encountered at surgery.

Unless orbital or intracranial complications are pending, it is preferable to avoid operating in the setting of acute symptom exacerbations in order to minimize the risks of complications such as perioperative bleeding. Also, the use of aspirin and other nonsteroidal anti-inflammatory drugs is discouraged within 2 weeks of surgery. The usual preoperative studies, including laboratory studies, chest radiography, electrocardiography, and cardiac/pulmonary consultation, are obtained as indicated. Finally, the potential complications of FESS are discussed with the patient, and informed consent is obtained.

Intraoperative Procedure

After the administration of general anesthesia or sedation, topical anesthetics and vasoconstrictors are applied. Under endoscopic visualization, lidocaine with epinephrine is injected submucosally at key points. This provides vasoconstriction and obviates the need for deeper planes of systemic anesthesia.

When it is deemed that septal deviation contributes to ostial obstruction, a septoplasty (straightening of the septum) is performed. In some instances, septoplasty is necessary to allow surgical access (passage of the endoscope and forceps) to posterior areas in the nasal cavity. Also, the middle turbinate may be collapsed onto the lateral nasal wall and must be fractured medially, or even partially resected, for access to the OMC. The same situation can exist if the turbinate is hypertrophic or pneumatized concha bullosa.

Any NPs are removed, and the uncinate process is resected to open the infundibulum. Pus and/or allergic mucin are suctioned or irrigated from the cavities. Removal of diseased tissue almost always can be accomplished via endonasal endoscopic approaches, although adjunctive external incisions are sometimes indicated. Representative steps are depicted in Fig. 12.6. The goal of FESS is to resect the inflamed ethmoidal tissue and to reestablish ventilation in the diseased larger sinuses by enlargement of their natural ostia, thus breaking the cycle of inflammation described above. Bony and mucosal septations between ethmoid cells are removed to create an unobstructed cavity. The ostia of the maxillary, sphenoid, and/or frontal sinuses can be enlarged, and NPs or inspissated mucous can be extracted.

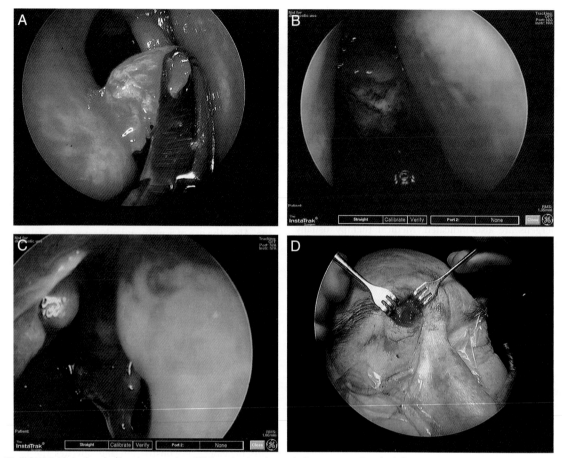

■ **FIGURE 12.6** Surgical instrumentation. (**A**) Standard endoscopic forcep removing the left uncinate process. (**B**) The microdebrider has suction and an oscillating cutting window at its tip. This instrument is ideal for polyp resection. (**C**) Allergic fungal mucin encountered in the ethmoid cavity, with associated polypoid changes of the adjacent mucosa. This mucin will have a "peanut butter-like" consistency. (**D**) Although sinus surgery is performed via endonasal endoscopic approaches in the vast majority of cases, external approaches are occasionally necessary to manage tumor or pending complications, such as orbital extension.

Subsequent mucous membrane recovery reestablishes mucociliary clearance via the newly enlarged physiologic ostia (Fig. 12.7). Any purulent material encountered intraoperatively may be sent for culture to guide future antibiotic therapy, and resected tissue is sent to pathology for histologic evaluation.

The operation may be performed unilaterally or bilaterally, and the extent of dissection is tailored according to the extent of disease severity. Although earlier reports suggested that each side could be dissected in as little as 5 to 20 minutes, recent practice has elucidated the importance of meticulously maintaining the mucosal lining of the neo-ethmoid cavity, often prolonging the procedure. In children, the frontal and sphenoid sinuses are often underdeveloped; therefore, only limited anterior ethmoid and maxillary work is generally necessary. As a consequence of the smaller anatomy, pediatric FESS requires a more meticulous technique (22).

Postoperative Management

The patient may be discharged on the evening of surgery or observed overnight in the hospital. Antibiotic prophylaxis against toxic shock syndrome is necessary if nasal tampons are placed. Approximately 1 to 7 days after the operation, any tampons are removed and the postsurgical cavity is cleaned of crusted secretions and blood under endoscopic guidance in the office. The role for sinonasal endoscopy therefore extends into the postoperative period. This debridement is repeated two or three more times during the first postoperative weeks, at which time the ethmoid cavity begins to mucosalize. The larger sinuses may require up to 6 weeks to heal, particularly in the setting of nasal polyposis (20,23). During recovery, topical nasal steroid sprays and saline sprays often are recommended. Patients are told to refrain from exercise and heavy lifting for 1 week to 2 weeks postoperatively. After the

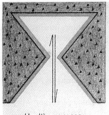

Healthy mucosa:
passage open

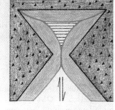

Diseased mucosa:
passage disturbed

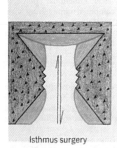

Isthmus surgery

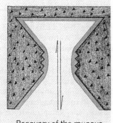

Recovery of the mucous
membrane

■ **FIGURE 12.7** Principle of FESS. After mucosal recovery, the result is a dilated natural ostium. (Reprinted from Wigand ME. *Endoscopic surgery of the paranasal sinuses and anterior skull base.* New York: Thieme, 1990; with permission.)

initial series of debridements, further office visits for diagnostic rhinoscopy are performed at 3-month intervals (18).

Complications

The incidence of major complications from FESS ranges from 0% to 5%. Examples include cerebrospinal fluid (CSF) leak, nasolacrimal duct injury, hemorrhage requiring transfusion, blindness, and meningitis. Minor complications occur in 4% to 29% of cases and include synechiae, orbital entry, ecchymosis, orbital emphysema, and minor hemorrhage (24).

Synechiae are considered the most common complication overall and occur in up to 8% of patients. Of the affected patients, however, only 15% experience persisting symptoms as a result. These scar bands are usually found between the anterior portion of the middle turbinate and the lateral nasal wall, where they may cause functional stenosis of the middle meatus (20).

The incidence and severity of postoperative hemorrhage is reported to be increased in patients with acquired immunodeficiency syndrome and diffuse polyp disease, and in revision cases (20). Fortunately, intraoperative bleeding is usually controlled by local anesthetic or cautery and is seldom a problem. If bleeding impairs the surgeon's visualization, however, the procedure is terminated and the nose is packed. Generally the average blood loss is less than 30 mL (20).

Orbital penetration occurs in 2% to 4% of cases, and in up to one-third of these cases there is also orbital

emphysema. Blindness, fortunately, is rare, with an incidence as low as zero in several large series (19,20,24). CSF leakage may occur in up to 1.4% of cases (20), but in skilled hands the incidence is lower than 0.01% in large series (20,24).

Prognosis

Overall, FESS is considered successful in 80% to 90% of cases after at least 2 years of follow-up (19,20). However, FESS is only a palliative procedure in patients with diffuse polyp disease. One study reported that 55% of patients with preoperative NPs had persistent disease at long-term follow-up, average 3 years and 5 months (19). Nonetheless, it is clear that surgery has a definite role in these patients because over half of the patients were asymptomatic or significantly improved and none was worse. As may be expected, however, results were better in those with a lesser degree of preoperative NP disease (19).

Most experts believe there is a link between asthma and CRS, although the details of this relationship are unclear. Recent studies have reported that CRS patients with steroid-dependent asthma have dramatically reduced steroid requirements after FESS. The patients studied required an average of 1,300 mg less prednisone and 21 fewer days of treatment in the year after FESS compared with the year before (63 days versus 84 days) (25). Antibiotic use also was significantly reduced after FESS in these patients (25). Other trials have reported similar results. For example, in one study 40% of patients with asthma were able to discontinue steroids after intranasal polypectomy (26), and another group demonstrated that 90% of patients had improvement in asthma symptoms 6.5 years after FESS (27). In some cases, it has been speculated that the removal of bacterial biofilms during FESS may be partially responsible for patient improvement (28).

■ SUMMARY

CRS is a clinical syndrome associated with persistent, symptomatic inflammatory changes in the sinonasal mucosa. Rhinoscopy and sinus CT scans may demonstrate associated mucus outflow obstruction. The role of surgery is primarily reserved for the management of patients who fail medical therapy necessitating reversal of congenital and acquired sinus outflow obstruction and restoration of normal nasal physiology. Technologic advances in rhinoscopic instrumentation have improved the accuracy of the office diagnosis and the precision of the surgery. Prior to the advent of surgical telescopes, sinus procedures were destructive in nature, with permanent alteration of sinus physiology. The precision afforded by the current technology permits less invasive surgical intervention that restores normal function to obstructed sinus cavities.

■ REFERENCES

1. Kern RC, Conley DB. Management of sinusitis: current perspectives. *Allergy Proc.* 1994;15:201–202.
2. Messerklinger W. Background and evolution of endoscopic sinus surgery. *Ear Nose Throat J.* 1994;73:449–450.
3. Bolger WE, Kennedy DW. Changing concepts in chronic rhinosinusitis. *Hosp Pract.* 1992;27:20–22, 26–28.
4. McCaffrey TV. Functional endoscopic sinus surgery: an overview. *Mayo Clin Proc.* 1993;68:571–577.
5. Benninger MS, Marple BF, Ferguson BJ, et al. Adult chronic rhinosinusitis: Definitions, diagnosis, epidemiolgy, and pathophysiology. *Otolaryngol Head Neck Surg.* 2003;129 (Suppl): S1–S32.
6. Patou J, Gevaert P, van Zele T. Staphylococcus aureus enterotoxin B, protein A, and lipoteichoic acid stimulations in nasal polyps. *J Allergy Clin Immunol.* 2007; e-publication. Available at http://www.mosby.com/jaci. Accessed December 7, 2007.
7. Fairbanks DNF, ed. *Antimicrobial Therapy in Otolaryngology-Head and Neck Surgery.* 9th ed. Alexandria, VA: American Academy of Otolaryngology-Head and Neck Surgery Foundation, 1999.
8. Brook I, Thompson DH, Frazier EH. Microbiology and management of chronic maxillary sinusitis. *Arch Otolaryngol Head Neck Surg.* 1994;120:1317–1320.
9. Ferguson BJ, Mabry RL. Laboratory diagnosis. *Otolaryngol Head Neck Surg.* 1997;117(suppl):12–26.
10. Stammberger H. Surgical treatment of nasal polyps: past, present, and future. *Allergy.* 1999;54(suppl 53):7–11.
11. Johnson JT, Kohut RI, Pillsbury HC, et al., eds. *Byron J. Bailey Head and Neck Surgery-Otolaryngology.* 1st ed. Philadelphia: JB Lippincott, 1993.
12. Osguthorpe JD, Derebery MJ, eds. Allergy management for the otolaryngologist. *Otolaryngol Clin North Am.* 1998;38(1):1–219.
13. Sasama J, Sherris DA, Shin SH, et al. New paradigm for the roles of fungi and eosinophils in chronic rhinosinusitis. *Curr Opin Otolaryngol Head Neck Surg.* 2005;13:2–8.
14. Min YG, Oh SJ, Won TB, et al. Effects of staphylococcal enterotoxin on ciliary activity and histology of the sinus mucosa. *Acta Otolaryngol.* 2006;941–947(7).
15. Ooi EH, Wormald PJ, Tan LW. Innate immunity in the paranasal sinuses: a review of nasal host defenses. *Am J Rhinol.* 2008;22:13–19.
16. Meltzer EO, Hamilos DL, Hadley JA, et al. Rhinosinusitis: developing guidance for clinical trials. *J Allergy Clin Immunol.* 2006;118(5 Suppl):S17–61.
17. Zinreich SJ. Rhinosinusitis: radiologic diagnosis. *Otolaryngol Head Neck Surg.* 1997;117(suppl):27–34.
18. Lund VJ, Kennedy DW. Staging for rhinosinusitis. *Otolaryngol Head Neck Surg.* 1997;117(suppl):35–40.
19. Danielsen A, Olofsson J. Endoscopic endonasal surgery—a long-term follow-up study. *Acta Otolaryngol.* 1996;116:611–619.
20. Stammberger H, Posawetz W. Functional endoscopic sinus surgery. Concept, indications, and results of the Messerklinger technique. *Eur Arch Otorhinolaryngol.* 1990;247:63–76.
21. Cook PR, Nishioka GJ, Davis WE, et al. Functional endoscopic sinus surgery in patients with normal computed tomography scans. *Otolaryngol Head Neck Surg.* 1994;110:505–509.
22. Lusk RP, Stankiewicz JA. Pediatric rhinosinusitis. *Otolaryngol Head Neck Surg.* 1997;117(suppl):53–57.
23. Chen B, Antunes MF, Claire SE, et al. Reversal of chronic rhinosinusitis-associated sinonasal ciliary dysfunction. *Am J Rhinol.* 2007;21(3):346–353.
24. Ramadan HH, Allen GC. Complications of endoscopic sinus surgery in a residency training program. *Laryngoscope.* 1995;105:376–379.
25. Palmer JN, Conley DB, Dong DG, et al. Efficacy of endoscopic sinus surgery in the management of patients with asthma and chronic rhinosinusitis. *Am J Rhinol.* 2001;15:49–53.
26. English G. Nasal polypectomy and sinus surgery in patients with asthma and aspirin idiosyncrasy. *Laryngoscope.* 1986;96:374–380.
27. Senior BA, Kennedy DW, Tanabodee J, et al. Long-term impact of functional endoscopic sinus surgery on asthma. *Otolaryngol Head Neck Surg.* 1999;121:66–68.
28. Sanclement JA, Webster P, Thomas J, et al. Bacterial biofilms in surgical specimens of patients with chronic rhinosinusitis. *Laryngoscope.* 2004;115:578–582.

CHAPTER 13

Principles of Immunologic Management of Allergic Diseases Due to Extrinsic Antigens

LESLIE C. GRAMMER AND KATHLEEN E. HARRIS

Three principal modalities are available to treat allergic diseases: avoidance of allergens, pharmacologic intervention, and immunotherapy. Pharmacologic intervention is discussed in the chapters relating to specific allergic diseases and in the chapters devoted to specific pharmacologic drug classes. The immunologic interventions, avoidance of allergens, and administration of immunotherapy are the subjects of this chapter.

■ ALLERGEN EXPOSURE RISK

Sensitization to a variety of allergens has been associated with asthma among children and young adults in numerous studies, with odds ratios ranging from 3 to 19 (1). The particular associated allergen varies with geographic location. Sensitization to house dust mite as a risk factor for asthma has been reported in Georgia, Virginia, Australia, New Zealand, and the United Kingdom (2). In drier climates such as Sweden (3) and New Mexico (4), sensitization to cat and dog dander has been associated with increased risk for asthma. Children in the inner city who become sensitized to cockroach allergens are at increased risk for asthma (5). All of these studies suggest that avoidance of sensitization might reduce the predisposition to asthma. Unfortunately, avoidance is not always simple. For instance, even if cockroaches and pets can be avoided at home, school dust may have very high levels of these allergens (6,7), resulting in sensitization.

■ AVOIDANCE OF ANTIGENS

Allergic diseases result from antigen–antibody interaction that subsequently results in release of mediators and cytokines that affect target organs. If exposure to the antigen or allergen can be avoided, no antigen–antibody interaction takes place, and, thus, there are no allergic disease manifestations. Consequently, the first tenet of allergic management is to remove the allergen if possible.

In the case of certain allergens, removal can be accomplished fairly well (8). For instance, an individual who is sensitive to cat or dog dander or other animal protein should not have the animal in the home if complete control of symptoms is the goal of management. Individualized, comprehensive, home-based environmental interventions to reduce exposure to indoor allergens have been reported to result in reduced asthma associated morbidity (9).

House Dust Mite

In the case of house dust mite allergy, complete avoidance is not possible in most climates, but the degree of exposure to this allergen can be diminished. House dust mite control measures that are evidence based are listed in Table 13.1.

The effectiveness of controlling mite allergens in beds by using encasings is well established (10). Covers should be chosen that are sturdy and easily cleaned. Washing linens in hot water (>130°F) or tumble-drying at a temperature of more than 130°F for 10 minutes will essentially kill all mites (14,15). It is well recognized that carpet is a reservoir for mites; polished floors are preferable, especially in the bedroom. Several studies have reported the association between indoor humidity and dust mite allergen levels (10). For this reason, the relative humidity in the home should be kept below 50%.

Relative to ionizers or filtration devices, including HEPA filters, the data are conflicting. Although steam cleaning of carpets or use of acaricides can kill mites, the reduction tends to be incomplete and short lived. Freezing stuffed animals, blankets, or clothes will kill mites. However, washing is required to remove the allergen from these items. Vacuum cleaning does help

TABLE 13.1 CONTROL MEASURES TO REDUCE HOUSE DUST MITE EXPOSURE

Encase pillows in allergen nonpermeable cover (<10 micron pore fine woven).

Encase mattress in vapor permeable or plastic cover.

Encase box springs in vinyl or plastic cover.

Wash bed linens weekly in water ≥130°F or tumble dry linens at ≥130°F for 10 minutes.

Reduce indoor humidity to ≤50%.

Vacuum clean weekly; wear mask and leave room for 20 minutes after vacuuming.

Ensure that vacuum cleaner has good quality bags (high efficiency particulate air filter).

Inform patients that carpets are reservoirs for mites; polished floors (e.g., linoleum, hardwood, terrazzo) are not and are therefore the flooring of choice, if feasible. This is especially important in the bedroom.

Do not sleep on upholstered furniture.

to reduce the overall allergen burden but is not likely to result in control of allergen from reservoirs like carpet and stuffed furniture (10).

Mold Spores

Exposure to mold spores may also be reduced by environmental precautions (11). The patient should avoid entering barns, mowing grass, and raking leaves because high concentrations of mold spores may be found there. Indoor molds are particularly prominent in humid environments. Bathrooms, kitchens, and basements require adequate ventilation and frequent cleaning. If the patient's home has a humidifier, it should be cleaned regularly so that mold does not have an opportunity to grow. Humidity should ideally be 25% to 50%. Water-damaged furnishings or structural elements should be completely replaced to avoid mold growth. Certain foods and beverages, such as aged cheese, canned tomatoes, and beer, may produce symptoms in some mold-sensitive patients. These foods and beverages should be avoided in highly sensitive subjects.

Cockroach Allergens

Control of cockroach allergen exposure may be very difficult, especially in the inner city. The National Co-operative Inner-City Asthma Study Group reported that intervention using abamectin applied by professional exterminators resulted in decreased Bla g 1 levels in the kitchen, only for a short time. Moreover, even the reduced levels were above those considered clinically significant (12). In another study of the effect of professional extermination using 0.05% abamectin and

house-cleaning measures, there was also a decrease in the cockroach population in inner-city homes of Baltimore. However, at the end of the 8-month study, levels of Bla g 1 were still above the clinically significant level of 20 units per gram of house dust (13). In a study of cockroach extermination with hydramethylnon, there was persistence of elevated Bla g 1 and Bla g 2 6 months after treatment (14). Taken together, the results of these studies indicate that pesticides applied by professional pest control technicians are not effective. Sustained cockroach elimination in the inner city will therefore likely require regular extermination in all rooms, coupled with cleaning measures such as addressing reservoirs of allergen in carpets and furniture and keeping food sources such as leftovers, snacks, pet food, and garbage in tightly sealed containers.

Animal Dander

Compared with house dust mite and cockroach allergen, animal aeroallergens are associated with smaller particles that remain airborne for hours; thus, there is a rationale for using air filtration. However, the extent to which exposure to cat allergen can be effectively controlled by methods such as removing reservoirs like carpet and HEPA filtration is not clear. There are conflicting studies. Some studies have reported clinical efficacy using the combination of removal of reservoirs, keeping the cat or dog out of one room (preferably the bedroom), air filtration, and washing the pet (15,16).

Other Inhalant Allergens

Other airborne allergens, such as tree, grass, and ragweed pollens, cannot be avoided except by staying out of geographic areas where they pollinate. For most individuals, this is impractical socially and economically. Air-conditioning and air-filtration systems reduce but do not eliminate exposure to these pollens.

■ IMMUNOTHERAPY

Immunotherapy is known by various other names: "allergy shots" to the lay public; hyposensitization or desensitization in older medical literature. These terms are not strictly correct in that they imply a mechanism that has not been proved. Desensitization applies to clinical situations in which antigens are administered in a few hours in sufficient quantity to neutralize available immunoglobulin E (IgE) antibody rapidly (17). This type of true desensitization may be necessary in treating patients with allergy to an antibiotic. It is not the operative mechanism in immunotherapy.

Immunotherapy, a term introduced by Norman and co-workers (18), does not imply a mechanism. It consists of injections of increasing amounts of allergen to which the patient has type I immediate hypersensitivity.

As a result of these injections, the patient is able to tolerate exposure to the allergen with fewer symptoms. The mechanism by which this improvement occurs has not been definitely established. However, over the years, several mechanisms have been postulated to account for the improvement. Immunotherapy was first used by Noon and Freeman, who observed that pollen was the etiologic agent of seasonal rhinitis and that immunization was effective in the treatment of various infectious diseases, including tetanus and diphtheria.

Immunotherapy was used empirically by physicians over the ensuing 40 years. Cooke (19) observed that cutaneous reactivity was not obliterated by allergy injections. Cooke also discovered a serum factor, which he called *blocking antibody*, in the serum of patients receiving immunotherapy (20). This serum factor could inhibit the passive transfer of allergic antibody described by Prausnitz and Küstner. However, there was not a constant relationship between blocking antibody titers and symptom relief.

The first controlled study of the efficacy of immunotherapy by Bruun was published in 1949 (21). Within a short time *in vitro* techniques were developed to assess objectively the immunologic results of immunotherapy. Many immunologic changes occur as a result of immunotherapy (22) (Table 13.2). Which changes are responsible for the efficacy of immunotherapy is unknown.

In general, immunotherapy is indicated for clinically significant disease when the usual methods of avoidance and medication are inadequate to control symptoms (23) (Table 13.3). It is considered to be effective in ameliorating symptoms of allergic rhinitis, allergic asthma, and Hymenoptera sensitivity. These topics are discussed in Chapters 9, 22, and 12, respectively. There are many examples of studies reporting the efficacy of immunotherapy in treating allergic rhinitis or allergic asthma caused by various inhalants, including ragweed, grass, and tree pollens, mold spores, and house dust

TABLE 13.3 INDICATIONS FOR ALLERGEN IMMUNOTHERAPY

IgE-mediated disease (allergic rhinitis or allergic asthma)

Significant symptomatology, in terms of duration and severity

Avoidance not possible

Pharmacologic therapy unsatisfactory

Availability of high-potency extract, appropriate dosage schedule, and compliant patient

mites (24) (Table 13.4). Assessment of efficacy in these studies is difficult because the diseases being treated are chronic and have variations based on geography, climate, and individuals. Assessments are generally made from subjective daily symptom and medication reports by the patient. In some studies, objective clinical evaluation by physicians or by nasal or bronchial challenge was also a part of the assessment. In several studies, children who received allergen immunotherapy developed fewer new sensitivities and less asthma than those who did not receive immunotherapy (25). Several meta-analyses of immunotherapy studies in asthma concluded that immunotherapy was efficacious, including a *Cochrane Systematic Review* in 2003 (24,26).

There are limited studies that suggest allergen immunotherapy might be beneficial in patients with atopic dermatitis who also have aeroallergen hypersensitivity; there are also studies that report some benefit in oral allergy syndrome after allergen immunotherapy (27). At the present time, clinical studies do not support the use of allergen immunotherapy for food allergy, chronic urticaria, or angioedema (27).

Choice of Allergens

The aeroallergens that are commonly used in immunotherapy of allergic rhinitis or allergic asthma include extracts of house dust mites, mold spores, and pollen from trees, grasses, and weeds. The pollen species vary with geographic location, and this information concerning regional aerobiology can be obtained from Chapter 7 and on websites such as the National Allergy Bureau (http://www.aaaai.org/nab). Because the population is quite mobile, it is usual practice to perform a skin test and treat with common, important allergens outside a physician's geographic location as well as those in the local environment. For instance, there is no Bermuda grass in Chicago. However, it is a potent allergen in the southern United States, Hawaii, Mexico, and the Caribbean, where people often vacation. Thus, it is used in skin testing and treatment of patients in Chicago. In the allergic evaluation, a patient undergoes skin testing with various allergens. Radioallergosorbent

TABLE 13.2 IMMUNOLOGIC CHANGES WITH IMMUNOTHERAPY

Increase in allergen-specific IgG

Decreased allergen-specific IgE after prolonged therapy

Decrease in seasonal rise of specific IgE

Increase in antiidiotypic antibodies

Decreased allergen-induced basophil histamine release

Increased regulatory T cells (CD4$^+$CD25$^+$FoxP3$^+$)

Decrease in histamine-releasing factors

Change of CD4$^+$ cells from the T$_H$2 to the T$_H$1 phenotype

TABLE 13.4   EXAMPLES OF DOUBLE-BLIND PLACEBO-CONTROLLED ALLERGEN IMMUNOTHERAPY STUDIES REPORTING EFFICACY

INVESTIGATOR, YEAR	ALLERGEN	PATIENTS	CONTROLS
Allergic rhinitis			
Van Metre et al., 1982 (36)	Ragweed	33	11
Ortolani et al., 1984 (60)	Grass	8	7
Pence et al., 1976 (61)	Mountain cedar	17	15
Des Roches et al., 1997 (62)	House dust mite	22	22
Horst et al., 1990 (63)	Alternaria	13	11
Dreborg et al., 1986 (64)	Cladosporium	14	16
Asthma			
Reid et al., 1986 (65)	Grass	9	9
Rak et al., 1990 (66)	Birch	20	20
Bousquet et al., 1988 (67)	House dust mite	171	44
Haugaard et al., 1993 (68)	House dust mite	55	19
Malling et al., 1986 (69)	Cladosporium	11	11
Dreburg et al., 1986 (64)	Cladosporium	14	16

tests (RAST) and other *in vitro* assays are less sensitive and more expensive than skin testing; therefore, skin tests are preferred for the diagnosis of IgE-mediated sensitivity (28). If the patient's history of exacerbations temporally corresponds to the skin test reactivity, the patient probably will benefit from immunotherapy. For example, a patient having a positive grass skin test, rhinorrhea, and palatal itching in May and June in the Midwest will benefit from grass pollen immunotherapy. In contrast, a patient with an isolated positive grass skin test and with perennial symptoms of rhinorrhea and nasal congestion probably has vasomotor rhinitis and will not benefit from immunotherapy.

Many patients have allergic rhinitis or allergic asthma from various types of animal dander. Avoidance is the most appropriate therapeutic maneuver for such patients. In some instances, avoidance is unacceptable; for example, a blind person with a guide dog or a veterinarian whose livelihood depends on animal exposure cannot be expected to avoid these animals. In these and other instances, immunotherapy with animal dander may be given. Patients who are very sensitive to dander extracts may have problems with local or systemic reactions, such that it is difficult to attain clinically efficacious doses (29).

Technical Aspects

Allergen Extract Potency and Dosage Schedules

The preparation and distribution of allergen extracts, also called *vaccines*, is regulated by the U.S. Food and Drug Administration (FDA), Center for Biologics Evaluation and Research (CBER). This agency has developed reference standards for a number of allergen vaccines and reference serum pools to be used by manufacturers to standardize their vaccines. The potency is initially established by an end-point titration technique called the ID_{50} *EAL method*. Based on these results, the extract is assigned a biologic allergy unit (BAU) potency. Subsequently, allergen extract manufacturers use *in vitro* assays to compare their extracts to the CBER references, and a BAU potency is assigned on the basis of these tests, most commonly RAST inhibition or enzyme-linked immunosorbent assay (ELISA) inhibition (30,31). Two dust mite extracts and eight grass extracts are standardized in this way. Short ragweed and cat extracts (both hair and pelt) are standardized by major allergen content, unit per milliliter of *Amb a 1* or unit per milliliter of *Fel d 1*, respectively. Other aeroallergen preparations made in the United States are currently not required to be standardized. Several unitage systems are currently in use (Table 13.5).

Neither of the common unitages, protein nitrogen unit (PNU) or weight per volume (W/V), is necessarily an indicator of potency. Potency can be measured in a number of ways: cutaneous end-point titration, radioimmunoassay inhibition, or content of a known major allergen like antigen E (*Amb a 1*) in ragweed, or *Fel d 1* in cat extracts (30). Standard extracts, including short ragweed and *Dermatophagoides pteronyssinus*, have been developed by the Allergen Standardization Subcommittee of the International Union of Immunologic Societies (32). These extracts have been extensively

TABLE 13.5   ALLERGY EXTRACT UNITAGE

UNITAGE	DERIVATION OF UNIT
Weight-to-volume ratio (W/V)	Weight (in grams) extracted per volume (in milliliters)
Protein nitrogen unit (PNU)	0.01 μg of protein nitrogen
Biologic allergy unit (BAU)	Based on average skin test end point of allergic individuals
Major allergen unit	Based on the amount of a major allergen in the extract
Biologic unit (BU)	Based on skin tests end point relative to histamine
International unit (IU)	Based on *in vitro* assays relative to World Health Organization standard allergenic preparations

tested for allergen content and immunologic properties and have been assigned an arbitrary unitage, international units (IU). Until reference standards and exact quantitation of potency can be established for all extracts, less exact methods such as W/V will continue to be used.

Allergen extracts may be given individually or may be mixed in one vial. That is, a patient receiving immunotherapy to grass pollen and tree pollen could receive two injections, one of grass and one of tree, or could receive one injection containing both grass and tree pollens. The latter is almost always preferable for patient comfort. Because mold extracts contain proteases that may influence other extracts like pollens and dust mite, some recommend giving mold as a separate injection. Most clinicians in the United States administer allergen immunotherapy subcutaneously, beginning with weekly or twice-weekly injections (33). Current evidence suggests that treatment with higher doses of pollen extracts results in better long-term reduction of clinical symptoms and greater immunologic changes than low-dose therapy. There is evidence that dosage based on the Rinkel technique, a low-dose protocol, is not effective (34).

There are no clear data on the optimal length of time immunotherapy should be continued (35). Most patients who are maintained on immunotherapy and show improvement through three annual pollen seasons continue to maintain improvement even when their injections are discontinued. Patients who do not respond after receiving maintenance doses of immunotherapy for 1 year are unlikely to improve with further treatment. Therefore, immunotherapy should be discontinued in patients who have not had appreciable improvement after an entire year of maintenance doses.

The most common method of administering perennial immunotherapy is subcutaneously using a dose schedule similar to that in Table 13.6. Very sensitive patients must begin at 1:100,000 W/V. The injections are given weekly until the patient reaches the maintenance dose of 0.50 mL of 1:100 W/V. At that point, the interval between injections may be gradually increased

to 2 weeks, 3 weeks, and ultimately monthly. When a new vial of extract is given to a patient receiving a maintenance dose of 0.50 mL of 1:100 W/V, the volume should be reduced to about 0.35 mL and increased by 0.05 mL each injection to 0.50 mL. The reason for this is that the new vial may be more potent. There are patients whose achievable maintenance dose is lower than the standard shown in Table 13.6.

Other types of dosage schedules have also been published. In *rush immunotherapy* schedules, the starting doses are similar to those in Table 13.6, but patients receive injections more frequently, at least twice a week. In *cluster immunotherapy* schedules, the initial dosages are similar to those in Table 13.6, and the visit frequency is usually weekly; however, at each visit, more than one injection is administered, with the interval between injections varying from 30 minutes to 2 hours. The advantage of both rush and cluster regimens is that the maintenance dose can be achieved more quickly; the cluster regimen can be especially useful in treating a patient who resides at a significant distance from the physician's office. The disadvantage of both cluster and rush regimens is that the reaction rate is probably somewhat higher than with more conventional schedules (36). For patients on those regimens, initial doses from new vials should also be reduced. Allergen extracts should be kept refrigerated at 4°C for retention of maximum potency. If a vial freezes or heats above 4°C, it should be discarded because the allergens may be altered.

A RAST-based method for determining patient sensitivity and first injection doses has been proposed. However, there is not sufficient evidence to support the use of this expensive technique instead of history and properly interpreted skin tests (37). In position statements by the American Academy of Allergy, Asthma and Immunology (38) and the American College of Allergy, Asthma and Immunology (28), it was noted that *in vitro* tests may be used inappropriately. Abuses of particular concern include the screening of unselected populations, remote formulation of allergen extracts, and the use of *in vitro* test results for translation into

TABLE 13.6   EXAMPLE OF AN ALLERGY TREATMENT TENTATIVE DOSAGE SCHEDULE

DATE	EXTRACT CONCENTRATION (W/V) (APPROX.)	EXTRACT CONCENTRATION (BAU/ML)	VOLUME	REMARKS
	1:100,000	1	0.1	
			0.2	
			0.4	
			0.8	
	1:10,000	10	0.05	
			0.10	
			0.15	
			0.20	
			0.30	
			0.40	
			0.50	
	1:1,000	100	0.05	
			0.10	
			0.20	
			0.30	
			0.40	
			0.50	
	1:100	1000	0.05	
			0.10	
			0.15	
			0.20	
			0.25	
			0.30	
			0.35	
			0.40	
			0.45	
			0.50	

BAU, biologic allergy unit; W/V, weight-to-volume ratio.

immunotherapy prescriptions without an appropriate clinical evaluation.

Procedures for Injections

Immunotherapy injections should be given only after the patient, the patient's dose schedule, and the patient's vial have been carefully identified because improper dose is a common cause of allergic reactions to immunotherapy. Injections should be given with a 1-mL syringe so that the appropriate dose can be given accurately. The injection should be subcutaneous with a 26-gauge needle. Before injecting material, the plunger of the syringe should be withdrawn; if blood appears, the needle and syringe should be withdrawn and discarded. Another needle and syringe should be used for the injection. Patients should be observed at least 30 minutes after their injections for evidence of reactions.

Reactions

Small local reactions with erythema and induration less than 20 mm are common and are of no consequence. Large local reactions and generalized reactions (e.g., rhinitis, conjunctivitis, urticaria, angioedema, bronchospasm, and hypotension) are cause for concern. Large local reactions generally can be treated with antihistamines and local application of ice. Rarely, significant swelling occurs such that 2 days of oral steroids are

TABLE 13.7   MANAGEMENT OF REACTIONS TO IMMUNOTHERAPY

Local reactions

| 1. Oral antihistamine |
| 2. Local application of cold |
| 3. Review of dosage schedule |

Systemic reactions (including generalized erythema, urticaria, angioedema, bronchospasm, laryngeal edema, shock, and cardiac arrest)

| 1. 0.01 mL/kg up to 0.2 mL aqueous adrenalin, 1:1,000 intramuscularly, at site of immunotherapy injection to slow absorption of antigen |
| 2. 0.01 mL/kg up to 0.3 mL aqueous adrenalin, 1:1,000 intramuscularly, at another site |
| 3. Diphenhydramine intravenously or intramuscularly, 1.25 mg/kg upto 50 mg |
| 4. Tourniquet above the site of injection of allergen |
| 5. Specific reaction |
| a. Bronchospasm: inhaled β-adrenergic bronchodilator. Intravenous aminophylline 4 mg/kg up to 500 mg given over 20 min, aqueous hydrocortisone 5 mg/kg up to 200 mg; oxygen |
| b. Laryngeal edema: oxygen, intubation, tracheostomy |
| c. Hypotension: vasopressors, fluids, corticosteroids |
| d. Cardiac arrest: resuscitation, sodium bicarbonate, defibrillation, antiarrhythmia medications |
| 6. Review of dosage schedule |

indicated. Generalized reactions consisting of bronchospasm, angioedema, or urticaria usually respond to 0.3 mL of 1:1,000 epinephrine subcutaneously. The dose for children weighing up to 30 kg is 0.01 mL/kg. This may be repeated every 10 or 15 minutes for up to three doses.

Practice parameters for the diagnosis and management of anaphylaxis have been published (39). If the patient has laryngeal edema and is unresponsive to epinephrine, intubation or tracheostomy is necessary. If the patient has hypotension unresponsive to epinephrine, the administration of intravenous fluids and pressors is necessary. Any physician who administers allergen injections must be prepared to treat serious anaphylactic reactions should they occur. If a patient has a large local reaction, the subsequent dose should be reduced or repeated, based on clinical judgment. If a systemic reaction occurs, the dose should be reduced to one-half to one-tenth the dose at which the reaction occurred before proceeding with subsequent slow increase. The management of local and systemic reactions is outlined in Table 13.7. Because of local or systemic reactions, there are patients who are unable to tolerate usual maintenance doses and must be maintained on a smaller dose, for instance, 0.20 mL of 1:100 W/V.

The safety of immunotherapy has been questioned. In one report, five of nine patients who developed polyarteritis nodosa had received immunotherapy (40). Asthma, however, may be the first symptom of polyarteritis nodosa, and the latter disease may have been present subclinically before the start of the injection therapy. If the polyarteritis nodosa were directly related to immunotherapy, an immunologic mechanism must be postulated, the likely one being antigen–antibody complex damage. However, the amount of antigen used in standard immunotherapy is far less than that producing antigen–antibody complex damage in experimental animals.

Another study compared a group of atopic patients receiving immunotherapy for at least 5 years with a group of atopic patients not on injection therapy (41). The treated group did not show an increased incidence of autoimmune, collagen vascular, or lymphoproliferative disease. There were no adverse effects on immunologic reactivity as measured by several laboratory immunologic tests. Appropriate immunotherapy is accepted as a safe therapy.

Special Considerations

Pregnancy

Patients doing well on maintenance doses of immunotherapy who become pregnant can be continued on immunotherapy (42). However, if a pregnant patient is not on immunotherapy, the risks and benefits need to be evaluated and the decision when to initiate immunotherapy individualized.

Medications

Because patients who receive immunotherapy may require treatment with epinephrine, the risks and benefits of concomitant drug therapy must be considered.

For example, the *Physician's Desk Reference* cautions that monoamine oxidase inhibitors should not be administered in conjunction with sympathomimetics (43). Also, β-blocking agents and possibly angiotensin-converting enzyme inhibitors could make the treatment of anaphylaxis more difficult in some cases, but a large study of β-blocking agents could not confirm an increased risk of systemic reactions (39).

Failure

If a patient has been on maintenance doses of immunotherapy for 12 months and has no improvement, the clinical allergy problem should be reassessed. Perhaps a new allergen such as an animal has been introduced into the environment. Possibly the patient has developed new sensitivities for which he or she is not receiving immunotherapy or perhaps the patient's disease is not allergic in origin but is nonallergic rhinitis or nonallergic asthma, neither of which is altered by immunotherapy. It is possible the patient may have misunderstood the benefits of immunotherapy. That is, symptom reduction, not symptom eradication, is all that can be expected from immunotherapy. It is important that the patient understand this at the initiation of therapy.

Alternate Administration Routes

In addition to the administration of allergen through the subcutaneous route, several other routes have been suggested. Local nasal immunotherapy (LNIT) consists of extracts that are sprayed into the nasal cavity by the patient at specified dosages at specified time intervals. There are reported clinical successes, but local side effects may be very bothersome and make LNIT relatively unpalatable (44). Pretreatment with nasal cromolyn does reduce the severity of the local reaction (45).

The efficacy of sublingual-swallow and oral immunotherapy are undergoing trials in the United States. Results to date have been conflicting; there is no consistent relationship between clinical efficacy, allergen dose, or treatment duration. There is no FDA-approved formulation for sublingual or oral immunotherapy at this time and therefore both are considered investigational at present (46).

Modified Allergens

Except for in the United States, most immunotherapy in industrialized nations is given as some type of modified allergen. Although immunotherapy with aqueous antigens has demonstrated efficacy, it is still a long, expensive process with a risk for severe systemic reactions. Therefore, polymerized allergens, formaldehyde-treated allergens, allergens conjugated to alginate, and other forms of modified immunotherapy are used, except in the United States, where such allergens could not be characterized to the satisfaction of FDA/CBER.

Administration of purified antigens, for instance, antigen E of short ragweed, was tried as a possible improvement of immunotherapy. Improvements similar to those obtained with whole extracts but with fewer reactions and injections were found with antigen E. The expense of the antigen E purification process has made this sort of administration impractical. Recombinant allergens have also been produced (47). Mixtures of recombinant allergens could be used for allergen immunotherapy but would be unlikely to improve safety or efficacy of current immunotherapy. Recombinant allergens can be engineered to produce proteins that no longer bind IgE but do retain T-cell epitopes that could result in efficacy with improved safety (48).

At present, there are two basic avenues of research to improve immunotherapy. The first is to attempt to inhibit IgE antibody production to a given allergen. Several compounds devised individually by Katz, Sehon, and Ishizaka et al. have been successful in animal models, but not in humans. Immunotherapy with T-cell epitope containing peptides has been reported to induce T-cell anergy and clinical efficacy, but trials have been discontinued for commercial reasons (49).

Administration of a neuropeptide, substance P with allergens, has been shown to reduce immediate cutaneous and airway responses in a subhuman primate model (50). Mechanistic studies are underway to assess this promising therapy. Others have reported that substance P and allergen can cause a switch from the helper T-cell subtypes T_H2 to T_H1 cytokines (51).

The other avenue is to reduce allergenicity of allergens while maintaining immunogenicity (52). The absorption of the antigen from the injection site can be slowed by using an aluminum-precipitated, buffered, aqueous extract of pollen antigen. Patients receiving this extract have shown significant clinical response and immunologic changes with fewer injections and reactions (53). This is the only modified immunotherapy available in the United States.

Aqueous antigens were used in a mineral oil emulsion to delay the absorption of antigen from the injection site. Problems with this method of treatment include persistent nodules, sterile abscesses, and granulomas. Mineral oil induces tumors in animals, and mineral oil emulsions are not licensed in the United States for human use (54). Use of liposomes as a form of repository therapy has been considered (55).

Norman et al. treated allergens with formalin to alter antigenic determinants. This reduced the allergenicity of the original extract and the skin test reactivity (56). There are data that demonstrate an efficacy of formaldehyde-treated grass allergens equivalent to that of standard allergy therapy in grass rhinitis. This therapy is available in countries other than the United States.

Patterson et al. polymerized ragweed and other pollen proteins with glutaraldehyde. Because there are fewer molecules of polymer on a weight basis compared with monomer allergens, there are fewer molecules to react with histamine-containing cells. There are data that demonstrate an efficacy of polymer equivalent to that of monomer with fewer injections and fewer systemic reactions (57). There are also data demonstrating efficacy of polymerized ragweed in double-blind histamine placebo-controlled trials. This therapy is also available in countries other than the United States.

In contrast to polymerized allergens, glutaraldehyde-modified tyrosine–adsorbed short ragweed extracts have been reported to result in only a modest reduction in symptoms (58).

Novel Therapies

Novel therapies, such as anti-IgE, anti–interleukin-5 (anti–IL-5), sIL-4, other human recombinant engineered proteins, immunostimulatory sequences of DNA, and peptide immunotherapy are discussed in Chapter 38. The addition of omalizumab to a rush immunotherapy protocol reduced the number of serious systemic reactions from 15% to 2.6% (59).

■ REFERENCES

1. Mullol J, Valero A, Alobid I. The nose—from symptoms to evidence-based medicine. *Allergy.* 2007;62:339–343.
2. Peden DB, Bush RK. Advances in environmental and occupational disorders 2006. *J Allergy Clin Immunol.* 2007;119:1127–1132.
3. Ronmark E, Lundback B, Jonsson E, et al. Asthma, type-1 allergy and related conditions in 7- and 8-years-old children in Northern Sweden: prevalence rates and risk factor patterns. *Respir Med.* 1998; 92:316–324.
4. Sporik R, Ingram JM, Price W, et al. Association of asthma with serum IgE and skin-test reactivity to allergens among children living at high altitude: tickling the dragon's breath. *Am J Respir Crit Care Med.* 1995;151:1388–1392.
5. Rosenstreich DL. The role of cockroach allergy and exposure to cockroach allergen causing morbidity among inner-city children with asthma. *N Engl J Med.* 1997;336:1356–1363.
6. Sarpong SB, Wood RA, Karrison T, et al. Cockroach allergen (Bla g 1) in school dust. *J Allergy Clin Immunol.* 1997;99:486–492.
7. Warner JA. Environmental allergen exposure in homes and schools. *Clin Exp Allergy.* 1992;22:210–216.
8. van Schayck OCP, Maas T, Kaper J, et al. Is there any role for allergen avoidance in the primary prevention of childhood asthma? *J Allergy Clin Immunol.* 2007;119:1323–1328.
9. Morgan WJ, Crain EF, Gruchalla RS, et al. Results of a home-based environmental intervention among urban children with asthma. *N Engl J Med.* 2004; 351:1068–1080.
10. Arlian LG, Platts-Mills TAE. The biology of dust mites and the remediation of mite allergens in allergic disease. *J Allergy Clin Immunol.* 2001;107:S406–S413.
11. Barnes CSD, Van Osdol P, Portnoy J. Comparison of indoor fungal spore levels before and after professional home remediation. *Ann Allergy Asthma & Immunol.* 2007;98:262–268.
12. Gergen PJ, Mortimer KM, Eggleston PA, et al. Results of the National Cooperative Inner-city Asthma Study (NCICAS) environmental intervention to reduce cockroach allergen exposure in inner-city homes. *J Allergy Clin Immunol.* 1999;103:501–506.
13. Eggleston PA, Wood RA, Rand C, et al. Removal of cockroach allergen from inner city homes. *J Allergy Clin Immunol.* 1999;104:842–846.
14. Williams LW, Reinfried P, Brenner RJ. Cockroach extermination does not rapidly reduce allergen in settled dust. *J Allergy Clin Immunol.* 1999;104:702–703.
15. Chapman MD, Wood RA. The role and remediation of animal allergens in allergic diseases. *J Allergy Clin Immunol.* 2001;107:S414–421.
16. Koren LGH, Janssen E, Willemse A. Cat allergen avoidance: a weekly cat treatment to keep the cat at home. *J Allergy Clin Immunol.* 1995;95:322.

17. Patterson R, Mellies CJ, Roberts M. Immunologic reactions against insulin. II. IgE anti-insulin, insulin allergy and combined IgE and IgG immunologic insulin resistance. *J Immunol.* 1973;110:1135–1145.
18. Norman P. The clinical significance of IgE. *Hosp Pract.* 1975;10:41–49.
19. Cooke RA. Studies in specific hypersensitiveness. IX. On the phenomenon of hyposensitization (the clinically lessened sensitiveness of allergy). *J Immunol.* 1922;7:219–242.
20. Cooke RA, Barnard JH, Hebald S, et al. Serologic evidence of immunity with coexisting sensitization in a type of human allergy (hayfever). *J Exp Med.* 1935;62:733–750.
21. Bruun E. Control examination of the specificity of specific desensitization in asthma. *Acta Allergologica.* 1949;2:122–128.
22. Cox L, Li JT, Nelson HS, et al. Mechanisms of immunotherapy. allergen immunotherapy: a practice parameter second update. *J Allergy Clin Immunol.* 2007;120:S38.
23. Cox L, Li JT, Nelson HS, et al. Patient selection. allergen immunotherapy: a practice parameter second update. *J Allergy Clin Immunol.* 2007;120:S46–S47.
24. Cox L, Li JT, Nelson HS, et al. Efficacy of immunotherapy. allergen immunotherapy: a practice parameter second update. *J Allergy Clin Immunol.* 2007;120: S41–S42.
25. Cox L, Li JT, Nelson HS, et al. Allergen immunotherapy in children. allergen immunotherapy: a practice parameter second update. *J Allergy Clin Immunol.* 2007;120: S63–S64.
26. Abramson MJ, Puy RM, Weiner JM. Allergen immunotherapy for asthma. *Cochrane Database Sys Rev.* 2003;CD001186.
27. Cox L, Li JT, Nelson HS, et al. Food allergy, urticaria and atopic dermatitis. allergen immunotherapy: a practice parameter second update. *J Allergy Clin Immunol.* 2007;120: S42–S43.
28. Bernstein IL, Storms WW. Practice parameters for allergy diagnostic testing. *Ann Allergy Asthma Immunol.* 1995;75:543–615.
29. Varney VA, Edward J, Tabbah K. Clinical efficacy of specific immunotherapy to cat dander, a double-blind placebo controlled trial. *Clin Exp Allergy.* 1997;27:860–867.
30. Slater JE. Standardized allergen extracts in the United States: In: Lockey RF, Bukantz SC, Bousquet J, eds. *Allergens and Allergen Immunotherapy.* 3rd ed. New York: Marcel Dekker; 2004:421–432.
31. deVore NC, Slater JE. Quantitation and standardization of allergens. In: Detrick B, Hamilton RG,Folds JD, eds. *Manual of Molecular and Clinical Laboratory Immunology.* 7th ed. Washington, DC: American Society for Microbiology; 2006:937–946.
32. Larsen JN, Houghton CG, Lowenstein H, et al. Manufacturing and standardizing Allergen Extracts in Europe. In Lockey RF, Bukantz SC, Bousquet J., eds. *Allergens and allergen immunotherapy.* 3rd ed. New York: Marcel Dekker, 2004:433–455.
33. Cox L, Li JT, Nelson HS, et al. Immunotherapy schedules and doses. allergen immunotherapy: a practice parameter second update. *J Allergy Clin Immunol.* 2007;120:S53–S59.
34. Hirsch SR, Kalbfleisch JH, Golbert TM, et al. Rinkel injection therapy: a multicenter controlled study. *J Allergy Clin Immunol.* 1981;68:133–155.
35. Durham SR, Walker SM, Varga EM, et al. Long-term clinical efficacy of grass-pollen immunotherapy. *N Engl J Med.* 1999;341:468–475.
36. Van Metre TE Jr, Adkinson NF Jr, Amodio FJ, et al. A comparison of immunotherapy schedules for injection treatment of ragweed hay fever. *J Allergy Clin Immunol.* 1982;69:181–193.
37. Adkinson NR Jr. The radioallergosorbent test: uses and abuses. *J Allergy Clin Immunol.* 1980;65:1–4.
38. American Academy of Allergy and Immunology. The use of in vitro tests for IgE antibody in the specific diagnosis of IgE mediated disorders and in the formulation of allergen immunotherapy. *J Allergy Clin Immunol.* 1992;90:263–267.
39. The diagnosis and management of anaphylaxis: an updated practice parameter. *J Allergy Clin Immunol.* 2005;115:S483–S523.
40. Phanupak P, Kohler PF. Recent advances in allergic vasculitis. *Adv Allergy Pulmonary Dis.* 1978;5:19–28.
41. Levinson AI, Summers RJ, Lawley TJ, et al. Evaluation of the adverse effects of long term hyposensitization. *J Allergy Clin Immunol.* 1978;62:109–114.
42. Metzger WJ, Turner E, Patterson R. The safety of immunotherapy during pregnancy. *J Allergy Clin Immunol.* 1978;61:268–272.
43. *Physician's Desk Reference.* 62nd ed. Montvale, NJ: Thomson Healthcare, 2008.
44. Passalacqua G, Albano M, Ruffoni S, et al. Nasal immunotherapy to prietaria: evidence of reduction of local allergic inflammation. *Am J Respir Crit Care Med.* 1995;152:461–466.
45. Hasegawa M, Saito Y, Watanabe K. The effects of sodium cromoglycate on the antigen induced nasal reaction in allergic rhinitis as

measured by rhinomanometry and symptomology. *Clin Allergy.* 1976;6:359–363.

46. Cox L, Li JT, Nelson HS, et al. Alternative routes of immunotherapy. allergen immunotherapy: a practice parameter second update. *J Allergy Clin Immunol.* 2007;120: S64–S66.

47. Smith AM, Chapman MD. Allergen-specific immunotherapy: new strategies using recombinant allergens. In: Bousquet J, Yssel H, eds. *Immunotherapy in Asthma.* New York: Marcel Dekker; 1999:99–118.

48. Schramm G, Kahlert H, Suck R, et al. "Allergen engineering": variants of the timothy grass pollen allergen Ph1 p 5b with reduced IgE-binding capacity but conserved T cell reactivity. *J Immunol.* 1999;162:2406–2414.

49. Norman PS, Ohman Jr, JL, Long AA, et al. Treatment of cat allergy with T cell reactive peptides. *Am J Respir Crit Care Med.* 1996;154:1623–1628.

50. Patterson R, Harris KE, Grammer LC, et al. Potential effect of the administration of substance P and allergen therapy on immunoglobulin E-mediated allergic reactions in human subjects. *J Lab Clin Med.* 1999;133:189–199.

51. Carucci JA, Herrick CA, Durkin HG. Neuropeptide-mediated regulation of hapten-specific IgE responses in mice. II. Mechanisms of substance P-mediated isotype-specific suppression of BPO-specific IgE antibody-forming cell responses induced in vitro. *J Neuroimmunol.* 1994;49:89–95.

52. Grammer LC, Shaughnessy MA. Immunotherapy with modified allergens. *Immunol Allergy Clin N Amer.* 1992;12:95–105.

53. Tuft L. Treatment of hay fever with alum precipitated pyridine (Allpyral) ragweed pollen extracts-a clinical reappraisal. *Ann Allergy.* 1980;44:279–282.

54. Norman PS. Controlled evaluations of repository therapy in ragweed hay fever. *J Allergy.* 1967; 39:82–92.

55. Gangal SV, Arora N, Chugh L, et al. Immunomodulation and immunotherapy using liposome entrapped allergens. *Arb Paul Ehrlich Inst Bundesamt Sera Impfstroffe Franf A M.* 1999;93:267–273.

56. Norman PS, Lichtenstein LM, Kagey-Sobotka A, et al. Controlled evaluation of allergoid in the immunotherapy of ragweed hay fever. *J Allergy Clin Immunol.* 1982;70:248–260.

57. Hendrix SG, Patterson R, Zeiss C, et al. A multi-institutional trial of polymerized whole ragweed for immunotherapy of ragweed allergy. *J Allergy Clin Immunol.* 1980;66:486–

58. Ko HS, Chen SJ, Jaworska E. IgG and IgE antibody response following Pollinex-R immunotherapy. *Annals Allergy.* 1987;59:441–449.

59. Klunker S, Saggar LR, Seyfert-Margolis V, et al.Combination treatment with omalizumab and rush immunotherapy for ragweed-induced allergic rhinitis: Inhibition of IgE-facilitated allergen binding. *J Allergy Clin Immunol.* 2007;120:688–695.

60. Ortolani C, Pestorello E, Moss RB. Grass pollen immunotherapy: a single year double blind placebo controlled study in patients with grass pollen induced asthma and rhinitis. *J Allergy Clin Immunol.* 1984;73:283–290.

61. Pence HL, Mitchell DQ, Greely RL, et al. Immunotherapy for mountain cedar pollinosis: a double-blind controlled study. *J Allergy Clin Immunol.* 1976;58:39–50.

62. Des Roches A, Paradis L, Menardo J-L, et al. Immunotherapy with a standardized *Dermatophagoides pteronyssinus* extract. VI. Specific immunotherapy prevents the onset of new sensitizations in children. *J Allergy Clin Immunol.* 1997;99:450–453.

63. Horst M, Hejjaoui A, Horst V, et al. Double-blind placebo controlled rush immunotherapy with a standardized *Alternaria* extract. *J Allergy Clin Immunol.* 1990;85:460–472.

64. Dreborg S, Agrell B, Foucard T, et al. A double-blind, multicenter immunotherapy trial in children, using a purified and standardized *Cladosporium Herbarum* preparation. *Allergy.* 1986;41:131–140.

65. Reid MJ, Moss RB, Hsu YP, et al. Seasonal asthma in northern California: allergic causes and efficacy of immunotherapy. *J Allergy Clin Immunol.* 1986;78:590–600.

66. Rak S, Hakanson L, Venge P. Immunotherapy abrogates the generation of eosinophil and neutrophil chemotactic activity during pollen season. *J Allergy Clin Immunol.* 1900;86:706–713.

67. Bousquet J, Hejjaoui A, Clauzel A-M, et al. Specific immunotherapy with a standardized *Dermatophagoides pteronyssinus* extract. II. Prediction of efficacy of immunotherapy. *J Allergy Clin Immunol.* 1988;82:971–977.

68. Haugaard L, Dahl R, Jacobsen L. A controlled dose-response study of immunotherapy with standardized, partially purified extract of house dust mite: Clinical efficacy and side effects. *J Allergy Clin Immunol.* 1993;91:709–722.

69. Malling HJ, Dreborg S, Weeke B. Diagnosis and immunotherapy of mould allergy. V. Clinical efficacy and side effects of immunotherapy with *Cladosporium herbarum. Allergy.* 1986;41:507–519.

SECTION IV

Anaphylaxis and Other Generalized Hypersensitivity

CHAPTER 14

Anaphylaxis

KRIS G. MCGRATH

■ HISTORY AND DEFINITION

Anaphylaxis is the clinical manifestation of immediate hypersensitivity. The definition of anaphylaxis is, "a serious allergic reaction that is rapid in onset and may cause death." This adverse event occurs rapidly, often dramatically, and is unanticipated. Anaphylaxis is the most severe form of allergy and is a true medical emergency. Death may occur suddenly through airway obstruction or irreversible vascular collapse. Anaphylaxis is a modern disease with sparse case reports from the 17th to the19th centuries. In the 20th century anaphylaxis predominately occurred in health care settings from injections of biological agents, such as tetanus and diphtheria antitoxins. In the 1950s and 1960s anaphylaxis was from medications, diagnostic agents, insect venoms, and food (1–4). Publications of idiopathic anaphylaxis (IA) occurred in the 1970s, followed in the 1980s by anaphylaxis triggered by exercise, exercise and food, and by natural rubber latex. Contemporary reports of anaphylaxis are from biologicals including cetuximab and omalizumab (1–4).

In 1902 Portier and Richet observed that injecting a previously tolerated sea anemone antigen into a dog produced a fatal reaction as opposed to the anticipated prophylaxis. They called this phenomenon *anaphylaxis*, the antonym of prophylaxis (Greek *ana*, backward, and *phylaxis*, protection). They observed two factors likely essential for anaphylaxis: increased sensitivity to a toxin after previous injection of the same toxin and an incubation period of at least 2 weeks to 3 weeks. Richet was recognized as the founder of the new science of allergy and was awarded the Nobel Prize in 1913 and honored on a French stamp issued in 1987 (5–7).

Anaphylaxis is caused by rapid release of mediators from mast cells and peripheral blood basophils. Classic terminology included anaphylaxis as IgE-mediated and anaphylactoid (anaphylaxis-like, pseudoallergic) as non-IgE-mediated. The World Allergy Organization's nomenclature eliminates the term *anaphylactoid* and classifies anaphylactic events as *immunologic* and *non-immunologic* (8). Immunologic anaphylaxis includes IgE fixing to FcεRI receptors on surface membranes of tissue mast cells and blood basophils. Receptor-bound IgE molecules aggregate on allergen re-exposure resulting in cellular activation and mediator response. This is the immediate hypersensitivity response

(IgE-dependent). IgE also enhances the expression of FcεRI on mast cells and basophils. Immunologic-induced anaphylaxis can also occur through activation of complement by immune complexes containing IgG or IgM; anaphylotoxins including C3a, C4a, and C5a are thereby produced. Nonimmunologic anaphylaxis (IgE-independent) occurs from factors acting directly on mast cells with exact mechanisms not fully understood. These include radiocontrast media (RCM), opioids, vancomycin, radiation, exercise, cold water or air exposure, and ethanol. Anaphylaxis may involve more than one mechanism as with insect venom constituents, which can act through specific IgE as well as complement activation. IA occurs spontaneously and is not caused by an unknown allergen; autoimmunity may be involved. Munchausen anaphylaxis is a purposeful self-induction of true anaphylaxis. All forms

of anaphylaxis present the same, requiring similar rigorous diagnostic and therapeutic intervention (8). Refer to Table 14.1 for examples and types of anaphylaxis.

The development of modern drugs, biological and diagnostic agents, and the use of herbal and natural remedies have resulted in increased incidence of anaphylaxis. These agents used by physicians, pharmacists, and the general public require acute awareness of the problem and knowledge of preventative and therapeutic measures.

The following factors are associated with the incidence of anaphylaxis. Studies are limited discussing the role of genetics factors in anaphylaxis (10–15).

- The nature of the antigen affects the risk for anaphylaxis (certain antigens more often are the cause of anaphylaxis, e.g., in drugs: β-lactam antibiotics and

TABLE 14.1   SOME CAUSES OF ANAPHYLAXIS IN HUMANS

Immune-Mediated IgE Examples

Drugs: β-Lactam antibiotics, sulfonamides, teracyclines, cisplatinum/carboplatinum thiopental/thioamyl

Biologics: vaccines, enzymes, hormones, OKT3 monoclonal antibody, cetuximab, horse antilymphocyte globulin, botox, herbals, bee products

Foods: Peanuts, tree nuts, cow's milk, hen's eggs, soy, wheat, fish, shellfish, grains, and seeds

Food additive: Carmine

Insect stings/bites and other bites:
Venoms: Hymenoptera, fire ants, jellyfish, scorpions, snakes
Insect saliva: mosquitoes, deer fly, pigeon ticks, triatomid bugs, green ants

Inhalents: grass pollen; peanut; horse, cat, and hamster dander

Seminal fluid

Natural rubber latex: gloves, condoms

Immunotherapy extracts: pollens, dust mite, mold, animal, venoms

Nonimmune-Mediated: direct release of mediators from mast cells and basophils or unknown mechanisms

Drugs: acetylsalicylic acid, COX 1 & COX 2 nonsteroidal anti-inflamatory agents, opiates, ethanol

Diagnostic agents: radiocontrast media, sulfobromophthalein

Physical: exercise, cold (air, water), heat, UV radiation

Combination of Mechanisms: Immune-IgE; immune-non-IgE: complement activation, immune complex, immune aggregates, cytotoxic; and nonimmune-direct mast cell mediator release, contact system

Drugs: vancomycin, protamine sulfate, succinylcholine, thiopental, d-Tubocurarine, pancuronium, atracurium, vecuronium (direct mast cell release and/or IgE mediated)

Colloid plasma expanders: dextran, hydroxyethyl starch (direct mast cell release and complement mediated-immune aggregates possible with dextran)

Blood products (blood, plasma, cells, IVIG) and transfusions: anti IgA antibody, immune complex, complement activation by serum protein aggregates. Cellular element anaphylaxis (Cytotoxic IgG, IgM)

Dialysis exposure: AN69 membrane (contact system/bradykinin mediated)

Psychogenic: Munchausen, factitious, undifferentiated somatoform idiopathic anaphylaxis

Autoimmune: Idiopathic

Miscellaneous: mechanism unclear: Exercise-induced, food-dependent exercise-induced (FDEIA), FDEIA+Aspirin/NSAID neuromuscular blockers, and in foods: peanuts, tree nuts, finned fish, shellfish, sesame, eggs, and milk).

- Parenteral administration of a drug is more likely to result in anaphylaxis than its oral ingestion.
- An atopic history is a risk factor for anaphylaxis to latex, ingested antigens, exercise, and radiographic contrast media. IA patients have a higher prevalence of atopy. Atopic persons are not at increased risk for anaphylaxis from insulin, penicillin, and Hymenoptera stings.
- Repeated interrupted courses of treatment with a specific substance increases the risk. There is less risk the longer the duration since the last antigen exposure.
- Immunotherapy extract injection to an asthmatic, especially if symptomatic or a forced expiratory volume in 1 second FEV_1 greater than or equal to 70% predicted.
- Gender: Males are at greater risk of anaphylaxis below the age of 15 and females are at greater risk above the age of 15. Females have a higher risk for latex, muscle relaxant, radio contrast media, idiopathic, and overall anaphylaxis. The male to female ratio for insect anaphylaxis is 60:40.
- Anaphylaxis is more common in community than health care settings.
- Anaphylaxis has increased in individuals of higher socioeconomic status.
- Age and anaphylaxis fatality: Fatalities from food-induced anaphylaxis are higher in adolescents and young adults. Fatalities predominate in middle-aged and older adults from anaphylaxis triggerd by insect stings, diagnostic agents, and medications.
- Stinging insect anaphylaxis risk is increased by stinging insect species, recent stings causing mast cell or basophil priming, comorbidity of asthma, COPD or mastocytosis, and concurrent use of β-adrenergic antagonists.
- A history of prior anaphylaxis.

Comorbidities that increase the risk of anaphylactic fatality include asthma, cardiovascular disease, mastocytosis, thyroid disease, hyperhistaminemia, acute infection, decreased host defenses, reduced level of platelet-activating factor acetylhydrolase activity, and activating Kit mutations (1,2,11,14). Psychiatric disease and emotional stress may impair recognition of the clinical presentation. Multiple concurrent factors may be in play such as an elderly patient with cardiovascular disease taking a new medication. Concurrent triggers may also have to be present, such as food plus exercise (11).

■ EPIDEMIOLOGY

The incidence of anaphylaxis in the general population has been underestimated because it is under reported, under recognized, and under diagnosed by physicians and patients. Contributing to the under recognition and

under treatment of the disease is frequent inability to confirm the clinical diagnosis. Mild episodes, although potentially fatal, often are not evaluated by a physician, especially an allergist-immunologist, and may even resolve spontaneously with the patient not reporting the episode to a physician. The International Classification of diseases coding may fail to identify all individuals with anaphylaxis. Differences in reports of anaphylaxis event frequency is likely due to the lack of standardized diagnostic criteria and studies involving selected groups, rather than the general population. Despite these limitations, the lifetime prevalence of anaphylaxis appears to be increasing from all triggers and is estimated to be 0.05% to 2%, with an average annual incidence of 21 per 100,000 person-years (16). The estimated case-fatality rate is 0.65%. Incidence based on prescriptions for automatic epinephrine injectors was an estimated 1% of the population of Manitoba, Canada (17). Further evidence of an increasing incidence is based on routine United Kingdom hospital admission data suggesting a 700% increase in severe anaphylaxis between 1991 and 2004 (18).

In the community, food-induced anaphylaxis is the leading cause of anaphylactic events treated in hospital emergency departments and estimates of incidence vary widely. Estimates range from 1,080 to 30,000 emergency department visits per year in the United States (19). Americans that have food-related anaphylaxis each year experience 2,000 hospitalizations and 150 deaths; the annual incidence of food-related anaphylaxis is between 7.6 and 10.8 cases per 100,000 person years (19,20).

Hospitalized patients are at increased risk of anaphylaxis over the general population. An international multicenter study of 481,752 patients estimated that in-hospital anaphylaxis occurs in 1 of every 5,100 admissions; smaller study estimates anaphylaxis initiates or complicates 1 of every 2,700 hospital admissions.(21) The Boston Collaborative Drug Surveillance Program reported 0.87 anaphylactic fatalities per 10,000 patients in 1973 (22). Other hospital studies estimate anaphylaxis to occur in one of every 3,000 patients and is responsible for more than 500 deaths per year. Weiler estimated that of 300 individuals expected to have anaphylaxis each year in a community of 1 million, 3 are expected to die (17).

In the hospital setting, medications are the most common cause of immunologic-induced anaphylaxis and radiocontrast media (RCM) is the most commom cause of nonimmunologic-induced anaphylaxis. Within medications, β-lactam antibiotics are the most common cause. Penicillin has been reported to cause fatal anaphylaxis at a rate of 0.002% (23). Life-threatening reactions after administration of RCM occur in approximately 0.1% of procedures. Fatal reactions occur in about 1:10,000 to 1:50,000 intravenous procedures. As many as 500 deaths per year occurred after RCM administration when high osmolality agents were used; the incidence of anaphylaxis and fatality is less if low osmolality agents are used (24,25). The history of a previous RCM reaction is a strong risk factor for a subsequent reaction with risk ranging from 16% to 44% (24,25). Seafood or shellfish allergy is not related to RCM allergy. These two iodine-containing entities have become falsely associated. RCM, iodine, and iodide do not cause IgE-mediated allergy, while shellfish allergens are tropomyosin proteins which cause IgE-mediated allergy.

The next most common cause of anaphylaxis is Hymenoptera stings, with an incidence of 23 deaths per 150 million stings. The National Office of Vital Statistics estimated an average death rate of 0.28 per 1 million persons per year from Hymenoptera stings (26).

Fatalities from allergen immunotherapy and skin testing are rare, with 6 fatalities from allergen skin testing and 24 fatalities (1:2.8 million injections) from immunotherapy reported from 1959 to 1984 (27). In another study, 17 fatalities (1:2 million injections) associated with immunotherapy occurred from 1985 to 1989 (28). In 2004 Bernstein et al. identified 41 immunotherapy fatalities spanning a 12-year period (1990–2001) or an average of 3.4 fatal immunotherapy reactions per year and a fatality rate of 1 per 2.5 million injections (29). Fatality due to skin testing is extremely rare with 6 reported deaths from intradermal testing where all but one patient were asthmatic (27). There was one reported death from percutaneous testing following skin-prick testing with 90 commercial foods (29).

The number of cases of IA in the United States was estimated by Patterson to be between 20,592 and 47,024 (30). IA in the series by Yocum et al. was 32%, similar to 37% in a review by Kemp et al. (16).

Occupation, race, season of the year, and geographic location are not predisposing factors for anaphylaxis. However, they may provide the nature of the inciting agent and circumstances of the event. There are gender differences in the risk for anaphylaxis. Males are at greater risk below the age of 15 and females above the age of 15. Anaphylaxis occurs more frequently in women exposed to intravenous muscle relaxants, RCM, latex, and aspirin; IA has a female predominance (31). The male to female ratio for insect sting anaphylaxis is 60:40 as discussed in Chapter 15. Most studies conclude that an atopic person is at no greater risk than the nonatopic person for developing IgE-mediated anaphylaxis from penicillin, insect stings, insulin, and muscle relaxants (1,2,32). Atopy is a risk factor for anaphylaxis from ingested antigens, latex, exercise anaphylaxis, IA, and RCM (1,2,33–35). The frequency of anaphylaxis is thought to be increased during pollen season for atopic individuals receiving immunotherapy (57,70). In the population-based study of Yocum et al., 53% of Olmstead County residents with an anaphylactic episode from all causes were atopic (16). The authors concluded that atopy is probably more prevalent among individuals having anaphylaxis than the general population. Generally, a cause is suspected in two-thirds of anaphylaxis cases, with the remaining one-third being idiopathic (1,2,16).

Not all persons who have had anaphylaxis have it again on reexposure to the same substance. Those who do may react less severely than at the initial event. Factors suggested to explain this include the interval between exposures, the route of exposure, and the amount of the substance received. The percentage of persons at risk for recurrent anaphylactic reactions has been estimated to be 10% to 20% for penicillins, 16% to 44% for RCM, and 40% to 60% for insect stings (23,36,37).

■ CLINICAL MANIFESTATIONS OF ANAPHYLAXIS

Humans vary greatly in the onset and course of anaphylaxis. Symptoms typically occur within 5 to 60 minutes of the inciting event. Many, up to 40, possible signs and symptoms may occur and differ among individuals and from one episode to another. Anaphylaxis is the most severe form of allergy and is appropriately called the killer allergy (2). Death may occur suddenly through upper airway edema and asphyxiation, intractable bronchospasm, or irreversible vascular collapse (1,38,39).

The skin, respiratory tract, cardiovascular system, and gastrointestinal tract may be affected solely or in combination. In order of frequency the clinical manifestations of anaphylaxis are as follows: cutaneous, >90%; respiratory, 55% to 60%; cardiovascular, 30% to 35%; gastrointestinal, 25% to 30%; and miscellaneous, 5.8% (40,41). Cutaneous manifestations include urticaria and angioedema, usually lasting less than 24 hours, often preceeded by pruritus, flushing, "skin burning," and a sense of impending doom. The respiratory manifestations include dyspnea, wheezing, and chest tightness. Difficulty swallowing or speaking are the result of oropharyngeal and/or laryngeal edema. Early laryngeal edema may manifest as hoarseness, dysphonia, or "lump in the throat," and may be followed by stridor resulting in suffocation. Respiratory failure may occur from airflow obstruction, pulmonary edema, or from the acute respiratory distress syndrome (ARDS), in which case, an initially elevated cardiac output becomes depressed, the vascular permeability increases, resulting in hypovolemia and cardiovascular collapse. Shock occurs in 30% of anaphylaxis cases (1,2,16). The progression of shock from the onset to the severe state is as follows: declining blood pressure, increasing pulse, declining cardiac output, and diminished intravascular volume. During shock, blood flow may be diverted away from the skin resulting in the initial absence of cutaneous manifestations (14). In a patient presenting with unexplained shock, urticaria may occur with restoration of the blood pressure, leading to the diagnosis of anaphylaxis. The cardiovascular changes are associated with complaints of "being lightheaded" and "feeling faint." In one series of anaphylactic deaths, 70% died of respiratory complications and 24% of cardiovascular failure (42). Gastrointestinal manifestations include nausea, vomiting, intense diarrhea (rarely bloody), and cramping pain in the abdomen. Neurological manifestations of confusion, dizziness, syncope, seizures, and loss of consciousness may occur as a result of cerebral hypoperfusion or as a direct toxic effect of mediator release (23).

Anaphylaxis from an ingested antigen can occur immediately, usually occurs within the first 2 hours and, occasionally, can be delayed for several hours (19). Initial signs and symptoms may include cutaneous erythema, angioedema, and pruritus, especially of the hands, feet, and groin. There can be a sense of oppression, impending doom, cramping abdominal pain, and a feeling of faintness or light headedness. The skin findings of urticaria and angioedema are the most frequent manifestations, and typically last less than 24 hours. Respiratory symptoms, the next most common manifestation, may progress to include mild airway obstruction from laryngeal edema and, more severely, to asphyxia. Early laryngeal edema may manifest as hoarseness, dysphonia, or "lump in the throat." Edema of the larynx, epiglottis, or surrounding tissues can result in stridor and suffocation. Grave concern is the concurrent appearance of airway obstruction and cardiovascular symptoms. Myocardial infarction may be a complication of anaphylaxis (43). Other manifestations include nasal, ocular, and palatal pruritus; sneezing; diaphoresis; disorientation; and fecal or urinary urgency or incontinence. The initial manifestation of anaphylaxis may even be loss of consciousness; death may follow in minutes (1). Sudden fatality has also been attributed to postural change during anaphylaxis, such as sitting or standing as opposed to remaining recumbent with elevated lower extremities (90). Late deaths may occur days to weeks after anaphylaxis, and are often manifestations of reperfusion injury experienced early in the course of anaphylaxis (1,2,16). In general, the later the onset of anaphylaxis, the less severe the reaction (16,24). In some patients, anaphylaxis resolves spontaneously or with treatment only to be followed by another episode of anaphylaxis, termed *biphasic anaphylaxis*. Protracted anaphylaxis may occur with persistence of symptoms for up to 48 hours despite therapy (44,45).

Biphasic anaphylaxis incidence ranges from less than 1% to 20% and occurs 1 hour to 78 hours after the initial event. It is more common for the second response to occur within 8 hours after the resolution of the original episode. The initial trigger can be immunologic, nonimmunologic, or idiopathic. The oral route appears to be a predisposing factor; however, biphasic responses can occur after parenteral or inhaled antigen exposure. This second response may be less severe, similar to, or more severe than the initial episode; death can occur. Possible risk factors include hypotension or laryngeal edema during the initial episode, delay of more than 30 minutes between exposure to offending antigen and the appearance of initial symptoms, oral antigen trigger, elderly individuals with cardiovascular disease, and patients taking β-adrenergic antagonists. Studies vary on whether therapeutic intervention of the initial event affects the incidence of the second. Therapeutic intervention variables include a delay or inadequate dosing of epinephrine and absence or too small a dose of corticosteroids with the initial event (44,45).

Persistent, also referred to as protracted or recurrent, anaphylaxis lasts 5 hours to 48 hours despite therapy. The estimated rate of persistent anaphylaxis is 23% to 28%, though other investigators suggest it is less common. Protracted anaphylaxis and biphasic anaphylaxis cannot be predicted from the severity of the initial event necessitating an appropriate duration of observation and communication with the patient (46). Spontaneous recovery frequently occurs, likely from endogenous compensatory mechanisms, particularly from increased secretion of angiotensin II and epinephrine (2,47).

Concurrent chemical or medication use may affect recognition of anaphylaxis including ethanol, recreational drugs, sedatives, and narcotics. Psychiatric disease, central nervous system diseases, and vision or hearing impairment may also impede the recognition of clinical manifestations of anaphylaxis (11).

■ PATHOLOGIC FINDINGS

The anatomic and microscopic findings must be examined relative to the underlying illness for which the patient was being treated, the drugs administered, and the effect of secondary changes related to hypoxia, hypovolemia, and postanaphylaxis therapy (1,2). Anaphylactic death is usually caused by respiratory arrest with or without cardiovascular collapse (48). The prominent pathologic features of fatal anaphylaxis in humans are acute pulmonary hyperinflation, laryngeal edema, upper airway submucosal transudate, pulmonary edema and intraalveolar hemorrhage, visceral congestion, urticaria, and angioedema. In some patients no specific pathologic findings are found, especially if death is from rapid cardiovascular collapse.

Microscopic examination reveals noninflammatory fluid in the lamina propria of the areas just described, increased airway secretions, and eosinophilic infiltrates in bronchial walls, the laminae propria of the gastrointestinal tract, and sinusoids of the spleen (2,48). Sudden vascular collapse usually is attributed to vessel dilation or cardiac arrhythmia, but myocardial infarction may be sufficient to explain the clinical findings. Myocardial damage may occur in up to 80% of fatal cases. During prolonged anaphylaxis, activation of the contact system can occur with the formation of kinins, coagulation pathway, and complement cascade activation which may prompt either blood clotting, lysis, and even disseminated intravascular coagulation (DIC) as a cause of death (14,49).

The diagnosis of anaphylaxis is clinical, but the following laboratory findings may assist in unusual cases or in ongoing management. A complete blood count may show an elevated hematocrit secondary to hemoconcentration. Blood chemistries may reveal elevated creatinine phosphokinase, troponin, aspartate aminotransferase, or lactate dehydrogenase if myocardial damage has occurred. Acute elevation of plasma or urine histamine and serum tryptase can occur, and complement abnormalities have been observed. Plasma histamine is elevated within 5 minutes to 10 minutes of mast cell activation and returns to baseline within 30 to 60 minutes. This short half-life limits the reliability for anaphylaxis diagnosis unless collection occurs within 15 to 60 minutes of onset. Urinary histamine metabolites, including methyl-histamine, may be found for up to 24 hours after the onset of anaphylaxis. Mast cell–derived tryptase with a half-life of several hours achieves a peak level at 1 hour and remains elevated for up to 6 hours following anaphylaxis. Optimal times for collecting serum tryptase levels range from 15 to 180 minutes of the onset of anaphylaxis. The peak tryptase level (typically within 1 hour of anaphylaxis onset) usually correlates with with severity of symptoms, particularly with the nadir of mean arterial pressure. Larger releases of tryptase can be detected longer and have been reported to be elevated for many hours after severe anaphylaxis. Tryptase is not elevated in other causes of death; however it is elevated in individuals with excessive number of mast cells, such as in mastocytosis. The β-tryptase level is more specific than total tryptase; however, this assay is not widely available. The ratio of total tryptase to β-trypyase is helpful in differentiating anaphylaxis from mastocytosis. A ratio of 10 or less suggests anaphylaxis and a ratio of 20 or greater indicates mastocytosis. This differentiation is very helpful when anaphylaxis occurs in a patient with mastocytosis who has a high baseline tryptase level. A normal serum total tryptase does not exclude anaphylaxis. Food-induced anaphylaxis is seldom associated with elevation of serum tryptase, possibly due to basophil predominance over mast cells. Serum tryptase may not be detected within the first 15 to 30 minutes of onset of anaphylaxis; therefore, persons with sudden fatal anaphylaxis may not have elevated tryptase in their postmortem sera. Unfortunately, even with optimal timed sampling, plasma histamine and tryptase levels remain within normal limits. If available comparison to stored or post event serum tryptase levels may be useful as well as serial tryptase levels. Future availability of measuring other mast cell and basophil activation markers will be useful. These include: mature β-tryptase, mast cell carboxypeptidase A3, chymase, platelet-activating factor (PAF), PAF-acetylhydrolase activity, as well as an anaphylaxis panel of such markers (11,50,51). The ImmunoCap (Phadia AB, Uppsala, Sweden) may be used on postmortem serum to measure specific IgE to antigens such as Hymenoptera or suspected foods. Together the postmortem serum tryptase and the determination of specific IgE may elucidate the cause of an unexplained death. Serum should be obtained preferably antemortem or within 15 hours of postmortem for tryptase and specific IgE assays, with sera frozen and stored at $-20°C$ (1,2). A chest radiograph may show hyperinflation, atelectasis, or pulmonary edema. The most common electrographic changes other than sinus tachycardia or infarction include T-wave flattening and inversion, bundle branch blocks, supraventricular arrhythmia, and intraventricular conduction defects (1).

■ PATHOPHYSIOLOGY OF ANAPHYLAXIS

Anaphylaxis is initiated when a host interacts with a foreign material. This foreign material can be almost anything as long as it is able to trigger the release of mediators from tissue mast cells and circulating basophils. The exposure can be topical, inhaled, ingested, or parenteral. Immunologic anaphylaxis includes IgE fixing to FcεRI receptors on surface membranes of tissue mast cells and blood basophils. Receptor-bound IgE molecules aggregate and cross-link upon allergen reexposure resulting in cell activation and mediator release. Immunologic and nonimmunologic initiation of anaphylaxis may involve other receptor activation than FcεRI receptors, such as G protein-coupled receptors or Toll-like receptors (16,40). This type of receptor is a heptahelical transmembrane molecule that can transduce extracellular signals by way of G proteins to intracellular second messenger systems (52,53). Mast cells and basophils initiate as well as amplify the acute allergic response. Activated mast cells are regulated by a balance of positive and negative intracellular molecular events extending beyond kinases and phosphatases, such as lyn and syk kinases which initiate a signal transduction analogous to that induced by T- and B-cell receptors. Sphingosine kinase is a determinate of mast cell responsiveness. Mast cell and basophil activation leads to rapid release of inflammatory mediators including histamine, proteases such as tryptase, mast cell carboxypeptidase A3 and chymase, PAF, prostaglandins (PGD2), leukotrienes, chemokines, and cytokines. In addition, stem cell factor and its c-kit receptor, are important in IgE-antigen-induced mast cell degranulation and cytokien production. Sialic acid-binding immunoglobulin-like lectins (Siglecs) are expressed on mast cells and are inhibitory. Basophil activation, control, and involvement are not as well understood with a recent discovery of a mAb directed against an intermediate form of pro-major basic protein 1 (11,54–56).

Preformed mast cell and basophil granule mediators are released by exocytosis within minutes. Arachidonic acid metabolite synthesis occurs within minutes including prostaglandins and leukotrienes. Activation of inflammatory cytokines and chemokines takes hours. Histamine is the most important preformed and stored vasoactive mediator in mast cell and basophil cytoplasmic granules. On its release, histamine acts on histamine receptors (H1>H2) on target organs to increase vascular permeability, causing flushing, itching, urticaria, angioedema, and vasodilation with lowered peripheral resistance and shift in fluid to the extravascular space. Histamine also enhances glandular secretions causing rhinorrhea and bronchorrhea. H1 increases mucous viscosity. H2 increases mucous production, gastrointestinal smooth muscle constriction, increased heart rate, and increased cardiac contraction. The heart is a shock organ in anaphylaxis as the chemical mediators act directly on the myocardium.

The H1 receptors mediate coronary artery vasoconstriction and increase vascular permeability. H2 receptors increase atrial and ventricular contractile forces, atrial rate, and coronary artery vasodilation. H1 and H2 receptor interaction likely mediates decreased diastolic pressure and increased pulse pressure. PAF decreases coronary blood flow, delays atrioventricular conduction, and has depressor effects on the heart (46,57). H1 receptor stimulation may cause coronary artery vasospasm and resultant myocardial infarction even if the coronary arteries are normal. Mast cell accumulation occurs at coronary plaque sites contributing to thrombosis. Antibodies attached to mast cell receptors causing degranulation have potential for plaque disruption (58). Flushing, headache, increased pulse pressure, and reduced diastolic pressure are better controlled with both H1 and H2 antagonists. Pruritus may be from brain H3 receptor stimulation (59). Other mast cell preformed mediators include neutral proteases (tryptase, chymase, carboxypeptidase A3), acid hydrolase (arylsulphatase), oxidative enzymes (superoxide, peroxidase), chemotactic factors (eosinophils, neutrophils), and proteoglycans (heparin). Circulating tryptase levels increase only after massive mast cell activation as seen in anaphylaxis or mastocytosis.

Along with tryptase, mast cell kininogenase and basophil kallikrein activation of multiple inflammatory cascades occur which are involved in anaphylaxis. These include the contact system, clotting system, and complement system. Tryptase activation of the contact (kallikrein-kinin) system decreases high molecular weight kininogen, formation of activation complexes, and bradykinin production, causing angioedema (60). Tryptase can also inactivate procoagulant proteins promoting fibrin clot lysis and may lead to DIC (60).

Chymase can activate the angiotensin system converting angiotensin I to angiotensin II to compensate intravascular volume loss from increased vascular permeability (61). Released heparin (a proteoglycan) also may play a compensatory role by binding to antithrombin III inhibiting the clotting cascade as well as inhibiting the arachidonic acid cascade's generated chemoattractants for eosinophils.

Mast cells generate and release eicosanoid lipid mediators such as prostaglandins and leukotrienes. Prostaglandin PGD2 causes bronchoconstriction, peripheral vasodilation, and coronary and pulmonary artery vasoconstriction and inhibits platelet aggregation. PGD2 is chemotactic for basophils, eosinophils, dendritic cells, and T_H2 cells, and enhances histamine release from basophils. Skin mast cells mainly produce PG2, whereas mast cells from the lung, heart, and GI tract secrete predominately PGD2 and LTC4. Cysteinyl leukotrienes are synthesized by mast cells, basophils, and eosinophils. The cysteinyl leukotrienes stimulate smooth muscle contraction independent of histamine. They also cause smooth muscle contraction and mucous secretion, increase vascular permeability, cause arteriolar constriction, recruit inflammatory cells, modulate cytokine production, influence neural transmission, and contribute to structural changes in the airway. LTB4 is chemotactic and may possibly contribute to the late phase of protracted anaphylaxis. PAF synthesized from membrane phospholipids causes bronchoconstriction (1,000 times more potent then histamine), increased vascular permeability, chemotaxis, and degranulation of eosinophils and neutrophils. Mast cells also release chemokines and cytokines which contribute to anaphylaxis. These mediators contribute predominantly to the late phase of biphasic anaphylaxis. TNF-α is released activating neutrophls, monocyte chemotaxis, and enhances other cytokine production by T cells. Other cytokines released include G-CSF, M-CSF, GM-CSF, IL-1, IL-3, IL-4, IL-6, IL-8, IL-10, IL-16, IL-18, IL-22, and TNF-α Basophils are a major source of IL-4, IL-13, and chemokines (46,52,61–63).

Large quantities of nitric oxide are produced during anaphylaxis. Nitric oxide is synthesized from L-arginine through the action of nitric oxide synthase (NOS). Three isoforms of NOS exist, two constituitive (cNOS), and one inducible (iNOS). cNOS is found in endothelium, myocardium, endocardium, skeletal muscle, platelets, and neural tissue. iNOS is in macrophages, fibroblasts, neutrophils, and smooth muscle. Mediators which enhance cNOS are the same mediators of anaphylaxis: histamine, PAF, several leukotrienes, and bradykinin. Synthesis is further enhanced by hypoxia within minutes and protracted synthesis may occur over hours. Nitric oxide has the potential to be both protective (relax bronchial smooth muscle) and harmful (enhancing vascular permeability). The sum affect is detrimental with vasodilation and enhanced permeability contributing to shock (14, 64). Nitric oxide has the potential to be both protective (relax bronchial smooth muscle) and harmful (enhances vascular permeability). The sum effect is detrimental with the molecule causing vasodilation, enhancing vascular permeability contributing further to shock (14, 64).

The biphasic response, especially characterized by severe hypotension and shock, follows initial mast cell degranulation resulting in activation of other inflammatory cascades including the complement system and clotting and clot lysis pathways. This is supported by falls in complement and activation of clotting and clot lysis in human episodes of severe anaphylaxis (45, 49).

Diagnosis and Differential Diagnosis

Criteria for the diagnosis of anaphylaxis were established by a multinational group of participants in 2005. Having any one of the three criteria are expected to capture more than 95% of the cases of anaphylaxis. These criteria are outlined in Table 14.2. More than 80% of anaphylactic episodes include skin symptoms. However, cutaneous symptoms are absent in up to 20% of anaphylaxis in children with food and insect sting allergy. In patients with a known allergen history and possible exposure, criterion 2 provides evidence of anaphylaxis. Gastrointestinal symptoms have been associated with severe outcomes in anaphylaxis, an important criterion 2 component. Criterion 3 identifies rare patients with an acute hypotensive episode following an exposure to a known allergen. Anaphylaxis is highly likely when any one of these three criteria are fulfilled (65).

Many individuals with anaphylaxis never develop hypotension or shock, an observation addressed by these criteria, supported by the latest definition of anaphylaxis, "Anaphylaxis is a serious allergic reaction that is rapid in onset and may cause death" (65). Because of the profound and dramatic presentation, the diagnosis of anaphylaxis is usually readily apparent, especially in a medical environment where medications and diagnostic agents are administered. Rapid onset of cutaneous manifestations with concurrent respiratory complaints typically prompt rapid diagnosis and therapeutic intervention. Unless shock is present, the absence of cutaneous signs and symptoms cast doubt on the diagnosis of anaphylaxis. Other diagnoses must be considered. These include cardiac arrhythmia, myocardial infarction, other types of shock (hemorrhagic, cardiogenic, endotoxic), severe cold urticaria, aspiration of food or foreign body, insulin reaction, pulmonary embolism, seizure disorder, vasovagal (vasodepressor) reaction, hyperventilation, globus hystericus, and factitious allergy. The most common is vasodepressor collapse after an injection or a painful stimulation. This is exhibited by hypotension, pallor, weakness, diaphoresis, nausea, and occasionally vomiting. The characteristic finding of bradycardia typically differentiates from anaphylaxis; however, relative bradycardia has been reported with insect sting anaphylaxis (66). There is no pruritus or cyanosis. Respiratory difficulty does not occur and symptoms are almost immediately reversed by recumbency and lower extremity elevation. Hereditary angioedema or acquired C1 inhibitor deficiency must be considered when laryngeal edema is accompanied by significant abdominal pain. This disorder usually has a slower onset, lacks urticaria and hypotension. There often is a family history of similar reactions. Noteworthy is a relative resistance to epinephrine.

"Restaurant syndromes" may mimic anaphylaxis from monosodium glutamate, sulfites, and "histamine" fish poisoning (Scombroidosis, Saurinosis). This latter

---

TABLE 14.2   CLINICAL CRITERIA FOR DIAGNOSING ANAPHYLAXIS

1. Acute onset of an illness (minutes to several hours) with involvement of the skin, mucosal tissues, or both (e.g., generalized hives, pruritus, or flushing, swollen lips-tongue-uvula), *and at least one of the following*:
   a. Respiratory compromise (e.g., dyspnea, wheeze-bronchospasm, stridor, reduced PEF, hypoxemia)
   b. Reduced BP or associated symptoms of end-organ dysfunction (e.g., hypotonia [collapse], syncope, incontinence)
2. Two or more of the following that occur rapidly after exposure to a *likely* allergen for that patient (minutes to several hours):
   a. Involvement of the skin-mucosal tissue (e.g., generalized hives, itch–flush, swollen lips-tongue-uvula)
   b. Respiratory compromise (e.g., dyspnea, wheeze-bronchospasm, stridor, reduced PEF, hypoxemia)
   c. Reduced BP or associated symptoms (e.g., hypotonia [collapse], syncope, incontinence)
   d. Persistent gastrointestinal symptoms (e.g., crampy abdominal pain, vomiting)
3. Reduced BP after exposure to *known* allergen for that patient (minutes to several hours):
   a. Infants and children: low systolic BP (age specific) or greater than 30% decrease in systolic BP[*]
   b. Adults: systolic BP of less than 90mm Hg or greater than 30% decrease from that person's baseline

PEF, peak expiratory flow; BP, blood pressure

[*]Low systolic blood pressure for children is defined as less than 70mm Hg from 1 month to 1 year, less than 70mm Hg + [2 X age] from 1 to 10 years, and less than 90 mm Hg from 11 to 17 years.

J Allergy Clin Immunol 1995; 96:894: with permission

reaction is from the histamine-like chemicals, saurine and cis-urocanic acid, bacterial byproducts from spoiled fish (67). Post prandial flush reactions mimic anaphylaxis casting false blame on monosodium glutamate and sulfites. Flushing also occurs from carcinoid, menopause, chlorpropamide, alcohol, medullary carcinoma of the thyroid, autonomic epilepsy, vasointestinal polypeptide secreting tumors, and idiopathic (14,67). Excessive endogenous production of histamine may mimic anaphylaxis from systemic mastocytosis, urticaria pigmentosa, basophilic leukemia, tretinoin treated acute promyelocytic leukemia, and ruptured hydatid cyst (46). Other differential diagnoses include panic attacks, vocal cord dysfunction syndrome, Munchausen stridor, undifferentiated somatoform anaphylaxis, and other factitious allergy (14,67,68).

The following laboratory findings assist in confirming the diagnosis, especially in unusual cases or in ongoing management. A complete blood count may show an elevated hematocrit from hemoconcentration. Blood chemistries may reveal elevated creatinine phosphokinase, troponin, aspartate aminotransferase, or lactate dehydrogenase when myocardial damage occurrs. Acute elevation of plasma or urine histamine and serum tryptase can occur, and complement abnormalities have been observed. Plasma histamine is elevated within 5 to 10 minutes of mast cell activation and returns to baseline within 30 to 60 minutes. This short half-life limits the reliability for anaphylaxis diagnosis unless collection occurs within 15 to 60 minutes of onset. Urinary histamine metabolites, including methyl-histamine, may be found up to 24 hours after the onset of anaphylaxis. Mast cell-derived tryptase with a half-life of several hours achieves a peak level at 1 hour and remains elevated for up to 6 hours following anaphylaxis. This necessitates collecting serum tryptase levels within 15 to 180 minutes of the onset of anaphylaxis. Larger releases of tryptase can be detected longer and have been reported to be elevated for up to 24 hours after death from anaphylaxis. It is not elevated in other causes of death; however, it is elevated in individuals with excessive number of mast cells, such as in mastocytosis. The mature β-tryptase level is more specific then total tryptase, however this assay is not widely available. The ratio of total tryptase to β-tryptase is helpful in differentiating anaphylaxis from mastocytosis. A ratio of 10 or less suggests anaphylaxis and a ratio of 20 or greater indicates mastocytosis. This is useful when anaphylaxis occurs in a patient with mastocytosis with a high baseline tryptase level. A normal serum total tryptase dose not exclude anaphylaxis.

Food-induced anaphylaxis is seldom associated with elevation of serum tryptase, possibly due to basophil predominance over mast cells. Serum tryptase may not be detected within the first 15 to 30 minutes of onset of anaphylaxis; therefore, persons with sudden fatal anaphylaxis may not have elevated tryptase in their postmortem sera. Unfortunately, even with optimal timed sampling plasma histamine and tryptase levels remain within normal limits. If available, comparison to stored or post-event serum tryptase levels may be useful as well as serial tryptase levels. Future availability of measuring other mast cell and basophil activation markers will be useful. These include: mature β-tryptase, mast cell carboxypeptidase A3, chymase, PAF, PAF-acetylhydrolase activity, as well as an anaphylaxis panel of such markers (11,49,50). The ImmunoCap may be used on postmortem serum to measure specific IgE to antigens such as Hymenoptera or suspected foods. Together the postmortem serum tryptase and the determination of specific IgE may elucidate the cause of an unexplained death. Serum should be obtained preferably antemortem or within 15 hours of postmortem for tryptase and specific IgE assays, with sera frozen and stored at −20°C (69).

Blood serotonin and the urinary 5-hydroxyindoleacetic acid level will be elevated in carcinoid syndrome. During controlled studies of immunotherapy for insect hypersensitivity, in patients experiencing shock the investigators noted dramatic increases in plasma histamine concentrations and a decrease in concentration levels of factor V, factor VIII, fibrinogen, and high-molecular-weight kininogen. In one patient a decrease in C3 and C4 occurred (1,2). Another study demonstrated an increase in C3a, a cleaved product of C3 of the complement cascade (70). A chest radiograph may show hyperinflation, atelectasis, or pulmonary edema. The most common electrographic changes other than sinus tachycardia or infarction include T-wave flattening and inversion, bundle branch blocks, supraventricular arrhythmia, and intraventricular conduction defects (1).

Munchausen stridor patients can be distracted from their vocal cord adduction by maneuvers such as asking the patient to cough. If carried out, the cough is preceeded by a nonstridorous inspiratory ausculatation especially over the neck. There are no cutaneous signs. In vocal cord dysfunction patients, the involuntary vocal cord adduction can be confirmed by video laryngoscopy during episodes and absence of cutaneous signs (67,68).

A history of recent antigen or substance exposure and clinical suspicion are the most important diagnostic tools. Initiate treatment and confirm patient stability and then obtain a detailed allergy based history. It is imperative to obtain the circumstances surrounding the event. One must start with the time of the event, the sequence of complaints, and physical findings observed by the patient. Take great effort to confirm these findings by witnesses, photographs, and medical personnel involved. Carefully review the medical records. Work backward regarding the timing of exposure to food, drugs (prescriptions, over-the-counter, illicit, alcohol, herbs, natural remedies, transferred/hidden/malicious), activities, diagnostic/surgical procedures, recent/concurrent illness, and any past history of anaphylaxis to known allergens. Activity history in addition to food ingestion must include eating followed by exercise and medication(s) before the meal or before exercise. IgE antibody can be demonstrated *in vivo* by skin-prick testing. Skin-prick testing can be useful in predicting anaphylactic sensitivity to many antigens. Caution must be exercised, beginning with very dilute antigens. Anaphylaxis has followed skin-prick testing with penicillin, insect sting extract, and foods. If the cause was obvious and episode severe, skin testing may offer more harm then benefit. The ImmunoCap is useful in those patients/physicians who may be fearful of skin testing or extensive skin disease is present. Absent IgE may justify a carefully observed oral graded food challenge. Immuno may be useful on postmortem serum to measure specific IgE to antigens such as Hymenoptera or suspected foods.

Other *in vitro* techniques that have been explored include the release of histamine from basophils of sensitive individuals on antigen challenge, and the ability of a patient's serum to passively sensitize normal tissues such as leukocytes for subsequent antigen-induced release of mediators (17). Complement consumption has not yet been used routinely to define anaphylactic mechanisms. The only currently reliable test for agents that alter arachidonic acid metabolism such as aspirin and other nonsteroidal anti-inflammatory agents and other suspected non–IgE-mediated agents is carefully graded oral challenge with close clinical observation and measurement of pulmonary function, nasal patency, and vital signs, following informed patient consent. Substances that can directly release histamine from mast cells and basophils may be identified *in vitro* using washed human leukocytes or by *in vivo* skin testing. These agents must release histamine in the absence of IgG or IgE antibody (1,2).

■ FACTORS INCREASING THE SEVERITY OF ANAPHYLAXIS OR INTERFERING WITH TREATMENT

There are many factors that increase the severity of anaphylaxis or interfere with treatment (Table 14.3). Rapid intravenous infusion of an allergen in a patient with a preexisting cardiac disorder may increase the risk for severe anaphylaxis. Concomitant therapy with β-adrenergic antagonist drugs or the presence of asthma exacerbate the responses of the airways in anaphylaxis, impede epinephrine response and inhibit resuscitative efforts (71,72). Epinephrine use in patients on β-adrenergic antagonists may theoretically induce unopposed α-adrenergic effects, resulting in severe hypertension. However, profound shock is more likely to be caused by severe anaphylaxis. Individuals taking β-adrenergic antagonists orally or topically may experience severe anaphylaxis associated with paradoxical bradycardia, profound hypotension, and severe bronchospasm.

TABLE 14.3 FACTORS THAT INTENSIFY ANAPHYLAXIS OR INTERFERE WITH TREATMENT

Presence of asthma
Underlying cardiac disease, especially with rapid infusion of allergen, older individual
Concomitant therapy with: β-adrenergic   antagonists (β1 & β2)   Monoamine oxidase inhibitors   Tricyclic antidepressants   Angiotensin converting enzyme inhibitors   Angiotensin receptor blockers
Delay or inadequate dose of epinephrine administration
Psychiatric disease

β-adrenergic antagonists should be used with caution, and preferably avoided in patients receiving immunotherapy and for patients with IA. The difficulty in reversing anaphylaxis may occur in part from underlying cardiac disease for which β-adrenergic antagonists have been given. Both β1 and β2 antagonists may inhibit the β-adrenergic receptor (71). Most patients on β-adrenergic antagonists are typically not completely blocked and epinephrine therapy should not be withheld.

Increased vascular permeability during anaphylaxis may result in a 50% shift of intravascular fluid into the extravascular space within 10 minutes. This shift in effective blood volume activates the rennin-angiotensin-aldosterone system causing a compensatory catecholamine response. Angiotensin converting enzyme (ACE) inhibitors may prevent or inhibit this response, the mobilization of angiotensin II, an endogenous compensatory mechanism, and these drugs can cause life-threatening tongue or pharyngeal edema (47,73,74). Monoamine oxidase inhibitors can increase the hazards of epinephrine by interfering with its degradation (1).

It is thought that systemic reactions occur more frequently in undertreated asthma patients receiving immunotherapy. Though not a standard practice, it has been recommended that measurements of FEV_1 be performed before immunotherapy, with injections withheld if the FEV_1 is below 70% of the predicted volume (75).

■ CAUSES OF ANAPHYLAXIS

Many substances have been reported to cause anaphylaxis in humans. Any agent that can activate mast cell or basophils has the potential to trigger anaphylaxis. Antigens are subdivided into proteins, polysaccharides, and haptens. A hapten is a low-molecular-weight organic compound that becomes antigenic when it or one of its metabolites forms a stable bond with a host protein. With penicillin, both the parent hapten and nonenzymatic transformation products may form bonds with host proteins to form an antigen. In cetuximab anaphylaxis patients, specific IgE has been demonstrated for the sugar galactose-α-1,3-galactose expressed, in the cell line to produce this biologic agent (3).

The route of agent exposure causing human anaphylaxis may be oral, parenteral, topical, or inhalational. An example of an agent that can cause anaphylaxis by any of four ways of entry is penicillin. The most common causes of anaphylaxis are foods, medications, insect stings, and allergen immunotherapy injections. Drugs can cause IgE- and non-IgE-mediated anaphylaxis. Previous drug exposure is required for formation of IgE; however, non-IgE-drug-induced anaphylaxis may happen on first exposure. IA is very common, accounting for an estimated one-third of cases (16,76,77). Table 14.1 lists common causes and mechanisms of anaphylaxis. This list is not all-inclusive. The following discussion is a review of some important and interesting causes of anaphylaxis.

Anaphylaxis to Drugs

Drugs and medications are the most common cause of anaphylaxis in health care environments. IgE-specific antibodies occur from a preceeding sensitization to the drug or a cross-reacting compound. Low molecular weight compounds typically bind to serum or tissue carrier proteins and become a multivalent antigen. A parent drug's metabolites covalently bind to host proteins and induce IgE antibody production. This limits the knowledge of relevent metabolites and allergenic determinants for skin testing utility. Penicillins are the most common cause of drug-induced anaphylaxis. Cephalosporins share with penicillin a common β-lactam ring and are also a frequent cause of anaphylaxis. Cross-reactivity between penicillin and cephalosporins range from 3% to 18% of patients with previous penicillin allergy (77). Estimates of nonfatal penicillin allergic reactions vary, ranging from 0.7% to 10%, and fatal reactions are estimated at a frequency of 0.002%, or 1 fatality per 7.5 million injections, and 1 per 50,000 to 100,000 penicillin courses (78). Penicillin degrades into two main reactive intermediates termed *major* and *minor antigenic determinants*. Skin testing reagents are not currently commercially available. Selected universities prepare minor determinates for skin testing. Minor determinant sensitivity, in some patients, is associated with more severe anaphylaxis. The patient's history is a poor predictor of risk of true penicillin allergy, with 90% of patients with a history of penicillin allergy having negative penicillin skin tests and tolerating penicillin (79). The positive predictive value of penicillin skin testing is 97% to 99%.

Only a small percentage of positive penicillin history patients with a positive penicillin skin test have adverse allergic events when given a cephalosporin. Anaphylactic deaths have occurred in penicillin allergic individuals not skin tested and administered a cephalosporin antibiotic. Patients who have a penicillin allergy history and negative penicillin skin tests to major and minor determinants are at no greater risk and may receive cephalosporins, though cautious graded challenges are typically performed. Monobactam antibiotics such as aztreonam does not cross-react with penicillins or other β-lactams, except ceftazadime. Skin test studies suggest cross-reactivity between carbapenems and penicillin necessitating penicillin skin testing before considering administration of carbapenems. However, the rate of clinical reactions in penicillin skin test positive patients is much lower than anticipated, suggesting a low rate of cross-reactivity.

In patients with non-IgE-mediated penicillin allergy, such as Stevens Johnson syndrome or toxic epidermal necrolysis, penicillin skin testing should not performed because penicillin is almost strictly contraindicated. Anaphylaxis to non-β-lactam antibiotics is less common. Skin testing using a nonirritating concentration of the parent drug at times may yield useful information, however the predictive value is uncertain. Unfortunately, this limits the diagnosis to the patient's history (80,81).

After penicillin, aspirin and other nonsteroidal anti-inflammatory drugs (NSAIDs) are the second most common cause of drug-induced anaphylaxis. Anaphlaxis from these agents is thought to be agent specific, with patients tolerating other NSAIDS (82). The cause is unknown with lack of drug specific IgE detection by skin and *in vitro* testing. Caution is advised if administering nonselective NSAIDs; COX-2 antagonists are usually tolerated.

Cancer chemotherapeutic drug induced anaphylaxis occurs, especially from the platinum containing drugs such as cisplatinum and carboplatinum and skin testing may be useful, especially if desensitization is required. A chemotherapy solvent, Cremophor-L may be nonimmunologic (83).

Insect Stings

Insect stings or bites are well known to cause anaphylaxis. The most common are from members of the order Hymenoptera; yellow jackets, hornets, bees, wasps, fire and harvester ants. Less commonly implicated insects include the Triatoma; kissing bugs or assassin bugs. Systemic allergic reactions to insect stings occur in an estimated 3.3% of the population, and an estamated 40 deaths occur annually in the United States from Hymenoptera stings (37,84). Fire ant stings also cause human anaphylaxis, particularly in the southern United States, at an estimated annual rate of 0.6% to 16%, with >80 fatalities (85–87).

Victims may not accurately identify the specific insect necessitating confirmation of hypersensitivity by skin testing with purified venoms or whole-body fire ant extracts. *In vitro* tests, such as ImmunoCap can be used to confirm a clinical history of Hymenoptera or fire ant hypersensitivity. The risk of anaphylaxis with any event is dependent on the nature of the most severe previous experience. The following is a breakdown of frequency of occurrence: unknown history 3%, large local 10%, child cutaneous anaphylaxis 10%, child systemic anaphylaxis 50% to 60%, adult anaphylaxis 50% to 60%, and receiving venom immunotherapy 2%. Severe reactions to insect stings with confirmed positive skin tests warrant the physician to advise highly effective Hymenoptera venom or whole-body fire ant extract immunotherapy. Additionally the patient should carry self-injectable epinephrine and practice avoidance (87).

Food

In the United States an estimated 150 food allergy-related deaths occur each year. In food-related fatalities reported by Bock, 87% of the subjects had a prior history of a reaction to the responsible food (20). Food is the leading cause of outpatient anaphylaxis accounting for one-third to one-half of anaphylaxis visits to emergency departments in North America, Europe, Asia and Australia (76,88). In children anaphylaxis is most commonly from cow's milk, egg, wheat, soy, peanuts, tree nuts, fish, and shellfish. In adulthood the most common food-induced anaphylaxis is from peanuts, tree nuts, fish, and shellfish (89). Any food can cause anaphylaxis with dietary factors affecting the prevalence. Peanut allergy is the most common food allergy in the United States, with seafood in Hong Kong and sesame in Israel (90). Food-induced anaphylaxis most frequently occurs at home with nearly one-fifth at school (91). In a United Kingdom study of 202 anaphylactic deaths, 45 (30%) were from food. Over one-half were attributable to nuts; one-third occurred at home, 25% at restaurants, and 15% at work or school (92). Food-induced anaphylaxis onset can occur within seconds to a few hours after ingestion. Fatalities may occur within 30 minutes (12). The food trigger may not always be obvious, such as hidden, trace, malicious or cross-contaminating food in a meal or snack. Other potential triggers may include hormonally or genetically modified food, substituted food, a hidden food ingredient or food additive. As seen below, concomitant exercise may be involved (93,94).

Diagnostic confirmation of food-induced anaphylaxis can be challenging. A lack of serum tryptase elevation occurs in the majority of cases (95). This may be due to basophil as opposed to mast cell mediation, as well as slower or biphasic onset. A better marker for food-induced anaphylaxis may be serum levels of platelet-activating factor acetylhydrolase activity (PAF-AH)

and mast cell carboxypeptidase (95). If the cause of anaphylaxis is not apparent from the patient's history (ingredient list from package/manufacture/recipe/chef), IgE-specific skin testing with food extracts or by ImmunoCap may demonstrate the food-specific IgE antibody responsible (96). Food selection for skin-prick or *in vitro* testing must be guided by the patient's history because up to 60% of the general population has food sensitization of which the majority will not develop anaphylaxis. Intradermal food testing is contraindicated. Not all commercial food allergens are standardized, frequently necessitating testing with fresh foods.

Skin testing with foods, rarely, may cause anaphylaxis, necessitating the use of diluted solutions, the skin-prick technique, physician presence, not necessarily applying all suspected foods simultaneously, and availability of emergency materials and equipment. Food-specific IgE levels with greater than 95% predictive risk values for clinical reactivity by ImmunoCap have been defined as follows for adults: cow's milk $\geq$15kU/L, egg $\geq$7kU/L, peanut $\geq$14kU/L, tree nuts $\geq$15kU/L, and fish $\geq$20kU/L; for infants, the levels are cow's milk $\geq$5kU/L and egg $\geq$2kU/L. The rate of decrease in food-specific IgE levels over time also has predictive value.

Oral food challenges are most often used to eliminate incriminated foods that are highly unlikely to have caused the event or to document tolerance to a past food which caused anaphylaxis following years of abstinence and lack of sensitization by IgE testing. Physician-monitored graded oral food challenge in an emergency equipped environment is, at times, required to exclude anaphylaxis. These challenges are time consuming, are not without risk, and should be guided by follow-up measurements of specific IgE-levels and skin-prick testing. In those who tolerate double-blind placebo controlled food challenges, recurrence of allergy occurs in 8% of peanut allergic individuals. This risk may be elevated when peanut is avoided after a negative challenge, suggesting regular consumption to maintain peanut tolerance. In the future, specific IgE-binding epitopes on an allergen may potentially increase predictive risk; examples include peanut and cow's milk (11,94,97).

Latex Anaphylaxis

The incidence of anaphylaxis to latex appears to be decreasing. Between 1988 and 1992 the U.S. Food and Drug Administration received more than 1,000 reports of latex anaphylaxis, 15 of which were fatal (98). With the development of powder-free, low-protein gloves, a reduction of latex sensitization has occurred and the incidence may be decreasing with time. Latex anaphylaxis is IgE-mediated from a number of antigens from the latex source, *Hevea brasiliensis*. Sensitization is present in up to 75% of spina bifida patients and 6.5% of the general population. It is the second leading cause of intraoperative anaphylaxis after neuromuscular agents. Latex-induced anaphylaxis can present in the operating room in patients, surgeons, nurses, or anesthesiologists, accounting for 17% of intraoperative anaphylaxis. Latex exposure is through aerosolization, inhalation, and direct contact (dermal, mucosal). Groups at risk for anaphylaxis to latex include: chronic bladder care, neural tube defects, spina bifida, myelomeningocele, spinal cord trauma, urogenital malformations, neurogenic bladder, health care workers (greatest for operating room), multiple surgical procedures, and atopy (99). Latex allergy continues to be observed with three groups at higher risk—health care workers, children with spina bifida and urogenital abnormalities, and workers with occupational exposure to latex. Anaphylaxis has been observed following exposure to latex containing medical and dental supplies such as gloves (dental and gynecologic exams), catheters, IV tubing/ports, vial stoppers, dental dams. Other triggers include condoms, balloons, topical adhesives, hair glue, and plastic balls with latex pits. Patients rarely react to hard/extruded rubber products such as automobile tires (93,100). Risk factors for health care workers include a personal history of atopy, frequent use of disposable latex gloves, and hand dermatitis (33). Clinical differences have been observed between surgical and nonsurgical latex induced anaphylaxis. Cutaneous, respiratory, and cardiovascular manifestations can occur in both. Cardiovascular collapse is a feature of surgical procedures, with dizziness or syncope more frequent in nonsurgical procedures. IgE detection by skin tests are more sensitive than ELISA or Immuno-Cap serologic tests (highly variable and sensitive, sensitivity 50% to 100%). No approved skin test reagent is available in the United States. Extracts have been made from raw latex (sap) and latex glove extracts (allergen content highly variable). Systemic reactions to latex skin testing have been reported; thus, care must be exercised when skin testing with uncharacterized extracts (101). When a patient tests positive for latex-specific IgE or has a history of latex anaphylaxis, the patient and medical record must be labeled as latex allergic. Latex must be avoided by these individuals, and when in the hospital, a latex-free environment should be provided. Inadvertent exposure may occur necessitating carrying of self-injectable epinephrine.

Anaphylaxis during and following General Anesthesia

Anaphylaxis, either immunologic or nonimmunologic, occurs during general anesthesia in 1:5000 to 1:25,000 administrations with death ranging from 0.05% to 4% to 6%. Most episodes of surgical anaphylaxis occur during the induction procedure when muscle relaxants, sedatives, and opiates are administered. Latex reactions typically occur during maintenance anesthesia with a delay from 30 to 60 minutes. It is often difficult to differentiate between immune and nonimmune mast/basophil cell-mediated reactions and pharmacologic effects from a variety of medications administered during general anesthesia (16,93,102). Clinical recognition of anaphylaxis in this setting may be modified by a multitude of anesthesia-related physiological changes. Clinical manifestations include flushing, urticaria, laryngeal edema or bronchospasm interfering with intubation, increased ventilatory pressure, and hypotension. Peri-anesthesia anaphylaxis diagnosis may be hindered by the patient's limited ability to describe symptoms of pruritus, shortness of breath, lightheadedness, urticaria, or angioedema. The observation of physical findings may be masked by surgical drapes. Cardiovascular collapse is the sole presentation in nearly 50% of cases. Anaphylaxis must always be considered if immediate hypotension occurs associated with or without bronchospasm following parenteral administration of a therapeutic agent or the induction of anesthesia. Muscle relaxant induced anaphylaxis is associated with bradycardia in 12% to 30% of cases (103–105).

In order of frequency, the causes of anaphylaxis related to anesthesia are muscle relaxants, latex, antibiotics (particularly β-lactam), induction/hypnotic agents, opiods, colloids (dextran, mannitol, hydroxyethyl starch), and blood products (105). Other less common causes are protamine, aprotinin, isosulfan blue dye, gelatin solution, chlorhexidine, ethylene oxide, radiocontrast media, streptokinase, methylmethacrylate, and chymopapain (1,2,105). The causes may vary related to the type of surgery. In cardiovascular surgery anaphylaxis is more likely from cephalosporins, gelatin solution, or protamine rather than from muscle relaxants.

Muscle relaxants account for 60% to 70% (99) of anaphylaxis during anesthesia. Succinylcholine is the most common. Mediation of muscle relaxant anaphylaxis can be IgE or non-IgE. Succinylcholine facilitates cross-linking of specific IgE on the mast cell and basophil membranes. The tertiary or quaternary ammonium group, common to all muscle relaxants are likely the immunodominant determinant recognized by IgE. Three out of 4 cases of anaphylaxis to muscle relaxants occur in females, suggesting cross-reactivity with ammonium compounds in personal care products (106). Serial dilution skin testing with specific muscle relaxants has been useful in determining the safest agent for subsequent surgery following anesthesia-related anaphylaxis. Latex is the second most common cause of anesthesia/intraoperative anaphylaxis and is discussed above in a separate section.

Hypnotic induction agents are the third common cause of anesthesia anaphylaxis. Intravenous barbiturates are most common, though the rate is <1:25,000.

Mixing barbiturates with neuromuscular blocking agents in the same intravenous line may increase the risk. Women are three times more likely than men to react to thiopental. Most anaphylaxis to barbiturates, particularly thiopental is caused by specific IgE; however, direct release of histamine may also occur. Propofol, a nonbarbiturate induction agent, is a useful substitute in the barbiturate sensitive patient. Propofol anaphylaxis can occur generally through direct mast cell activation, however specific IgE to propofol has been reported (107). Narcotics and opioids very rarely cause anaphylaxis, more commonly causing flushing and urticaria, which are lessened by reducing the intravenous rate. Narcotics and opioids, with the exception of fentanyl, cause direct release of mast cell mediators (93). Antibiotics are frequently administered perioperatively and are responsible for anaphylaxis at a rate of 0.001%. The most common implicated antibiotics are β-lactams and vancomycin. Intravenous administration of penicillin results in more severe anaphylaxis. Vancomycin induced anaphylaxis is typically nonimmunologic and rarely IgE mediated. Vancomycin's anaphylaxis potential is infusion rate related leading to direct release of histamine and direct myocardial depression. This risk can be reduced by a slower infusion rate and/or pre infusion of a slowly infused diluted dose of vancomycin (93).

Colloid plasma expanders such as dextran and hydroxyethyl starch (HES) are responsible for anaphylaxis at rates of 0.008% to 0.08% for dextran and 0.08% for HES. The clinical significance of reported specific antibodies to dextran and HES is unknown (108).

Blood transfusion reactions may be hemolytic from complement activation or from anti-IgA antibodies in a IgA-deficient patient receiving IgA antibody in nonwashed packed red blood cells or whole blood from a normal donor. These IgA antibodies typically are IgG, some may be an IgE isotype (109).

The differential of peri-anesthetic anaphylaxis includes asthma, arrythmias, hemorrhage, hereditary angioedema, Jarish-Herxheimer reaction, mastocytosis, myocardial infarction, vasoactive drug overdose, pericardial tamponade, postextubation stridor, pulmonary edema, pulmonary embolus, sepsis, tension pneumothorax, vasodepressor response, and venous air or fat embolism. Anaphylaxis occurring during general anesthesia—during or after surgery—necessitates collecting serum tryptase levels within 1 to 4 hours of the onset to assist in confirming the diagnosis. A sample can also be obtained postmortem if necessary. Comparison to a control is optimal, obtaining a control preoperatively or 24 hours after the event. The tryptase sampling times should be recorded in relation to the onset of anaphylaxis (110). An extensive review of suggested skin-prick and intradermal skin tests to perianesthetic agents is available in a review by Ebo et al. 2007 (111). Other useful *in vitro* tesing to elucidate

mechanisms of action include: basophil allergen challenge, leucocyte histamine release, and flow cytometric analysis of *in vitro*-activated basophils (112).

Blood Components, Seminal Fluid, and Biologic Agents

Blood transfusions have induced anaphylaxis through several mechanisms. These include: cytotoxic reactions from IgG or IgM, inadvertent transfusion of small amounts of IgA to IgA-deficient patients, and passive transfusion of IgE antibodies from allergic donors transiently sensitizing recipients' mast cells and basophils. An estimated 25% of blood donors have IgE antibodies to common allergens and an estimated one-third of these donors have allergen-specific IgE >10kU/L. A nonatopic recipient may be passively sensitized by transfusion of donor blood containing elevated titers of IgE (113). Conversely, in rare cases, transfusion of an allergen or drug into an atopic recipient has caused plasma anaphylaxis.

Antihuman IgA antibodies are present in about 40% of individuals with selective IgA deficiency. Some of the patients have allergic reactions varying from mild urticaria to fatal anaphylaxis, usually after numerous transfusions. These antibodies are usually IgG-mediated but may be from an IgE isotype. These reactions can be prevented by using sufficiently washed red blood cells or by using blood from IgA-deficient donors (109).

Serum protein aggregates (nonimmune complex) such as human albumin, human γ globulin, and horse antihuman lymphocyte globulin can cause anaphylaxis. These complexes apparently activate complement, resulting in release of bioactive mediators (114).

Cryoprecipitate and factor VIII concentrate have been reported as causes of anaphylaxis. An IgE-mediated mechanism was demonstrated in one patient by leukocyte histamine release; positive skin test results to factor VIII, factor IX, and cryoprecipitate; and positive RAST results to factor VIII. An attempt at pretreatment with corticosteroids and diphenhydramine and an attempt to desensitize did not prevent future reactions (114,115). The incidence of horse antilymphocyte globulin anaphylaxis is near 2%. Skin testing should precede use of such preparations to identify the presence of IgE antibodies (116).

Anaphylaxis from human seminal fluid by coital exposure rarely occurs with >30 cases reported since the initial report in 1958. It is IgE-mediated from seminal proteins of varying molecular weight. Exogenous allergens may also be transferred in seminal fluid to a woman from a male partner's ingestion of food or drug to which the woman is sensitized. Artificial insemination with sperm devoid of seminal plasma induced pregnancy in a woman with human seminal plasma atopy. Immunotherapy with seminal plasma fractions of the male partner have been successful in those couples wishing to conceive. Anaphylaxis can also be avoided by abstinence, regular use of condoms, as well as artificial insemination to achieve pregnancy (117,118).

Biologic agents are being introduced into the drug market at an increasing rate. This recent emergence has not allowed an estimated incidence of anaphylaxis. The use of omalizumab, a recombinate murine based anti-IgE antibody is therapeutic for severe allergic asthma. The rate of anaphylaxis from omalizumab is estimated between 0.09% and ≤0.2%. Anaphylaxis occured in 48 cases from an estimated 39,510 omalizumab exposed patients. Anaphylaxis can occur after any dose, even if a previous dose was well tolerated. Anaphylaxis occurred after the first dose in 40% of cases and after repeat administration in 56% of cases. Some patients experienced anaphylaxis after 2 years of chronic treatment. Anaphylaxis occurred within 2 hours in 71% of cases with delayed onset between 2 hours to more than 24 hours after injection (119). Anaphylaxis to cetuximab is from IgE against the sugar galactose-α-1,3-galactose expressed in the cell line used in production (1,2).

EXERCISE-INDUCED ANAPHYLAXIS AND FOOD DEPENDENT EXERCISE-INDUCED ANAPHYLAXIS

Exercise-induced anaphylaxis (EIA) occurs with vigorous exercise and may produce shock or loss of consciousness. Patients tend to have a personal or family history of atopy. Jogging is the most common activity; however, it has also been attributed to brisk walking, bicycling, racquet sports, skiing, and aerobics. Symptoms may include warmth, pruritus, erythema, urticaria, angioedema, nausea, vomiting, abdominal cramps, diarrhea, laryngeal edema, bronchospasm, respiratory distress, and vascular collapse. Symptoms last 30 minutes to hours. The reaction typically begins during or after exercise is completed and may occur only when exercise is performed shortly after a meal or a medication such as aspirin or nonsteroidal anti-inflammatory agent. Unlike cholinergic urticaria, exercise-induced anaphylaxis is not from elevated body core temperature. EIA does not occur with each period of exercise, and the same amount of exercise on each occasion may not lead to anaphylaxis. About two-thirds of patients with EIA have a family history of atopy, and about half have a personal history of atopy. Familial EIA also has been reported. Dyspnea with a choking sensation occurs in 60% of patients and loss of consciousness occurs in 30% patients. At least one death has been reported from EIA. The effectiveness of H1 and H2 antagonists is controversial and may reduce the severity or intensity of the attack. It is best for the patient to recognize his or her threshold as well as early manifestations necessitating prompt cessation of exercise. These patients should carry self-injectable epinephrine and exercise with a companion familiar with this disorder and emergency treatment measures.

Food dependent exercise-induced anaphylaxis (FDEIA) is a distinct form of food allergy induced by physical exercise. Aspirin is an additional exacerbating factor. Specific foods that have been linked to FDEIA include celery, shellfish, wheat, buckwheat, cuttlefish, nuts, apples, squid, abalone, hazelnuts, grapes, eggs, oranges, cheese, cabbage, mushrooms, corn, garlic, beef, pork, rice, and chicken. In Japan wheat is the most common cause. These foods are tolerated without exercise, and exercising without eating these foods does not cause anaphylaxis. Nonspecific food dependent EIA also can occur. Eighty per cent of the patients have symptoms within 2 hours of eating.

The mechanism of action likely involves IgE mediation with positive food skin-prick, RAST, and CAP tests in most patients. Enhanced mast cell degranulation has been observed following exercise challenges. Some evidence supports the hypothesis that exercise enhances the absorption of incompletely or undigested allergen proteins from the gastrointestinal tract (92). When aspirin is combined with food to trigger exercise induced anaphylaxis it has been hypothesized that aspirin may activate mast cells in combination with IgE cross-linking. Aspirin and exercise may both facilitate gastrointestinal absorption. Along with standard anaphylaxis treatment, patients with FDEIA, should be told not to exercise 4 to 6 hours after eating (120–122).

IDIOPATHIC ANAPHYLAXIS

Idiopathic anaphylaxis was described three decades ago, and in the following 15 years IA was classified, treatment regimens were established, and remission was induced in most cases. Fortunately, the majority of patients improve with time, with complete remission in most. At least 3 fatalities have been reported from IA and the number of cases of IA in the United States was estimated to be 33,000 in 1995. Patients with frequent episodes have multiple emergency service visits and hospitalizations and typically are very frightened. IA is not limited to the United States and is likely to be worldwide in distribution. When IA is identified and the treatment regimens are instituted, the prognosis for control is excellent. Fortunately, the diagnostic methodology and treatment regimens are successful and the alert physician who is aware of IA as the explanation for single or recurrent episodes of anaphylaxis with no apparent external cause can competently and successfully manage IA in pediatric or adult populations (123,124).

IA is an immediate-type, life-threatening event with no external allergen triggering the onset through an IgE antibody-mediated reaction. It is a diagnosis of exclusion after eliminating other causes, such as anaphylaxis from food, exercise, food and exercise, medications,

TABLE 14.4   CLASSIFICATION OF IDIOPATHIC ANAPHYLAXIS

DISEASE	SYMPTOMS
IA-generalized-infrequent (IA-G-I)	Urticaria or angioedema with bronchospasm, hypotension, syncope, or gastrointestinal symptoms with or without upper airway compromise with infrequent episodes (fewer than 6 episodes occurring per year)
IA-generalized-frequent (IA-G-F)	Clinical manifestations as for IA-G-I but occurring more than 6 times per year
IA-angioedema-infrequent (IA-A-I)	Urticaria or angioedema with upper airway compromise such as laryngeal edema, severe pharyngeal edema, or massive tongue edema without other systemic manifestations with infrequent episodes (fewer than 6 episodes occurring per year)
IA-angioedema-frequent (IA-A-F)	Clinical manifestations as for IA-A-I but occurring more than 6 times per year
IA-questionable (IA-Q)	This diagnosis is applied for a patient who is referred for management with a presumptive diagnosis of IA for which repeated attempts at documentation of objective findings are unsuccessful, response to appropriate doses of prednisone do not occur, and the diagnosis of IA becomes uncertain.
IA-variant (IA-V)	This diagnosis is applied when symptoms and physical findings of IA vary from classic findings of IA; IA-V may subsequently be classified as IA-Q or IA-excluded or IA-A or IA-G.
Undifferentiated somatoform IA	Symptoms mimic IA but no objective findings are seen and there is no response to the regimen for IA

diagnostic agents, insect stings and bites, and illnesses such as mastocytosis and C1 esterase inhibitor deficiency and/or dysfunction (31). The symptoms of IA are identical to known causes of anaphylaxis. Foods, drugs, venoms, and specific activities are not related to the onset of episodes of IA. These are typical triggers of anaphylaxis but must be excluded during initial evaluation and re-excluded following recurrent episodes, especially in the difficult-to-control patient. The two major types of IA are IA-angioedema (IA-A), in which airway obstruction occurs, or IA-generalized (IA-G), in which the various other systemic manifestations of anaphylaxis occur. Both types may exhibit urticaria. The classification of IA relative to clinical manifestations and frequency is shown in Table 14.4. The differential diagnosis for IA are listed in Table 14.5. Treatment regimens initially evolved from treating or preventing anaphylactic-type reactions such as those due to radiographic contrast media (123).

Acute management of IA begins at the onset of urticaria, abdominal pain, generalized pruritus, or other anaphylaxis symptoms. Initially the patient should self-inject epinephrine 0.3 mg intramuscularly in the upper lateral thigh and ingest prednisone 50 mg and a H1 antagonist, such as cetirizine 10 mg. Other H1 antagonists are acceptable. This is referred to as triple therapy. The patient then should seek medical care depending on the circumstances; contact a physician for advice, call 911, or proceed to an emergency department where

additional intensive therapy may be required. IA is a corticosteroid-responsive condition and patients with frequent episodes of IA who have more than 6 episodes in 1 year or more than 2 episodes per month require daily H1 agonist and have their triple therapy ready. Empiric treatment to control the disease and reduce frequency and severity include prednisone 60 mg to 100 mg each morning for 7 days followed by 60 mg on alternate mornings. This is continued for 2 weeks and reduced by 5 mg to 10 mg every 2 weeks assuming there are no episodes, including urticaria or angioedema. Cetirizine or alternative H1 antagonist therapy is continued. In one series of IA patients treated with this regimen the rate of remission was 48% in patients with IA-G and 40% in patients with IA-A (31,125). Patients who are unable to

TABLE 14.5   DIFFERENTIAL DIAGNOSIS OF IDIOPATHIC ANAPHYLAXIS

Hereditary and aquired angioedema
Systemic mastocytosis
Hidden allergen (e.g., latex, food, drug)
Munchausen anaphylaxis (purposeful self-exposure to antigen)
Undifferentiated somatoform idiopathic anaphylaxis

discontinue prednisone have corticosteroid-dependent IA (CSD-IA) and additional medications may be useful. These include ketotifen 2 mg, two to three times daily, oral cromolyn concentrate (100 mg/5 mL/ampoule) 2 ampoules pre-meals and at bedtime along with H1 and H2 antagonist (126). These additional agents may allow reduction and eventual discontinuation of prednisone, and possibly induce a remission. Alternatively, these medications may not alter the prednisone requirement, in which case they should be tapered and discontinued, and the diagnosis would remain CSD-IA. Leukotriene antagonists may be of benefit (31).

After initiation of a regimen for IA-GF, consisting of prednisone, H1/H2 antagonist, and albuterol, the episodes of IA should cease while the patient is receiving daily prednisone. This may require 1 to 6 weeks of daily prednisone. If longer daily prednisone is required, the diagnosis of IA becomes questionable and alternate diagnoses must be considered, including those in the differential diagnosis of IA (Table 14.5). If the patient's condition is not controlled by prednisone (adult dose of 60 mg daily) for 2 weeks and alternate day for an additional 4 weeks, the diagnosis is likely not IA and undifferentiated somatoform IA (127) must be considered seriously. Alternatively, panic disorder and prednisone nonadherance should be considered.

After IA is controlled with daily prednisone, an alternate-day regimen of prednisone at a higher dose is initiated, and if the IA remains controlled, the dose of prednisone is reduced cautiously. If, after a reduction of alternate-day prednisone, an episode of IA occurs, daily prednisone must be resumed followed by alternate-day prednisone at a higher dose and slower reduction. The long-term result of this regimen will be an induction of remission, and in most patients the use of prednisone can then be terminated. If a dose of alternate-day prednisone is reached below which episodes of IA recur, this is corticosteroid-dependent IA (CSD-IA). Various other treatment protocols have been published using other H1 antagonist, H2 antagonist and β-agonists. In summary, frequent episodes of IA and some cases of very severe single episode IA generally require a 3-month empiric course of prednisone and H1 antagonist with or without oral albuterol, and readily available emergency triple therapy of epinephrine, H1 antagonist, and prednisone. Infrequent episodes are managed with readily available triple therapy.

A major goal in management of IA has to be the education of the patient, family, and sometimes the referring physician. It is important that they understand several aspects of the disease. First, there is not an external agent; therefore, attention must be given to pharmacologic induction of a remission. Second, patients should understand the risks and benefits of prednisone so that they will be able to make informed choices about their management. Finally, it is important to explain to patients that research continues into

IA etiology such as evidence of mast cell activation by detection of urinary histamine, urinary methylimidazole acetic acid, plasma histamine, serum tryptase, and IA patients with an increased number of skin mast cells. IA patients have an increased cutaneous response to codeine. Lymphocyte activation in IA patients has been demonstrated by increase in the numbers of CD3$^+$ HLA$^-$DR$^+$T cells. Additionally an elevation of CD19$^+$ (B cells) was observed. These finding suggest activated T lymphocytes during acute episodes of IA. IA patients also have a greater number of activated B cells (31). Additionally, FcεRI receptors may be aggregated through autoimmune mechanisms.

Undifferentiated somatoform idiopathic anaphylaxis is the term applied when patients describe symptoms consistent with IA but medical records are void of any objective evidence of anaphylaxis. In reports of 9 cases (127), the following general characteristics have been observed. The referring physician generally has not recognized the nonorganic nature of the problem. The medical costs of hospitalizations, emergency service visits, and laboratory tests can be extremely high, and these patients may be treated excessively with unnecessary corticosteroids. When the managing physician arrives at this conclusion, further management may become difficult. Approaching the basis of the problem as psychologic in origin with referral to a psychiatrist is the logical approach. Psychologic diagnoses include generalized anxiety disorder, somatization, globus hystericus, panic disorder, or conversion reactions. This may be accepted by the patient. Alternatively, the patient may reject the concept of a psychologic disorder as the explanation, often with hostility. Some of these cases can be managed by the allergist and primary care physician with safe, low doses of antihistamines and supportive ambulatory visits at increasing intervals. Other patients may continue appearing at hospital emergency services and be admitted.

The ratio of pediatric IA to adult IA cases is about 1 pediatric IA case to 20 adult cases. For this reason, the diagnosis of IA in children may be more delayed than would the diagnosis in adults. Fortunately, the response to the regimen for IA (with adjustment of doses for the pediatric population) appears equally successful and the prognosis equally favorable as in the majority of adults. Long-term follow-up studies and a cost analysis for IA patients estimates that $11 million per year can be saved in the United States (128,129). The primary issues of concern from referring physicians include severity, guidance for treatment, and advice to local physicians (130).

■ ANAPHYLAXIS TREATMENT AND PREVENTION

The treatment of anaphylaxis should follow established principles for emergency resuscitation. Anaphylaxis has a highly variable presentation, and treatment must be individualized for a patient's particular underlying medical conditions, symptoms, and their severity. Treatment recommendations are based on clinical experience, understanding pathologic mechanisms, and the known action of various drugs (131). Management recommendations are subject to physician discretion and variations in sequence and performance rely on physician judgment (93). Recommendations depend on site resources and proximity to additional emergency assistance. Prompt recognition followed by rapid therapy is of utmost importance including a treatment log to accurately record progress. Medical facilities should be stocked with anaphylaxis supplies with expiration dates recorded, available injectable epinephrine, intravenous fluids, needles, oxygen canula and mask, oral airways device, stethoscope, and a sphygmomanometer as minimal essentials. The approach outlined in Table 14.6 is required to counteract the effects of mediator release, support vital functions, and prevent further release of mediators.

At the first sign of anaphylaxis the patient should be treated with epinephrine. Next, the clinician should determine whether the patient is dyspneic or hypotensive. Airway patency must be assessed, and if the patient has suffered cardiopulmonary arrest, basic cardiopulmonary resuscitation must be instituted immediately. If shock is present or impending, the patient should not attempt to sit or stand, the lower extremities should be elevated and intravenous fluids administered. Epinephrine is the most important single agent in the treatment of anaphylaxis, and its delay or failure to be administered is more problematic than its administration. There are no absolute contraindications to the use of epinephrine, including patients with heart disease who experience anaphylaxis. However, several anaphylaxis fatalities have been attributed to injudicious intravenous epinephrine administration (46). Administer aqueous epinephrine 1:1000 dilution, 0.3 mL to 0.5 mL (0.01 mg/kg in children to a maximum 0.3 mg) intramuscularly in the thigh every 5 to 10 minutes as necessary. Alternatively, an epinephrine autoinjector may be administered through

---

TABLE 14.6 MANAGEMENT OF ANAPHYLAXIS

1. *Immediate:* Aqueous epinephrine 1:1000 dilution, 0.3 mL to 0.5 mL (0.01mg/kg in children; maximum 0.3 mg) IM in thigh. May repeat every 5 to 10 minutes if necessary. IV epinephrine only in dire situations when severe hypotension or cardiac collapse is unresponsive to IM doses using 5 μg to 10 μg IV bolus (0.2 μg/kg) for hypotension and 0.1mg to 0.5 mg IV for cardiovascular collapse with toxicity monoriting; children: 0.01 mg/kg (0.1mL/kg of a 1:10,000 solution). Consider continous low-dose epinephrine IV infusion at 4 μg/min to 10 μg/min.
2. If sting: tourniquet proximal to site releasing every 1 to 2 minutes every 10 minutes, injecting one-half dose aqueous epinephrine into site (0.1 mg to 0.2 mg)
3. Record blood pressure, pulse, and O_2 saturation
4. Depending on severity, degree of response and the individual patient:
   a. Diphenhydramine, IV slowly: 25mg to 50mg for adults; 1mg/kg up to 50mg maximum for children
      Ranitidine: 50 mg for adults, 12.5 mg to 50 mg children (1 mg/kg) IV over 5 to 10 minutes
   b. Nasal oxygen or high-flow oxygen through nonrebreather mask or endotracheal tube
5. Methylprednisolone 1 mg/kg/d to 2 mg/kg/d IV or hydrocortisone 5 mg/kg (200 mg max) every 4 to 6 hrs or prednisone 0.5 mg/kg/d PO (exact doses of corticosteroids not established)
6. Be prepared for intubation; hypotension
7. For severe bronchospasm:
   inhaled β2-agonist: nebulized; albuterol 2.5 mg/3 mL to 5 mg/3 mL saline or levalbuterol 0.63 mg to 1.25mg, unit dose. If not responsive, IV aminophyline 5mg/kg over 30 minutes
8. For systolic blood pressure <90 mm Hg adult <50mm Hg children:
   a. 2 IV lines wide open
   b. Dopamine, norepinephrine, metaraminol. Aortic balloon counterpulsation for myocardial dysfunction
9. For patients taking β-adrenergic antagonists:
   a. Glucagon 1 mg to 5 mg IV slowly, then titrate at 5 μg/min to 15 μg/min infusion, emesis precaution
   b. Atropine if bradycardia; 0.3 mg to 0.5 mg IM or IV every 10 minutes, to a maximum of 2 mg.
10. Observation for protracted or biphasic anaphylaxis in emergency department observation unit, hospital admission or intensive care unit. Observation period individualized on patient's severity, reliability and access to care.
11. Obtain serum tryptase within 3 hours of onset of anaphylaxis, mark time of blood draw.
12. Discharge with emergency preparedness plan: avoid trigger if known, 2 epinephrine autoinjectors. Omit (2 pack), anaphylaxis action plan (www.aaaai.org), medical identification, referral to allergy-immunology specialist.
13. IM, intramuscular; IV, intravenous

clothing into the anterolateral thigh. Intravenous epinephrine should be used only in patients with severe hypotension-cardiovascular collapse or terminal or grave clinical status not responding to intramuscular epinephrine and aggressive fluid replacement, including colloid-containing solutions if necessary. A suggested, though not established, intravenous dose of aqueous epinephrine for hypotension is a 5 μg to 10 μg intravenous bolus (0.2 μg/kg) and for cardiovascular collapse 0.1 mg to 0.5 mg intravenously. In children, 0.01 mg/kg (0.1 mL/kg of a 1:10,000 solution) repeated every 3 to 5 minutes for an ongoing arrest. For safety, titratability, and avoidance of accidental bolus dosing, continuous low-dose epinephrine, at 4 μg/min to 10 μg/min infusion, may be the most effective in the more severe individual (46,65).

If anaphylaxis resulted from an injection or sting, as long as the sting is not on the head, neck, hands, or feet, a second injection of aqueous epinephrine 1:1000, one-half dose (0.1 mg to 0.2 mg), may be given at the injection or sting site to reduce antigen absorption. A tourniquet can be placed proximal to the injection site (not if injection or sting in head, hands, feet), releasing every 1 to 2 minutes every 10 minutes (131).

Oxygen should be given in patients with cyanosis, dyspnea, or wheezing with oximetric monitoring. High-flow oxygen is administered through a nonrebreather mask or endotracheal tube. Caution must be exercised if the patient has preexisting chronic obstructive pulmonary disease. If bronchospasm is refractory to epinephrine, inhaled β-agonists may be useful. These include nebulized albuterol, 2.5 mg to 5 mg in 3 mL of saline or levalbuterol in an albuterol intolerant subject, 0.63 mg to 1.25 mg unit dose, repeating as necessary. Aminophyline may be used if bronchospasm is not responsive to albuterol or levalbuterol, 5 mg/kg over 30 minutes intravenously adjusting the dose based on age, concurrent medications, and underlying disease state. Use atropine and transcutaneous pacing if asystole or pulseless electrical activity are present (46).

Antihistamines, including H1 and H2 antagonist are useful for symptomatic relief of urticaria, angioedema, and pruritus. They have a slower onset of action then epinephrine and have little effect on blood pressure. The combination of H1 and H2 have been reported to be more effective in reducing the cutaneous manifestations of anaphylaxis than treatment with H1 antagonist alone. The H1 antagonist diphenhydramine can be administered intravenously (slowly over 20 seconds), intramuscularly, or orally, 50 mg or more in divided doses every 6 hours for 48 hours, longer if needed with maximum daily dose of 300 mg (5 mg/kg) for children and 400 mg for adults. The H2 antagonist ranitidine, 50 mg in adults and 12.5 mg to 50 mg (1 mg/kg) in children, may be diluted in 5% dextrose to a total volume of 20 mL and injected intravenously over 5 minutes. Other rapidly absorbed antihistamines (H1 and H2) may be substituted.

If the patient does not respond to the above measures and remains hypotensive or in persistent respiratory distress, hospitalization in an intensive care unit is essential. In these circumstances, intravenous fluids should be given through the largest gauge line available at a rate necessary to maintain a systolic blood pressure above 90 mm Hg in adults and 50 mm Hg in children (132). If intravenous fluids are not effective, potent vasopressors such as noradrenaline, vasopressin, or metaraminol may be necessary. Corticosteroids are not helpful in the acute management of anaphylaxis due to a slow onset of action. Their effectiveness has never been determined in placebo-controlled studies. Their usefulness is well established in other allergic diseases leading to their incorporation into anaphylaxis management. They should be used promptly in moderate or severe reactions in hope of preventing protracted or biphasic anaphylaxis (133,134). If given, the dose of intravenous corticosteroid should be equivalent to 1.0 mg/kg to 2.0 mg/kg per dose of methylprednisolone every 6 hours. Oral prednisone can be given for milder episodes at 1.0 mg/kg, up to 50 mg.

Glucagon may be the drug of choice for adult patients taking β-adrenergic antagonists. Glucagon is thought to reverse refractory hypotension and bronchospasm by activating adenylate cyclase independent of the β-receptor. The recommended intravenous dose of glucagon is 1 mg to 5 mg (children 20 μg/kg to 30 μg/kg; maximal dose 1 mg) over 5 minutes followed by 5 μg/kg to 15μg/min titration to clinical response. Protection of airway is necessary during glucacons infusion due to frequently observed emesis (1,2).

After the patient's condition has been stabilized, supportive therapy should be maintained with fluids, drugs, and ventilation as long as it is needed to support vital signs and functions. Biphasic reactions occur in 1% to 20% of patients with anaphylaxis, 20% of fatal or near-fatal food-induced episodes. The second phase occurs ranging 1 to 72 hours after the first. A reasonable postanaphylactic observation time is 4 to 6 hours in most patients, lengthening the time in hospitalized patients or those with severe or refractory symptoms. Additional caution and observation is required for patients with anaphylaxis and a history of asthma, because most fatalities associated with anaphylaxis occur in this group.

At discharge following anaphylaxis three steps are recommended: a prescription for self-injectable epinephrine with instructions on usage and demonstration with trainer device; patient education, including how to avoid the precipitating agent, if known; follow-up evaluation preferably with an allergist. In addition the patient can be informed about national organizations that provide important information and educational materials, such as the Food Allergy and Anaphylaxis Network, www.foodallergy.org; the American Academy of Allergy, Asthma and Immunology, www.aaaai.org; the American College of Allergy, Asthma and Immunology,

---

TABLE 14.7   RULES TO REDUCE THE RISK OF ANAPHYLAXIS

1. Know the patient's allergy and medical history, especially comorbidities, with medical record documentation. *Consider cross-reacting agents that could trigger anaphylaxis.*
2. Know the patient's concurrent therapy.
3. Administer drugs orally rather than parenterally if possible.
4. Observe immunotherapy patients in the physician's office 30 minutes after the injection.
5. Hold immunotherapy in the presence of undertreated asthma.
6. The patient should carry, at all times, a statement of allergy in the form of a bracelet, necklace, or wallet card.
7. Patients with a history of an anaphylactoid reaction, such as radiographic contrast media should be pretreated if use of the agent is essential.
8. Patients with exercise and idiopathic anaphylaxis or those at risk of accidental exposure to known trigger should carry an emergency treatment kit. Exercise with a companion/buddy.

J Allergy Clin Immunol 2006; 117:393: with permission

---

www.acaai.org; and the American Latex Allergy Association, www.latexallergyresources.org.

A careful history of previous anaphylaxis to suspected antigens is mandatory. As in all allergic diseases, avoidance of a known antigen is the single most effective prophylactic measure. Avoidance of a known food should be advised, but accidental exposure may still occur from food mixtures or utensils. General measures include avoidance, repellents, and protective clothing to help avoid some stinging insect reactions. Drug avoidance is paramount based on a detailed history. Alternative drugs must be used. If the drug is documented as absolutely essential, skin testing, graded test dosing, desensitization, or premedication may be attempted with great caution, depending on the drug's allergic mechanisms of action. Substances requiring pretreatment regimens include RCM, flouroscein, protamine sulfate, and etoposide. Skin testing before drug use may be required, such as with penicillin, succinylcholine, and local anesthetics. Oral food and substance challenge was discussed earlier in this chapter. Washed red blood cells, predeposited blood, and IgA-deficient blood are choices for IgA-deficient patients requiring blood products. Skin testing, ELISA, and ImmunoCap were discussed earlier in this chapter. Latex-induced anaphylaxis should be treated as any other cause of anaphylaxis; however, efforts of prevention by latex avoidance is imperative. A latex-free workplace is required for the latex-sensitive health care worker. For the latex-sensitive patient, a latex-free examination and procedure environment is necessary. Emergency equipment and medications should be readily available in both environments. General rules to reduce the risk for anaphylaxis are listed in Table 14.7.

■ EMERGENCY DRUGS AVAILABLE TO PATIENTS AND FAMILY EDUCATION

Certain patients are at risk for unpredictable anaphylaxis. This includes stinging insect exposure, food allergy, latex allergy, exercise-induced, food-dependent exercise-induced, and IA. These patients (parents or guardians of children and adolescents) should carry at all times self-injectable epinephrine, an oral antihistamine, 30 mg to 50 mg of prednisone, and a tourniquet (for stinging insects). Examples of self-injectable epinephrine are EpiPen regular or junior (Dey, Nappa, CA), a prefilled automatic injection device with 0.3 mg or 0.15 mg aqueous epinephrine, and Twinject (Sciele Pharma, Inc., Atlanta, GA), also an automatic injection device with 0.3 mg or 0.15 mg aqueous epinephrine. Two doses should be available with a second dose required in up to one-third of cases. A second dose may be administered if no improvement within 10 minutes. After taking these actions the patient should go to the nearest medical facility and seek further definitive therapy. A medic alert card or jewelry may be useful (MedicAlert, Turlock, CA, www.medicalert.co.us) as well as a folding wallet card from the American Academy of Allergy, Asthma and Immunology anaphylaxis educational materials (www.aaaai.org). The first episode of anaphylaxis may be fatal necessitating increased awareness of this *killer allergy* among teachers, coaches, camp directors, child care providers, and food industry workers. Patient education and individual action plans are suggested; however, at times these are associated with therapeutic complexity and ethical dilemmas (135,136). Landmark legislation was implemented in 2006 with the National Food Allergy Labeling Consumer Protection Act in the United States mandating clear food labeling and in Ontario, Canada, an Act to Protect Anaphylactic Pupils (Sabrina's Law), establishing minimum standards for managing anaphylaxis in schools (2).

■ REFERENCES

1. James LP Jr, Austen KF. Fatal systemic anaphylaxis in man. *N Engl J Med.* 1964;270:597–603.
2. Simons FER. Anaphylaxis, killer allergy: long-term management in the community. *J Allergy Clin Immunol.* 2006;117:367–377.

3. Chung CH, Mirakhur B, Chan E, et al. Cetuximab-induced anaphylaxis and IgE specific for galactose-α-1,3-galactose. *N Engl J Med.* 2008;358:1109–1117.

4. Cox L, Platts-Mills TAE, Finegold I. American Academy of Allergy, Asthma & Immunology/American College of Allergy, Asthma and Immunology Joint Task Force Report on omalizumab-associated anaphylaxis. *J Allergy Clin Immunol.* 2007;120(6):1373–1377.

5. Wasserman SI. The allergist in the new millennium. *J Allergy Clin Immunol.* 2000;105:3–8

6. Portier P, Richet C. De l'action anaphylactique de certaines venins. *Compt Rend Soc Biol.* 1902;54:170–172.

7. Shafrir E. Pioneers in allergy and anaphylaxis. *Isr J Med Sci.* 1999;32:344.

8. Simons FER. Anaphylaxis. *J Allergy Clin Immunol.* 2008; 121(2): S402–S407.

9. Johansson SG, Hourihane JO, Bousquet J, et al. A revised nomenclature for allergy: an EAACI position statement from the EAACI nomenclature task force. *Allergy.* 2001;56:813–824.

10. Johansson SGO, Bieber T, Dahl R, et al. Revised nomenclature for allergy for global use: report of the Nomenclature Review Committee of the World Allergy Organization, October 2003. *J Allergy Clin Immunol.* 2004;113:832–836.

11. Simons FER, Frew AJ, Ansotegui JJ, et al. Risk assessment in anaphylaxis: current and future approaches. *J Allergy Clin Immunol.* 2007;120:S2–S24.

12. Greenberger PA, Rotskoff BD, Lifschultz B. Fatal anaphylaxis: postmortem findings and associated comorbid diseases. *Ann Allergy Asthma Immunol.* 2007;98:252–257.

13. Pumphrey RSH, Gowland MH. Further fatal allergic reactions to food in the United Kingdom, 1999–2006. *J Allergy Clin Immunol.* 2007;119:1018–1019.

14. Lieberman P. Anaphylaxis. *Med Clin North Am.* 2006; 90:77–95.

15. Golden DBK, Breisch NL, Hamilton RG, et al. Clinical and entomological factors influence the outcome of sting challenge studies. *J Allergy Clin Immunol.* 2006;121:S402–407.

16. Yocum MW, Butterfield JH, Klein JS, et al. Epidemiology of anaphylaxis in Olmstead County: a population-based study. *J Allergy Clin Immunol.* 1999;104:452–456.

17. Weiler JM. Anaphylaxis in the general population: a frequent and occasionally fatal disorder that is underrecognized. *J Allergy Clin Immunol.* 1999;104:271–273.

18. Gupta R, Sheikh A, Strachan DP, et al. Time trends in allergic disorders in the UK. *Thorax* 2007;62:91–96.

19. Lieberman P, Camargo CA Jr, Bohlke K, et al. Epidemiology of anaphylaxis: findings of the American College of Allergy, Asthma and Immunology Epidemiology of Anaphylaxis Working Group. *Ann Allergy Asthma Immunol.* 2006;97:596–602.

20. Bock SA, Munoz-Furlong A, Sampson HA. Further fatalities caused by anaphylactic reactions to food 2001–2006. *J Allergy Clin Immunol.* 2007;119:1016–1018.

21. Ross MP, Ferguson M, Street D, et al. Analysis of food-allergic and anaphylactic events in the National Electronic Injury Surveillance System. *J Allergy Clin Immunol.* 2008;121(1):166–171.

22. Boston Collaborative Drug Surveillance Program. Drug-induced anaphylaxis. *JAMA* 1973;224:613–615.

23. International Collaborative study of severe anaphylaxis. An epidemiologic study of severe anaphylactic and anaphylactoid reactions among hospital patients: methods and overall risks. *Epidemiology.* 1998;9:141–146.

24. Lieberman P. Anaphylactoid reactions to radiocontrast material. *Immunol Allergy Clin North Am.* 1992;12:649–658.

25. Morcoc SK, Thomsen HS, Webb JA. Prevention of generalized reactions to contrast media: a consensus report and guidelines. *Eur Radiol.* 2001;11:1720–1728.

26. Valentine MD. Anaphylaxis and stinging insect hypersensitivity. *JAMA.* 1992;268:2830–2833.

27. Lockey RF, Benedict IM, Turkeltauk PC, et al. Fatalities from immunotherapy (IT) and skin testing (ST). *J Allergy Clin Immunol.* 1987;79:660–677.

28. Reid MJ, Lockey RF, Turkeltaub PC, et al. Survey of fatalities from skin testing and immunotherapy 1985–1989. *J Allergy Clin Immunol.* 1993;92:6–15.

29. Bernstein DI, Wanner M, Borish L, et al. Twelve-year survey of fatal reactions to allergen injections and skin testing: 1990–2001. *J Allergy Clin Immunol.* 2004;113(6):1129–1136.

30. Patterson R, Hogan MB, Yarnold PR, et al. Idiopathic anaphylaxis: an attempt to estimate the incidence in the United States. *Arch Intern Med.* 1995;155:869–871.

31. Greenberger PA. Idiopathic anaphylaxis. *Immunol Allergy Clin N Am.* 2007;27:273–293.

32. Lieberman P, Patterson R, Metz R, et al. Allergic reactions to insulin. *JAMA.* 1971;215:1106–1112.

33. Slater J. Latex allergies. *Ann Allergy.* 1993;70:1–2.

34. Horan RF, Sheffer AL. Exercise-induced anaphylaxis. *Immunol Allergy Clin North Am.* 1992;12:559–570.

35. Orfan NA, Stoffoff RS, Harris KE, et al. Idiopathic anaphylaxis: total experience with 225 patients. *Allergy Proc.* 1992;13:35–43.

36. Weiss ME, Adkinson NF. Immediate hypersensitivity reactions to penicillin and related antibiotics. *Clin Allergy.* 1988;18:515–540.

37. Hunt KJ, Valentine MD, Sobotka AK, et al. A controlled trial of immunotherapy in insect hypersensitivity. *N Engl J Med.* 1978;299:157–161.

38. Wade JP, Liang MH, Sheffer AL. Exercise-induced anaphylaxis: epidemiological observations. *Prog Clin Biol Res.* 1989;297:175–182.

39. Ditto A, Harris K, Krasnick J, et al. Idiopathic anaphylaxis: a series of 335 cases. *Ann Allergy Asthma Immunol.* 1996;77:285–291.

40. Sampson HA, Munoz-Furlong A, Bock SA, et al. Symposium on the definition and management of anaphylaxis. *J Allergy Clin Immunol.* 2005;115(3):584–591.

41. Golden DB. Patterns of anaphylaxis: acute and late phase features of allergic reactions. *Novartis Foundation Symposium.* 2004; 257: 101

42. Barnard JH. Studies of 400 hymenoptera sting deaths in the United States. *J Allergy Clin Immunol.* 1973;52:525–530.

43. Levine HD. Acute myocardial infarction following wasp sting: report of two cases and critical survey of the literature. *American Heart J.* 1976;91:365–374.

44. Douglas DM, Sukenick E, Andrade WP, et al. Biphasic systemic anaphylaxis: an inpatient and outpatient study. *J Allergy Clin Immunol.* 1994;93:977–985.

45. Tole JW, Lieberman P. Biphasic anaphylaxis: review of incidence, clinical predictors, and observation recommendations. *Immunol Allergy Clin N Am.* 2007;27:309–326.

46. Kemp SF, Lockey RF. Anaphylaxis: a review of causes and mechanisms. *J Allergy Clin Immunol.* 2002;110(3):341–348.

47. van der Linden PW, Struyvenberg A, Kraaijenhagen RJ, et al. Anaphylactic shock after insect-sting challenge in 138 persons with a previous insect-sting reaction. *Ann Intern Med.* 1993;118:161–168.

48. Hunt EL. Death from allergic shock. *N Engl J Med.* 1993;228:502–504.

49. DeSousa RL, Short T, Warmin GR, et al. Anaphylaxis with associated fibrinolysis reversed with tranexamic acid and demonstrated by thromboelastography. *Anaesth Intensive Care.* 2004; 32: 580–587.

50. Schwartz LB. Diagnostic value of tryptase in anaphylaxis and mastocytosis. *Immunol Allergy Clin North Am.* 2006;26:451–463.

51. Vadas P, Gold M, Perelman B, et al. Platelet-activating factor, PAF-acetylhydrolase and severe anaphylaxis. *N Engl J Med.* 2008; 358:28–35.

52. Yoshiko O, Grant JA. Mediators of anaphylaxis. *Immunol Allergy Clin N Am.* 2007;27:249–260.

53. Simons EFR. Advances in H1-antihistamines. *N Engl J Med.* 2004;351:2203–2217.

54. Prussin C, Metcalfe DD. IgE, mast cells, basophils, and eosinophils. *J Allergy Clin Immunol.* 2006;117:S450–S456.

55. Jensen BM, Metcalfe DD, Gilfillan AM. Targeting kit activation: a potential therapeutic approach in the treatment of allergic inflammation. *Inflamm Allergy Drug Targets.* 2007;6:57–62.

56. Yokoi H, Meyers A, Matsumoto K, et al. Alteration and acquisition of Siglecs during in vitro maturation of CD34+ progenitors into human mast cells. *Allergy.* 2006;61: 769–776.

57. Chrusch C, Sharma S, Unruh H, et al. Histamine H3 receptor blockade improves cardiac function in canine anaphylaxis. *Am J Respir Crit Care Med.* 1999;160:142–149.

58. Kovanen PT, Kaartinen M, Paavonen T. Infiltrates of activated mast cells at the site of coronary atheromatous erosion or rupture in myocardial infarction. *Circulation.* 1995;92:1084–1088.

59. Sugimoto Y, Iba Y, Nakamura Y, et al. Pruritos-associated response mediated by cutaneous histamine H3 receptors. *Clin Exp Allergy.* 2004;34:456–459.

60. Stack MS, Johnson DA. Human mast cell tryptase activates single-chain urinary-type plasminogen activator (pro-urokinase). *J Biol Chem.* 1994;269:9416–9419.

61. Castells M. Mast cell mediators in allergic inflammation and mastocytosis. *Immunol Allergy Clin North Am.* 2006;26:465–485.

62. Cauwels A, Janssen B, Buys E, et al. Anaphylactic shock depends on PI3K and eNOS-derived NO. *J Clin Invest.* 2006; 116(8):2244–2251.

63. Prussin C, Metcalfe DD. IgE, mast cells, basophils, and eosinophils. *J Allergy Clin Immunol.* 2006;117:S450–456.

64. Rolla G, Nebiol F, Guida G, et al. Level of exhaled nitric oxide during human anaphylaxis. *Ann of Allergy, Asthma Immunol.* 2006; 97:264–265.

65. Sampson HA, Munoz-Furlong A, Campbell RL, et al. Second symposium on the definition and management of anaphylaxis: summary report-second national institute of allergy and infectious disease/food allergy and anaphlaxis network symposium. *J Allergy Clin Immunol.* 2006;117:391–397.

66. Brown SGA, Blackman KE, Stenleke V, et al. Insect sting anaphylaxis: prospective evaluation of treatment with intravenous adrenaline and volume resuscitation. *Emerg Med.* 2004;21:149–154.

67. Lieberman P. Distinguishing anaphylaxis from other serious disorders. *J Respir Dis.* 1995;16:411–420.

68. McGrath KG, Greenberger PA, Zeiss CR. Factitious allergic disease: multiple factitious illness and familial Munchausen's stridor. *Immunol Allergy Pract.* 1984;6:41–47.

69. Becker A, Mactavrish G, Frith E, et al. Postmortem tryptase and immunoglobulin E [Abstract]. *J Allergy Clin Immunol.* 1995;95:369.

70. van der Linden PW, Hack CE, Kerckhaert J, et al. Preliminary report: complement activation in wasp-sting anaphylaxis. *Lancet.* 1990;336:904–906.

71. Muller UR, Haeberli G. Use of beta-blockers during immunotherapy for Hymenoptera venom allergy. *J Allergy Clin Immunol.* 2005;115:606–610.

72. Toogood JH. Risk of anaphylaxis in patients receiving beta-blocker drugs. *J Allergy Clin Immunol.* 1988;81:1–5.

73. Horan RF, Sheffer AL. Exercise-induced anaphylaxis. *Immunol Allergy Clin North Am.* 1992;12:559–570.

74. Kemp SF, Lieberman P. Inhibitors of angiotensin II: potential hazards for patients at risk for anaphylaxis? *Ann Allergy Immunol.* 1997;78:527–529.

75. Bousquet J, Hejjaeni A, Dhivert H, et al. Immunotherapy with a standardized *Dermatophagoides pteronyssinus* extract IV. Systemic reactions according to the immunotherapy schedule. *J Allergy Clin Immunol.* 1990;85:473–479.

76. Shortened version of a World Health Organization/International Union of Immunological Societies Working Group Report. Current status of allergen immunotherapy. *Lancet.* 1989;1:259.

77. Apter AJ, Kinman JL, Bilker WB, et al. Is there cross-reactivity between penicillins and cephalosporins? *Am J Med.* 2006;119:354.

78. Idsoe O, Guthe T, Willcox RR, et al. Nature and extent of penicillin side-reactions, with particular reference to fatalities from anaphylactic shock. *Bull WHO.* 1968;38:159–188.

79. Sogn DD, Evans R, Sheppard GM, et al. Results of the National Institute of Allergy and Infectious Diseases collaborative clinical trial to test the predictive value of skin testing with major and minor penicillin derivatives in hospitalized adults. *Arch Intern Med.* 1992;152:1025–1032.

80. Bernstien IL, Gruchalla RS, Lee RE, et al. Disease management of drug hypersensitivity: a practice parameter. *Ann Allergy Asthma Immunol.* 1999;83:665–700.

81. Saxon A, Hassner A, Swabb EA, et al. Lack of cross-reactivity with penicillin in humans. *J Allergy Clin Immunol.* 1988;82:213–217.

82. Stevenson DD. Aspirin and NSAID sensitivity. *Immunol Allergy Clin N Am.* 2004;24:491–505.

83. Choi J, Hartnett P, Fulcher DA. Carboplatin desensitization. *Ann Allergy Asthma Immunol.* 2004;93:137–141.

84. Golden DBK. Epidemiology of allergy to insect venoms and stings. *Allergy Proc.* 1989;10:103–107.

85. Stafford CT. Hypersensitivity to fire ant venom. *Ann Allergy Asthma Immunol.* 1996;77:87–95.

86. Kemp SF, deShazo RD, Moffit JE, et al. Expanding habitat of the imported fire ant (*Solenopsis invecta*): a public health concern. *J Allergy Clin Immunol.* 2000;105:683–691.

87. Duplantier JE, Freeman TM, Bahna SL, et al. Successful rush immunotherapy for anaphylaxis to imported fire ants. *J Allergy Clin Immunol.* 1998;101:855–856.

88. Wang J, Sampson HA. Food anaphylaxis. *Clin Exp Allergy.* 2007;37(5):651–660.

89. Burks, W, Bannon GA, Sicherer S, et al. Peanut-induced anaphylactic reactions. *Int Arch Allergy Immunol.* 1999;119:165–172.

90. Smit de V, Cameron PA, Rainer TH. Anaphylaxis presentations to an emergency department in Hong Kong: incidence and predictors of biphasic reactions. *J Emerg Med.* 2005;28:381–388.

91. Lee JM, Greenes DS. Biphasic anaphylactic reactions in pediatrics. *Pediatrics.* 2000;106:762–766.

92. Pumphrey R. Anaphylaxis: can we tell who is at risk of a fatal reaction? *Curr Opin Allergy Clin Immunol.* 2004;4:285–290.

93. Joint Task Force on Practice Parameters, American Academy of Allergy Asthma and Immunology, Joint Council of Allergy Asthma and Immunology. The diagnosis and management of anaphylaxis: an updated practice parameter. *J Allergy Immunol.* 2005;115(suppl):S483–S523.

94. Sampson HA. Update on food allergy. *J Allergy Clin Immunol.* 2004;113:805–819.

95. Sampson HA, Mendelson L, Rosen JP. Fatal and near-fatal anaphylactic reactions to food in children and adolescents. *N Eng J Med.* 1992;327:380–384.

96. Stricker WE, Anorve-Lopez E, Reed CE. Food skin testing in patients with idiopathic anaphylaxis. *J Allergy Clin Immunol.* 1986;77:516–519.

97. Sicherer SH, Sampson HA. Food Allergy. *J Allergy Clin Immunol.* 2006;117:S470–S475.

98. Nicklas RA, Bernstein IL, Li JT, et al. The diagnosis and management of anaphylaxis. *J Allergy Clin Immunol.* 1998;101(suppl):S465–5497.

99. Allmers H, Schmengler J, John SM. Decreasing incidence of occupational contact urticaria caused by natural rubber latex in German health care workers. *J Allergy Clin Immunol.* 2004;114:347.

100. Sussman GL, Beezhold DH, Krup VP. Allergens and natural rubber proteins. *J Allergy Clin Immunol.* 2002;110:S33–S39.

101. Polen GE Jr, Slater JE. Latex allergy. *J Allergy Clin Immunol.* 2000;105:1054–1062.

102. Lieberman P. Anaphylactic reactions during surgical and medical procedures. *J Allergy Clin Immunol.* 2002;110(2 Suppl.): S64–S69.

103. Levy JH, Adkinson NK. Anaphylaxis during cardiac surgery: implications for clinicians. *Anesth Analg.* 2008;106:392–403.

104. Bani D, Nistri S, Mannaioni PF, et al. Cardiac anaphylaxis: pathophysiology and therapeutic perspectives. *Curr Allergy Asthma Rep.* 2006;6:14–19.

105. Mertes PM, Laxenaire MC. Adverse reactions to neuromuscular blocking agents. *Curr Allergy Asthma Rep.* 2004;4:7–16.

106. Peng CH, Tan PH, Lin HY, et al. Fatal anaphylactoid shock associated with protamine for heparin reversal during anesthesia. *Acta Anaesthesiol Sin.* 2000;38:97–102.

107. Koppert W, Blunk JA, Petersen LJ, et al. Different patterns of mast cell activation by muscle relaxants in human skin. *Anesthesiology.* 2001;95:659–667.

108. Laxenaire MC, Charpentier C, Feldman L. Anaphylactoid reactions to colloid plasma substitutes incidence risk factors, mechanisms: a French multicenter prospective study. *Ann Fr Anesh Reanim.* 1994;13:301–310.

109. Martinez-Sanz R, Marsal L, De La Llana R, et al. Anaphylactic reaction associated with anti-IgA antibodies. Description of one case successfully treated by means of extracorporeal circulation. *J Cardiovasc Surg.* 1990;31:247–248.

110. Fisher MM, Baldo BA. Mast cell tryptase in anaesthetic anaphylactoid reactions. *Br J Anaesth.* 1998;80:26–29.

111. Ebo DG, Fisher MM, Hagendorens MM, et al. Anaphylaxis during anaesthesia: diagnostic approach. *Allergy.* 2007;62:471–487.

112. Kroigaard M, Garvey LH, Gillberg L, et al. Scandinavian clinical practice guidelines on the diagnosis, management and follow-up of anaphylaxis during anaesthesia. *Acta Anaesthesiol Scand.* 2007;51:655–670.

113. Johansson SGO, Nopp A, Florvaag E, et al. High prevalence of IgE antibodies among blood donors in Sweden and Norway. *Allergy.* 2005;60:1312–1315.

114. Burman D, Hodson AK, Wood CBS, et al. Acute anaphylaxis, pulmonary edema and intravascular hemolysis due to cryoprecipitate. *Arch Dis Child.* 1973;48:483–485.

115. Helmer RE, Alperin JR, Yunginger JW, et al. Anaphylactic reactions following infusion of factor VIII in a patient with classic hemophilia. *Am J Med.* 1980;69:953–957.

116. Ring J, Seifert J, Lob G, et al. Allergic reactions to horse globulin therapy and their prevention by induction of immunologic tolerance. *Allergol Immunopathol.* 1974;2:93–121.

117. Bernstein JA, Sugumaran R, Bernstein DI, et al. Prevalence of human seminal plasma hypersensitivity among symptomatic women. *Ann Allergy Asthma Immunol.* 1997;78:54–58.

118. Iwahashi K, Miyasaki T, Kuji N, et al. Successful pregnancy in a woman with human seminal plasma allergy. A case report. *J Reprod Med.* 1999;44:391–393.

119. Limb SL, Starke PR, Lee CE, et al. Delayed onset and protracted progression of anaphylaxis after omalizumab administration in patients with asthma. *J Allergy Clin Immunol.* 2007;120(6):1378–1381.

120. Shadick MA, Liang MH, Partridge B, et al. The natural history of exercise-induced anaphylaxis: survey results from a 10 year follow-up study. *J Allergy Clin Allergy.* 1999;104:123–127.

121. Harada S, Horikawa T, Ashida M, et al. Aspirin enhances the induction of type 1 allergic symptoms when combined with food and exercise in patients with food–dependent exercise-induced anaphylaxis. *Br J Dermatol*. 2001;145:336–339.

122. Aihara M, Miyazawa M, Osuna H, et al. Food-dependent exercise-induced anaphylaxis: influence of concurrent aspirin administration on skin testing and provocation. *Br J Dermatol*. 2002;146:466–472.

123. Patterson R, Booth BH, Clayton DE, et al. Fatal and near fatal idiopathic anaphylaxis. *Allergy Proc*. 1995;16:103–108.

124. Krasnick J, Patterson R, Meyers GL. A fatality from idiopathic anaphylaxis. *Ann Allergy Asthma Immunol*. 1996;76:376–378.

125. Wong S, Yarnold PR, Yango C, et al. Outcome of prophylactic therapy for idiopathic anaphylaxis. *Ann Intern Med*. 1991;114(2):133–136.

126. Wong S, Patterson R, Harris, et al. Efficacy of ketotifen in corticosteroid-dependent idiopathic anaphylaxis. *Ann Allergy*. 1991;67:359–364.

127. Choy AC, Patterson R, Patterson DR, et al. Undifferentiated somatoform idiopathic anaphylaxis: non-organic symptoms mimicking idiopathic anaphylaxis. *J Allergy Clin Immunol*. 1995;96:893–900.

128. Ditto AM, Krasnick J, Greenberger PA, et al. Pediatric idiopathic anaphylaxis: experience with 22 patients. *J Allergy Clin Immunol*. 1997;100:320–326.

129. Krasnick J, Patterson R, Harris KE. Idiopathic anaphylaxis: long-term follow-up, cost, and outlook. *Allergy*. 1996;51:724–731.

130. Patterson R, Harris KE. Ideopathic anaphylaxis. In: Grammer LC, Greenberger PA, eds. *Patterson's Allergic Diseases*. 6th ed. Philadelphia: Lippincott Williams & Wilkins. 2002:437–443.

131. Bonner JR. Anaphylaxis. Part I. Etiology and pathogenesis. *Alabama J Med Sci*. 1988;25:283–287.

132. Gavalas M, Sadana A, Metcalf S. Guidelines for the management of anaphylaxis in the emergency department. *J Accid Emerg Med*. 1998;15:96–98.

133. Sampson HA, Mendelson LM, Rosen JP. Fatal and near-fatal anaphylactic reactions to food in children and adolescents. *N Engl J Med*. 1992;327:380–384.

134. Lieberman P. Biphasic anaphylactic reactions. *Ann Allergy Asthma Immunol*. 2005;95:217–226.

135. Sicherer SH, Simons FER. Quandaries in prescribing an emergency action plan and self-injectable epinephrine for first-aid management of anaphylaxis in the community. *J Allergy Clin Immunol*. 2005;115:575–583.

136. Hu W, Kemp AS, Kerridge I. Making clinical decisions when the stakes are high and the evidence unclear. *BMJ*. 2004;329:852–854.

CHAPTER 15

Allergy to Stinging Insects

ROBERT E. REISMAN

Allergic reactions to insect stings constitute a major medical problem, resulting in about 50 recognized fatalities annually in the United States (1), and are likely responsible for other unexplained sudden deaths. People at risk often are very anxious about future stings and modify their daily living patterns and lifestyles. Clinical observations correlated with the application of immunologic measurements have led to understanding of the natural history of insect sting allergy and the appropriate diagnosis and treatment for people at risk for insect sting anaphylaxis. For many affected people this is a self-limited disease; for others, treatment results in a "permanent cure."

■ THE INSECTS

The stinging insects are members of the order Hymenoptera of the class Insecta. They may be broadly divided into two families: the vespids, which include the yellow jacket, hornet, and wasp; and the apids, which include the honeybee and the bumblebee. People may be allergic to one or all of the stinging insects. The identification of the culprit insect responsible for the reactions is thus important in terms of specific advice and specific venom immunotherapy (VIT) discussed later.

The honeybee and bumblebee are quite docile and tend to sting only when provoked. The bumblebee is a rare offender although it has become an occupational hazard in greenhouse workers in Europe (2). Because of the common use of the honeybee for the production of honey and in plant fertilization, exposure to this insect is quite common. Multiple stings from honeybees may occur, particularly if their hive, which may contain thousands of insects, is in danger. The honeybee usually loses its stinging mechanism in the sting process, thereby inflicting self-evisceration and death.

The problem of many simultaneous insect stings has been intensified by the introduction of the Africanized honeybee, the so-called killer bee, into the southwestern United States (3). These bees are much more aggressive than the domesticated European honeybees which are found throughout the United States. Massive sting incidents have occurred, resulting in death from venom toxicity. The Africanized honeybees entered south Texas in 1990 and are now present in Arizona and California. It is anticipated that these bees will continue to spread throughout the southern United States. They are unable to survive in colder climates but may make periodic forays into the northern United States during the summer months.

The yellow jacket is the most common cause of allergic insect sting reactions. These insects nest in the ground and are easily disturbed in the course of activities, such as lawn mowing and gardening. They are also attracted to food and commonly found around garbage and picnic areas. They are present in increasing numbers in late summer and fall months of the year. Hornets, which are closely related to the yellow jacket, nest in shrubs and are also easily provoked by activities such as hedge clipping. Wasps usually build honeycomb nests under eaves and rafters and are relatively few in number in such nests. However, in some parts of the country, such as Texas, they are the most common cause for insect stings.

In contrast to stinging insects, biting insects such as mosquitos rarely cause serious allergic reactions. These insects deposit salivary gland secretions, which have no relationship to the venom deposited by stinging insects. Anaphylaxis has occurred from bites of the deer fly, kissing bug, black fly, and bed bug. Isolated reports also suggest that, on a rare occasion, mosquito bites have caused anaphylaxis. It is much more common, however, for insect bites to cause large local reactions, which may have an immune pathogenesis (4).

■ REACTIONS TO INSECT STINGS

Normal Reaction

The usual reaction after an insect sting is mild erythema and swelling at the sting site. This reaction is transient and disappears within several hours. Little treatment is needed other than analgesics and cold compresses.

Insect stings, in contrast to insect bites, always cause pain at the sting site.

Large Local Reactions

Extensive swelling and erythema, extending from the sting site over a large area, is a fairly common reaction. The swelling usually reaches a maximum in 24 to 48 hours and may last as long as 10 days. On occasion, fatigue, nausea, and malaise may accompany the large local reaction. Aspirin and antihistamines are usually adequate treatment. When severe or disabling, administration of steroids, such as prednisone, 40 mg daily for 2 to 3 days, may be very helpful. These large local reactions have been confused with infection and cellulitis. Insect sting sites are rarely infected and antibiotic therapy rarely indicated.

Most people who have had large local reactions from insect stings will have similar large local reactions from subsequent re-stings (5). The risk for generalized anaphylaxis is very low, less than 5%. Thus, people who have had large local reactions are usually not considered candidates for VIT (discussed later) and do not require venom skin tests. Recently, Kelly et al. have successfully used VIT to decrease local reactions in people frequently exposed (6). This decision to use immunotherapy for treatment of people with large local reactions should be dependent on the frequency and severity of the reaction and the therapeutic response to steroids administered shortly after the sting.

Anaphylaxis

The most serious reaction that follows an insect sting is anaphylaxis. Retrospective population studies suggest that the incidence of this acute allergic reaction from an insect sting ranges between 0.4% and 3.0% (7–9). Allergic reactions can occur at any age; most have occurred in individuals younger than 20 years of age, and with a male-to-female ratio of 2:1. These factors may reflect exposure rather than any specific age or sex predilection. Several clinical studies suggest that about one-third of individuals suffering systemic reactions have a personal history of atopic disease. Stings around the head and neck most commonly cause allergic reactions, but reactions may occur from stings occurring on any area of the body (10–14).

In most patients, anaphylactic symptoms occur within 15 minutes after the sting, although there have been rare reports of reactions developing later. Clinical observations suggest that the sooner the symptoms occur, the more severe the reactions may be. The clinical symptoms vary from patient to patient and are typical of anaphylaxis from any cause. The most common symptoms involve the skin and include generalized urticaria, flushing, and angioedema. More serious symptoms are respiratory and cardiovascular. Upper airway edema involving the pharynx, epiglottis, and trachea has been responsible for numerous fatalities. Circulatory collapse with shock and hypotension also has been responsible for mortality. Other symptoms include bowel spasm and diarrhea and uterine contractions (12,15).

Severe anaphylaxis, including loss of consciousness, occurs in all age groups. In one large study (16), the incidence of severe anaphylaxis was similar throughout all ages. Most deaths from sting anaphylaxis occur in adults. The reason for this increased mortality rate in adults might be the presence of cardiovascular disease or other pathologic changes associated with age. Adults may have less tolerance for the profound biochemical and physiologic changes that accompany anaphylaxis (17–19).

There are no clinical, absolute criteria that will identify people at risk for acquiring venom allergy. Most people who have venom anaphylaxis have tolerated stings without any reaction before the first episode of anaphylaxis. Even individuals who have died from insect sting anaphylaxis usually had no history of prior allergic reactions (1). The occurrence of venom anaphylaxis after first known insect sting exposure is another confusing observation, raising the issue of the etiology of prior sensitization of the pathogenesis of this initial reaction. People who have had large local reactions usually have positive venom skin tests and often very high titers of serum venom-specific immunoglobulin E (IgE); thus, these tests do not discriminate the few potential anaphylactic reactors. Anecdotal observations suggest that the use of β-blocking medication, which certainly potentiates the seriousness of any anaphylactic reaction, may also be a risk factor for subsequent occurrence of anaphylaxis in people who have had large local reactions.

Many simultaneous stings (greater than 100) may sensitize a person, who then might be at risk for anaphylaxis from a subsequent single sting. Exposure to this large amount of venom protein can induce IgE production. This potential problem is now recognized more often because of the many stings inflicted by the so-called killer bees. After experiencing a large number of stings with or without a toxic clinical reaction, people should be tested to determine the possibility of potential venom allergy. After an uneventful insect sting, some people may develop a positive skin test, which is usually transient in occurrence. Currently, skin testing of people who do not have an allergic reaction from a single sting is not recommended.

The natural history of insect sting anaphylaxis has now been well studied and is most intriguing. People who have had insect sting anaphylaxis have an approximate 60% recurrence rate of anaphylaxis after subsequent stings (20). Viewed from a different perspective, not all people presumed to be at risk react to re-stings. The incidence of these re-sting reactions is influenced by age and severity of the symptoms of the initial reaction. In general, children are less likely to have re-sting reactions as compared to adults. The more severe the anaphylactic symptoms the more likely it is to reoccur. For example, children who have had dermal symptoms (hives, angioedema) as the only manifestation of anaphylaxis have a remarkably low re-sting reaction rate (20,21). On the other hand individuals of any age who have had severe anaphylaxis have an approximate 70% likelihood of repeat reactions (16,20). When anaphylaxis does reoccur, the severity of the reaction tends to be similar to the initial reaction. No relationship has been found between the occurrence and degree of anaphylaxis and the intensity of venom skin test reactions. Thus, factors other than IgE antibodies modulate clinical anaphylaxis.

Unusual Reactions

Serum sickness type reactions, characterized by urticaria, joint pain, malaise, and fever, have occurred approximately 7 days after an insect sting. On occasion these reactions have also been associated with an immediate anaphylactic reaction. People who have this serum sickness type reaction are subsequently at risk for acute anaphylaxis after repeat stings and thus are considered candidates for VIT (22).

There have been isolated reports of other reactions such as vasculitis, nephritis, neuritis, and encephalitis occurring in a temporal relationship to an insect sting. The basic etiology for these reactions has not been established (23).

Toxic Reactions

Toxic reactions may occur as a result of many simultaneous stings. Insect venom contains a number of potent pharmacologic agents, and as a result of the properties of these substances, vascular collapse, shock, hypotension, and death may occur (24). The differentiation between allergic and toxic reactions sometimes can be difficult. As noted, after toxic reactions, individuals may develop IgE antibody and then be at risk for subsequent allergic sting reactions following a single sting.

■ IMMUNITY

Studies of immunity to insect venoms were initially carried out with beekeepers, who are stung frequently and generally have minor or no local reactions (25). Beekeepers have high levels of serum venom-specific IgG, correlating to some extent with the amount of venom exposure (stings). These IgG antibodies are capable of blocking in vitro venom-induced histamine release from basophils of allergic individuals. In addition, administration of hyperimmune gammaglobulin obtained from beekeepers provided temporary immunity from venom anaphylaxis in sensitive individuals (26). Successful VIT is accompanied by the production of high titers of venom-specific IgG. These observations suggest that IgG antibodies reacting with venom have a protective function, although there are other factors which appear to influence the lack of an allergic reaction in people who have detectable venom-specific IgE.

■ DIAGNOSTIC TESTS

Individual honeybee (Apis mellifera), yellow jacket (Vespula species), yellow hornet (Vespula arenaria), bald-face hornet (Vespula maculata), and wasp (Polistes species) extracts are available for the diagnosis and therapy of stinging insect allergy. Honeybee venom is obtained by electric stimulation. The vespid venoms (yellow jacket, hornet, and wasp) are obtained by dissecting and crushing the individual venom sacs. People with relevant stinging insect histories should undergo skin tests with the appropriate dilutions of each of the available five single Hymenoptera venom preparations. Venom dilutions must be made with a special diluent that contains human serum albumin. Testing is usually initiated with venom concentrations of 0.01 µg/mL to 0.0001 µg/mL. The initial studies of venom skin tests concluded that an immunologically specific reaction suggesting that the patient is sensitive is a reaction of 1+ or greater at a concentration of 1 µg/mL or less, provided the 1+ reaction is greater than that of a diluent control (27). Venom concentrations higher than 1 µg/mL cause nonspecific or irritative reactions and do not distinguish the insect-nonallergic from the insect-allergic population.

In vitro tests have been used for the diagnosis of stinging insect allergy. IgE antibodies have been measured by the radioallergosorbent test (RAST) (28,29) in vitro enzymatic assay (CAP, Phadia), and by histamine release from leukocytes (30). In general, about 15% to 20% of people who had positive venom skin tests do not react in the RAST or CAP assay. This may be a reflection of the sensitivity of the test. Also, the RAST results are affected by other factors, including the type and concentration of venom used for coupling and the presence of serum venom-specific IgG that could interfere by competing for the radiolabeled antisera. The in vitro test remains an excellent procedure for quantifying antibody titers over time. Histamine release from leukocytes is basically a laboratory procedure too cumbersome for routine diagnostic evaluation.

People have been described who have a history of venom anaphylaxis, have negative venom skin tests and reacted to a subsequent intentional skin challenge (31). The majority of these people had detectable serum venom specific IgE (RAST) usually in the low titer and several had positive venom skin test reactions when tested at a later date. This observation has raised the issue of the accuracy of the venom skin test. It is important to emphasize that those individuals represent a very small percentage of people who have had allergic reactions to insect stings (32).

From a clinical viewpoint, people who have had severe anaphylaxis following an insect sting and have negative venom skin tests, should have a venom *in vitro* test. If negative, epinephrine availability is advisable. If both the skin test and *in vitro* results are negative, it seems reasonable to repeat the skin tests at periodic intervals, which really need to be defined. An initial repeat test at 3 months seems reasonable, but there is no good evidence to suggest which time interval would be appropriate in the absence of further venom exposure.

Baseline serum tryptase levels have been found to be elevated in some people who had insect sting anaphylaxis, particularly in people who have had more severe symptoms. This has led to a search for occult mastocytosis in these people. It is postulated that with an increased number of mast cells, venom may release mediators on either an immunologic or a nonimmunologic basis and lead to more severe symptoms. These people may require more intensive VIT, as discussed later (33).

■ THERAPY

People who have a history of systemic reactions after an insect sting and have detectable venom-specific IgE (positive skin tests or RAST) are considered at risk for subsequent reactions. Recommendations for therapy include measures to minimize exposure to insects, availability of emergency medication for medical treatment of anaphylaxis, and specific VIT.

Avoidance

The risk of insect stings may be minimized by the use of simple precautions. Individuals at risk should protect themselves with shoes and long pants or slacks when in grass or fields, and should wear gloves when gardening. Cosmetics, perfumes, and hair sprays, which attract insects, should be avoided. Black and dark colors also attract insects; individuals should choose white or light colored clothes. Food and odors attract insects; thus garbage should be well wrapped and covered and care should be taken with outdoor cooking and eating. Insect repellents are not effective against stinging insects (34).

Medical Therapy

Acute allergic reactions from the insect stings are treated in the same manner as anaphylaxis from any cause. See Chapter 14 for specific recommendations. Patients at risk are taught to self-administer epinephrine and are advised to keep epinephrine and antihistamine preparations available. Epinephrine is available in preloaded syringes (Twinject, Verus Pharmaceuticals, San Diego, CA; EpiPen, Dey LP, Napa, CA) and can be administered easily. Consideration should be given to having an identification bracelet describing their insect allergy.

At the present time, studies are being done with a fast-disintegrating tablet of sublingual epinephrine (35). Plasma concentrations of epinephrine 40 mg sublingually are similar to those obtained after intramuscular injection of 0.3 mg of epinephrine, which is the usual therapeutic dose. With further development, sublingual epinephrine tablets may replace intramuscular injections providing a more feasible alternative for the medical treatment of anaphylaxis.

Venom Immunotherapy

Venom immunotherapy (VIT) has been shown to be highly effective in preventing subsequent sting reactions (36,37). Successful therapy is associated with the production of venom-specific IgG, which appears to be the immunologic corollary to clinical immunity. Current recommendations are to administer VIT to individuals who have had sting anaphylaxis and have positive venom skin tests. As discussed previously, recent studies of the natural history of the disease process in untreated patients have led to observations that modify this recommendation. The presence of IgE antibody in an individual who has had a previous systemic reaction does not necessarily imply that a subsequent reaction will occur on re-exposure. Observations relevant to the decision to use VIT include age, interval since the sting reaction, the nature of the anaphylactic symptoms, and anticipated exposures. Immunotherapy guidelines are summarized in Tables 15.1 through 15.3.

Patient Selection

Children who have dermal reactions (generalized urticaria and/or angioedema that was not life-threatening) as the sole signs of anaphylaxis do not require VIT and can be treated with keeping symptomatic medication available (Table 15.1). This recommendation is based on the very low incidence of reactions to subsequent re-stings and the continued mild nature of most reactions, which are dermal only when they do occur. More severe re-sting reactions have occurred but are rare (20,21). A 20-year follow-up of these children (38) confirmed this benign prognosis. The incidence of repeat systemic reactions was 13% in those children who did not receive VIT and no reactions occurred in 21 people who had received immunotherapy. In contrast, a higher incidence of systemic reactions did occur in people who had more severe anaphylaxis during childhood. VIT in childhood in this group did lower the subsequent adult re-sting reaction rate.

Adults who have had mild symptoms of anaphylaxis such as dermal reactions only, probably could be managed with symptomatic medication only. However, because the documentation for the benign prognosis in adults has not been as well substantiated, this decision requires full patient discussion and concurrence.

TABLE 15.1   INDICATIONS FOR VENOM IMMUNOTHERAPY IN PATIENTS WITH POSITIVE VENOM SKIN TESTS[a]

INSECT STING REACTION	VENOM IMMUNOTHERAPY
"Normal"—transient pain, swelling	No
Extensive local swelling	No[b]
Anaphylaxis—severe	Yes
Anaphylaxis—moderate	Yes
Anaphylaxis—mild; dermal only	
Children	No
Adults	Yes[c]
Serum sickness	Yes
Toxic	Yes

[a]Venom immunotherapy is not indicated for individuals with negative venom skin tests.
[b]Recent studies suggest venom immunotherapy may be effective.
[c]Patients in this group might be managed without immunotherapy. See text.

The recommendation to have epinephrine available is not a benign one. There is often great concern, justifiably so, that epinephrine is always available, such as in school, the work environment, and recreational areas, and that personnel have been trained to administer the medication. An equally important aspect is the duration of this recommendation, especially in children. The question remains: how long is it necessary to prescribe epinephrine? The results of venom skin tests may resolve this question. If venom skin tests become negative, there should be no risk for anaphylaxis, and epinephrine availability should be unnecessary. It is reasonable to repeat skin tests every 2 to 3 years when epinephrine availability is recommended.

People of all ages who have had moderate to severe symptoms of anaphylaxis, such as respiratory distress, hypotension, or upper airway edema, regardless of the time interval since the sting reaction and have positive venom skin tests or detectable serum venom-specific IgE, should receive VIT. For people who have had severe anaphylaxis and have negative venom skin tests

and undetectable venom-specific IgE, it is prudent to recommend epinephrine availability. While the majority of such people probably are no longer allergic, there are reports of rare people who continue to have systemic reactions. People with histories of mild to moderate anaphylaxis who have negative skin tests and RASTs are most likely no longer allergic and will not need epinephrine. Furthermore, if a reaction did occur, it most likely would be similar to and not more severe than the initial reaction.

As mentioned previously, after uneventful stings, a small percentage of people have positive skin tests which are usually transient. VIT is not recommended.

Because of this discrepancy in the actual incidence of re-sting reactions as compared with the number of individuals who are considered at risk—history of sting anaphylaxis and positive venom skin test—a diagnostic sting challenge has been suggested as a criterion for initiating VIT. In several large studies (39,40,41) sting challenges elicit reactions in 25% to 60% of people potentially at risk. Unfortunately, there were no clinical

TABLE 15.2   GENERAL VENOM IMMUNOTHERAPY DOSING GUIDELINES

Initial dose	Dose of 0.01 µg to 0.1 µg, depending on degree of skin test reaction
Incremental doses	Schedules vary from "rush" therapy, administering multiple venom injections over several days, to traditional once-weekly injections
Maintenance dose	Dose of 50 µg to 100 of single venoms, 300 µg of mixed vespid venom
Maintenance interval	4 weeks, 1st year 6 weeks, 2nd year 8 weeks, 3rd year May be extended after 3rd year
Duration of therapy	Stop if (1) skin test becomes negative, (2) finite time; 3 to 5 years (see text).

TABLE 15.3   REPRESENTATIVE EXAMPLES OF VENOM IMMUNOTHERAPY DOSING SCHEDULES[a]

	TRADITIONAL	MODIFIED RUSH	RUSH	
Day				
1	0.1	0.1	0.1[b]	3.0
		0.3	0.3	5.0
		0.6	0.6	10
			1.0	
			20.0	
2			35.0	
			50.0[c]	
			75.0	
3			100.0	
Week				
1	0.3	1.0		
		3.0		
2	1.0	5.0	100.0	
		10.0	Repeat every 4 wks	
3	3.0	20.0		
4	5.0	35.0		
5	10.0	50.0[c]		
6	20.0	65.0		
7	35.0	80.0		
8	50.0[c]	100.0		
9	65.0			
10	80.0	100.0		
11	100.0	Repeat every 4 wks		
12				
13	100.0			
	Repeat every 4 wks			

[a]Starting dose may vary depending on patient's skin test sensitivity. Subsequent doses modified by local or systemic reactions. Doses expressed in micrograms.

[b]Sequential venom doses administered on same day at 20- to 30-minute intervals.

[c]50 µg may be used as top dose.

or immunologic data from these challenge studies that reliably identified potential reactors or nonreactors.

Safety, reliability, and practicality are pertinent to the general application of sting challenges. Observations from both field stings and intentional sting challenges have shown that 20% of potentially allergic individuals who initially tolerate an insect re-sting will react to a subsequent re-sting (20,41). Thus, the predictive value of a single sting challenge result can be questioned. Safety is a serious concern because life threatening anaphylactic reactions have occurred with intentional diagnostic sting challenges. Testing must be carefully monitored and treatment available for severe anaphylaxis. The issue is further confused by observations suggesting differences in the incidence of sting challenge reactions induced by stings of two different yellow jacket species (42). In addition to these reliability and safety issues, sting challenges are impractical for routine application.

VIT is also very effective treatment for people with systemic mastocytosis and who have had anaphylaxis from Hymenoptera stings (43–45). These people have a higher risk of severe anaphylaxis, and VIT is, most importantly, well tolerated and confers protection. Several people were reported who received VIT although they had negative skin tests.

Venom Selection

The commercial venom product brochure recommends immunotherapy with each venom to which the patient is sensitive, as determined by the skin test reaction. Applying this criterion, one or multiple venoms may be administered. A mixed vespid venom preparation composed of equal parts of yellow jacket, yellow hornet, and bald-faced hornet venoms, is available.

The area of venom selection is also controversial. The issue is whether multiple positive skin tests indicate specific individual venom allergy or reflect cross-reactivity among venoms. Extensive studies have been carried out concerning the cross-reactivity among venoms. The honeybees (apids) and yellow jackets, hornets, and wasps (vespids) are in different families. Within the vespid family, there is extensive cross-reactivity between the hornet venoms (46), extensive cross-reaction between the yellow jacket and hornet venoms (47), and limited cross-reactivity between wasp venom and other vespid venoms (48). In this author's experience, most patients who have had yellow jacket sting reactions also have positive skin test reactions to hornet venom and occasionally to *Polistes* species venom. Thus it is very common to find multiple vespid skin test reactions in individuals who have reacted to one of the vespids. The product brochure recommends treatment with each of these vespid venoms. When the causative insect can be positively identified (particularly, the yellow jacket), single vespid venom may be given with excellent protection from subsequent restings (37).

The relationship between honeybee venom and yellow jacket venom is more complex (49). RAST-inhibition studies using sera from patients with co-existing elevated titers of honeybee venom and yellow jacket venom-specific IgE have shown different patterns of reactivity ranging from no cross-reaction to fairly extensive cross-reaction. For an individual patient, this procedure is too tedious and not available to define the pattern. Knowledge of these results, however, may help suggest that single venom therapy would be adequate.

Bumblebees are very docile and nonaggressive. Field stings are very uncommon. Bumblebees are used extensively in greenhouses for plant fertilization. Reports from the Netherlands summarized by deGroot (2) describe the clinical issues of bumblebee venom allergy, the relationships between bumblebee and honeybee venoms, and successful desensitization with locally collected bumblebee venom, not commercially available. Two categories of patients are suggested. There are nonprofessionally exposed people who were initially sensitized to honeybee venom and then react to bumblebee stings as a result of earlier exposure. These people are reacting to cross-reactive allergens in honeybee and bumblebee venoms and can be successfully treated with honeybee immunotherapy. Skin tests with honeybee venom should be positive (2,50). The second group are workers sensitized to bumblebee venom as a result of frequent stings. Their bumblebee venom-specific IgE reacts poorly with honeybee venom. Immunotherapy with bumblebee venom, not honeybee venom, can be protective. DeGroot recommends these people change jobs and avoid further exposure.

Dosing Schedule

The basic approach to VIT is similar to other forms of allergy immunotherapy (Tables 15.2 and 15.3). Therapy is initiated in small doses, usually from 0.01 to 0.1 µg and incremental doses are given until a recommended dose of 100 µg is reached. Several dosing schedules have been used. A common schedule is to administer two or three injections during early visits, with doses being doubled or tripled at 30 minute intervals. When higher doses are reached, a single dose is given each week. Other schedules call for more traditional dosing, with one injection per week throughout the build-up period. At the other end of the spectrum, rush desensitization has been given, with multiple doses administered to patients in a hospital setting over a period of 2 to 3 days to 1 week. The most important goal of VIT is to reach the recommended 100 µg dose of a single venom or 300 µg of mixed vespid venom. Maintenance doses are given every 4 weeks during the first year. Thereafter, the maintenance interval usually can be extended to 6 and even 8 weeks with no loss of clinical effectiveness or increase in immunotherapy reactions (51,52).

In this author's experience, 50 µg may be used as the top venom dose. Using this maximum dose and primarily single-venom therapy, results with immunotherapy have been excellent, with an approximate 98% success rate (37). The more rapid schedules appear to be accompanied by a more rapid increase in venom-specific IgG production, and thus this schedule might provide protection earlier (53). Reaction rates to venom administered by both rapid and slower schedules vary in different studies, but are not significantly different.

Reactions to Therapy

As with other allergenic extracts, reactions can occur from VIT. The usual reactions are fairly typical large local reactions lasting several days, and immediate systemic reactions. These reactions may present more of a problem, however. To ensure clinical protection, it is necessary to reach full maintenance doses of venom. With other allergenic extracts, such as pollen, doses are usually decreased and maintained at lower levels. Treatment of local reactions includes splitting of doses (limiting the amount of venom delivered at one site), cold compresses, and antihistamines.

In the large study of insect sting allergy conducted by the American Academy of Allergy, Asthma and Immunology, the incidence of venom-induced systemic reactions was about 10% (54). There were no identifiable factors predicting these reactions. After a systemic reaction, the next dose is reduced by about 25% to 50%, depending on the severity of the reaction, and subsequent doses are slowly increased. If patients are receiving multiple venom therapy, it might be useful to give individual venom on separate days. This may help identify the specific venom responsible for the reaction.

Severe anaphylaxis, often difficult to treat, has occurred in patients on β-adrenergic blocking drugs. Because of this risk of anaphylaxis, it has been recommended that patients receiving allergen immunotherapy not receive these drugs. The issue is more complex when VIT, which is remarkably effective, is needed to prevent potentially serious anaphylaxis. Müller and Haeberli reported observations of allergic patients with cardiovascular disease receiving VIT and β-blocker medications (55). Of 25 patients on β-blockers during immunotherapy, 3 (12%) developed allergic side effects; this compared with 23 (16.7%) of 117 patients with cardiovascular disease not receiving β-blockers. Systemic allergic symptoms following re-stings were observed in 1 of 7 (14.3%) patients receiving and 4 of 29 (13.8%) patients not receiving β-blockers. No severe reactions occurred in the patients on β-blockers, either from immunotherapy or re-stings. This author's clinical experience is similar. If β-blocker treatment is needed and cannot be substituted, VIT can be administered safely. This author suggests a slower initial venom build-up dosing schedule and at least a 30-minute observation period after each venom injection.

There are several case reports of serious anaphylaxis due to VIT occurring in patients taking angiotensin-converting enzyme (ACE) inhibitors (56). There are possible biochemical mechanisms for this occurrence. The authors of one report suggest that patients not take their ACE inhibitor within 24 hours of receiving their venom injection. At present, this author does not believe that available evidence strongly supports stopping or withholding ACE inhibitors.

Another adverse reaction occasionally noted after injections of other allergenic extracts but more frequently with venom, is the occurrence of generalized fatigue and aching often associated with large local swelling. Prevention of these reactions can usually be accomplished with aspirin 650 mg given about 30 minutes before the venom injection and repeated every 4 hours as needed. If this therapy is ineffective, steroids have been used, administered at the same time as venom injection.

Fortunately, most people who have had reactions to VIT are ultimately able to reach maintenance doses. On rare occasions, systemic reactions have necessitated cessation of treatment. There have been no identified adverse reactions from long-term VIT. Venom injections appear to be safe during pregnancy, with no adverse effect to either the mother or the fetus (57).

Monitoring Therapy

VIT is associated with immunologic responses, which include rising titers of serum venom-specific IgG and, over a period of time, decreasing titers of serum venom-specific IgE. One criterion for stopping VIT (discussed later) is the conversion to a negative venom skin test. For this reason, venom-treated patients should have repeat venom skin tests about every 2 to 3 years.

As discussed earlier, serum venom-specific IgG is associated with the development of immunity to insect stings. Initial evidence for the role of venom-specific IgG came from studies of beekeepers, who are a highly immune population, the antithesis of the allergic individual. More specific documentation of this protective role was provided by the results of passive administration of hyperimmune gammaglobulin, obtained from beekeepers, to honeybee allergic people and the subsequent inhibition of allergic reactions following a venom challenge. Studies of people receiving VIT have suggested that, at least in early months, this antibody might be responsible for the loss of clinical sensitivity.

Golden et al. (58) compared people who failed VIT treatment and continued to have sting-induced systemic reactions with successfully treated people and suggested that the difference was related to lower titers of serum venom-specific IgG. A group of patients with a serum IgG antibody level greater than 3 µg/mL had a 1.6% re-sting reaction rate, compared with a group of patients with serum levels less than 3 µg/mL that had a 16% reaction rate. These data applied only to yellow jacket venom-allergic people treated for less than 4 years. There was no correlation between honeybee-specific IgG- and re-sting reaction rates. The authors recommended periodic monitoring of serum venom-specific IgG to detect potential treatment failures, which then would dictate an increase in the VIT dose. Careful review of the individual data suggested, however, that there was not a close relationship between treatment failure and IgG response (59). There was a lack of reproducible reactions to sting challenges in people with low antibody titers. There was no documentation that increased antibody responses induced by higher venom doses were clinically effective. The data could not be applied to yellow jacket-allergic people treated for more than 4 years or to honeybee-allergic people. Thus, taken in total, review of this study and other relevant data, particularly the remarkable success rate of VIT, does not support the routine measurement of venom-specific IgG. From a practical viewpoint, there is little clinical reason to measure venom-specific IgG as part of the overall management and treatment of venom-allergic people.

Treatment Failure

VIT is remarkably effective, protecting about 98% of treated patients. Re-sting reactions while receiving maintenance VIT are rare. If a re-sting reaction does occur, it is initially important to determine if the treatment venom(s) is the same as the venom responsible for the reaction. In addition to historical details, further testing may be indicated. If the treatment venom(s) is correct, then the immunotherapy maintenance dose should be raised 50% to 100% (60).

Cessation of Venom Immunotherapy

The adequate duration of VIT (i.e., the timing of its cessation) is probably the most common concern and question raised by allergists. Germane to this question are two major observations. First, for many individuals, insect sting allergy is a self-limiting process. This is the only explanation for the 50-year-old belief that whole insect body extracts, now recognized as impotent, seemed to be effective treatment. Second is the clinical observation that not all individuals with positive venom skin tests and a history of venom-induced anaphylaxis will continue to have clinical reactions when re-stung. Thus, in analyzing the appropriate criteria for discontinuing therapy, this spontaneous loss of clinical allergy must be appreciated.

Two major criteria have been suggested as guidelines for discontinuing treatment:

1. Conversion to a negative skin test.
2. A finite period of VIT, usually 3 to 5 years, despite the persistence of a positive venom skin test.

The second criterion is influenced by a number of issues such as the nature of the initial anaphylactic symptoms, reactions during VIT, perhaps the specific insect causing the reaction, and the general physical health of the individual, particularly the presence of significant cardiovascular disease. These issues are reviewed in detail in a *Practice Parameter Update* from a joint task force representing the American Academy of Allergy, Asthma, and Immunology, the American College of Allergy, Asthma and Immunology, and the Joint Council of Allergy, Asthma and Immunology (61).

Conversion to a negative skin venom test should be an absolute criterion for stopping immunotherapy. This conclusion is supported by several studies and is obviously a rational decision. If the immunologic mediator of venom anaphylaxis, an IgE antibody, is no longer present, there should no longer be any risk for

anaphylaxis. In individuals who have had severe anaphylactic reactions, the lack of specific IgE can be confirmed with a serum antibody assay. As noted, there have been rare anecdotal reports of individuals who apparently had allergic reactions from insect stings despite a negative venom skin test. The conversion to a negative skin test while receiving VIT is a different clinical and immunologic issue.

Because a positive skin test does not necessarily imply continued clinical sensitivity, a number of studies have explored the efficacy of a finite period of treatment, usually 3 to 5 years in the presence of a persistently positive skin test. The skin test is a very sensitive test, as exemplified by people with a remote history of ragweed hayfever who continue to have a positive test indefinitely. In venom studies, the re-sting reaction rate after cessation of VIT in this setting is low, generally in the range of 5% to 10%. Four of the studies that reported re-sting reactions after cessation of VIT are summarized in Table 15.4. Lerch and Müller (62), Haugaard et al. (63), and Golden et al. (64) reported the results of intentional sting challenges in patients off immunotherapy, usually for 1 to 2 years. The re-sting reaction rates ranged from 0% to 12.5%. Our studies used field re-stings and found a 9% re-sting reaction rate; these data were further analyzed in relationship to the severity of the initial anaphylactic reaction (65). There were 25 patients who had initial mild anaphylaxis; no reactions occurred after re-stings. Forty-one patients had had initial moderate reactions; three had re-sting reactions. In the group of 47 patients who had severe anaphylaxis, as defined by loss of consciousness, respiratory distress, hypotension, or upper airway edema, there was a 15% re-sting reaction rate. Unfortunately, the severity of the allergic reaction, when it did occur, was often the same as the initial reaction preceding VIT. In our study (65) and that of Lerch and Müller (62), no re-sting reactions occurred in the presence of a negative venom skin test, confirmed by a negative RAST. For most individuals, the loss of clinical sensitivity is permanent, with no reactions to subsequent re-stings once therapy is stopped for the appropriate reasons.

In one study (66) in which we examined a decrease in venom-specific IgE levels to insignificant levels as a criterion for stopping treatment, the control group included patients who stopped by self-choice. It was interesting to see that the average time of therapy was about 2 years, both in patients who stopped because of a decreased RAST and in those patients who stopped by self-choice. The re-sting reaction rate was very close in both groups, about 10%. Thus, 2 years of treatment may significantly reduce the risk for reactions from about 60% in untreated individuals to only 10%.

Other factors have been suggested as related to increased risk for a re-sting reaction after stopping therapy and are outlined in Table 15.5. There is no association with gender or presence of atopy. As already noted, more severe initial reactions are associated with

TABLE 15.4   RE-STING REACTIONS AFTER STOPPING VENOM IMMUNOTHERAPY—SELECTED REPORTS

INVESTIGATORS (REF.)	NO. OF PATIENTS	RESULTS (VENOM IMMUNOTHERAPY DURATION)	REACTION
Lerch & Müller (62)	200	>3 years	25 (12.5%)
Haugaard et al. (63)	25	3 to 7 years	0
Golden et al. (64)	74	5 years	7 (10%)
Reisman (65)	113	2 to 5 years	10 (9%)

increased risk. Re-sting reaction risk may be higher in adults, in honeybee-allergic people, in people who have had systemic reactions to VIT, and in people whose degree of skin test reactivity is unchanged during immunotherapy.

This author's current three recommendations for stopping treatment are as follows:

1. Conversion to a negative venom skin test is an absolute criterion for stopping treatment. This may occur at any time whether treatment has been given for 1 or 5 years.

2. For people who have had mild to moderate anaphylactic symptoms and retain positive venom skin tests, 3 to 5 years of VIT is sufficient. This decision is influenced by consideration of other medical problems, concomitant medication, patient lifestyle, and patient preference.

3. For people who have severe anaphylaxis as exemplified by hypotension, loss of consciousness, or upper airway edema, therapy is administered indefinitely as long as the skin test remains positive. It is important to point out that maintenance VIT can be given every 8 weeks and even at longer intervals after 3 years of treatment.

■ FIRE ANT AND HARVESTER ANT STINGS

Systemic reactions to the stings of the fire ant have been reported with increasing frequency (67,68). This insect is present in growing numbers in the southeastern United States, particularly in states bordering the Gulf Coast, and has now spread into Virginia and California. The fire ant attaches itself to its victim by biting with its jaws and then pivots around its head, stinging in multiple sites in a circular pattern with a stinger located on the abdomen. Within 24 hours of the sting, a sterile pustule develops that is diagnostic of the fire ant sting. Allergic symptoms occurring after stings are typical of acute anaphylaxis. Fatalities have occurred in children and adults. Indoor massive sting attacks by fire ants have been reported (69).

Skin tests with extracts prepared from whole bodies of fire ants appear to be reliable in identifying allergic individuals, with few false-positive reactions in nonallergic controls. Fire ant venom, not commercially available at present, has been collected and compared with fire ant whole-body extract. The results of skin tests and *in vitro* tests show that the venom is a better diagnostic antigen. Whole-body extracts can be prepared, however, that apparently contain sufficient allergen and are reliable for

TABLE 15.5   POTENTIAL RISK FACTORS RELATED TO RISK OF RE-STING REACTION AFTER STOPPING THERAPY

PARAMETER	RE-STING RISK
Age	Increased in adults
Atopy	No association
Sex	No association
Insect species	Increased with honeybee
Initial anaphylaxis	Increased with more severe reaction
Venom immunotherapy tolerance	Increased with reactions to therapy
Skin test reactivity	Increased if unchanged during therapy

skin test diagnosis. These results suggest that the antigens responsible for allergic reactions can be preserved in the preparation of whole-body extracts. Unfortunately, the potency of different commercial fire ant whole-body extracts has been variable. Future availability of fire ant venom will provide a potent, reliable extract.

Fire ant venom has been well studied, and differs considerably from other Hymenoptera venoms. Studies have shown four allergenic fractions in the fire ant venom (70). Immunotherapy with whole-body fire ant extract appears to be quite effective. Because the whole-body fire ant extract can be a good diagnostic agent, this therapeutic response might be anticipated. It is important, however, that control observations studying the response of subsequent stings in allergic individuals not receiving VIT have been limited. There has been one study comparing the results of fire ant re-stings in whole-body extract treated patients and untreated patients (71). In the treated group, there were 47 re-stings, with one systemic reaction. In contrast, of the 11 untreated patients, 6 patients had 11 re-stings, all of which resulted in systemic reactions. Serologic studies defining the nature of the immunity to fire ant stings have not been conducted.

Dosing schedules for fire ant whole-body extract are not as well defined as those for Hymenoptera venoms. Initial doses are in the range of 0.1 mL 1 to 10,000 wt/vol with a weekly incremental dose reaching 0.5 mL 1 to 100 wt/vol (61,72). A successful rush immunotherapy protocol has not been published (73). The adequate duration of fire ant immunotherapy has not been established, but should be similar to the guidelines established for VIT.

In vitro studies suggest there is some cross-reaction between the major allergens in fire ant venom and the winged Hymenoptera venoms. The clinical significance of this observation is still unclear; there appears to be limited clinical application. Individuals allergic to bees and vespids do not appear to be at major risk for fire ant reactions, and similarly, fire ant allergic individuals are not at major risk for reactions from the winged Hymenoptera.

Anaphylaxis from the sting of the harvester ant, another nonwinged Hymenoptera present in the southwestern United States, has been described (74). Specific IgE antibodies have been detected with direct skin tests and leukocyte histamine release using harvester ant venom.

In summary, hypersensitivity reactions to ants, especially fire ants, have become clinically important. Fire ant venom has been analyzed and many of the antigens are cross-reactive among the species. Fire ant whole-body extract has also been characterized and is known to contain venom antigens. Fire ant allergy will likely become a more important clinical problem as the ants spread, as the human population grows in the southern United States, and as the land is cultivated to favor their habitation.

■ REFERENCES

1. Barnard JH. Studies of 400 Hymenoptera sting deaths in the United States. *J Allergy Clin Immunol.* 1973;52:259–264.
2. deGroot H. Allergy to bumblebees. *Curr Opin Allergy Clin Immunol.* 2006:6(4):299–297.
3. McKenna WR. Killer bees: what the allergist should know. *Ped Asthma Allergy Immunol.* 1992;4:275–285.
4. Simons FER, Peng Z. Mosquito allergy. In: Levine MI, Lockey RE, eds. *Monograph on Insect Allergy.* American Academy of Allergy Asthma and Immunology; 2003:175–203.
5. Mauriello PM, Barde SH, Georgitis JW, et al. Natural history of large local reactions (LLR) to stinging insects. *J Allergy Clin Immunol.* 1984;74:494–498.
6. Kelly D, Golden DBK, Hamilton RG, et al. Venom immunotherapy (VIT) reduces large local reactions (LLR) to insect stings. *J Allergy Clin Immunol.* 2007;119:579.
7. Golden DBK. Epidemiology of allergy to insect venoms and stings. *Allergy Proc.* 198;10:103–107.
8. Chaffee FH. The prevalence of bee sting allergy in an allergic population. *Acta Allergol.* 1979;25:292–293.
9. Settipane GA, Boyd GK. Prevalence of bee sting allergy in 4,992 Boy Scouts. *Acta Allergol.* 1970;25:286–287.
10. Brown H, Bernton HS. Allergy to the Hymenoptera. *Arch Intern Med.* 1970;125:665–660.
11. Frazier CA. Allergic reactions to insect stings: a review of 180 cases. *South Med J.* 1964:57:1028–1034.
12. Mueller HL. Further experiences with severe allergic reactions to insect stings. *N Engl J Med.* 1959;261:374–377.
13. Mueller HL, Schmid WH, Rubinsztain R. Stinging insect hypersensitivity. A 20 year study of immunologic treatment. *Pediatrics.* 1975;55:530–535.
14. Schwartz HJ, Kahn B. Hymenoptera sensitivity: II. The role of atopy in the development of clinical hypersensitivity. *J Allergy.* 1970;45:87–91.
15. Barnard JH. Nonfatal results in third degree anaphylaxis from Hymenoptera stings. *J Allergy.* 1970;45:92–96.
16. Lantner R, Reisman RE. Clinical and immunologic features and subsequent course of patients with severe insect sting anaphylaxis. *J Allergy Clin Immunol.* 1989;84:900–906.
17. Jensen OM. Sudden death due to stings from bees and wasps. *Acta Pathol Microbiol Immunol Scand* (A). 1962;54:9–29.
18. O'Connor R, Stier RA, Rosenbrook W Jr, et al. Death from "wasp" sting. *Ann Allergy.* 1964;22:385–393.
19. Schenken JR, Tamisiea J, Winter FD. Hypersensitivity to bee sting. *Am J Clin Pathol.* 1953;23:1216–1221.
20. Reisman RE. Natural history of insect sting allergy: relationship of severity of symptoms of initial sting anaphylaxis to re-sting reactions. *J Allergy Clin Immunol.* 1992;90:335–339.
21. Valentine MD, Schuberth KC, Kagey-Sobotka A, et al. The value of immunotherapy with venom in children with allergy to insect stings. *N Engl J Med.* 1991;23:1601–1603.
22. Reisman RE, Livingston A. Late onset reactions including serum sickness, following insect stings. *J Allergy Clin Immunol.* 1989;84:331–337.
23. Light WC, Reisman RE, Shimizu M, et al. Unusual reactions following insect stings. *J Allergy Clin Immunol.* 1977;59:391–397.
24. Hoffman DR. Hymenoptera venoms: composition, standardization, stability. In: Levine MI, Lockey RF, eds. *Monograph on Insect Allergy.* American Academy of Allergy Asthma and Immunology; 2003:37–53.
25. Light WC, Reisman RE, Wypych JI, et al. Clinical and immunological studies of beekeepers. *Clin Allergy.* 1975;5:389–395.
26. Lessof MH, Sobotka AK, Lichtenstein LM. Effects of passive antibody in bee venom anaphylaxis. *Johns Hopkins Med J.* 1978;142:1–7.
27. Hunt KJ, Valentine MD, Sobotka AK, et al. Diagnosis of allergy to stinging insects by skin testing with Hymenoptera venoms. *Ann Intern Med.* 1976;85:56–59.
28. Reisman RE, Wypych JI, Arbesman CE. Stinging insect allergy: detection and clinical significance of venom IgE antibodies. *J. Allergy Clin Immunol.* 1975;56:443–449.
29. Sobotka AK, Adkinson NF Jr, Valentine MD, et al. Allergy to insect stings: V. Diagnosis by radioallergosorbent tests (RAST). *J Immunol.* 1978;121:2477–2484.
30. Sobotka AK, Valentine MD, Benton AW, et al. Allergy to insect stings: I. Diagnosis of IgE-mediated Hymenoptera sensitivity by venom induced histamine release. *J Allergy Clin Immunol.* 1974;53:170–184.
31. Golden DBK, Kagey-Sobotka A, Norman PS, et al. Insect sting allergy with negative venom skin test responses. *J Allergy Clin Immunol.* 2001;107:897–901.

32. Reisman RE. Insect sting allergy: the dilemma of the negative skin test reactor. *J Allergy Clin Immunol.* 2001;107:781–782.

33. Ludolph-Hauser JD, Ruëff F, Fries C, et al. Constituitively raised serum concentrations of mast-cell tryptase and severe anaphylactic reactions to Hymenoptera stings, *Lancet.* 2001;357;361–362.

34. Buckingham BB, Levine MI. Protective measures against insect stings and bites. In: Levine MI, Lockey RD, eds. *Monograph on Insect Allergy.* American Academy of Allergy Asthma and Immunology; 2003:153–160.

35. Rawas-Qalaji MM, Simons FE, Simons KJ. Sublingual epinephrine tablets versus intramuscular injection of epinephrine: dose equivalence for potential treatment of anaphylaxis. *J Allergy Clin Immunol.* 2006;17:398–403.

36. Valentine MD. Insect venom allergy: diagnosis and treatment. *J Allergy Clin Immunol.* 1984:73:299–304.

37. Reisman RE, Livingston A. Venom immunotherapy (VIT): ten years experience with administration of single venoms and fifty micrograms maintenance doses. *J Allergy Clin Immunol.* 1992;89:1185–1189.

38. Golden DBK, Kagey-Sobotka A, Norman PS, et al. Outcomes of allergy to insect stings in children with and without venom immunotherapy. *N Engl J Med.* 2004;351:668–674.

39. Parker JL, Santrach PJ, Dahlberg MJE, et al. Evaluation of Hymenoptera sting sensitivity with deliberate sting challenges: the inadequacy of present diagnostic methods. *J Allergy Clin Immunol.* 1982; 69:200–207.

40. van derLinden PWH, Hack CE, Struyvenberg A, et al. Insect-sting challenge in 324 subjects with a previous anaphylactic reaction: current criteria for insect-venom hypersensitivity do not predict the occurrence and severity of anaphylaxis. *J Allergy Clin Immunol.* 1994;94:151–159.

41. Franken HH, DuBois EAJ, Minkema HJ, et al. Lack of reproducibility of a single negative sting challenge response in the assessment of anaphylactic risk in patient with suspected yellow jacket hypersensitivity. *J Allergy Clin Immunol.* 1994;93:431–435.

42. Golden DBK, Breisch NL, Hamilton RG, et al. Clinical and entomological factors influence the outcome of sting challenge studies. *J Allergy Clin Immunol.* 2006;117:670–675.

43. Fricker M, Helbling A, Schwartz L, et al. Hymenoptera sting anaphylaxis and urticaria pigmentosa: clinical findings and results of venom immunotherapy in ten patients. *J Allergy Clin Immunol.* 1997;100:11–15.

44. Haeberli G, Bronnimann M, Hunziker T, et al. Elevated basal serum tryptase and Hymenoptera venom allergy: relation of severity of sting reactions and to safety and efficacy of immunotherapy. *Clin Exp Allergy.* 2003;33:1216–1220.

45. Bonadonna P, Zanotti R, Caruso B, et al. Allergen specific immunotherapy is safe and effective in patients with systemic mastocytosis and Hymenoptera allergy. *J Allergy Clin Immunol.* 2008;121:256–257.

46. Mueller U, Elliott W, Reisman RE, et al. Comparison of biochemical and immunologic properties of venoms from the four hornet species. *J Allergy Clin Immunol.* 1981;67:290–298.

47. Reisman RE, Mueller U, Wypych J, et al. Comparison of the allergenicity and antigenicity of yellow jacket and hornet venoms. *J Allergy Clin Immunol.* 1982;69:268–274.

48. Reisman RE, Wypych JI, Mueller UR, et al. Comparison of the allergenicity and antigenicity of Polistes venom and other vespid venoms. *J Allergy Clin Immunol.* 1982;70:281–287.

49. Reisman RE, Mueller UR, Wypych JI, et al. Studies of coexisting honeybee and vespid venom sensitivity. *J Allergy Clin Immunol.* 1983;73:246–252.

50. Hoffman DR, El-Choutani SE, Smith MM, deGroot H. Occupational allergy to bumblebees: allergens of Bombus terrestris. *J Allergy Clin Immunol.* 2001;108:855–860.

51. Goldberg A, Reisman RE. Prolonged interval maintenance venom immunotherapy. *Ann Allergy.* 1988:61:177–179.

52. Golden DBK, Kagey-Sobotka A, Valentine MD, et al. Prolonged maintenance interval in Hymenoptera venom immunotherapy. *J Allergy Clin Immunol.* 1987;67:482–484.

53. Golden DBK, Valentine MD, Sobotka AK, et al. Regimens of Hymenoptera venom immunotherapy. *Ann Intern Med.* 1980;92:620–624.

54. Lockey RF, Turkeltaub PC, Olive ES, et al. The hymenoptera venom study III: safety of venom immunotherapy. *J Allergy Clin Immunol.* 1990;86:775–780.

55. Müller UR, Haeberli G. Use of β-blockers during immunotherapy for Hymenoptera venom allergy. *J Allergy Clin Immunol.* 2005;115:666–610.

56. Ober AI, MacLean JH, Hannaway PJ. Life-threatening anaphylaxis to venom immunotherapy in a patient taking an angiotensin-converting enzyme inhibitor. *J Allergy Clin Immunol.* 2003;112:1008–1009.

57. Schwartz HJ, Golden DBK, Lockey RF. Venom immunotherapy in the Hymenoptera allergic pregnant patient. *J Allergy Clin Immunol.* 1990;85:709–712.

58. Golden DBK, Lawrence ID, Hamilton RH, et al. Clinical correlations of the venom specific IgG antibody level during maintenance venom immunotherapy. *J Allergy Clin Immunol.* 1992;90:386–393.

59. Reisman RE. Should routine measures of serum venom specific IgG be a standard of practice in patients receiving venom immunotherapy? *J Allergy Clin Immunol.* 1992;90:282–284.

60. Ruëff F, Wenderoth A, Przybilla B. Patients still reacting to a sting challenge while receiving conventional Hymenoptera venom immunotherapy are protected by increased venom doses. *J Allergy Clin Immunol.* 2001;108:1027–1032.

61. Moffitt JE, Golden DBK, Reisman RE, et al. Stinging insect hypersensitivity: a practice parameter update. *J Allergy Clin Immunol.* 2004;114:869–886.

62. Lerch E, Müller UR. Long-term protection after stopping venom immunotherapy: results of restings in 200 patients. *J Allergy Clin Immunol.* 1998;101:606–612.

63. Haugaard L, Norregaard OFH, Dahl R. In-hospital sting challenge in insect venom-allergic patients after stopping venom immunotherapy. *J Allergy Clin Immunol.* 1991;87:699–702.

64. Golden DBK, Kwiterovich KD, Kagey-Sobotka A, et al. Discontinuing venom immunotherapy extended observations. *J Allergy Clin Immunol.* 1988;101:298–305.

65. Reisman RE. Duration of venom immunotherapy: relationship to the severity of symptoms of initial insect sting anaphylaxis. *J Allergy Clin Immunol.* 1993;92:831–836.

66. Reisman RE, Lantner R. Further observations on discontinuation of venom immunotherapy: Comparisons of patients stopped because of a fall in serum venom specific IgE to insignificant levels with patients stopped "prematurely" by self-choice. *J Allergy Clin Immunol.* 1989;83:1049–1054.

67. Stafford CT. Hypersensitivity to fire ant venom. *Ann Allergy.* 1996;77:87–99.

68. Kemp SF, deShazo RD, Moffitt JE, et al. Expanding habitat of the imported fire ant (Solenopsis invicta): a public health concern. *J Allergy Clin Immunol.* 2000;105:683–691.

69. deShazo RD, Kemp SF, deShazo MD, et al. Fire ant attacks on patients in nursing homes: an increasing problem. *Am J Med.* 2004;116:843–846.

70. Hoffman DR. Fire ant venom allergy. *Allergy.* 1995;50:535–544.

71. Freeman TM, Hylander RD, Ortiz A, et al. Imported fire ant immunotherapy; Effectiveness of whole body extracts. *J Allergy Clin Immunol.* 1992;90:210–215.

72. Moffitt J, Barker J, Stafford C. Management of imported fire ant allergy: results of a survey. *Ann Allergy.* 1997;79:125–130.

73. Tankersley MS, Walker RL, Butler WK, et al. Safety and efficacy of an imported fire ant rush immunotherapy protocol with and without prophylactic treatment. *J Allergy Clin Immunol.* 2002;109:556–562.

74. Pinnas JL, Strunk RC, Wang TM, et al. Harvester ant sensitivity: in vitro and in vivo studies using whole body extracts and venom. *J Allergy Clin Immunol.* 1977;59:10–16.

CHAPTER 16

Erythema Multiforme, Stevens-Johnson Syndrome, and Toxic Epidermal Necrolysis

ANJU T. PETERS AND NEILL T. PETERS

Erythema multiforme (EM), Stevens-Johnson syndrome (SJS), and toxic epidermal necrolysis (TEN) represent a spectrum of immunologically mediated diseases most often due to hypersensitivity to drugs or infections. There is no uniformly accepted definition or classification of these diseases, and understanding of their exact immunologic basis is lacking.

■ HISTORICAL BACKGROUND

Erythema multiforme (EM) is a term originally attributed to Ferdinand von Hebra. In 1866, he wrote about "erythema exudativum multiforme," a single cutaneous eruption with multiple evolving stages of lesions (1). Von Hebra described EM as a mild cutaneous syndrome featuring symmetric acral lesions, which resolved without sequelae, and had a tendency to recur. In 1922, Stevens and Johnson described a generalized eruption in two children characterized by fever, erosive stomatitis, and severe ocular involvement (2). This eruption became known as Stevens-Johnson syndrome. Thomas, in 1950, proposed that the milder von Hebra form of EM be called EM minor, and the more severe mucocutaneous eruption of SJS be called EM major (3). According to Thomas, fever and severe ocular involvement were the main points of distinction between the two types. The term *toxic epidermal necrolysis* was first introduced in 1956 by Lyell to describe patients with extensive epidermal necrosis that resembled scalded skin (4).

In 1993, an international consensus conference attempted to classify severe EM, SJS, and TEN on the basis of skin lesions and the extent of epidermal detachment (5). Using an illustrated atlas to standardize the diagnosis of acute severe bullous disorders attributed to drugs and infectious agents, the researchers defined bullous EM, SJS, SJS-TEN overlap, and TEN (Table 16.1).

Unfortunately, the ultimate classification of severe forms of EM remains a matter of debate and confusion for both primary care physicians and specialists. Given the rarity of SJS and TEN, it has been difficult to create a universally accepted standard of care for the management of these patients. Nonetheless, several concepts regarding EM, SJS, and TEN and their therapy have been proposed. It is well accepted that SJS and TEN represent varying severity of the same disease spectrum, with TEN being the most severe form (6,7).

■ ERYTHEMA MULTIFORME

Erythema multiforme, or the classic von Hebra type of EM, is a symmetric eruption with a predilection for the extremities. The characteristic primary lesion is a "target" comprised of three zones (8) (Figs. 16.1 and 16.2). Centrally there is a disk surrounded by an elevated, pale ring. A zone of erythema then borders the pale ring (5). Mucosal involvement occurs in a majority of cases of EM; however, it is usually limited to the oral or ocular mucosa and typically is not severe (9,10). EM is often associated with herpes simplex virus (HSV) infections and follows an outbreak of HSV by 1 to 3 weeks (11,12). The eruption is self-limited, lasts 1 to 4 weeks, and requires **only** symptomatic management. HSV-induced EM may be recurrent, and in such cases, recurrences can be prevented with suppressive antiherpetic therapy (13,14). More severe variants of EM have been also described and are often caused by infections including HSV and *Mycoplasma pneumoniae* (15,16). Drugs may cause a small proportion of EM cases (17,18). Discontinuation of the implicated medication and supportive therapy results in complete resolution of the skin eruption. Short courses of oral corticosteroids have been used in treatment protocols without any significant side effects (16). In some cases of EM, no obvious cause may be elicited (18).

TABLE 16.1   CLASSIFICATION OF ERYTHEMA MULTIFORME, STEVENS-JOHNSON SYNDROME AND TOXIC EPIDERMAL NECROLYSIS

	SKIN LESIONS	EXTENT OF SKIN DETACHMENT
Bullous erythema multiforme	Typical targets or raised atypical targets	<10%
SJS	Erythematous or purpuric macules or flat atypical targets	<10%
Overlap SJS/TEN	Purpuric macules or flat atypical targets	10% to 30%
TEN with spots	Purpuric macules or flat atypical targets	>30%
TEN without spots	Detachment of large epidermal sheets without any macules or targets	>10%

Adapted from Bastuji-Garin S, Rzany B, Stern RS, et al. Clinical classification of cases of toxic epidermal necrolysis, Stevens-Johnson syndrome, and erythema multiforme. *Arch Dermatol* 1993;129:92–96.

■ STEVENS-JOHNSON SYNDROME AND TOXIC EPIDERMAL NECROLYSIS

SJS and TEN are severe, mucocutaneous eruptions involving two or more mucosal surfaces, with or without visceral involvement (Figs. 16.3 and 16.4). Both SJS and TEN are rare, with an incidence of 1.89 cases per million people per year (19). The majority of the cases are attributed to drug exposures (18–26) (Table 16.2). Infections, especially with *Mycoplasma pneumoniae*, are also known to produce SJS (27,28). Vaccines and viral infections such as varicella zoster virus have also been reported to cause SJS (29–31). TEN has significant morbidity, and a mortality rate of about 30% (23,25,32). Most deaths are attributed to sepsis (22,25,32).

The eruption classically starts 7 to 21 days after initiation of the drug. Reexposure of a sensitized individual to a drug that had previously induced SJS/TEN may result in an acute recurrence of the eruption in 1 to 2 days (33). Constitutional symptoms such as fever and malaise are often present (22). The eruption typically starts on the face and the upper torso and extends rapidly; individual lesions include flat, atypical targets with dusky centers and purpuric macules (5). Flaccid blisters also may form. SJS and TEN feature extensive mucosal involvement in over 90% of patients. Oral, ocular, genitourinary, respiratory, and gastrointestinal mucosae all may be involved, and therefore require appropriate evaluation (27,34,35). Nearly 69% to 81% of patients have ocular manifestations ranging from mild conjunctivitis to corneal ulcerations (9,36). The skin lesions may be painful and the epidermis may slough off in large sheets. Up to 10% of total body surface area (TBSA) epidermal detachment is classified as SJS, 10% to 30% detachment is classified as SJS/TEN overlap, and greater than 30% as TEN (5). Nikolsky's sign that is characterized by detachment of the superficial skin by rubbing is present in involved areas of TEN.

Clinicians familiar with SJS/TEN usually have little difficulty recognizing a fully developed case. A skin biopsy, and in some cases a direct immunofluoresence study, can help confirm a diagnosis of SJS/TEN and exclude other diagnostic considerations.

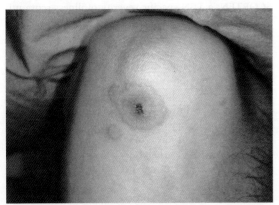

■ **FIGURE 16.1** Target lesion characteristic of erythema multiforme. (Courtesy of Dana Sachs, MD.)

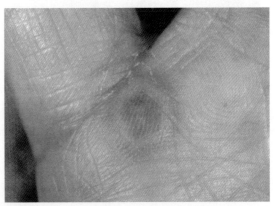

■ **FIGURE 16.2** Target lesion. (Courtesy of Dana Sachs, MD.)

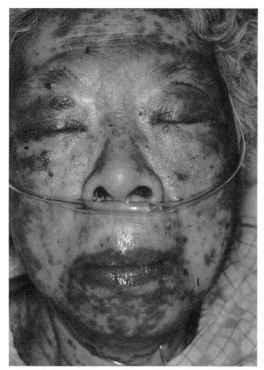

■ **FIGURE 16.3** Stevens-Johnson syndrome secondary to trimethoprim-sulfamethoxazole.

TABLE 16.2 MEDICATIONS COMMONLY IMPLICATED IN STEVENS-JOHNSON SYNDROME AND TOXIC EPIDERMAL NECROLYSIS

Sulfonamides	Allopurinol
Carbamazepine	Penicillins
Phenytoin	Nonsteroidal anti-inflammatory agents
Phenobarbital	Fluoroquinolones
Chlormezanone[a]	Cephalosporins
Acetaminophen (Paracetamol)	Valproic acid

[a]muscle relaxant-sedative
Data from references 18–26.

Treatment

Hospital admission is necessary in patients presenting with SJS/TEN. The extent of skin and mucosal involvement and laboratory findings need to be evaluated emergently. The extent of epidermal detachment is considered both a prognostic factor and a guide to therapy (32). If greater than 10% TBSA epidermal detachment is present, the patient has SJS/TEN overlap or TEN and requires different therapy (see discussion below on treatment of TEN). The laboratory investigation should include a complete blood cell count with differential, serum electrolytes, liver function tests, and urinalysis. The possible precipitating drug must be identified and discontinued. If a patient is on multiple medications, all nonessential drugs should be discontinued. Early discontinuation of the etiologic drug has been reported to improve survival in patients with SJS and TEN (37). Ophthalmologic consultation should be obtained early in all patients with ocular involvement. Further diagnostic evaluation is dictated by the patient's condition. SCORTEN, a TEN specific severity of illness score utilizes independent variables to predict mortality in patients with SJS/TEN (Table 16.3) (38).

In addition to supportive care and removal of the potential precipitating cause, early use of systemic corticosteroids may be beneficial in SJS. For mild cases, oral prednisone at doses of 1 mg/kg/day may be sufficient (16,33). Intravenous methylprednisolone, at doses of 1 mg/kg/day to 4 mg/kg/day, may be necessary for severe SJS. The dose of corticosteroids should be gradually reduced as the eruption resolves. An exacerbation of the eruption may occur if corticosteroids are withdrawn too rapidly.

The use of systemic corticosteroids for SJS remains controversial with some groups reporting benefit with corticosteroids while others suggest an increased risk of

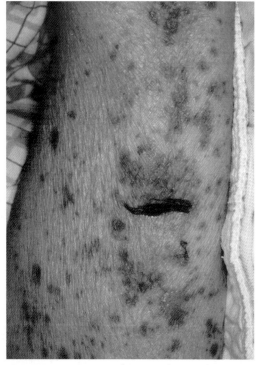

■ **FIGURE 16.4** Stevens-Johnson syndrome. Same patient as shown in Fig. 16.3.

TABLE 16.3   THE SCORTEN SCORING SYSTEM (BASED ON THE FIRST 24 HOURS OF ADMISSION)

Age > 40 years
History of malignancy
Heart rate >120/min
Blood urea nitrogen >27 mg/dL
Serum bicarbonate <20 mEq/L
Serum glucose >252 mg/dL
Epidermal detachment >10% of body surface area at day 1

Mortality can be predicted by the total score: 0–1 points = 3.2%; 2 points = 12.1%; 3 points = 35.3%; 4 points = 58.3%; >5 points = 90% mortality

Adapted from Bastuji-Garin S, Rouchard N, Bertocchi M, et al. SCORTEN: a severity of illness score for toxic epidermal necrolysis. *J Invest Dermatol* 2000;114:149–153.

complications (39–43). In a series of patients with SJS, complete recovery was observed in all patients with SJS who were diagnosed early and in whom the precipitating cause was removed and corticosteroids were used promptly and in adequate doses (33–35,44,45). Three of the 67 patients in the series died; however, their deaths were not attributable to either SJS or corticosteroid therapy (33–35).

In general, systemic corticosteroid therapy has been avoided in TEN and has not shown a benefit in the treatment of patients (46,47). A recent, uncontrolled series of patients with SJS, SJS/TEN overlap, and TEN suggests reduced mortality with dexamethasone pulse therapy; however, this was based on a small study of 12 patients (48). Therapy for TEN is supportive. Patients with TEN need aggressive fluid and electrolyte correction, local skin care, and fastidious infection precautions. This is best achieved in a burn unit (46,49).

Intravenous immunoglobulin (IVIG) has been used in treatment of SJS and TEN with variable success. Some groups have shown reduction in healing time as well as improved survival (50–52). Others, however, have suggested no benefit with IVIG and, possibly, increased mortality (53). Cyclosporin, and cyclophosphamide have been reported to improve outcomes in TEN (54,55). These results are based on small series of patients, and at the present time, the use of these agents in TEN is not universally accepted.

Pathogenesis

The exact immunologic basis for SJS and TEN is unknown. SJS/TEN is thought to occur through cell-mediated responses. $CD8^+$ T cells, the predominant cells found in the epidermis in bullous exanthems, SJS,

and TEN, are thought to mediate keratinocyte destruction (55–58). One study identified increased expression of adhesion molecules in the epidermis of patients with EM (59). Expression of these molecules, such as intracellular adhesion molecule type 1, on the surface of keratinocytes facilitates the cell trafficking of T lymphocytes into the epidermis. Perforin, a cytoplasmic peptide found in cytotoxic T cells, also has been detected in the dermis of SJS patients (60). Perforin can damage target cell membranes and therefore facilitate the entry of other granules such as granzymes into the target cell. These granules are known to trigger a series of reactions culminating in apoptosis (61). Histopathologic specimens from patients with SJS and TEN exhibit apoptosis (60,62).

Another mechanism involved in keratinocyte apoptosis in SJS and TEN may involve Fas-Fas ligand interactions. Studies have identified high concentrations of soluble Fas ligand in the sera of SJS/TEN patients (50,63). Others have reported that cells of the monocyte-macrophage lineage also play a role in SJS. These cells act as antigen-presenting cells and may mediate keratinocyte destruction through the release of cytokines such as tumor necrosis factor α (64).

Genetic links have been described for severe drug reactions. For example, association between certain medications and SJS/TEN has been described with HLA-B*1502 and HLA-B*5801 in Asian populations. However further research is necessary to define the role of the HLA region in SJS/TEN pathogenesis (65,66).

■ CONCLUSION

SJS and TEN are severe cutaneous reactions most commonly due to medications. Early recognition and withdrawal of the causative drug decreases the risk of death. Patients should be labeled allergic to the potential causative agent and counseled on strictly avoiding that drug in the future.

■ REFERENCES

1. von Hebra F. *On diseases of the Skin Including the Exanthemata*. Vol. 1. Fogge CH, trans. London: New Sydenham Society; 1866:285–289.
2. Stevens AM, Johnson FC. A new eruptive fever associated with stomatitis and ophthalmia. *Am J Dis Child.* 1992;24:526–533.
3. Thomas BA. The so-called Stevens-Johnson syndrome. *BMJ.* 1950;1:1393–1397.
4. Lyell A. Toxic epidermal necrolysis: an eruption resembling scalding of the skin. *Br J Dermatol.* 1956;68:355–361.
5. Bastuji-Garin S, Rzany B, Stern RS, et al. Clinical classification of cases of toxic epidermal necrolysis, Stevens-Johnson syndrome, and erythema multiforme. *Arch Dermatol.* 1993;129:92–96.
6. Roujeau JC. Stevens-Johnson syndrome and toxic epidermal necrolysis are severity variants of the same disease which differs from erythema multiforme. *J Dermatol.* 1997;24:726–729.
7. Auquier-Dunant A, Mockenhaupt M, Naldi L, et al. Correlations between clinical patterns and causes of erythema multiforme majus, Stevens-Johnson syndrome, and toxic epidermal necrolysis. *Arch Dermatol.* 2002;138:1019–1024.
8. Huff JC, Weston WL, Tonnesen ME. Erythema multiforme: a critical review of characteristics, diagnostic criteria, and causes. *J Am Acad Dermatol.* 1983;8:763–775.

9. Chang YS, Huang FC, Tseng SH, et al. Erythema multiforme, Stevens-Johnson syndrome, and toxic epidermal necrolysis: acute ocular manifestations, causes, and management. *Cornea*. 2007;26: 123–129.

10. Schofield JK, Tatnall FM, Leigh IM. Recurrent erythema multiforme: clinical features and treatment in a large series of patients. *Br J Dermatol*. 1993;128:542–545.

11. Anderson NP. Erythema multiforme: its relationship to herpes simplex. *Arch Dermatol*. 1945;5:10–16.

12. Shelley WB. Herpes simplex virus as a cause of erythema multiforme. *JAMA*. 1967;201:153–156.

13. Kerob D, Assier-Bonnet H, Esnault-Gelly P, et al. Recurrent erythemata multiforme unresponsive to acyclovir prophylaxis and responsive to valacyclovir continuous therapy. *Arch Dermatol*. 1998;134: 876–877.

14. Lemak MA, Duric M, Bean SF. Oral acyclovir for the prevention of herpes associated erythema multiforme. *J Am Acad Dermatol*. 1986;15:50–54.

15. Auquier-Dunant A, Mockenhaupt M, Naldi L, et al. Correlations between clinical patterns and causes of erythema multiforme majus, Stevens-Johnson Syndrome, and toxic epidermal necrolysis. *Arch Dermatol*. 2002;138:1019–1024.

16. Lam NS, Yang Y, Wang LD, et al. Clinical characteristics of childhood erythema multiforme, Stevens-Johnson syndrome, and toxic epidermal necrolysis in Taiwanese children. *J Microbiol Immunol Infect*. 2004;37:366–370.

17. Howland WW, Golitz LE, Weston WL, et al. Erythema multiforme, clinical, histopathologic and immunologic study. *J Am Acad Dermatol*. 1984;10:438–446.

18. Assier M, Bastuji-Garin S, Revuz J, et al. Erythema multiforme with mucous membrane involvement and Stevens-Johnson syndrome are clinically different disorders with distinct causes. *Arch Dermatol*. 1995;131:539–543.

19. Rzany B, Mockenhaupt M, Baur S, et al. Epidemiology of erythema exudativum multiforme majus, Stevens-Johnson syndrome, and toxic epidermal necrolysis in Germany (1990–1992): structure and results of a population-based registry. *J Clin Epidemiol*. 1996;49:769–773.

20. Roujeau JC, Kelly JP, Naldi L, et al. Medication use and the risk of Stevens-Johnson syndrome and toxic epidermal necrolysis. *N Engl J Med*. 1995;333:1600–1607.

21. Roujeau JC, Stern RS. Severe adverse reactions to drugs. *N Engl J Med*. 1994;331:1272–1284.

22. Ruiz-Maldonado R. Acute disseminated epidermal necrosis types 1, 2, and 3. Study of sixty cases. *J Am Acad Dermatol*. 1985;13:623–635.

23. Roujeau JC, Guillaume JC, Fabre JP, et al. Toxic epidermal necrolysis (Lyell syndrome): incidence and drug etiology in France, 1981–1985. *Arch Dermatol*. 1990;127:839–842.

24. Guillaume JC, Roujeau JC, Revuz J, et al. The culprit drugs in 87 cases of toxic epidermal necrolysis (Lyell's syndrome). *Arch Dermatol*. 1987;123:1166–1170.

25. Schöpf E, Stühmer A, Rzany B, et al. Toxic epidermal necrolysis and Stevens-Johnson syndrome: an epidemiologic study from West Germany. *Arch Dermatol*. 1991;127:839–842.

26. Rzany B, Hering O, Mockenhaupt M, et al. Histopathological and epidemiological characteristics of patients with erythema exudativum multiforme major, Stevens-Johnson syndrome and toxic epidermal necrolysis. *Br J Dermatol*. 1996;135:6–11.

27. Tay YK, Fluff JC, Weston WL. *Mycoplasma pneumoniae* infection is associated with Stevens-Johnson syndrome, not erythema multiforme (von Hebra). *J Am Acad Dermatol*. 1996;35:757–760.

28. Leaute-Labreze C, Lamireau T, Chawki D, et al. Diagnosis, classification, and management of erythema multiforme and Stevens-Johnson syndrome. *Arch Dis Child*. 2000;831:347–352.

29. Ball R, Ball LK, Wise RP, et al. Stevens-Johnson syndrome and toxic epidermal necrolysis after vaccinations: reports to the vaccine adverse event reporting system. *Pediatr Infect Dis J*. 2001;20:219–223.

30. Chopra A, Drage LA, Hanson EM, et al. Stevens-Johnson syndrome after immunization with smallpox, anthrax, and tetanus vaccines. *Mayo Clin Proc*. 2004;79(9):1193–1196.

31. Bay A, Akdeniz N, Calka O, et al. Primary varicella infection associated with Stevens-Johnson syndrome in a Turkish child. *J Dermatol*. 2005;32:745–750.

32. Ruiz J, Penso D, Roujeau J-C, et al. Toxic epidermal necrolysis. Clinical findings and prognosis factors in 87 patients. *Arch Dermatol*. 1987;123:1160–1165.

33. Tripathi A, Ditto AM, Grammer LC, et al. Corticosteroid therapy in an additional 13 cases of Stevens-Johnson syndrome: a total series of 67 cases. *Allergy Asthma Proc*. 2000;21:101–105.

34. Patterson R, Dykewicz MS, Gonzalzles A, et al. Erythema multiforme and Stevens-Johnson syndrome descriptive and therapeutic controversy. *Chest*. 1990;98:331–336.

35. Patterson R, Miller M, Kaplan M, et al. Effectiveness of early therapy with corticosteroids in Stevens-Johnson syndrome: experience with 41 cases and a hypothesis regarding pathogenesis. *Ann Allergy*. 1994;73:27–34.

36. Power WJ, Ghoraishi M, Merayo-Lloves J, et al. Analysis of the acute ophthalmic manifestations of the erythema multiforme/Stevens-Johnson syndrome/toxic epidermal necrolysis disease spectrum. *Ophthalmology*. 1995;102:1669–1676.

37. Garcia DI, LeCleach L, Bocquet H, et al. Toxic epidermal necrolysis and Stevens-Johnson syndrome. Does early withdrawal of causative drugs decrease the risk of death? *Arch Dermatol*. 2000; 136:323–327.

38. Bastuji-Garin S, Rouchard N, Bertocchi M, et al. SCORTEN: a severity of illness score for toxic epidermal necrolysis. *J Invest Dermatol*. 2000;114:149–153.

39. Rasmussen JE. Erythema multiforme in children: response to treatment with systemic corticosteroids. *Br J Dermatol* 1976;95:181–186.

40. Halebian P, Shires T. Burn unit treatment of acute severe exfoliating disorders. *Annu Rev Med*. 1989;40:137–147.

41. Ginsberg CM. Stevens-Johnson syndrome in children. *Pediatr Infect Dis*. 1982;1:155–158.

42. Kakourou T, Klonza D, Soteropoulou F, et al. Corticosteroid treatment of erythema multiforme major (Stevens-Johnson syndrome) in children. *Eur J Pediatr*. 1997;156:90–93.

43. Nethecott JR, Choi BCK. Erythema multiforme (Stevens-Johnson syndrome) chart review of 123 hospitalized patients. *Dermatology*. 1985;171:383–396.

44. Patterson R, Grammer LC, Greenberger PA, et al. Stevens-Johnson Syndrome (SJS): effectiveness of corticosteroids in management and recurrent SJS. *Allergy Proc*. 1992;2:89–95.

45. Cheriyan S, Patterson R, Greenberger PA, et al. The outcome of Stevens-Johnson syndrome treated with corticosteroids. *Allergy Proc*. 1995;16:151–155.

46. Palmieri TL, Greenhalgh DG, Saffle JR, et al. A multicenter review of toxic epidermal necrolysis treated in U.S. burn centers at the end of the twentieth century. *J Burn Care Rehabil*. 2002;23:87–96.

47. Kim PS, Goldfard IW, Gaisford JC, et al. Stevens-Johnson syndrome and toxic epidermal necrolysis: a physiologic review with recommendations for a treatment protocol. *J Burn Care Rehabil*. 1983;4:91–100.

48. Kardaun SH, Jonkman MF. Dexamethasone pulse therapy for Stevens-Johnson syndrome/toxic epidermal necrolysis. *Acta Derm Venereol*. 2007;87:144–148.

49. Heimbach DM, Engrau LH, Marvin JA, et al. Toxic epidermal necrolysis: a step forward in treatment. *JAMA*. 1987;257:2171–2175.

50. Viard I, Wehrli P, Bullani R, et al. Inhibition of toxic epidermal necrolysis by blockade of CD95 with human intravenous immunoglobulin. *Science*. 1998;282:490–493.

51. Prins C, Kerdel FA, Padilla RS, et al. Treatment of toxic epidermal necrolysis with high dose intravenous immunoglobulins. *Arch Dermatol*. 2003;139:26–32.

52. Trent JT, Kirsner RS, Romanelli P, et al. Analysis of intravenous immunoglobulin for the treatment of toxic epidermal necrolysis using SCORTEN. *Arch Dermatol*. 2003;139:39–43.

53. Bachot N, Revuz J, Roujeau JC. Intravenous immunoglobulin treatment for Stevens-Johnson syndrome and toxic epidermal necrolysis. *Arch Dermatol*. 2003;139:33–36.

54. Hewitt J, Onerod AP. Toxic epidermal necrolysis treated with cyclosporin. *Clin Exp Dermatol*. 1992;19:264–265.

55. Heng MCY, Allen SG. Efficacy of cyclophosphamide in toxic epidermal necrolysis. Clinical and pathophysiologic aspects. *J Am Acad Dermatol*. 1991;25:773–786.

56. Margolis RJ, Tonneson MG, Harrist TJ, et al. Lymphocyte subsets and Langerhans cells/indeterminate cells in erythema multiforme. *J Invest Dermatol*. 1983;81:403–406.

57. Miyauchi H, Losokawa H, Akaeda T, et al. Cell subsets in drug induced toxic epidermal necrolysis. *Arch Dermatol*. 1991;127: 851–855.

58. Hertl M, Bohlem H, Jugert F, et al. Predominance of epidermal CD8$^+$ T lymphocytes in bullous cutaneous reactions caused by β-lactam antibiotics. *J Invest Dermatol*. 1993;101:794–799.

59. Shiohara T, Chiba M, Tanaka Y, et al. Drug induced photosensitive erythema multiforme-like eruptions: possible role for cell adhesion molecules in a flare induced by rhus dermatitis. *J Am Acad Dermatol*. 1990;22:647–650.

60. Inachi S, Mizutani H, Shimizu M. Epidermal apoptotic cell death in erythema multiforme and Stevens-Johnson syndrome. *Arch Dermatol.* 1997;133:845–849.

61. Cohen JJ, Duke RC. Apoptosis and programmed cell death in immunity. *Annu Rev Immunol.* 1992;10:167–193.

62. Paul C, Wolkenstein P, Adle H, et al. Apoptosis as a mechanism of keratinocyte death in toxic epidermal necrolysis. *Br J Dermatol.* 1996;134:710–714.

63. Abe R, Shimizu T, Shibaki A, et al. Toxic epidermal necrolysis and Stevens-Johnson syndrome are induced by soluble Fas ligand. *Am J Pathol.* 2003;162:1515–1520.

64. Pacquet P, Nikkels A, Arrese J, et al. Macrophages and tumor factor in toxic epidermal necrolysis. *Arch Dermatol.* 1994;130:605–608.

65. Lonjou C, Borot N, Sekula P, et al. A European study of HLA-B in Stevens-Johnson syndrome and toxic epidermal necrolysis related to five high-risk drugs. *Pharmacogenet Genomics.* 2008;18:99–107.

66. Chung WH, Hung SI, Hong HS, et al. A marker for Stevens-Johnson syndrome. *Nature.* 2004;428:486.

Drug Allergy

PART A

Introduction, Epidemiology, Classification of Adverse Reactions, Immunochemical Basis, Risk Factors, Evaluation of Patients with Suspected Drug Allergy, Patient Management Considerations

ANNE MARIE DITTO

In the fifth edition of this text, the subject of drug allergy was extensively reviewed (1). Although a reasonably comprehensive overview of this important topic is addressed in the sixth edition (2) and in the current edition, an effort has been made to focus more sharply on clinically applicable information. An even more concise, practical review is published elsewhere (3). Other reviews of drug allergy are also recommended (4). Further, although specific recommendations are suggested regarding drug challenges and desensitization protocols, it is advisable, if possible, for those inexperienced in such matters to consult with physicians who regularly evaluate and manage hypersensitivity phenomena.

■ EPIDEMIOLOGY

A consequence of the rapid development of new drugs to diagnose and treat human illness has been the increased incidence of adverse reactions to these agents, which may produce additional morbidity and, on occasion, mortality. Their occurrence violates a basic principle of medical practice, *primum non nocere* (above all, do no harm). It is a sobering fact that adverse drug reactions are responsible for most iatrogenic illnesses. This should serve to remind physicians not to select potent and often unnecessary drugs to treat inconsequential illnesses. Many patients have come to expect drug treatments for the most trivial of symptoms. On the other hand, a physician should not deprive a patient of necessary medication for fear of a reaction. Fortunately, most adverse reactions are not severe, but the predictability of seriousness is usually not possible in the individual case or with the individual drug.

An *adverse drug reaction* (ADR) may be defined as any undesired and unintended response that occurs at doses of an appropriate drug given for the therapeutic, diagnostic, or prophylactic benefit of the patient. The reaction should appear within a reasonable time after administration of the drug. This definition excludes therapeutic failure, which the patient may perceive as an adverse drug reaction. A *drug* may be defined as any substance used in diagnosis, therapy, and prophylaxis of disease.

Although the exact incidence of adverse drug reactions is unknown, some estimates of their magnitude are available. Reported estimates of the incidence of adverse drug reactions leading to hospitalization vary and this is complicated by inconsistency with definitions used, with methods used to collect and analyze data, and with some studies measuring prevalence while others measure incidence. One study based on a computerized surveillance system determined that 2%

of hospital admissions were a result of adverse drug reactions (5). A meta-analysis of 33 prospective studies from 1966 to 1996 in the United States showed an incidence of 3.1% to 6.2% of hospital admissions were due to ADRs (6). Other studies from various countries including Switzerland, Australia, and Germany showed that ADRs were the reason for 2% to 6.1% of hospital admissions (7–11). As many as 15% to 30% of medical inpatients experience an adverse drug reaction (12). Drug-attributed deaths occur in 0.01% of surgical inpatients and in 0.14% to 0.17% of medical inpatients (7,10,13–15). Most of these fatalities occurred among patients who were terminally ill (16); in a study of ADR and hospital admissions in Australia, admissions for ADRs increased with patient age (10). Most deaths were due to a small number of drugs that, by their nature, are known to be quite toxic.

Information regarding outpatient adverse drug events is scant by comparison because most are not reported to pharmaceutical companies and appropriate national registries. Such surveys are complicated by the problem of differentiating between signs and symptoms attributable to the natural disease and those related to its treatment. Adverse drug reactions may mimic virtually every disease, including the disease being treated. The challenge of monitoring adverse drug reactions is further complicated by multiple drug prescribing and the frequent use of nonprescription medications. Despite these limitations, such monitoring did identify the drug-induced skin rash that often follows ampicillin therapy.

Although most drug safety information is obtained from clinical trials before drug approval, premarketing studies are narrow in scope and thus cannot uncover adverse drug reactions in all patient populations. Adverse effects that occur over time or that are less frequent than 1 in 1,000, such as drug hypersensitivity, will not be detected until used by large numbers of patients after drug approval (17).

Thus, postmarketing surveillance is essential to the discovery of unexpected adverse drug effects. However, one estimate is that only 1% of adverse drug reactions are voluntarily reported to pharmaceutical companies and the U.S. Food and Drug Administration (FDA) (18). In an attempt to ensure the timely collection of adverse drug reactions, the FDA introduced a simplified medical products reporting program in 1993, MedWatch (19). Although the FDA had an ADR reporting system in place before MedWatch, it was awkward to use and understandably discouraged health professionals' participation. Using MedWatch, the reporting individual does not have to prove absolutely an association between the drug and the adverse reaction. When reported, the information becomes part of a large database and can be investigated further. A simple, self-addressed, one-page form is available and can be sent by mail, fax, or electronically (http://www.fda.gov/medwatch). The Web site also has an e-list where one can sign up to receive safety information

TABLE 17A.1   REPORTING ADVERSE REACTIONS TO MEDWATCH

By Mail
- Use postage-paid MedWatch form 3500

By Phone
- 1-800-FDA-1088 to report by phone, to receive copies of form 3500 or a copy of *FDA Desk Guide for Adverse Event and Product Problem Reporting*
- 1-800-FDA-0178 to FAX report
- 1-800-FDA-7967 for a Vaccine Adverse Event Reporting System (VAERS) form for vaccines

By Internet
- http://www.fda.gov/medwatch

reports directly by e-mail. Table 17A.1 summarizes how to report ADRs to MedWatch. Voluntary reporting led to the observation that ventricular arrhythmias, such as torsades de pointes, may occur when terfenadine is administered with erythromycin or ketoconazole (20).

Most ADRs do not have an allergic basis. What follows is a discussion that primarily focuses on those reactions that are, or possibly could be, mediated by immunologic mechanisms.

Allergic drug reactions account for 6% to 10% of all observed adverse drug reactions. It has been suggested that the risk for an allergic reaction is about 1% to 3% for most drugs. It is estimated that about 5% of adults may be allergic to one or more drugs. However, as many as 15% believe themselves to be or have been incorrectly labeled as being allergic to one or more drugs and, therefore, may be denied treatment with an essential medication. At times, it may be imperative to establish the presence or absence of allergy to a drug when its use is necessary and there are no safe alternatives. Although many patients with a history of reacting to a drug could safely receive that drug again, the outcome could be serious if that patient is truly allergic. Hence, a suspicion of drug hypersensitivity must be evaluated carefully.

■ CLASSIFICATION OF ADVERSE DRUG REACTIONS

Before proceeding with a detailed analysis of drug hypersensitivity, it is appropriate to attempt to place it in perspective with other adverse drug reactions. Physicians should carefully analyze ADRs to determine their nature because this will influence future use. For example, a drug-induced side effect may be corrected by simply reducing the dose. On the other hand, an allergic reaction to a drug may mean that drug cannot be used or may require special considerations before future administration.

Adverse drug reactions may be divided into two major groups: (a) *predictable adverse reactions,* which are (i) often dose-dependent, (ii) related to the known pharmacologic actions of the drug, (iii) occur in otherwise normal patients, and (iv) account for 80% or more of adverse drug effects; and (b) *unpredictable adverse reactions,* which are (i) usually dose-independent, (ii) usually unrelated to the drug's pharmacologic actions, and (iii) often related to the individual's immunologic responsiveness or, on occasion, to genetic differences in susceptible patients.

Not included in this classification are those reactions that are unrelated to the drug itself but are attributable to events associated with and during its administration. Such events are often mistakenly ascribed to the drug, and the patient is inappropriately denied that agent in the future. Particularly after parenteral administration of a drug, *psychophysiologic reactions* in the form of hysteria, hyperventilation, or vasovagal response may ensue. Some of these reactions may be manifestations of underlying psychiatric disorders (21). Even anaphylactoid symptoms have been observed in placebo-treated patients (22). Another group of signs and symptoms is considered a *coincidental reaction.* They are a result of the disease under treatment and may be incorrectly attributed to the drug, for example, the appearance of viral exanthems and even urticaria during the course of a treatment with an antibiotic. Although it may be difficult to characterize a particular drug reaction, a helpful classification is shown in Table 17A.2, followed by a brief description of each.

TABLE 17A.2 CLASSIFICATION OF ADVERSE DRUG REACTIONS

Predictable Adverse Reactions Occurring in Normal Patients

Overdosage: toxicity
Side effects • Immediate expression • Delayed expression
Secondary or indirect effects • Drug-related • Disease-associated
Drug–drug interactions

Unpredictable Adverse Reactions Occurring in Susceptible Patients

Intolerance
Idiosyncratic reactions
Allergic (hypersensitivity) reactions
Pseudoallergic reactions

Overdosage: Toxicity

The toxic effects of a drug are directly related to the systemic or local concentration of the drug in the body. Such effects are usually predictable on the basis of animal experimentation and may be expected in any patient provided a threshold level has been exceeded. Each drug tends to have its own characteristic toxic effects. Overdosage may result from an excess dose taken accidentally or deliberately. It may be due to accumulation as a result of some abnormality in the patient that interferes with normal metabolism and excretion of the drug. The toxicity of morphine is enhanced in the presence of liver disease (inability to detoxify the drug) or myxedema (depression of metabolic rate). The toxicity of chloramphenicol in infants is due to immaturity of the glucuronide conjugating system, allowing a toxic concentration to accumulate. In the presence of renal failure, drugs such as the aminoglycosides, normally excreted by this route, may accumulate and produce toxic reactions.

Side Effects

Side effects are the most frequent adverse drug reactions. They are therapeutically undesirable, but often unavoidable, pharmacologic actions occurring at usual prescribed drug dosages. A drug frequently has several pharmacologic actions, and only one of those may be the desired therapeutic effect. The others may be considered side effects. The first-generation antihistamines commonly cause adverse central nervous system effects, such as sedation. Their anticholinergic side effects include dry mouth, blurred vision, and urinary retention.

Other side effects may be delayed in expression and include teratogenicity and carcinogenicity. Methotrexate, which has been used in some steroid-dependent asthmatic patients, is teratogenic and should not be used during pregnancy. Immunosuppressive agents can alter host immunity and may predispose the patient to malignancy (23).

Secondary or Indirect Effects

Secondary effects are indirect, but not inevitable, consequences of the drug's primary pharmacologic action. They may be interpreted as the appearance of another naturally occurring disease rather than being associated with administration of the drug. Some appear to be due to the drug itself, creating an ecologic disturbance and permitting the overgrowth of microorganisms. In the presence of antimicrobial (notably ampicillin, clindamycin, or cephalosporins) exposure, *Clostridium difficile* can flourish in the gastrointestinal tract in an environment in which there is reduced bacterial competition. Toxins produced by this organism may result in the development of pseudomembranous colitis (24).

Antimicrobial agents may be associated with another group of reactions that may mimic hypersensitivity, but appear to be disease associated. The *Jarisch-Herxheimer* phenomenon involves the development of fever, chills, headaches, skin rash, edema, lymphadenopathy, and often an exacerbation of preexisting skin lesions. The reaction is believed to result from the release of microbial antigens, endotoxins, or both (25). This has usually followed penicillin treatment of syphilis and leptospirosis, but also has been observed during treatment of parasitic and fungal infections. With continued treatment, the reaction subsides, thus confirming it is not an allergic response. Unfortunately, treatment is often discontinued and the drug blamed for the reaction. Another example would include the high incidence of skin rash in patients with the Epstein-Barr virus treated with ampicillin.

Drug–Drug Interactions

A drug–drug interaction is generally regarded as the modification of the effect of one drug by prior or concomitant administration of another. Fortunately, drug–drug interactions of major clinical consequence are relatively infrequent (26). It is also important to recall that not all drug interactions are harmful, and some may be used to clinical advantage.

As the number of drugs taken concurrently increases, the greater the likelihood of an adverse drug interaction. When an interaction is reported, an average of between four and eight drugs are being taken by the patient. Therefore, the largest risk group are elderly patients, who often receive polypharmacy. The danger of an interaction also escalates when several physicians are treating a patient, each for a separate condition. It is the physician's responsibility to determine what other medications the patient is taking, even nonprescription drugs.

Several widely prescribed agents used to treat allergic rhinitis and asthma interacted significantly with other drugs. The second-generation antihistamines, terfenadine and astemizole, were metabolized by cytochrome P-450 mixed-function oxidase enzymes. These antihistamines, in combination with drugs that inhibited the P-450 enzyme system, such as the imidazole antifungals ketoconazole and itraconazole or the macrolide antibiotics erythromycin and clarithromycin, resulted in increased concentrations of the antihistamines. This caused potential for prolongation of the QT interval, sometimes producing torsades de pointes or other serious cardiac arrhythmias (19). These antihistamines are no longer available in the United States. Although plasma concentrations of loratadine increased with concomitant administration of ketoconazole, this did not cause prolongation of the QT interval and the risk for torsades de pointes (27).

An excellent review of other adverse drug interactions may be found in a looseleaf publication authored by Hansten and Horn (28).

Intolerance

Intolerance is a characteristic pharmacologic effect of a drug which is quantitatively increased, and often is produced, by an unusually small dose of medication. Most patients develop tinnitus after large doses of salicylates and quinine, but few experience it after a single average dose or a smaller dose than usual. This untoward effect may be genetically determined and appears to be a function of the recipient, or it may occur in individuals lying at the extremes of dose–response curves for pharmacologic effects.

In contrast to intolerance, which implies a quantitatively increased pharmacologic effect occurring among susceptible individuals, *idiosyncratic and allergic reactions* are qualitatively aberrant and inexplicable in terms of the normal pharmacology of the drug given in usual therapeutic doses.

Idiosyncratic Reactions

Idiosyncrasy is a term used to describe a qualitatively abnormal, unexpected response to a drug, differing from its pharmacologic actions and thus resembling hypersensitivity. However, this reaction does not involve a proven, or even suspected, allergic mechanism.

A familiar example of an idiosyncratic reaction is the hemolytic anemia occurring commonly in African and Mediterranean populations and in 10% to 13% of African American males (sex-linked) exposed to oxidant drugs or their metabolites. About 25% of African American females are carriers, and of these, only one-fifth have a sufficiently severe expression of the deficiency to be clinically important. A more severe form of the deficiency occurs in Caucasian Americans, primarily among people of Mediterranean origin. The erythrocytes of such individuals lack the enzyme glucose-6-phosphate dehydrogenase (G6PD) that is essential for aerobic metabolism of glucose and, consequently, cellular integrity (29). Although the original observations of this phenomenon were among susceptible individuals receiving primaquine, more than 50 drugs are known that induce hemolysis in G6PD-deficient patients. Clinically, the three classes of drugs most important in terms of their hemolytic potential are sulfonamides, nitrofurans, and water-soluble vitamin K analogues. If G6PD deficiency is suspected, simple screening tests dependent on hemoglobin oxidation, dye reduction, or fluorescence generation provide supporting evidence. The study of genetic G6PD deficiency and other genetic defects leading to adverse drug reactions has been termed *pharmacogenetics* (30).

Allergic Reactions

Allergic drug reactions occur in only a small number of individuals, are unpredictable and quantitatively abnormal, and are unrelated to the pharmacologic action of the drug. Unlike idiosyncrasy, allergic drug reactions are the result of an immune response to a drug following previous exposure to the same drug or to an immunochemically related substance that had resulted in the formation of specific antibodies, of sensitized T lymphocytes, or of both. Ideally, the term *drug allergy* or *hypersensitivity* should be restricted to those reactions proved, or more often presumed, to be the result of an immunologic mechanism.

The establishment of an allergic mechanism should be based on the demonstration of specific antibodies, sensitized lymphocytes, or both. This is not often possible for many reactions ascribed to drug allergy. The diagnosis is usually based on clinical observations and, in selected instances, reexposure to the suspected agent under controlled circumstances. Even in the absence of direct immunologic evidence, an allergic drug reaction often is suspected when certain clinical and laboratory criteria are present, as suggested in Table 17A.3. Obviously, none of these is absolutely reliable (31).

Immediate reactions occurring within minutes often include manifestations of anaphylaxis. Accelerated reactions taking place after 1 hour to 3 days frequently are manifested as urticaria and angioedema and occasionally as other rashes, especially exanthems with fever. Delayed or late reactions do not appear until 3 days or longer after drug therapy is initiated and commonly include a diverse group of skin rashes, drug fever, and serum sickness–like reactions and, less commonly, hematologic, pulmonary, hepatic, and renal reactions, vasculitis, and a condition resembling lupus erythematosus.

Because clinical criteria are often inadequate, specific immunologic testing is desirable. Until this is accomplished, at best the relationship can be considered only presumptive. With few exceptions, safe, reliable *in vivo* tests and simple, rapid, predictable *in vitro* tests for the absolute diagnosis of drug allergy are unavailable. The most conclusive test is cautious readministration of the suspected drug, but usually the risk is not justified.

Pseudoallergic Reactions

Pseudoallergy refers to an immediate generalized reaction involving mast cell mediator release by an immunoglobulin E (IgE)-independent mechanism (32). Although the clinical manifestations often mimic or resemble IgE-mediated events (anaphylaxis), the initiating event does not involve an interaction between the drug or drug metabolites and drug-specific IgE antibodies. A differential point is that these reactions may occur in patients without a previous exposure to these substances.

Such reactions appear to result from nonimmunologic activation of effector pathways. Certain drugs, such as opiates, vancomycin, polymyxin B, and D-tubocurarine, may directly release mediators from mast cells, resulting in urticaria, angioedema, or even a clinical picture resembling anaphylaxis. In general, these reactions can be prevented by pretreatment with

---

TABLE 17A.3   CLINICAL CRITERIA OF ALLERGIC DRUG REACTIONS

1. Allergic reactions occur in only a small percentage of patients receiving the drug and cannot be predicted from animal studies.
2. The observed clinical manifestations do not resemble known pharmacologic actions of the drug.
3. In the absence of prior exposure to the drug, allergic symptoms rarely appear before 1 week of continuous treatment. After sensitization, even years previously, the reaction may develop rapidly on reexposure to the drug. As a rule, drugs used with impunity for several months or longer are rarely the culprits. This temporal relationship is often the most vital information in determining which of many drugs being taken needs to be considered most seriously as the cause of a suspected drug hypersensitivity reaction.
4. The reaction may resemble other established allergic reactions, such as anaphylaxis, urticaria, asthma, and serum sickness–like reactions. However, a variety of skin rashes (particularly exanthems), fever, pulmonary infiltrates with eosinophilia, hepatitis, acute interstitial nephritis, and lupus syndrome have been attributed to drug hypersensitivity.
5. The reaction may be reproduced by small doses of the suspected drug or other agents possessing similar or cross-reacting chemical structures.
6. Eosinophilia may be suggestive if present.
7. Rarely, drug-specific antibodies or T lymphocytes have been identified that react with the suspected drug or relevant drug metabolite.
8. As with adverse drug reactions in general, the reaction usually subsides within several days after discontinuation of the drug.

corticosteroids and antihistamines, as outlined for radiographic contrast media (RCM) (33). IgE-mediated allergic reactions, however, cannot.

Summary

The classification of ADRs presented here must be considered tentative. At times, it may be impossible to place a particular drug reaction under one of these headings. However, the common practice of labeling any ADR as "allergic" should be discouraged.

■ IMMUNOCHEMICAL BASIS OF DRUG ALLERGY

Drugs as Immunogens

The allergenic potential of drugs is largely dependent on their chemical properties. Increases in molecular size and complexity are associated with an increased ability to elicit an immune response. Hence, high-molecular-weight drugs, such as heterologous antisera, and recombinant proteins (e.g., infliximab and etanercept), streptokinase, L-asparaginase, and insulin, are complete antigens that can induce immune responses and elicit hypersensitivity reactions. Immunogenicity is weak or absent when substances have a molecular weight of less than 4,000 daltons (34).

Most drugs are simple organic chemicals of low molecular weight, usually less than 1,000 daltons. For such low-molecular-weight drugs to become immunogenic, the drug or a drug metabolite must be bound to a macromolecular carrier, often by covalent bonds, for effective antigen processing. The simple chemical (hapten), nonimmunogenic by itself, becomes immunogenic in the presence of the carrier macromolecule and now directs the specificity of the response.

β-Lactam antibiotics are highly reactive with proteins and can directly haptenate carrier macromolecules. However, most drugs are not sufficiently reactive to form a stable immunogenic complex. It is likely that haptens derived from most drugs are *reactive metabolites* of the parent compound, which then bind to carrier macromolecules to become immunogenic. This requirement for metabolic processing may help to explain the low incidence of drug allergy, the predisposition of certain drugs to cause sensitization as they are prone to form highly reactive metabolites, and the inability of skin testing and other immunologic tests with the unaltered drug to predict or identify the reaction as being allergic in nature.

Another model describing immunogenicity of low-molecular-weight compounds is the pharmacologic interactive (p-i) model in which nonreactive drugs form noncovalent bonds with MHC receptors and directly stimulate T cells (35,36). A third model proposed by Matzinger is the danger model which states that an antigen presenting cell becomes activated when it receives "danger signals" from damaged or stressed cells, thus forming necessary co-stimulatory molecules and cytokines that propagate as well as determine the immunogenic response (37,38).

Penicillin allergy has received the most attention as a model of drug haptenization (39). Unfortunately, relevant drug haptens have not been identified for most allergic drug reactions. Recent studies of human IgE and IgG to sulfonamides have established the N^4-sulfonamidoyl determinant to be the major sulfonamide haptenic determinant (40).

It should be noted that an antigen must have multiple combining sites (multivalent) to elicit hypersensitivity reactions. This requirement permits bridging of IgE- and IgG-antibody molecules or antigen receptors on lymphocytes. Conjugation of the free drug or metabolite (hapten) with a macromolecular carrier to form a multivalent hapten-carrier conjugate is necessary to initiate an immune response and elicit a hypersensitivity reaction. The univalent ligand (free drug or metabolite), in large excess, may inhibit the response by competing with the multivalent conjugates for the same receptors. Therefore, the relative concentration of each will determine the frequency, severity, and rate of allergic drug reactions. Also, removal of haptens from carrier molecules by plasma enzymes (dehaptenation) will influence the likelihood of such reactions (41).

Finally, some low-molecular-weight drugs, such as quaternary ammonium muscle relaxants and aminoglycosides, have enough distance between determinants to act as bivalent antigens without requiring conjugation to a carrier (42).

Immunologic Response to Drugs

Drugs often induce an immune response, but only a small number of patients actually experience clinical hypersensitivity reactions. For example, most patients exposed to penicillin and insulin develop demonstrable antibodies; however, in most instances, these do not result in allergic reactions or reduced effectiveness of the drug.

Mechanisms of Drug-induced Immunopathology

An immunologic response to any antigen may be quite diverse and the attendant reactions quite complex. Drugs are no exception and have been associated with all of the immunologic reactions proposed by Coombs and Gell (43) subsequently modified by Janeway (44) and Kay (45). It is likely that more than one mechanism may contribute to a particular reaction, but often one will predominate. Table 17A.4 is an attempt to provide an overview of the immunopathology of allergic drug reactions based on the original Coombs and Gell classification.

TABLE 17A.4   IMMUNOPATHOLOGY OF ALLERGIC REACTIONS TO DRUGS

CLASSIFICATION	IMMUNOREACTANTS	CLINICAL PRESENTATION
Type I	Mast cell-mediated IGR • IgE-dependent (anaphylactic) • IgE-independent (pseudo allergic or anaphylactoid)	Anaphylaxis, urticaria, angio-edema, asthma, rhinitis
Type IIa	Antibody-mediated cytotoxic reactions—IgG and IgM antibodies Complement often involved	Immune cytopenias Some organ inflammation
Type III	Immune complex–mediated reactions Complement involved	Serum sickness, vasculitis
Type IVa$_1$	T lymphocyte-mediated reactions (CD4 and T$_H$1) type 1 cytokines	Contact dermatitis Some exanthems

IGR, immediate generalized reactions; IgE, immunoglobulin E; IgM, immunoglobulin M.

Adapted from Kay AB. Concepts of allergy and hypersensitivity. In: Kay AB, ed. *Allergy and allergic diseases.* Oxford, UK: Blackwell Science, 1997:23.

Penicillin alone has been associated with many of these reactions. Anaphylaxis and urticaria following penicillin administration are examples of type I reactions. The hemolytic anemia associated with high-dose penicillin therapy is a type II reaction. A serum sickness–like reaction, now most commonly associated with penicillin treatment, is a type III reaction. Finally, the contact dermatitis that occurred when penicillin was used topically in the past is an example of a type IV reaction.

■ RISK FACTORS FOR DRUG ALLERGY

Several factors have been identified that may influence the induction of drug-specific immune responses and the elicitation of clinical reactions to these agents (46,47) (Table 17A.5).

Drug- and Treatment-related Factors

Nature of the Drug

Macromolecular drugs, such as heterologous antisera and insulin, are complex antigens and have the potential to sensitize any patient. As noted earlier, most drugs have molecular weights of less than 1,000 daltons and are not immunogenic by themselves. Immunogenicity is determined by the potential of the drug or, more often, a drug metabolite to form conjugates with carrier proteins.

β-Lactam antibiotics, aspirin and nonsteroidal anti-inflammatory drugs (NSAIDs), and sulfonamides account for 80% of allergic or pseudoallergic reactions.

Drug Exposure

Cutaneous application of a drug is generally considered to be associated with the greatest risk for sensitizing patients (47). In fact, penicillin, sulfonamides, and antihistamines are no longer used topically because of this potential. The adjuvant effect of some intramuscular preparations may increase the risk for sensitization; for example, the incidence of reactions to benzathine penicillin is higher than other penicillin preparations. The intravenous route may be the least likely to sensitize patients.

Once a patient is sensitized, the difference in reaction rates between oral and parenteral drug administration is likely related to the rate of drug administration. Anaphylaxis is less common after oral administration of a drug, although severe reactions have occurred. For other allergic drug reactions, the evidence supporting oral administration is less clear.

The dose and duration of treatment appear to affect the development of a drug-specific immunologic response. In drug-induced lupus erythematosus (DIL), the dose and duration of hydralazine therapy are important factors. Penicillin-induced hemolytic anemia follows high, sustained levels of drug therapy.

There is currently evidence that the frequency of drug administration affects the likelihood of sensitization (48). Thus, frequent courses of treatment are more likely to elicit an allergic reaction as is interrupted therapy. The longer the intervals between therapy, the less likely there will be an allergic reaction.

Patient-related Factors

Age and Gender

There is a general impression that children are less likely to become sensitized to drugs than adults. However, serious allergic drug reactions do occur in children. Some confusion may arise in that the rash associated with a viral illness in children may incorrectly be ascribed to an antibiotic being administered as

TABLE 17A.5   RISK FACTORS FOR DRUG ALLERGY

Drug- and Treatment-Related Factors

Nature of the drug
  Immunologic reactivity
  Nonimmunologic activity

Drug exposure
  Route of administration
  Dose, duration, and frequency of treatment

Patient-Related Factors

Age and gender

Genetic factors
  Role of atopy
  Acetylator status
  Human leukocyte antigen type
  Familial drug allergy

Prior drug reactions
  Persistence of drug-immune response
  Cross-sensitization
  Multiple drug allergy syndrome

Concurrent medical illness

Asthma
Cystic fibrosis
Epstein-Barr viral infection
Human immunodeficiency virus-infected
  patients

Concurrent medical therapy

β-Adrenergic receptor blocking agents

---

treatment. Women are reported to have a higher incidence of ADRs than men (49,50).

Genetic Factors

Allergic drug reactions occur in only a small percentage of individuals treated with a given drug. It is likely that many factors, both genetic and environmental, are involved in determining which individuals in a large random population will develop an allergic reaction to a given drug.

Patients with a history of allergic rhinitis, asthma, or atopic dermatitis (*the atopic constitution*) are not at increased risk for being sensitized to drugs compared with the general population (47). However, it does appear that atopic patients are more likely to develop pseudoallergic reactions, especially to RCM (51).

The rate of metabolism of a drug may influence the prevalence of sensitization. Individuals who are genetically *slow acetylators* are more likely to develop DIL associated with the administration of hydralazine and procainamide (52,53). Adverse reactions to sulfonamides may be more severe among slow acetylators (54).

Specific *human leukocyte antigen (HLA)* genes have been associated with the risk for drug allergy. The susceptibility for drug-induced nephropathy in patients with rheumatoid arthritis treated with gold salts or penicillamine is associated with the HLA-DRw3 and HLA-B8 phenotypes respectively (55). In addition, specific HLA genes have been associated with hydralazine-induced lupus erythematosus, levamisole-induced agranulocytosis, and sulfonamide-induced toxic epidermal necrolysis (TEN) (56). In a Han Chinese population, studies have shown a strong association between carbamazapime-induced SJS and HLA-B*1502 (57) as well as a strong association between HLA-B*5801 and severe cutaneous drug reactions (SJS and TEN) due to allopurinol (58). An association between HLA-B*5201 and hypersensitivity to abacavir, a potent reverse transcriptase inhibitor, was shown in an HIV population in Western Australia (59). This has been confirmed in several other cohort studies (60–62); however, this association has not been found in black populations (61).

The possibility of *familial drug allergy* has been reported recently (56). Among adolescents whose parents had sustained an allergic reaction to antibiotics, 25.6% experienced an allergic reaction to an antimicrobial agent, whereas only 1.7% reacted when their parents tolerated antibiotics without an allergic reaction.

Prior Drug Reactions

Undoubtedly, the most important risk factor is a history of a prior hypersensitivity reaction to a drug being considered for treatment or one that may be immunochemically similar. However, drug hypersensitivity may not persist indefinitely. It is well established that, after an allergic reaction to penicillin, the half-life of antipenicilloyl IgE antibodies in serum ranges from 55 days to an indeterminate, long interval in excess of 2,000 days (47). Ten years after an immediate-type reaction to penicillin, only about 20% of individuals are still skin test positive.

There may be *cross-sensitization* between drugs. The likelihood of cross-reactivity among the various sulfonamide groups (antibacterials, sulfonylureas, diuretics) is an issue that has not been resolved. There is little supporting evidence in the medical literature that cross-sensitization is a significant problem. Patients who have demonstrated drug hypersensitivity in the past appear to have an increased tendency to develop sensitivity to new drugs. Penicillin-allergic patients have about a 10-fold increased risk for an allergic reaction to non–β-lactam antimicrobial drugs (63,64). The reactions were not restricted to immediate-type hypersensitivity. Fifty-seven percent reacted to a sulfonamide. With the exception of the aminoglycosides, reaction rates were much higher than expected in all other antibiotic classes, including erythromycin. Among children with multiple antibiotic sensitivities by history, 26% had positive penicillin skin tests (65). These observations suggest that such patients are prone to react to haptenating drugs during an infection (66), possibly due to the "danger" signals induced by infection. Obviously, such patients present difficult clinical management problems.

Concurrent Medical Illness

Although atopy does not predispose to the development of IgE-mediated drug hypersensitivity, it appears to be a risk factor for more severe reactions once sensitivity has occurred, especially in asthmatic patients (46,47). Children with cystic fibrosis are more likely to experience allergic drug reactions, especially during drug desensitization (67). Maculopapular rashes following the administration of ampicillin occur more frequently during Epstein-Barr viral infections and among patients with lymphatic leukemia (68).

Immune deficiency is associated with an increased frequency of adverse drug reactions, many of which appear to be allergic in nature. Patients who are immunosuppressed may become deficient in regulatory T lymphocytes that control IgE-antibody synthesis.

In recent years, much attention has been given to adverse drug reactions, in particular hypersensitivity, which occur with a much higher frequency among human immunodeficiency virus (HIV)-infected patients than among patients who are HIV seronegative (69,70). A retrospective study comparing *Pneumocystis carinii* pneumonia (PCP) in patients with acquired immunodeficiency syndrome (AIDS) to a similar pneumonia in patients with other underlying immunosuppressive conditions reported adverse reactions to trimethoprim-sulfamethoxazole (TMP-SMX) in 65% of AIDS patients compared with 12% of patients with other immunosuppressive diseases, suggesting the abnormality may be due to the HIV infection (71). Slow acetylator phenotype is a risk factor for TMP-SMX in HIV-negative patients but not HIV-positive patients (72–74). TMP-SMX has been associated with rash, fever, and hematologic disturbances and, less frequently, with more severe reactions such as Stevens-Johnson syndrome (SJS), toxic epidermal necrolysis, and anaphylactic reactions. Also, pentamidine, antituberculosis regimens containing isoniazid and rifampin, amoxicillin-clavulanate, and clindamycin have been associated with an increased incidence of adverse drug reactions, some of which may involve an allergic mechanism. It also appears that progression of HIV disease to a more advanced stage confers an increased risk for hypersensitivity reactions (69).

Concurrent Medical Therapy

Some medications may alter the risk and severity of reactions to drugs. Patients treated with β-adrenergic blocking agents, even timolol maleate ophthalmic solution, may be more susceptible to, and prove to be more refractory to, treatment of drug-induced anaphylaxis, requiring greater fluid resuscitation and possibly more epinephrine to overcome the β blockade (75).

■ CLINICAL CLASSIFICATION OF ALLERGIC REACTIONS TO DRUGS

A useful classification is based primarily on the clinical presentation or manifestations of such reactions. The presumption of allergy is based on clinical criteria cited earlier (Table 17A.3). Table 17A.6 provides an overview of a clinical classification based on organ systems involved; namely, generalized multisystem involvement and predominantly organ-specific responses.

What follows is a brief discussion of each of these clinical entities, including a list of most commonly implicated drugs. Detailed lists of implicated drugs appear in periodic literature reviews (76,77).

Generalized or Multisystem Involvement

Immediate Generalized Reactions

The acute systemic reactions are among the most urgent of drug-related events. Greenberger has used the term *immediate generalized reactions* to underscore the fact that many are not IgE-mediated (78). Drug-induced *anaphylaxis* should be reserved for a systemic reaction proved to be IgE-mediated. Drug-induced *anaphylactoid reactions* are clinically indistinguishable from anaphylaxis but occur through IgE-independent mechanisms. Both ultimately result in the release of potent vasoactive and inflammatory mediators from mast cells and basophils.

In a series of 32,812 continuously monitored patients, such reactions occurred in 12 patients (0.04%), and there were 2 deaths (79). Because anaphylaxis is more likely to be reported when a fatality occurs, its prevalence may be underestimated. Drug-induced anaphylaxis does not appear to confer increased risk for such generalized reactions to allergens from other sources (80).

Most reactions occur within 30 minutes, and death may ensue within minutes. In a retrospective study by Pumphrey in the United Kingdom investigating fatalities associated with anaphylaxis, more than one-half of the fatal reactions were iatrogenic. The majority of these reactions were due to intravenous (IV) medications and took 5 minutes or less from the time of administration to the time of arrest (81). Anaphylaxis occurs most commonly after parenteral administration, but it has also followed oral, percutaneous, and respiratory exposure. Symptoms usually subside rapidly with

TABLE 17A.6   CLINICAL CLASSIFICATION OF ALLERGIC REACTIONS TO DRUGS

Generalized or multisystem involvement

Immediate generalized reactions
  Anaphylaxis (IgE-mediated reactions)
  Anaphylactoid reactions (IgE-independent)

Serum sickness and serum sickness–like reactions

Drug fever

Drug-induced autoimmunity
  Reactions simulating systemic lupus
    erythematosus
  Other reactions

Hypersensitivity vasculitis

Reactions predominantly organ-specific

Dermatologic manifestations[a]

Pulmonary manifestations
  Asthma
  Pulmonary infiltrates with eosinophilia
  Pneumonitis and fibrosis
  Noncardiogenic pulmonary edema

Hematologic manifestations

  Eosinophilia

  Drug-induced immune cytopenias
    Thrombocytopenia
    Hemolytic anemia
    Agranulocytosis

Hepatic manifestations
  Cholestasis
  Hepatocellular damage
  Mixed pattern

Renal manifestations
  Glomerulonephritis
  Nephrotic syndrome
  Acute interstitial nephritis

Lymphoid system manifestations
  Pseudolymphoma
  Infectious mononucleosis–like syndrome

Cardiac manifestations

Neurologic manifestations

[a]A separate listing of dermatologic manifestations is included in that section (Table 17A.8).

IgE, immunoglobulin E.

TABLE 17A.7   DRUGS IMPLICATED IN IMMEDIATE GENERALIZED REACTIONS

Anaphylaxis (IgE-mediated)

β-Lactam antibiotics

Allergen extracts

Heterologous antisera

Insulin

Vaccines (egg-based)

Streptokinase

Chymopapain

L-Asparaginase

Cisplatin

Carboplatin

Latex[a]

Anaphylactoid (IgE-independent)

Radiocontrast material

Aspirin

Nonsteroidal anti-inflammatory drugs

Dextran and iron dextran

Anesthetic drugs
  Induction agents[b]
  Muscle relaxants[b]

Protamine[b]

Vancomycin[b]

Ciprofloxacin

Paclitaxel (Taxol)

[a]Not a drug per se, but often an important consideration in a medical setting.

[b]Some reactions may be mediated by IgE antibodies.

IgE, immunoglobulin E.

appropriate treatment, but may last 24 hours or longer, and recurrent symptoms may appear several hours after apparent resolution of the reaction. As a rule, the severity of the reaction decreases with increasing time between exposure to the drug and onset of symptoms. Death is usually due to cardiovascular collapse or respiratory obstruction, especially laryngeal or upper airway edema. Although most reactions do not terminate fatally, the potential for such must be borne in mind, and the attending physician must respond immediately with appropriate treatment.

Table 17A.7 summarizes agents most frequently associated with immediate generalized reactions. In some situations, drugs, such as general anesthetic agents and vancomycin, which are primarily direct mast cell mediator releasers, can produce an IgE-mediated reaction (42,82). This distinction has clinical relevance in that IgE-independent reactions may be prevented or modified by pretreatment with corticosteroids and antihistamines, whereas such protection from drug-induced IgE-mediated reactions is less likely. In the latter situation, when the drug is medically necessary, desensitization is an option.

The β-lactam antibiotics, notably penicillin, are by far the most common causes of drug-induced anaphylaxis. Essentially all β-lactam anaphylactic reactions are IgE-mediated. Immediate generalized reactions to other antibiotics occur but are relatively uncommon. Recently, anaphylactoid reactions have been reported after the administration of ciprofloxacin and norfloxacin (83).

Cancer chemotherapeutic agents have been associated with hypersensitivity reactions, most commonly type I immediate generalized reactions (84). L-Asparaginase has the highest risk for such reactions. Serious anaphylactic reactions with respiratory distress and hypotension occur in about 10% of patients treated. It is likely that most of these reactions are IgE-mediated. However, skin testing appears to be of no value in predicting a reaction because there are both false-positive and false-negative results. Therefore, one must be prepared to treat anaphylaxis with each dose. For those reacting to L-asparaginase derived from *Escherichia coli*, one derived from *Erwinia chyoanthermia* (a plant pathogen) or a modified asparaginase (pegaspargase) may be a clinically effective substitute. Cisplatin and carboplatin are second only to L-asparaginase in producing such reactions. Skin testing with these agents appears to have predictive value, and desensitization has been successful when these drugs are medically necessary (85). The initial use of paclitaxel (Taxol) to treat ovarian and breast cancer was associated with a 10% risk for anaphylactoid reactions. However, with premedication and lengthening of the infusion time, the risk is significantly reduced (86). All other antitumor drugs, except altretamine, the nitrosoureas, and dactinomycin, have occasionally been associated with hypersensitivity reactions (84). Some appear to be IgE mediated, but most are probably IgE independent.

Anaphylactic and anaphylactoid reactions occurring during the perioperative period have received increased attention. The evaluation and detection of these reactions is complicated by the use of multiple medications and the fact that patients are often unconscious and draped, which may mask the early signs and symptoms of an immediate generalized reaction (87). During anesthesia, the only feature observed may be cardiovascular collapse (88) or airway obstruction. Cyanosis due to oxygen desaturation may be noted. One large multicenter study indicated that 70% of cases were due to muscle relaxants and 12% were due to latex (89). Other agents, such as intravenous induction drugs, plasma volume expanders (dextran), opioid analgesics and antibiotics, also require consideration. With the increased use of cardiopulmonary bypass surgery, the incidence of protamine-induced immediate life-threatening reactions has risen (90). Anaphylaxis to ethylene oxide-sterilized devices has been described; hence, such devices used during anesthesia could potentially cause anaphylaxis (91).

Psyllium seed is an active ingredient of several bulk laxatives, and has been responsible for asthma following inhalation and anaphylaxis after ingestion, particularly in atopic subjects (92). Anaphylactoid reactions following IV fluorescein may be modified by pretreatment with corticosteroids and antihistamines (93). Of patients reacting to iron-dextran, 0.6% had a life-threatening anaphylactoid reaction (94). Anaphylactoid reactions may also be caused by blood and blood products through the activation of complement and the production of anaphylatoxins. Adverse reactions to monoclonal antibodies include immediate generalized manifestations, but the mechanism for such remains unclear (95). Most appear not to be IgE mediated (96) and protocols including rapid desensitization have been established for managing these reactions (97,98).

If one surveys the medical literature, one will find that virtually all drugs, including corticosteroids, tetracycline, cromolyn, erythromycin, and cimetidine, have been implicated in such immediate generalized reactions. However, these infrequent reports should not be a reason to withhold essential medication.

Serum Sickness and Serum Sickness–like Reactions

Serum sickness results from the administration of heterologous (often equine) antisera and is the human equivalent of immune complex-mediated serum sickness observed in experimental animals (99). A serum sickness–like illness has been attributed to a number of nonprotein drugs, notably the β-lactam antibiotics. These reactions are usually self-limited and the outcome favorable, but H_1 blockers and prednisone may be needed.

With effective immunization procedures, antimicrobial therapy, and the availability of human antitoxins, the incidence of serum sickness has declined. Currently, heterologous antisera are still used to counteract potent toxins such as snake venoms, black widow and brown recluse spider venom, botulism, and gas gangrene toxins as well as to treat diphtheria and rabies. Equine and rabbit antisera, used as antilymphocyte or antithymocyte globulins and as monoclonal antibodies for immunomodulation and cancer treatment, may cause serum sickness (100). Serum sickness has also been reported in patients receiving streptokinase (101).

β-Lactam antibiotics are considered to be the most common nonserum causes of serum sickness–like reactions (102). One literature review did not support this assertion (103). In fact, such reactions appear to be quite infrequent, with an incidence of 1.8 per 100,000 prescriptions of cefaclor and 1 per 10 million for amoxicillin and cephalexin (104). Other drugs occasionally incriminated include ciprofloxacin, metronidazole, streptomycin, sulfonamides, allopurinol, carbamazepine, hydantoins, methimazole, phenylbutazone, propanolol, and thiouracil. It should be noted that the criteria for diagnosis might not be uniform for each drug.

The onset of serum sickness typically begins 6 to 21 days after administration of the causative agent. The latent period reflects the time required for the production of antibodies. The onset of symptoms coincides with the development of immune complexes. Among previously immunized individuals, the reaction may begin within 2 to 4 days following administration of the inciting agent. The manifestations include fever and malaise, skin eruptions, joint symptoms, and lymphadenopathy.

There is no laboratory finding specific for the diagnosis of serum sickness or serum sickness–like reactions. Laboratory abnormalities may be helpful, if present. The erythrocyte sedimentation rate may be elevated, although it has been noted to be normal or low (102). There may be a transient leukopenia or leukocytosis during the acute phase (79,105.) Plasmacytosis may occasionally be present; in fact, serum sickness is one of the few illnesses in which plasma cells may be seen in the peripheral blood (106). The urinalysis may reveal slight proteinuria, hyaline casts, hemoglobinuria, and microscopic hematuria. However, nitrogen retention is rare. Transaminases and serum creatinine may be transiently elevated (100).

Serum concentrations of C3, C4, and total hemolytic complement are depressed, providing some evidence that an immune complex mechanism is operative. These may rapidly return to normal. Immune complex and elevated plasma concentrations of C3a and C5a anaphylatoxins have been documented (107).

The prognosis for complete recovery is excellent. The symptoms may be mild, lasting only a few days, or quite severe, persisting for several weeks or longer.

Antihistamines control urticaria. If symptoms are severe, corticosteroids (e.g., prednisone, 40 mg/day for 1 week and then taper) are indicated. However, corticosteroids do not prevent serum sickness, as noted in patients receiving antithymocyte globulin (100). Skin testing with foreign antisera is routinely performed to avoid anaphylaxis with future use of foreign serum.

Drug Fever

Fever is a well-known drug hypersensitivity reaction. An immunologic mechanism is often suspected. Fever may be the sole manifestation of drug hypersensitivity and is particularly perplexing in a clinical situation in which a patient is being treated for an infection.

The height of the temperature does not distinguish drug fever, and there does not appear to be any fever pattern typical of this entity. Although a distinct disparity between the recorded febrile response and the relative well-being of the patient has been emphasized, clearly such individuals may be quite ill with high fever and shaking chills. Drug fever may be the sole manifestation of a drug allergy but is commonly seen with other signs of drug hypersensitivity such as rash, elevated liver enzymes, and eosinophils.

Laboratory studies usually reveal leukocytosis with a shift to the left, thus mimicking an infectious process.

Mild eosinophilia may be present. An elevated erythrocyte sedimentation rate and abnormal liver function tests are present in most cases.

The most consistent feature of drug fever is prompt defervescence, usually within 48 to 72 hours after withdrawal of the offending agent. Subsequent readministration of the drug produces fever, and occasionally chills, within a matter of hours.

In general, the diagnosis of drug fever is one of exclusion after eliminating other potential causes of the febrile reaction. Prompt recognition of drug fever is essential. If not appreciated, patients may be subjected to multiple diagnostic procedures and inappropriate treatment. Of greater concern is the possibility that the reaction may become more generalized with resultant tissue damage. Autopsies on patients who died during drug fever show arteritis and focal necrosis in many organs, such as myocardium, lung, and liver.

Drug-induced Autoimmunity

Drug-induced Lupus Erythematosus

DIL is the most familiar drug-induced autoimmune disease, in part because systemic lupus erythematosus (SLE) remains the prototype of autoimmunity. DIL is termed *autoimmune* because of its association with the development of antinuclear antibodies (ANAs). However, these same autoantibodies are found frequently in the absence of frank disease. An excellent review of drug-induced autoimmunity appears elsewhere (108) as well as a comprehensive review of the medications implicated (109).

Convincing evidence for DIL first appeared in 1953 after the introduction of hydralazine for treatment of hypertension (110) although it was first described in 1945 associated with sulfadiazine (111). Procainamide-induced lupus was first reported in 1962 and is now the most common cause of DIL in the United States (112). These drugs have also been the best studied. Other agents for which there has been definite proof of an association include isoniazid, chlorpromazine, methyldopa, quinidine, and minocycline. Another group of drugs probably associated with the syndrome includes many anticonvulsants, β blockers, antithyroid drugs, penicillamine, sulfasalazine, and lithium. There have been case reports of DIL associated with monoclonal antibodies such as infliximab and etanercept (113,114) and an ANA-negative, anti-histone-positive DIL has been described with lisinopril (115). There are case reports linking statins such as lovastatin, fluvastatin, and atorvastatin with DIL but with varying clinical manifestations including pneumonitis, and cutaneous manifestations (116).

The incidence of DIL is not precisely known. In a recent survey of patients with lupus erythematosus seen in a private practice, 3% had DIL (117). The estimated incidence is 15,000 to 20,000 cases per year (118). In contrast to SLE, patients with DIL tend to be older and males and females are equally affected (119). Patients with idiopathic SLE do not appear to be at increased risk from drugs implicated in DIL (120). Identified risk factors for developing DIL include HLA-DR4 (121), HLA-DR*0301 (122), slow acetylator status (123), and complement C4 null allele (124).

Fever, malaise, arthralgias, myalgias, pleurisy, and slight weight loss may appear acutely in a patient receiving an implicated drug. Pleuropericardial manifestations, such as pleurisy, pleural effusions, pulmonary infiltrates, pericarditis, and pericardial effusions, are more often seen in patients taking procainamide. Unlike idiopathic SLE, the classic butterfly malar rash, discoid lesions, oral mucosal ulcers, Raynaud phenomenon, alopecia, and renal and central nervous system disease are unusual in DIL. Glomerulonephritis has occasionally been reported in hydralazine-induced lupus. As a rule, DIL is a milder disease than idiopathic SLE. Because many clinical features are nonspecific, the presence of ANAs (homogenous pattern) or antihistone antibodies is essential in the diagnosis of drug-induced disease.

Clinical symptoms usually do not appear for many months after institution of drug treatment. Clinical features of DIL usually subside within days to weeks after the offending drug is discontinued. In an occasional patient, the symptoms may persist or recur over several months before disappearing. ANAs often disappear in a few weeks to months but may persist for 1 year or longer. Mild symptoms may be managed with NSAIDs; more severe disease may require corticosteroid treatment.

If no satisfactory alternative drug is available and treatment is essential, the minimum effective dose of the drug and corticosteroids may be given simultaneously with caution and careful observation. With respect to procainamide, DIL can be prevented by giving N-acetylprocainamide, the major acetylated metabolite of procainamide. In fact, remission of procainamide-induced lupus has occurred when patients were switched to N-acetylprocainamide therapy (125,126). Finally, there are no data to suggest that the presence of ANAs necessitates discontinuance of the drug in asymptomatic patients. The low probability of clinical symptoms in seroreactors and the fact that major organs are usually spared in DIL support this recommendation (127).

Other Drug-induced Autoimmune Disorders

In addition to DIL, D-penicillamine has been associated with several other autoimmune syndromes, such as myasthenia gravis, polymyositis and dermatomyositis, pemphigus and pemphigoid, membranous glomerulonephritis, Goodpasture syndrome, and immune cytopenias (128). It has been suggested that by binding to cell membranes as a hapten, penicillamine could induce an autologous T-cell reaction, B-cell proliferation, autoantibodies, and autoimmune disorders (129).

Hypersensitivity Vasculitis

Vasculitis is a condition that is characterized by inflammation and necrosis of blood vessels. Organs or systems with a rich supply of blood vessels are most often involved. Thus, the skin is often involved in vasculitic syndromes. In the systemic necrotizing vasculitis group (polyarteritis nodosa, allergic granulomatosis of Churg-Strauss) and granulomatous vasculitides (Wegener's granulomatosis, lymphomatoid granulomatosis, giant cell arteritides), cutaneous involvement is not as common a presenting feature as seen in the hypersensitivity vasculitides (HSV). Also, drugs do not appear to be implicated in the systemic necrotizing and granulomatous vasculitic syndromes.

Drugs appear to be responsible for or associated with a significant number of cases of HSV (130). These may occur at any age, but the average age of onset is in the fifth decade (131). The older patient is more likely to be taking medications that have been associated with this syndrome, for example, diuretics and cardiac drugs. Other frequently implicated agents include penicillin, sulfonamides, thiouracils, hydantoins, iodides, and allopurinol. Allopurinol administration, particularly in association with renal compromise and concomitant thiazide therapy, has produced a vasculitic syndrome manifested by fever, malaise, rash, hepatocellular injury, renal failure, leukocytosis, and eosinophilia. The mortality rate approaches 25% (132). However, in many cases of HSV, no cause is ever identified. Fortunately, idiopathic cases tend to be self-limited.

The most common clinical feature of HSV is palpable purpura, and the skin may be the only site where vasculitis is recognized. The lesions occur in recurrent crops of varying size and number and are usually distributed in a symmetric pattern on the lower extremities and sacral area. Fever, malaise, myalgia, and anorexia may accompany the appearance of skin lesions. Usually, only cutaneous involvement occurs in drug-induced HSV, but glomerulonephritis, arthralgias or arthritis, abdominal pain and gastrointestinal bleeding, pulmonary infiltrates, and peripheral neuropathy are occasionally present.

The diagnosis of HSV is established by skin biopsy of a lesion demonstrating characteristic neutrophilic infiltrate of the blood vessel wall terminating in necrosis, leukocytoclasis (nuclear dust or fragmentation of nuclei), fibrinoid changes, and extravasation of erythrocytes. This inflammation involves small blood vessels, predominantly postcapillary venules. Recent studies indicate that in drug-induced vasculitis, multispecific antinuclear cytoplasmic antibody (ANCA) (ANCA positive to several neutrophil antigens) is commonly found. This is distinguished from ANCA to only one neutrophil antigen as is seen with idiopathic vasculitis and may serve to distinguish between the two (133).

When a patient presents with palpable purpura and has started a drug within the previous few months, consideration should be given to stopping that agent. Generally, the prognosis for HSV is excellent, and elimination of the offending agent, if one exists, usually suffices for therapy. For a minority of patients who have persistent lesions or significant involvement of other organ systems, corticosteroids are indicated.

Predominantly Organ-specific Reactions

Dermatologic Manifestations

Cutaneous eruptions are the most frequent manifestations of adverse drug reactions and occur in 2% to 3% of hospitalized inpatients (134). The offending drug could be identified in most cases and in one study was confirmed by drug challenges in 62% of patients (135). Frequently implicated agents include β-lactam antibiotics (especially ampicillin and amoxicillin), sulfonamides (especially TMP-SMX), NSAIDs, anticonvulsants, and central nervous system depressants (136).

Drug eruptions are most often exanthematous or morbilliform in nature. Most are of mild or moderate severity, often fade within a few days, and pose no threat to life or subsequent health. On rare occasions, such drug eruptions may be severe or even life-threatening, for example, SJS and toxic epidermal necrolysis. Some more typical features of a drug-induced eruption include an acute onset within 1 to 2 weeks after drug exposure, symmetric distribution, predominant truncal involvement, brilliant coloration, and pruritus. Features that suggest that a reaction is serious include the presence of urticaria, blisters, mucosal involvement, facial edema, ulcerations, palpable purpura, fever, lymphadenopathy, and eosinophilia (137). The presence of these usually necessitates prompt withdrawal of the offending drug.

Table 17A.8 provides a list of recognizable cutaneous eruptions frequently induced by drugs, presumably on an immunologic basis.

Exanthematous or Morbilliform Eruptions

Exanthematous or morbilliform eruptions are the most common drug-induced eruptions and may be difficult to distinguish from viral exanthems. The rash may be predominantly erythematous, maculopapular, or morbilliform (measles-like), and often begins on the trunk or in areas of pressure, for example, the backs of bedridden patients. Pruritus is variable or minimal. Occasionally, pruritus may be an early symptom, preceding the development of cutaneous manifestations. Gold salts and sulfonamides have been associated with pruritus as an isolated feature. This rarely progresses to overt

TABLE 17A.8 DRUG-INDUCED CUTANEOUS MANIFESTATIONS

Most Frequent

Exanthematous or morbilliform eruptions

Urticaria and angioedema

Contact dermatitis[a]
  Allergic eczematous contact dermatitis
  Systemic eczematous "contact-type" dermatitis

Less Frequent

Fixed drug eruptions

Erythema multiforme–like eruptions
  Stevens-Johnson syndrome

Generalized exfoliative dermatitis

Photosensitivity

Uncommon

Purpuric eruptions

Toxic epidermal necrolysis (Lyell syndrome)

Erythema nodosum

Acute generalized exanthematous pustulosis

[a]Contact dermatitis is still listed among the top three, but there is evidence that this problem may be decreasing with the purposeful avoidance of topical sensitizers.

exfoliation, although this is possible (138). Usually, this drug-induced eruption appears within a week or so after institution of treatment. Unlike the generally benign nature of this adverse drug reaction, a syndrome with a similar rash and fever, often with hepatitis, arthralgias, lymphadenopathy, and eosinophilia, has been termed *hypersensitivity syndrome* (137), now referred to as drug rash with eosinophilia and systemic symptoms (DRESS) (139). It has a relatively later onset (2 to 6 weeks after initiation of treatment), evolves slowly, and may be difficult to distinguish from drug-induced vasculitis. Anticonvulsants, sulfonamides, and allopurinol are the most frequent causes of DRESS although other drugs such as antituberculous medication has been reported (140). Recovery is usually complete, but the rash and hepatitis may persist for weeks.

Urticaria and Angioedema

Urticaria with or without angioedema is the second most frequent drug-induced eruption. It may occur alone or may be part of an immediate generalized reaction, such as anaphylaxis, or serum sickness. An allergic IgE-mediated mechanism is often suspected, but it may be the result of a pseudoallergic reaction. One study reported that β-lactam antibiotics (through an allergic mechanism) accounted for one-third, and NSAIDs (through a pseudoallergic mechanism) accounted for another third, of drug-induced urticarial reactions (141).

Often, urticaria appears shortly after drug therapy is initiated, but its appearance may be delayed for days to weeks. Usually, individual urticarial lesions do not persist much longer than 24 hours, but new lesions may continue to appear in different areas of the body for 1 to 2 weeks. If the individual lesions last longer than 24 hours, or if the rash persists for much longer than 2 weeks, the possibility of another diagnosis such as urticarial vasculitis should be considered. A drug etiology should be considered in any patient with chronic urticaria, which is defined as lasting more than 6 weeks.

Angioedema is most often associated with urticaria, but it may occur alone. Angiotensin-converting enzyme (ACE) inhibitors are responsible for most cases of angioedema requiring hospitalization (142). The risk for angioedema is estimated to be between 0.1% and 0.2% in patients receiving such therapy (143). Patients with ididopathic angioedema are at increased risk of ACE inhibitor-induced angioedema as are African Americans and women; therefore, caution should be used in treating these populations (144,145). The angioedema commonly involves the face and oropharyngeal tissues and may result in acute airway obstruction necessitating emergency intervention. Most episodes occur within the first week or so of therapy, but there are occasional reports of angioedema as long as 2 years after initiation of treatment (146). The mechanism of angioedema is probably ACE inhibitor potentiation of bradykinin production (147), although this is unclear as angioedema has been reported with angiotensin II receptor blockers (ARBs) as well (148,149). Because treatment with epinephrine, antihistamines, and corticosteroids may be ineffective, the physician must be aware of the potential for airway compromise and the possible need for early airway intervention measures. When angioedema follows the use of any one of these agents, treatment with any ACE inhibitor should be avoided. ARBs may be a good alternative. Angioedema has been reported with these although the incidence is much lower (148,149).

Allergic Contact Dermatitis

Allergic contact dermatitis is produced by medications or by components of the drug delivery system applied topically to the skin and is an example of a type IV cell-mediated immune reaction (Table 17A.4). Following topical sensitization, the contact dermatitis may be elicited by subsequent topical application. The appearance of the skin reaction and diagnosis by patch testing is similar to allergic contact dermatitis from other causes. The diagnosis should be suspected when the condition for which the topical preparation is being applied, such as eczema, fails to improve or worsens. Patients at increased risk for allergic contact dermatitis include those with stasis dermatitis, leg ulcers, perianal dermatitis, and hand eczema (150). Common offenders include neomycin, benzocaine, and ethylenediamine. Less common sensitizers include paraben esters, thimerosal, antihistamines, bacitracin, and, rarely, sunscreens and topical corticosteroids (151).

Neomycin is the most widely used topical antibiotic and has become the most sensitizing of all antibacterial preparations. Other aminoglycosides (e.g., streptomycin, kanamycin, gentamicin, tobramycin, amikacin, and netilmicin) may cross-react with neomycin, but this is variable (152). Neomycin-allergic patients may develop a systemic "contact-type" dermatitis when exposed to some of these drugs systemically. Many neomycin-allergic patients also react to bacitracin. In addition to neomycin, other topical antibiotics that are frequent sensitizers include penicillin, sulfonamides, chloramphenicol, and hydroxyquinolones. For this reason, they are seldom prescribed in the United States.

Benzocaine, a para-aminobenzoic acid (PABA) derivative, is the most common topical anesthetic associated with allergic contact dermatitis. It is found in many nonprescription preparations, such as sunburn and poison ivy remedies, topical analgesics, throat lozenges, and hemorrhoid preparations. In some benzocaine-sensitive patients, there may be cross-reactivity with other local anesthetics that are based on PABA esters, such as procaine, butacaine, and tetracaine. Suitable alternatives are the local anesthetics based on an amide structure, such as lidocaine, mepivacaine, and bupivacaine. Such individuals may also react to other para-amino compounds, such as some hair dyes (paraphenylenediamine), PABA-containing sunscreens, aniline dyes, and sulfonamides.

Ethylenediamine, a stabilizer used in some antibiotics, corticosteroids, and nystatin-containing combination creams, is a common sensitizer. Once sensitized to ethylenediamine topically, a patient may experience widespread dermatitis following the systemic administration of medicaments that contain ethylenediamine, such as aminophylline, hydroxyzine, and tripelennamine (153), however this is not common.

Among the less-frequent topical sensitizers, paraben esters, used as preservatives in topical corticosteroid creams, were thought to be important; however, a recent study failed to support this assertion (154). Thimerosal (Merthiolate) is used topically as an antiseptic and also as a preservative. In one study, 7.5% of patients had a positive patch test with this material. Not all such patients are mercury allergic; many react to the thiosalicylic moiety. Local and even systemic reactions have been ascribed to thimerosal used as a preservative in some vaccines (155). However, if a patient's allergic history to thimerosal is topical sensitization only, skin testing to the vaccine followed by cautious test dosing may be considered. Systemic administration of BB: antihistamines is rarely, if ever, associated with an allergic reaction; however, topical antihistamines are potential sensitizers, and their use should be avoided. Most instances of allergic contact dermatitis attributed to topical corticosteroids are due to the vehicle, not to the

steroid itself. Patch testing with the highest concentration of the steroid ointment may help identify whether
the steroid itself or the vehicle constituent is responsible. Some attention has already been focused on systemic eczematous contact-type dermatitis.

In summary, physicians should attempt to avoid or
minimize the use of common sensitizers, such as neomycin and benzocaine, in the treatment of patients with
chronic dermatoses such as stasis dermatitis and hand
eczema. A more comprehensive review of drug-induced
allergic contact dermatitis is found elsewhere (156) and
in Chapter 30.

Fixed Drug Eruptions

Fixed drug eruptions, in contrast to most other drug-
induced dermatoses, are considered to be pathognomonic of drug hypersensitivity. Men are more frequently affected than women, and ages 20 to 40 are
most common (157,158), but children may also be
affected (159,160). The term *fixed* relates to the fact that
these lesions tend to recur in the same sites each time
the specific drug is administered. On occasion, the dermatitis may flare with antigenically related and even
unrelated substances.

The characteristic lesion is well delineated and
round or oval; it varies in size from a few millimeters to
25 cm to 30 cm. Edema appears initially, followed by
erythema, which then darkens to become a deeply colored, reddish purple, dense raised lesion. On occasion,
the lesions may be eczematous, urticarial, vesiculobul-
lous, hemorrhagic, or nodular. Lesions are most common on the lips and genitals but may occur anywhere
on the skin or mucous membranes (161,162). Usually,
a solitary lesion is present, but the lesions may be more
numerous, and additional ones may develop with subsequent administration of the drug. The length of time
from reexposure to the drug to the onset of symptoms
is 30 minutes to 8 hours (mean, 2.1 hours). The lesions
usually resolve within 2 to 3 weeks after drug withdrawal, leaving transient desquamation and residual
hyperpigmentation.

The mechanism is unknown, but the histopathology
is consistent with T cell-mediated destruction of epidermal cells, resulting in keratinocyte damage (163).
Recent studies point to a possible role for $CD8^+$ T cell
infiltration mediating keratinocyte apoptosis through a
Fas/Fas ligand mechanism (164). Commonly implicated drugs include phenolphthalein, barbiturates, sulfonamides, tetracycline, and NSAIDs although many
drugs have been implicated such as antifungals, antie-
leptics, narcotics, and many antibiotics (165). Drugs
most commonly implicated vary depending on the
country, the availability of drugs, and their pattern of
use (166,167). In addition, some authors believe the
location of lesions may be specific to the drug (168).

Treatment is usually not required after the offending
drug has been withdrawn because most fixed drug

eruptions are mild and not associated with significant
symptoms. Corticosteroids may decrease the severity of
the reaction without changing the course of the dermatitis (159).

Acute Generalized Exanthematous Pustulosis

Acute generalized exanthematous pustulosis (AGEP) is
an acute eruption of numerous small (less than 5mm),
sterile, mostly nonfollicular pustules in conjunction
with fever more than 38°C and peripheral neutrophil
count greater than $7 \times 10^3/\mu l$. The pustules are subcor-
neal or intraepidermal and appear on an erythemetous,
edematous base, most commonly involve the trunk,
upper extremeties, and main skinfolds such as the neck,
axilla, and groin. Transient renal failure and hypocalce-
mia are not uncommon (169). AGEP can be distinguished histologically from pustular psoriasis and focal
keratinocyte necrosis, vasculitis, perivascular eosin-
phils, as well as dermal edema can be seen on biopsy
(170,171). AGEP is rare and for years was classified as
pustular psoriasis and in 1968 was first thought to be a
separate entity (172) and then better characterized in
1980 (173). Unlike pustular psoriasis, AGEP is most
commonly due to drug hypersensitivity, with antibiotics, in particular aminopenicillins, and diltiazem most
commonly implicated (174). It is self-limited, with skin
eruptions occurring soon after the medication is first
administered (less than 2 days) followed by superficial
desquamation and spontaneous resolution in less than
15 days (171). AGEP is a predominantly neutrophilic
inflammatory process in which drug specific T cells
have been found to play a role (175,176).

Erythema Multiforme–like Eruptions

A useful classification for the heterogeneous syndrome
of erythema multiforme has been suggested (177).
Additional details can be found in Chapter 16. It is often a benign cutaneous illness with or without minimal
mucous membrane involvement and has been designated *erythema multiforme minor* (EM minor). A more
severe cutaneous reaction with marked mucous membrane (at least two mucosal surfaces) involvement and
constitutional symptoms has been termed *erythema
multiforme major* (EM major). SJS has become synonymous with EM major. In addition, some have considered TEN to represent the most severe form of this
disease process, but others believe it should be considered as a separate entity.

EM minor is a mild, self-limited cutaneous illness
characterized by the sudden onset of symmetric erythematous eruptions on the dorsum of the hands and
feet and on the extensor surfaces of the forearms and
legs; palms and soles are commonly involved. Lesions
rarely involve the scalp or face. Truncal involvement is
usually sparse. The rash is minimally painful or pruritic.
It is a relatively common condition in young adults 20 to
40 years of age and is often recurrent in nature. Mucous

membrane involvement is usually limited to the oral cavity. Typically, the lesions begin as red, edematous papules that may resemble urticaria. Some lesions may develop concentric zones of color change, producing the pathognomonic "target" or "iris" lesions. The rash usually resolves in 2 to 4 weeks, leaving some residual postinflammatory hyperpigmentation but no scarring or atrophy. Constitutional symptoms are minimal or absent. The most common cause is believed to be herpes simplex infection, and oral acyclovir has been used to prevent recurrence of EM minor (178).

Most instances of drug-induced erythema multiforme result in more severe manifestations, classified as EM major or SJS. This bullous-erosive form can result in skin loss of up to 10% of the total body surface area (TBSA) and is often preceded by constitutional symptoms of high fever, headache, and malaise. Involvement of mucosal surfaces is a prominent and consistent feature. The cutaneous involvement is more extensive than in EM minor, and there is often more pronounced truncal involvement. Painful oropharyngeal mucous membrane lesions may interfere with nutrition. The vermilion border of the lips becomes denuded and develops serosanguinous crusts, a typical feature of this syndrome. Eighty-five percent of patients develop conjunctival lesions, ranging from hyperemia to extensive pseudomembrane formation. Serious ocular complications include the development of keratitis sicca, corneal erosions, uveitis, and even bulbar perforation. Permanent visual impairment occurs in about 10% of patients. Mucous membrane involvement of the nares, anorectal junction, vulvovaginal region, and urethral meatus is less common. The epithelium of the tracheobronchial tree and esophagus may be involved, leading to stricture formation. EM major has a more protracted course, but most cases heal within 6 weeks (177). The mortality rate approaches 10% among patients with extensive disease. Sepsis is a major cause of death. Visceral involvement may include liver, kidney, or pulmonary disease.

The pathogenesis of this disorder is uncertain; however, the histopathologic features are similar to graft-versus-host disease and suggest an immune mechanism. Deposition of C3, IgM, and fibrin can be found in the upper dermal blood vessels (179). Upregulation of intercellular adhesion molecule 1, an adhesion molecule that facilitates recruitment of inflammatory cells, has been found in the epidermis of patients with erythema multiforme (180). However, unlike immune complex-mediated cutaneous vasculitis in which the cell infiltrate is mostly polymorphonuclear leukocytes, a mononuclear cell infiltrate (mostly lymphocytes) is present around the upper dermal blood vessels (181,182). Activated lymphocytes, mainly CD8$^+$ cells, are present, and there is increasing evidence that they are responsible for keratinocyte destruction (182–185). Epidermal apoptosis has also been reported in patients with SJS and TEN (182–186), and the role of the T cell

in apoptosis is well established. It is possible that a drug or drug metabolite may bind to the cell surface, after which the patient then develops lymphocyte reactivity directed against the drug-cell complex.

Genetic susceptibility likely also plays a role. Recently, in a Han Chinese population, HLA-B*5801 was found to have a strong association with development of SJS and TEN to allopurinol (58) and HLA-B*1502 with development of SJS to carbamazapime (57). Other studies have shown a possible susceptibility to ocular involvement with HLA-Bw44 (part of HLA-B12) and HLA-oq81*0601 (187).

Drugs are the most common cause of SJS, accounting for at least half of cases (137). Drugs most frequently associated with this syndrome and also TEN include sulfonamides (especially TMP-SMX), anticonvulsants (notably carbamazepine), barbiturates, phenylbutazone, piroxicam, allopurinol, and the aminopenicillins. Occasional reactions have followed the use of cephalosporins, fluoroquinolones, vancomycin (188), antituberculous drugs, and NSAIDs and proton pump inhibitors (PPIs) have been reported as a cause of SJS (189,190). Typically, symptoms begin 1 to 3 weeks after initiation of therapy.

Although there is some disagreement based on a series of 67 patients, early management of SJS with high-dose corticosteroids (160 mg to 240 mg methylprednisolone a day initially) should be implemented (191,192). Corticosteroids hastened recovery, produced no major side effects, and were associated with 100% survival and full recovery with no significant residual complications. This recommendation does not apply to the management of TEN. Drug challenges to establish whether a patient can safely tolerate a drug following a suspected reaction should not be considered with serious adverse reactions such as SJS, TEN, and exfoliative dermatitis.

Generalized Exfoliative Dermatitis

Exfoliative dermatitis is a serious and potentially life-threatening skin disease characterized by erythema and extensive scaling in which the superficial skin is shed over virtually the entire body. Even hair and nails are lost. Fever, chills, and malaise are often prominent, and there is a large extrarenal fluid loss. Secondary infection frequently develops, and on occasion, a glomerulonephritis has developed. Fatalities occur most often in elderly or debilitated patients. Laboratory tests and skin biopsy are helpful only to exclude other causes, such as psoriasis or cutaneous lymphoma. High-dose systemic corticosteroids and careful attention to fluid and electrolyte replacement are essential.

Exfoliative dermatitis may occur as a complication of pre-existing skin disorders (e.g., psoriasis, seborrheic dermatitis, atopic dermatitis, and contact dermatitis); in association with lymphomas, leukemias, and other internal malignancies; or as a reaction to drugs. At times, a predisposing cause is not evident. The

TABLE 17A.9   DIFFERENTIAL FEATURES OF PHOTOSENSITIVITY

FEATURE	PHOTOTOXIC	PHOTOALLERGIC
Incidence	Common	Uncommon
Clinical picture	Sunburn-like	Eczematous
Reaction possible with first drug exposure	Yes	Requires sensitization period of days to months
Onset	4 to 8 hours after exposure	12 to 24 hours after exposure once sensitized
Chemical alteration of drug	No	Yes
Ultraviolet range	2,800 nm to 3,100 nm	3,200 nm to 4,500 nm
Drug dosages	Dose-related	Dose-independent once sensitized
Immunologic mechanism	None	T cell-mediated
Flares at distant previously involved sites	No	May occur
Recurrence from exposure to ultraviolet light alone	No	May occur in persistent eruptions

drug-induced eruption may appear abruptly or may follow an apparently benign, drug-induced exanthematous eruption. The process may continue for weeks or months after withdrawal of the offending drug.

Many drugs have been implicated in the development of exfoliative dermatitis, but the most frequently encountered are sulfonamides, penicillins, barbiturates, carbamazepine, phenytoin, phenylbutazone, allopurinol, and gold salts (193). No immunologic mechanism has been identified. The diagnosis is based on clinical grounds, the presence of erythema followed by scaling, and drug use compatible with this cutaneous reaction. The outcome is usually favorable if the causative agent is identified and then discontinued and corticosteroids are initiated. However, an older study reported a 40% mortality rate, reminding us of the potential seriousness of this disorder (194).

Photosensitivity

Photosensitivity reactions are produced by the interaction of a drug present in the skin and light energy. The drug may be administered topically, orally, or parenterally. Although direct sunlight (ultraviolet spectrum 2,800 nm to 4,500 nm or 280 mm to 450 mm) is usually required, filtered or artificial light may produce reactions. African Americans have a lower incidence of drug photosensitivity, presumably because of greater melanin protection. The eruption is limited to light-exposed areas, such as the face, the V area of the neck, the forearms, and the dorsa of the hands. Often, a triangular area on the neck is spared because of shielding by the mandible. The intranasal areas and the groove of the chin are also spared. Although symmetric involvement is usual, unilateral distribution may result from

activities such as keeping an arm out of the window while driving a car.

Photosensitivity may occur as a phototoxic nonimmunologic phenomenon and, less frequently, as a photoallergic immunologic reaction. Differential features are shown in Table 17A.9. Phototoxic reactions are nonimmunologic, occurring in a significant number of patients on first exposure when adequate light and drug concentrations are present. The drug absorbs light, and this oxidative energy is transferred to tissues, resulting in damage. The light absorption spectrum is specific for each drug. Clinically, the reaction resembles an exaggerated sunburn developing within a few hours after exposure. On occasion, vesiculation occurs, and hyperpigmentation remains in the area. Most phototoxic reactions are prevented if the light is filtered through ordinary window glass. Tetracycline, fluoroquinolones, and amiodarone are some of the many agents implicated in phototoxic reactions (195).

Photoallergic reactions, in contrast, generally start with an eczematous phase and more closely resemble contact dermatitis. Here, the radiant energy presumably alters the drug to form reactive metabolites that combine with cutaneous proteins to form a complete antigen, to which a T cell-mediated immunologic response is directed. Such reactions occur in only a small number of patients exposed to the drug and light. The sensitization period may be days or months. The concentration of drug required to elicit the reaction can be very small, and there is cross-reactivity with immunochemically related substances. Flare-ups may occur at lightly covered or unexposed areas and at distant, previously exposed sites. The reaction may recur over a period of days or months after light exposure, even without further drug administration. As a rule, longer ultraviolet light waves are involved, and window glass does not protect against a reaction. The photoallergic reaction may be detected by a positive photo patch test, which involves application of the suspected drug as an ordinary patch test for 24 hours, followed by exposure to a light source. Drugs implicated include the sulfonamides (antibacterials, hypoglycemics, diuretics), phenothiazines, NSAIDs, and griseofulvin (196).

Purpuric Eruptions

Purpuric eruptions may occur as the sole expression of drug allergy, or they may be associated with other severe eruptions, notably erythema multiforme. Purpura caused by drug hypersensitivity may be due to thrombocytopenia.

Simple, nonthrombocytopenic purpura has been described with sulfonamides, barbiturates, gold salts, carbromal, iodides, antihistamines, and meprobamate. Phenylbutazone has produced both thrombocytopenic and nonthrombocytopenic purpura. The typical eruption is symmetric and appears around the feet and ankles or on the lower part of the legs, with subsequent spread upward. The face and neck usually are not involved. The eruption is composed of small, well-defined macules or patches of a reddish brown color. The lesions do not blanch on pressure and often are quite pruritic. With time, the dermatitis turns brown or grayish brown, and pigmentation may persist for a relatively long period. The mechanism of simple purpura is unknown.

A very severe purpuric eruption, often associated with hemorrhagic infection and necrosis with large sloughs, has been associated with coumarin anticoagulants. Although originally thought to be an immune-mediated process, it is now believed to be the result of an imbalance between procoagulant and fibrinolytic factors (197,198).

Toxic Epidermal Necrolysis

TEN (Lyell syndrome) induced by drugs is a rare, fulminating, potentially lethal syndrome characterized by the sudden onset of widespread blistering of the skin, extensive epidermal necrosis, and exfoliation of the skin involving more than 30% of the TBSA. *Overlap syndrome* (199) is the term used for 10% to 30% loss associated with severe constitutional symptoms. It has been suggested that TEN may represent the extreme manifestation of EM major, but this position has been contested by others who cite the explosive onset of widespread blistering, the absence of target lesions, the peridermal necrosis without dermal infiltrates, and the paucity of immunologic deposits in the skin in TEN (200).

However, it has generally been assumed that TEN is an immunologically mediated disease because of its association with graft-versus-host disease, reports of immunoreactants in the skin, drug-dependent antiepidermal antibodies in some cases, and altered lymphocyte subsets in peripheral blood and the inflammatory infiltrate (200). An increased expression of HLA-B12 has been reported in TEN cases (56), and in a Han Chinese population, a very strong association has been shown with HLA-B*5801 and SJS and TEN to allopurinol (58). High concentrations of soluble Fas ligand have been found in the sera of patients with TEN (201). Recent evidence suggests that Fas-FasL interaction on keratinocytes is responsible for apoptosis seen in TEN. Conserved levels of Fas are found on keratinocytes along with increased levels of bound FasL in lesional skin of patients with TEN. FasL on keratinocytes had been shown to be cytolytic in TEN and can be blocked with antibodies that interfere with Fas/FasL binding (201–203). TEN usually affects adults and is not to be confused with the staphylococcal scalded-skin syndrome seen in children. The latter is characterized by a staphylococcal elaborated epidermolytic toxin, a cleavage plane high in the epidermis, and response to appropriate antimicrobial therapy. Features of TEN include keratinocyte necrosis and cleavage at the basal layer with loss of the entire epidermis (204). In addition, the mucosa of the respiratory and gastrointestinal tracts may be affected.

These patients are seriously ill with high fever, asthenia, skin pain, and anxiety. Marked skin erythema progresses over 1 to 3 days to the formation of huge bullae, which peel off in sheets, leaving painful denuded areas. Detachment of more than 30% of the epidermis is expected, whereas detachment of less than 10% is compatible with SJS (199) and 10% to 30% is considered overlap syndrome. A positive Nikolsky sign (i.e., dislodgment of the epidermis by lateral pressure) is present on erythematous areas. Mucosal lesions, including painful erosions and crusting, may be present on any surface. The complications of TEN and extensive thermal burns are similar. Unlike SJS, high-dose corticosteroids are of no benefit (191,192). Mortality may be reduced from an overall rate of 50% to less than 30% by early transfer to a burn center (205). Intravenous immunoglobulin (IVIG) contains antibodies to Fas and is therefore able to block Fas-FasL interaction (201). To date, most case reports of using IVIG in the treatment of TEN suggests that it may be beneficial clinically (206,207) particularly when used in doses greater than 2 g/kg (208). The drugs most frequently implicated in TEN include sulfonamides (20% to 28%; especially TMP-SMX), allopurinol (6% to 20%), barbiturates (6%), carbamazepine (5%), phenytoin (18%), and NSAIDs (especially oxyphenbutazone, 18%; piroxicam, isoxicam, and phenylbutazone, 8% each) (209,210).

Erythema Nodosum

Erythema nodosum–like lesions are usually bilateral, symmetric, ill-defined, warm, and tender subcutaneous nodules involving the anterior aspects (shins) of the legs. The lesions are usually red or sometimes resemble a hematoma and may persist for a few days to several weeks. They do not ulcerate or suppurate, and usually resemble contusions as they involute. Mild constitutional symptoms of low-grade fever, malaise, myalgia, and arthralgia may be present. The lesions occur in association with streptococcal infections, tuberculosis, leprosy, deep fungal infections, cat scratch fever, lymphogranuloma venereum, sarcoidosis, ulcerative colitis, and other illnesses.

There is some disagreement whether drugs may cause erythema nodosum. Because the etiology of this disorder is unclear, its occurrence simultaneously with drug administration may be more coincidental than causative. Drugs most commonly implicated include sulfonamides, bromides, and oral contraceptives. Several other drugs, such as penicillin, barbiturates, and salicylates, are often suspected but seldom proved as causes of erythema nodosum. Treatment with corticosteroids is effective but is seldom necessary after withdrawal of the offending drug.

Pulmonary Manifestations

Bronchial Asthma

Pharmacologic agents are a common cause of acute exacerbations of asthma, which, on occasion, may be severe or even fatal. Drug-induced bronchospasm most often occurs in patients with known asthma but may unmask subclinical reactive airways disease. It may occur as a result of inhalation, ingestion, or parenteral administration of a drug. Although asthma may occur in drug-induced anaphylaxis or anaphylactoid reactions, bronchospasm is usually not a prominent feature; laryngeal edema is far more common as is shock (81).

Airborne exposure to drugs during manufacture or during final preparation in the hospital or at home has resulted in asthma. Parents of children with cystic fibrosis have developed asthma following inhalation of pancreatic extract powder in the process of preparing their children's meals (211). Occupational exposure to some of these agents has caused asthma in nurses, for example, psyllium in bulk laxatives (212), and in pharmaceutical workers following exposure to various antibiotics (213). Spiramycin used in animal feeds has resulted in asthma among farmers, pet shop owners, and laboratory animal workers who inhale dusts from these products. NSAIDs account for more than two-thirds of drug-induced asthmatic reactions, with aspirin being responsible for more than half of these (214).

Both oral and ophthalmic preparations that block β-adrenergic receptors may induce bronchospasm among individuals with asthma or subclinical bronchial hyperreactivity. This may occur immediately after initiation of treatment, or rarely after several months or years of therapy. Metoprolol, atenolol, and labetalol are less likely to cause bronchospasm than are propranolol, nadolol, and timolol (215). Timolol has been associated with fatal bronchospasm in patients using this ophthalmic preparation for glaucoma. Occasional subjects without asthma have developed bronchoconstriction after treatment with β-blocking drugs (216). One should also recall that β blockers may increase the occurrence and magnitude of immediate generalized reactions to other agents (75), make resuscitation with epinephrine more difficult, and lead to larger volume loss.

Cholinesterase inhibitors, such as echothiophate ophthalmic solution used to treat glaucoma, and neostigmine or pyridostigmine used for myasthenia gravis, have produced bronchospasm. For obvious reasons, methacholine is no longer used in the treatment of glaucoma.

Although ACE inhibitors have been reported to cause acute bronchospasm or aggravate chronic asthma (217), a harsh, at times disabling, cough is a more likely side effect that may be confused with asthma. This occurs in 10% to 25% of patients taking these drugs, usually within the first 8 weeks of treatment, although it may develop within days or may not appear for up to 1 year (218). Switching from one agent to another is of no benefit. The cough typically resolves within 1 to 2 weeks after discontinuing the medication; persistence longer than 4 weeks should trigger a more comprehensive diagnostic evaluation. The mechanism of ACE inhibitor-induced cough is unclear. Cough may be avoided with the use of an ARB (219,220). As stated previously, ACE inhibitors may cause angioedema and may be a source of cough and dyspnea (221).

Sulfites and metabisulfites can provoke bronchospasm in a subset of asthmatic patients. The incidence is probably low but may be higher among those who are steroid-dependent (222). These agents are used as preservatives to reduce microbial spoilage of foods, as inhibitors of enzymatic and nonenzymatic discoloration of foods, and as antioxidants that are often found in bronchodilator solutions. The mechanism responsible for sulfite-induced asthmatic reactions may be the result of the generation of sulfur dioxide from stomach acid, which is then inhaled. However, sulfite-sensitive asthmatic patients are not more sensitive to inhaled sulfur dioxide than are other asthmatic patients (223). The diagnosis of sulfite sensitivity may be established on the basis of sulfite challenge. There is no cross-reactivity between sulfites and aspirin (224). Bronchospasm in these patients may be treated with metered-dose inhalers or nebulized bronchodilator solutions containing negligible amounts of metabisulfites. Although epinephrine contains sulfites, its use in an emergency situation even among sulfite-sensitive asthmatic patients should not be discouraged (223).

Pulmonary Infiltrates with Eosinophilia

An immunologic mechanism is probably operative in two forms of drug-induced acute lung injury, namely hypersensitivity pneumonitis and pulmonary infiltrates associated with peripheral eosinophilia. Peripheral eosinophilia syndrome has been associated with the use of a number of drugs, including sulfonamides, penicillin, NSAIDs, methotrexate, carbamazepine, nitrofurantoin, phenytoin, cromolyn sodium, imipramine, and L-tryptophan (163). Although a nonproductive cough is the main symptom, headache, malaise, fever, nasal symptoms, dyspnea, and chest discomfort may occur. The chest radiograph may show diffuse or migratory focal infiltrates. Peripheral blood eosinophilia is usually present. Pulmonary function testing reveals restriction with decreased carbon dioxide diffusing capacity (DLCO). A lung biopsy demonstrates interstitial and alveolar inflammation consisting of eosinophils and mononuclear cells. The outcome is usually excellent, with rapid clinical improvement on drug cessation and corticosteroid therapy. Usually, the patient's pulmonary function is restored with little residual damage.

Nitrofurantoin may also induce an acute syndrome, in which peripheral eosinophilia is present in about one-third of patients. However, this reaction differs from the drug-induced pulmonary infiltrates with peripheral eosinophilia syndrome just described because tissue eosinophilia is not present, and the clinical picture frequently includes the presence of a pleural effusion (225). Adverse pulmonary reactions occur in less than 1% of those taking the drug. Typically, the onset of the acute pulmonary reaction begins a few hours to 7 to 10 days after commencement of treatment. Typical symptoms include fever, dry cough, dyspnea (occasional wheezing), and, less commonly, pleuritic chest pain. A chest radiograph may show diffuse or unilateral involvement, with an alveolar or interstitial process that tends to involve lung bases. A small pleural effusion, usually unilateral, is seen in about one-third of patients. With the exception of DIL, nitrofurantoin is one of the only drugs producing an acute drug-induced pleural effusion. Knowledge of this reaction can prevent unnecessary hospitalization for suspected pneumonia. Acute reactions have a mortality rate of less than 1%. On withdrawal of the drug, resolution of the chest radiograph findings occurs within 24 to 48 hours.

Although the acute nitrofurantoin-induced pulmonary reaction is rarely fatal, a chronic reaction that is uncommon has a higher mortality rate of 8%. Cough and dyspnea develop insidiously after 1 month or often longer of treatment. The chronic reaction mimics idiopathic pulmonary fibrosis clinically, radiologically, and histologically. Although somewhat controversial, if no improvement occurs after the drug has been withdrawn for 6 weeks, prednisone, 40 mg/day, should be given and continued for 3 to 6 months (225, 226).

Of the cytotoxic chemotherapeutic agents, methotrexate is the most common cause of a noncytotoxic pulmonary reaction in which peripheral blood, but not tissue, eosinophilia may be present (227). In recent years, this drug has also been used to treat nonmalignant conditions, such as psoriasis, rheumatoid arthritis, and asthma. Symptoms usually begin within 6 weeks after initiation of treatment. Fever, malaise, headache, and chills may overshadow the presence of a nonproductive cough and dyspnea. Eosinophilia is present in 40% of cases. The chest radiograph demonstrates a diffuse interstitial process, and 10% to 15% of patients develop hilar adenopathy or pleural effusions. Recovery is usually prompt on withdrawal of methotrexate, but fatalities can occur. The addition of corticosteroid therapy may hasten recovery time. Although an immunologic mechanism has been suggested, some patients who have recovered may be able to resume methotrexate without adverse sequelae. Bleomycin and procarbazine, chemotherapeutic agents usually associated with cytotoxic pulmonary reactions, have occasionally produced a reaction similar to that of methotrexate.

Pneumonitis and Fibrosis

Slowly progressive pneumonitis or fibrosis is usually associated with cytotoxic chemotherapeutic drugs, such as bleomycin. However, some drugs, such as amiodarone, may produce a clinical picture similar to hypersensitivity pneumonitis without the presence of eosinophilia. In many cases, this category of drug-induced lung disease is often dose-dependent.

Amiodarone, an important therapeutic agent in the treatment of many life-threatening arrhythmias, has produced an adverse pulmonary reaction in about 6% of patients, with 5% to 10% of these reactions being fatal (228). Symptoms rarely develop in a patient receiving less than 400 mg/day for less than 2 months. The clinical presentation is usually subacute with initial symptoms of nonproductive cough, dyspnea, and occasionally low-grade fever. The chest radiograph reveals an interstitial or alveolar process. Pulmonary function studies demonstrate a restrictive pattern with a diffusion defect. The sedimentation rate is elevated, but there is no eosinophilia. Histologic findings include the intraalveolar accumulation of foamy macrophages, alveolar septal thickening, and occasional diffuse alveolar damage (229). Amiodarone has the unique ability to stimulate the accumulation of phospholipids in many cells, including type II pneumocytes and alveolar macrophages. It is unclear whether these changes cause interstitial pneumonitis, as these findings are seen in most patients receiving this drug without any adverse pulmonary reactions. Although an immunologic mechanism has been suggested, the role of hypersensitivity in amiodarone-induced pneumonitis remains speculative (230). Most patients recover completely after cessation of therapy, although the addition of corticosteroids may be required. Further, when the drug is absolutely required to control a potentially fatal cardiac arrhythmia, patients may be able to continue treatment at the lowest dose possible when corticosteroids are given concomitantly (231).

Gold-induced pneumonitis is subacute in onset, occurring after a mean duration of therapy of 15 weeks and a mean cumulative dose of 582 mg (232). Exertional dyspnea is the predominant symptom, although a nonproductive cough and fever may be present. Radiographic findings include interstitial or alveolar infiltrates, whereas pulmonary function testing reveals findings compatible with a restrictive lung disorder. Peripheral blood eosinophilia is rare. Intense lymphocytosis is the most common finding in bronchoalveolar lavage. The condition is usually reversible after discontinuation of the gold injections, but corticosteroids may be required to reverse the process. Although this pulmonary reaction is rare, it must not be confused with rheumatoid lung disease.

Drug-induced chronic fibrotic reactions are probably nonimmunologic in nature, but their exact mechanism is unknown. Cytotoxic chemotherapeutic agents (azathioprine, bleomycin sulfate, busulfan, chlorambucil, cyclophosphamide, hydroxyurea, melphalan, mitomycin, nitrosoureas, and procarbazine hydrochloride) may induce pulmonary disease that is manifested clinically by the development of fever, nonproductive cough, and progressive dyspnea of gradual onset after treatment for 2 to 6 months or, rarely, years (233). It is essential to recognize this complication because such reactions may be fatal and could mimic other diseases, such as opportunistic infections. The chest radiograph reveals an interstitial or intraalveolar pattern, especially at the lung bases. A decline in carbon monoxide diffusing capacity may even precede chest radiograph changes. Frequent early etiologic findings include damage to type I pneumocytes, which are the major alveolar lining cells, and atypia and proliferation of type II pneumocytes. Mononuclear cell infiltration of the interstitium may be seen early, followed by interstitial and alveolar fibrosis, which may progress to honeycombing. The prognosis is often poor, and the response to corticosteroids is variable. Even those who respond to treatment may be left with clinically significant pulmonary function abnormalities. Although an immunologic mechanism has been suspected in some cases (234), it is now generally believed that these drugs induce the formation of toxic oxygen radicals that produce lung injury.

Noncardiogenic Pulmonary Edema

Another acute pulmonary reaction without eosinophilia is drug-induced noncardiogenic pulmonary edema. This develops very rapidly and may even begin with the first dose of the drug. The chest radiograph is similar to that caused by congestive heart failure. Hydrochlorothiazide is the only thiazide associated with this reaction (234). Most of the drugs associated with this reaction are illegal, including cocaine, heroin, and methadone (235,236). Salicylate-induced noncardiogenic pulmonary edema may occur when the blood salicylate level is over 40 mg/dL (237). In most cases,

the reaction resolves rapidly after the drug is stopped. However, some cases may follow the clinical course of acute respiratory distress syndrome, notably with chemotherapeutic agents, such as mitomycin C or cytosine arabinoside (238), and rarely 2 hours after administration of RCM (239). The mechanism is unknown.

Hematologic Manifestations

Many instances of drug-induced thrombocytopenia and hemolytic anemia have been unequivocally shown by *in vitro* methods to be mediated by immunologic mechanisms. There is less certainty regarding drug-induced agranulocytosis. These reactions usually appear alone, without other organ involvement. The onset is usually abrupt, and recovery is expected within 1 to 2 weeks after drug withdrawal.

Eosinophilia

Eosinophilia may be present as the sole manifestation of drug hypersensitivity (240). More commonly, it is associated with other manifestations of drug allergy. Its recognition is useful because it may give early warning of hypersensitivity reactions that could produce permanent tissue damage or even death. However, most would agree that eosinophilia alone is not sufficient reason to discontinue treatment. In fact, some drugs, such as digitalis, may regularly produce eosinophilia, yet hypersensitivity reactions to this drug are rare.

Drugs that may be associated with eosinophilia in the absence of clinical disease include gold salts, allopurinol, aminosalicylic acid, ampicillin, tricyclic antidepressants, capreomycin sulfate, carbamazepine, digitalis, phenytoin, sulfonamides, vancomycin, and streptomycin. There does not appear to be a common chemical or pharmacologic feature of these agents to account for the development of eosinophilia. Although the incidence of eosinophilia is probably less than 0.1% for most drugs, gold salts have been associated with marked eosinophilia in up to 47% of patients with rheumatoid arthritis and may be an early sign of an adverse reaction (241). Drug-induced eosinophilia does not appear to progress to a chronic eosinophilia or hypereosinophilic syndrome. However, in the face of a rising eosinophil count, discontinuing the drug may prevent further problems.

Thrombocytopenia

Thrombocytopenia is a well-recognized complication of drug therapy. The usual clinical manifestations are widespread petechiae and ecchymoses and occasionally gastrointestinal bleeding, hemoptysis, hematuria, and vaginal bleeding. Fortunately, intracranial hemorrhage is rare. On occasion, there may be associated fever, chills, and arthralgia. Bone marrow examination shows normal or increased numbers of normal-appearing megakaryocytes. With the exception of gold-induced immune thrombocytopenia, which may continue for months because of the persistence of the antigen in the reticulo-endothelial system, prompt recovery within 2 weeks is expected on withdrawal of the drug (242). Fatalities are relatively infrequent. Readministration of the drug, even in minute doses, may produce an abrupt recrudescence of severe thrombocytopenia, often within a few hours.

Although many drugs have been reported to cause immune thrombocytopenia, the most common offenders in clinical practice today are quinidine, the sulfonamides (antibacterials, sulfonylureas, thiazide diuretics), gold salts, and heparin.

The mechanism of drug-induced immune thrombocytopenia is thought to be the "innocent bystander" type. Shulman suggested the formation of an immunogenic drug–plasma protein complex to which antibodies are formed; this antibody drug complex then reacts with the platelet (the innocent bystander), thereby initiating complement activation with subsequent platelet destruction (243). Some studies indicate that quinidine antibodies react with a platelet membrane glycoprotein in association with the drug (244). Patients with HLA-DR3 appear to be at increased risk for gold-induced thrombocytopenia.

Because heparin has had more widespread clinical use, the incidence of heparin-induced thrombocytopenia is about 5% (245). Some of these patients simultaneously develop acute thromboembolic complications. A heparin-dependent IgG antibody has been demonstrated in the serum of these patients. A low-molecular-weight heparinoid can be substituted for heparin in patients who previously developed heparin-induced thrombocytopenia (246).

The diagnosis is often presumptive because the platelet count usually returns to normal within 2 weeks (longer if the drug is slowly excreted) after the drug is discontinued. Many in vitro tests are available at some centers to demonstrate drug-related platelet antibodies. A test dose of the offending drug is probably the most reliable means of diagnosis, but this involves significant risk and is seldom justified. Treatment involves stopping the suspected drug and observing the patient carefully over the next few weeks. Corticosteroids do not shorten the duration of thrombocytopenia but may hasten recovery because of their capillary protective effect. Platelet transfusions should not be given because transfused platelets are destroyed rapidly and may produce additional symptoms.

Hemolytic Anemia

Drug-induced immune hemolytic anemia may develop through three mechanisms: (a) immune complex type; (b) hapten or drug adsorption type; and (c) autoimmune induction (108). Another mechanism involves nonimmunologic adsorption of protein to the red blood cell membrane, which results in a positive Coombs test but seldom causes a hemolytic anemia. Hemolytic anemia after drug administration accounts for about 16% to 18% of acquired hemolytic anemias.

The *immune complex mechanism* accounts for most cases of drug-induced immune hemolysis. The antidrug antibody binds to a complex of drug and a specific blood group antigen, for example, Kidd, Kell, Rh, or Ii, on the red blood cell membrane (247). Drugs implicated include quinidine, chlorpropamide, nitrofurantoin, probenecid, rifampin, and streptomycin. Of note is that many of these drugs have also been associated with immune complex-mediated thrombocytopenia. The serum antidrug antibody is often IgM, and the direct Coombs test is usually positive.

Penicillin is the prototype of a drug that induces a hemolytic anemia by the *hapten or drug absorption mechanism* (248). Penicillin normally binds to proteins on the red blood cell membrane, and among patients who develop antibodies to the drug hapten on the red blood cell, a hemolytic anemia may occur. In sharp contrast to immune complex-mediated hemolysis, penicillin-induced hemolytic anemia occurs only with large doses of penicillin, at least 10 million units daily intravenously. Anemia usually develops after 1 week of therapy, more rapidly in patients with pre-existing penicillin antibodies. The antidrug antibody is IgG, and the red blood cells are removed by splenic sequestration independent of complement. About 3% of patients receiving high-dose penicillin therapy develop positive Coombs test results, but only some of these patients actually develop hemolytic anemia. The anemia usually abates promptly, but mild hemolysis may persist for several weeks. Other drugs occasionally associated with hemolysis by this mechanism include cisplatin and tetracycline.

Methyldopa is the most common cause of an *autoimmune* drug-induced hemolysis. A positive Coombs test develops in 11% to 36% of patients, depending on drug dosage, after 3 to 6 months of treatment (249). However, less than 1% of patients develop hemolytic anemia. The IgG autoantibody has specificity for antigens related to the Rh complex. The mechanism of autoantibody production is not clear. Hemolysis usually subsides within 1 to 2 weeks after the drug is stopped, but the Coombs test may remain positive for up to 2 years. These drug-induced antibodies will react with normal red blood cells. Because only a small number of patients actually develop hemolysis, a positive Coombs test alone is not sufficient reason to discontinue the medication. Several other drugs have induced autoimmune hemolytic disease, including levodopa, mefenamic acid, procainamide, and tolmetin.

A small number of patients treated with cephalothin develop a positive Coombs test as a result of *nonspecific adsorption of plasma proteins* onto red blood cell membranes. This does not result in a hemolytic anemia but may provide confusion in blood bank serology. Finally, several other drugs have been associated with hemolytic disease, but the mechanism is unclear. Such agents include chlorpromazine, erythromycin, ibuprofen, isoniazid, mesantoin, paraaminosalicylic acid, phenacetin, thiazides, and triamterene.

Agranulocytosis

Most instances of drug-induced neutropenia are due to bone marrow suppression, but they can also be mediated by immunologic mechanisms (250). The process usually develops 6 to 10 days after initial drug therapy; readministration of the drug after recovery may result in a hyperacute fall in granulocytes within 24 to 48 hours. Patients frequently develop high fever, chills, arthralgias, and severe prostration. The granulocytes disappear within a matter of hours, and this may persist 5 to 10 days after the offending drug is stopped. The role of drug-induced leukoagglutinins in producing the neutropenia has been questioned because such antibodies have also been found in patients who are not neutropenic. The exact immunologic mechanism by which some drugs induce neutropenia is unknown (251). Although many drugs have been occasionally incriminated, sulfonamides, sulfasalazine, propylthiouracil, quinidine, procainamide, phenytoin, phenothiazines, semisynthetic penicillins, cephalosporins, and gold are more commonly reported offenders. After withdrawal of the offending agent, recovery is usual within 1 to 2 weeks, although it may require many weeks or months. Treatment includes the use of antibiotics and other supportive measures. The value of leukocyte transfusions is unclear. Hematopoietic growth factors appears to be of value (252).

Hepatic Manifestations

The liver is especially vulnerable to drug-induced injury because high concentrations of drugs are presented to it after ingestion and also because it plays a prominent role in the biotransformation of drugs to potentially toxic reactive metabolites. These reactive metabolites may induce tissue injury through inherent toxicity, or possibly on an immunologic basis (253). Drug-induced hepatic injury may mimic any form of acute or chronic hepatobiliary disease; however, these hepatic reactions are more commonly associated with acute injury.

Some estimates of the frequency of liver injury due to drugs follow (254):

- >2%: Aminosalicylic acid, troleandomycin, dapsone, chenodeoxycholate
- 1% to 2%: Lovastatin, cyclosporine, dantrolene
- 1%: Isoniazid, amiodarone
- 0.5% to 1%: Phenytoin, sulfonamides, chlorpromazine
- 0.1% to 0.5%: Gold salts, salicylates, methyldopa, chlorpropamide, erythromycin estolate
- <0.01%: Ketoconazole, contraceptive steroids
- <0.001%: Hydralazine, halothane
- <0.0001%: Penicillin, enflurane, cimetidine

Drug-induced liver injury due to intrinsic toxicity of the drug or one of its metabolites is becoming less common. Such toxicity is often predictable because it is frequently detected in animal studies and during the early phases of clinical trials. A typical example of a drug producing such hepatotoxicity follows massive doses of acetaminophen (255). The excess acetaminophen is shunted into the cytochrome P-450 system pathway, resulting in excess formation of the reactive metabolite that binds to subcellular proteins, which in turn leads to cellular necrosis.

Although there is little direct evidence that an immunologic mechanism (hepatocyte-specific antibodies or sensitized T lymphocytes) is operative in drug-induced hepatic injury, such reactions are often associated with other hypersensitivity features. Injury attributed to hypersensitivity is suspected when there is a variable sensitization period of 1 to 5 weeks; when the hepatic injury is associated with clinical features of hypersensitivity such as seen with DRESS; when histologic features reveal an eosinophil-rich inflammatory exudate or granulomas in the liver; when hepatitis-associated antigen is absent; and when there is prompt recurrence of hepatic dysfunction following the readministration of small doses of the suspected drug (not usually recommended). After withdrawal of the offending drug, recovery is expected unless irreversible cell damage has occurred. Such liver injury may take the form of cholestatic disease, hepatocellular injury or necrosis, or a mixed pattern.

Drug-induced cholestasis is most often manifested by icterus, but fever, skin rash, and eosinophilia may also be present. The serum alkaline phosphatase levels are often elevated 2 to 10 times normal, whereas the serum aminotransferases are only minimally increased. Occasionally, antimitochondrial antibodies are present. Liver biopsy reveals cholestasis, slight periportal mononuclear and eosinophilic infiltration, and minimal hepatocellular necrosis. After withdrawal of the offending drug, recovery may take several weeks. Persistent reactions may mimic primary biliary cirrhosis; however, antimitochondrial antibodies are usually not present. The most frequently implicated agents are the phenothiazines (particularly chlorpromazine), the estolate salt of erythromycin, and less frequently, nitrofurantoin and sulfonamides (256).

Drug-induced hepatocellular injury mimics viral hepatitis but has a higher morbidity rate. In fact, 10% to 20% of patients with fulminant hepatic failure have drug-induced injury. The serum aminotransferases are increased, and icterus may develop, the latter associated with a higher mortality rate. The histologic appearance of the liver is not specific for drug-induced injury. Drugs commonly associated with hepatocellular damage are halothane, isoniazid, phenytoin, methyldopa, nitrofurantoin, allopurinol, and sulfonamides. It is now clear that damage from isoniazid is due to metabolism of the drug to a toxic metabolite, acetylhydrazine (257).

Only halothane-induced liver injury has reasonably good support for an immune-mediated process, primarily on the basis of finding circulating antibodies that react with halothane-induced hepatic neoantigen in a significant number of patients with halothane-induced hepatitis (258). In the United States, enflurane and isoflurane have largely replaced halothane (except in children) because the incidence of hepatic injury appears to be less. However, cross-reacting antibodies have been identified in some patients (259).

Mixed pattern disease denotes instances of drug-induced liver disease that do not fit exactly into acute cholestasis or hepatocellular injury. There may be moderate abnormalities of serum aminotransferases and alkaline phosphatase levels with variable icterus. Among patients with phenytoin-induced hepatic injury, the pattern may resemble infectious mononucleosis with fever, lymphadenopathy, lymphoid hyperplasia, and spotty necrosis. Granulomas in the liver with variable hepatocellular necrosis are a hallmark of quinidine-induced hepatitis (260). Other drugs associated with hepatic granulomas are sulfonamides, allopurinol, carbamazepine, methyldopa, and phenothiazines.

Drug-induced chronic liver disease is rare but may also mimic any chronic hepatobiliary disease. Drug-induced chronic active hepatitis has been associated with methyldopa, isoniazid, and nitrofurantoin (261). Some of these patients may develop antinuclear and smooth muscle antibodies. Also, the chronic liver injury may not improve after withdrawal of the offending drug.

Renal Manifestations

The kidney is especially vulnerable to drug-induced toxicity because it receives, transports, and concentrates within its parenchyma a variety of potentially toxic substances. Tubular necrosis may follow drug-induced anaphylactic shock or drug-induced immunohemolysis. Immune drug-induced renal disease is rare, but glomerulonephritis, nephrotic syndrome, and acute interstitial nephritis (AIN) occasionally have been ascribed to drug hypersensitivity.

Glomerulitis is a prominent feature of experimental serum sickness but is rarely of clinical significance in drug-induced, serum sickness–like reactions in humans. In all probability, it is a transient, completely reversible phenomenon that subsides entirely once the offending drug has been discontinued. Although spontaneously occurring SLE is frequently associated with glomerulonephritis, drug-induced SLE rarely manifests significant renal involvement. As a rule, cutaneous involvement is the prominent feature of drug-induced vasculitis, but occasionally glomerulonephritis may be present. Chronic glomerulonephritis was described in a patient with Munchausen syndrome who repeatedly injected herself with DPT vaccine (262). Among heroin addicts, there is a 10% incidence of chronic glomerulonephritis at autopsy. It is suggested that this may be due to immune complexes developing as a result of an immune response to contaminants acquired in the "street" processing of the drug (263). A case of Goodpasture syndrome (pulmonary hemorrhage and progressive glomerulonephritis) was associated with D-penicillamine treatment of Wilson disease—the first case report of a drug being implicated in the etiology of this syndrome (264).

Nephrotic syndrome induced by drugs occurs primarily from immunologic processes that result in membranous glomerulonephritis. This has been more commonly associated with heavy metals (especially gold salts), captopril, heroin, NSAIDs, penicillamine, and probenecid, and less commonly with anticonvulsants (mesantoin, trimethadione, paramethadione), sulfonylureas, lithium, ampicillin, rifampin, and methimazole. An immune complex mechanism is probably responsible for this drug-induced nephropathy (265,266). Proteinuria usually resolves when these agents are discontinued.

AIN, thought to be due to drug hypersensitivity, has been recognized with many agents (267). More frequently reported drugs include the β-lactam antibiotics (especially methicillin), NSAIDs, rifampin, sulfonamide derivatives, captopril, allopurinol, methyldopa, anticonvulsants, cimetidine, ciprofloxacin and PPIs. Drug-induced AIN should be suspected when acute renal insufficiency is associated with fever, skin rash, arthralgias, eosinophilia, mild proteinuria, microhematuria, and eosinophiluria beginning days to weeks after initiation of therapy. However, the classic triad of fever, rash, and eosinophilia is not so common, seen only in 10% to 30% of patients diagnosed with AIN (268). NSAID-induced AIN usually develops in elderly patients months after initiating therapy and is often associated with massive proteinuria and rapidly progressive renal failure (269). Fever and eosinophilia are not usually present. Although the pathogenesis of this drug-induced nephropathy is uncertain, a number of immunologic findings have been documented in methicillin-induced AIN (270). These include the detection of penicilloyl haptenic groups and immunoglobulin deposition along glomerular and tubular basement membranes, circulating antitubular basement-membrane antibodies, a positive delayed skin test reaction to methicillin, and a positive lymphocyte transformation test to methicillin. Also, the lymphocytes infiltrating the renal interstitium are cytotoxic T cells. The prognosis is excellent following discontinuation of the drug, with full recovery expected within 12 months. After recovery, the offending drug or a chemically related one should be avoided because there have been several cases of cross-reactivity between methicillin and another β-lactam drug, or among various NSAIDs.

Lymphoid System Manifestations

Lymphadenopathy is a common feature of the serum sickness syndrome and may be present in drug-induced SLE. Lymphadenopathy associated with prolonged treatment with anticonvulsants, notably phenytoin, is a rare but well-established disorder that may mimic clinically and pathologically a malignant lymphoma (271), and is often referred to as drug-induced pseudolymphoma. Cervical lymphadenopathy is most frequent, but may be generalized; hepatomegaly and splenomegaly are uncommon. Other features may include fever, a morbilliform or erythematous skin rash, and eosinophilia (DRESS). Rarely, arthritis and jaundice may be present. The pathogenesis of this syndrome is unknown. However, phenytoin may induce immunosuppression, which then leads to lymphoreticular malignancies. The reaction usually subsides within several weeks after the drug is stopped and reappears promptly on readministration of the offending drug. However, not all patients recover after drug withdrawal, and some develop Hodgkin disease and lymphoma (272). An infectious mononucleosis–like syndrome has been described with phenytoin, aminosalicylic acid, and dapsone (273).

Cardiac Manifestations

Hypersensitivity myocarditis is rarely identified as a clinical entity. Although endomyocardial biopsy has, on occasion, suggested hypersensitivity myocarditis, reported cases are usually diagnosed at autopsy (274). Many drugs have been implicated, but the main offenders are the sulfonamides, methyldopa, penicillin, and its derivatives. Many of these drugs have also been associated with hypersensitivity vasculitis. In most cases diagnosed at autopsy, the patients died suddenly and unexpectedly while being treated for an unrelated and nonlethal illness (275).

The diagnosis should be considered when new electrocardiographic changes appear in association with unexpected tachycardia, mildly elevated cardiac enzymes, and cardiomegaly in a patient with an allergic drug reaction, usually with evidence of eosinophilia (276). Confirmation is usually obtained by a biopsy of the endomyocardium that demonstrates diffuse interstitial infiltrates rich with eosinophils.

Because cellular necrosis is less prominent than in other forms of myocarditis, permanent cardiac damage is less if the entity is recognized and the offending drug eliminated. Most patients recover in a few days to a few weeks. Aggressive treatment with corticosteroids or immunosuppressives may be necessary if myocarditis is severe and persistent. The diagnosed cases probably represent only the tip of the iceberg, with many cases presumably self-limited and unrecognized. This reaction should not be confused with other types of chronic eosinophilic myocardiopathy, which often lead to permanent cardiac damage and impairment of function.

Neurologic Manifestations

An allergic etiology for drug-induced damage to the central and peripheral nervous system is unusual. Postvaccinal encephalomyelitis does resemble experimental encephalomyelitis in animals. A peripheral neuritis has been reported in patients receiving gold salts, colchicine, nitrofurantoin, and sulfonamides; although such reactions have not been analyzed sufficiently to implicate an immunologic mechanism, this has been suggested.

■ EVALUATION OF PATIENTS WITH SUSPECTED DRUG HYPERSENSITIVITY

The investigation and identification of a drug responsible for a suspected allergic reaction still depends largely on circumstantial evidence and clinical skills of the physician. Absolute proof that a drug is the actual offender is usually lacking because, with few exceptions, conventional methods to diagnose allergic disorders are either unavailable, unreliable, or unsafe.

Knowledge of the clinical criteria (Table 17A.3) and clinical manifestations ascribed to drug hypersensitivity is helpful in evaluation. None of these clinical manifestations is unique for drug allergy, but physicians should consider this very treatable condition along with other diagnostic possibilities.

The complexity and heterogeneity of immune responses induced by drugs, the variety of immunologic tests needed for their detection, and the fact that the relevant drug antigens are in most cases not able to be prepared *in vitro*, but rather are the result of complex metabolic interactions occurring *in vivo*, have largely prevented the development of clinically applicable *in vivo* and *in vitro* diagnostic tests. Table 17A.10 provides an overview of useful approaches available to evaluate and diagnose allergic drug reactions.

Detailed History

The most important consideration in the evaluation of patients for possible drug allergy is a suspicion by the physician that an unexplained symptom or sign may be due to a drug currently being administered. Next in importance is obtaining a complete history of *all* drugs taken currently, and within the past month or so, as well as a history of any drug reactions in the past. It is helpful to be aware of those drugs most frequently implicated in allergic reactions (Table 17A.11).

The clinical features of the reaction may suggest drug hypersensitivity, although morphologic changes associated with drug allergy are often protean in nature and usually not agent specific. It is obviously helpful to know whether the presenting manifestations have been reported previously as features of a reaction to the drug being taken.

TABLE 17A.10   OVERVIEW OF METHODS USED TO EVALUATE PATENTS WITH SUSPECTED DRUG HYPERSENSITIVITY

Detailed history[a]—basis for diagnosis in most cases

- Consider the possibility
- Complete history of *all* drugs taken and any prior reactions
- Compatible clinical manifestations
- Temporal eligibility

***In vivo* testing**—clinically indicated in some cases

- Cutaneous tests for IgE-mediated reactions[a]
- Patch tests[a]
- Incremental provocative test dosing[a]

***In vitro* testing**—rarely helpful clinically

- Drug-specific IgE antibodies (RAST)
- Drug-specific IgG and IgM antibodies
- Lymphocyte blast transformation
- Others: mediator release, complement activation, immune complex detection

Withdrawal of the suspected drug—presumptive evidence if symptoms clear

- Eliminate any drug not clearly indicated
- Use alternate agents if possible

[a]These methods are clinically most available and useful in evaluating allergic drug reactions.

IgE, immunoglobulin E; IgM, immunoglobulin M; RAST, radioallergosorbent test.

The history should establish temporal eligibility of the suspected drug. Unless the patient has been sensitized previously to the same or a cross-reacting drug, there should be an interval between initiation of treatment and the subsequent reaction. For most medications, this interval is rarely less than 1 week, and reactions generally appear within a month or so following initiation of therapy. It is unusual for a drug taken for long periods of time to be incriminated. This information has proved especially useful in deciding which drug is the likely offender when patients are receiving multiple medications. It is helpful to construct a graph denoting times when drugs were added and discontinued, along with the time of onset of clinical manifestations. For patients previously sensitized to a drug, allergic reactions may occur within minutes or hours after institution of therapy.

In Vivo Testing

In vivo testing for drug hypersensitivity involves skin testing or cautious readministration of the suspected provocative agent, test dosing. Such an approach may be clinically indicated in selected cases.

Immediate Wheal-and-Flare Skin Tests

Prick (puncture) and intradermal cutaneous tests for IgE-mediated drug reactions may be quite helpful in some clinical situations. Tests must be performed in the absence of medications that interfere with the wheal-and-flare response, such as antihistamines and tricyclic antidepressants. Positive (histamine) and negative (diluent) control skin tests should be performed. For safety, prick tests must be negative before proceeding with intradermal tests. A wheal without surrounding erythema is clinically insignificant (277).

For high-molecular-weight agents that have multiple antigenic determinants, such as foreign antisera,

TABLE 17A.11   DRUGS FREQUENTLY IMPLICATED IN ALLERGIC DRUG REACTIONS

Aspirin and nonsteroidal anti-inflammatory drugs	Radiocontrast media
β-Lactam antibiotics	Antihypertensive agents (angiotensin-converting enzyme inhibitors, methyldopa)
Sulfonamides (antibacterial, hypoglycemics, diuretics)	Antiarrhythmia drugs (procainamide, quinidine)
Antituberculous drugs (isoniazid, rifampicin)	Heavy metals (gold salts)
Nitrofurans	Organ extracts (insulin, other hormones)[a]
Anticonvulsants (hydantoin, carbamazepine)	Antisera (antitoxins, monoclonal antibodies)[a]
Anesthetic agents (muscle relaxants, thiopental)	Enzymes (L-asparaginase, streptokinase, chymopapain)[a]
Allopurinol	Vaccines (egg-based)[a]
Antipsychotic tranquilizers	Latex[a,b]
Cisplatin	

[a]Complete antigens.

[b]Not a drug per se, but frequently present in a medical setting.

hormones (e.g., insulin), enzymes, egg-containing vaccines, monoclonal antibodies, other recombinant proteins, and latex, positive immediate wheal-and-flare skin test reactions identify patients at risk for anaphylaxis. With low-molecular-weight drugs, skin testing has a role in the evaluation of IgE-mediated reactions to β-lactam antibiotics and at times has been helpful in the detection of IgE antibodies to muscle relaxants, aminoglycosides, sulfamethoxazole, cephalosporins, and monobactams.

There are occasional reports of immediate wheal-and-flare skin tests to other drugs implicated in immediate generalized reactions, but their significance is uncertain. However, this should not deter one from attempting such with dilute solutions of the suspected drug (278). It is theoretically possible that a drug may bind to high-molecular-weight carriers at the skin test site, thus permitting the required IgE antibody cross-linking for mast cell mediator release and the attendant wheal-and-flare response. When such testing is attempted with drugs that have not been previously validated, normal controls must also be tested to eliminate the possibility of false-positive responses. A positive skin test suggests that the patient may be at risk for an IgE-mediated reaction; however, a negative skin test reaction does not eliminate that possibility.

Patch Tests

Patch and photo patch tests are of value in cases of contact dermatitis to topically applied medicaments, even if the eruption was provoked by systemic administration of the drug. In photoallergic reactions, the patch test may become positive only after subsequent exposure to an erythemic dose of ultraviolet light (photo patch testing). The value of the patch test as a diagnostic tool in systemic drug reactions is unclear. However, some patients who have developed maculopapular or eczematous rashes after the administration of carbamazepine, practolol, and diazepam have consistently demonstrated positive patch tests to these drugs (279).

Incremental Provocative Test Dosing

Direct challenge of the patient with a test dose of the drug (provocative test dosing) remains the only absolute method to establish or exclude an etiologic relationship between most suspected drugs and the clinical manifestations produced. In certain situations, it is essential to determine whether a patient reacts to the drug, especially if there are no acceptable substitutes. Provocative testing only to satisfy the patient's curiosity or physician's academic interest is not justified. The procedure is potentially dangerous and is inadvisable without appropriate consultation and considerable experience in management of hypersensitivity phenomena. In fact, in one large series, patients were rechallenged with a drug suspected of producing a cutaneous reaction; 86% recurred, 11% of which were severe reactions (135).

The principle of incremental test dosing, also known as *graded challenge*, is to administer sufficiently small doses that would not cause a serious reaction initially, and to increase the dose by safe increments (usually 2-fold to 10-fold) over a matter of hours or days until a therapeutic dose is achieved (2). Generally, the initial starting dose is 1% of the therapeutic dose; it is 100-fold to 1,000-fold less if the previous reaction was severe. If the prior reaction was acute (e.g., anaphylaxis), the increased doses may be given at 15- to 30-minute intervals, with the entire procedure completed in 4 hours or less. When the previous reaction was delayed (e.g., morbilliform dermatitis), the interval between doses may be 24 to 48 hours and requires several weeks or longer for completion. Such slow test dosing may not be feasible in urgent situations, such as the need for TMP-SMX in AIDS patients with life-threatening *Pneumocystis carinii* pneumonia. If a reaction occurs during test dosing, a decision must be made as to whether the drug should be terminated or desensitization attempted.

Provocative test dosing should not be confused with desensitization (3). With respect to test dosing, the probability of a true allergic reaction is low, but the clinician is concerned about the possibility of such a reaction. It is likely that many of these patients could have tolerated the drug without significant risk, but for safety, reassurance, and medicolegal concerns, this cautious administration has merit. Desensitization is the procedure employed to administer a drug to a patient in whom true allergy has been reasonably well established, specifically IgE-mediated, immediate hypersensitivity.

Before proceeding with drug challenges, informed consent must be obtained and the information recorded in the medical record. It is advisable to explain the risks of giving as well as withholding the drug. Appropriate specialty consultation to underscore the need for the drug is desirable, if available. Hospitalization is usually required, and emergency equipment to treat anaphylaxis must be available. The drug challenge is performed immediately before treatment, not weeks or months in advance of therapy. Also, prophylactic treatment with antihistamines and corticosteroids before drug challenges is not recommended because these mask more mild reactions that may occur at low doses, risking a more serious reaction at higher doses. Drug rechallenges should not be considered when the previous reaction resulted in erythema multiforme major (SJS), TEN, exfoliative dermatitis, and drug-induced immune cytopenias.

In Vitro Testing

Testing *in vitro* to detect drug hypersensitivity has the obvious advantage of avoiding the inherent dangers in challenging patients with the drug. Although the demonstration of the drug-specific IgE is usually considered significant, the presence of other drug-specific immunoglobulin classes or cell-mediated allergy correlates poorly with a clinical adverse reaction. Drug-specific immune responses occur more frequently than clinical allergic drug reactions.

Drug-specific Immunoglobulin E Antibodies

The *in vitro* detection of drug-specific IgE antibodies is generally less sensitive than skin testing with the suspected agent. Further, this approach, as was true for skin testing with drugs, is hampered by the lack of information regarding relevant drug metabolites that are immunogenic.

A solid-phase radioimmunoassay, the radioallergosorbent test (RAST) has been validated mainly for the detection of IgE antibodies to the major (penicilloyl) determinant of penicillin and correlates reasonably well with skin tests using penicilloyl-polylysine. A RAST for penicillin minor determinant sensitivity remains elusive. In addition to penicillin, specific IgE antibodies have been detected in the sera of patients who sustained generalized immediate reactions to other β-lactam antibiotics, sulfamethoxazole, trimethoprim, sodium aurothiomalate, muscle relaxants, insulin, chymopapain, and latex (280). If positive, these tests may be helpful in identifying patients at risk; if negative, they do not exclude the possibility.

Drug-specific Immunoglobulin G and Immunoglobulin M Antibodies

With the exception of drug-induced immune cytopenias, there is often little correlation between the presence of drug-specific IgG and IgM antibodies and other drug-induced immunopathologic reactions. It has been reported that the presence of IgG antibodies to protamine in diabetic patients treated with NPH insulin increased the risk for immediate generalized reactions to protamine sulfate (281).

Drug-induced immune cytopenias afford an opportunity to test affected cells *in vitro*. Such testing should be performed as soon as the suspicion arises because the antibodies may disappear rapidly after withdrawal of the drug. For drug-induced immune hemolysis, a positive Coombs test is a useful screening procedure and may be followed by tests for drug-specific antibodies if available. Antiplatelet antibodies are best detected by the complement fixation test and the liberation of platelet factor 3. *In vitro* tests for drug-induced immune agranulocytosis are often disappointing because leukoagglutinins disappear very rapidly and are occasionally present in neutropenic conditions where no drug is involved.

Lymphocyte Blast Transformation

T lymphocyte-mediated reactions (delayed hypersensitivity) have been suspected in some patients with drug allergy. Lymphocyte blastogenesis (lymphocyte transformation test) has been suggested as an *in vitro* diagnostic test for such reactions. This test detects *in vitro* proliferation of the patient's lymphocytes in response to drugs (282). A variation on this assay measures the T lymphocyte-cytokine production rather than proliferation (283). There is disagreement regarding the value of this procedure in the diagnosis of drug allergy. However, because there appears to be a high incidence of false-negative and false-positive results, these tests have little clinical relevance (284).

Other Tests

The measurement of mast cell mediator release during drug-induced anaphylaxis or anaphylactoid reactions appears to be promising. Tryptase is a neutral protease that is specifically released by mast cells and remains in the serum for at least 3 hours after the reaction (285). It is a relatively stable protein that may be measured in stored serum samples. After a reaction, several serum samples should be obtained during the first 8 to 12 hours. A positive test for tryptase is helpful, but a negative result does not rule out an immediate generalized reaction.

Complement activation and immune complex assays are other tests that may be helpful in the evaluation of drug-induced serum sickness–like reactions. Immunoglobulins and complement have been demonstrated in drug-induced immunologic nephritis, but it is often unclear whether the drugs themselves are present in the immune complexes (286).

Withdrawal of the Suspected Drug

With a reasonable history suggesting drug allergy and the usual lack of objective tests to support the diagnosis, further clinical evaluation involves withdrawal of the suspected drugs, followed by prompt resolution of the reaction, often within a few days or weeks. This is presumptive evidence of drug allergy and usually suffices for most clinical purposes.

Typically, patients are taking several medications. Those drugs that are not clearly indicated should be stopped. For drugs that are necessary, an attempt should be made to switch to alternative, noncross-reacting agents. After the reaction subsides, resumption of treatment with the drug least likely to have caused the problem may be considered, if that drug is sufficiently important. However, there may be risk for anaphylaxis if the causative agent is resumed after interruption of therapy. Therefore, this should be considered before any therapy is discontinued.

There may be circumstances in which it would be detrimental to discontinue a drug when there is no suitable alternative available. The physician must then consider whether the drug reaction or the disease poses a greater risk. If the reaction is mild and does not appear to be progressive, it may be desirable to treat the reaction symptomatically and continue therapy. For example, in patients being treated with a β-lactam antibiotic, the appearance of urticaria may be managed with antihistamines or low-dose prednisone. Anaphylaxis has not developed in this setting (4). However, interruption of therapy for 24 to 48 hours may result in anaphylaxis if treatment is resumed.

■ PATIENT MANAGEMENT CONSIDERATIONS: TREATMENT, PREVENTION, AND REINTRODUCTION OF DRUGS

Treatment of Allergic Drug Reactions

General Principles

Withdrawal of the suspected drug is the most helpful diagnostic maneuver. At the same time, it is also the treatment of choice. Frequently, no additional treatment is necessary, and the clinical manifestations often subside within a few days or weeks without significant morbidity. If the reaction is not severe, and more than one drug is a candidate, withdrawal of one drug at a time may clarify the situation.

There may be clinical situations in which continued use of the suspected drug is essential. Here, the risk of continuing the drug may be less than the risk of not treating the underlying disease, particularly if no suitable alternative drug is available. Careful observation of the patient to detect any progression of the reaction, for example, a morbilliform rash becoming exfoliative in nature, and use of antihistamines and prednisone, may permit completion of the recommended course of therapy. Some physicians may elect to treat through milder reactions, but this is not without risk and should be supervised by physicians with experience. There are also situations in which a manifestation, often cutaneous, appears during the treatment but is due to the basic illness and not the drug.

Symptomatic Treatment

Pharmacologic management of allergic drug reactions is aimed at alleviating the manifestations until the reaction subsides. For mild reactions, therapy is usually not required. Treatment of more severe reactions depends on the nature of the skin eruption and the degree of systemic involvement.

Drug-induced anaphylaxis and anaphylactoid reactions, urticaria, angioedema, and asthma are treated in a manner described in other chapters in this text dealing with these entities.

For most patients with drug-induced serum sickness or serum sickness–like reactions, treatment with antihistamines and NSAIDs is all that is required. More severe manifestations require treatment with prednisone, 40 mg to 60 mg daily to start, with tapering over 7 to 10 days. Occasionally, plasmapheresis has been used to remove immune reactants.

The treatment of SJS includes high-dose corticosteroid therapy (191,192). For milder ambulatory cases, a minimum of 80 mg of prednisone daily is advised. Severe cases require hospitalization and administration of 60 mg of intravenous methylprednisolone every 4 to 6 hours until the lesions show improvement. Corticosteroids should then be tapered slowly over 2 to 3 weeks because tapering prematurely may result in recurrence of the lesions (191,192). For TEN, corticosteroids will not suppress the severe cutaneous involvement, and such patients are most efficiently managed in a burn unit. IVIG in doses totaling 2 g/kg appear to decrease mortality and time to recovery (287,288). Sepsis is the principal cause of death in affected patients.

For other drug-induced immune reactions, such as drug fever, DRESS, DIL, and vasculitis, and for reactions involving circulating blood elements and solid organs, corticosteroids accelerate resolution of these adverse drug effects and may prevent irreparable damage or even fatalities.

Prevention of Allergic Drug Reactions

Drug Considerations

The best way to reduce the incidence of allergic drug reactions is to prescribe only those medications that are clinically essential. Of 30 penicillin anaphylactic deaths, only 12 patients had clear indication for penicillin administration (289). A survey of patients with allopurinol hypersensitivity syndrome reported that the drug was given correctly in only 14 of 72 cases, and there were 17 deaths (290). Also, using many drugs when fewer would be adequate will complicate identification of the offending drug should a reaction occur. The use of drugs in Scotland is about half that in the United States, and not surprisingly, the incidence of adverse drug reactions is considerably less (291). Interruption of therapy increases risk for allergy and should be avoided. The physician must be well informed regarding adverse reactions to drugs being prescribed.

Patient Considerations

The patient or a responsible person must be questioned carefully about a previous reaction to any drug about to be prescribed, and information should also be obtained about all other drugs previously taken. If available, a review of the patient's medical records may uncover essential information regarding prior drug reactions. Unfortunately, studies have demonstrated that many health care professionals do not obtain adequate drug histories and document them in the medical record. This incomplete documentation did not appear to be related to the patients' inability to provide accurate information (292). Failure to follow these simple procedures not only may harm patients but also may result in significant malpractice claims (293).

Although overdiagnosis may be a problem, it is generally advisable to accept what the patient believes or has been advised without the need for further documentation. Fortunately, there are alternative, noncross-reacting agents available for most clinical situations. However, there may be situations in which one might choose an alternative drug when there is a chance of cross-reactivity; for example, selecting a cephalosporin in a penicillin-allergic patient to avoid using a more toxic drug, such as an aminoglycoside. In this situation, the patient should be skin tested for penicillin, and if test results are positive, the cross-reacting drug should be administered with a desensitization protocol in a monitored setting. Although cross-reactivity risk may be low, reactions may be severe (294).

Available Screening Tests

For acute generalized reactions, immediate wheal-and-flare skin tests are sensitive indicators for the detection of specific IgE antibodies to proteins. Skin testing is mandatory before administration of foreign antisera to reduce the likelihood of anaphylaxis.

Immediate wheal-and-flare skin tests with nonprotein, haptenic drugs have been validated for penicillin, thus permitting identification of patients with a history of penicillin allergy who are no longer at significant risk for readministration of this agent. For other haptenic drugs, such testing may detect drug-specific IgE antibodies when positive at concentrations that do not result in false-positive reactions in normal subjects. However, negative skin tests do not eliminate the possibility of clinically significant allergic sensitivity. None of the available *in vitro* tests for assessment of drug hypersensitivity qualify as screening procedures. Obviously, the simplicity, rapidity, and sensitivity of skin testing make it a logical choice for clinical purposes.

Methods of Drug Administration

Although there is some disagreement (47), the oral route of drug administration is perhaps preferable to parenteral administration because allergic reactions are less frequent and generally less severe. Clearly, topical use of drugs carries the highest risk for sensitization. For drugs given parenterally, an extremity should be used if possible to permit placement of a tourniquet if a reaction occurs. Close observation is required as one study noted that most severe reactions involving IV medications resulted in the patient arresting in less than 5 minutes

(81). In addition, patients should be kept under observation for 30 minutes after parenteral administration of a drug. If the patient is likely to develop a vasovagal reaction after an injection, the drug may be given while the patient is sitting or in a recumbent position.

Prolonged exposure to a drug increases the likelihood of sensitization. The frequency of drug usage increases the chance of eliciting an allergic response. The risk for a reaction appears to be greater during the first few months after a preceding course of treatment.

Follow-up After an Allergic Drug Reaction

The responsibility to a patient who has sustained an adverse drug reaction does not end with discontinuation of the agent and subsequent management of the reaction. The patient or responsible people must be informed of the reaction and advised how to avoid future exposure to the suspected agent and any agents that may cross-react with the offending drug. It is also helpful to mention alternative drugs that may be useful in the future. The patient should be educated regarding the importance of alerting other treating physicians about drugs being taken and any past adverse drug reactions. A retrospective cohort study by Apter et al. found that represcription of penicillin to patients with previous reactions is more common than anticipated (295).

All medical records must prominently display this information in a conspicuous location. The patient could carry a card (296) or wear an identification tag or bracelet (MedicAlert Emblems, Turlock, CA) noting those drugs to be avoided if possible.

Reintroduction of Drugs to Patients with a History of a Previous Reaction

If the patient has had a previous documented or suspected allergic reaction to a medication, and now requires its use again, the physician must consider the risks and benefits of readministration of that drug. Cautious reintroduction of that medication may be considered when there are no acceptable alternatives available or when the alternative drug produces unacceptable side effects, is clearly less effective, or requires limited use because of resistance (e.g., increased vancomycin use leading to vancomycin-resistant enterococci). Physicians specializing in hypersensitivity reactions have developed a number of management strategies that permit many patients to receive appropriate drug therapy safely or to undergo an essential diagnostic evaluation (3). These procedures include premedication protocols, desensitization schedules, and test-dosing regimens (Fig. 17A.1).

Because these approaches constitute reintroduction of an agent previously implicated in an allergic reaction and thereby carry a risk for a potentially severe, even fatal,

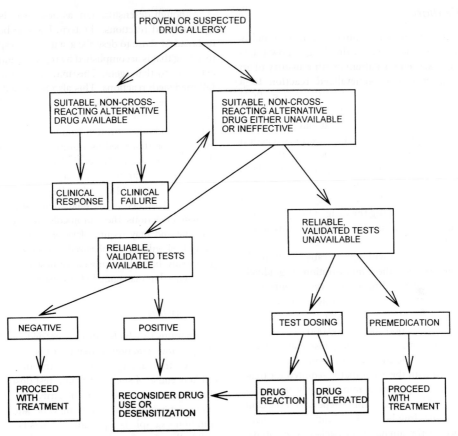

■ **FIGURE 17A.1** This algorithm provides guidelines for the reintroduction of drugs to patients with a history of a previous drug reaction.

reaction, consultation should be obtained from the appropriate specialist (e.g., infectious disease specialist) to underscore the essentiality of the drug and its subsequent readministration. The medical record must contain this information in writing as well as informed consent from the patient or other responsible individuals. Informed consent must include a statement of potential risks of the procedure as well as risks that may develop without the treatment. Further, the medical setting should provide arrangements for emergency treatment of an acute reaction. Ideally, patients should not be receiving β-blocking drugs (even timolol ophthalmic solution), and asthma, if present, must be under optimal control.

Desensitization is best performed by an experienced allergist. Medical supervision is required throughout the procedure which should be done in an intensive care unit setting. Patients are often frightened by the risks of these procedures, and symptoms of anxiety may make evaluation difficult. The physicians must quickly decide whether to continue or abandon the procedure. In general, the presence of symptoms without objective findings suggests that the reaction may be psychological in nature, and treatment should be continued.

Premedication

The prophylactic administration of antihistamines and corticosteroids alone or in combination with β-adrenergic agonists has been effective in reducing the incidence and severity of anaphylactoid reactions to RCM among patients with a previous history of such reactions. A similar approach has been used to minimize the likelihood of an anaphylactoid reaction following the administration of intravenous muscle relaxants, opiates, iron dextran, and protamine (3,297) as well as many chemotherapeutic agents (98). It appears likely that drug-induced anaphylactoid events and possibly other situations in which reaction mechanisms are unknown may be amenable to medication by such pretreatment regimens. Such premedication protocols are ineffective in blocking drug-induced IgE-mediated anaphylaxis. For this reason, prophylactic therapy before desensitization or test dosing to drugs is not recommended (3). Pretreatment may mask a mild reaction occurring at low doses of the drug and risk a more serious reaction at higher doses, which may be more difficult to manage.

Desensitization

Desensitization involves the conversion from a highly sensitive state to one in which the drug is now tolerated. This is reserved for patients with a history of an IgE-mediated immediate generalized reaction to a drug, confirmed by skin testing if available (e.g., PCN skin testing). Ideally, the term *desensitization* should be reserved for those reactions that have an established immunologic basis, and the cautious reaction with, and elimination of, IgE antibody as the goal. This produces a temporary, nonresponsive state lasting as long as therapy is uninterrupted. If therapy is interrupted, anaphylactic sensitivity may return within 48 hours of stopping the drug. Thus, continuation of an agent, such as insulin, after desensitization, is appropriate.

Acute desensitization with agents causing IgE-mediated reactions involves the administration of gradually increasing doses of the drug over several hours (e.g., penicillin) or days (e.g., insulin), often starting with amounts as low as $\frac{1}{1,000,000}$ to $\frac{1}{100,000}$ of the therapeutic dose. The initial desensitizing dose may be based on the results of skin testing or test dosing. This process is accomplished with the agent that is required for treatment. Both oral and parenteral routes have been used for desensitization. The choice of route depends on the clinical condition, the drug being given, and the experience or preference of the attending physician. The intravenous dose is then doubled every 15 minutes while carefully monitoring the patient. Using such a protocol, anaphylaxis has not been reported during desensitization, or with continued uninterrupted treatment using a reduced dose. However, mild systemic reactions, notably urticaria and pruritus, occur in about one-third of patients during desensitization. These mild reactions may subside spontaneously; they usually respond to symptomatic treatment, dosage adjustment, or both.

This approach has been used successfully to permit treatment with β-lactam antibiotics among patients with a history of penicillin allergy and positive tests for the major and minor haptenic determinants of penicillin, among diabetic patients with systemic insulin allergy, and among patients with positive skin tests for heterologous antisera. Desensitization to these IgE-mediated reactions renders mast cells specifically unresponsive to only the drug antigen used for desensitization. In many patients, successful desensitization is accompanied by a marked decrease or disappearance of the cutaneous wheal-and-flare response. Similar changes in skin test responses have been reported after successful desensitization to aminoglycosides and vancomycin (298,299). This is temporary; within 48 hours of discontinuing the drug, the skin tests are again positive. The patient is then at risk for anaphylaxis if the drug is resumed.

Although desensitization, as described, is limited to IgE-mediated reactions, the term has also been used in its broadest sense to describe a state of unresponsiveness to a drug that is accomplished by repeated and increasing exposure to that agent. This may include delayed, not IgE-mediated, reactions. This also is applied to patients who have had undeniable reactions to these drugs in the past. However, this does not involve elimination of available IgE antibodies through "controlled anaphylaxis" and may best be described as cautious readministration of the offending agent. Protocols have been described for the cautious administration of aspirin, sulfonamides (especially TMP-SMX and sulfasalazine), allopurinol (300), and others (3). Unlike desensitization to IgE-mediated reactions, these protocols are often more cumbersome and may require days or even weeks to complete. It should be emphasized that desensitization is a potentially hazardous procedure best left to physicians experienced in managing hypersensitivity reactions.

Test Dosing

In situations in which a drug is needed and the history of a previous reaction to that agent is vague, the possibility of true allergy is low, or the drug itself is an unlikely cause of such a reaction, test dosing or graded challenge is a method used to clarify the situation and safely determine whether it may be administered. A common example is a patient who has been advised to avoid all "caines," and now requires the use of a local anesthetic agent. True systemic allergy to local anesthetics is very rare. Test dosing provides reassurance to the patient, physician, or dentist that this agent can be given safely.

The principle of test dosing is to select a dose of the drug below that which would potentially cause a serious reaction, and then proceed with relatively large incremental increases to full therapeutic doses. Using this technique, one can determine whether a reaction occurs before proceeding to the next dose. If a reaction occurs, it can be easily treated. If the drug is necessary, a desensitization protocol may then be considered.

The starting dose, incremental increase, and interval between challenges depend on the drug and the urgency of reaching therapeutic doses. For oral drugs, a usual starting dose is 0.1 mg or 1.0 mg, and then proceeds to 10 mg, 50 mg, 100 mg, and 200 mg. For parenteral drugs, the initial dose is less, for example, 0.01 mg or 0.001 mg. If the suspected reaction was immediate, a 30-minute interval between doses is appropriate, and the procedure is usually completed in 3 to 5 hours or less. For late-onset reactions, such as dermatitis, the dosing interval may be as long as 24 to 48 hours, with the procedure requiring 1 to 2 weeks or longer to complete. Although there is always the possibility of a severe reaction, the risk of test dosing appears to be very low (3).

■ REFERENCES

1. Deswarte RD. Drug allergy. In: Patterson R, Grammer LC, Greenberger PA, eds. *Allergic Diseases: Diagnosis and Management.* 4th ed. Phladelphia: JB Lippincott; 1993:395.

2. Ditto AM, Greenberger PA, Grammer LC. Drug allergy. In: Grammer LC, Greenberger PA, eds. *Patterson's Allergic Diseases.* 5th ed. Philadelphia: Lippincott, Williams & Wilkins; 1997:295.

3. Greenberger PA, Grammer LC, eds. *Drug Allergy and Protocols for Management of Drug Allergies.* 3rd ed. Providence, RI: Oceanside; 2003.

4. Adkinson NF. Drug allergy. In: Adkinson NF, Yunginger JW, Busse WW, eds. *Middleton's Allergy: Principles and Practice.* Philadelphia: Mosby; 2003:1679.

5. Classen DC, Pestotnik SL, Evans RS, et al. Computerized surveillance of adverse drug events in hospital patients. *JAMA.* 1991;266(20): 2847–2851.

6. Lazarou J, Pomeranz BH, Corey PN. Incidence of adverse drug reactions in hospitalized patients: a meta-analysis of prospective studies. *JAMA.* 1998;279(15): p.1200–1205.

7. Fattinger K, Fattinger K, Roos M, et al. Epidemiology of drug exposure and adverse drug reactions in two swiss departments of internal medicine. *Br J Clin Pharmacol.* 2000;49(2):158–167.

8. Olivier P, Boulbés O, Tubery M, et al. Assessing the feasibility of using an adverse drug reaction preventability scale in clinical practice: a study in a French emergency department. *Drug Saf.* 2002;25(14):1035–1044.

9. Dormann H, Criegee-Rieck M, Neubert A, et al. Lack of awareness of community-acquired adverse drug reactions upon hospital admission: dimensions and consequences of a dilemma. *Drug Saf.* 2003;26(5):353–362.

10. Runciman WB, Roughead EE, Semple SJ, et al. Adverse drug events and medication errors in Australia. *Int J Qual Health Care.* 2003;15(Suppl 1):i49–59.

11. Hardmeier B, Braunschweig S, Cavallaro M, et al. Adverse drug events caused by medication errors in medical inpatients. *Swiss Med Wkly.* 2004;134(45–46):664–670.

12. Jick H. Adverse drug reactions: the magnitude of the problem. *J Allergy Clin Immunol.* 1984;74(4 Pt 2):555–557.

13. Armstrong B, Dinan B, Jick H. Fatal drug reactions in patients admitted to surgical services. *Am J Surg.* 1976;132(5):643–645.

14. Porter J, Jick H. Drug-related deaths among medical inpatients. *JAMA.* 1977;237(9):879–881.

15. Pirmohamed M, James S, Meakin S, et al. Adverse drug reactions as cause of admission to hospital: prospective analysis of 18 820 patients. *BMJ.* 2004;329(7456):15–19.

16. Jick H. Drugs—remarkably nontoxic. *N Engl J Med.* 1974; 291(16):824–828.

17. Spilker B. *Guide to Clinical Trials.* New York: Raven; 1991.

18. Scott HD, Rosenbaum SE, Waters WJ, et al. Rhode Island physicians' recognition and reporting of adverse drug reactions. *R I Med J.* 1987;70(7):311–316.

19. Kessler DA. Introducing MEDWatch. A new approach to reporting medication and device adverse effects and product problems. *JAMA.* 1993;269(21):2765–2768.

20. Honig PK, Wortham DC, Zamani K, et al. Terfenadine-ketoconazole interaction. Pharmacokinetic and electrocardiographic consequences. *JAMA.* 1993;269(12):1513–1518.

21. Schatz M, Patterson R, DeSwarte R. Nonorganic adverse reactions to aeroallergen immunotherapy. *J Allergy Clin Immunol.* 1976;58(1 PT. 2):198–203.

22. Wolf S. The pharmacology of placebos. *Pharmacol Rev.* 1959;11: 689–704.

23. Penn I. Cancers following cyclosporine therapy. *Transplant Proc.* 1987;19(1 Pt 3):2211–2213.

24. Kelly CP, Pothoulakis C, LaMont JT. Clostridium difficile colitis. *N Engl J Med.* 1994;330(4):257–262.

25. Gelfand JA, Elin RJ, Berry FW Jr, et al. Endotoxemia associated with the Jarisch-Herxheimer reaction. *N Engl J Med.* 1976;295(4):211–213.

26. McInnes GT, Brodie MJ. Drug interactions that matter. A critical reappraisal. *Drugs.* 1988;36(1):83–110.

27. Affrime MB, Lorber R, Danzig M, et. al. Three month evaluation of electrocardiographic effects of loratadine in humans. *J Allergy Clin Immunol.* 1993;91(1 Pt 2):259.

28. Hansten PD, Horn JR. *The top 100 Drug Interactions: A Guide to Patient Management.* 2008 ed. Edmonds, WA: H & H Publications; 2008.

29. Beutler E. Glucose-6-phosphate dehydrogenase deficiency. *N Engl J Med.* 1991;324(3):169–174.

30. Du BN Jr. Pharmacogenetics. *Med Clin North Am.* 1969; 53(4):839–855.

31. DeSwarte RD. Drug allergy: an overview. *Clin Rev Allergy.* 1986; 4(2):143–169.

32. Ring J. Pseudoallergic drug reactions. In: Korenblat PE, ed. *Allergy: Theory and Practice.* Philadelphia: WB Saunders; 1992.

33. Greenberger PA, Patterson R. The prevention of immediate generalized reactions to radiocontrast media in high-risk patients. *J Allergy Clin Immunol.* 1991;87(4): p. 867–872.

34. deWeck AL. Pharmacologic and immunochemical mechanisms of drug hypersensitivity. *Immunol Allergy Clin North Am.* 1991;11:461–474.

35. Pichler WJ. Delayed drug hypersensitivity reactions. *Ann Intern Med.* 2003;139(8):683–693.

36. Pichler WJ. Pharmacological interaction of drugs with antigen-specific immune receptors: the p-i concept. *Curr Opin Allergy Clin Immunol.* 2002;2(4):301–305.

37. Matzinger P. Tolerance, danger, and the extended family. *Annu Rev Immunol.* 1994;12: 991–1045.

38. Seguin B, Uetrecht J. The danger hypothesis applied to idiosyncratic drug reactions. *Curr Opin Allergy Clin Immunol.* 2003;3(4): 235–242.

39. Levine BB. Immunologic mechanisms of penicillin allergy. A haptenic model system for the study of allergic diseases of man. *N Engl J Med.* 1966;275(20):1115–1125.

40. Carrington DM, Earl HS, Sullivan TJ. Studies of human IgE to a sulfonamide determinant. *J Allergy Clin Immunol.* 1987;79(3):442–447.

41. Sullivan TJ. Dehaptenation of albumin substituted with benzylpenicillin G determinants. *J Allergy Clin Immunol.* 1988;81:222.

42. Didier A, Cador D, Bongrand P, et al. Role of the quaternary ammonium ion determinants in allergy to muscle relaxants. *J Allergy Clin Immunol.* 1987;79(4):578–584.

43. Coombs RRA, Gell PGH. Classification of allergic reactions responsible for clinical hypersensitivity and disease. In: Gell PGH, Coombs RRA, Lachman PJ, eds. *Clinical Aspects of Immunology.* 3rd ed. Oxford: Blackwell Scientific Publications; 1975.

44. Janeway CA, Travers P. Immune responses in the absence of infection. In: Janeway CA, Travers P, eds. *Immunobiology: The Immune System in Health and Disease.* 2nd ed. 1995, London: Garland Press.

45. Kay AB. Concepts of allergy and hypersensitivity. In: Kay AB, ed. *Allergy and Allergic Diseases.* Malden, MA: Blackwell Science; 1997.

46. Van Arsdel PP Jr. Classification and risk factors for drug allergy. *Immunol Allergy Clin North Am.* 1991;11:475–492.

47. Adkinson NF Jr. Risk factors for drug allergy. *J Allergy Clin Immunol.* 1984;74(4 Pt 2): 567–572.

48. Gomes ER, Demoly P. Epidemiology of hypersensitivity drug reactions. *Curr Opin Allergy Clin Immunol.* 2005;5(4):309–316.

49. Barranco P, Lopez-Serrano MC. General and epidemiological aspects of allergic drug reactions. *Clin Exp Allergy.* 1998;28(Suppl 4):61–62.

50. Haddi E, Charpin D, Tafforeau M, et al. Atopy and systemic reactions to drugs. *Allergy.* 1990;45(3):236–239.

51. Enright T, Chua-Lim A, Duda E, et al. The role of a documented allergic profile as a risk factor for radiographic contrast media reaction. *Ann Allergy.* 1989;62(4):302–305.

52. Perry HM Jr, Tan EM, Carmody S, et al. Relationship of acetyl transferase activity to antinuclear antibodies and toxic symptoms in hypertensive patients treated with hydralazine. *J Lab Clin Med.* 1970;76(1):114–125.

53. Woosley RL, Drayer DE, Reidenberg MM, et al. Effect of acetylator phenotype on the rate at which procainamide induces antinuclear antibodies and the lupus syndrome. *N Engl J Med.* 1978; 298(21):1157–1159.

54. Rieder MJ, Uetrecht J, Shear NH, et al. Diagnosis of sulfonamide hypersensitivity reactions by in-vitro "rechallenge" with hydroxylamine metabolites. *Ann Intern Med.* 1989;110(4):286–289.

55. Wooley PH, Griffin J, Panayi GS, et al. HLA-DR antigens and toxic reaction to sodium aurothiomalate and D-penicillamine in patients with rheumatoid arthritis. *N Engl J Med.* 1980;303(6):300–302.

56. Roujeau JC, Huynh TN, Bracq C, et al. Genetic susceptibility to toxic epidermal necrolysis. *Arch Dermatol.* 1987;123(9):1171–1173.

57. Chung WH, Hung SI, Hong HS, et al. Medical genetics: a marker for Stevens-Johnson syndrome. *Nature.* 2004;428(6982):486.

58. Hung SI, Chung WH, Liou LB, et al. HLA-B*5801 allele as a genetic marker for severe cutaneous adverse reactions caused by allopurinol. *Proc Natl Acad Sci USA.* 2005;102(11):4134–4139.

59. Mallal S, Nolan D, Witt C, et al. Association between presence of HLA-B*5701, HLA-DR7, and HLA-DQ3 and hypersensitivity to HIV-1 reverse-transcriptase inhibitor abacavir. *Lancet.* 2002;359(9308): 727–732.

60. Hetherington S, Hughes AR, Mosteller M, et al. Genetic variations in HLA-B region and hypersensitivity reactions to abacavir. *Lancet.* 2002;359(9312):1121–1122.

61. Hughes AR, Mosteller M, Bansal AT, et al. Association of genetic variations in HLA-B region with hypersensitivity to abacavir in some, but not all, populations. *Pharmacogenomics.* 2004;5(2):203–211.

62. Hughes DA, Vilar FJ, Ward CC, et al. Cost-effectiveness analysis of HLA B*5701 genotyping in preventing abacavir hypersensitivity. *Pharmacogenetics.* 2004;14(6):335–342.

63. Sullivan TJ, Ong RC, Gilliam LK. Studies of the multiple drug allergy syndrome. *J Allergy Clin Immunol.* 1989;83:270.

64. Moseley EK, Sullivan TJ. Allergic reactions to antimicrobial drugs in patients with a history of prior drug allergy. *J Allergy Clin Immunol.* 1991;87:226.

65. Kamada MM, Twarog F, Leung DY. Multiple antibiotic sensitivity in a pediatric population. *Allergy Proc.* 1991;12(5):347–350.

66. Sullivan TJ. Management of patients allergic to antimicrobial drugs. *Allergy Proc.* 1991;12(6):361–364.

67. Moss RB. Sensitization to aztreonam and cross-reactivity with other beta-lactam antibiotics in high-risk patients with cystic fibrosis. *J Allergy Clin Immunol.* 1991;87(1 Pt 1):78–88.

68. Bierman CW, Pierson WE, Zeitz SJ, et al. Reactions associated with ampicillin therapy. *JAMA.* 1972;220(8):1098–1100.

69. Harb GE, Jacobson MA. Human immunodeficiency virus (HIV) infection. Does it increase susceptibility to adverse drug reactions? *Drug Saf.* 1993;9(1):1–8.

70. Bayard PJ, Berger TG, Jacobson MA. Drug hypersensitivity reactions and human immunodeficiency virus disease. *J Acquir Immune Defic Syndr.* 1992;5(12):1237–1257.

71. Kovacs JA, Hiemenz JW, Macher AM, et al. Pneumocystis carinii pneumonia: a comparison between patients with the acquired immunodeficiency syndrome and patients with other immunodeficiencies. *Ann Intern Med.* 1984;100(5):663–671.

72. Alfirevic A, Stalford AC, Vilar FJ, et al. Slow acetylator phenotype and genotype in HIV-positive patients with sulphamethoxazole hypersensitivity. *Br J Clin Pharmacol.* 2003;55(2):158–165.

73. Wolkenstein P, Loriot MA, Aractingi S, et al. Prospective evaluation of detoxification pathways as markers of cutaneous adverse reactions to sulphonamides in AIDS. *Pharmacogenetics.* 2000;10(9):821–828.

74. Pirmohamed M, Alfirevic A, Vilar J, et al. Association analysis of drug metabolizing enzyme gene polymorphisms in HIV-positive patients with co-trimoxazole hypersensitivity. *Pharmacogenetics.* 2000;10(8):705–713.

75. Toogood JH. Risk of anaphylaxis in patients receiving beta-blocker drugs. *J Allergy Clin Immunol.* 1988;81(1):1–5.

76. Aronson JK, ed. *Meyler's Side Effects of Drugs: The International Encyclopedia of Adverse Drug Reactions and Interactions.* 15th ed. Amsterdam: Elsevier Science; 2006:4192.

77. Aronson JK. *Side Effects of Drugs, Annual 29.* Vol 29. Amsterdam-Oxford: Elsevier; 2007.

78. Greenberger PA. Drug allergies. In: Rich RR, Fleisher TA, Schwarz BD, et al., eds. *Clinical Immunology: Principles and Practice.* St. Louis: Mosby-Year Book; 1996:988.

79. Porter J, Jick H. Drug-induced anaphylaxis, convulsions, deafness, and extrapyramidal symptoms. *Lancet.* 1977;1(8011):587–588.

80. Herrera AM, deShazo RD. Current concepts in anaphylaxis. *Immunol Allergy Clin North Am.* 1992;12:517.

81. Pumphrey RS. Fatal anaphylaxis in the UK, 1992–2001. *Novartis Found Symp.* 2004;257:116–128; discussion 128–132,157–160,276–285.

82. Weiss ME, Adkinson NF Jr, Hirshman CA. Evaluation of allergic drug reactions in the perioperative period. *Anesthesiology.* 1989; 71(4):483–486.

83. Davis H, McGoodwin E, Reed TG. Anaphylactoid reactions reported after treatment with ciprofloxacin. *Ann Intern Med.* 1989; 111(12):1041–1043.

84. Weiss RB. Hypersensitivity reactions. *Semin Oncol.* 1992;19(5): 458–477.

85. Windom HH, et al. Anaphylaxis to carboplatin—a new platinum chemotherapeutic agent. *J Allergy Clin Immunol.* 1992;90(4 Pt 1):681–683.

86. Weiss RB, Donehower RC, Wiernik PH, et al. Hypersensitivity reactions from taxol. *J Clin Oncol.* 1990;8(7):1263–1268.

87. Weiss ME. Drug allergy. *Med Clin North Am.* 1992;76(4):857–882.

88. Lenchner KI, Ditto AM. A 62-year-old woman with 3 episodes of anaphylaxis. *Ann Allergy Asthma Immunol.* 2005;95(1):14–18.

89. Laxenaire MC. Drugs and other agents involved in anaphylactic shock occurring during anaesthesia. A French multicenter epidemiological inquiry. *Ann Fr Anesth Reanim.* 1993;12(2):91–96.

90. Weiler JM, Gellhaus MA, Carte JG, et al. A prospective study of the risk of an immediate adverse reaction to protamine sulfate during cardiopulmonary bypass surgery. *J Allergy Clin Immunol.* 1990;85(4): 713–719.

91. Grammer LC, Paterson BF, Roxe D, et al. IgE against ethylene oxide-altered human serum albumin in patients with anaphylactic reactions to dialysis. *J Allergy Clin Immunol.* 1985;76(3):511–514.

92. Seggev JS, Ohta K, Tipton WR. IgE mediated anaphylaxis due to a psyllium-containing drug. *Ann Allergy.* 1984;53(4):325–326.

93. Rohr AS, Pappano JE Jr. Prophylaxis against fluorescein-induced anaphylactoid reactions. *J Allergy Clin Immunol.* 1992;90(3 Pt 1):407–408.

94. Hamstra RD, Block MH, Schocket AL. Intravenous iron dextran in clinical medicine. *JAMA.* 1980;243(17):1726–1731.

95. Dykewicz MS, Rosen ST, O'Connell MM, et al. Plasma histamine but not anaphylatoxin levels correlate with generalized urticaria from infusions of anti-lymphocyte monoclonal antibodies. *J Lab Clin Med.* 1992;120(2):290–296.

96. Cheifetz A, Smedley M, Martin S, et al. The incidence and management of infusion reactions to infliximab: a large center experience. *Am J Gastroenterol.* 2003;98(6):1315–1324.

97. Lenz HJ. Management and preparedness for infusion and hypersensitivity reactions. *Oncologist.* 2007;12(5):601–609.

98. Castells MC, Tennant NM, Sloane DE, et al. Hypersensitivity reactions to chemotherapy: outcomes and safety of rapid desensitization in 413 cases. *J Allergy Clin Immunol.* 2008;122(3):574–580.

99. Dixon FJ, et al. Pathogenesis of serum sickness. *AMA Arch Pathol.* 1958;65(1):18–28.

100. Bielory L, Gascon P, Lawley TJ, et al. Human serum sickness: a prospective analysis of 35 patients treated with equine anti-thymocyte globulin for bone marrow failure. *Medicine (Baltimore).* 1988;67(1):40–57.

101. Davidson JR, Bush RK, Grogan EW, et al. Immunology of a serum sickness/vasculitis reaction secondary to streptokinase used for acute myocardial infarction. *Clin Exp Rheumatol.* 1988;6(4):381–384.

102. Tatum AJ, Ditto AM, Patterson R. Severe serum sickness-like reaction to oral penicillin drugs: three case reports. *Ann Allergy Asthma Immunol.* 2001;86(3):330–334.

103. Erffmeyer JE. Serum sickness. *Ann Allergy.* 1986;56(2):105–109.

104. Platt R, Dreis MW, Kennedy DL, et al. Serum sickness-like reactions to amoxicillin, cefaclor, cephalexin, and trimethoprim-sulfamethoxazole. *J Infect Dis.* 1988.;158(2):474–477.

105. Naguwa SM, Nelson BL. Human serum sickness. *Clin Rev Allergy.* 1985;3(1):117–126.

106. Barnett EV, Stone G, Swisher SN, et al. Serum sickness and plasmacytosis. a clinical, immunologic and hematologic analysis. *Am J Med.* 1963;35:113–122.

107. Lawley TJ, Bielory L, Gascon P, et al. A prospective clinical and immunologic analysis of patients with serum sickness. *N Engl J Med.* 1984;311(22):1407–1413.

108. Gilliland BC. Drug-induced autoimmune and hematologic disorders. *Immunol Allergy Clin North Am.* 1991;11:525.

109. Sarzi-Puttini P, Atzeni F, Iaccarino L, et al. Environment and systemic lupus erythematosus: an overview. *Autoimmunity.* 2005;38(7):465–472.

110. Morrow JD, Schroeder HA, Perry HM Jr. Studies on the control of hypertension by hyphex. II. Toxic reactions and side effects. *Circulation.* 1953;8(6):829–839.

111. Hoffman BJ. Sensitivity to sufadiazine resembling acute disseminated lupus erythematosus. *Arch Dermatol Syphilol.* 1945;51:190–192.

112. Ladd AT. Procainamide-induced lupus erythematosus. *N Engl J Med.* 1962;267:1357–1358.

113. Abunasser J, Forouhar FA, Metersky ML. Etanercept-induced lupus erythematosus presenting as a unilateral pleural effusion. *Chest.* 2008;134(4):850–853.

114. Benucci M, Nenci G, Cappelletti C, et al. (Lupus like syndrome induced by treatment with anti TNF alpha (infliximab): report of three cases. *Recenti Prog Med.* 2008;99(7–8):363–366.

115. Carter JD, Valeriano-Marcet J, Kanik KS, et al. Antinuclear antibody-negative, drug-induced lupus caused by lisinopril. *South Med J.* 2001;94(11):1122–1123.

116. Graziadei IW, Obermoser GE, Sepp NT, et al. Drug-induced lupus-like syndrome associated with severe autoimmune hepatitis. *Lupus.* 2003;12(5):409–412.

117. Pistiner M, Wallace DJ, Nessim S, et al. Lupus erythematosus in the 1980s: a survey of 570 patients. *Semin Arthritis Rheum.* 1991;21(1):55–64.

118. Atzeni F, Marrazza MG, Sarzi-Puttini P, et al. [Drug-induced lupus erythematosus]. *Reumatismo.* 2003;55(3):147–154.

119. Kale SA. Drug-induced systemic lupus erythematosus. Differentiating it from the real thing. *Postgrad Med.* 1985;77(3):231–235,238–239,242.

120. Steinberg AD, Gourley MF, Klinman DM, et al. NIH conference. Systemic lupus erythematosus. *Ann Intern Med.* 1991;115(7):548–559.

121. Batchelor JR, Welsh KI, Tinoco RM, et al. Hydralazine-induced systemic lupus erythematosus: influence of HLA-DR and sex on susceptibility. *Lancet.* 1980;1(8178):1107–1109.

122. Gunnarsson I, Nordmark B, Hassan Bakri A, et al. Development of lupus-related side-effects in patients with early RA during sulphasalazine treatment-the role of IL-10 and HLA. *Rheumatology (Oxford).* 2000;39(8): 886–893.

123. Mansilla-Tinoco R, Harland SJ, Ryan PJ, et al. Hydralazine, antinuclear antibodies, and the lupus syndrome. *Br Med J (Clin Res Ed).* 1982;284(6320):936–939.

124. Speirs C, Fielder AH, Chapel H, et al. Complement system protein C4 and susceptibility to hydralazine-induced systemic lupus erythematosus. *Lancet.* 1989;1(8644):922–924.

125. Lahita R, Kluger J, Drayer DE, et al. Antibodies to nuclear antigens in patients treated with procainamide or acetylprocainamide. *N Engl J Med.* 1979;301(25): 1382–1385.

126. Stec GP, Lertora JJ, Atkinson AJ Jr, et al. Remission of procainamide-induced lupus erythematosus with N-acetylprocainamide therapy. *Ann Intern Med.* 1979;90(5):799–801.

127. Blomgren SE, Condemi JJ, Bignall MC, et al. Antinuclear antibody induced by procainamide. A prospective study. *N Engl J Med.* 1969;281(2):64–66.

128. Finegold I. Oral desensitization to trimethoprim-sulfamethoxazole in a patient with AIDS. *J Allergy Clin Immunol.* 1985;75:137.

129. Gleichmann E, Pals ST, Rolink AG, et al. Graft-versus-host reactions: clues to the etiopathology of a spectrum of immunological disease. *Immunol Today.* 1984;5:324.

130. Fauci AS. Vasculitis. *J Allergy Clin Immunol.* 1983;72(3):211–223.

131. Hunder GG, Arend WP, Bloch DA, et al. The American College of Rheumatology 1990 criteria for the classification of vasculitis. Introduction. *Arthritis Rheum.* 1990;33(8):1065–1067.

132. Arellano F, Sacristan JA. Allopurinol hypersensitivity syndrome: a review. *Ann Pharmacother.* 1993;27(3):337–343.

133. Wiik A. Laboratory diagnostics in vasculitis patients. *Isr Med Assoc J.* 2001;3(4):275–277.

134. Bigby M, Jick S, Jick H, et al. Drug-induced cutaneous reactions. A report from the Boston Collaborative Drug Surveillance Program on 15,438 consecutive inpatients, 1975 to 1982. *JAMA.* 1986;256(24): 3358–3363.

135. Kauppinen K. Rational performance of drug challenge in cutaneous hypersensitivity. *Semin Dermatol.* 1983;2:227–230.

136. Kauppinen K, Stubb S. Drug eruptions: causative agents and clinical types. A series of in-patients during a 10-year period. *Acta Derm Venereol.* 1984;64(4):320–324.

137. Roujeau JC, Stern RS. Severe adverse cutaneous reactions to drugs. *N Engl J Med.* 1994;331(19):1272–1285.

138. Levenson DE, Arndt KA, Stern RS. Cutaneous manifestations of adverse drug reactions. *Immunol Allergy Clin North Am.* 1991;11:493.

139. Bocquet H, Bagot M, Roujeau JC. Drug-induced pseudolymphoma and drug hypersensitivity syndrome (drug rash with eosinophilia and systemic symptoms: DRESS). *Semin Cutan Med Surg.* 1996;15(4):250–257.

140. Story RE, Ditto AM. A 32-year-old man with tuberculosis, fever, and rash. *Ann Allergy Asthma Immunol.* 2004;92(5):495–499.

141. Alanko K, Stubb S, Kauppinen K. Cutaneous drug reactions: clinical types and causative agents. A five-year survey of in-patients (1981–1985). *Acta Derm Venereol.* 1989;69(3):223–226.

142. Hedner T, Samuelsson O, Lunde H, et al. Angio-oedema in relation to treatment with angiotensin converting enzyme inhibitors. *BMJ.* 1992;304(6832):941–946.

143. Orfan N, Patterson R, Dykewicz MS. Severe angioedema related to ACE inhibitors in patients with a history of idiopathic angioedema. *JAMA.* 1990;264(10):1287–1289.

144. Miller DR, Oliveria SA, Berlowitz DR, et al. Angioedema incidence in US veterans initiating angiotensin-converting enzyme inhibitors. *Hypertension.* 2008;51(6): 1624–1630.

145. Kostis JB, Kim HJ, Rusnak J, et al. Incidence and characteristics of angioedema associated with enalapril. *Arch Intern Med.* 2005. 165(14):1637–1642.

146. Chin HL, Buchan DA. Severe angioedema after long-term use of an angiotensin-converting enzyme inhibitor. *Ann Intern Med.* 1990;112(4):312–313.

147. Anderson MW, deShazo RD. Studies of the mechanism of angiotensin-converting enzyme (ACE) inhibitor-associated angioedema: the effect of an ACE inhibitor on cutaneous responses to bradykinin, codeine, and histamine. *J Allergy Clin Immunol.* 1990;85(5):856–858.

148. Sharma PK, Yium JJ. Angioedema associated with angiotensin II receptor antagonist losartan. *South Med J.* 1997;90(5):552–553.

149. Rupprecht R, Vente C, Grafe A, et al. Angioedema due to losartan. *Allergy.* 1999; 54(1):81–82.

150. Angelini G, Vena GA, Meneghini CL. Allergic contact dermatitis to some medicaments. *Contact Dermatitis.* 1985;12(5):263–269.

151. Storrs FJ. Contact dermatitis caused by drugs. *Immunol Allergy Clin North Am.* 1991;11:509.

152. Rudzki E, Zakrzewski Z, Rebandel P, et al. Cross reactions between aminoglycoside antibiotics. *Contact Dermatitis.* 1988;18(5): 314–16.

153. Elias JA, Levinson AI. Hypersensitivity reactions to ethylenediamine in aminophylline. *Am Rev Respir Dis.* 1981;123(5):550–552.

154. Storrs FJ, Rosenthal LE, Adams RM, et al. Prevalence and relevance of allergic reactions in patients patch tested in North America—1984 to 1985. *J Am Acad Dermatol.* 1989;20(6):1038–1045.

155. Rietschel RL, Adams RM. Reactions to thimerosal in hepatitis B vaccines. *Dermatol Clin.* 1990;8(1):161–164.

156. Fisher AA. Contact dermatitis from topical medicaments. *Semin Dermatol.* 1982;1:49.

157. Shukla SR. Drugs causing fixed drug eruptions. *Dermatologica.* 1981;163(2):160–163.

158. Pandhi RK, Kumar AS, Satish DA, et al. Fixed drug eruptions on male genitalia: clinical and etiologic study. *Sex Transm Dis.* 1984;11(3):164–166.

159. Stubb S, Heikkila H, Kauppinen K. Cutaneous reactions to drugs: a series of in-patients during a five-year period. *Acta Derm Venereol.* 1994;74(4):289–291.

160. Sharma VK, Dhar S. Clinical pattern of cutaneous drug eruption among children and adolescents in north India. *Pediatr Dermatol.* 1995;12(2):178–183.

161. Cohen HA, Barzilai A, Matalon A, et al. Fixed drug eruption of the penis due to hydroxyzine hydrochloride. *Ann Pharmacother.* 1997;31(3):327–329.

162. Gruber F, Stasic A, Lenkovic M, et al. Postcoital fixed drug eruption in a man sensitive to trimethoprim-sulphamethoxazole. *Clin Exp Dermatol.* 1997;22(3): 144–145.

163. Shiohara T. The interaction between keratinocytes and T cells—an overview of the role of adhesion molecules and the characterization of epidermal T cells. *J Dermatol.* 1992;19(11): 726–730.

164. Choi HJ, Ku JK, Kim MY, et al. Possible role of Fas/Fas ligand-mediated apoptosis in the pathogenesis of fixed drug eruption. *Br J Dermatol.* 2006;154(3):419–425.

165. Sehgal VN, Srivastava G. Fixed drug eruption (FDE): changing scenario of incriminating drugs. *Int J Dermatol.* 2006.;45(8):897–908.

166. Mahboob A, Haroon TS. Drugs causing fixed eruptions: a study of 450 cases. *Int J Dermatol.* 1998;37(11):833–838.

167. Lee AY. Topical provocation in 31 cases of fixed drug eruption: change of causative drugs in 10 years. *Contact Dermatitis.* 1998;38(5):258–260.

168. Thankappan TP, Zachariah J. Drug-specific clinical pattern in fixed drug eruptions. *Int J Dermatol.* 1991;30(12):867–870.

169. Roujeau JC, Bioulac-Sage P, Bourseau C, et al. Acute generalized exanthematous pustulosis. Analysis of 63 cases. *Arch Dermatol.* 1991;127(9):1333–1338.

170. Roujeau JC. Neutrophilic drug eruptions. *Clin Dermatol.* 2000;18(3):331–337.

171. Sidoroff A, Halevy S, Bavinck JN, et al. Acute generalized exanthematous pustulosis (AGEP)—a clinical reaction pattern. *J Cutan Pathol.* 2001;28(3):113–119.

172. Baker H, Ryan TJ. Generalized pustular psoriasis. A clinical and epidemiological study of 104 cases. *Br J Dermatol.* 1968;80(12): 771–793.

173. Beylot C, Bioulac P, Doutre MS. [Acute generalized exanthematic pustuloses (four cases) (author's transl)]. *Ann Dermatol Venereol.* 1980;107(1–2):37–48.

174. Roujeau JC. Clinical heterogeneity of drug hypersensitivity. *Toxicology.* 2005;209(2): 123–129.

175. Britschgi M, Pichler WJ. Acute generalized exanthematous pustulosis, a clue to neutrophil-mediated inflammatory processes orchestrated by T cells. *Curr Opin Allergy Clin Immunol.* 2002;2(4):325–331.

176. Schmid S, Kuechler PC, Britschgi M, et al. Acute generalized exanthematous pustulosis: role of cytotoxic T cells in pustule formation. *Am J Pathol.* 2002;161(6):2079–2086.

177. Huff JC, Weston WL, Tonnesen MG. Erythema multiforme: a critical review of characteristics, diagnostic criteria, and causes. *J Am Acad Dermatol.* 1983;8(6):763–775.

178. Brice SL, Krzemien D, Weston WL, et al. Detection of herpes simplex virus DNA in cutaneous lesions of erythema multiforme. *J Invest Dermatol.* 1989;93(1):183–187.

179. Finan MC, Schroeter AL. Cutaneous immunofluorescence study of erythema multiforme: correlation with light microscopic patterns and etiologic agents. *J Am Acad Dermatol.* 1984;10(3):497–506.

180. Shiohara T, Chiba M, Tanaka Y, et al. Drug-induced, photosensitive, erythema multiforme-like eruption: possible role for cell adhesion

molecules in a flare induced by Rhus dermatitis. *J Am Acad Dermatol.* 1990;22(4):647–650.

181. Tonnesen MG, Harrist TJ, Wintroub BU, et al. Erythema multiforme: microvascular damage and infiltration of lymphocytes and basophils. *J Invest Dermatol.* 1983;80(4):282–286.

182. Margolis RJ, Tonnesen MG, Harrist TJ, et al. Lymphocyte subsets and Langerhans cells/indeterminate cells in erythema multiforme. *J Invest Dermatol.* 1983;81(5):403–406.

183. Heng MC, Allen SG. Efficacy of cyclophosphamide in toxic epidermal necrolysis. Clinical and pathophysiologic aspects. *J Am Acad Dermatol.* 1991;25(5 Pt 1):778–786.

184. Miyauchi H, Hosokawa H, Akaeda T, et al. T-cell subsets in drug-induced toxic epidermal necrolysis. Possible pathogenic mechanism induced by CD8-positive T cells. *Arch Dermatol.* 1991;127(6):851–855.

185. Hertl M, Bohlen H, Jugert F, et al. Predominance of epidermal CD8+ T lymphocytes in bullous cutaneous reactions caused by beta-lactam antibiotics. *J Invest Dermatol.* 1993;101(6):794–799.

186. Correia O, Delgado L, Ramos JP, et al. Cutaneous T-cell recruitment in toxic epidermal necrolysis. Further evidence of CD8+ lymphocyte involvement. *Arch Dermatol.* 1993;129(4):466–468.

187. Power WJ, Saidman SL, Zhang DS, et al. HLA typing in patients with ocular manifestations of Stevens-Johnson syndrome. *Ophthalmology.* 1996;103(9): 1406–1409.

188. Cheriyan S, Rosa RM, Patterson R. Stevens-Johnson syndrome presenting as intravenous line sepsis. *Allergy Proc.* 1995;16(2):85–87.

189. Mockenhaupt M, Viboud C, Dunant A, et al. Stevens-Johnson syndrome and toxic epidermal necrolysis: assessment of medication risks with emphasis on recently marketed drugs. The EuroSCAR-study. *J Invest Dermatol.* 2008;128(1):35–44.

190. Severino G, Chillotti C, De Lisa R, et al. Adverse reactions during imatinib and lansoprazole treatment in gastrointestinal stromal tumors. *Ann Pharmacother.* 2005;39(1):162–164.

191. Cheriyan S, Patterson R, Greenberger PA, et al. The outcome of Stevens-Johnson syndrome treated with corticosteroids. *Allergy Proc.* 1995;16(4):151–155.

192. Tripathi A, Ditto AM, Grammer LC, et al. Corticosteroid therapy in an additional 13 cases of Stevens-Johnson syndrome: a total series of 67 cases. *Allergy Asthma Proc.* 2000;21(2):101–105.

193. Adam JE. Exofoliative dermatitis. *Can Med Assoc J.* 1968;99(13): 660–666.

194. Nicolis GD, Helwig EB. Exfoliative dermatitis. A clinicopathologic study of 135 cases. *Arch Dermatol.* 1973;108(6):788–797.

195. Bigby M, Stern RS, Arndt KA. Allergic cutaneous reactions to drugs. *Prim Care.* 1989;16(3):713–727.

196. Epstein JH, Wintroub BU. Photosensitivity due to drugs. *Drugs.* 1985;30(1):42–57.

197. Nalbandian RM, Mader IJ, Barrett JL, et al. Petechiae, ecchymoses, and necrosis of skin induced by coumarin congeners: rare, occasionally lethal complication of anticoagulant therapy. *JAMA.* 1965;192:603–608.

198. Bauer KA. Coumarin-induced skin necrosis. *Arch Dermatol.* 1993;129(6):766–768.

199. Bastuji-Garin S, Rzany B, Stern RS, et al. Clinical classification of cases of toxic epidermal necrolysis, Stevens-Johnson syndrome, and erythema multiforme. *Arch Dermatol.* 1993;129(1):92–96.

200. Goldstein SM, Wintroub BW, Elias PM, et al. Toxic epidermal necrolysis. Unmuddying the waters. *Arch Dermatol.* 1987;123(9):1153–1156.

201. Viard I, Wehrli P, Bullani R, et al. Inhibition of toxic epidermal necrolysis by blockade of CD95 with human intravenous immunoglobulin. *Science.* 1998;282(5388):490–493.

202. Nassif A, Bensussan A, Boumsell L, et al. Toxic epidermal necrolysis: effector cells are drug-specific cytotoxic T cells. *J Allergy Clin Immunol.* 2004;114(5):1209–1215.

203. Ito K, Hara H, Okada T, et al. Toxic epidermal necrolysis treated with low-dose intravenous immunoglobulin: immunohistochemical study of Fas and Fas-ligand expression. *Clin Exp Dermatol.* 2004;29(6):679–680.

204. Amon RB, Dimond RL. Toxic epidermal necrolysis. Rapid differentiation between staphylococcal- and drug-induced disease. *Arch Dermatol.* 1975;111(11):1433–1437.

205. Heimbach DM, Engrav LH, Marvin JA, et al. Toxic epidermal necrolysis. A step forward in treatment. *JAMA.* 1987;257(16):2171–2175.

206. Mittmann N, Chan B, Knowles S, et al. Intravenous immunoglobulin use in patients with toxic epidermal necrolysis and Stevens-Johnson syndrome. *Am J Clin Dermatol.* 2006;7(6):359–368.

207. Khalili B, Bahna SL. Pathogenesis and recent therapeutic trends in Stevens-Johnson syndrome and toxic epidermal necrolysis. *Ann Allergy Asthma Immunol.* 2006;97(3):272–280; quiz 281–283,320.

208. French LE, Trent JT, Kerdel FA. Use of intravenous immunoglobulin in toxic epidermal necrolysis and Stevens-Johnson syndrome: our current understanding. *Int Immunopharmacol.* 2006;6(4):543–549.

209. Guillaume JC, Roujeau JC, Revuz J, et al. The culprit drugs in 87 cases of toxic epidermal necrolysis (Lyell's syndrome). *Arch Dermatol.* 1987;123(9):1166–1170.

210. Stern RS, Chan HL. Usefulness of case report literature in determining drugs responsible for toxic epidermal necrolysis. *J Am Acad Dermatol.* 1989;21(2 Pt 1):317–322.

211. Twarog FJ, Weinstein SF, Khaw KT, et al. Hypersensitivity to pancreatic extracts in parents of patients with cystic fibrosis. *J Allergy Clin Immunol.* 1977;59(1):35–40.

212. Pozner LH, Mandarano C, Zitt MJ, et al. Recurrent bronchospasm in a nurse. *Ann Allergy.* 1986;56(1):14–15, 44–47.

213. Coutts II, Dally MB, Taylor AJ, et al. Asthma in workers manufacturing cephalosporins. *Br Med J (Clin Res Ed).* 1981;283(6297):950.

214. Hunt LW, Rosenow EC 3rd. Asthma-producing drugs. *Ann Allergy.* 1992;68(6): 453–462.

215. Meeker DP, Wiedemann HP. Drug-induced bronchospasm. *Clin Chest Med.* 1990;11(1):163–175.

216. Fraley DS, Bruns FJ, Segel DP, et al. Propranolol-related bronchospasm in patients without history of asthma. *South Med J.* 1980;73:238–240.

217. Lunde H, Hedner T, Samuelsson O, et al. Dyspnoea, asthma, and bronchospasm in relation to treatment with angiotensin converting enzyme inhibitors. *BMJ.* 1994;308:18–21.

218. Simon SR, Black HR, Moser M, et al. Cough and ACE inhibitors. *Arch Intern Med.* 1992;152:1698–1700.

219. Pylypchuk GB. ACE inhibitor- versus angiotensin II blocker–induced cough and angioedema. *Ann Pharmacother.* 1998;32(10):1060–1066.

220. Lacourciere Y, Lefebvre J, Nakhle G, et al. Association between cough and angiotensin converting enzyme inhibitors versus angiotensin II antagonists: the design of a prospective, controlled study. *J Hypertens Suppl.* 1994;12:S49–53.

221. Israili ZH, Hall WD. Cough and angioneurotic edema associated with angiotensin-converting enzyme inhibitor therapy. A review of the literature and pathophysiology. *Ann Intern Med.* 1992;117(3):234–242.

222. Bush RK, Taylor SL, Holden K, et al. Prevalence of sensitivity to sulfiting agents in asthmatic patients. *Am J Med.* 1986;81:816–820.

223. Goldfarb G, Simon RA. Provocation of sulfite sensitive asthma. *J Allergy Clin Immunol.* 1984;73:135.

224. Simon RA, Stevenson DD. Lack of cross sensitivity between aspirin and sulfite in sensitive asthmatics. *J Allergy Clin Immunol.* 1987;79:257.

225. Holmberg L, et al. Adverse reactions to nitrofurantoin. Analysis of 921 reports. *Am J Med.* 1980;69(5):733–738.

226. Pisani RJ, Rosenow EC III. Drug-induced pulmonary disease. In: Simmons DH, Tierney DF, eds. *Current Pulmonology.* St. Louis: Mosby–Year Book; 1992:311.

227. Sostman HD, Matthay RA, Putman CE, et al. Methotrexate-induced pneumonitis. *Medicine (Baltimore).* 1976;55:371–388.

228. Martin WJ 2nd, Rosenow EC 3rd, Amiodarone pulmonary toxicity. Recognition and pathogenesis (Part I). *Chest.* 1988;93(5):1067–1075.

229. Kennedy JI Jr. Clinical aspects of amiodarone pulmonary toxicity. *Clin Chest Med.* 1990; 11(1):119–129.

230. Manicardi V, et al. Low-dose amiodarone-induced pneumonitis: evidence of an immunologic pathogenetic mechanism. *Am J Med.* 1989;86(1):134–135.

231. Kennedy JI, Myers JL, Plumb VJ, et al. Amiodarone pulmonary toxicity. Clinical, radiologic, and pathologic correlations. *Arch Intern Med.* 1987;147:50–55.

232. Evans RB, Ettensohn DB, Fawaz-Estrup F, et al. Gold lung: recent developments in pathogenesis, diagnosis, and therapy. *Semin Arthritis Rheum.* 1987;16:196–205.

233. Cooper JA Jr, White DA, Matthay RA. Drug-induced pulmonary disease. Part 1: Cytotoxic drugs. *Am Rev Respir Dis.* 1986;133(2):321–340.

234. Holoye PY, Luna MA, MacKay B, et al. Bleomycin hypersensitivity pneumonitis. *Ann Intern Med.* 1978;88:47–49.

235. Kline JN, Hirasuna JD. Pulmonary edema after freebase cocaine smoking—not due to an adulterant. *Chest.* 1990;97(4):1009–1010.

236. Brashear RE. Effects of heroin, morphine, methadone, and propoxyphene on the lung. *Semin Respir Med.* 1980;2:59.

237. Heffner JE, Sahn SA. Salicylate-induced pulmonary edema. Clinical features and prognosis. *Ann Intern Med.* 1981;95(4):405–409.

238. Andersson BS, Luna MA, Yee C, et al. Fatal pulmonary failure complicating high-dose cytosine arabinoside therapy in acute leukemia. *Cancer.* 1990;65:1079–1084.

239. Ramesh S, Reisman RE. Noncardiogenic pulmonary edema due to radiocontrast media. *Ann Allergy Asthma Immunol.* 1995;75(4):308–310.

240. Spry CJ. Eosinophilia and allergic reactions to drugs. *Clin Haematol.* 1980;9(3):521–534.

241. Davis P, Hughes GR. Significance of eosinophilia during gold therapy. *Arthritis Rheum.* 1974;17(6):964–968.

242. Stafford BT, Crosby WH. Late onset of gold-induced thrombocytopenia. With a practical note on the injections of dimercaprol. *JAMA.* 1978;239(1):50–51.

243. Shulman NR. A Mechanism of cell destruction in individuals sensitized to foreign antigens and its implications in auto-immunity. combined clinical staff conference at the National Institutes of Health. *Ann Intern Med.* 1964;60:506–521.

244. Stricker RB, Shuman MA. Quinidine purpura: evidence that glycoprotein V is a target platelet antigen. *Blood.* 1986;67(5):1377–1381.

245. Chong BH. Heparin-induced thrombocytopenia. *Blood Rev.* 1988.;2(2):108–114.

246. Chong BH, Ismail F, Cade J, et al. Heparin-induced thrombocytopenia: studies with a new low molecular weight heparinoid, Org 10172. *Blood.* 1989;73:1592–1596.

247. Salama A. Mueller-Eckhardt C. On the mechanisms of sensitization and attachment of antibodies to RBC in drug-induced immune hemolytic anemia. *Blood.* 1987;69(4):1006–1010.

248. Swanson MA, Chanmougan D, Schwartz RS. Immunohemolytic anemia due to antipenicillin antibodies. Report of a case. *N Engl J Med.* 1966;274(4):178–181.

249. Worlledge SM, Carstairs KC, Dacie JV. Autoimmune haemolytic anaemia associated with alpha-methyldopa therapy. *Lancet.* 1966;2(7455):135–139.

250. Vincent PC. Drug-induced aplastic anaemia and agranulocytosis. Incidence and mechanisms. *Drugs.* 1986;31(1):52–63.

251. Kaufman DW, Kelly JP, Jurgelon JM, et al. Drugs in the aetiology of agranulocytosis and aplastic anaemia. *Eur J Haematol Suppl.* 1996;60:23–30.

252. Andres E, Maloisel F. Idiosyncratic drug-induced agranulocytosis or acute neutropenia. *Curr Opin Hematol.* 200;15(1):15–21.

253. Willson RA. The liver: its role in drug biotransformation and as a target of immunologic injury. *Immunol Allergy Clin North Am.* 1991;11:555.

254. Lewis JH, Zimmerman HJ. Drug-induced liver disease. *Med Clin North Am.* 1989;73(4): 775–792.

255. Black M. Acetaminophen hepatotoxicity. *Annu Rev Med.* 1984;35:577–593.

256. Zimmerman HJ, Lewis JH. Drug-induced cholestasis. *Med Toxicol.* 1987;2(2):112–160.

257. Mitchell JR, Zimmerman HJ, Ishak KG, et al. Isoniazid liver injury: clinical spectrum, pathology, and probable pathogenesis. *Ann Intern Med.* 1976;84:181–192.

258. Kenna JG, Neuberger J, Williams R. Evidence for expression in human liver of halothane-induced neoantigens recognized by antibodies in sera from patients with halothane hepatitis. *Hepatology.* 1988;8(6):1635–1641.

259. Christ DD, Kenna JG, Kammerer W, et al. Enflurane metabolism produces covalently bound liver adducts recognized by antibodies from patients with halothane hepatitis. *Anesthesiology.* 1988;69:833–838.

260. Knobler H, Levij IS, Gavish D, et al. Quinidine-induced hepatitis. A common and reversible hypersensitivity reaction. *Arch Intern Med.* 1986;146:526–528.

261. Zimmerman HJ. Drug-induced chronic hepatic disease. *Med Clin North Am.* 1979;63(3): 567–582.

262. Boulton-Jones JM, et al. Self-induced glomerulonephritis. *Br Med J.* 1974;3(5927):387–390.

263. Treser G, Cherubin C, Longergan ET, et al. Renal lesions in narcotic addicts. *Am J Med.* 1974;57:687–694.

264. Sternlieb I, Bennett B, Scheinberg IH. D-penicillamine induced Goodpasture's syndrome in Wilson's disease. *Ann Intern Med.* 1975;82(5):673–676.

265. Silverberg DS, et al. Gold nephropathy. A clinical and pathologic study. *Arthritis Rheum.* 1970;13(6):812–825.

266. Case DB, Atlas SA, Mouradian JA, et al. Proteinuria during long-term captopril therapy. *JAMA.* 1980;244:346–349.

267. Kleinknecht D, et al. Acute interstitial nephritis due to drug hypersensitivity. An up-to-date review with a report of 19 cases. *Adv Nephrol Necker Hosp.* 1983;12:277–308.

268. Baker RJ, Pusey CD. The changing profile of acute tubulointerstitial nephritis. *Nephrol Dial Transplant.* 2004;19(1):8–11.

269. Porile JL, Bakris GL, Garella S. Acute interstitial nephritis with glomerulopathy due to nonsteroidal anti-inflammatory agents: a review of its clinical spectrum and effects of steroid therapy. *J Clin Pharmacol.* 1990;30(5):468–475.

270. Galpin JE, Shinaberger JH, Stanley TM, et al. Acute interstitial nephritis due to methicillin. *Am J Med.* 1978;65:756–765.

271. Charlesworth EN. Phenytoin-induced pseudolymphoma syndrome: an immunologic study. *Arch Dermatol.* 1977;113(4):477–480.

272. McCarthy LJ, Aguilar JC, Ransburg R. Fatal benign phenytoin lymphadenopathy. *Arch Intern Med.* 1979;139(3):367–368.

273. Tomecki KJ, Catalano CJ. Dapsone hypersensitivity. The sulfone syndrome revisited. *Arch Dermatol.* 1981;117(1):38–39.

274. Fenoglio JJ Jr, McAllister HA Jr, Mullick FG. Drug related myocarditis. I. Hypersensitivity myocarditis. *Hum Pathol.* 1981;12(10):900–907.

275. Taliercio CP, Olney BA, Lie JT. Myocarditis related to drug hypersensitivity. *Mayo Clin Proc.* 1985;60(7):463–468.

276. Kounis NG, Zavras GM, Soufras GD, et al. Hypersensitivity myocarditis. *Ann Allergy.* 1989;62:71–74.

277. Ten RM, Klein JS, Frigas E. Allergy skin testing. *Mayo Clin Proc.* 1995;70(8): 783–784.

278. Adkinson NF. Diagnosis of immunologic drug reactions. *N Engl Rev Allergy Proc.* 1984;5:104.

279. Calkin JM, Maibach HI. Delayed hypersensitivity drug reactions diagnosed by patch testing. *Contact Dermatitis.* 1993;29(5):223–233.

280. Baldo BA, Harle DG. Drug allergenic determinants. *Monogr Allergy.* 1990;28:11–51.

281. Weiss ME, Nyhan D, Peng ZK, et al. Association of protamine IgE and IgG antibodies with life-threatening reactions to intravenous protamine. *N Engl J Med.* 1989;320:886–892.

282. Dobozy A, Hunyadi J, Kenderessy AS, et al. Lymphocyte transformation test in detection of drug hypersensitivity. *Clin Exp Dermatol.* 1981;6:367–372.

283. Livni E, Halevy S, Stahl B, et al. The appearance of macrophage migration-inhibition factor in drug reactions. *J Allergy Clin Immunol.* 1987;80:843–849.

284. Kalish RS, LaPorte A, Wood JA, et al. Sulfonamide-reactive lymphocytes detected at very low frequency in the peripheral blood of patients with drug-induced eruptions. *J Allergy Clin Immunol.* 1994;94:465–472.

285. Schwartz LB. Tryptase, a mediator of human mast cells. *J Allergy Clin Immunol.* 1990;86(4 Pt 2):594–598.

286. Appel GB. A decade of penicillin related acute interstitial nephritis—more questions than answers. *Clin Nephrol.* 1980;13(4):151–154.

287. French LE. Toxic epidermal necrolysis and Stevens Johnson syndrome: our current understanding. *Allergol Int.* 2006;55(1):9–16.

288. Mittmann N, Chan BC, Knowles S, et al. IVIG for the treatment of toxic epidermal necrolysis. *Skin Therapy Lett.* 2007;12:7–9.

289. Rosenthal A. Followup study of fatal penicillin reactions. *JAMA.* 1959;167:118.

290. Singer JZ, Wallace SL. The allopurinol hypersensitivity syndrome. Unnecessary morbidity and mortality. *Arthritis Rheum.* 1986;29(1):82–87.

291. Lawson DH, Jick H. Drug prescribing in hospitals: an international comparison. *Am J Public Health.* 1976;66(7):644–648.

292. Pau AK, Morgan JE, Terlingo A. Drug allergy documentation by physicians, nurses, and medical students. *Am J Hosp Pharm.* 1989;46(3):570–573.

293. Kuehm SL, Doyle MJ. Medication errors: 1977 to 1988. Experience in medical malpractice claims. *N J Med.* 1990;87(1):27–34.

294. Blanca M, Fernandez J, Miranda A, et al. Cross-reactivity between penicillins and cephalosporins: clinical and immunologic studies. *J Allergy Clin Immunol.* 1989;83:381–385.

295. Apter AJ, Kinman JL, Bilker WB, et al. Represcription of penicillin after allergic-like events. *J Allergy Clin Immunol.* 2004;113:764–770.

296. Hannaford PC. Adverse drug reaction cards carried by patients. *Br Med J (Clin Res Ed).* 1986;292(6528):1109–1112.

297. Altman LC, Petersen PE. Successful prevention of an anaphylactoid reaction to iron dextran. *Ann Intern Med.* 1988;109(4):346–347.

298. Chandler MJ, Ong RC, Grammer LC, et al. Detection, characterization, and desensitization of IgE to streptomycin. *J Allergy Clin Immunol.* 1992;89:178.

299. Anne S, Middleton E Jr, Reisman RE. Vancomycin anaphylaxis and successful desensitization. *Ann Allergy.* 1994;73(5):402–404.

300. Webster E, Panush RS. Allopurinol hypersensitivity in a patient with severe, chronic, tophaceous gout. *Arthritis Rheum.* 1985;28(6): 707–709.

PART B
Allergic Reactions to Individual Drugs: Low Molecular Weight

PAUL A. GREENBERGER

The approach described in this part of the chapter has been used successfully to permit treatment with both low- and high-molecular-weight drugs: β-lactam antibiotics among patients with a history of penicillin allergy and positive tests for the major and minor haptenic determinants of penicillin; among diabetic patients with systemic insulin allergy; and among patients with positive skin tests for heterologous antisera. Desensitization to these IgE-mediated reactions renders mast cells specifically unresponsive to only the drug antigen used for desensitization. In many patients, successful desensitization is accompanied by a marked decrease or transient disappearance of the cutaneous wheal-and-flare response. Similar changes in skin test responses have been reported following successful desensitization to vancomycin (1), aminoglycosides (2), and carboplatin (3).

The term *desensitization* has been used in its broadest sense to describe a state of unresponsiveness to a drug that is accomplished by repeated and increasing exposure to that agent (4,5). Similar to acute desensitization for IgE-mediated reactions, these patients have had undeniable reactions to these drugs in the past. In the absence of positive immediate skin test reactions converting to negative during the administration of the incriminated medication, the terms *test dosing* (4) or *graded drug challenge* (6) are recommended. For billing purposes, the only term is desensitization. Protocols have been described for the cautious administration of aspirin (7,8), sulfonamides (especially TMP-SMX and

sulfasalazine) (9–12), allopurinol (13), tobramycin (14), and antiretroviral medications (10,15,16). Unlike desensitization to IgE-mediated reactions, these protocols are often more cumbersome and may require hours or days to complete (10). Finally, one should be reminded that graded dose challenges or true desensitization are potentially hazardous procedures best left to physicians experienced in managing hypersensitivity reactions (17). Highly trained nurses or other health care providers can participate in the monitoring of patients during challenges.

■ TEST DOSING/GRADED DOSE CHALLENGES

In situations in which a drug is needed and the history of a previous reaction to that agent is vague, and the possibility of true allergy is low, or the drug itself is an unlikely cause of such a reaction, test dosing or graded drug challenge is a method used to clarify the situation and safely determine whether it may be administered (17). A common example is a patient who has been advised to avoid all "caines," and now requires the use of a local anesthetic agent. True systemic allergy to local anesthetics essentially is unheard of. Test dosing provides reassurance to the patient, physician, or dentist that this agent can be safely given. Alternatively, when the test dosing results in symptoms such as instantaneous throat closure without objective findings, it helps to confirm the level of anxiety involved without demonstrating true allergy.

The principle of test dosing (graded drug challenge) is to select a dose of the drug below that which would potentially cause a serious reaction, and then proceed with increasingly larger incremental doses to full therapeutic doses. Using this technique, one can determine whether a reaction has occurred before proceeding to the next dose. If a reaction occurs, it can be easily treated. If the drug is necessary, a desensitization protocol then may be performed. In this setting, *controlled anaphylaxis* can be carried out.

The starting dose, incremental increase, and interval between challenges depend on the drug and the urgency of reaching therapeutic doses (10). For oral drugs, a usual starting dose is 0.1 mg or 1.0 mg, and then proceeds to 10 mg, 50 mg, 100 mg, and 200 mg (10). For parenteral drugs, the initial dose is less, for example, 0.01 mg or 0.001 mg. When the suspected reaction was immediate, a 20- to 30-minute interval between doses is appropriate, and the procedure is usually completed in 3 to 5 hours or less. For late-onset reactions, such as a nonblistering or nonexfoliating dermatitis, the dosing interval may be as long as 24 to 48 hours, with the same protocols requiring 1 to 2 weeks or longer. Although there is always the possibility of a severe anaphylactic reaction, the risk of test dosing appears to be very low. Nevertheless, graded drug challenge of patients with a history of a bullous reaction to a medication or a serum sickness reaction (severe urticaria and arthralgia) (18) would have to be considered in rare patients, otherwise not attempted (10,17).

■ SPECIAL CONSIDERATIONS FOR PROVEN OR SUSPECTED ALLERGIC REACTIONS TO INDIVIDUAL DRUGS

In this section, specific recommendations as they pertain to important drugs commonly used in clinical practice are reviewed. For each agent, relevant background information is provided. Table 17B.1 summarizes useful strategies for administering agents, once indication for the agent to be administered has been verified.

Penicillins and Other β-Lactam Antibiotics

Background

β-Lactam antibiotic hypersensitivity deserves special consideration because of its medical importance. Penicillin has been studied extensively and has become a prototype for the study of allergic drug reactions. As many as 10% of hospitalized patients report a history of penicillin allergy. In a study of 1,893 consecutive adult patients who had an order written for an antimicrobial agent while hospitalized, 470 (25%) patients reported an allergy to at least one drug (19). Two hundred and ninety-five (15.6%) patients listed penicillin. A manual

review of the charts revealed that just 32% of records specified the details of the allergic reaction. Some patients have been labeled falsely as penicillin allergic and are denied this useful, remarkably nontoxic agent. The reasons for this discrepancy are either a previously incorrect diagnosis or the frequently evanescent nature of penicillin allergy. Following an acute allergic reaction, there is a time-dependent decline in the rate of positive skin tests to penicillin. In the first year, 90% to 100% retain sensitivity after a convincing allergic reaction, but that percentage drops to about 30% at 10 years (20). It may be even lower in terms of cross-sectional studies of varying time periods. For example, penicillin allergy, confirmed by skin testing, can be 18% in penicillin allergic subjects (17,21). Some patients, however, maintain the penicillin-specific IgE antibody for 30 to 40 years. It is therefore highly desirable to predict which patients are at risk for a penicillin reaction. It is important to recognize that penicillin allergic patients, who have current penicillin sensitization by skin testing, may not have an "impressive" history of urticaria, angioedema, acute wheezing, etc. In a literature review, 347 of 1,063 (33%) patients, who tested positive on penicillin skin testing, had vague histories of penicillin allergy (22). These patients may well have had their level of risk from penicillin minimized.

The overall prevalence of β-lactam allergy is estimated to range from as high as 2% per course of treatment (23) to as low as 0.05% (24). The incidence of anaphylaxis has been reported to be as low as about 1:100,000 (24). The most frequent manifestations of penicillin allergy are cutaneous, notably morbilliform, and urticarial eruptions; the most serious is anaphylaxis. For historical comparison from the 1960s, penicillin-induced anaphylaxis occurred in about 0.01% to 0.05% (1 per 5,000 to 10,000) of patient treatment courses, with a fatal outcome in 0.0015% to 0.002% (1 death per 50,000 to 100,000 treatment courses) (25).

An atopic background (allergic rhinitis, asthma, atopic dermatitis) does not predispose an individual to the development of penicillin hypersensitivity, but once sensitized, such individuals are at increased risk for severe or fatal anaphylactic reactions (26). Anaphylaxis occurring in patients with asthma may result in acute severe respiratory failure. Also, atopic patients with *Penicillium* species "mold" allergy can receive penicillin unless specifically allergic to penicillin.

Patients with a history of prior penicillin reaction have a fourfold to sixfold increased risk for subsequent reactions to β-lactam antibiotics (27), but not necessarily as high to carbapenems, e.g., imipenem and meropenem (28,29). Among penicillin-allergic individuals who are skin test positive, the unmodified (regular infusion of the therapeutic dose) administration of β-lactam antibiotics causes acute reactions in about two-thirds of patients (30). If desensitization is performed, the incidence of reactions is very much lower (17,21). Graded

TABLE 17B.1   EXAMPLES OF USEFUL EVALUATION TECHNIQUES AND MANAGEMENT STRATEGIES FOR SELECTED DRUGS AND AGENTS

DRUGS OR AGENTS	SKIN TESTS OF VALUE	PREMEDICATION USEFUL	TEST DOSING INDICATED	DESENSITIZATION IF ESSENTIAL	ADDITIONAL COMMENTS
Immediate Generalized Reactions (IgE-Mediated)					
β-Lactam antibiotics	√		See comments	√	Test the dose in absence of penicillin.
					Use MDM or validated cephalosporin skin tests.
Insulin	√			√	Use least reactive insulin by skin test for desensitization.
Immune sera	√			√	Is risky in atopic patients allergic to horse dander.
Egg-containing vaccines	√			√	May be unnecessary for MMR vaccine.
Tetanus toxoid	√			√	If serum antitoxin levels adequate, desensitization not required.
Latex	See comments				No standardized skin test is available.
					Avoidance is only effective treatment.
Protamine		See comments			There are no studies to validate premedication.
Streptokinase	√				Substitute urokinase or tissue plasminogen activator.
Chymopapain	√				Consider laminectomy.
Immediate Generalized Reactions (IgE-Independent)					
Aspirin and non-steroidal anti-inflammatory drugs			√	See comments	Term *desensitization* used, although reaction is not IgE-mediated.
Contrast media		√			Is also useful for nonvascular studies.
					Lower osmolality media is a better choice.
Opioid analgesics			√		Pentazocaine or fentanyl are less active histamine releasers.
Cancer chemotherapy		√			Slow infusion and premedication have been useful.

TABLE 17B.1   EXAMPLES OF USEFUL EVALUATION TECHNIQUES AND MANAGEMENT STRATEGIES FOR SELECTED DRUGS AND AGENTS (*CONTINUED*)

DRUGS OR AGENTS	SKIN TESTS OF VALUE	PREMEDICATION USEFUL	TEST DOSING INDICATED	DESENSITIZATION IF ESSENTIAL	ADDITIONAL COMMENTS
Allergy Presumed Mechanism Unclear					
Sulfonamides			√	See comments	Term *desensitization* often used, but reaction is usually IgE independent.
Local anesthetics			√		True systemic reactions are rare.
					Reassurance is primary goal.
Anticonvulsants			√		Is a potentially dangerous procedure.
Other rarely incriminated drugs or agents			√		Seek consultation with experienced allergist.

MDM, minor determinant mixture; MMR, measles, mumps, and rubella.
Adapted from Reference 5.

test challenge with imipenem and meropenem to patients with a history of penicillin allergy and positive immediate skin tests to penicillin or a determinant can be carried out safely when the skin tests to imipenem are nonreactive and the first dose of the antibiotic is 0.01 of the target dosage (28,29).

Although this discussion focuses primarily on the evaluation of and strategies to deal with IgE-mediated reactions, this group of agents has also been associated with other adverse, IgE-independent immunologic events that are briefly noted here and have been extensively reviewed elsewhere (11,16,17). *Immediate reactions* occur within the first hour following administration of the β-lactam drug, are IgE-mediated, and may present a serious threat to life. *Accelerated reactions* develop 1 to 72 hours after drug administration, are IgE-mediated, usually present as urticaria and angioedema, and are rarely life endangering. *Delayed or late reactions* occur after 3 days, are IgE-independent, and usually present as benign morbilliform skin eruptions. Exfoliative dermatitis and Stevens-Johnson syndrome may occur. Late reactions include serum sickness-like reactions (18) and drug fever (31,32). Unusual late reactions are immune cytopenias, acute interstitial nephritis, pulmonary infiltrates with eosinophilia, and hypersensitivity vasculitis.

In general, the previously described adverse events are common to all β-lactam antibiotics, such as the natural penicillins (penicillin G, penicillin V), the penicillinase-resistant penicillins (methicillin, nafcillin, dicloxacillin),

the aminopenicillins (ampicillin, amoxicillin), and the extended spectrum penicillins (carbenicillin, ticarcillin, mezlocillin, azlocillin, piperacillin). Hypersensitivity reactions are less with the cephalosporins (10,11,17,33–35) and carbapenems (28,29). However, this statement is based on group mean statistics; the individual patient, who is destined to experience anaphylaxis from the antibiotic administration, is a "direct hit." The data for carbapenems included graded challenges such as beginning with 1/100 then 1/10 of the target dose for imipenem (28).

Individual β-lactam antibiotics have been associated more commonly with certain types of reactions. For instance, ampicillin and amoxicillin therapy is associated with a higher incidence (about 10%) of nonpruritic maculopapular rash than are other penicillins (about 2%) (36). The rash usually appears after at least 1 week of therapy, initially develops on the knees and elbows, and then spreads symmetrically to cover the entire body (37). If the patient has infectious mononucleosis, the incidence approaches 90%. The incidence of this cutaneous reaction is increased in patients with HIV and cytomegalovirus (CMV) infection, chronic lymphatic leukemia, non-Hodgkin lymphoma, SLE, and hyperuricemia (38). This eruption does not appear to be allergic in nature, but if there is an urticarial component, it may represent true IgE-mediated penicillin allergy, and rechallenge could result in a severe immediate generalized allergic reaction.

Cephalosporins produce reactions similar to those described for penicillins. The more common reactions include maculopapular or morbilliform skin eruption, drug fever, and a positive Coombs test (clinical hemolysis is unusual). Less common reactions are urticaria, serum sickness-like reactions (especially with cefaclor in children) (34,39–43), and anaphylaxis (34,44–48). Drug-induced cytopenias and acute interstitial nephritis are rare. Compared with the first-generation cephalosporins (e.g., cephalothin, cefazolin, cephalexin,* cefadroxil,* cefaclor*) and second-generation cephalosporins (e.g., cefamandole, cefuroxime, cefuroxime axetil*), the third-generation cephalosporins (e.g., cefotaxime, ceftizoxime, ceftriaxone, ceftazidime, cefixime*) have a lower incidence of immediate, presumably IgE-mediated, generalized allergic reactions (34).

Some degree of cross-reactivity (or independent sensitivity to non-β-lactam ring moieties) among the different classes of β-lactam antibiotics is well established (49). Because the semisynthetic penicillins contain the same 6-aminopenicillanic acid nucleus as natural penicillin G, it is not surprising that cross-allergenicity among these agents exists, albeit to various degrees. Individuals have been identified who have reacted to ampicillin and amoxicillin but not to penicillin (50–52). It is presumed that this is related to hypersensitivity to the side chains that differentiate the antibiotic from the parent compound. The incidence and clinical significance of these side-chain–specific reactions remains unknown. However, at this time, if a patient reports a history of penicillin allergy, it is prudent to assume that the individual is allergic to all penicillins (10,11,16,17). Because 9% to 25% of patients receiving antibiotics report a penicillin allergy (19,53–55), the impact of penicillin allergy in hospitalized patients remains significant.

Cephalosporins share a common β-lactam ring with penicillin but have a six-member dihydrothiazine ring instead of the five-membered thiazolidine ring of the penicillin molecule. Shortly after the introduction of the cephalosporins into clinical use, allergic reactions, including anaphylaxis, were reported, and the question of cross-reactivity between cephalosporins and penicillins was raised. Data suggest that the extent is not that high (56–59). Significant *in vitro* and *in vivo* cross-reactivity with penicillin has been demonstrated with first-generation cephalosporins (5% to 16.5%) (17,56–57). Fortunately, clinically relevant cross-reactivity between penicillin and the cephalosporins (especially second and third generation) is about 10% (17) and 2% to 3% (17), respectively. A literature review of patients with a history of penicillin allergy and positive skin tests to penicillin determinants challenged with cephalosporins revealed allergic reactions in 8.1% of patients compared with 1.9% among those with negative penicillin skin tests (59). A provocative review suggested that penicillin-allergic patients, who are identified by either history or positive penicillin skin tests, are not at increased risk compared with the general population, and they may be safely treated with cephalosporin antibiotics (35). However, cautious administration of cephalosporins to penicillin-allergic patients is advisable, especially when the history is that of acute urticaria or other anaphylactic reaction. Regrettably, in a report of six penicillin-allergic patients, three experienced fatal anaphylactic reactions from the first dose of a cephalosporin (47).

Primary cephalosporin allergy, including anaphylaxis, has occasionally been reported in both penicillin-allergic and penicillin-nonallergic patients and may be fatal (47). Most investigators have studied tolerance to the cephalosporins in penicillin-allergic patients, but little information is available regarding tolerance to other β-lactam antibiotics in patients with primary cephalosporin allergy. Such studies are limited by the lack of reliable cephalosporin determinants for skin testing. It appears that antibodies directed against unique side chains rather than against the common ring structure are more important in the immune response to cephalosporins (34,56–58). This would explain the low cross-reactivity among different cephalosporins, which share the same nucleus but have different side chains (34,56–59). Also, it may help to explain the low cross-reactivity between cephalosporins and penicillins, which share the same β-lactam ring in the nucleus but have different side chains. Until better information is available, it is best to avoid the use of β-lactam antibiotics in cephalosporin-allergic patients; if essential, cautious graded drug challenge is advisable. Although skin testing with the parent cephalosporin has not been used widely, initial reports of skin testing with the parent cephalosporin (2 mg/mL prick test, then 0.02 mL, intradermal) describe high negative predictive value (60).

The carbapenems (imipenem, meropenem), monobactams (aztreonam), and carbacephems (loracarbef) are three classes of antibiotics that possess β-lactam ring structures. There is significant cross-reactivity between penicillin and imipenem (61) and meropenem based on structure and using the specific determinants of impenem for example (61). Graded challenges were not carried out, but 47% of penicillin-allergic subjects had positive skin test reactions to imipenem determinants (61). Immediate skin reactivity to imipenem (1 mg/mL) by prick test was demonstrated in a patient who experienced shock and cardiac arrest from imipenem (62). Unexpectedly, there is much less actual, clinical cross-reactivity than anticipated between penicillin and the carbapenems, when the carbapenems are administered by graded challenge (28,29). Aztreonam is the prototypical monobactam antibiotic. It is very weakly cross-reactive in the penicillin-allergic patient and may be administered safely to most patients allergic to other β-lactam antibiotics (17,63). The antibodies generated are specific to the side chain rather than the β-lactam ring. It should be noted, however, that

---

* Oral agents.

ceftazidime, a third-generation cephalosporin, shares an identical side chain with aztreonam. It may be prudent not to use ceftazidime in rare subjects allergic to aztreonam. Loracarbef, a carbacephem, structurally resembles cefaclor, but the degree of cross-reactivity with penicillins and cephalosporins is unknown. Finally, clavulanic acid is also a β-lactam antibiotic with weak antibacterial activity but is a potent inhibitor of β-lactamase. It is often combined with amoxicillin to enhance antimicrobial activity. There is a report of two immediate generalized allergic reactions attributed to clavulanic acid (64).

Diagnostic Testing

Although obtaining and recording a past history of penicillin allergy is essential, one cannot completely rely on that information to predict who is allergic. The history may be inaccurate, and many patients lose their sensitivity over time. The failure to elicit this information has resulted in fatalities following the administration of these drugs to patients with a convincing history of β-lactam hypersensitivity. To help clarify this situation, when the drug is essential, skin testing with penicillin has been useful to identify those patients at risk for anaphylaxis and other, milder IgE-mediated reactions. When appropriate skin testing reagents are either unavailable or have not been validated, test dosing (graded drug challenge) with the desired β-lactam antibiotic is recommended.

Benzylpenicillin (BP) has a molecular weight of 300 and transforms (is not metabolized) in large part (about 95%) into a penicilloyl hapten moiety. This transformation product is referred to as the major determinant and has been conjugated to poly-D-lysine to form penicilloyl-polylysine (PPL), which had been commercially available as Pre-Pen (Hollister-Stier, Spokane, WA) for skin testing until 2004. Other penicillin transformation products, including BP itself, constitute 5% or less of administered penicillin and are collectively referred to as the *minor determinant mixture* (MDM). They are minor in name only but are responsible for some penicillin anaphylactic reactions. A standardized MDM is not available commercially for skin testing. Therefore, a fresh solution of BP (10,000 units/mL) has been used for skin testing purposes. Skin testing with both PPL and freshly prepared BP (as the sole minor determinant) should detect 85% to 88% of potential reactors (10,11,16,17,21). Almost all patients (99%) with negative skin tests to PPL and MDM reagents can be treated safely with penicillin (17,21). If PPL is not used but MDM is, from 34% to 60% of skin test-positive patients would be missed (17). Thus, the major determinant identifies a significant proportion of skin test–positive patients, and its use improves safety during testing and desensitization. With the PPL and MDM, the negative predictive value of skin testing with major and minor determinants is as high as

99% (17,21) compared with about 40% to 66% with MDM only (17).

In general, skin testing with BP-derived reagents, PPL and MDM, is also predictive of reactions to other β-lactam antibiotics (17); however, there are occasional patients with reactions to ampicillin, amoxicillin, and cephalosporin side chains who may not be detected by skin testing (50–52). Although skin testing with the β-lactam antibiotic of therapeutic choice has been advocated to detect additional potential reactors, skin test reagents prepared from other penicillins, cephalosporins, imipenem, and aztreonam have not been standardized, and the results are not validated. A positive skin test using these materials suggests the potential for an IgE-mediated reaction, but a negative test does not eliminate this concern. The incidence of such reactions to other β-lactam antibiotics when skin tests are negative to penicillin major and minor determinant reagents is probably low (17). Some minor determinant mixtures are not as sensitive as others and have led to confusion about the need to detect side-chain–specific IgE.

In practice, penicillin skin testing to evaluate the potential of or current risk for an IgE-mediated reaction should be reserved for patients with a history suggesting penicillin allergy when administration of the drug is essential or when confusion about penicillin interferes with optimal antibiotic selection. Such testing is of no value in predicting the occurrence of non–IgE-mediated reactions and is contraindicated when the previous reaction was Stevens-Johnson syndrome, toxic epidermal necrolysis (TEN), or exfoliative dermatitis. Elective penicillin skin testing followed by an oral challenge and subsequent 10-day course of treatment with penicillin or amoxicillin in skin test–negative subjects has been recommended, particularly in children with a history suggesting penicillin allergy (65). It was hoped that this procedure would eliminate the need to carry out such testing when the child is ill and in need of penicillin therapy. Using this approach, the risk for resensitization was about 1%. In one small study of 19 patients, 16% of penicillin history–positive, but skin test–negative adults receiving intravenous penicillin therapy became skin test positive 1 to 12 months after completion of treatment (66). In another study, none of 33 penicillin history–positive, skin test–negative adults had evidence of IgE-mediated reactions, suggesting loss of antipenicillin IgE antibodies (67). In a series of 568 patients with penicillin allergy and negative skin tests, only 1 of 33 patients, who were tested after the initial therapeutic course that resulted in a reaction, was skin test positive (68). These data suggest that reactions are not always IgE-mediated and that resensitization appears to be very low. The overall data support the use of penicillin skin tests in managing patients with a history of penicillin allergy, regardless of the severity of the previous reaction. Penicillin skin testing is rapid, and the risk for a serious reaction is minimal when

TABLE 17B.2   β-LACTAM ANTIBIOTIC SKIN TESTS

SKIN TEST REAGENTS	DRUG TEST ROUTE	SKIN TEST CONCENTRATION	VOLUME	DOSE
Penicilloyl-polylysine[a] (Pre-Pen) (6 × 10⁻⁵ M)	Prick Intradermal	Full strength Full strength	1 drop 0.02 mL	
Penicillin G[a] potassium (freshly prepared)	Prick Intradermal (serial 10-fold dilutions optional)[d]	10,000 U/mL 10,000 U/mL	1 drop 0.02 mL	200 units
Penicillin minor determinant mixture[b] (10⁻² M)	Prick Intradermal (serial 10-fold dilutions optional)[d]	Full strength Full strength	1 drop 0.01 mL to 0.02 mL	
Cephalosporins and other penicillins[c]	Prick Intradermal (serial 10-fold dilutions optional)[d]	3 mg/mL 3 mg/mL	1 drop 0.02 mL	60 μg
Aztreonam[c]	Prick Intradermal (serial 10-fold dilutions optional)[d]	3 mg/mL 3 mg/mL	1 drop 0.02 mL	60 μg
Imipenem[c]	Prick Intradermal (serial 10-fold dilutions optional)[d]	1 mg/mL 1 mg/mL	1 drop 0.02 mL	20 μg
Histamine (Histatrol)—positive control	Prick Intradermal	1 mg/mL 0.1 mg/mL	1 drop 0.02 mL	
Saline or diluent—negative control	Prick Intradermal	NA NA	1 drop 0.02 mL	

[a]Testing validated.

[b]Testing validated; reagents not available (except at some medical centers).

[c]Testing not validated. Negative tests do not rule out possibility of a reaction.

[d]Serial skin tests may be prudent when previous reaction was anaphylactic in nature.

performed by trained personnel, using recommended drug concentrations, and completing skin-prick tests before attempting intradermal skin tests. Testing should be completed shortly before administration of the drug. However, in the absence of commercially available penicillin skin test reagents, the only option is to identify patients at higher risk than the normal population and perform graded drug challenges with caution.

Table 17B.2 summarizes the reagents used for β-lactam antibiotic skin tests and the recommended starting concentrations of these reagents, which are adequately sensitive but have a low risk for provoking a systemic or nonspecific irritant reaction. In patients with a history of a life-threatening reaction to penicillin, it may be advisable to dilute the skin test reagents 100-fold for initial testing. Skin-prick testing is accomplished by pricking through a drop of the reagent placed on the volar surface of the forearm and observing for 15 to 20 minutes. A significant reaction is a wheal 4 mm or larger than the control with surrounding erythema. If negative, proceed with intradermal skin tests. Using a tuberculin or allergy syringe, inject 0.01 mL to 0.02 mL of the reagent, sufficient to raise a 2-mm to 3-mm bleb on the volar surface of the forearm. After 15 to 20 minutes, a positive test produces a wheal of 4 mm or larger with surrounding erythema. If the results are equivocal or difficult to interpret, the tests should be repeated. It should be noted that there is some disagreement among investigators as to what constitutes an acceptable positive skin test (20). A 4-mm wheal with surrounding erythema is positive; a 4-mm or greater wheal without erythema is "indeterminate" and usually not representative of antipenicillin IgE antibodies. Caution is required on test dose challenges though.

Because penicillin PPL and MDM are not commercially available in the United States, and skin testing with other β-lactam antibiotics has not been standardized, nor have the results been validated, test dosing (graded drug challenge) is recommended in patients with a past history of penicillin allergy. How one approaches this procedure depends on the severity of the previous reaction and the experience of the managing physician. After documenting the need for the drug, obtaining informed verbal or written consent, and being prepared to treat anaphylaxis, a graded dose challenge protocol may be initiated with a physician in constant attendance; 0.001 mg (1 unit) of the therapeutic β-lactam antibiotic is administered by the desired (oral, intravenous) route. The patient is observed for signs of pruritus, flushing, urticaria, dyspnea, and hypotension. In the absence of these signs, at 15-minute intervals, subsequent doses are given as outlined in Table 17B.3. If a reaction occurs during this procedure, it is treated with epinephrine intramuscularly and antihistamines; the need for the drug should be reevaluated and actual desensitization considered if this agent is essential. This is a rather conservative test dosing schedule. More experienced physicians may elect to shorten this procedure; one suggestion has been to test dose with 1/100 of the therapeutic dose (1/1000 of the therapeutic dose if the previous reaction was severe), and then increase toward the full therapeutic dose if there is no evidence of urticaria, flushing, wheezing, or hypotension (10).

Because there is a small risk associated with skin testing and test dosing, in vitro tests have obvious appeal. Solid-phase immunoassays, such as the radioallergosorbent test (RAST) and the enzyme-linked immunosorbent assay (ELISA), have been developed to detect serum IgE antibodies against the major penicilloyl determinant. The RAST or fluorescent immunoassay generally correlates with skin testing to PPL. RAST and fluorescent immunoassays for cephalosporins and other antimicrobial drugs have been reported but are available only for research. At present, in vitro tests have limited-to-no clinical usefulness.

Management of Patients with a History of Penicillin Allergy

Preferable management of patients with a history of penicillin or other β-lactam antibiotic allergy is the use of an equally effective, non–cross-reacting antibiotic. In most situations, adequate substitutes are available, and consultation with infectious disease experts is valuable. Aztreonam, a monocyclic β-lactam antibiotic, has no clinical cross-reactivity with penicillins or cephalosporins and can be administered to patients with prior anaphylactic reactions to penicillin.

If alternative drugs fail, or if there is known antibiotic resistance by suspected pathogens, skin testing and graded dose challenge with the β-lactam antibiotic of choice should be performed. If skin tests are positive, if the patient reacts to test doses, or if such testing is not done, administration of the β-lactam antibiotic, using a graded dose challenge protocol, is advised (10,17). One begins with a subanaphylactic dose so that if anaphylaxis occurs, it can be controlled. For example, doses less than 1 mg would not be expected to induce anaphylaxis.

Some infections in which this approach becomes necessary include enterococcal infections, brain abscess, bacterial meningitis, sepsis with staphylococci, *Neisseria* or *Pseudomonas* species organisms, *Listeria* infections, endocarditis, osteomyelitis, neurosyphilis, and syphilis in pregnant women. In fact, penicillin desensitization is indicated for pregnant women with syphilis who demonstrate immediate hypersensitivity to that drug (10). Also, at present, there are no data to support the use of alternatives to penicillin for treatment of neurosyphilis and all stages of syphilis among HIV/AIDS-infected patients (10). With a target dose of 2,400,000 units of benzylpenicillin G, the starting dose is 0.1 unit subcutaneously, followed by 1 unit, 10 units, 100 units, 1,000 units, 10,000 units and 100,000 units. Then 200,000 units are administered intramuscularly followed by 2,100,000 units by the same route (10). This protocol delivers the 2,400,000 units for the initial dose (10).

The usual scenario involves a patient who presents with a convincing history of penicillin allergy and the physician has no available skin tests such as Pre-Pen and MDM. Therefore, graded penicillin challenge, as

TABLE 17B.3   SUGGESTED TEST DOSING SCHEDULE FOR β-LACTAM ANTIBIOTICS

DOSE (MG)[a]	DOSE (UNITS)[a]
0.001	1
0.005	10
0.01	20
0.05	100
0.10	200
0.50	800
1	1,600
10	16,000
50	80,000
100	160,000
200	320,000

Full dose may be administered

[a]400,000 units penicillin G potassium is roughly equivalent to 250 mg of other β-lactam antibiotics (1 μg = 1.8 units).

previously outlined, is recommended. If a reaction occurs at any test dose, the need for the drug should be reevaluated. If essential, an actual desensitization protocol should be considered. A more unusual scenario is a patient with a positive history and available penicillin skin tests. Penicillin history–positive patients are at significant risk for anaphylaxis, but the risk can be clarified by the presence or absence of positive immediate skin tests for penicillin determinants. Desensitization protocols significantly reduce the risk for anaphylaxis in skin test–positive patients, whereas deliberate infusion of a β-lactam antibiotic at the usual rate could cause a severe or fatal anaphylactic reaction.

While graded drug challenges can be performed in an outpatient facility, acute β-lactam antibiotic desensitization should be performed in a monitored or intensive care setting. Informed consent (verbal or written) is advised. Patients with asthma or congestive heart failure should be under optimal control. Premedication with antihistamines and corticosteroids is not recommended, because these drugs have not proved effective in suppressing anaphylaxis and could mask mild allergic manifestations that may have resulted in a modification of the desensitization protocol. It is believed that the early recognition of flushing and limited urticarial lesions during desensitization (or graded drug challenge) would alert the physician to the evidence of mast cell activation and risks involved. Suppression of the flushing or limited urticaria might result in a more serious, subsequent allergic reaction.

Before initiation of desensitization, two intravenous lines or one line in a large vein is established; baseline vital signs are recorded. The clinical state of the patient is assessed. A baseline electrocardiogram, spirometry have been advocated by some as well as continuous electrocardiographic monitoring depending on the patient's comorbidities. During desensitization, vital signs and the clinical state of the patient are noted before each dose, and at 10- to 20-minute intervals following each dose. A physician must be in close attendance during the entire procedure so that unexpected reactions such as hypotension can be reversed quickly.

Desensitization has been accomplished successfully using either the oral or intravenous routes of administration (69–73). Oral desensitization is favored by some who believe that the risk for a serious reaction is less. The intravenous route is chosen by others, including myself, who prefer absolute control of the drug concentration used and its rate of administration. Unfortunately, there is no completely standardized regimen, and there have been no direct comparative studies between oral and intravenous desensitizing protocols.

Regardless of the method chosen for desensitization, the basic principles are similar. The initial dose is typically $\frac{1}{10,000}$ of the therapeutic dose. Oral desensitization may begin with the dose that is tolerated during oral test dosing. Intravenous desensitization should begin with 1/10 or 1/100 (if the previous reaction was severe) of the dose producing a positive skin test or intravenous test dose response. The dose is then usually doubled at 7- to 15-minute intervals until full therapeutic doses are achieved, typically within 4 to 5 hours. Representative protocols for intravenous (Table 17B.4) and oral (Table 17B.5) desensitization are presented.

Table 17B.4 outlines an intravenous desensitization protocol for penicillin G potassium or any other β-lactam antibiotic (10). The dose to be administered is placed in a small volume of 5% dextrose in water for piggyback delivery into the already established intravenous line. It is administered slowly at first, then more rapidly if no warning signs, such as pruritus or flushing, appear. If symptoms develop during the procedure, the flow rate is slowed or stopped and the patient treated appropriately, using the other intravenous site if necessary. After symptoms subside, the flow rate is slowly increased once again. Once the patient has received and tolerated 800,000 units of penicillin G or 800 mg of any other β-lactam antibiotic, the full therapeutic dose may be given and therapy continued without interruption.

Table 17B.5 provides a protocol for oral desensitization with β-lactam antibiotics. If the patient is unable to take oral medication, it may be administered through a feeding tube. Mild reactions during desensitization, such as pruritus, fleeting urticaria, mild rhinitis, or wheezing, require the dose to be repeated until tolerated. If a more serious reaction occurs, such as hypotension, laryngeal edema, or severe asthma, the next dose should be decreased to at least one-third of the provoking dose and withheld until the patient is stable. If an oral form of the desired β-lactam agent is unavailable, intravenous desensitization should be considered. Once desensitized, treatment must not lapse. Regardless of the route selected for desensitization, mild reactions, usually pruritic rashes, may be expected in about 0 to 30% of patients during and after the procedure. These reactions usually subside with continued treatment, but symptomatic therapy may be necessary.

After successful desensitization, some individuals may have predictable needs for future exposures to β-lactam antibiotics. Patients with cystic fibrosis, chronic neutropenia, or occupational exposure to these agents may benefit from chronic twice-daily oral penicillin therapy to sustain a desensitized state between courses of high-dose parenteral therapy (71). However, some investigators are concerned about the ability to maintain 100% compliance among cystic fibrosis patients in an outpatient setting and therefore prefer to perform intravenous desensitization each time β-lactam antibiotic therapy is required (72).

TABLE 17B.4   PROTOCOL FOR INTRAVENOUS DESENSITIZATION WITH β-LACTAM ANTIBIOTICS

β-LACTAM CONCENTRATION (MG/ML)	PENICILLIN G CONCENTRATION (U/ML)	DOSE NO.[a]	AMOUNT GIVEN (ML)	DOSE GIVEN (MG/UNITS)
0.1	160	1	0.10	0.01/16
		2	0.20	0.02/32
		3	0.40	0.04/64
		4	0.80	0.08/128
1	1,600	5	0.15	0.15/240
		6	0.30	0.30/480
		7	0.60	0.06/960
		8	1.00	1/1,600
10	16,000	9	0.20	2/3,200
		10	0.40	4/6,400
		11	0.80	8/12,800
100	160,000	12	0.15	15/24,000
		13	0.30	30/48,000
		14	0.60	60/96,000
		15	1.00	100/160,000
1,000	1,600,000	16	0.20	200/320,000
		17	0.40	400/640,000
		18	0.80	800/1,280,000

Observe patient for 30 minutes; administer full therapeutic dose intravenously.

[a]Dose approximately doubled every 7 to 15 min.

Adapted from Adkinson NF Jr. Drug allergy. In: Middleton EJ, Reed CE, Ellis EF, et al., eds. *Allergy: principles and practice*. 5th ed. St. Louis: CV Mosby, 1998:1212–1224.

In summary, β-lactam antibiotics can be administered by desensitization with relatively little risk in most patients with a history of allergy to these drugs and a positive reaction to skin testing. Once successfully desensitized, the need for uninterrupted therapy is advisable until treatment has been completed. Any lapse in therapy greater than 12 hours may permit such sensitivity to return. Mild reactions during and after desensitization are not an indication to discontinue treatment. Many such reactions resolve spontaneously or may require symptomatic therapy.

Among successfully desensitized patients with a positive history of β-lactam allergy and a positive response to skin testing or graded challenge, this same approach may be repeated before a future course of therapy. There appears to be little risk for resensitization following an uneventful course of therapy among patients with positive histories and negative skin tests or after uneventful test dosing (67,68). Desensitization does require an essential indication for the incriminated antibiotic (74,75) and preparedness for anaphylaxis and its treatment. In the absence of skin testing, which helps to place the patient at high risk (if positive) and very low risk (if negative), patients with penicillin allergy are often undergoing graded drug challenges as opposed to actual desensitization. Nevertheless, when beginning the graded challenge, without skin test results, the risk is based on the history and patient's co-morbidities, including ineffectively controlled asthma or sepsis, as opposed to more precise data such as presence or absence of antipenicillin major determinant, Pre-Pen, or MDM, IgE antibodies.

Non–β-Lactam Antimicrobial Agents

Allergic reactions to non–β-lactam antimicrobial drugs, most commonly cutaneous eruptions, are common causes of morbidity and, rarely, mortality. Anaphylaxis to these agents is a rare event. The estimated overall incidence of a hypersensitivity-type reaction to

TABLE 17B.5   PROTOCOL FOR ORAL DESENSITIZATION WITH β-LACTAM ANTIBIOTICS

β-LACTAM CONCEN-TRATION (MG/ML)[a]	DOSE NO.[b]	AMOUNT GIVEN[c] (ML)	DOSE GIVEN (MG)
0.5	1	0.10	0.05
	2	0.20	0.10
	3	0.40	0.20
	4	0.80	0.40
	5	1.60	0.80
	6	3.20	1.60
	7	6.40	3.20
5	8	1.20	6
	9	2.40	12
	10	4.80	24
50	11	1.00	50
	12	2.00	100
	13	4.00	200
	14	8.00	400

Observe patient for 30 minutes; give full therapeutic dose by route of choice.

[a]Dilutions prepared from antibiotic syrup, 250 mg/5 mL.

[b]Dose approximately doubled every 15 min.

[c]Drug amount given in 30 mL water or flavored beverage.

Adapted from Sullivan TJ. Drug Allergy. In: Middleton EJ, Reed CE, Ellis EF, et al., eds. *Allergy: principles and practice.* 4th ed. St. Louis: CV Mosby, 1993:1726.

non–β-lactam drugs is about 1% to 3%. Some antimicrobial agents, however, such as TMP-SMX, produce reactions more commonly; in contrast, others, such as tetracycline, are much less likely to do so.

Unlike the β-lactam antimicrobials, other antibiotics have been less well studied and also include a wide variety of chemical agents. Research has been hampered by the lack of information regarding the immunochemistry of most of these drugs and, therefore, the unavailability of proven immunodiagnostic tests to assist the physician. Although skin testing with the free drug and some *in vitro* tests have been described for sulfonamides, aminoglycosides, and vancomycin, there are no large series reported to validate their clinical usefulness. Use of pharmacogenomic data prospectively should permit more precise "personalized medicine" and result in fewer adverse reactions.

Despite these shortcomings, when such agents, notably TMP-SMX, are medically necessary, protocols have been developed to administer these drugs (4,10,16). With the exception of sulfonamides and occasionally other non–β-lactam drugs, urgent administration is usually not required. Slow, cautious test dosing is generally a safe and effective method to determine whether the

drug is now tolerated. An example is with TMP-SMX, where one can use the suspension containing 40 mg trimethoprim and 200 mg sulfamethoxazole per 5 mL (4,10,16). The first dose is with 0.1 mg orally of the dose for sulfamethoxazole and, at 30- to 60-minute intervals, administer 1 mg, 10 mg, and 50 mg. If there is no reaction, on the following day, 100 mg and 200 mg may be given. On occasion, particularly in life-threatening Pneumocystis or toxoplasma infections in HIV/AIDS patients, an every-4-hour dosing schedule may be required. Because most reactions to non–β-lactam antimicrobial agents are nonanaphylactic (IgE-independent), desensitization is indicated rarely and may be quite dangerous, as described later.

Sulfonamides

Background

The stimulus for continued attention to sulfonamide and trimethoprim hypersensitivity is due to their utility in treatment of a wide variety of gram-positive and gram-negative bacterial infections and to their importance in the acute or empiric treatment of infectious complications in patients with HIV/AIDS. In patients infected with HIV and living in poor countries, TMP-SMX may be used as prophylaxis and primary therapy for Pneumocystis pneumonia, and as prophylaxis for *Toxoplasma gondii* infections, and as treatment for *Isospora belli* gastroenteritis. The combination of sulfadiazine and pyrimethamine is available for treatment of chorioretinitis and encephalitis due to toxoplasmosis in HIV-positive patients. Another sulfonamide, sulfasalazine, may be used in the management of inflammatory bowel disease, although the alternatives, olsalazine and mesalamine are considerably safer alternatives.

The most common reaction ascribed to sulfonamide hypersensitivity is a generalized rash, usually maculopapular in nature, developing 7 to 12 days after initiation of treatment. Fever may be associated with the rash. Urticaria is occasionally present, but anaphylaxis is a rare event. The TMP-SMX may have been associated with acute urticaria or other immediate reaction; while it is often considered to be from SMX, anaphylaxis and allergic reactions have been attributable to TMP (76–79). In addition, severe cutaneous reactions, such as Stevens-Johnson syndrome and toxic epidermal necrolysis, may occur. Hematologic reactions, notably thrombocytopenia and neutropenia, serum sickness–like reactions, as well as hepatic and renal complications may occur occasionally.

Diagnostic Testing

There are no *in vivo* or *in vitro* tests available to evaluate the presence of sulfonamide allergy. However, there is evidence that some of these reactions are mediated by an IgE antibody directed against its immunogenic metabolite, N^4-sulfonamidoyl (80). Further, studies using multiple N^4-sulfonamidoyl residues attached to polytyrosine carrier as a skin test reagent have been reported (81), but additional studies are necessary to evaluate its clinical usefulness. Also, it appears that most sulfonamide reactions are not IgE-mediated. One notion is that most adverse reactions are due to hydroxylamine metabolites, which induce *in vitro* cytotoxic reactions in peripheral blood lymphocytes of patients with sulfonamide hypersensitivity (82–84). Pharmacogenetics explain some adverse reactions as there are wide variations in acetylation, e.g., slow acetylators experiencing more adverse reactions. The enzyme arylamine N-acetyltransferase 2 (NAT2) has multiple polymorphisms that account for variations in acetylation status (85). From 45% to 70% of sulfamethoxazole is acetylated to N-acetylsulfamethoxazole, with little oxidized to hydroxylamine (86). The hydroxylamine becomes nitrosulfamethoxazole and can result in cytotoxic effects (82–84,86). It is thought that low glutathione stores facilitate cellular injury because of an inability to limit the effects of reactive nitroso metabolites (86).

Clinical confirmation of sulfonamide reaction is accomplished graded drug challenge (10,16,17). This is

of concern particularly when treating HIV-positive patients with TMP-SMX and also with the use of sulfasalazine in the management of inflammatory bowel disease.

Management of Sulfonamide Reactions in Patients with HIV/Acquired Immunodeficiency Syndrome

Patients infected with HIV/AIDS are at increased risk for hypersensitivity reactions to certain drugs (86–89). The best-known example of a drug that produces hypersensitivity reactions in such patients is TMP-SMX. Before the highly active anti-retroviral therapy (HAART) era and in areas of the world where TMP-SMX is used widely, the following data are noteworthy: cutaneous eruptions from TMP-SMX occur in 3.4% of medical inpatients and in 29% to 65% of patients with HIV/AIDS being treated for Pneumocystis pneumonia with this drug (89). The frequency of reactions to TMP-SMX has been reported also as 5% in HIV-negative subjects and up to 60% in HIV-positive subjects (87). Adverse reactions to TMP-SMX have been reported to be more likely when the CD4 count is greater than 20×10^6 cells/L, the CD4/CD8 is less than 0.10 and acetylation status is slow (86). The pathogenesis of these reactions is multifactorial (86). It is recognized that the sulfamethoxazole moiety is responsible for most of the cutaneous reactions, although trimethoprim may be a cause of acute urticaria or anaphylaxis (76–79).

With a reasonable or definite history of a previous reaction, the preferred approach is to use alternative drugs (HAART). The recognized hyperallergic state of HIV regarding allergic-type medication reactions has been documented for various HAART modalities such as mevirapine and atazanavir (86). Pentamidine is a much less desirable alternative and is also associated with serious adverse reactions such as pancreatitis. Cautious readministration of antiviral medications becomes an important consideration. Some protocols for HAART involve graded drug challenge over 36 hours to 5 days as opposed to full dose rechallenge.

When TMP-SMX is indicated, one graded schedule SMX begins with administration of 1/100 of the full dose on day 1, 1/10 on day 2, 3/10 on day 3, and the full dose on day 4 (10,16,17). By taking several days to complete, delayed reactions may become evident. When more urgent administration is necessary, TMP-SMX has been given intravenously in doses of 0.8 mg, 7.2 mg, 40 mg, 80 mg, 400 mg, and 680 mg (based on the SMX component) at 20-minute intervals (90). Desensitization may be performed with the pediatric suspension of TMP-SMX (5 mL contains 40 mg TMP and 200 mg of SMX) (4). The first dose is 0.05 mL (0.01 of a reduced adult dose). More prolonged courses of oral test dosing, such as 10 and 26 days, have been described (91,92). Delayed reactions may be treated with 30 mg to 50 mg of prednisone daily and antihistamines to permit completion of the course of therapy for PCP. In one study, when the history was rash or rash and fever, a 5-day oral course was successful in 14 of 17 patients (93).

Test dosing with intravenous pentamidine has been successfully performed in the face of a previous reaction to this agent. A stock solution containing 200 mg pentamidine in 250 mL dextrose in water (0.8 mg/mL) is prepared. Starting with a 1:10,000 dilution of this solution, 2 mL is given intravenously over 2 minutes. At 15-minute intervals, 2 mL of 1:1,000, 2 mL of 1:100, and 2 mL of 1:10 dilution are administered. After this, 250 mL full-strength solution is given over 2 hours. Successful treatment with aerosolized pentamidine in patients with adverse reactions to systemic pentamidine has been reported using a rapid test dosing schedule (94).

There are reports of anaphylactic-like reactions in patients with previous TMP-SMX–induced cutaneous reactions. Oral desensitization with TMP-SMX has been described, beginning with 0.00001 mg (SMX component) and progressing to full-dose treatment in 7 hours. This procedure is rarely indicated and is dangerous.

TMP-SMX may be indicated in some HIV/AIDS patients. If there has been a previous reaction to this agent, oral graded challenge such as over 36 hours to 5 days followed by daily administration has been effective but may reintroduce a rash. In such cases, prednisone is utilized to minimize the rash and continue the TMP-SMX. Bullous lesions are a contraindication to continuing the TMP-SMX.

Sulfadiazine, together with pyrimethamine, may be indicated for treatment of toxoplasmosis in HIV-infected patients. Among patients who react to sulfadiazine, clindamycin and pyrimethamine are less satisfactory alternatives for treatment of *T. gondii* encephalitis or chorioretinitis. Should this fail, rapid test dosing with sulfadiazine can be accomplished by using 1 mg; 10 mg; 100 mg; 500 mg; 1,000 mg; and 1,500 mg at 4-hour intervals (95). Delayed cutaneous reactions can be treated with prednisone in an effort to complete the recommended course of therapy.

A history of Stevens-Johnson syndrome is nearly always an absolute contraindication to test dosing or desensitization with TMP-SMX (4,10,17). Two patients with previous Stevens-Johnson syndrome were successfully treated with TMP-SMX after an 8-day protocol beginning with 1 mL of 1:1,000,000 dilution of TMP-SMX suspension (96). Only in extreme circumstances should such a procedure be performed.

Management of Sulfasalazine Reactions in Patients with Inflammatory Bowel Disease

The active therapeutic component in sulfasalazine is 5-aminosalicylic acid (5-ASA), which is linked by an azobond to sulfapyridine. After oral ingestion, sulfasalazine is delivered intact to the colon, where bacteria split the azobond to release 5-ASA, which acts topically on inflamed colonic mucosa. (5-ASA may be administered as a suppository for ulcerative proctitis.) The sulfapyridine component is absorbed systemically and accounts for most of the adverse effects attributed to sulfasalazine. The drug has been used for mildly or moderately active ulcerative colitis, for maintaining remission of inactive ulcerative colitis and for some cases of Crohn disease. Oral 5-ASA preparations (e.g., olsalazine, mesalamine, or its prodrug balsalazide) are preferred as first-line agents because of their superior side-effect profile and equivalent therapeutic efficacy compared with sulfasalazine (97). These medications also have a role in Crohn disease and possibly as a chemoprotective agent for colorectal cancer (97).

For the occasional patient with possible drug allergy who requires sulfasalazine, a slow graded challenge has been published (98). This approach starts with a dilute suspension of the drug (liquid sulfasalazine suspension diluted with simple syrup) and advancing the dose slowly, as shown in Table 17B.6 (98). If a rash or fever develops, the dose may be reduced and then advanced more slowly. This approach is ineffective for nonallergic toxicity (headache, nausea, vomiting, abdominal pain) and should not be considered in patients who have had severe reactions, such as Stevens-Johnson syndrome, TEN, agranulocytosis, or fibrosing alveolitis. Most patients were able to achieve therapeutic doses, although some patients did require several trials.

TABLE 17B.6 TEST DOSING WITH SULFASALAZINE[a]

DAY	DOSE (MG)
1	1
2	2
3	4
4	8
5–11	10
12	20
13	40
14	80
15–21	100
22	200
23	400
24	800
25–31	1,000
32 on	2,000

[a]Patients should have failed newer anti-inflammatory agents.

Adapted from Purdy BH, Philips DM, Summers RW. Desensitization for sulfasalazine rash. *Ann Intern Med* 1984;100:512.

With aminosalicylate preparations and corticosteroid enemas (budesonide), the use of other immunosuppressive drugs or immunomodulators, the medical management of inflammatory bowel disease will continue to improve, and, consequently, the need for sulfasalazine should continue to decrease.

Other Antimicrobial Agents

Aminoglycosides

Despite the introduction of newer, less toxic antimicrobial agents, the aminoglycosides continue to be useful with multiple indications. These agents have considerable intrinsic toxicity, namely nephrotoxicity and ototoxicity.

Hypersensitivity-type reactions to aminoglycosides are infrequent and minor, usually taking the form of benign skin rashes or drug-induced fever. Anaphylactic reactions are rare but have been reported after tobramycin and streptomycin administration. Intravenous tobramycin has caused acute respiratory failure requiring intubation. Successful desensitization to tobramycin (14,99,100) and streptomycin (2) has been accomplished. In a case report, desensitization to tobramycin occurred with nebulized administration (14).

Vancomycin

Vancomycin is an important treatment for serious infections in patients with hypersensitivity reactions to β-lactams or in whom there is suspected or known bacterial resistance to β-lactam antibiotics.

Except for the "red-man" or "red-neck" syndrome, adverse reactions to vancomycin are relatively rare. Red-man syndrome is characterized by pruritus and erythema or flushing involving the face, neck, and upper torso, occasionally accompanied by hypotension. This has been attributed to the nonimmunologic release of histamine (101). This complication may be minimized by administering vancomycin, 1,000 mg, over at least a 1- to 2-hour period. Otherwise 1,000 mg of vancomycin administered over 30 minutes or less will cause mast cell histamine release (101). When a patient has ongoing pruritus from chronic renal failure or a dermatologic condition, a slower infusion (over 5 hours) of 500 mg or 1 g is recommended (102). In addition, pretreatment with antihistamines (e.g., cetirizine) may be protective.

Vancomycin has been reported to cause Stevens-Johnson syndrome (103,104) and exfoliative dermatitis (105,106). The exfoliative dermatitis is widespread (generalized) erythroderma with desquamation. Test dosing or desensitization should be avoided in such patients except in the most demanding circumstances. Vancomycin associated Stevens-Johnson syndrome should be differentiated from linear IgA bullous dermatosis (104).

Fluoroquinolones

Fluoroquinolones are valuable antimicrobial agents with a broad range of activity against both gram-negative and gram-positive organisms. Skin rashes and pruritus have been reported in less than 1% of patients receiving these drugs. Phototoxicity may occur. Rarely, Achilles tendon inflammation or rupture occurs. Anaphylactoid reactions, following the initial dose of fluoroquinolones or within the first 3 days of treatment, have been described (24,107–109).

Tetracyclines

Tetracyclines are bacteriostatic agents with broad-spectrum antimicrobial activity. Hypersensitivity-type reactions, including morbilliform rashes, urticaria, and anaphylaxis, occur very rarely with tetracycline drugs. Doxycycline and demeclocycline may produce a mild-to-severe phototoxic dermatitis; minocycline does not. Photosensitivity may occur with all tetracycline drugs.

Chloramphenicol

With the availability of numerous alternative agents and the concern about toxicity, this drug is used infrequently. In patients with bacterial meningitis and a history of severe β-lactam hypersensitivity, chloramphenicol is an alternative choice, after ceftriaxone test dosing. For treatment of rickettsial infections in young children or pregnant women, when tetracycline is contraindicated, chloramphenicol has been utilized.

Bone marrow aplasia is the most serious toxic effect. Believed to be idiosyncratic, occurring in 1 in 40,000 cases of therapy, it tends to occur in patients who undergo prolonged treatment, particularly if the drug has been administered on multiple occasions. This might suggest an immunologic mechanism, but this has not been established. Skin rash, fever, and eosinophilia are observed rarely. Anaphylaxis has been reported (110,111) even from topical, ophthalmologic application (111).

Macrolides

Erythromycin is one of the oldest antibiotics and is infrequently prescribed. Side effects include nausea and vomiting. Hypersensitivity-type reactions are uncommon, and they consist of usually benign skin rashes, fever, eosinophilia, or acute urticaria and angioedema. Anaphylaxis to oral erythromycin, 500 mg, has been reported (112). Cholestatic hepatitis occurs infrequently, most often in association with erythromycin estolate. Recovery is expected on withdrawal of the drug, although it may require a month or so to resolve.

The newer macrolides, azithromycin and clarithromycin, are better tolerated and less toxic. Cholestatic hepatitis has been reported with clarithromycin (113,114). The ketolide, telithromycin has caused anaphylaxis (115). Some cases of hepatic failure have limited the use of this bactericidal macrolide.

Clindamycin

This drug is active against most anaerobes, most gram-positive cocci, and certain protozoa. The main concern with clindamycin use is *Clostridium difficile* pseudomembranous colitis. Adverse drug reactions to clindamycin occurred in less than 1% of hospitalized patients (116). Urticaria, drug fever, eosinophilia, and erythema multiforme have been reported occasionally. Anaphylactic shock is extremely rare (117).

Metronidazole

Metronidazole is useful against most anaerobes, certain protozoa, and *Helicobacter pylori*. The most common adverse reactions are gastrointestinal. Hypersensitivity reactions, including urticaria, pruritus, and erythematous rash, have been reported as has anaphylaxis (118). There is a case report of successful oral desensitization in a patient after what appeared to be an anaphylactic event (119).

Antifungal Agents

Allergic reactions to amphotericin B are quite rare. A report described a patient with amphotericin B–induced anaphylaxis (120). The patient was successfully challenged intravenously with amphotericin, using a desensitization-type protocol. Acute stridor during testing with amphotericin B may occur and require racemic epinephrine (121). Liposomal amphotericin is not necessarily safer than amphotericin B in terms of nephrotoxic effects. Anaphylactic reactions have been reported in patients receiving liposomal preparations (122–124) including a fatality (124).

Hypersensitivity-type reactions, notably rash and pruritus, occur with azoles such as from ketoconazole. A case of anaphylactic shock on the fourth day of administration has been reported with a tryptase concentration of 35 ng/mL (125). Itraconazole has been associated with generalized maculopapular rash. There is a report of successful oral desensitization to itraconazole in a patient with localized coccidioidomycosis (126). Overall, the adverse effects from the azoles (itraconazole, ketoconazole, voriconazole, and posaconazole) consist of the possibility of drug interactions (potentiation of effects), hepatotoxicity, and occasional visual change (127). Rarely, urticaria occurs (128).

The echinocandin class of antifungals (caspofungin, micafungin) can result in infusion associated flushing or urticaria (127).

Antiviral Agents

Hypersensitivity reactions to HAART agents are very common among HIV-infected patients (86). There is a report of a patient who was successfully desensitized to zidovudine using a protocol requiring 37 days (129) and a shorter, 10-day protocol (130).

In a patient with allergic type cutaneous reactions to both acyclovir and fancyclovir, successful graded challenge with acyclovir was reported. The starting dose was 2 mg with doubling to reach 200 mg (131).

The neuraminidase inhibitors, oseltamivir and zanamivir, inhibit both influenza A and B viruses and infrequently cause rashes. Life threatening bronchoconstriction can occur with zanamivir. Patients with asthma should receive zanamivir with caution (132) if at all.

Acute tongue and pharyngeal swelling with urticaria, stridor, and hypotension has been reported with another antiviral agent, lamivudine (133).

Antituberculous Agents

Many manifestations of hypersensitivity resulting from antituberculous drugs usually appear within 3 to 7 weeks after initiation of treatment. The most common signs are fever and rash, and the fever may be present alone for a week or more before other manifestations develop. The skin rash is usually morbilliform but may be urticarial, purpuric, or rarely exfoliative. Less common manifestations include a lupus-like syndrome (especially with isoniazid). Anaphylaxis rarely has been associated with streptomycin and ethambutol.

A common approach is to discontinue all drugs (usually isoniazid, rifampin, pyrazinamide) and allow the reaction (usually a rash) to subside. Subsequently, each drug is reintroduced by test dosing to identify the responsible agent. Another drug then may be substituted for the causative agent. Another approach has been to suppress the reaction with an initial dose of 40 mg to 80 mg of prednisone daily while antituberculous therapy is maintained. This has resulted in prompt clearing of the hypersensitivity reaction, and with adequate chemotherapy, steroids do not appear to affect the course of tuberculosis unfavorably. After taking prednisone for several weeks, the corticosteroid preparation may be discontinued, and the reaction may not reappear.

Adverse drug reactions often may be attributable to isoniazid, rifampin, and ethambutol, as these medications can cause severe hypersensitivity reactions (134,135). There is a case report of drug reaction with eosinophilia and systemic symptoms (DRESS) with streptomycin (135).

Multiple Antibiotic Sensitivity Syndrome

Patients who have reacted to any antimicrobial drug in the past have as high as a 10-fold increased risk for an allergic reaction to another antimicrobial agent (136). The physician should be aware of this possibility and be prepared for such and institute prompt treatment. Alternatively, patients with chronic neurodermatitis (purigo nodularis), chronic or sporadic idiopathic urticaria, dermatographism, or high levels of anxiety may confuse pruritus or idiopathic urticaria with new onset of drug hypersensitivity.

Aspirin and Other Nonsteroidal Anti-inflammatory Drugs

Background

Aspirin (ASA) and nonselective nonsteroidal anti-inflammatory drugs (NSAIDs) rank second or third to the β-lactam antibiotics in producing "allergic-type" drug reactions. Unpredictable reactions to these agents include: (a) acute bronchoconstriction in some patients with nasal polyps and persistent asthma (aspirin exacerbated respiratory disease (AERD), formerly Aspirin Triad or Sampter syndrome; (b) an exacerbation of urticaria in 20% to 30% of patients with idiopathic urticaria or angioedema; (c) anaphylactic reactions with a threat to life, and (d) acute urticaria and/or angiodema (137). When patients are challenged, the reaction occurs with less than 100 mg of aspirin within 3 hours of ingestion (138). During aspirin challenge, between 66% to 97% AERD patients will have positive responses (138). Among otherwise normal individuals, anaphylactic and urticarial reactions have occurred within minutes after the ingestion of a full dose of ASA or a nonselective NSAID. For some patients, it is a particular, single NSAID that causes the reaction (137). Although ASA has been recommended to treat indolent mastocytosis, there is a subset of patients with this disorder who experience either acute urticaria/angioedema or anaphylactoid reactions after the ingestion of ASA and nonselective NSAIDs.

The typical AERD patient is an adult with chronic rhinosinusitis, often with nasal polyps, and persistent allergic asthma. Often, asthma began in childhood. In other words, such patients have had established persistent asthma for years before the first clear episode of an ASA-induced respiratory reaction occurs in adulthood. Such reactions usually occur within 2 hours after the ingestion of ASA or NSAIDs, and may be quite severe and rarely fatal. The reaction may be associated with profound nasal congestion, rhinorrhea, and ocular injection.

Currently, one of the more attractive hypotheses to explain these ASA- and NSAID-induced respiratory reactions stems from the observation that these drugs share the property of inhibiting the generation of cyclo-oxygenase-1 products, thereby permitting the synthesis of lipoxygenase products, most notably leukotriene-D_4 (LTD_4). LTD_4 causes acute bronchoconstriction and increases vascular permeability. To support this assertion, the 5-lipoxygenase inhibitor, zileuton, has been shown to block the decline in forced expiratory volume at 1 second (FEV_1) after ASA ingestion among ASA-sensitive asthmatic patients (139). Also, after aspirin challenge, there is a 10-fold increase in urine LTE_4 concentration, reflecting heightened synthesis of LTD_4 (140). Furthermore, patients with ASA-sensitive asthma are hyperresponsive to LTE_4 given during bronchoprovocation; indeed, they are hypersensitive by a

factor of 13 compared with ASA-tolerant patients with asthma (138,141). Drugs that block cyclooxygenase-1 reduce production of prostaglandin E_2, originally recognized as a bronchodilator. However, it has a critical "braking" effect on the generation of leukotrienes by inhibiting 5-lipoxygenase (5-LO) and 5-lipoxygenase-acting protein (FLAP) (138). Thus, nonselective NSAIDs reduce the production of this critical "braking" prostaglandin.

The selective cyclooxygenase-2 antagonists, celecoxib and refecoxib, have been tolerated uneventfully in nearly all aspirin-intolerant patients with asthma to date (137,138,142). Test challenges in a supervised setting do not appear necessary.

A subpopulation of patients with *chronic idiopathic urticaria or angioedema* experience an exacerbation of urticaria after ingesting ASA or nonselective NSAIDs (143). Using appropriate challenge techniques, the prevalence is between 20% and 30% (137). A reaction is much more likely to occur when the urticaria is active at the time of challenge (143). Avoidance of these agents eliminates acute exacerbations of urticaria following their ingestion but appears to have little effect on the ongoing chronic idiopathic urticaria.

The prevalence of *anaphylactic* (formerly called *anaphylactoid*) *reactions* after the ingestion of both ASA or specific NSAIDs is unknown. Characteristically, such patients appear to be normal and react to only one NSAID or to ASA (137). Cross-reactivity within the entire class of cyclooxygenase-1 inhibitors is rare in these patients. Further, some such reactions occur after two or more exposures to the same NSAID. These features suggest the possibility of an IgE-mediated response, but specific IgE against ASA or any NSAID has not been demonstrated. On occasion, urticaria or angioedema alone may occur after the ingestion of ASA or a nonselective NSAID in patients without ongoing chronic urticaria. It is advisable to have patients avoid all nonselective NSAIDs (and aspirin) unless it has been demonstrated that a specific nonselective NSAID is the sole cause of anaphylaxis or urticaria or angioedema (10,11,17).

Diagnostic Tests

The diagnosis can usually be established by history and does not require confirmatory testing. On occasion, there may be circumstances in which the diagnosis is unclear or a specific diagnosis is required. Skin tests are of no value in the diagnosis of ASA or NSAID sensitivity. Also, there are currently no reliable *in vitro* tests available for the detection of ASA sensitivity. The only definitive diagnostic test is oral test dosing (7,10,11,137,138).

Among patients with asthma, test dosing with ASA or nonselective NSAIDs can provoke a severe acute respiratory reaction and should be attempted only by experienced physicians capable of managing acute, severe asthma in an appropriate medical setting. The asthma should be under optimal control before test dosing is begun. The high risk for this procedure must be considered in relation to its potential benefit. The FEV_1 should be at least 70% of predicted and the respiratory status of the patient stable. A detailed description of a 3-day test dosing protocol may be found elsewhere (144). A typical starting dose of ASA is 3 mg, and progresses to 30 mg, 60 mg, 100 mg, 150 mg, 325 mg, and 650 mg at 3-hour intervals if there is no reaction (144). If a reaction occurs, subsequent ASA challenges are suspended, and the reaction is treated vigorously. After an ASA-induced respiratory reaction, there is a 2- to 5-day refractory period during which the patient may tolerate ASA and all other nonselective NSAIDs (145). Although not currently available in the United States, ASA-lysine has been used for inhalation challenge to verify ASA-sensitive asthmatic patients in Europe (146). Considering the potential difficulties with test dosing and the fact that ASA and other nonselective NSAIDs can be avoided, such diagnostic challenges should be reserved for research purposes or for patients with suspected sensitivity to ASA or NSAIDs who now require those agents for management of chronic conditions.

For patients with chronic idiopathic urticaria, test dosing may be performed in an outpatient setting for patients with coronary or carotid artery disease. For those with ongoing urticarial lesions, treatment of the condition should be continued to avoid false-positive results. If the urticaria is intermittent, test dosing can be accomplished during a remission. One approach is to begin the challenge with 10 mg. If there is no urticaria or symptoms in the first 30 minutes, then administer 30 mg and 41 mg at 30 minute intervals. At this point, the patient is observed for 90 minutes and if no objective evidence of urticaria or angioedema (or bronchoconstriction) has occurred, the patient can be released to home. If the target dosage is 81 mg daily, the patient continues that dosage. Otherwise, the dosage of aspirin can be 81 mg on day 2, 162 mg on day 3, 243 mg on day 4, and 325 mg on day 5, and thereafter. If the patient develops urticaria, it is difficult to "treat through" or desensitize. Depending on the essentiality of aspirin therapy, a decision would be made as to whether such desensitization should be attempted.

Test dosing for anaphylactic reactions is seldom indicated and can be dangerous. However, as previously noted, anaphylactic reactions are limited usually to either ASA or a single nonselective NSAID. Therefore, test dosing with another NSAID may demonstrate its safety for use in treating a medical condition. When ASA administration is essential, other NSAIDs are unacceptable alternatives as platelet inhibitors. For this reason, the above suggested protocol is used during the oral ASA test challenge to reach an initial final dose of 81 mg.

Management of Aspirin- and Other Nonsteroidal Anti-inflammatory Drug-sensitive Patients

Once ASA and other NSAID sensitivity develops, it may last for years. Therefore, strict avoidance of these drugs is critical. Patients should be attentive to the variety of commonly available nonprescription preparations that contain ASA or nonselective NSAIDs, such as "cold," headache, and analgesic remedies. All nonselective NSAIDs that inhibit the cyclooxygenase-1 pathway cross-react to varying degrees with ASA in causing respiratory reactions among ASA-sensitive asthmatic patients and in triggering urticarial reactions among patients with chronic idiopathic urticaria who react to ASA. A current list of NSAIDs that cross-react with ASA is provided in Table 17B.7.

Among ASA-sensitive patients, acetaminophen is most commonly recommended as an alternative and is almost always tolerated uneventfully. However, in one study, high doses of acetaminophen, such as 1,000 mg, were reported to provoke acute bronchoconstriction (decreases in FEV_1) in about one-third of ASA-sensitive asthmatic patients (147). In general, acetaminophen-induced respiratory reactions are much milder and of shorter duration than those induced by ASA. When asthma is stable, if necessary, test dosing with acetaminophen may be attempted starting with 325 mg. If there is no reaction after 2 to 3 hours, 650 mg is given. After 3 more hours, if there has been no adverse reaction, 1,000 mg of acetaminophen may be given (147). Salsalate is also a weak cyclooxygenase inhibitor, which has caused a decrease in FEV_1 in up to 20% of ASA-sensitive asthmatic patients when 2,000 mg is given (148). Salsalate and choline magnesium trisalicylate have no effect on cyclooxygenase-1 in vitro and do not cause acute bronchoconstriction in ASA-sensitive asthmatic patients in recommended doses. Although there was a report of a bronchoconstrictive reaction to hydrocortisone sodium succinate (Solu-Cortef) in 1 of 45 ASA-sensitive asthmatic patients (149), this occurrence seems exceedingly rare. Also, tartrazine (FD & C yellow dye) does not cross-react with ASA in ASA-sensitive patients or induce acute respiratory reactions, as was thought at one time (138).

A practical problem is what advice to give to historically non–ASA-sensitive asthmatic patients regarding the use of ASA and other nonselective NSAIDs. One approach is to caution such patients about the potential for such a reaction, particularly if they have nasal polyps and are prednisone-dependant. There is a low incidence of ASA sensitivity in patients with asthma with normal computed tomography scans of the sinuses and in patients with clear evidence of IgE-mediated asthma. Treatment with ASA or other nonselective NSAIDs may be medically necessary in some patients with AERD, such as the management of a rheumatoid or osteoarthritis

TABLE 17B.7   STRONG INHIBITORS, WEAK INHIBITORS, AND NONINHIBITORS OF CYCLOOXYGENASE-1

Strong Inhibitors of Cyclooxygenase-1

Diclofenac (Voltaren, Arthrotec, Cataflam)

Diflunisal (Dolobid)

Etodolac (Lodine)

Fenoprofen (Nalfon)

Flubiprofen (Ansaid)

Ibuprofen (Motrin, Advil, Nuprin, Haltran, Medipren)

Indomethacin (Indocin)

Ketoprofen (Orudis, Oruvail)

Ketorolac (Toradol)

Meclofenamate (Meclomen)

Mefanamic acid (Ponstel)

Meloxicam (Mobic)

Nabumetone (Relafen)

Naproxen (Naprosyn, Anaprox, Aleve, Naprelan)

Oxaprozin (Daypro)

Piroxicam (Feldene)

Sulindac (Clinoril)

Tolmetin (Tolectin)

Weak Inhibitors of Cyclooxygenase-1 (suitable, initial alternatives)

Acetaminophen (Tylenol, Datril, Excedrin, Midol, Percogesic)

Salsalate (Disalcid)

Noninhibitors of Cyclooxygenase-1

Choline magnesium trisalicylate (Trilisate)

Celecoxib (Celebrex)

Hydroxychloroquine (Plaquenil)

Refecoxib (Vioxx)

or to inhibit platelet aggregation for coronary artery or carotid disease. The term *desensitization* has been applied to this procedure, although many would prefer that this term be reserved for IgE-mediated reactions. The process is identical to oral graded challenge with ASA for diagnostic purposes, except that the challenge continues following a positive respiratory reaction. The dose of ASA that caused the reaction is reintroduced after the patient has recovered. If no further reaction occurs, at 3-hour intervals, the dose is gradually increased until either another reaction occurs or the patient can tolerate 650 mg of ASA without a reaction. Once successfully desensitized, cross-desensitization between ASA and all other nonselective

NSAIDs is complete. This state can be maintained indefinitely if the patient takes at least one ASA dose daily; if ASA is stopped, it persists for only 2 to 5 days.

ASA desensitization followed by long-term ASA treatment has been advocated for treatment of AERD including for the chronic rhinosinusitis (7,138,144). Such treatment has resulted in improvement in rhinosinusitis with prevention of nasal polyp reformation and improved sense of smell, as well as allowing a significant reduction in the need for systemic and inhaled corticosteroids. Nevertheless, as with other antiasthma treatments, ASA desensitization does not induce a remission of persistent asthma. The target dosage is 650 mg twice daily and this dosage may result in gastritis or gastrointestinal bleeding. Nevertheless, patients may benefit if they can tolerate the long-term aspirin at this dosage (7,138,144).

Unlike AERD, ASA-sensitive urticaria and angioedema do not appear to respond to ASA desensitization (143). Aspirin desensitization has been employed to prevent synthesis of mast cell–derived prostaglandin D_2, a cyclooxygenase-1 product thought to be largely responsible for systemic reactions, among patients with indolent mastocytosis, who in fact, have experienced anaphylactic reactions after the ingestion of ASA or nonselective NSAIDs.

Acetaminophen

In contrast to the rare AERD patient who develops a 25% to 33% decrease in FEV_1 with a 1,000 mg challenge with acetaminophen (147), true anaphylactic reactions to acetaminophen have been reported (150–153). The provoking doses necessary to induce shock were described as 125 mg, 191 mg, and 300 mg (150–152). Elevated plasma or urine histamine concentrations were demonstrated (150,152). These patients were not ASA-sensitive and had anaphylactic reactions, as compared with the rare AERD patient who has a moderate bronchoconstrictive response to 1,000 mg of acetaminophen.

Concurrent acetaminophen and aspirin sensitivity was reported in a 13-year-old girl with asthma (154). She experienced acute urticaria, angioedema, and dyspnea within 10 minutes of ingesting 650 mg of acetaminophen. Aspirin, 325 mg, and indomethacin, 300 mg, caused acute urticaria (154). Such sensitivity must be exceedingly rare. For practical purposes, AERD patients can use acetaminophen in recommended doses (650 mg) without initial test dosing.

Radiographic Contrast Media

Background

Radiographic contrast media (RCM) are clear solutions and should not be called "dyes." Nonfatal immediate generalized reactions (most commonly urticaria) occur in 2% to 3% of patients receiving conventional ionic high-osmolality RCM and in less than 0.5% of patients receiving the lower-osmolality agents. A large prospective study reported severe life-threatening (often anaphylactic) reactions occurring in 0.22% of those receiving the high-osmolality media compared with only 0.04% of those receiving lower-osmolality preparations (155). It is clear that the lower-osmolality RCM causes significantly fewer adverse reactions (156–159), but severe or fatal reactions may occur (160,161). In fact, the risk for a fatal reaction may be the same with either class of RCM and is estimated to be 0.9 cases per 100,000 infusions (157). Deaths have occurred with all types of RCM (157). The volume infused in fatal reactions may be less than 10 mL in some cases (157).

The overall prevalence of reactions to the noniodinated, gadolinium-based contrast agents for magnetic resonance imaging (MRI) is about 1% to 2%. Allergic type reactions occur in about 1:1451 injections (0.07%) (162,163). Severe systemic reactions to these agents were reported in 1:19, 588 injections (162). Pretreatment with prednisone-diphendydramine does not always prevent reactions to gadolinium-based contrast agents (162).

Clearly, there are patients at increased risk for an immediate generalized (anaphylactic) reaction to RCM. The most obvious and important risk factor is a history of a previous reaction to these agents. The exact reaction rate is unknown, but with ionic hyperosmolality RCM, it ranges between 17% and 60% (159). The administration of nonionic lower-osmolality agents to such patients reduces the risk to 4% to 5.5% (164,165). Severe coronary artery disease, unstable angina, advanced age, female sex, and receipt of large volumes of contrast media are also risk factors (157). Atopic individuals and asthmatic patients appear to be more susceptible to anaphylactic reactions to RCM (155,157,166). There is some disagreement about the risk for an anaphylactic reaction to RCM among patients receiving β-adrenergic blocking agents (167,168). The risk was not found to be increased in frequency or severity in a prospective study (167); however, reactions may be more severe and less responsive to treatment in patients with cardiac impairment. Among such patients, the use of lower-osmolality RCM and possibly pretreatment with antihistamines and corticosteroids (discussed later) may be advisable. The data that patients who have reacted to topical iodine cleansing solutions and iodides and those allergic to shellfish are at slightly increased risk for RCM reactions were based on use of older, higher osmolality RCM (169). The history of allergic disorders does not justify use of lower-osmolality RCM in the absence of a previous anaphylactic reaction to RCM or very high anxiety about the procedure. In facilities, where lower-osmolality RCM are standard practice, patients with a history of shellfish allergy or "iodine" allergy do not have to be pretreated (170,171) unless

there is a high level of anxiety about the procedure. This approach is different from the American College of Radiology (157) which recommends pretreatment.

Typically, most anaphylactic reactions from RCM begin within 1 to 3 minutes after intravascular administration, very rarely after 20 minutes. Nausea, emesis, and flushing are most common and may be due to vagal stimulation. Such reactions are to be distinguished from anaphylactic reactions, which include pruritus, urticaria, angioedema, bronchospasm, hypotension, and syncope. Urticaria is the most common reaction. Most of these reactions are self-limited and respond promptly to the administration of epinephrine and antihistamines. However, the potential for a fatal outcome must not be ignored, and trained personnel must be available to recognize and treat hypotension and cardiac or respiratory arrest. Sudden-onset grand mal seizure likely reflects cerebral hypoperfusion and not epilepsy.

The mechanism of RCM-induced immediate generalized reactions remains incompletely understood. These reactions are not IgE-mediated but involve mast cell activation with release of histamine, tryptase, and other mediators (157).

Diagnostic Testing

There are no *in vivo* or *in vitro* tests to identify potential reactors to RCM. Severe and fatal reactions have occurred after an intravenous test dose of 1 mL to 2 mL. Also, severe reactions have followed a negative test dose. Graded test dosing has been abandoned.

As noted previously, a history of a previous reaction to RCM is the most essential information necessary to assess the risk for a repeat reaction (157,159).

Management of Patients at Increased Risk for a Repeat Radiographic Contrast Media Reaction

Among patients with a previous reaction to RCM, the incidence and severity of subsequent reactions has been reduced using pretreatment regimens of corticosteroids, antihistamines, and adrenergic agents. Using older higher-osmolality RCM, pretreatment with prednisone and diphenhydramine reduced the prevalence of repeat reactions to about 10%, whereas the addition of ephedrine to this protocol reduced it further to 5% (172). The addition of lower-osmolality RCM to the prednisone-diphenhydramine regimen decreased the incidence of repeat reactions even further to 0.5% (159). Most repeated reactions tended to be quite mild. Unfortunately, the higher cost of these lower-osmolality RCM remains an issue for some hospitals and physicians.

The following summarizes a useful approach that can be recommended when patients with a history of a RCM-associated anaphylactic reaction require a repeated study (157,159):

1. Document in the medical record the need for the procedure and that alternative procedures are unsatisfactory.
2. Document in the record that the patient or responsible person understands the need for the test and that the pretreatment regimen may not prevent all adverse reactions.
3. Recommend the use of lower-osmolality RCM if available.
4. Pretreatment medications (157,159) are as follows:
   A. Prednisone, 50 mg orally, 13 hours, 7 hours, and 1 hour before the RCM procedure.
   B. Diphenhydramine, 50 mg intramuscularly or orally, 1 hour before the RCM procedure.
   C. Albuterol, 4 mg orally, 1 hour before the RCM procedure (withhold if the patient has unstable angina, cardiac arrhythmia, or other cardiac risks).
5. Proceed with the RCM study and have emergency therapy available.

There may be situations in which high-risk patients require an emergency RCM study. The following emergency protocol is recommended (10,159):

1. Administer hydrocortisone, 200 mg intravenously, immediately and every 4 hours until the study is completed.
2. Administer diphenhydramine, 50 mg intramuscularly, immediately before or 1 hour before the procedure.
3. Administer albuterol, 4 mg orally, immediately before or 1 hour before the procedure (optional).
4. Recommend the use of lower-osmolality RCM if available.

Because several hours are required for corticosteroids to be effective, it is best to avoid the emergency administration of RCM unless absolutely necessary. The medical record should note that there has not been time for conventional pretreatment and that there is limited experience with such abbreviated programs.

It is also important to be aware that anaphylactic reactions to RCM may occur when these agents are administered by nonvascular routes, for example, retrograde pyelograms, hysterosalpingograms, myelograms, and arthrograms. Previous reactors undergoing those procedures should receive pretreatment as described previously.

Finally, it should be noted that the pretreatment protocols are useful only for the prevention of anaphylactic reactions, but not for other types of life-threatening reactions, such as ventricular tachycardia or fibrillation, the adult respiratory tract distress syndrome or noncardiogenic pulmonary edema.

Patients with asthma should have their respiratory status stable under ideal circumstances. Similarly, isotonic hydration and perhaps acetylcysteine should be employed to prevent acute renal failure or increases in serum creatinine (173).

Local Anesthetics

Background
Patients who experience adverse reactions of virtually any type following the injection of a local anesthetic may be advised erroneously that they are allergic to these agents and should never receive "caines" in the future. Such patients may be denied the benefit of dental care or a surgical procedure. A patient may experience a respiratory or cardiac arrest after receiving a local anesthetic with epinephrine injection for routine dental care. The likely explanation is acute cardiac ischemia from the 1:100,000 epinephrine being absorbed quickly into the sublingual veins. The patient then may develop apparent noncardiogenic "flash" pulmonary edema. Such patients are not truly reacting to the local anesthetic.

More commonly, adverse effects are vasovagal reactions, toxic reactions, hysterical reactions, or as noted, epinephrine-related effects. Allergic contact dermatitis is the most common immunologic reaction to local anesthetics. On occasion, clinical manifestations suggestive of anaphylactic reactions are described, but most reported series have shown that such reactions occur rarely, if ever (174–176). In one study, reproducible reactions were noted for articane and lidocaine (176).

As shown in Table 17B.8, local anesthetics may be classified as benzoic acid esters (group I) or others (group II). On the basis of local anesthetic contact dermatitis and patch testing studies, the benzoic acid esters often cross-react with each other but do not cross-react with those agents in group II. Also, drugs in group II do not cross-react with each other and appear to be less sensitizing.

It has been suggested that sulfites and parabens, which are used as preservatives in local anesthetics, may be responsible for allergic-like reactions. However, such reactions are so rare as to be reportable (177). When confronted with this remote possibility, the pragmatic approach is to avoid preparations containing them. On the other hand, latex-containing products, such as gloves and rubber dams, are often used in dental and surgical practices. Local or systemic reactions may occur in latex-sensitive patients, and this possibility should be considered in the differential diagnosis of adverse reactions attributed to local anesthetic agents.

Diagnostic Testing
Initial skin testing as a part of a test dosing protocol is the preferred approach. Prick tests are usually negative. Positive intradermal skin tests are often found in otherwise healthy controls and do not correlate with the outcome of test dosing (10,11,174–176). *In vitro* testing is not applicable.

TABLE 17B.8 CLASSIFICATION OF LOCAL ANESTHETICS

Benzoic Acid Esters (group I)

Benzocaine[a]
Butamben picrate (Butesin)[a]
Chloroprocaine (Nesacaine)
Cocaine[a]
Procaine (Novocain)
Proparacaine[a]
Tetracaine (Pontocaine)

Amide or Miscellaneous Structures (group II)

Bupivacaine (Marcaine, Sensorcaine)[b]
Dibucane (Nupercaine)[b]
Dyclonine (Dyclone)[a]
Etiodocaine (Duranest)[b]
Levobupivacaine (Chirocaine)[b]
Lidocaine (Xylocaine)[b]
Mepivacaine (Carbocaine, Polocaine)[b]
Pramoxine (Tronothane)[a]
Prilocaine (Citanest)[b]
Roprivacaine (Naropin)[b]

[a]Primarily topical agents.
[b]Contains amide structure.

Management of Patients with a History of Reactions to Local Anesthetics

If the local anesthetic agent causing the previous reaction is known, a different local anesthetic agent should be selected for administration for reassurance. For example, if the drug is an ester, an amide may be chosen. If the drug is an amide, another amide may be used.

The use of diphenhydramine may provide reasonable anesthesia required for suturing, but clearly this is inadequate for dental anesthesia.

Unfortunately, the local anesthetic agent is often unknown, and the clinical details of the previous reaction are often vague, unavailable, or of uncertain significance. For this reason, the following protocol has been effective in identifying a local anesthetic agent that the patient will tolerate (10,11):

1. Obtain consent.
2. Determine the local anesthetic agent to be used by the dentist or physician. It must not contain epinephrine. These are usually available as ampules.
3. At 15-minute intervals:
   A. Perform a skin-prick test using the undiluted local anesthetic.
   B. If negative, inject 0.1 mL of a 1:100 dilution subcutaneously in an extremity.
   C. If there is no local reaction, inject 0.1 mL of a 1:10 dilution of local anesthetic subcutaneously.
   D. If there is no local reaction, inject 0.1 mL of undiluted local anesthetic agent.
   E. If there is no local reaction, inject 1 mL and then 2 mL of the undiluted local anesthetic agent.
4. Following this procedure, a letter is given to the patient indicating that the patient has received 3 mL of the respective local anesthetic with no reaction and is at no greater risk for a subsequent allergic reaction than the general population.
5. Such test dosing should be undertaken by individuals with training and experience in such tests, and also in treatment of anaphylactic reactions.

This regimen should be completed before the anticipated procedure, and in some cases, it can be done to help exclude local anesthetic "allergy." To date, we are not aware of any patient with negative test dosing who reacted later when the local anesthetic agent was used for a procedure, with the exception of hysterical reactions. The success of this approach is undoubtedly related to the extreme rarity of true allergic reactions to local anesthetic agents. However, at the least, the protocol serves to allay some or all of the anxiety of patients and referring dentists and physicians, and at the most, it may permit one to identify safely that rare patient truly at risk for an allergic reaction to subsequent local anesthetic administration.

Angiotensin-converting Enzyme Inhibitors and Angiotensin II Receptor Antagonists

Angiotensin-converting enzyme (ACE) inhibitors have efficacy in treatment of patients with left ventricular systolic dysfunction or congestive heart failure, as secondary prevention in patients who have experienced a myocardial infarction, in diabetic patients, and as antihypertensive agents. ACE inhibitors have been reported to cause a nonproductive cough in 1% to 39% of patients; this cough subsides in a few days or in less than 4 weeks in exceptional cases (178). Angioedema has been recognized in other patients, perhaps with an incidence of 0.1% to 0.3% (179,180). The angioedema may cause marked tongue or pharyngeal swelling such that intubation is required. It has a predilection for the tongue, pharynx, and face as opposed to gastrointestinal tract or as isolated dysphagia (179). It has been reported that first episodes occurred in the first 4 weeks of ACE inhibitor use in 22% of patients, and 77% occurred after that time, with an overall mean duration until presentation of 11 months (181,182). In another study, the mean time was 19 months, with a range of 3 days to 6.3 years (183). African Americans appear to be at increased risk for experiencing angioedema from ACE inhibitors (179,182). Because 7 of 9 patients in one series were using aspirin, it has been hypothesized that aspirin could be a cofactor in ACE inhibitor angioedema (180). Nonselective NSAIDs also may be a cofactor (179). Complement is not consumed during these reactions.

ACE inhibitors have been reported to induce anaphylactic reactions during hemodialysis, especially when the dialysis membrane is polyacrilonitrile but not cuprophane or polysulfone (184–186).

ACE inhibitors have 3 substrates: bradykinin, Substance P, and angiotensin I. The mechanism of acute angioedema is thought to be attributable to production of excessive bradykinin in that ACE inhibitors, which block generation of angiotensin II from angiotensin I, also inhibit inactivation of bradykinin and Substance P. Accumulation of bradykinin is thought to cause cough and angioedema and contribute to anaphylactic reactions by causing vasodilation. The major pathways for bradykinin degradation utilize ACE (bradykininase) and aminopeptidase P. ACE inhibitors decrease the metabolism of aminopeptidase P (179,187). There is a minor pathway for bradykinin degradation into des-Arg-bradykinin via action of carboxypeptidase N (179). Genetic differences in reactors appear to explain some episodes (187). It remains to be determined whether this understanding is the correct explanation because acute angioedema from angiotensin II receptor blockers also occurs (180). These drugs do not inhibit ACE so that accumulation of bradykinin does not occur. Reactions to losartan have occurred within 1 day to 16 months after beginning therapy (188). Some patients have never received an ACE inhibitor. Angiotensin II receptor blockers are not contraindicated in patients who have experienced angioedema from an ACE inhibitor, but physician awareness of potential future episodes is warranted (179).

In patients with idiopathic anaphylaxis, hereditary angioedema, or acquired C1 esterase inhibitor deficiency, ACE inhibitors (and β-adrenergic antagonists) are contraindicated at least on a relative basis until our understanding of these reactions improves.

Opiates

Opiates have their historical basis traced back 1,800 years ago related to opium (189). Opioid receptors have been identified as μ, δ, κ, and nociceptin/orphanin FQ (189). The classic opioid actions are mediated by μ-receptor stimulation which results in analgesia, decreased gastrointestinal transit time, contraction of the sphincter of Oddi, respiratory depression, decreased cough, and pupillary constriction. Analgesia is caused by activation of μ, δ, and κ receptors. However, μ receptors are present in ascending nerves in the spinal tract and in the brain, whereas κ receptors are present only in spinal nerves. Morphine activates μ and κ receptors while fentanyl acts on μ, δ, and κreceptors.

Morphine and codeine are most likely to activate mast cells and cause flushing or acute urticaria. Intravenous morphine could cause symptoms consistent with an anaphylactic reaction. Meperidine, tramadol, and fentanyl are ineffective triggers of mast cells. Meperidine is out of favor because of sharp rises and falls in serum concentrations; although it can cause diaphoresis, it is an unlikely cause of urticaria.

Patients may have confused opioid effects for hypersensitivity, but when there is a history of codeine- or morphine-induced urticaria, alternative agents may be selected if narcotics are required. For example, fentanyl can be administered intravenously or transdermally. Lower doses of long-acting formulations of morphine may be tried as well.

Chemotherapy for Neoplastic Diseases

Many chemotherapeutic agents result in bone marrow suppression or other particular adverse effects including serious cutaneous eruptions. Interstitial lung disease, infiltrates, or pulmonary fibrosis can occur with use of bleomycin, methotrexate, cyclophosphamide, busulfan, carmustine (BCNU), platinum derivatives (cisplatin and oxaliplatin), docetaxel, placitaxel, and all trans-retinoic acid as examples (10,190–195). The latter has been associated with basophil-derived histamine release causing acute bronchoconstriction when administered to patients with acute promyelocytic leukemia. The promyelocytes resemble basophils! Capillary leak syndromes occur with IL-2, cytosine arabinoside, the combination of mitomycin and vinca alkaloids and other agents. L-asparaginase, docetaxel, and placitaxel can cause anaphylactic type reactions (10). The stabilizer, Cremophor El is like Tween 80 and can be the explanation for the reactions (10). Premedication with corticosteroids and antihistamines can reduce the number of reactions from paxlitaxel (10) and some other chemotherapeutic agents. Reducing the rate of infusion may be of value.

Anaphylaxis has occurred with various chemotherapeutic agents but fortunately is rare. Cisplatin and carboplatin can cross-react, are potent sensitizers (193,194), and can cause anaphylactic type reactions (193,194,196). Because some of these reactions are IgE-mediated, prednisone-diphenhydramine pretreatment is not expected to be successful. If either of these agents is truly essential and the patient agrees, skin testing can be carried out with prick tests of 0.1 mg/mL concentration with intradermals of 0.001 mg/mL, 0.01 mg/mL, and 0.1 mg/mL (194). Desensitization should begin with 0.01 mg or less depending on the skin test results. In some cases, desensitization will be successfully carried out, but not in all cases. Indeed, as little as 3.5 mg of cisplatin has caused anaphylaxis (194). The physician must be in attendance with epinephrine available as described with desensitization protocols (3,5)

Anticonvulsants

The anticonvulsant hypersensitivity syndrome is rare but typically begins within 2 months of initiation of phenytoin, carbamazepine, phenobarbital or lamotrigine or other anticonvulsants (197–206). In a few cases, the onset is in the third month of therapy. Reactions consist of fever, marked erythematous papules that may blister or demonstrate necrosis from vasculitis, and desquamate. Other findings include tender lymphadenopathy, liver enlargement, and oral ulcerations. The term *anticonvulsant hypersensitivity syndrome* clinically is referred to as DRESS. This author believes that such patients have sufficient criteria for the diagnosis of Stevens-Johnson syndrome, but DRESS is recognized as its own entity. In fact, in a series of patients with Stevens-Johnson syndrome, phenytoin, carbamazepine, valproic acid, lamotrigine, and phenobarbital all were identified among culprit medications. Associated laboratory findings may include atypical lymphocytes, eosinophilia, elevation of serum creatinine, and liver function test abnormalities. Leukopenia may occur in some patients. Pulmonary eosinophilia with respiratory failure has been reported. The name of *anticonvulsant hypersensitivity syndrome* had been suggested because of the combination of fever, severe pruritic rash, and lymphadenopathy associated with multisystem involvement (207), but DRESS is preferred now. Some cases are familial (203). Carbamazepine may be more likely to cause the DRESS syndrome or Stevens-Johnson syndrome based on HLA-B genotypes (HLA-B*1502) primarily in Southeast Asians (200,201). This finding has not been confirmed in Caucasians (202). Because of shared structures and metabolism, it is thought that when a patient develops the DRESS syndrome to either phenytoin or carbamazepine, that neither of these medications or phenobarbital should be re-administered. When the diagnosis has not been clear or an error occurs, even a single additional dose of phenytoin or carbamazepine may elicit the DRESS or Stevens-Johnson syndrome in a susceptible patient. However, phenobarbital is not automatically contraindicated in patients allergic to phenytoin or carbamazepine (203). Challenges must be carried out in exceptional cases and with very small doses. However, when the rash was not necessarily part of DRESS syndrome, alternative anticonvulsants often are prescribed. The rate of cross-reactivity has been reported as follows: rash to phenytoin implied a rash to carbamazepine in 42%, phenobarbital in 19.5%, and lamotrigine in 18.9%; rash to carbamazepine implied a rash to phenytoin in 57.6%, to phenobarbital in 26.7%, and to lamotrigine in 20% (206).

The mechanism may relate to inadequate detoxification by epoxide hydrolase of hepatic microsome-generated metabolites of phenytoin and carbamazepine (197,198,202,203). The relatives of affected patients who are themselves nonepileptic and nonexposed to phenytoin may have findings of delayed metabolism (203). The metabolites are thought to cause either apoptosis or neoantigen formation with the clinical hypersensitivity syndrome (197–199,203). Sensitized $CD4^+$ T_H2 lymphocytes, $CD8^+$ lymphocytes, and presence of the skin-homing receptor, CLA, have been reported as findings in skin rashes and/or blistering (200,204). Genetic polymorphisms predispose Southeast Asians positive for HLA-B*1502 for carbamazepine Stevens-Johnson syndrome and HLA-B*5701 for carbamazepine Stevens-Johnson syndrome/TEN (200,201). This genotype has not been reproduced in some Caucasian people (202). Whatever the mechanism, systemic corticosteroids should be administered and anticonvulsants discontinued (10) (see Chapter 16).

Alternative anticonvulsants, if necessary, should be selected, such as valproic acid, divalproex, phenobarbital, benzodiazepines, or gabapentin. Valproic acid and divalproex are hepatotoxic, so caution is advised in patients with liver involvement. Appropriate neurologic consultation is advisable because of the high frequency of cutaneous reactions (206).

Muscle Relaxants

The neuromuscular blocking agents are divided into depolarizing (succinylcholine) and nondepolarizing (vecuronium, pancuronium) categories. Acute anaphylactic reactions present as sudden onset hypotension, shock, or acute bronchoconstriction with difficulty in ventilation by the anesthesiologist. Emergent intubation and cardiopulmonary resuscitation may be necessary. Generalized urticaria may or may not be reported but flushing or angioedema may be observed on the face. Serum tryptase concentrations may be elevated as evidence of mast cell activation. The neuromuscular blocking agents may cause an IgE-mediated reaction or induce mast cell activation independent of IgE antibodies. Improvements in synthesis have resulted in agents with little ability to activate mast cells. In some cases, very rapid infusion of the agent causes an immediate reaction, whereas administration over 30 to 60 seconds does not. The incidence of anaphylactic reactions during general anesthesia may be in the range from about 1:5,000 to 1:25,000 (208). Up to 25% of reactions occur on the initial anesthetic exposure, which might be explained by the presence of quaternary and tertiary ammonium ions being present in cosmetics, disinfectants, foods, and other medications.

The nondepolarizing neuromuscular blocking agents have tertiary and quaternary ammonium groups that are considered to be the antigenic sites for IgE. Cross-reactivity exists based on skin test results. Skin testing begins with prick tests and then intradermal testing (10,208–212). The neuromuscular blocking agents must be diluted (208–211). For prick (epicutaneous) testing, dilutions for testing are as follows:

Pancuronium   1 mg/mL

Succinylcholine   20 mg/mL

Vecuronium   1 mg/mL

For intradermal testing, dilutions begin as follows:

Pancuronium   0.002 mg/mL.....0.02 mg/
                     mL......0.2 mg/mL

Succinylcholine   0.001 mg/mL.....0.01 mg/
                     mL......0.1 mg/mL

Vecuronium   0.004 mg/mL....0.04 mg/
                     mL......0.4 mg/mL

If the prick test is negative, begin with the weakest dilution for intradermal testing. If the first intradermal skin test is negative, continue with step-wise skin testing until the highest strength is used. If it also is negative, the agent can be considered for administration. Incriminated agents include vecuronium, pancuronium, atracurium, cisatracurium, rocuronium, d-tubocurarine, and succinylcholine. Skin testing will identify cross-reactive agents, but some patients have immediate cutaneous reactivity to a single agent. Negative skin tests help identify the agents that can be administered safely.

Latex allergy, empiric antibiotics such as cefazolin (208), fentanyl (213), and protamine are in the differential diagnosis of anaphylactic reactions during anesthesia. Other agents such as benzodiazepines, thiopental, propofol, and even chlorhexidine rarely are proven to be etiologic (211,212). The hypnotic agent ketamine, which has sympathetic stimulating actions, caused acute severe pulmonary edema in an 8-year-old child (214).

Proton Pump Inhibitors/Histamine₂ Receptor Antagonists

Proton pump inhibitors and histamine$_2$ receptor antagonists usually are tolerated uneventfully except for patients who experience diarrhea or other gastrointestinal side effects. Anaphylaxis has been reported with omeprazole (215,216) as well as desensitization to omeprazole (216). Cross-reactivity by skin testing has been demonstrated between omeprazole and lansoprazole (215). Severe erythroderma, erythema multiforme, and even TEN from proton pump inhibitors have been reported (217).

Stevens-Johnson syndrome has been described from ranitidine (218). In one patient, the target lesions, sublingual ulcers and conjunctivitis, began one day after a single raniditine tablet (218). The history was of uneventful exposure 2 years previously during a month of treatment and "itchy skin eruptions" on the forearms and legs 1 year previously. This patient's case reinforces the point that a single tablet of medication can induce Stevens-Johnson syndrome when the patient is sensitized (see Chapter 16).

Antiplatelet Therapy

Antiplatelet therapy is indicated for patients with coronary artery disease who may require coronary artery bypass grafting, insertion of a bare metal stent (1 month of clopidogrel with aspirin) or drug eluting stent (12 months of clopidogrel with aspirin) (219). Ticlopidine administration has recognized adverse effects such as neutropenia and thrombocytopenic purpura. Clopidogrel has reduced incidence of such adverse effects but may cause pruritus, rash, angioedema, or anaphylaxis. Often, the pruritic rash from clopidogrel begins within the first 3 days to 1 month of therapy. It may be necessary to perform desensitization. Approaches include a protocol of 0.005 mg, 0.010 mg, 0.020 mg, 0.040 mg, 0.080 mg, 0.160 mg, 0.30 mg, 0.60 mg, 1.20 mg, 2.50 mg, 5.0 mg, 10 mg, 20 mg, 40 mg (220–222). Alternatively, it may be possible to begin with 0.30 mg and proceed every 30 minutes with an accumulated target dose of 75 mg. Depending on the rash that may occur during desensitization, prednisone and antihistamines may be required. In some cases, desensitization is not possible as the cutaneous eruption does not allow for continued clopidogrel administration.

■ REFERENCES

1. Anné S, Middleton E Jr, Reisman RE. Vancomycin anaphylaxis and successful desensitization. *Ann Allergy.* 1994;73:402–404.
2. Chandler MJ, Ong RC, Grammer LC, et al. Detection, characterization, and desensitization of IgE to streptomycin. *J Allergy Clin Immunol.* 1992;89:178.
3. Lee C-W, Matulonis UA, Castells MC. Carboplatin hypersensitivity: a 6-h 12-step protocol effective in 35 desensitizations in patients with gynecologic malignancies and mast cell/IgE-mediated reactions. *Gynecol Oncol.* 2004;95:370–376.
4. Greenberger PA. Desensitization and test-dosing for the drug-allergic patient. *Ann Allergy Asthma Immunol.* 2000;85:250–251.
5. Castells MC, Tennant NM, Sloanne DE, et al. Hypersensitivity reactions to chemotherapy: outcomes and safety of rapid desensitization in 413 cases. *J Allergy Clin Immunol.* 2008;122:574–580.
6. Adkinson FA Jr. Desensitization for drug hypersensitivity. *J Allergy Clin Immunol.* 2008;122:581–582.
7. Macy E, Bernstein JA, Castells MC, et al. Aspirin challenge and desensitization for aspirin-exacerbated respiratory disease: a practice paper. *Ann Allergy Asthma Immunol.* 2007;9 8:172–174.
8. Williams AN, Simon RA, Woessner KM, et al. The relationship between historical aspirin-induced asthma and severity of asthma induced during oral aspirin challenges. *J Allergy Clin Immunol.* 2007; 120:273–277.
9. Lin D, Li WK, Rieder MJ. Cotrimoxazole for prophylaxis or treatment of opportunistic infections of HIV/AIDS in patients with previous history of hypersensitivity to cotrimoxazole. *Cochrane Database Syst Rev.* 2007 April 18;(2):CD005646. Review.
10. Grammer LC, Greenberger PA. *Drug Allergy and Protocols for Management of Drug Allergies.* 3rd ed. Providence, RI: Oceanside Pubs; 2003:1–42.
11. Bernstein IL, Gruchalla RS, Lee RE, et al. Disease management of drug hypersensitivity: a practice parameter. *Ann Allergy Asthma Immunol.* 1999;83:665–700.
12. Stelzle RC, Squire EN. Oral desensitization to 5-aminosalicylic acid medications. *Ann Allergy Asthma Immunol.* 1999;83:23–24.
13. Schumacher MJ, Copeland JG. Intravenous desensitization to allopurinol in a heart transplant patient with gout. *Ann Allergy Asthma Immunol.* 2004;92:374–376.
14. Spigarelli MG, Hurwitz ME, Nasr SZ. Hypersensitivity to inhaled TOBI® following reaction to gentamicin. *Ped Pulmonol.* 2002;33: 311–314.
15. Shahar E, Moar C, Pollack S. Successful desensitization of enfuvirtide-induced skin hypersensitivity reaction. *AIDS.* 2005;19:451–452.

16. Patterson R, DeSwarte RD, Greenberger PA, et al. Drug allergy and protocols for management of drug allergies. *Allergy Proc.* 1994;15:239–264.

17. Greenberger PA. 8. Drug allergy. *J Allergy Clin Immunol.* 2006;117 (2 Suppl Mini Primer):S464–S470.

18. Jerath Tatum A, Ditto AM, Patterson R. Severe serum sickness-like reaction to oral penicillin drugs: three case reports. *Ann Allergy Asthma Immunol.* 2001;86:330–334.

19. Lee CE, Zembower TR, Fotis MA, et al. The incidence of antimicrobial allergies in hospitalized patients: implications regarding prescribing patterns and emerging bacterial resistance. *Arch Intern Med.* 2000;160:2819–2899.

20. Sullivan TJ, Wedner HJ, Shatz GS, et al. Skin testing to detect penicillin allergy. *J Allergy Clin Immunol.* 1981;68:171–180.

21. Sogn D, Evans R III, Shepherd GM, et al. Results of the National Institute of Allergy and Infectious Diseases collaborative clinical trial to test the predictive value of skin testing with major and minor penicillin derivatives in hospitalized adults. *Arch Intern Med.* 1992;15:1025–1032.

22. Solensky R, Earl HS, Gruchalla RS. Penicillin allergy: prevalence of vague history in skin test-positive patients. *Ann Allergy Asthma Immunol.* 2000;85:195–199.

23. Shepherd GM. Allergy to B-Lactam antibiotics. *Immunol Allergy Clin North Am.* 1991;11:611.

24. Johannes CB, Ziyadeh N, Seeger JD, et al. Incidence of allergic reactions associated with antibacterial use in a large, managed care organization. *Drug Saf.* 2007;30:705–713.

25. Idsoe O, Guthe T, Willcox RR, et al. Nature and extent of penicillin side-reactions with particular reference to fatalities from anaphylactic shock. *Bull WHO.* 1968;38:159.

26. Weiss ME, Adkinson NF Jr. Immediate hypersensitivity reactions to penicillin and related antibiotics. *Clin Allergy.* 1988;18:515.

27. Apter AJ, Kinman JL, Bilker WB, et al. Is there cross-reactivity between penicillins and cephalosporins? *Am J Med.* 2006;119:354,311–354.e20.

28. Romano A, Viola M, Gueant-Rodriquez R-M, et al. Imipenem in patients with immediate hypersensitivity to penicillins. *N Engl J Med.* 2006;354:2835–2837.

29. Romano A, Viola M, Gueant-Rodriquez R-M, et al. Brief communication: tolerability of meropenem in patients with IgE-mediated hypersensitivity to penicillins. *Ann Intern Med.* 2007;146:266–269.

30. Levine BB, Zolov DM. Prediction of penicillin allergy by immunologic tests. *J Allergy.* 1969;43:231–244.

31. Mackowiak PA, LeMaistre CF. Drug fever: a critical appraisal of conventional concepts. An analysis of 51 episodes in two Dallas hospitals and 97 episodes reported in the English literature. *Ann Intern Med.* 1987;106:728–733.

32. Roush MK, Nelson KM. Understanding drug-induced febrile reactions. *Am Pharm.* 1993;NS33–NS39.

33. Fonacier L, Hirschberg R, Gerson S. Adverse drug reactions to a cephalosporins in hospitalized patients with a history of penicillin allergy. *Allergy Asthma.* 2005;26:135–141.

34. Kelkar PS, Li J T-C. Cephalosporin allergy. *N Engl J Med.* 2001;345:804–809.

35. Annè S, Reisman RE. Risk of administering cephalosporin antibiotics to patients with histories of penicillin allergy. *Ann Allergy Asthma Immunol.* 1995;74:167–170.

36. Gonzalez-Delgado P, Blanes M, Soriano V, et al. Erythema multiforme to amoxicillin with concurrent infection by Epstein-Barr virus. *Allergol Immunopathol (Madr).* 2006;34:76–78.

37. Jappe U. Amoxicillin-induced exanthema in patients with infectious mononucleosis: allergy or transient immunostimulation? *Allergy.* 2007;62:1474–1475.

38. Hernandez-Salazar A, Rosales SP, Rangel-Frausto S, et al. Epidemiology of adverse cutaneous drug reactions. A prospective study in hospitalized patients. *Arch Med Res.* 2006;37:899–902.

39. Platt R, Dreis MW, Kennedy DL, et al. Serum sickness-like reactions to amoxicillin, cefaclor, cephalexin, and trimethoprim-sulfamethoxazole. *J Infect Dis.* 1988;158:474.

40. Joubert GI, Hadad K, Matsui D, et al. Selection of treatment of cefaclor-associated urticarial, serum sickness-like reactions and erythema multiforme by emergency pediatricians: lack of a uniform standard of care. *Can J Clin Pharmacol.* 1999;6:197–201.

41. Isaacs D. Serum sickness-like reaction to cefaclor. *J Paediatr Child Health.* 2001;37:298–299.

42. Isaacs D. Serum sickness-like reaction to cefaclor. *J Paediatr Child Health.* 2001;37:298–299.

43. Romano A, Gaeta F, Valluzzi RL, et al. Diagnosing hypersensitivity reactions to cephalosporins in children. *Pediatrics.* 2008;122:521–527.

44. Grouhi M, Hummel D, Roifman CM. Anaphylactic reaction to oral cefaclor in a child. *Pediatrics.* 1999;103:e50.

45. Pumphrey RS. Anaphylaxis: can we tell who is at risk of a fatal reaction? *Curr Opin Allergy Immunol.* 2004;4:285–290.

46. Greenberger PA, Rotskoff BD, Lifschultz B. Fatal anaphylaxis: postmortem findings and associated comorbid diseases. *Ann Allergy Asthma Immunol.* 2007;98:252–257.

47. Pumphrey RS, Roberts IS. Postmortem findings after fatal anaphylactic reactions. *J Clin Pathol.* 2000;53:273–276.

48. Tayman C, Mete E, Bayrak O, et al. Unexpected cefazolin anaphylaxis in a 5-month-old girl. *Pediatr Emerg Care.* 2008;24:344–345.

49. Hasdenteufel F, Luyasu S, Renaudin J-M, et al. Anaphylactic shock associated with cefuroxime axetil: structure-activity relationships. *Ann Pharmacother.* 2007;41:1069–1072.

50. Silviu-Dan F, McPhillips S, Warrington RJ. The frequency of skin test reactions to side-chain penicillin determinants. *J Allergy Clin Immunol.* 1993;91:694–701.

51. Gonzalez J, Miranda A, Martin A, et al. Sensitivity to amoxycillin with good tolerance to penicillin. *J Allergy Clin Immunol.* 1988;81:222(abst).

52. Fernandez T, Torres MJ, R-Pena R, et al. Decrease of selective immunoglobulin E response to amoxicillin despite repeated administration of benzylpenicillin and penicillin V. *Clin Exp Allergy.* 2005;35:1645–1650.

53. Harris AD, Sauberman L, Kabbash L, et al. Penicillin skin testing: a way to optimize antibiotic utilization. *Am J Med.* 1999;107:166–168.

54. Arroliga ME, Wagner W, Bobek MB, et al. A pilot study of penicillin skin testing in patients with a history of penicillin allergy admitted to a medical ICU. *Chest.* 2000;188:1106–1108.

55. DePestel DD, Benniger MS, Danzinger L, et al. Cephalosporin use in treatment of patients with penicillin allergies. *J Am Pharm Assoc (2003).* 2008:48:530–550.

56. Petz L. Immunologic cross-reactivity between penicillins and cephalosporins: a review. *J Infect Dis.* 1978;137:574.

57. Blanca M, Fernandez J, Miranda A, et al. Cross-reactivity between penicillins and cephalosporins: clinical and immunological studies. *J Allergy Clin Immunol.* 1989;83:381–385.

58. Antunez C, Blanca-Lopez N, Torres MJ, et al. Immediate allergic reactions to cephalosporins: evaluation of cross-reactivity with a panel of penicillins and cephalosporins. *J Allergy Clin Immunol.* 2006;117:404–410.

59. Lin RY. A perspective on penicillin allergy. *Arch Intern Med.* 1992;152:930–937.

60. Romano A, Gueart-Rodriguez RM, Viola M, et al. Cross-reactivity and tolerability of cephalosporins in patients with immediate hypersensitivity to penicillins. *Ann Intern Med.* 2004;141:16–22.

61. Saxon A, Adelman DC, Patel A, et al. Imipenem cross-reactivity with penicillin in humans. *J Allergy Clin Immunol.* 1988;82:213–217.

62. Chen Z, Baur X, Kutscha-Lissberg F, et al. IgE-mediated anaphylactic reaction to imipenem. *Allergy.* 2000;55:92–99.

63. Sodhi M, Axtell SS, Callahan J, et al. Is it safe to use carbapenems in patients with a history of allergy to penicillin? *J Antimicrobial Chemotherapy.* 2004;54:1155–1157.

64. Fernandez-Rivas M, Carral CP, Cuevas M, et al. Selective allergic reactions to clavulanic acid. *J Allergy Clin Immunol.* 1995;95:748–750.

65. Mendelson LM, Ressler C, Rosen JP, et al. Routine elective penicillin allergy skin testing in children and adolescents: study of sensitization. *J Allergy Clin Immunol.* 1984;73:76–81.

66. Parker PJ, Parrinello JT, Condemi JJ, et al. Penicillin resensitization among hospitalized patients. *J Allergy Clin Immunol.* 1991;88:213–217.

67. Bittner A, Greenberger PA. Incidence of resensitization after tolerating penicillin treatment in penicillin-allergic patients. *Allergy Asthma Proc.* 2004;25:161–164.

68. Macy E, Mangat R, Burchette RJ. Penicillin skin testing in advance of need: Multiyear follow-up of 568 test result-negative subjects exposed to oral penicillins. *J Allergy Clin Immunol.* 2003;111:1111–1115.

69. Sullivan T, Yecies L, Shatz G, et al. Desensitization of patients allergic to penicillin using orally administered B-lactam antibiotics. *J Allergy Clin Immunol.* 1982;69:275–82.

70. Borish L, Tamir R, Rosenwasser L. Intravenous desensitization to beta-lactam antibiotics. *J Allergy Clin Immunol.* 1987;80:314–319.

71. Stark BJ, Earl HS, Gross GN, et al. Acute and chronic desensitization of penicillin-allergic patients using oral penicillin. *J Allergy Clin Immunol.* 1987;79:523–532.

72. Brown LA, Goldberg ND, Shearer WT. Long-term ticarcillin desensitization by the continuous oral administration of penicillin. *J Allergy Clin Immunol.* 1982;69:51.

73. Yates AB. Management of patients with a history of allergy to beta-lactam antibiotics. *Am J Med.* 2008;121:572–576.

74. Gruchalla RS, Pirmohamed M. Clinical practice. Antibiotic allergy. *N Engl J Med.* 2006;354:601–609.

75. Berdal J-A, Eskensen A. Short-term success, but long-term treatment failure with linezolid for enterococcal endocarditis. *Scand J Infect Dis.* 2008;40:765–766.

76. Nordstrand IA. Anaphylaxis to trimethoprim: an under-appreciated risk in acute medical care. *Emerg Med Australas.* 2004;16:82–85.

77. Bijl AM, Van Der Klauw MM, Van Vliet AC, et al. Anaphylactic reactions associated with trimethoprim. *Clin Exp Allergy.* 1998;28:510–512.

78. Cabañas R, Caballero MT, Veta A, et al. Anaphylaxis to trimethoprim. *J Allergy Clin Immunol.* 1996;97:137–138.

79. Alonso MD, Marcos C, Dávila I, et al. Hypersensitivity to trimethoprim. *Allergy.* 1992;47:340–342.

80. Carrington DM, Earl HS, Sullivan TJ. Studies of human IgE to a sulfonamide determinant. *J Allergy Clin Immunol.* 1987;79:442–447.

81. Gruchalla RS, Sullivan TJ. Detection of human IgE to sulfamethoxazole by skin testing with sulfamethoxazoyl-poly-L-tyrosine. *J Allergy Clin Immunol.* 1991;88:784–792.

82. Shear NH, Spielberg SP, Grant DM, et al. Differences in metabolism of sulfonamides predisposing to idiosyncratic toxicity. *Ann Intern Med.* 1986;105:179–184.

83. Rieder MJ, Vetrecht J, Shear NH, et al. Diagnosis of sulfonamide hypersensitivity reactions by *in vitro* "rechallenge" with hydroxylamine metabolites. *Ann Intern Med.* 1989;110:286–289.

84. Carr A, Tindall B, Penny R, et al. *In vitro* cytotoxicity as a marker of hypersensitivity to sulphamethoxazole in patients with HIV. *Clin Exp Immunol.* 1993;94:21.

85. Garcia-Martin E. Interethnic and intraethnic variability of NAT2 single nucleotide polymorphisms. *Curr Drug Metab.* 2008;9:87–97.

86. Davis CM, Shearer WT. Diagnosis and management of HIV drug hypersensitivity. *J Allergy Clin Immunol.* 2008;121:826–832.

87. Phillips E, Mallal S. Drug hypersensitivity in HIV. *Curr Opin Allergy Clin Immunol.* 2007;7:324–330.

88. Lin D, Li WK, Rieder MJ. Cotrimoxazole for prophylaxis or treatment of opportunistic infections of HIV/AIDS in patients with previous history of hypersensitivity to cotrimoxazole. *Cochrane Database Syst Rev.* 2007;Apr 18;(2):CD 005646.

89. Carr A, Cooper DA, Penny R. Allergic manifestations of human immunodeficiency virus infection. *J Clin Immunol.* 1991;11:52–64.

90. Greenberger PA, Patterson R. Management of drug allergy in patients with acquired immunodeficiency syndrome. *J Allergy Clin Immunol.* 1987;79:484–488.

91. Absar N, Daneshvar H, Beall G. Desensitization to trimethoprim/sulfamethoxazole in HIV-infected patients. *J Allergy Clin Immunol.* 1994;93:1001–1005.

92. White MV, Haddad ZH, Brunner E, et al. Desensitization to trimethoprim-sulfamethoxazole in patients with acquired immunodeficiency syndrome and *Pneumocystis carinii* pneumonia. *Ann Allergy.* 1989;62:177–179.

93. Yoshizawa S, Yasuoka A, Kikuchi Y, et al. A 5-day course of oral desensitization to trimethoprim/sulfamethoxazole (T/S) is successful in patients with human immunodeficiency virus type-1 infection who were previously intolerant to T/S but had no sulfamethoxazole-specific IgE. *Ann Allergy Asthma Immunol.* 2000;85:241–244.

94. Baum CG, Sonnabend JA, O'Sullivan M. Prophylaxis of AIDS-related *Pneumocystis carinii* pneumonia with aerosolized pentamidine in a patient with hypersensitivity to systemic pentamidine. *J Allergy Clin Immunol.* 1992;90:268–289.

95. Boxer MB, Dykewicz MS, Patterson R, et al. The management of patients with sulfonamide allergy. *N Engl Reg Allergy Proc.* 1988;9:219–223.

96. Douglas R, Spelman D, Czarny D, et al. Successful desensitization of two patients who previously developed Stevens-Johnson syndrome while receiving trimethoprim-sulfamethoxazole. *Clin Infect Dis.* 1997;25:1480.

97. van Bodegraven AA, Mulder CJ. Indications for 5-aminosalicylate in inflammatory bowel disease: is the body of evidence complete? *World J Gastroenterol.* 2006;12:6115–6123.

98. Purdy BH, Philips DM, Summers RW. Desensitization for sulfasalazine rash. *Ann Intern Med.* 1984;100:512–514.

99. Earl HS, Sullivan TJ. Acute desensitization of a patient with cystic fibrosis allergic to both B-lactam and aminoglycoside antibiotics. *J Allergy Clin Immunol.* 1987;79:477–483.

100. Schretlen-Doherty JS, Troutman WG. Tobramycin-induced hypersensitivity reaction. *Ann Pharmacother.* 1995;29:704–706.

101. Polk RE, Healy DP, Schwartz LB, et al. Vancomycin and the red man syndrome: pharmacodynamics of histamine release. *J Infect Dis.* 1988;157:502–507.

102. Lin RY. Desensitization in the management of vancomycin hypersensitivity. *Arch Intern Med.* 1990;150:2197–2198.

103. Alexander II, Greenberger PA. Vancomycin-induced Stevens-Johnson syndrome. *Allergy Asthma Proc.* 1996;17:75–78.

104. Jones DH, Todd M, Craig TJ. Early diagnosis is key in vancomycin-induced linear IgA bullous dermatosis and Stevens-Johnson syndrome. *J Am Osteopath Assoc.* 2004;104:157–163.

105. Forrence EA, Goldman MP. Vancomycin-associated exfoliative dermatitis. *DICP Ann Pharmacother.* 1990;24:369–371.

106. Richards Al, Cleland H. Exfoliative dermatitis, fever and acute renal failure in a 60% burns patient. *Burns.* 2005;31:1056–1060.

107. Davis H, McGoodwin E, Reed TG. Anaphylactoid reactions reported after treatment with ciprofloxacin. *Ann Intern Med.* 1989;111:1041–1043.

108. Smythe MA, Cappelletty DM. Anaphylactoid reaction to levofloxacin. *Pharmacotherapy.* 2000;20:1520–1523.

109. Sachs B, Riegel S, Seebeck J, et al. Fluoroquinolone-associated anaphylaxis in spontaneous adverse drug reaction reports in Germany: differences in reporting rates between individual fluoroquinolones and occurrence after first-ever use. *Drug Saf.* 2006;29:1087–1100.

110. Palchick BA, Fink EA, McEntire JE, et al. Anaphylaxis due to chloramphenicol. *Am J Med Sci.* 1984;288:43.

111. Liphshitz I, Loewenstein A. Anaphylactic reaction following application of chloramphenicol eye ointment. *Br J Ophthalmol.* 1991;75:64.

112. Jorro G, Morales C, Brasó JV, et al. Anaphylaxis to erythromycin. *Ann Allergy Asthma Immunol.* 1996;77:456–458.

113. Yeu WW, Chau CH, Lee J, et al. Cholestatic hepatitis in a patient who received clarithromycin therapy for a *M. chelonae* lung infection. *Clin Infect Dis.* 1994;18:1025.

114. Giannattasio A, D'Ambrosi M, Volpicelli M. Steroid therapy for a case of severe drug-induced cholestasis. *Ann Pharmacother.* 2006;40:1196–1199.

115. Bottenberg MM, Wall GC, Hicklin GA. Apparent anaphylactoid reaction after treatment with a single dose of telithromycin. *Ann Allergy Asthma Immunol.* 2007;98:89–91.

116. Mazur N, Greenberger PA, Regalado J. Clindamycin hypersensitivity appears to be rare. *Ann Allergy Asthma Immunol.* 1999;82:443–445.

117. Chiou CS, Lin SM, Lin SP, et al. Clindamycin-induced anaphylactic shock during general anesthesia. *J Chin Med Assoc.* 2006;69:549–551.

118. Asensio Sanchez T, Davila I, Moreno E, et al. Anaphylaxis due to metronidazole with positive skin prick test. *J Investig Allergol Clin Immunol.* 2008;18:138–139.

119. Kurohara ML, Kwong FK, Lebherz TB, et al. Metronidazole hypersensitivity and oral desensitization. *J Allergy Clin Immunol.* 1991;88:279–280.

120. Kemp SF, Lockey RF. Amphotericin B: emergency challenge in a neutropenic, asthmatic patient with fungal sepsis. *J Allergy Clin Immunol.* 1995;96:425–427.

121. Lowery MM, Greenberger PA. Amphotericin-induced stridor: a review of stridor, amphotericin preparations, and their immunoregulatory effects. *Ann Allergy Asthma Immunol.* 2003;91:460–466.

122. Vaidya SJ, Seydel C, Patel SR, et al. Anaphylactic reaction to liposomal amphotericin B. *Ann Pharmacother.* 2002;36:1480–1481.

123. Kauffman CA, Wiseman SW. Anaphylaxis upon switching lipid-containing amphotericin B formulations. *Clin Infect Dis.* 1998;26:1237–1238.

124. Schneider P, Klein RM, Dietze L, et al. Anaphylactic reaction to liposomal amphotericin (Ambisome). *Br J Haematol.* 1998;102:1107–1111.

125. Liu PY, Lee CH, Lin LJ, et al. Refractory anaphylactic shock associated with ketoconazole treatment. *Ann Pharmacother.* 2005;39:547–550.

126. Bittleman DB, Stapleton J, Casale TB. Report of successful desensitization to itraconazole. *J Allergy Clin Immunol.* 1994;94:270–271.

127. Kauffman CA. Clinical efficacy of new antifungal agents. *Curr Opin Microbiol.* 2006;9:483–488.

128. Greenberg RN, Mullane K, van Burik JA, et al. Posaconazole as salvage therapy for zygomycosis. *Antimicrob Agents Chemother.* 2006;50:126–133.

129. Carr A, Penny R, Cooper DA. Allergy and desensitization to zidovudine in patients with acquired immunodeficiency syndrome (AIDS). *J Allergy Clin Immunol.* 1993;91:683–685.

130. Duque S, de la Puente J, Rodríguez F. Zidovudine-related erythroderma and successful desensitization: a case report. *J Allergy Clin Immunol.* 1996;98:234–235.

131. Kawsar M, Parkin JM, Forster G. Graded challenge in an aciclovir allergic patient. *Sex Transm Infect.* 2001;77:204–205.

132. Williamson JC, Pegram PS. Neuraminidase inhibitors in patients with underlying airways disease. *Am J Resp Med.* 2002;1:85–90.
133. Kainer MA, Mijch A. Anaphylactoid reaction, angioedema and urticaria associated with lamivudine. *Lancet.* 1996;348:1519.
134. Wurtz RM, Abrams D, Becker S, et al. Anaphylactoid drug reactions due to ciprofloxacin and rifampicin in HIV-infected patients. *Lancet.* 1989;1:955–956.
135. Hmouda H, Laouani-Kechrid C, Nejib Karoui M, et al. A rare case of streptomycin-induced toxic epidermal necrolysis in a patient with tuberculosis: a therapeutic dilemma. *Ann Pharmacother.* 2005;39:165–168.
136. Moseley EK, Sullivan TJ. Allergic reactions to antimicrobial drugs in patients with a history of prior drug allergy. *J Allergy Clin Immunol.* 1991;87:226.
137. Gollapudi RR, Teirstein PS, Stevenson DD, et al. Aspirin sensitivity: implications for patients with coronary artery disease. *JAMA.* 2004;292:3017–3023.
138. Stevenson DD, Szczeklik A. Clinical and pathologic perspectives on aspirin sensitivity and asthma. *J Allergy Clin Immunol.* 2006;118:773–786.
139. Israel E, Fischer AR, Rosenberg MA, et al. The pivotal role of 5-lipoxygenase products in the reaction of aspirin-sensitive asthmatics to aspirin. *Am Rev Respir Dis.* 1993;148:1447–1451.
140. Christie PE, Tagari P, Ford Hutchinson AW, et al. Urinary LTE$_4$ concentrations increase after aspirin challenge in aspirin-sensitive asthmatic subjects. *Am Rev Respir Dis.* 1991;143:1025–1029.
141. Stevenson DD. Adverse reactions to nonsteroidal anti-inflammatory drugs. *Immunol Allergy Clin North Am.* 1998;18:773–798.
142. Dahlen B, Szczeklik A, Murray JJ. Celecoxib in patients with asthma and aspirin intolerance. *N Engl J Med.* 2001;344:142.
143. Mathison DA, Lumry WR, Stevenson DD, et al. Aspirin in chronic urticaria and/or angioedema: studies of sensitivity and desensitization. *J Allergy Clin Immunol.* 1982;69:135.
144. Williams AN, Simon RA, Woessner KM, et al. The relationship between historical aspirin-induced asthma and severity of asthma induced during oral aspirin challenges. *J Allergy Clin Immunol.* 2007;120:273–277.
145. Pleskow WW, Stevenson DD, Mathison DA, et al. Aspirin desensitization in aspirin-sensitive asthmatic patients: clinical manifestations and characterization of the refractory period. *J Allergy Clin Immunol.* 1982;69:11–19.
146. Makowska JS, Grzegoczyk J, Bienkiewicz B, et al. Systemic responses after bronchial aspirin challenge in sensitive patients with asthma. *J Allergy Clin Immunol.* 2008;121:348–354.
147. Settipane RA, Schrank PJ, Simon RA, et al. Prevalence of cross-reactivity with acetaminophen in aspirin-sensitive asthmatic subjects. *J Allergy Clin Immunol.* 1995;96:480–485.
148. Stevenson DD, Hougham AJ, Schrank PJ, et al. Salsalate cross-sensitivity in aspirin-sensitive asthmatic patients. *J Allergy Clin Immunol.* 1990;86:749–758.
149. Feigenbaum BA, Stevenson DD, Simon RA. Hydrocortisone sodium succinate does not cross-react with aspirin in aspirin-sensitive patients with asthma. *J Allergy Clin Immunol.* 1995;96:545–548.
150. Van Diem L, Grilliat JP. Anaphylactic shock induced by paracetamol. *Eur J Clin Pharmacol.* 1990;38:389–390.
151. Vidal C, Pérez-Carral C, González-Quintela A. Paracetamol (acetaminophen) hypersensitivity. *Ann Allergy Asthma Immunol.* 1997;79:320–321.
152. Doan T, Greenberger PA. Nearly fatal episodes of hypotension, flushing, and dyspnea in a 47-year-old woman. *Ann Allergy.* 1993;70:439–444.
153. Gowrinath K, Balachandran C. Anaphylactic reaction due to paracetamol. *J Indian Med Assoc.* 2004;102:223,226.
154. Schwarz N, Ham Pong A. Acetaminophen anaphylaxis with aspirin and sodium salicylate sensitivity: a case report. *Ann Allergy Asthma Immunol.* 1996;77:473–474.
155. Katayama H, Yamaguchi K, Kozuka T, et al. Adverse reactions to ionic and nonionic contrast media: a report from the Japanese Committee on the safety of contrast media. *Radiology.* 1990;175:621–628.
156. Palmer FJ. The RACR survey of intravenous contrast media reactions: Final report. *Aust Radiol.* 1988;32:426–428.
157. Committee on Drugs and Contrast Media, American College of Radiology. *Manual on Contrast Media.* Version 5.0. Reston, VA: American College of Radiology; 2004:1–77.
158. Neugut AI, Ghatak AT, Miller RL. Anaphylaxis in the United States: an investigation into its epidemiology. *Arch Intern Med.* 2001;161:15–21.
159. Greenberger PA, Patterson R. The prevention of immediate generalized reactions to radiocontrast media in high-risk patients. *J Allergy Clin Immunol.* 1991;87:867–872.
160. Caro JJ, Trindale E, McGregor M. The risk of death and of severe nonfatal reactions with high-versus low-osmolality contrast media: a meta-analysis. *AJR Am J Roentgenol.* 1991;156:825–832.
161. Spring DB, Bettman MA, Barkan HE. Deaths related to iodinated contrast media reported spontaneously to the U.S. Food and Drug Administration 1978–1994: effect of the availability of low-osmolality contrast media. *Radiology.* 1997;204:333–337.
162. Dillman JR, Ellis JH, Cohan RH, et al. Allergic-like breakthrough reactions to gadolinium contrast agents after corticosteroid and antihistamine premedication. *AJR Am J Roentgenol.* 2008;190:187–190.
163. Dillman JR, Ellis JH, Cohan RH, et al. Frequency and severity of acute allergic-like reactions to gadolinium-containing i.v. contrast media in children and adults. *AJR Am J Roentgenol.* 2007;189:153–158.
164. Siegle RL, Halvosen R, Dillon J, et al. The use of iohexol in patients with previous reactions to ionic contrast material. *Invest Radiol.* 1991;26:411–416.
165. Schrott KM, Behrends B, Clauss W, et al. Iohexol in excretory urography: results of the drug monitoring programs. *Fortschr Med.* 1986;104:153–156.
166. Enright T, Chua-Lim A, Duda E, et al. The role of a documented allergic profile as a risk factor for radiographic contrast media reactions. *Ann Allergy.* 1989;62:302–305.
167. Greenberger PA, Meyers SN, Kramer BL, et al. Effects of beta-adrenergic and calcium antagonists on the development of anaphylactoid reactions from radiographic contrast media during cardiac angiography. *J Allergy Clin Immunol.* 1987;80:698–702.
168. Lang DM, Alpern MB, Visintainer PF, et al. Increased risk for anaphylactoid reaction from contrast media in patients on B-adrenergic blockers or with asthma. *Ann Intern Med.* 1991;115:270–276.
169. Witten DM, Hirsch FD, Hartman GW. Acute reactions to urographic contrast medium: Incidence, clinical characteristics and relationship to history of hypersensitivity states. *AJR Am J Roentgenol.* 1973;119:832–840.
170. Huang SW. Seafood and iodine: an analysis of a medical myth. *Allergy Asthma Proc.* 2005;26:468–469.
171. Beaty AD, Lieberman PL, Slavin RG. Seafood allergy and radiocontrast media: are physicians propagating a myth? *Am J Med.* 2008;121:158.e1–4.
172. Greenberger PA, Patterson R, Tapio CM. Prophylaxis against repeated radiocontrast media reactions in 857 cases. *Arch Intern Med.* 1985;145:2197–2200.
173. Weisbord SD, Mor MK, Resnick AL, et al. Prevention, incidence, and outcomes of contrast-induced acute kidney injury. *Arch Intern Med.* 2008;168:1325–1332.
174. deShazo RD, Nelson HS. An approach to the patient with a history of local anesthetic hypersensitivity: experience with 90 patients. *J Allergy Clin Immunol.* 1979;63:387–394.
175. Incaudo G, Schatz M, Patterson R, et al. Administration of local anesthetics to patients with a history of a prior reaction. *J Allergy Clin Immunol.* 1978;61:339–345.
176. Gall H, Kaufmann R, Kalveram CM. Adverse reactions to local anesthetics: analysis of 197 cases. *J Allergy Clin Immunol.* 1996;97:933–937.
177. Schwartz HJ, Sher TH. Bisulfite sensitivity manifesting as allergy to local dental anesthesia. *J Allergy Clin Immunol.* 1985;75:525–527.
178. Dicpinigaitis PV. Angiotensin-converting enzyme inhibitor-induced cough: ACCP evidence-based clinical practice guidelines. *Chest.* 2006;129:169S–173S.
179. Malde B, Regalado J, Greenberger PA. Investigation of angioedema associated with the use of angiotensin-converting enzyme inhibitors and angiotensin receptor blockers. *Ann Allergy Asthma Immunol.* 2007;98:57–63.
180. ONTARGET Investigators, Yusuf S, Teo KK, et al. Telmisartan, ramipril, or both in patients at high risk for vascular events. *N Engl J Med.* 2008;358:1547–1559.
181. Brown NJ, Snowden M, Griffin MR. Recurrent angiotensin-converting enzyme inhibitor-associated angioedema. *JAMA.* 1997;278: 232–233.
182. Brown NJ, Ray WA, Snowden M, et al. Black Americans have an increased rate of angiotensin converting enzyme inhibitor associated angioedema. *Clin Pharmacol Ther.* 1996;60:8–13.
183. Abbosh J, Anderson JA, Levine AB, et al. Antiotensin converting enzyme inhibitor-induced angioedema more prevalent in transplant patients. *Ann Allergy Asthma Immunol.* 1999;82:473–476.
184. Tielemans C, Madhoun P, Lenaers M, et al. Anaphylactoid reactions during hemodialysis on AN69 membranes in patients receiving ACE inhibitors. *Kidney Int.* 1990;38:982–984.
185. Alvarez-Lara MA, Martin-Malo A, Espinosa M, et al. ACE inhibitors and anaphylactoid reactions to high-flux membrane dialysis [Letter]. *Lancet.* 1991;337:370.

186. Tielemans C, Vanherweghem JL, Blumberg A, et al. ACE inhibitors and anaphylactoid reactions to high-flux membrane dialysis [Letter]. *Lancet.* 1991;337: 370–371.

187. Molinaro G, Duan QL, Chagnon M, et al. Kinin-dependent hypersensitivity reactions in hemodialysis: metabolic and genetic factors. *Kidney Int.* 2006;70:1823–1831.

188. van Rijnsoever EW, Kwee-Zuiderwijk WJM, Feenstra J. Angioneurotic edema attributed to the use of losartan. *Arch Intern Med.* 1998;158:2063–2065.

189. Gutstein HB, Akil H. Opioid analgesics. In: Brunton LL, Lazo JS, Parker KL, eds. *Goodman & Gilman's The Pharmacologic Basis of Therapeutics.* 11th ed. New York: McGraw Hill; 2006: Chapter 21. Accessed online 11/24/2008.

190. Mundt P, Mochmann HC, Ebhardt H, et al. Pulmonary fibrosis after chemotherapy with oxaliplatin and 5-fluorouracil for colorectal cancer. *Oncology.* 2007;73:270–272.

191. Reed WL, Mortimer JE, Picus J. Severe interstitial pneumonitis associated with docetaxel administration. *Cancer.* 2002;94:847–853.

192. Zitnik RJ. Drug-induced lung disease: cancer chemotherapy agents. *J Resp Dis.* 1995;16:855–865.

193. Shlebak AA, Clark PI, Green JA. Hypersensitivity and cross-reactivity to cisplatin and analogues. *Cancer Chemother Pharmacol.* 1995;35:349–351.

194. Goldberg A, Altaras MM, Mekori YA, et al. Anaphylaxis to cisplatin: diagnosis and value of pretreatment in prevention of recurrent allergic reactions. *Ann Allergy.* 1994;73:271–272.

195. Camus P, Costabel U. Drug-induced respiratory disease in patients with hematological diseases. *Semin Respir Crit Care Med.* 2005;26:458–481.

196. Vermorken JB, Mesia R, Rivera F, et al. Platinum-based chemotherapy plus cetuximab in head and neck cancer. *N Engl J Med.* 2008;359:1116–1127.

197. Bohan KH, Mansuri TF, Wilson NM. Anticonvulsant hypersensitivity syndrome: implications for pharmaceutical care. *Pharmacotherapy.* 2007;27:1425–1439.

198. Mansur AT, Pekcan Yascar S, Gotay F. Anticonvulsant hypersensitivity syndrome: clinical and laboratory features. *Int J Dermatol.* 2008;47:1184–1189.

199. Krivoy N, Taer M, Neuman MG. Antiepileptic drug-induced hypersensitivity syndrome reactions. *Curr Drug Saf.* 2006;1:289–299.

200. Chung WH, Hung SI, Chen YI. Human leukocyte antigens and drug hypersensitivity. *Curr Opin Allergy Clin Immunol.* 2007;7:317–323.

201. Yang C-W, Hung S-l, Juo CG, et al. HLA-B*1502-bound peptides: implications for the pathogenesis of carbamazepine-induced Stevens-Johnson syndrome. *J Allergy Clin Immunol.* 2007; 120:870–877.

202. Alfirevic A, Jorgensen AL, Williamson PR, et al. HLA-B locus in Caucasian patients with carbamazepine hypersensitivity. Pharmacogenomics. 2006;7:813–816.

203. Gennis MA, Vemuri R, Burns EA, et al. Familial occurrence of hypersensitivity to phenytoin. *Am J Med.* 1991;91:631–634.

204. Gonzalez FJ, Carvajal MJ, del Pozo V, et al. Erythema multiforme to phenobarbital: involvement of eosinophils and T cells expressing the skin homing receptor. *J Allergy Clin Immunol.* 1997;100:135–137.

205. Chopra S, Levell NJ, Cowley G, et al. Systemic corticosteroids in the phenytoin hypersensitivity syndrome. *Br J Dermatol.* 1996;134: 1109–1112.

206. Hirsch LJ, Arif H, Nahm EA, et al. Cross-sensitivity of skin rashes with antiepileptic drug use. *Neurology.* 2008;71:1527–1534.

207. Vittorio CC, Muglia JJ. Anticonvulsant hypersensitivity syndrome. *Arch Intern Med.* 1995;155:2285–2290.

208. Culp JA, Palis RI, Castells MC, et al. Perioperative anaphylaxis in a 44-year old man. *Allergy Asthma Proc.* 2007;28:602–605.

209. Mertes PM, Laxenaire MC, Lienhart A, et al. Reducing the risk of anaphylaxis during anesthesia during anesthesia: guidelines for clinic practice. *J Investig Allergol Clin Immunol.* 2005;15:91–101.

210. Matthey P, Wang P, Finegan BA, et al. Rocuronium anaphylaxis and multiple neuromuscular blocking drug sensitivities. *Can J Anesth.* 2000;47:890–893.

211. Chong YY, Caballero MR, Lukawska J, et al. Anaphylaxis during general anaesthesia: one-year survey from a British allergy clinic. *Singapore Med J.* 2008;49:483–487.

212. Harboe T, Guttormsen AB, Irgens A, et al. Anaphylaxis during anesthesia in Norway. *Anesthesiology.* 2005;102:897–903.

213. Cummings KC III, Arnaut K. Case report: Fentanyl-associated intraoperative anaphylaxis with pulmonary edema. *Can J Anesth.* 2007;54:301–306.

214. Kant Pandey C, Mathur N, Singh N, et al. Fulminant pulmonary edema after intramuscular ketamine. *Can J Anesth.* 2000;47:894–896.

215. Galindo PA, Borja J, Feo F, et al. Anaphylaxis to omeprazole. *Ann Allergy Asthma Immunol.* 1999;82:52–54.

216. Confino-Cohen R, Goldberg A. Anaphylaxis to omeprazole: diagnosis and desensitization protocol. *Ann Allergy Asthma Immunol.* 2006;96:33–36.

217. Cochayne SE, Glet RJ, Gawkrodger DJ, et al. Severe erythrodermic reactions to the proton pump inhibitors omeprazole and lansoprazole. *Brit J Dermatol.* 1999;141:173–174.

218. Lin C-C, Wu J-C, Huang D-F, et al. Ranitidine-related Stevens-Johnson syndrome in patients with severe liver diseases: A report of two cases. *J Gastro Hepatol.* 2001;16:481–483.

219. Becker RC, Meade TW, Berger PB, et al. The primary and secondary prevention of coronary artery disease: American College of Chest Physicians evidence-based clinical practice guidelines (8th edition). *Chest.* 2008;133:776S–814S.

220. Owen Ph, Garner J, Hergott L, et al. Clopidogrel desensitization: case report and review of published protocols. *Pharmacotherapy.* 2008;28:259–270.

221. Oppedijk B, Odekerken DAM, van der Wildt JJ, et al. Rapid oral desensitization procedure in clopidogrel hypersensitivity. *Neth Heart J.* 2008;16:21–23.

222. Camara MG, Almeda FQ. Clopidogrel (Plavix) desensitization: a case series. *Cathet Cardiovasc Intervent.* 2005;65:525–527.

PART C

Immunologic Reactions to High-Molecular-Weight Therapeutic Agents

LESLIE C. GRAMMER

Most therapeutic agents are small haptens, less than 1 kDa, which require conjugation to a large molecule, usually a protein, in order to be recognized by the human immunologic system. However, there are increasing numbers of therapeutic agents that are proteins, including humanized monoclonal antibodies such as infliximab and recombinant human proteins such as erythropoietin. Therapeutic agents that are proteins, either of human or nonhuman origin, greater than 3 kDa to 5 kDa, can be recognized by the human immunologic system and can cause sensitization and hypersensitivity reactions. Because these proteins are complete antigens, they can be used as skin testing reagents or as antigens in *in vitro* assays. Nonhuman protein hormones like porcine insulin and adrenocorticotropic hormone (ACTH) are well-recognized causes of hypersensitivity reactions (1). Nonhuman protein enzymes like chymopapain and streptokinase have been reported to cause anaphylaxis and other milder hypersensitivity reactions (2). Antithymocyte globulin (ATG), derived from rabbit or equine sources, has been reported to cause immediate type I hypersensitivity as well as type III immune complex–mediated hypersensitivity (3).

Human recombinant proteins are less likely than nonhuman proteins to result in hypersensitivity reactions, but they do occur. Factors influencing the immunogenicity of proteins include frequency and duration of treatment, route of administration, and genetic background of the patient (4). A likely explanation for this somewhat unexpected occurrence is that the hypersensitivity reactions are caused by B-cell recognition of alteration in tertiary or quaternary structure. The primary amino acid sequence, recognized by T cells, is an exact copy of the endogenously produced human protein and, therefore, cannot initiate immunologic processes such as hypersensitivity (5). Insulin was the first recombinant human protein to which hypersensitivity reactions were reported (1). Initially, most of the patients who were identified as allergic to human recombinant insulin had actually been sensitized to porcine or bovine insulin. Subsequently, however, there were reports of human recombinant proteins, such as granulocyte-macrophage colony-stimulating factor (GM-CSF), and soluble type I interleukin-1 (IL-1) receptor, causing hypersensitivity reactions with no prior sensitization to nonhuman analogue proteins (6).

■ INSULIN

Background

The exact incidence of insulin allergy is unknown; however, it appears to be on the decline (1). The increasing use of human recombinant DNA (rDNA) insulin may in part be responsible. However, it should be noted that human rDNA insulin has been associated with severe allergic reactions. Patients with systemic allergy to animal source insulins have demonstrated cutaneous reactivity to human rDNA insulin (7). In most patients, the anti-insulin antibody appears to be directed against a determinant present in all commercially available insulins (8). There has even been a report of systemic allergy to endogenous insulin during therapy with recombinant insulin (9).

While about 40% of patients receiving porcine insulin developed clinically insignificant skin test reactivity to insulin, the prevalence of cutaneous reactivity in patients receiving human rDNA insulin is unknown. Immunologic insulin resistance that is due to anti-insulin IgG antibodies may follow or occur simultaneously with IgE-mediated insulin allergy (7). The most common, clinically important, immunologic reactions to insulin are local and systemic allergic reactions and insulin resistance.

Local allergic reactions are common, usually appear within the first 1 to 4 weeks of treatment, and consist of mild erythema, induration, burning, and pruritus at the injection site. Immediate, delayed, and biphasic IgE-mediated reactions have been described. Although most local allergic reactions disappear in 3 to 4 weeks with continued insulin administration, they may persist and may precede a systemic reaction. Discontinuing insulin because of local reactions may increase the risk for a systemic allergic reaction when insulin therapy is resumed. Treatment of local reactions, which is occasionally indicated, involves the administration of antihistamines as needed; in some cases, it may be useful to switch to a different preparation.

Systemic allergic reactions to insulin are IgE-mediated and are characterized by urticaria, angioedema, bronchospasm, and hypotension; such reactions are rare (11). Most commonly, these patients have a history of interruption in insulin treatment. Systemic reactions occur most frequently within 2 weeks of resumption of insulin therapy and are often preceded by the development of progressively larger local reactions. It is most common to have a large urticarial lesion at the site of insulin injection.

Immunologic insulin resistance is even more rare than insulin allergy and is related to the development of anti-insulin IgG antibodies of sufficient titer and affinity to inactivate large amounts of exogenously administered insulin, generally in excess of 200 units daily. When non-immune causes of insulin resistance such as obesity, infection, and endocrinopathies have been excluded, treatment involves the use of corticosteroids, for example, 60 mg to 100 mg prednisone daily. This is effective in the majority of patients, and improvement is expected during the first 2 weeks of treatment. The dose of prednisone is decreased gradually once a response has occurred, but many patients may require small doses, such as 15 mg on alternate days, for up to 6 to 12 months (8).

Management of Patients with Systemic Insulin Allergy

After a systemic allergic reaction to insulin, and presuming insulin treatment is necessary, insulin should not be discontinued if the last dose of insulin has been given within 24 hours. The next dose should be reduced to about one-third to one-tenth of the dose that produced the reaction, depending on the severity of the initial reaction. Subsequently, insulin can be increased slowly by 2 to 5 units per injection until a therapeutic dose is achieved (1,12). Very slow subcutaneous infusion insulin is another approach (13).

If more than 24 hours has elapsed since the systemic allergic reaction to insulin, desensitization may be attempted cautiously if insulin is absolutely indicated. The least allergenic insulin may be selected by skin testing with commercially available insulins. Table 17C.1 provides a representative insulin desensitization schedule (8). When no emergency exists, slow desensitization over several days is appropriate. The schedule may require modifications if large local or systemic reactions occur. In addition to being prepared to treat anaphylaxis, the physician must also be prepared to treat hypoglycemia, which may complicate the frequent doses of insulin required for desensitization. More rapid desensitization may be required if ketoacidosis is present. The schedule suggested in Table 17C.1 may be used, but the doses are administered at 15- to 30-minute intervals.

■ PROTAMINE SULFATE

Protamine is a small polycationic polypeptide (4.5 kDa). It is derived from salmon sperm, and it is used to retard the absorption of insulins, such as neutral protamine Hagedorn (NPH), and to reverse heparin anticoagulation. This latter application has increased significantly with the increased use of cardiopulmonary bypass procedures, cardiac catheterization, hemodialysis, and leukopheresis. Increased reports of life-threatening adverse reactions have coincided with increased use.

Acute reactions to intravenous protamine may be mild and consist of rash, urticaria, and transient elevations in pulmonary artery pressure. Other reactions are more severe and include bronchospasm, hypotension, and at times, cardiovascular collapse and death (14). The exact incidence of these reactions is unknown. However, a prospective study of patients undergoing cardiopulmonary bypass surgery reported a reaction rate of 10.7%, although severe reactions were 1.6% (15).

Diabetic patients treated with protamine-containing insulins have a 40-fold increased risk (2.9% versus 0.07%) for sensitization to protamine (16). Previous exposure to intravenous protamine may increase the risk for reactions on subsequent exposures; neither vasectomy nor fish allergy are risk factors (17). The exact mechanisms by which protamine produces adverse reactions are not completely understood. Some appear to be IgE-mediated anaphylaxis, whereas others may be complement-mediated anaphylactoid reactions due to heparin–protamine complexes or protamine–antiprotamine complexes (18,19).

Although skin-prick tests have been recommended using 1 mg/mL of protamine, in normal volunteers, there

TABLE 17C.1 INSULIN DESENSITIZATION SCHEDULE

DAY	TIME[a]	INSULIN (UNITS)	ROUTE[b]
1	7:30 AM	0.00001[c]	Intradermal
	12:00 noon	0.0001	Intradermal
	4:30 PM	0.001	Intradermal
2	7:30 AM	0.01	Intradermal
	12:00 noon	0.1	Intradermal
	4:30 PM	1.0	Intradermal
3	7:30 AM	2.0	Subcutaneous
	12:00 noon	4.0	Subcutaneous
	4:30 PM	8.0	Subcutaneous
4	7:30 AM	12.0	Subcutaneous
	12:00 noon	16.0	Subcutaneous
5	7:30 AM	20.0[d]	Subcutaneous
6	7:30 AM	25.0[d]	Subcutaneous

[a]Increase by 5 units per day until therapeutic levels are achieved; In ketoacidosis, the doses may be given every 15 to 30 minutes.
[b]Some physicians prefer to give all doses subcutaneously.
[c]Days 1 through 4: regular insulin.
[d]Days 5 and 6: NPH or Lente insulin.

was an unacceptable rate of false-positive reactions (15). Using more dilute solutions did not appear to be predictive of an adverse reaction to protamine. Although serum antiprotamine IgE and IgG antibodies have been demonstrated *in vitro*, this has not been reported to be helpful in evaluating potential reactors (20).

There are no widely accepted alternatives to the use of protamine to reverse heparin anticoagulation. Allowing heparin anticoagulation to reverse spontaneously has been advocated, but at the risk of significant hemorrhage. Pretreatment with corticosteroids and antihistamines may be considered, but there are no studies to support this approach. Hexadimethrine (Polybrene®) has been used in the past to reverse heparin anticoagulation, but the potential for renal toxicity has led to its removal from general use. However, it may be available as a compassionate-use drug for patients who previously had a life-threatening reaction to protamine used as a heparinase. Test dosing may be valuable, but it is unproved. Emergency treatment for anaphylaxis should be immediately available.

■ **STREPTOKINASE AND OTHER THROMBOLYTICS**

A nonenzymatic protein produced by group C β-hemolytic streptococci, streptokinase has been used for thrombolytic therapy but is associated with allergic reactions. The reported reaction rate ranges from 1.7%

to 18%. The descriptions of allergic reactions have not been well characterized but have included urticaria, serum sickness, bronchospasm, and hypotension. Both *in vivo* and *in vitro* evidence for an IgE-mediated mechanism have been reported (21).

In the past, intradermal skin tests with 100 IU of streptokinase were recommended (22). Using this approach, patients who were at risk for anaphylaxis could be identified. If there is a negative skin test, streptokinase may be administered. However, such testing did not eliminate the possibility of a late reaction, such as serum sickness (22). If the skin test is positive, the more expensive treatment, recombinant tissue plasminogen activator (rt-PA) may be used. Currently, thrombolytic therapy can be performed with urokinase or rt-PA, which very rarely have been associated with acute urticaria, angioedema, or anaphylaxis (23,24).

■ **LATEX**

Latex is used in the manufacture of a variety of medical products, such as a urethral catheters and latex gloves. Latex is the natural milky rubber sap that is harvested from the rubber tree, *Hevea brasiliensis*. Latex allergy has been reported to cause contact dermatitis and IgE-mediated reactions during procedures involving latex exposure. Fortunately, the incidence of hypersensitivity reactions is declining (25).

During the manufacturing process, various accelerators, antioxidants, and preservatives are added to ammoniated latex. These agents are responsible for the type IV contact dermatitis (26). Latex gloves are then formed by dipping porcelain molds into the compounded latex. Subsequent steps include oven heating, leaching to remove water-soluble proteins and excess additives, curing by vulcanization, and finally powdering the gloves with cornstarch to decrease friction and provide comfort. Powder-free gloves are passed through a chlorination wash, which may also reduce the amount of water-soluble antigen. The natural rubber latex allergens are proteins present in raw latex and are not a result of the manufacturing process (25).

Since 1979, when the first case of rubber-induced contact urticaria was reported, many instances of IgE-mediated hypersensitivity reactions have been described, including contact urticaria, rhinitis, asthma, and anaphylaxis. Contact urticaria is the most common early manifestation of IgE-mediated rubber allergy, particularly in latex-sensitive health care workers, who report contact urticaria involving their hands. These symptoms are often incorrectly attributed to the powder in the gloves or frequent handwashing. Inhalation of latex-coated cornstarch particles from powdered gloves has evoked rhinitis and asthma in latex-sensitive people. Many of these individuals are atopic with a history of rhinitis due to pollens and asthma due to dust mites and animal dander (26). These reactions have been noted in both health care workers and people employed in factories that produce rubber products (27).

Latex anaphylaxis is usually associated with parenteral or mucosal exposure. Reactions have occurred after contact with rubber bladder catheters or condoms and during surgery, childbirth, and dental procedures. Patients with latex-induced anaphylaxis during anesthesia often have a prior history of contact urticaria or angioedema from rubber products, such as gloves or balloons. It should be noted that latex anaphylaxis has followed the blowing up of toy balloons. Fatal anaphylactic reactions have been reported with rubber balloon catheters used for barium enemas; this device is no longer available in the United States (28).

Currently, the diagnosis of latex allergy is primarily based on the clinical history. Patients should be questioned if they have ever noted erythema, pruritus, urticaria, or angioedema after contact with rubber products. Unexplained episodes of urticaria and anaphylaxis should be scrutinized. Also, the work history may uncover potential occupational exposure to latex. In some patients, contact dermatitis may precede IgE-mediated reactions.

In vivo and in vitro testing for the presence of latex-induced IgE antibodies has limited value. Skin prick tests using commercial latex reagents have been widely used in Europe and Canada. In the United States, there are no standardized, licensed latex extracts for diagnostic use.

Some investigators have used their own extracts prepared from latex gloves. However, latex gloves vary significantly in their allergen content, and systemic reactions have occurred with these unstandardized preparations. Intradermal skin testing for latex allergy is generally not recommended. However, experienced allergists may prepare latex allergens for cautious prick and then intradermal tests beginning with low and then increasing concentrations (25).

Once the diagnosis of latex allergy is established, avoidance is the only effective therapy. Natural rubber latex is ubiquitous, and avoidance is often difficult. Additional protective measures for individuals with known latex allergy include wearing a MedicAlert bracelet, having autoinjectable epinephrine (EpiPen) available, and keeping a supply of nonlatex gloves for emergencies. Because there has been association between latex allergy and allergy to certain foods, latex-sensitive patients should be queried about reactions to bananas, avocado, kiwi fruit, chestnuts, and passion fruit, and advised to be cautious when ingesting them.

Prevention of latex allergy is the goal. When the Mayo Clinic changed to low-latex nonpowdered gloves, the incidence of latex sensitization decreased significantly (29). Dr. Baur and his colleagues reported reduction of latex aeroallergens after removal of powdered latex gloves from their hospital (30). Other studies to address this strategy are ongoing.

■ BLOOD PRODUCTS

Transfusions of blood products (e.g., red cells, white cells, platelets, fresh frozen plasma) may elicit immediate generalized reactions in 0.1% to 0.2% of these administration procedures (31,32). Anaphylactic shock occurs in 1:20,000 to 1:50,000 (33). There are probably 4 different mechanisms that result in anaphylactic transfusion reactions: IgE-mediated against foreign protein, IgE-mediated against a hapten-self protein conjugate, complement activation with anaphylotoxin generation, and direct activation of mast cells (31).

Patients with IgA deficiency should receive preparations from IgA-deficient donors because they may have preexisting serum IgE or IgG antibodies to IgA; only a tiny minority of anaphylactic transfusion reactions are related to IgE anti-IgA. It has been suggested that pretreatment with corticosteroids and antihistamines may be helpful in some cases, but severe reactions may occur, and epinephrine must be readily available for treatment.

Other immunologically mediated reactions may occur with blood transfusions. If the antigens are leukocyte cell surface proteins, a reaction consisting of fever, chills, myalgias, and dyspnea, with or without hypotension, can occur (34). The treatment for this is supportive care. ABO red blood cell mismatching can result in severe hemolytic transfusion reactions, causing acute renal failure, shock, and death.

■ IMMUNE SERA THERAPY: HETEROLOGOUS AND HUMAN

Background

The two major allergic reactions that may follow an injection of heterologous antisera are anaphylaxis and serum sickness. Anaphylaxis is less common but is very likely to occur among patients who are atopic and have IgE antibodies directed against the corresponding animal dander, most commonly horse. For this reason, such individuals may react after the first injection of antisera. Serum sickness is more common and is dose-related.

Current immunization procedures and the availability of human immune serum globulin (ISG) and specific human immune serum globulin (SIG) preparations have reduced the need for heterologous antisera. However, equine antitoxins may still be required in the management of snakebite (pit vipers and coral snake), black widow spider bite, diphtheria, and botulism (35,36). Antilymphocyte and antithymocyte globulins, prepared in horses and rabbits, have been used to provide immunosuppression for transplants and to treat aplastic anemia. Where available and appropriate, human ISG preparations should be used in preference to animal antisera. Although infrequent, immediate generalized reactions have followed the administration of human ISG preparations. Intramuscular ISG preparations contain high-molecular-weight IgG aggregates that are biologically active and may activate serum complement to produce anaphylactoid reactions. Anaphylaxis has also followed the administration of both intramuscular and intravenous human ISG among IgA-deficient patients who may produce IgE and IgG antibodies directed against IgA. Such patients are at risk for anaphylaxis on infusion of IgA-containing blood products.

Tests before Heterologous Antisera Administration

Before administering heterologous antisera to any patient, regardless of history, skin testing, as indicated in the package insert, should be performed to determine whether there is the presence of IgE antibodies and thereby predict the likelihood of anaphylaxis. Most package inserts have suggested procedures. If not, skin prick tests using antisera diluted 1:10 with normal saline and a saline control are performed. If negative after 15 minutes, intradermal skin tests using 0.02 mL of a 1:100 dilution of antisera and a saline control are completed. If the history suggests a previous reaction, or if the patient has atopic symptoms after exposure to the corresponding animal, begin intradermal testing using 0.02 mL of a 1:1,000 dilution. A negative skin test virtually excludes significant anaphylactic sensitivity, but some would recommend giving a test dose of 0.5 mL of undiluted antisera intravenously before proceeding with recommended doses. It should be remembered that this approach does not exclude the possibility of a late reaction, notably serum sickness 8 to 12 days later.

Desensitization

When there is no alternative to the use of heterologous antisera, desensitization has occasionally been successful despite a positive skin test to the material. The procedure is dangerous and may be more difficult to accomplish in patients who are allergic to the corresponding animal dander. There are several protocols recommended for desensitization. The package insert often recommends at least one such schedule. An intravenous infusion should be established in both arms. A conservative schedule begins with the subcutaneous administration of 0.1 mL of a 1:100 dilution in an extremity, where a tourniquet may be placed proximally if required. The dose is doubled every 15 minutes. If a reaction occurs, it is treated, and desensitization is resumed using half the dose provoking the reaction. After reaching 1 mL of the undiluted antiserum, the remainder may be given by slow intravenous infusion.

At times, more rapid delivery of the antisera may be required. In that case, intravenous infusions are also established in both arms; one to administer the antisera, and the other for treatment of complications. Initiate a slow infusion of the antisera through one of the intravenous lines. If there is no reaction after 15 minutes, the infusion rate may be increased. If a reaction occurs, the antisera infusion is stopped and the reaction treated appropriately. After the reaction has been controlled, the slow infusion is reestablished. Most patients can be given 80 mL to 100 mL over 4 hours. If there is no reaction, it is possible to give that amount in the first hour. However, some patients do not tolerate desensitization despite adherence to the above procedure (37).

After successful desensitization, it is possible that serum sickness will develop in 8 to 12 days. If the dose of antisera is in excess of 100 mL, virtually all patients will experience some degree of serum sickness. Treatment with corticosteroids is effective, the prognosis is excellent, and long-term complications are rare.

■ BIOLOGIC AGENTS

As is reviewed extensively in Chapter 1, the human immune system is regulated by a variety of proteins including lymphokines, monokines, chemokines, hormones, and colony-stimulating factors. Many of those proteins, and their corresponding receptors, have been sequenced and cloned. In many cases, human recombinant proteins, antibodies against the proteins or their receptors have been produced for therapeutic purposes; it is hoped that these new therapeutic agents will favorably influence diseases characterized by neoplasia or inappropriate inflammation (38). These proteins have been collectively called "biologic response modifiers" or "biologic agents," which is the term used in this chapter.

Inasmuch as biologic agents are proteins, hypersensitivity reactions and other immunologic responses can be induced by biologic agents. To classify adverse events due to biologic agents, a five-category rubric for reactions, both immunologic and nonimmunologic has been proposed by Pichler and Campi (39). Type α reactions result in massive cytokine release, sometimes called "cytokine storm" or cytokine release syndrome; an example would be the severe, even fatal capillary leak syndrome that occurs with administration of a monoclonal antibody against CD3, a ubiquitous T cell surface marker. Type ß reactions are hypersensitivity reactions, which are the focus of this chapter; most hypersensitivity reactions are mediated by IgE, IgG, or T cells.

Type γ reactions result in immune imbalance, either immunodeficiency or autoimmunity; for example, anti-tumor necrosis factors (TNFs) can impair the immune system enough to predispose to escape of infections like tuberculosis and they can also result in generation of anti-nuclear antibodies, occasionally inducing clinically apparent lupus. Type δ reactions are due to cross-reactivity. For example, epidermal growth factor receptor (EGFR) is expressed on many types of carcinomas and is also found on normal skin. While anti-EGFRs reduce carcinoma size, they also commonly cause an acneiform eruption that is believed to be due to the action of anti-EGFRs on skin receptors. Finally, Type ε reactions occur when a given molecule is unexpectedly found to participate in a different physiologic function. For instance, when CD40 inhibitors were administered, they caused thrombosis in a significant number of patients. It was then discovered that CD40 and CD40L are present on platelets.

Another adverse event that occurs with biologic agents that is not included in the Pichler-Campi classification is the development of neutralizing antibodies. Perhaps, in a future classification, it can be referred to as a Type ζ reaction. Sometimes, the side effect is simply that the biologic agent is no longer effective, as occurs when antibodies to interferons develop and patients being treated for hepatitis C have relapses. Unfortunately, if the antibodies are very cross-reactive with endogenous protein, severe reactions can occur as has been reported in patients being treated with erythropoietin whose antibody development resulted in severe, red cell aplasia due to neutralization of their own endogenously produced erythropoeitin (40).

Monoclonal Antibodies

Clinical trials with monoclonal antibodies have reported their potential uses as diagnostic and therapeutic agents for malignant disease, inflammatory bowel disease, and various autoimmune diseases. However, various immunologic mechanisms can make their administration difficult. With the human monoclonal antibodies that are chimerized with some murine proteins, hypersensitivity may occur. Hypersensitivity reactions may include fever, chills, rigors, diaphoresis, malaise, pruritus, urticaria, nausea, dyspnea, and hypotension. Although rare, anaphylaxis has also been reported (41,42). Monoclonal antibodies may also cross-react with normal tissue, resulting in various adverse effects depending on the affected tissue (43). For example, both neuropathy and encephalopathy have been reported.

Edrecolomab is a mouse-derived monoclonal IgG2a antibody that recognizes the human tumor-associated antigen CO17-1A which is expressed on the cell surface of a wide variety of tumors and normal epithelial tissue. In patients with colorectal carcinoma treated with edrecolomab, immunologic reactions were reported that necessitated reducing the dose of the antibody; anaphylaxis has also been reported (44). One study reported that an anti-CD20, rituximab, was well tolerated by patients with non-Hodgkin lymphoma (45). However, in a study of patients with a different disease, chronic lymphocytic leukemia, cytokine release syndrome, a Type α reaction, was reported to occur in several patients after receiving rituximab (46). The elevated cytokine levels were associated with clinical symptoms, including fever, chills, nausea, vomiting, dyspnea, and hypotension. The severity and frequency of these events were associated with the number of circulating tumor cells at baseline.

Tumor necrosis factor (TNF) is a key cytokine in the inflammation of a variety of diseases including inflammatory bowel disease, psoriasis, and rheumatoid arthritis. TNF antagonists include infliximab and etanercept. Reports of significant Type γ reactions, both immunodeficiency and autoimmunity, have been published relative to these agents (47). In addition both IgE-mediated anaphylaxis and IgG-mediated serum sickness Type β hypersensitivity reactions have been reported.

In the previous edition, we reported that an anti-IL-2 receptor monoclonal antibody, basiliximab, had not been reported to cause hypersensitivity or other adverse immunologic events. During post marketing studies, both IgE-mediated anaphylaxis and Type α cytokine release syndrome have been reported. On the other hand, we reported similar safety with palivizumab, SB 209763, a monoclonal antibody against respiratory syncytial virus, and it still has not been associated with hypersensitivity or other adverse immunologic events (48).

Polyclonal sheep antidigoxin antibodies have proved useful when administered to patients with digoxin overdose. Unfortunately, significant hypersensitivity reactions, including severe anaphylaxis, have been described (49). Anti-CD3 monoclonal antibody has not been reported to cause mild Type α, cytokine release syndrome, reactions; patients may become resistant to treatment as a result of development of neutralizing antibody (50).

As mentioned previously, EGFR antagonists are associated with significant Type δ reactions, and, at the same time, have demonstrated activity against heretofore difficult to treat carcinomas such as lung, colon and pancreatic cancer. Agents include erlotinib, cetuximab, and panitumumab. A stepwise approach to characterizing and managing these adverse immunologic reactions has been developed by an international consensus (51). As new biologic agents with promising therapeutic potential and adverse reaction profiles are identified, it will be key to have allergist-immunologists involved in the development of strategies to characterize and manage adverse reactions to clinically effective biologic agents.

Human Recombinant Proteins

Recombinant human GM-CSF is used to accelerate myeloid recovery after bone marrow transplantation or high-dose chemotherapy. In a patient with pruritus, urticaria, and angioedema after GM-CSF administration, positive prick tests were reported with 100 μg/mL and 250 μg/mL. There are other reports of anaphylaxis in the literature (53). There are also reports of localized reactions and generalized maculopapular eruptions. The immunopathogenesis of the latter reactions has not been well characterized. GM-CSF has also been reported to induce antibodies that neutralize the biologic activity of GM-CSF, thus compromising its therapeutic efficacy (54). Recombinant G-CSF has not yet been reported to cause hypersensitivity reactions, nor are there reports of neutralizing antibody induction (55).

Although hypersensitivity reactions have not yet been reported with erythropoietin, antibodies, including neutralizing antibodies, have been reported. In one patient, antibody development was actually associated with red blood cell aplasia that resolved when erythropoietin was discontinued and the antibody titers declined (56). A rapid serologic method for detecting antirecombinant human erythropoietin antibodies has been published as a tool for the diagnosis of erythropoietin resistance. Antibody production against erythropoietin should be considered in the evaluation of patients whose anemia becomes refractory to erythropoietin therapy.

Recombinant interferon-α (rIFN-α) has been reported to be a useful therapy in patients with chronic hepatitis C, mastocytosis, chronic myelogenous leukemia, and chronic granulomatous disease. In some of these patients, development of antibody against rIFN-α has been reported (57). The prevalence varies from 1.2% to 20.2%, depending on the preparation. In some studies, the development of antibodies was associated with a relapse of disease, and it is presumed that the antibody was inactivating the rIFN-α. In the treatment of patients with chronic myelogenous leukemia,

neutralizing antibody has also been associated with relapse. It has been reported that the epitopes, which are recognized by neutralizing antibody, are located in the N-terminal function domain of rIFN-α (58).

Chronic granulomatous disease has been reported to be treated safely and effectively with rIFN-α. However, high-avidity IFN-neutralizing antibodies have been reported in pharmacologically prepared human immunoglobulin. In a patient receiving rIFN-α for systemic mastocytosis, anti-IFN antibodies were reported. Cessation of the rIFN-α therapy resulted in a decline of antibody titer (59).

With the increasing number of infertile couples deciding to pursue *in vitro* fertilization, the use of a variety of hormones has increased. Follicle-stimulating hormone (FSH) is one such hormone. Before the advent of recombinant FSH, it was recovered from human urine, purified, sterilized, and administered. One patient was reported who developed a severe anaphylactic reaction to urine-derived FSH (60). She had a positive intradermal test as corroborative evidence. She tolerated the administration of recombinant FSH and had establishment of a clinical pregnancy. There are other documented hypersensitivity reactions to urine-derived preparations while subsequently tolerating the recombinant protein (61). Whether these phenomena are explained by immunologic reactions to proteins other than FSH in the urine has not been studied.

Until recombinant factor VIII was available, patients with hemophilia were treated with factor VIII concentrates derived from human plasma. Because factor VIII is a "foreign protein" to patients with hemophilia, the development of an immunologic response is expected. There is one report of anaphylaxis to factor VIII concentrate (62). When that patient suffered another episode of hemorrhage, desensitization with pretreatment was attempted, but a moderately severe reaction occurred. No anaphylactic reactions definitely due to recombinant factor VIII have been reported (62). The major immunologic problem in hemophilia is not hypersensitivity to factor VIII, but developing inhibitors of factor VIII, namely neutralizing antibody (39–41). Several investigators predicted that the incidence of inhibitors in patients treated only with the recombinant product would be higher; however, the studies suggest that the prevalence is about the same, with most patients having a low level of inhibitor that does not significantly affect the efficacy (63).

Other Recombinant Proteins

Hirudin is a thrombin inhibitor found in the salivary glands of leeches. In a trial of use of recombinant hirudin as an anticoagulant, an IgE-mediated hypersensitivity reaction was reported (64). Although tissue plasminogen activator (tPA) is generally not a cause of hypersensitivity reactions, a case of anaphylaxis temporally related to its administration has been reported

(65). That patient also had IgE antibodies directed against tPA detected in the serum. In patients with cystic fibrosis treated with recombinant DNAase, a few patients developed antibody, but there have been no reports of anaphylaxis or other significant hypersensitivity reactions (66). In patients treated with humanized monoclonal antibody against IgE (rhuMAb-E25), patients have developed adverse effects, including the rare possibility of anaphylaxis (42,67).

■ VACCINES

Vaccine related adverse events, immunologic or otherwise, are infrequent, mild, and well tolerated (68). A variety of adverse reactions can result from vaccine administration: arthralgias from rubella vaccines, significant fever from pertussis vaccines, and fever with rash from live measles vaccine. A second risk of immunization is the possibility of reactions to vaccine components, such as eggs, gelatin, and neomycin. Another risk that occurs, for example, with frequent tetanus toxoid exposure, is development of IgE antibodies with resultant anaphylaxis or urticaria. As happened with killed rubeola and respiratory syncytial virus vaccines, the protective immunity declined with time. When natural exposure resulted in infection, it was often atypical and actually more severe than in individuals who had never been immunized (69).

Tetanus Toxoid

Although minor reactions, such as local swelling, are common after tetanus toxoid or diphtheria-tetanus (dT) toxoid vaccinations, true IgE-mediated reactions are rare. However, the 1994 Institute of Medicine Report concluded that there was a causative relationship between anaphylaxis and administration of tetanus toxoid with or without diphtheria (70). A number of case reports have been published, but surveys estimate the risk for a systemic reaction to be very small, 0.00001% (71). Because diphtheria toxoid is not available as a single agent, it is impossible to separate the true incidence of diphtheria-associated reactions from those due to tetanus toxoid.

When it appears necessary to administer tetanus toxoid to a patient with a history of a previous adverse reaction, a skin test–graded challenge may be performed (72). One recommended approach is to begin with a skin-prick test using undiluted toxoid. If negative, at 15-minute intervals, 0.02 mL of successive dilutions of toxoid 1:1,000 and 1:100 are injected intradermally. If the prick test was positive, begin with a 1:10,000 dilution. Subsequently, 0.02 mL and 0.20 mL of a 1:10 dilution are given subcutaneously. This may be followed by 0.05 mL, 0.10 mL, 0.15 mL, and 0.20 mL of full-strength toxoid given subcutaneously. Some would prefer to wait for 24 hours after 0.10 mL is given to detect delayed reactivity. After that, the balance of full-strength material may be given for a final total dose of 0.50 mL.

Pertussis and Rubella

The Institute of Medicine analyzed adverse effects of pertussis and rubella vaccines (73). With pertussis vaccines, reactions at the site are common, as is fever. Seizures occur in one in every 1,750 injections, as does the "collapse syndrome," hypotonic, hyporesponsive episodes. Encephalitis and other neurologic sequelae were once thought to be a consequence of pertussis vaccine, but the evidence does not report a causal association. Rubella vaccination results in arthritis and arthralgia in a significant percentage of adult and adolescent females. The incidence of arthralgia among children is very low.

Measles, Mumps, Rubella

Because the live attenuated virus used in the measles, mumps, rubella (MMR) vaccine is grown in cultured chick-embryo fibroblasts, concern has been raised regarding its administration to egg-allergic children. The fibroblast cultures used to produce MMR vaccine contain no or trivial amounts of egg allergen. For this reason, and also based on extensive clinical experience, it has been suggested that egg-allergic children be given MMR vaccine without preliminary skin testing with the vaccine (73). The Advisory Committee on Immunization Practices no longer recommends skin testing or test dosing in egg-allergic subjects who are to receive MMR (74). It should be noted that hypersensitivity reactions to MMR vaccine have been described in children who tolerate eggs. There are reports that indicate that those reactions are due to another component, gelatin (75). In addition to causing anaphylaxis in patients receiving MMR, anaphylaxis due to gelatin has been reported in patients receiving Japanese encephalitis vaccine (76).

If it is deemed necessary to test an egg-allergic patient for MMR vaccine, a prick test is performed with a 1:10 dilution of MMR vaccine in normal saline, and a normal saline control. Intradermal skin tests, following a negative skin-prick test, are probably unnecessary and may be misleading. After a negative prick test, the vaccine may be administered in the routine fashion.

After a positive skin-prick test for MMR vaccine, at 15-minute intervals, the following dilutions of vaccine are administered subcutaneously: 0.05 mL of a 1:100 dilution, 0.05 mL of a 1:10 dilution, and 0.05 mL of the undiluted vaccine. Subsequently, at 15-minute intervals, increasing amounts of the undiluted vaccine (0.10 mL, 0.15 mL, and 0.20 mL) are given until the total immunizing dose of 0.50 mL is received. Using this protocol, systemic reactions have been reported; hence, a physician must be prepared to treat anaphylaxis (77). After completion of the procedure, it is advisable to keep the patient under observation for an additional 30 minutes.

Influenza and Yellow Fever Vaccine in Egg-Allergic Patients

Allergic reactions to influenza vaccine are rare, and the vaccine may be given safely to people who are able to tolerate eggs by ingestion, even if they demonstrate a positive skin test to egg protein (78). Anaphylaxis to influenza vaccine has been reported at a rate of 0.024:100,000. The Advisory Committee on Immunization Practices does state that influenza vaccine should not be administered to people known to have anaphylactic hypersensitivity to eggs or other components of the vaccine without first consulting a physician. Among asthmatic patients, there was some concern about inducing bronchospasm after administration; however, there appears to be no evidence of asthmagenicity after influenza vaccine. Clearly, the patient with moderate-to-severe asthma is at risk from natural infection and will benefit from influenza vaccination.

Although yellow fever vaccine is not required in the United States, travelers to endemic areas may require immunization. Of the egg-based vaccines, yellow fever vaccine contains the most egg protein. Yellow fever vaccine also contains gelatin. In a review of 5,236,820 vaccinations, it was estimated that the risk for anaphylaxis was about 1 in 131,000 (79). In another study, two of 493 individuals with a positive history of egg allergy had anaphylaxis following yellow fever immunization; both of these patents had positive skin tests to both egg and the vaccine (80). The Centers for Disease Control and Prevention (CDC) lists egg hypersensitivity as one of the reasons that an individual should not receive yellow fever vaccine. It is suggested that the individual obtain a waiver letter from a consular or embassy official (81). For patients with a clear history of egg allergy or when in doubt, skin testing with the appropriate vaccine is a reliable method to identify the patients at risk. A prick test is performed with a 1:10 dilution of the vaccine in normal saline, and a normal saline control. If negative or equivocal, an intradermal skin test using 0.02 mL of a 1:100 dilution of the vaccine and a saline control are performed. If negative, the vaccine may be administered in a routine fashion.

After a positive skin test to the vaccine, if it is considered essential, administer 0.05 mL of a 1:100 dilution intramuscularly and, at 15- to 20-minute intervals, give 0.05 mL of a 1:10 dilution, 0.05 mL of undiluted vaccine, followed by 0.10 mL, 0.15 mL, and 0.20 mL of undiluted vaccine for a total dose of 0.50 mL. Using this format, patients develop adequate protective antibody titers (116).

Other Vaccines

Both typhoid and paratyphoid vaccines have been reported to cause anaphylaxis (83). In a study of 14,249 marines who received Japanese encephalitis vaccine, the reaction rate was 0.00267% (84). The reactions were primarily urticaria, angioedema, and pruritus. In a study of 1,198,751 individuals who received meningococcal vaccine, the rate of anaphylaxis was reported as 0.1 in 100,000, a very rare event (85). Because varicella vaccine contains neomycin, individuals with neomycin hypersensitivity would be at potential risk for an allergic reaction (86). There are case reports of anaphylactic episodes after hepatitis B vaccine (87). Until 1999, the only hepatitis B vaccines available contained thimerosal, making them difficult to administer to individuals with thimerosal allergy (88). In addition, hypersensitivity reactions may also occur due to a variety of vaccine components (89).

For the most current information on adverse reactions to vaccines, the CDC website is very useful (90). In addition, if you observe an adverse effect that happens after a patient receives a vaccine, the CDC has established a Vaccine Adverse Event Reporting System (VARES) that allows for reporting by fax, mail, or online (91).

■ REFERENCES

1. Heinzerling L, Raile K, Rochlitz H, et al. Insulin allergy: clinical manifestations and management strategies. *Allergy.* 2008;63:148–155.
2. Grammer LC, Patterson R. Proteins: chymopapain and insulin. *J Allergy Clin Immunol.* 1984;74:635–640.
3. Niblack G, Johnson K, Williams T, et al. Antibody formation following administration of antilymphocyte serum. *Transplant Proc.* 1987;19:1896–1897.
4. Schellekens H. Factors influencing the immunogenicity of therapeutic proteins. *Nephrol Dial Transplant.* 2005 20 [Suppl 6]: vi3–vi9.
5. Rodgers JR, Rich RR. Antigens and antigen presentation. In: Fleisher TA, Schwartz BD, Shearer WT, et al., eds. *Clinical Immunology.* St Louis: CV Mosby,1996:114–130.
6. Ballow M. Biologic immune modifiers: Trials and tribulations—are we there yet? *J Allergy Clin Immunol.* 2006;118:1209–1215.
7. Grammer LC, Metzger B, Patterson R. Cutaneous allergy to human (recombinant DNA) insulin. *JAMA.* 1984;251:1459.
8. Matheu V, Perez E, Hernandez M, et al. Insulin allergy and resistance successfully treated by desensitization with Aspart insulin. *Clin Mol Allergy.* 2005 3:16–21.
9. Alvarez-Thull L, Rosenwasser LJ, Brodie TD. Systemic allergy to endogenous insulin during therapy with recombinant DNA (rDNA) insulin. *Ann Allergy Asthma Immunol.* 1996;76:253–256.
10. deShazo R, Boehm T, Kumar D, et al. Dermal hypersensitivity reaction to insulin: correlations of three patterns to their histopathology. *J Allergy Clin Immunol.* 1982;69:229.
11. Fineberg SE, Kawabata TT, Finco-Kent D, et al. Immunological responses to exogenous insulin. *Endocr Rev.* 2007;28:625–652.
12. Bodtger U, Wittrup M. A rational clinical approach to suspected insulin allergy: status after five years and 22 cases. *Diabet Med.* 2005;22:102–106.
13. Castera V, Dutour-Meyer A, Koeppel M, et al. Systemic allergy to human insulin and its rapid and long acting analogs: successful treatment by continuous subcutaneous insulin lispro infusion. *Diabetes Metab.* 2005;31:391–400.
14. Park KW. Protamine and protamine reactions. *Int Anesthesiol Clin.* 2004;42:135–145.
15. Weiler JM, Gellhaus MA, Carter JG, et al. A prospective study of the risk of an immediate adverse reaction to protamine sulfate during cardiopulmonary bypass surgery. *J Allergy Clin Immunol.* 1990;85:713.
16. Gottschlich GM, Graulee GP, Georgitis JW. Adverse reactions to protamine sulfate during cardiac surgery in diabetic and non-diabetic patients. *Ann Allergy.* 1988;61:277–281.
17. Weiss ME, Adkinson NF Jr. Allergy to protamine. *Clin Rev Allergy.* 1991;9:339.
18. Weiss ME, Nyhan D, Peng Z, et al. Association of protamine IgE and IgG antibodies with life-threatening reactions to intravenous protamine. *N Engl J Med.* 1989;320:886–892.
19. Tan F, Jackman H, Skidgel RA, et al. Protamine inhibits plasma carboxypeptidase N, the inactivator of anaphylatoxins and kinins. *Anesthesiology.* 1989;70:267–275.

20. Horrow JC, Pharo GH, Levit LS, et al. Neither skin tests nor serum enzyme-linked immunosorbent assay tests provide specificity for protamine allergy. *Anesth Analg.* 1996;82:386–389.

21. McGrath KG, Patterson R. Anaphylactic reactivity to streptokinase. *JAMA.* 1984;252:1314–1317.

22. Dykewicz MS, McGrath KG, Davison R, et al. Identification of patients at risk for anaphylaxis due to streptokinase. *Arch Intern Med.* 1986;146:305–307.

23. Pechlaner C, Knapp E, Wiedermann CJ. Hypersensitivity reactions associated with recombinant tissue-type plasminogen activator and urokinase. *Blood Coagul Fibrinolysis.* 2001;12(6):491–494.

24. Franco S, Kelly M, Ushay M, et al. Highly probable anaphylactic reaction to systemic thrombolytic therapy with high dose urokinase in a child with a prosthetic valve. [Case Reports Letter] *J Pediatr Hematol Oncol.* 1998;20(2):181–182.

25. Charous BL, Blanco C, Tarlo S, et al. Natural rubber latex after 12 years: recommendations and perspectives. *J Allergy Clin Immunol.* 2002;109:31–34.

26. Suneja T, Belsito DV. Occupational dermatoses in health care workers evaluated for suspected allergic contact dermatitis. *Contact Derm.* 2008;58:285–290.

27. Sussman GL, Beezhold DH, Kurup VP. Allergens and natural rubber proteins. *J Allergy Clin Immunol.* 2002;110:S33–S39.

28. Gelfand DW. Barium enemas, latex balloons, and anaphylactic reactions. *AJR Am J Roentgenol.* 1991;156:1–2.

29. Hunt LW, Fransway AF, Reed CE, et al. An epidemic of occupational allergy to latex involving health care workers. *J Occup Environ Med.* 1995;37:1204–1209.

30. Latza U, Haamann F, Baur X. Effectiveness of a nationwide interdisciplinary preventive programme for latex allergy. *Int Arch Occup Environ Health.* 2005;78:394–402.

31. Gilstad CW. Anaphylactic transfusion reactions *Curr Opin Hematol.* 2003 10:419–423.

32. Norda R, Tynell E, Akerblom O. Cumulative risks of early fresh frozen plasma, cryoprecipitate and platelet transfusion in Europe. *J Trauma.* 2006;60:S41–45

33. Vamvakas EC, Pineda AA. Allergic and anaphylactic Reactions. In: Popovsky MA, eds. *Transfusion Reactions.* 2nd ed. Bethesda, MD: AABB Press; 2001:83–127.

34. Winkelstein A, Kiss JE. Immunohematologic disorders. *JAMA.* 1997;278:1982–1992.

35. Gupta RK, Siber GR. Use of in vitro Vero cell assay and ELISA in the United States potency test of vaccines containing adsorbed diphtheria and tetanus toxoids. *Dev Biol Stand.* 1996;86:207–215.

36. Shapiro RL, Hatheway C, Swerdlow DL. Botulism in the United States: a clinical and epidemiologic review. *Ann Intern Med.* 1998;129:221–228.

37. Millar MM, Grammer LC. Case reports of evaluation and desensitization for anti-thymocyte globulin hypersensitivity. *Ann Allergy Asthma Immunol.* 2000;85:311–316.

38. Campi P, Benucci M, Manfredi M, et al. Hypersensitivity to biologic agents with special emphasis on tumor necrosis factor-α antagonists. *Curr Opin Allergy Clin Immunol.* 207;7:393–403.

39. Pichler WJ, Campi P. Adverse side effects to biologic agents. In: Pichler WJ, ed. *Drug Hypersensitivity.* Basel: Karger; 2007:160–174.

40. Shankar G, Shores E, Wagner C, et al. Scientific and regulatory considerations on the immunogenicity of biologics. *Trends Biotechnol.* 2006;24:274–280.

41. Chavez-Lopez MA, Delgado-Villafana J, Gallaga A, et al. Severe anaphylactic reaction during the second infusion of infliximab in a patient with psoriatic arthritis. *Allergol Immunopathol.* 2005;33:291–292.

42. Cox L, Platts-Mills TAE, Finegold I, et al. American Academy of Allergy, Asthma and Immunology/American College of Allergy, Asthma and Immunology Joint Task Force Report on omalizumab-associated anaphylaxis. *J Allergy Clin Immunol.* 2007;120:1373–1377.

43. Klastersky J. Adverse effects of the humanized antibodies used as cancer therapeutics. *Curr Opin Oncol.* 2006;18:316–320.

44. Hjelm Skog A, Ragnhammar P, Fagerberg J, et al. Clinical effects of monoclonal antibody 17-1A combined with granulocyte/macrophage-colony-stimulating factor and interleukin-2 for treatment of patients with advanced colorectal carcinoma. *Cancer Immunol Immunother.* 1999;48:463–470.

45. Tsai D, Moore H, Hardy C, et al. Rituximab (anti-CD20 monoclonal antibody) therapy for progressive intermediate-grade non-Hodgkin's lymphoma after high-dose therapy and autologous peripheral stem cell transplantation. *Bone Marrow Transplant.* 1999;24:521–526.

46. Winkler U, Jensen M, Manzke O, et al. Cytokine-release syndrome in patients with B-cell chronic lymphocytic leukemia and high lymphocyte counts after treatment with an anti-CD20 monoclonal antibody (rituximab, IDEC-C2B8). *Blood.* 1999;94:2217–2224.

47. Weinberg JM. An overview of infliximab, etanercept, efalizumab and alefacept as biologic therapy for psoriasis. *J Derm Sci.* 2005;38: 75–87.

48. Feltes TF, Sondheimer HM. Palivizumab and the prevention of respiratory syncytial virus illness in pediatric patients with congestive heart failure. *Expert Opin Biolog Therapy.* 2007;7:1471–1480.

49. Ball WJ Jr, Kasturi R, Dey P, et al. Isolation and characterization of human monoclonal antibodies to digoxin. *J Immunol.* 1999;163:2291–2298.

50. Bisikirska BC, Herold KC. Use of Anti-CD3 monoclonal antibody to induce immune regulation in Type 1 Diabetes. *Ann NY Acad Sci.* 2004;1037:1–9.

51. Lynch TJ, Kim ES, Eaby B, et al. Epidermal growth factor receptor inhibitor-associated cutaneous toxicities: an evolving paradigm in clinical management. *The Oncologist.* 2007;12:610–621.

52. Frost H. Antibody-mediated side effects of recombinant proteins. *Toxicology.* 2005;209:155–160.

53. Stone HD Jr, DiPiro C, Davis PC, et al. Hypersensitivity reactions to *Escherichia coli*-derived polythylene glycolated-asparaginase associated with subsequent immediate skin test reactivity to *E. coli*-derived granulocyte colony-stimulating factor. *J Allergy Clin Immunol.* 1998; 101:429–431.

54. Wadhwa M, Skog AL, Bird C, et al. Immunogenicity of granulocyte-macrophage colony-stimulating factor (GM-CSF) products in patients undergoing combination therapy with GM-CSF. *Clin Cancer Res.* 1999;5:1353–1361.

55. Cheng AC, Stephens DP, Currie BJ. Granulocyte-Colony Stimulating Factor (G-CSF) as an adjunct to antibiotics in the treatment of pneumonia in adults. *Cochrane Database Syst Rev.* 2007Apr 12;(2):CD004400.

56. Cournoyer D, Toffelmire EB, Wells GA, et al. Anti-erythropoietin antibody-mediated pure red cell aplasia after treatment with recombinant erythropoietin products: recommendations for minimization of risk. *J Am Soc Nephrol.* 2004;15:2728–2734.

57. Freedman MS, Pachner AR. Neutralizing antibodies to biological therapies: a "touch of gray" vs a "black and white" story. *Neurology.* 2007;69(14):1386–1387

58. Nolte KU, Gunther G, von Wussow P. Epitopes recognized by neutralizing therapy-induced human anti-interferon-alpha antibodies are localized within the N-terminal functional domain of recombinant interferon-alpha 2. *Eur J Immunol.* 1996;26:2155–2159.

59. Prummer O, Fiehn C, Gallati H. Anti-interferon-γ antibodies in a patient undergoing interferon-γ treatment for systemic mastocytosis. *J Interferon Cytokine Res.* 1996;16:519–522.

60. Phipps WR, Holden D, Sheehan RK. Use of recombinant human follicle-stimulating hormone for in vitro fertilization-embryo transfer after severe systemic immunoglobulin E-mediated reaction to urofollitropin. *Fertil Steril.* 1996;66:148–150.

61. Whitman-Elia GF, Banks K, O'Dea LS. Recombinant follicle-stimulating hormone in a patient hypersensitive to urinary-derived gonadotropin. *Gynecol Endocrinol.* 1998;12:209–212.

62. Shopnick RI, Kazemi M, Brettler DB, et al. Anaphylaxis after treatment with recombinant factor VIII. *Transfusion.* 1996;36:358–361.

63. Rothschild C, Laurian Y, Satre EP, et al. French previously untreated patients with severe hemophilia A after exposure to recombinant factor VIII: incidence of inhibitor and evaluation of immune tolerance. *Thromb Haemost.* 1998;80:779–783.

64. Bircher AJ, Czendlik CH, Messmer SL, et al. Acute urticaria caused by subcutaneous recombinant hirudin: evidence for an IgE-mediated hypersensitivity reaction. *J Allergy Clin Immunol.* 1996;98:994–996.

65. Rudolf J, Grond M, Prince WS, et al. Evidence of anaphylaxis after alteplase infusion. *Stroke.* 1999;30:1142–1143.

66. Eisenberg JD, Aitken ML, Dorkin HL, et al. Safety of repeated intermittent courses of aerosolized recombinant human deoxyribonuclease in patients with cystic fibrosis. *J Pediatr.* 1997;131:118–124.

67. Miller CW, Krishnaswamy N, Johnston C, et al. Severe asthma and the omalizumab option. *Clin Mol Allergy.* 2008 May 20; 6:4.

68. Babl FE, Lewena S, Brown L. Vaccination-related Adverse events. *Ped Emerg Care.* 2006;22: 514–519.

69. Signore C. Rubeola. *Prim Care Update Ob/Gyns.* 2001;8:138-140.

70. Institute of Medicine. *Adverse events associated with childhood vaccines: evidence bearing on causality.* Washington, DC: National Academy of Sciences, 1994.

71. Mansfield LE, Ting S, Rawls DO, et al. Systemic reactions during cutaneous testing for tetanus toxoid hypersensitivity. *Ann Allergy.* 1986;57:135–137.

72. Turktas I, Ergenekon E. Anaphylaxis following diphtheria-tetanus-pertussis vaccination: a reminder. *Eur J Pediatr.* 1999;158:434.

73. James JM, Burks AW, Roberson PK, et al. Safe administration of the measles vaccine to children allergic to eggs. *N Engl J Med.* 1995; 332:1262–1266.

74. Advisory Committee on Immunization Practices, Update regarding administration of combination MMRV Vaccine *MMWR.* 2008;57:258–260.

75. Sakaguchi M, Hori H, Ebihara T, et al. Reactivity of the immunoglobulin E in bovine gelatin-sensitive children to gelatins from various animals. *Immunology.* 1999;96:286–290.

76. Sakaguchi M, Yoshida M, Kuroda W, et al. Systemic immediate-type reactions to gelatin included in Japanese encephalitis vaccines. *Vaccine.* 1997;15:121–122.

77. Trotter AC, Stone BD, Laszlo DJ, et al. Measles, mumps, rubella vaccine administration in egg-sensitive children: systemic reactions during vaccine desensitization. *Ann Allergy.* 1994;72:25–28.

78. James JM, Zeiger RS, Lester MR, et al. Safe administration of influenza vaccine to patients with egg allergy. *J Pediatr.* 1998;133: 624–628.

79. Kelso JM, Mootrey GT, Tsai TF. Anaphylaxis from yellow fever vaccine. *J Allergy Clin Immunol.* 1999;103:698–701.

80. *Yellow fever: disease and vaccine.* National Center for Infectious Diseases/Centers for Disease Control and Prevention, June 10, 1999.

81. Kletz MR, Holland CL, Mendelson JS, et al. Administration of egg-derived vaccines in patients with history of egg sensitivity. *Ann Allergy.* 1990;64:527–529.

82. Miller JR, Orgel A, Meltzer EO. The safety of egg-containing vaccines for egg-allergic patients. *J Allergy Clin Immunol.* 1983;71:568–573.

83. Kelleher PC, Kelley LR, Rickman LS. Anaphylactoid reaction after typhoid vaccination. *Am J Med.* 1990;89:822–824.

84. Berg SW, Mitchell BS, Hanson RK, et al. Systemic reactions in U.S. Marine Corps personnel who received Japanese encephalitis vaccine. *Clin Infect Dis.* 1997;24:265–266.

85. Yergeau A, Alain L, Pless R, et al. Adverse events temporally associated with meningococcal vaccines. *CMAJ.* 1996;154:503–507.

86. Ventura A. Varicella vaccination guidelines for adolescents and adults. *Am Fam Physician.* 1997;55:1220–1224.

87. Bohlke K, Davis RL, Marcy SM, et al. Risk of anaphylaxis after vaccination of children and adolescents. *Pediatrics.* 2003 112:815–820.

88. Availability of Hepatitis B vaccine that does not contain thimersol as a preservative. *MMWR Morb Mortal Wkly Rep.* 1999;48:780–782.

89. Heidary N, Cohen DE. Hypersensitivity Reactions to Vaccine Components. *Dermatitis.* 2005;16: 115–120.

90. Centers for Disease Control and Prevention. Web site. http://www.cdc.gov/vaccines.

91. Vaccine Adverse Events Reporting System. Web site. http://www.vaers.hhs.gov/reportable.htm.

CHAPTER 18

Food Allergies

JOHN JAMES AND WESLEY BURKS

■ INTRODUCTION

Valuable information concerning the basic science and clinical aspects of food allergy and other adverse reactions to foods has continued to be published over the past decade. The term adverse food reaction encompasses a variety of reactions to food, only some of which are the result of IgE-mediated food allergy. In an attempt to standardize nomenclature in the scientific literature, the American Academy of Allergy and Immunology and the National Institutes of Health have defined adverse food reactions (1). An adverse food reaction is defined as any untoward reaction to a food or food additive following ingestion. These reactions can be further subdivided into food allergy and food intolerance. Basically, food allergy is any adverse food reaction due to an immunologic mechanism (e.g., IgE-mediated and non-IgE-mediated). In contrast, food intolerance is any adverse reaction due to a nonimmunologic mechanism. These reactions may be the result of pharmacologic properties of the food (e.g., caffeine in irritable bowel syndrome; tyramine-induced nausea, emesis, and headache in patients with migraines), toxins in the food, usually from improper food handling (e.g., histamine generation in scombroid fish poisoning; bacterial food poisoning), foods that exacerbate reflux (peppermint, spicy or acidic food) or metabolic disorders (lactase deficiency; pancreatic insufficiency) (Table 18.1). This chapter will summarize several key areas related to food allergy including epidemiology, pathophysiology and mucosal immunity, food allergens and IgE, as well as non-IgE-mediated food reactions. Other areas that will be reviewed include the diagnosis, management, and treatment of food allergy; a review of the natural history of food allergy; and exciting new developments in food allergy treatment.

■ EPIDEMIOLOGY

The true incidence and prevalence of food allergy has been difficult to determine in the past. Despite this, significant progress has been made over the past 10 years. Recent epidemiological studies suggest that nearly 4%

of Americans are afflicted with food allergy (1) and children are more affected than adults. Using a randomized telephone survey and standardized questionnaire in 10 European nations, an approximate measure for food allergy prevalence was determined to be 3.75% with the most affected age group being 2- to 3-year-olds (2). Unfortunately, the overall prevalence of food allergy has traditionally been overestimated. For example, 28% of mothers in one investigation perceived their children to have had at least one adverse reaction to food (3), but only 8% or one-third of these children had reactions confirmed by double-blind, placebo-controlled food challenges (DBPCFC). A recent meta-analysis reviewed the prevalence of food allergy according to the method of assessment used (5). The prevalence of self-reported food allergy was very high, 3% to 35% for any food, compared with objective measures. There was a marked heterogeneity in the prevalence of food allergy that could be a result of differences in study design or methodology, or differences among populations.

Within the past few years, specific investigations have examined the prevalence rates of allergy to specific foods such as peanuts and seafood, which typically can be severe, lifelong, and potentially fatal allergies. First, in North America and the United Kingdom, the prevalence rates among schoolchildren are now in the excess of 1% (6). Second, physician-diagnosed and/or convincing seafood allergy has been reported by 2.3% of the general population, or approximately 6.6 million Americans (7).

The epidemiology of food allergy can certainly be influenced by the specific disease state (Table 18.2). For example, the prevalence of food allergy appears to be approximately 30% in children with moderate-severe, refractory atopic dermatitis (8). Likewise, an Australian investigation determined the relative risk of an infant with atopic dermatitis having an IgE-mediated food allergy was 5.9% for the most severely affected group (9).

Studies from the UK have determined the cumulative incidence of food hypersensitivity by 12 months to be 4% (95% confidence interval (CI), 2.9% to 5.5%) on the basis of open food challenges and 3.2% (95% CI,

TABLE 18.1 FOOD ALLERGY: DIFFERENTIAL DIAGNOSIS

1. **Gastrointestinal disorders**
   - Structural abnormalities
   - Enzyme deficiencies
   - Cystic fibrosis
2. **Contaminants and additives**
   - Flavorings, dyes, preservatives, contaminants
   - Infectious organisms
   - Seafood-associated disorders
3. **Pharmacological contaminants**
   - Caffeine, histamine, tyramine
4. **Psychological reactions**
   - Bulimia, anorexia, factitious

2.2% to 4.5%) on the basis of DBPCFC (10). The rate of parentally perceived food hypersensitivity was considerably higher than objectively assessed food hypersensitivity. In addition, the incidence of food allergy was found to be 5% to 6% in children by 3 years of age based on food challenges and a good clinical history (11).

■ PATHOPHYSIOLOGY/MUCOSAL IMMUNITY

Mucosal Barrier

The main function of the gastrointestinal tract is to process ingested food into a form that can be absorbed and utilized for energy and cell growth. This process requires that the intestinal immune system be capable of discriminating between harmful and harmless foreign proteins (12). Both nonimmunologic and immunologic mechanisms help to block harmful foreign antigens (bacteria, viruses, parasites, food proteins) from entering the interior of the body, thus forming the gastrointestinal "mucosal barrier." The developmental immaturity of these mechanisms in infants reduces the

TABLE 18.2 FOOD ALLERGY PREVALENCE IN SPECIFIC DISORDERS

DISORDER	FOOD ALLERGY PREVALENCE
Anaphylaxis	35%
Atopic dermatitis	37% in children (rare in adults)
Urticaria	20% in acute cases (rare in chronic)
Asthma	5% to 6% in children with asthma
Oral allergy syndrome	25% to 75% in pollen allergy
Chronic rhinitis	rare

efficiency of the infant mucosal barrier, and likely plays a major role in the increased prevalence of gastrointestinal infections and food allergy seen in the first few years of life. The relatively low concentrations of (secretory) S-IgA in the infant's intestine and the relatively large quantities of ingested proteins place a significant burden on the immature gut-associated immune system.

The gut-associated lymphoid tissue (GALT) must mount a significant response against potentially harmful foreign substances and pathogenic organisms, but must remain unresponsive to enormous quantities of nutrient antigens and about 10^{14} commensal organisms forming the normal gut flora. The GALT is comprised of four distinct lymphoid compartments: (a) Peyer's patches (PPs) and the appendix (aggregates of lymphoid follicles throughout the intestinal mucosa), (b) lamina propria lymphocytes and plasma cells, (c) intraepithelial lymphocytes interdigitated between enterocytes, and (d) mesenteric lymph nodes (12).

S-IgA, a dimeric form of IgA that is found in intestinal secretions, does not activate complement or bind to Fc receptors, and therefore does not induce inflammatory responses. S-IgA antibodies are directed against bacterial or viral surface molecules that can prevent their binding to the epithelium and/or facilitate agglutinating pathogens resulting in complexes that become trapped in the mucus barrier and pass out in the stool (13). Despite the evolution of this well developed barrier system, about 2% of ingested food antigens are absorbed and transported throughout the body in an "immunologically" intact form, even through the mature gut (14).

Oral Tolerance Induction

Oral tolerance is defined as the specific immunological unresponsiveness to antigens induced by their prior feeding (12). Intact food antigens penetrate the gastrointestinal tract and enter the circulation in both normal children and adults (15,16). These intact proteins do not normally cause clinical symptoms because most individuals develop tolerance to ingested antigens. In mucosal tissues, soluble antigens, such as food and inhaled antigens are usually poor immunogens, inducing a state of unresponsiveness known as oral tolerance. Unresponsiveness of T cells to ingested food proteins may be the result of three different mechanisms: induction of regulatory T cells, T-cell clonal deletion, or T-cell anergy.

Commensal gut flora take residence in the gastrointestinal tract within 24 hours of birth at a concentration that has been estimated to be between 10^{12} and 10^{14} bacteria per gram of colon tissue (17). The impact of gut flora on oral tolerance is supported by the finding that mice raised in germ-free environments following birth are unable to develop tolerance to orally administered ovalbumin (18).

Normal Immune Response to Ingested Antigens

Low concentrations of detectable serum IgG, IgM, and IgA food-specific antibodies are commonly found in normal individuals (19). In general, the younger an infant when a food antigen is introduced into the diet, the more pronounced the antibody response (20). Following the introduction of cow's milk, serum milk protein-specific IgG antibodies rise over the first month, achieving peak antibody levels after several months, and then generally decline, even though cow's milk proteins continue to be ingested (21). Individuals with various inflammatory gastrointestinal disorders (e.g., celiac disease, food allergy, inflammatory bowel disease) frequently have high levels of food-specific IgG and IgM antibodies. It is important to recognize that these antibodies do not indicate that the patient is allergic to these foods (22). The increased levels of food-specific antibodies (not IgE) appear to be secondary to increased gastrointestinal permeability to food antigens and simply reflect dietary intake.

■ ALLERGENS

Sensitization to food allergens may occur in the gastrointestinal tract, considered "traditional" or Class 1 food allergy, or as a consequence of an allergic sensitization to inhalant allergens, considered Class 2 food allergy (23). The major food allergens that have been identified in Class 1 allergy are water-soluble glycoproteins that have molecular weights ranging from 10 kilodaltons to 70 kilodaltons (kD) and are stable to treatment with heat, acid, and proteases (24) (Table 18.3). There are no consistent physicochemical properties common to the Class 2 food allergens. The majority of these generally plant-derived proteins are highly heat-labile and difficult to extract. A number of the Class 1 and 2 food allergens have been identified, cloned, sequenced, and expressed as recombinant proteins. Many of the plant-related allergens are homologous to pathogen-related proteins (PRs), which are expressed by the plant in response to infections or other stress factors, or comprise seed storage proteins, profilins, peroxidases, or protease inhibitors common to many plants (25).

Cow's Milk

Cow's milk is the most common food allergy in young children (if both IgE- and non-IgE-mediated hypersensitivities are considered) (1). IgE-mediated cow's milk allergy affects 2.5% of children less than 2 years of age and most patients become tolerant by 4 to 5 years of age. Cow's milk contains at least 20 protein components, which may lead to antibody production in man (26). The milk protein fractions are subdivided into casein (76% to 86%) and whey proteins. The casein fraction is precipitated from skim milk by acid at pH 4.6 and is comprised of four basic caseins (α_{s1}, α_{s2}, β, and κ comprising 32%, 10%, 28%, and 10% of the total milk protein, respectively). The noncasein fraction, or whey, consists of β-lactoglobulin, α-lactalbumin, bovine immunoglobulins, bovine serum albumin, and minute quantities of various proteins (e.g., lactoferrin, transferrin, lipases, esterases). Extensive heating will destroy several of the whey proteins. However, routine pasteurization is not sufficient to denature these proteins and has been reported to increase the allergenicity of some milk proteins, such as β-lactoglobulin (27). Sequential (linear) allergenic (IgE) epitopes have been mapped on the caseins, β-lactoglobulin and α-lactalbumin, and have been correlated with the persistence of cow's milk allergy (28–30). The most recent studies with more highly purified proteins suggest that the casein proteins are more allergenic (31).

IgE-immunoblotting techniques also have shown cross-reactivity among milk proteins in cows, goats, and sheep, due to the high degree of homology among these proteins. Oral challenge studies in cow's milk-allergic children indicated that at least 90% of cow's milk-allergic children will react to goat's milk (32). Interestingly, about 10% of milk-allergic children will react to beef, with a slightly higher number reacting to rare beef (33).

Chicken Egg

Chicken egg is another common IgE-mediated food allergy in children. The yolk is considered less allergenic than the white (34). The egg white contains 23 different glycoproteins with ovomucoid, ovalbumin and ovotransferin being identified as the major allergens (35,36). Although ovalbumin comprises the majority of the protein in egg white, ovomucoid has been shown to be the dominant allergen when highly purified egg white proteins are utilized (37). Ovomucoid (*Gal d 1*) is comprised of 186 amino acids arranged in three tandem domains, a set tertiary structure, and six sequential (linear) IgE-binding sites. Blinded oral food challenges with ovomucoid-depleted egg white demonstrated that

TABLE 18.3 ALLERGENS

1. Proteins (carbohydrate, not fat)
   - 10-70 kD glycoproteins
   - heat resistant, acid stable
2. Major allergenic foods (>85% of allergy)
   - Children: cow's milk, eggs, peanuts, soy, and wheat
   - Adults: peanuts, tree nuts, shellfish, and fish
3. Single food > many allergies
4. Characterization of epitopes underway
   - Linear versus conformational epitopes
   - B-cell versus T-cell epitopes

ovomucoid is responsible for clinical reactivity in the vast majority of egg allergic children (38). In addition, it was shown that about 70% of egg-allergic children may be able to ingest small amounts of egg protein in extensively heated (baked) products, e.g., breads, cakes, and cookies (39). These children appear to lack IgE antibodies to continuous epitopes, and since the prolonged high temperature destroys the tertiary structure (discontinuous or conformational epitopes) of the egg white proteins, the children fail to react (36,37).

Peanuts

The peanut, a member of the legume family, is the most common food allergy in individuals beyond the age of 4 years in most industrialized societies (40). Peanut proteins are traditionally classified as albumins (water-soluble) and globulins (saline-solution soluble), the latter of which is further subdivided into arachin and conarachin fractions (36). Three proteins with molecular weights of 63.5 kD (*Ara h 1*) (34, 41), 17 kD (*Ara h 2*) (42), and 64 kD (*Ara h 3*) (43) have been identified as major allergens. *Ara h 4-8* have also been identified (44). *Ara h 5* is a profilin, whereas *Ara h 4* appears to be an isoform of *Ara h 3*, and *Ara h 6* and *7* appear to be isoforms of *Ara h 2*. *Ara h 8* is a member of the pathogenesis-related PR-10 family, primarily involved in pollen-associated food allergy (45). *Ara h 1* belongs to the vicilin family of seed storage proteins, *Ara h 2* is a member of the conglutin family of storage proteins (46), and *Ara h 3* is a member of the glycinin family of storage of proteins (43). Refined peanut oil was found to be safe in all 60 peanut allergic individuals, whereas pressed (or extruded) oils were found to retain some of their allergenicity (47).

Soybean

Soybean is another member of the legume family that provokes a significant number of hypersensitivity reactions predominantly in infants and young children. Since soybeans provide an inexpensive source of high quality protein, soybean protein is used in many commercial foods. Approximately 10% of the seed proteins are water-soluble albumins and the remainder are salt-soluble globulins. Four major protein fractions have been separated by ultracentrifugation: 2S (contained in whey fraction), 7S (50% β-conglycinin), 11S (glycinin), and 15S (aggregated glycinin). A number of soy proteins have been isolated and characterized, particularly a 34 kD thiol protease-like protein (*Gly m Bd 30K*). Interestingly, the allergenic epitopes on glycinin G1 acidic chain are homologous to IgE-binding epitopes on peanut *Ara h 3* (48). Similar to highly refined peanut oil, refined soy oil did not provoke allergic reactions to soy in any of eight patients after ingesting up to 8 mL of soy oil (49).

Tree Nut

Tree nut allergies affect about 0.6% of the American population (50). In a national registry of peanut and nut allergic individuals, walnuts were the nut provoking the most allergic reactions (34%), followed by cashews (20%), almonds (15%), pecans (9%), and pistachios (7%). Hazel nuts, Brazil nuts, pine nuts, and macadamia nuts all account for less than 5%. Sesame seed allergy is becoming more commonly recognized in the United States (51,52). Skin testing reveals extensive cross-reactivity among tree nuts. While individuals allergic to one nut can clearly tolerate other nuts, too few patients have been systematically challenged to a variety of nuts to determine the extent of clinical cross-reactivity. Patients allergic to tree nuts do not necessarily need to avoid peanuts (a legume), and vice versa unless, for safety reasons, it is better to avoid all of them. However, surveys suggest that about 35% to 50% of peanut allergic patients are also reactive to at least one tree nut (53,54).

Fish

Fish are one of the most common causes of food allergic reactions in adults, and a common cause in children as well (7,55). The major allergen in cod, *Gad c 1*, is a parvalbumin that has been isolated from the myogen fraction of the white meat. It is heat-stable and resistant to proteolytic digestion, has a molecular weight of 12 kD, an isoelectric point of 4.75, and is composed of 113 amino acids (56). The 3-dimensional structure of *Gad c 1* has been defined and shown to be arranged in 3 domains, 2 of which bind calcium (57). Unlike many other food allergens, the fish protein fraction(s) responsible for clinical symptoms in some patients appear to be more susceptible to manipulation (e.g., heating, lyophilization) than other foods, since reactions occurred during open feedings of the fish in approximately 20% of those with negative DBPCFCs utilizing lyophilized fish (58). Furthermore, it was found that most patients allergic to fresh cooked salmon or tuna could ingest canned salmon or tuna without difficulty, indicating that preparation led to destruction of the major allergens. Nevertheless, allergic reactions following exposure to airborne allergen emitted during cooking are not uncommon (57).

Shellfish

Shellfish allergens are considered a major cause of food allergic reactions in adults, affecting up to 2.3% of the U.S. adult population (7). This group consists of a wide variety of mollusks (snails, mussels, oysters, scallops, clams, squid, and octopus) and crustacea (lobsters, crabs, prawns, and shrimp). Shrimp allergens have been most extensively studied. Tropomyosin, a protein found both in muscle and elsewhere, has been identified as the major allergen in shrimp (59). Considerable cross-reactivity among crustacea has been demonstrated by skin test and *in vitro* IgE analyses (60). Invertebrate tropomyosins are highly homologous and tend to be allergenic: crustaceans (e.g., shrimp, crab, crawfish, and lobster), arachnids (house dust mites); insects (cockroaches); and mollusks (squid, snails) (61). Vertebrate tropomyosin tends to be nonallergenic.

Wheat

Wheat (spelt) and other cereal grains share a number of homologous proteins and are not infrequently implicated in food allergic reactions in children. It has been suggested that the globulin and glutenin fractions are the major allergenic fractions in antibody-mediated reactions (e.g., gliadins in celiac disease and albumins in Baker's asthma) (62). Nonspecific binding to lectin fractions has been noted with each grain, and extensive immunologic cross-reactivity has been reported among the cereals, as was corroborated with skin-prick testing. In addition, homologies to allergenic proteins in grass pollens account for a large number of clinically irrelevant positive skin tests to wheat and other cereal grains. More recent studies have suggested that the water-insoluble gliadin fraction may be important in clinical reactivity to wheat, especially in cases of food-associated exercise-induced anaphylaxis (63–65).

Pathogenesis-related Proteins

Pathogenesis-related proteins (PRs) have been shown to comprise a large number of Class 2 allergenic proteins found in various vegetables and fruits (Table 18.4) (23,66,67). These proteins are induced when pathogens stress the plant; examples include wounding or certain environmental stresses, such as drought and heat. PRs have been classified into 14 families, although 6 PR families account for the majority of cross-reactivity among plant proteins. Two families of chitinases that are similar to the latex allergen, *Hev b 6.02*, have been identified as allergens in a number of vegetables: PR-3

type proteins are found in chestnut and avocado (*Pers a 1*) while PR-4 type proteins are wound-induced proteins found in tomato and potato (*Win 1* and *Win 2* proteins). PR-5 type thaumatin-like proteins have been identified as cross-reacting proteins found in apples (*Mal d 2*) and cherry (*Pru av 2*). The PR-10 type proteins are homologous to the major birch pollen allergen, *Bet v 1*, and account for cross-reactivity between birch pollen and fruits of the Rosaceae species: apple (*Mal d 1*), cherry (*Pru av 1*), apricot (*Pru ar 1*), pear (*Pyr c 1*); or vegetables of the Apiaceae species: carrot (*Dau c 1*), celery (*Api g 1*), and parsley (*pcPR 1* and 2); and hazel nut (*Cor a 1*). The lipid transfer proteins (LTPs), or PR-14 type proteins, form a family of 9 kD proteins distributed widely throughout the plant kingdom. LTPs have been identified as major allergenic proteins in Prunoideae species such as peach (*Pru p 1* in peach skin and *Pru p 3* in the fruit), apple (*Mal d 3*), apricot, plum, and cherries. *Gly m 1*, a major allergen in soybean, has been found to be a LTP.

Profilin

Profilin is an actin-binding protein that was first identified in birch pollen (*Bet v 2*) and is now recognized as an allergenic protein in a number of fruits and vegetables (23). Profilins are responsible for the celery-mugwort-spice syndrome and is responsible for oral allergy syndrome to apple, pear, carrot, celery (*Api g 4*), and potato in birch pollen-allergic patients. Profilins have also been identified in tomato, peanut (*Ara h 5*), and soybean (*Gly m 3*), but whether these proteins cause allergic reactions remains to be established.

■ IGE-MEDIATED FOOD REACTIONS

Immune responses mediated by specific IgE antibodies to food allergens are the most widely recognized mechanism for food-induced allergy symptoms (1). Atopic patients produce IgE antibodies to specific epitopes in the food allergen. These antibodies bind to high affinity

TABLE 18.4 PATHOGENESIS-RELATED PROTEINS

GROUP	PROTEIN CLASS	ALLERGEN SOURCE/ALLERGEN
PR-2	β-1,3 glucanases	fruits and vegetables
PR-3	Class 1 chitinases	avocado (*Pers a 1*), chestnut, and banana
PR-4	Chitinases	tomato, potato (*Win 1* and *Win 2* proteins), turnip, and elderberry
PR-5	Thaumatin-like	cherry (*Pru av 2*), apple (*Mal d 2*), bell pepper
PR-10	*Bet v 1* homologues	apple (*Mal d 1*), cherry (*Pru av 1*), pear (*Pyr c 1*), celery (*Api g 1*), carrot (*Dau c 1*), potato, apricot (*Pru ar 1*), parsley, hazelnut (*Cor a 1*)
PR-14	Lipid transfer proteins	peach skin (*Pru p 1*), peach pulp (*Pru p 3*), apple (*Mal d 3*), cherry (*Pru av 3*), apricot, plum, almond, soy (*Gly m 1*), barley

IgE receptors on basophils and tissue mast cells throughout the body. When antigen binds to multiple adjacent IgE antibodies on a mast cell or basophil, these cells become activated, degranulate, and release preformed mediators such as histamine and newly formed mediators such as leukotrienes and prostaglandins. These mediators are responsible for the immediate allergic reaction and the clinical symptoms observed. Eosinophils, monocytes, and lymphocytes are recruited to the area affected in the late-phase allergic response and release a variety of cytokines and inflammatory mediators. Mast cell-derived mediators can cause endothelial cells to increase expression of adhesion molecules for eosinophils, basophils, and lymphocytes. The following section will review the specific clinical manifestations of IgE-mediated food reactions.

Cutaneous Manifestations

Cutaneous manifestations are the most common clinical symptoms of food allergy (68). These cutaneous symptoms range from acute urticaria or angioedema to a morbilliform pruritic dermatitis. Chronic urticaria is almost never caused by food allergy (69). Cutaneous symptoms may present with signs and symptoms from other organ systems such as the gastrointestinal and respiratory systems (70). Urticaria can be elicited in approximately 12% of food challenges and overall, the incidence of acute food-dependent urticaria is about 1% to 2% (70). Contact dermatitis also has been reported to various foods (71). True allergic contact urticaria can proceed to a systemic reaction; therefore, a thorough diagnostic workup to rule out involvement of the immune system is important. In children with atopic dermatitis, food allergies have been confirmed by DBPCFC in about one-third of the children (72,73). In one study of 210 children evaluated and followed to determine a relationship between food allergy and exacerbations of their atopic dermatitis, 62% of children had a reaction to at least one food. Of all reactions that occurred within 2 hours of a DBPCFC, 75% were cutaneous (74). Cutaneous manifestations predominantly involved erythema and pruritus leading to scratching and exacerbation of the atopic dermatitis.

Sampson and Broadbent reported an increase in histamine releasabililty in patients with atopic dermatitis who repeatedly ingest a food allergen (75). This is probably due to the stimulation of mononuclear cells to secrete histamine-releasing factors (HRFs), some of which interact with IgE molecules bound to the surface of basophils. Increased HRF production has been associated with an increase in symptoms as well as increased lung and skin hyperreactivity.

Gastrointestinal Manifestations

Gastrointestinal symptoms are the second most frequently observed manifestation of food allergy. Clinical presentations include nausea, vomiting, diarrhea, and abdominal pain and cramping. As with cutaneous manifestations, gastrointestinal symptoms may occur alone or in combination with symptoms from other organ systems. There is considerable evidence that many of these symptoms result from the activation of mast cells (76).

Allergic eosinophilic gastroenteropathies are manifested by eosinophilic infiltration of the gastrointestinal tract. Symptoms depend on the layers of GI tract involved and are intermittent (77). Often this is associated with peripheral eosinophilia but rarely involves other organs. These patients do not meet criteria for hypereosinophilic syndrome (78). Eosinophilic infiltration of the mucosal layer is most common and can be seen in any part of the GI tract. Clinical symptoms include abdominal pain, postprandial nausea, vomiting, diarrhea, weight loss, failure to thrive, occult or gross blood loss in the stools, anemia, hypoalbuminemia, and peripheral edema (77,79). Involvement of the submucosal and muscular regions is more common in the prepyloric region of the gastric antrum and the distal small intestine. These patients also may have symptoms of gastric outlet obstruction, a mass lesion with epigastric tenderness, and even perforation of the intestinal wall (78,80). Rarely, eosinophilic infiltration involves the serosal surface, presenting with prominent ascites (78,79).

Over the past few years, there has been a dramatic increase in the number of publications related to eosinophilic esophagitis (EE) (81,82). Chapter 40 is devoted to EE and gastroesophageal reflux disease (GERD) and discusses them in additional detail. Typical clinical symptoms for EE depend on the age group involved. For example, young children with EE usually present with GERD that has not responded well to typical medical management and who have normal pH probes results. In contrast, adolescents present with dysphagia and adults present with dysphagia, food impaction, and strictures (81). There may be a significant delay between symptoms and confirmatory diagnosis by esophageal biopsy, which typically reveals greater than 15 to 20 intramucosal esosinophils per high-power field, preferably with multiple biopsy sites (77). Food allergens have been implicated as causative agents in more than 90% of patients with EE. A combination of skin-prick testing and atopy patch testing have been utilized to identify offending food allergens in patients with this disease (77,81–85). The more common food allergens that have been implicated in EE include cow's milk, eggs, soy, chicken, wheat, beef, peanuts, rice, and potatoes. The usefulness of the atopy patch test in the diagnostic workup of children with food allergy-related gastrointestinal symptoms is still unclear; its diagnostic accuracy appears to be higher with fresh foods than with commercial extracts (84). The medical management of EE has been investigated in detail (8). The three main dietary strategies that have been utilized and assessed include a strict elemental diet (e.g., amino acid-based formula), an elimination diet based on the results of the skin-prick test and atopy patch test findings or removal of the six most common food allergens (e.g., cow's milk, eggs, wheat, soy, nuts, and seafood). While up to 98% of patients experience significant improvement with a strict elemental dietary therapy, this response rate decreases with the other elimination diets (77). Another form of therapy that has been utilized in these patients involved the use of swallowed inhaled corticosteroid preparations and general guidelines have recommended (77,83).

Allergic eosinophilic gastroenteritis is another eosinophilic gastroenteropathy that is less common than EE (78). This condition can present in infancy through adolescence and typical clinical symptoms include abdominal pain, nausea/vomiting, diarrhea, poor appetite, weight loss, occult blood in the stool, and in some cases, a protein-losing enteropathy. Approximately 50% of these patients are atopic and 50% have a peripheral eosinophilia. The most common form of this disease is characterized by endoscopic biopsy findings of a significant eosinophilic infiltration of the gastric mucosa and submucosa. Resolution of clinical symptoms can be observed with the removal of the causal food within 6 weeks, and the most common offending foods include cow's milk, eggs, soy cereals, and fish. Oral cromolyn and ketotifen have been utilized with some success (77). Of note, most patients have an excellent response to use of an elemental diet such as an amino acid-based formula. While the clinical course can be prolonged, the natural history of this condition is not well understood (86).

Pollen-Food Syndrome (Oral Allergy Syndrome)

Patients allergic to certain airborne pollens can display adverse reactions on the ingestion of plant-derived foods as a result of IgE-cross-reactive structures shared by pollen and food allergen sources. This clinical entity is known as the pollen-food syndrome, PFS (also known as the oral allergy syndrome) and it is considered to be a form of contact urticaria with symptoms resulting from interaction of the food allergen with the oral mucosa (87,88). Symptoms include pruritus with or without angioedema of the lips, tongue, palate, and posterior oropharynx. Rarely, systemic anaphylaxis can be observed with this syndrome. Shared allergen sensitivities have been reported between ragweed and the gourd family (watermelon, cantaloupe, honeydew melon, zucchini, and cucumbers) and bananas (89). PFS has been described with ingestion of apples (90), carrots, parsnips, celery, hazelnuts, potatoes (91,92), celery (93), and kiwi (94) in patients sensitive to birch pollen, and with ingestion of apples, tree nuts, peaches, oranges, pears, cherries, fennel, tomatoes, and carrots in patients allergic to tree and grass pollens (95). PFS

symptoms resolve rapidly and rarely involve any other target organs. However, ingestion of celery tuber (celery root), which cross-reacts with birch pollen, may cause more severe systemic symptoms in pollen-allergic patients (93). This may be explained by the presence of both heat-labile and heat-stable proteins (96).

Respiratory Manifestations
Oral Ingestion of Food Allergens

Oral ingestion of food allergens is the primary route of exposure that can cause or exacerbate food hypersensitivity symptoms. Anaphylactic reactions to foods including significant respiratory symptoms and, in some cases, fatal and near fatal anaphylactic reactions have also been reported (68,97,98). Respiratory manifestations may include sneezing; rhinorrhea; ocular, otic, and palatal pruritus; bronchospasm; and laryngeal edema. Isolated airway symptoms as a manifestation of food allergy are exceedingly rare (99). Respiratory reactions including wheezing, throat tightness, and nasal congestion, were reported in 42% and 56% of respondents as part of their initial reactions to peanuts and tree nuts, respectively (52), and the presence of asthma was a risk factor for these patients to have more severe reactions (33% versus 21%; P<0.0001). Finally, respiratory symptoms including shortness of breath and throat tightness were reported by more than 50% of patients with fish or shellfish allergy in a recent published survey (7).

Asthma Induced by Food Allergy

The majority of information regarding food allergy and respiratory tract symptoms has focused on asthma (100–102). Asthma symptoms induced by food allergy have been typically accompanied by skin and gastrointestinal manifestations. In addition, patients with food allergy and asthma were generally younger and had a past medical history of atopic dermatitis. Other investigations have confirmed that food allergy, especially with cow's milk and eggs, can induce asthma in children, especially those with atopic dermatitis (103–105). Respiratory reactions induced by food challenges in children with pulmonary disease have been well documented (106,107). The most common foods that were responsible for these reactions included peanuts, cow's milk, eggs, and tree nuts. Interestingly, only five (2%) of these patients had wheezing as their only objective adverse symptom. The patients were highly atopic, had multiple allergic sensitivities to foods, and over one-half had a prior diagnosis of asthma. Overall, 17% to 24% of the children with positive food challenges developed wheezing as part of their overall clinical reaction. Furthermore, a subset of these patients was monitored with pulmonary function testing during positive and negative food challenges (107). Thirteen (15%) developed lower respiratory symptoms, including wheezing, however, only six patients had a greater than 20% decrease in forced expiratory volume in 1 second (FEV_1). Wheezing as the only manifestation of the respiratory reaction was a rare observation.

Airway Hyperresponsiveness Induced by Food Allergy

In a select subset of pediatric patients with asthma, the chronic ingestion of a food to which the patient is allergic may result in increased airway hyperreactivity despite the absence of acute symptoms following ingestion (108). Significant increases in airway hyperreactivity, demonstrated with methacholine inhalation challenges, were documented several hours after positive food challenges in patients who experienced adverse chest symptoms during these food challenges. This investigation suggested that food-induced allergic reactions may increase airway reactivity in a subset of patients with moderate to severe asthma. In contrast, a different investigation concluded that food allergy was an unlikely cause of increased airway reactivity in adult patients (109). Evaluation for food allergy should be considered among patients with: recalcitrant or otherwise unexplained acute severe asthma exacerbations, asthma triggered following ingestion of particular foods, and in patients with asthma and other manifestations of food allergy (e.g., anaphylaxis, moderate to severe atopic dermatitis).

Inhalation of Food Allergens

As opposed to the ingestion route, exposure to food allergens through inhalation can also cause food hypersensitivity reactions. Several published reports have highlighted cases of food hypersensitivity reactions that have been precipitated following the inhalation of airborne food allergens. For example, the inhalation of allergens from fish, shellfish, seeds, soybeans, cereal grains, chicken eggs, cow's milk, and many other foods have been implicated in these reactions. Symptoms have typically included respiratory manifestations such as rhinoconjunctivitis, coughing, wheezing, dyspnea, asthma, and even anaphylaxis.

In addition, there have been many published reports of occupational asthma following the inhalation of relevant food allergens. These reactions are most likely the result of IgE-mediated food reactions that result from inhalation of aerosolized antigens, usually in an occupational setting. While the resultant symptoms are the same as respiratory symptoms seen with aeroallergens (i.e., rhinoconjunctivitis and asthma), asthma is the most prominent symptom. Patients typically have IgE antibody to the food as demonstrated by skin tests or immunoassay. Occupational asthma is discussed in additional detail in Chapter 25.

Baker's asthma is caused by occupational exposure to airborne cereal grain dust and can result in chronic asthma (110). A significant percentage of bakers develop occupational asthma and chronic obstructive bronchitis. There was a positive methacholine test in 33% of bakers with atopic status, compared to 6.1% (P<0.01) of nonatopic bakers (111). Another investigation characterized exposure to inhalation dust, wheat flour, and alpha-amylase allergens in industrial and traditional bakeries (112). Likewise, bakery workers have been reported to develop IgE-mediated occupational asthma to soybean flour. The allergens involved are predominantly high molecular weight proteins that are present both in soybean hull and flour (113). Sensitization to this allergen is common in subjects who are repeatedly exposed to soybean dust inhalation (114). Asthma attacks and mortality due to inhalation of soybean antigens in Barcelona have also been documented (115). Implementation of stricter protective measures in silos for the soybean unloading process has reduced the concentration of soybean dust in the atmosphere demonstrating the effectiveness of these measures.

Occupational asthma due to fish inhalation, confirmed by specific bronchial challenge (SBC), has been reported in fish-processing workers with asthma (116,117). Other investigators have examined the prevalence, work-related symptoms, and possible risk factors for IgE-mediated sensitization in seafood processing workers (118–121). Presence of atopy, as well as the intensity and the duration of exposure, were found to be potential risk factors for sensitization. Therefore, the evaluation of food allergy should be considered among patients with histories of allergic reactions not only after the ingestion of a suspected food allergen(s), but also following relevant inhalational exposures. Prevention of exposure to certain aerosolized particles through inhalation in relevant environments (i.e., seafood restaurants and bakeries) is encouraged.

Anaphylaxis

Food-induced Anaphylactic Reactions

Food is the most common cause of outpatient anaphylaxis, but the actual prevalence of food-induced anaphylaxis, an under-recognized and under-treated medical emergency, is not known (122–124). Food allergens account for up to 30% of fatal cases of anaphylaxis; one-third of cases occur at home, 25% in restaurants, and 15% at school or work. Reactions to peanuts and tree nuts accounted for 94% of fatalities (122). The most commonly implicated foods responsible for food-induced anaphylaxis include peanuts, tree nuts, fish, and shellfish. Symptoms were reported in the first known exposure in 72% of tree nut and/or peanut allergic patients. In addition, sesame seeds have recently been identified as a cause of food-induced anaphylaxis. Compelling evidence exists that sesame allergy is becoming a serious public health problem in many countries around the globe (125,126). Sesame appears to be an internationally common food allergen (126). Sesame allergy has been identified mainly in populations where sesame is widely consumed: Israel, Asia, Australia, and Italy. The prevalence of sesame allergy appears to be rising in the United Kingdom and the United States, as well (126). Sesame allergy is often associated with systemic anaphylaxis similar to peanut and tree nut allergies (127), and sesame allergy is rarely outgrown.

Symptoms of food-induced anaphylaxis typically include pruritus in the oropharynx, angioedema (e.g., laryngeal edema), stridor, cough, dyspnea, wheezing, and dysphonia. In a survey of six fatal and seven near-fatal anaphylactic reactions following food ingestion, all patients had asthma and respiratory symptoms as part of their clinical presentation (68). The foods responsible for these serious reactions were peanuts, tree nuts, eggs, and cow's milk. Another report summarized acute allergic reactions to peanuts and/or tree nuts in 122 atopic children. In the group, 52% had lower respiratory tract symptoms as part of their overall reactions (54).

In summary, the presence of asthma and a short list of common food allergens are significant risk factors for serious and even fatal cases of food-induced anaphylaxis (97). Common themes associated with fatal food anaphylaxis include: (a) reactions to peanuts and tree nuts, (b) victims are typically teenagers or young adults, (b) patients have a known history of asthma, and (d) the failure to promptly administer epinephrine. Cutaneous symptoms are the most common, appearing in more than 90% of cases (122,128,129). Respiratory symptoms, especially shortness of breath, are another common manifestation.

■ FOOD-RELATED EXERCISE-INDUCED ANAPHYLAXIS

Exercise-induced anaphylaxis is a unique syndrome characterized by generalized body warmth, erythema, and pruritus, which can progress to fulminant anaphylaxis, including confluent urticaria, laryngeal edema, bronchospasm, GI symptoms, hypotension, and even vascular collapse (130). A subset of patients have these symptoms only if exercise is performed within 2 to 6 hours of food ingestion (131). With food alone or exercise alone, there is no anaphylaxis (131,132). For some patients, this postprandial exercise-induced anaphylaxis may occur with any food ingestion followed by exercise (131,132). Others have exercise-induced anaphylaxis only associated with the ingestion of specific foods, such as wheat (133), celery (131), or shellfish (123,134). Both high and low aerobic sports and physical activities have been associated with food-dependent exercise-induced anaphylaxis. Reports of fatalities are rare and restricted to adults. These patients have positive skin tests to the foods, yet they have no allergic reactions unless ingestion is followed by or preceded by rigorous exercise (131,134). For all food-related exercise-induced anaphylaxis, episodes are prevented with avoidance of food ingestion 4 to 6 hours prior to or following exercise (132). Treatment also includes carrying self-injectable epinephrine, exercising with a friend or "buddy," wearing Medic Alert identification, and exercising only if a medical facility is in reasonable proximity. If affordable, a cell phone should be carried. The mechanism of this type of anaphylaxis is not well understood, but it is thought to be mediated by mast cell degranulation (130). Other aspects of anaphylaxis are covered in more detail in Chapter 14.

■ NON-IgE-MEDIATED FOOD REACTIONS

Food Protein-induced Enterocolitis Syndrome (FPIES)

Food protein-induced enterocolitis syndrome (FPIES) typically occurs in formula-fed infants by 4 to 6 months of age (e.g., cow's milk and/or soy); it has not been reported in breastfed infants (86,135). Symptoms consist of profuse vomiting and diarrhea within 2 to 3 hours of eating the offending food protein, which can lead to profound dehydration and lethargy. With chronic exposure, failure to thrive and hypoalbuminemia can be observed. Removal of the causal food results in the resolution of clinical symptoms. Negative skin tests and serum food-specific IgE tests are common in this syndrome. Treatment of patients with FPIES consists of vigorous intravenous hydration and elimination of the offending food protein. Resolution of clinical reactivity occurs with age, typically by 3 years.

Food-induced Colitis

Otherwise known as allergic protocolitis or allergic colitis, food-induced colitis, usually presents by 6 months of age (136). Clinical symptoms include blood streaked, loose stools with or without diarrhea in an otherwise healthy appearing infant. This condition commonly occurs in breastfed infants (i.e., up to 60%) or in cow's milk or soy milk formula-fed infants. The diagnosis is made by clinical history; specific IgE measurements are negative. The differential diagnosis includes anal fissures, gastrointestinal infections, necrotizing enterocolitis, and intussusception. Treatment consists of elimination of the responsible protein, use of casein hydrolysate formulas, and in rare cases, the use of amino acid-based formulas. Clinical symptoms typically resolve by 1 year of age.

Celiac Disease

Celiac disease is characterized by small intestinal mucosal injury and nutrient malabsorption in genetically susceptible individuals in response to the dietary ingestion of gluten-containing grains, especially wheat, rye, and barley (137,138). Immune responses to key gliadin epitopes are recognized as important in celiac disease pathogenesis. There is a strong HLA association with HLA-DQ2 and HLA-DQ8 molecules, but human HLA-DQ risk factors do not explain the entire genetic susceptibility to gluten intolerance (139). Lesions of the small intestine are contiguous and most often involve the mucosa only, sparing the submucosa, muscularis, and serosa (140). There is flattening of the intestinal villi (141). The lamina propria is hypercellular, with a predominance of lymphocytes and plasma cells (140,141); there is a predominance of IgA-producing cells (142). In addition to the classic intestinal lesions, serologic markers are often present in this disease. There are IgA antibodies found against reticulin and smooth muscle endomysium (143). IgA-antitissue transglutaminase antibodies, recently known as antiendomysial antibodies, have been reported to be both sensitive and specific for the evaluation of celiac disease (144,145).

Clinical symptoms of celiac disease are those of malabsorption, and the severity of symptoms correlates directly with the amount of intestine involved. Patients have classic symptoms of malabsorption, but extraintestinal manifestations, such as glossitis and osteopenia reflecting severe malabsorption, may also be present (146). Increasing numbers of atypical or asymptomatic celiac disease are being diagnosed (138,147).

Dermatitis Herpetiformis

Dermatitis herpetiformis is a cutaneous manifestation of gluten sensitivity, occasionally associated with other autoimmune disorders and reportedly associated with an increased risk of lymphoproliferative disorders (148,149). It occurs most commonly in children 2 to 7 years of age. The rash is an erythematous, pleomorphic pruritic eruption involving predominantly the knees, elbows, shoulders, buttocks, and scalp; mucous membranes are spared. Celiac disease is present in most, and lesions respond to gluten elimination. Lesions can be urticarial, papular, vesicular, or bullous (150). Sulfones are the mainstay of therapy for the cutaneous lesions and may relieve pruritic symptoms within 24 hours (150).

■ DIAGNOSIS

The diagnostic approach to adverse food reactions begins with the medical history and physical examination and if indicated, laboratory studies. The value of the medical history is largely dependent on the patient's recollection of symptoms and the examiner's ability to differentiate between disorders provoked by food hypersensitivity and other etiologies. However, in several series less than 50% of reported food allergy could

be verified by DBPCFC. The information required to establish that a food allergic reaction occurred and to construct an appropriate blinded challenge to confirm the reaction if necessary, include the following: (a) the food presumed to have provoked the reaction, (b) the quantity of the suspected food ingested, (c) the length of time between ingestion and development of symptoms, (d) whether similar symptoms developed on other occasions when the food was eaten, (e) whether other factors (e.g., exercise) are necessary, and (f) how long since the last reaction to the food occurred. Although any food may cause an allergic reaction, a few foods account for about 90% of reactions: in adults—peanuts, nuts, fish, and shellfish; in young children—eggs, milk, peanuts, soy, and wheat (fish in Scandinavian countries). In chronic disorders (e.g., atopic dermatitis, asthma, chronic urticaria), history is often an unreliable indicator of the offending allergen.

Diet Diaries

Diet diaries are frequently discussed as an adjunct to history. Patients are instructed to keep a chronological record of all foods ingested over a specified period of time. Only occasionally does this method detect an unrecognized association between a food and a patient's symptoms. As opposed to the medical history, it collects information on a prospective basis and is not as dependent on a patient's memory.

Diagnostic Elimination Diets

Diagnostic elimination diets are frequently utilized both in diagnosis and management of adverse food reactions. Once certain foods are suspected of provoking allergic disorders, they are completely omitted from the diet. The success of these diets depends on the identification of the correct allergen(s), the ability of the patient to maintain a diet completely free of all forms of the offending allergen, and the assumption that other factors do not provoke similar symptoms during the period of study. Although avoidance of suspected food allergens is recommended prior to blinded challenges, elimination diets alone are rarely diagnostic of food allergy, especially in chronic disorders such as atopic dermatitis or asthma.

Skin-Prick Tests

Skin-Prick tests are reproducible (151) and frequently utilized to screen patients with suspected IgE-mediated food allergies. Glycerinated food extracts (1:10 or 1:20) and appropriate positive (histamine) and negative (saline) controls are applied by the prick or puncture technique. The criteria for interpreting skin-prick tests was established by Bock and May about 30 years ago (152). Any food allergens eliciting a wheal at least 3 mm greater than the negative control are considered positive; all others are considered negative. More recently investigators have been evaluating the utility of using the mean wheal diameter as a predictor of clinical reactivity. Recent studies have reported that skin-prick tests inducing mean wheal diameters > 8mm are diagnostic of milk, egg, and peanut allergies and are >95% predictive of clinical reactivity (153–155). A positive skin-prick test should be interpreted as indicating the *possibility* that the patient has symptomatic reactivity to the specific food, whereas negative skin tests confirm the absence of IgE-mediated reactions (negative predictive accuracy is greater than 95%), if good quality food extracts are utilized (152,156). Therefore, the skin-prick test may be considered an excellent means of excluding IgE-mediated food allergies, but only suggestive of the presence of clinical food allergies (157,158,159). There are some exceptions to this general statement: (a) IgE-mediated sensitivity to several fruits and vegetables (e.g., apples, oranges, bananas, pears, melons, potatoes, carrots, celery) are frequently not detected with commercially prepared reagents, presumably due to the lability of the responsible allergen (95); (b) commercial extracts sometimes lack the appropriate allergen to which an individual is reactive, as demonstrated by the use of fresh foods for skin test reagents (160); (c) children less than 1 year of age may have IgE-mediated food allergy in the absence of positive skin tests, and infants less than 2 years may have smaller wheals, presumably due to lack of skin reactivity (161); and conversely, (d) a positive skin test to a food, that when ingested in the absence of other foods, provokes a serious systemic anaphylactic reaction may be considered diagnostic.

Intradermal skin testing is more sensitive than the skin-prick test when detecting specific-IgE but is much less specific when compared to the DBPCFC (152). No patients with a positive intradermal skin test to a food and a concomitant negative skin-prick test have been shown to have a positive DBPCFC. In addition, intradermal skin testing can significantly increase the risk of inducing a systemic reaction compared to skin-prick testing, and therefore is not recommended.

Atopy Patch Test

In recent years there has been increasing interest in the use of the atopy patch test for the diagnosis of non-IgE-mediated food allergy (162–165). There is limited utility of this testing method at the present time. In a recent study of children with atopic dermatitis, the investigators concluded that the patch test added little diagnostic benefit compared to standard diagnostic tests (166).

In Vitro Allergen-specific IgE Tests

In vitro allergen-specific IgE tests (including RAST; ELISA; CAP System FEIA™ and UniCAP™ [Phadia;

TABLE 18.5 FOOD-SPECIFIC IgE ANTIBODIES: DIAGNOSTIC UTILITY

Peanut	
IgE ≥ 14:	95% PPV
IgE ≥ 57:	100% PPV
Cow's milk	
IgE ≥15:	95% PPV (age 4; atopic)
IgE ≥5:	95% PPV (infants)
Egg	
IgE ≥7:	95% PPV (age 4; atopic)
IgE ≥2:	95% PPV (infants)

Uppsala, Sweden]; Magic Lite™; ALK-Abello, Denmark) are utilized for measuring serum for IgE-mediated food allergies. While generally considered slightly less sensitive than skin tests, one study comparing Phadebas RAST™ with DBPCFCs found skin-prick tests and RASTs to have similar sensitivity and specificity to food challenge outcome when a Phadebas score of three or greater was considered positive (156). In the past 10 years the use of a quantitative measurement of food-specific IgE antibodies (CAP System FEIA™ or UniCAP™) has been shown to be predictive of symptomatic IgE-mediated food allergy (167,168) (Table 18.5). Food-specific IgE levels exceeding the diagnostic values established as cut-off points indicate that the patient is greater than 95% likely to experience an allergic reaction if he or she ingests the specific food. In addition, the IgE levels can be monitored and if they fall to less than 2 kU$_A$/L for eggs, milk, or peanuts, the patient should be re-challenged to determine whether he or she has "outgrown" their food allergy (168–171). Basophil histamine release assays are reserved for research settings.

The Double-blind Placebo-controlled Food Challenge

The double-blind placebo-controlled food challenge (DBPCFC) has been labeled the "gold standard" for the diagnosis of food allergies; it controls for the variability of chronic disorders like urticaria and other precipitating factors such as psychogenic (172). Many investigators have utilized DBPCFCs successfully in children and adults to examine a variety of food-related complaints (173–176). The selection of foods to be tested in DBPCFCs is generally based on history and/or skin test (*in vitro* IgE) results. Foods unlikely to provoke food allergic reactions may be screened by open or single-blind challenges. Importantly, for research studies positive reactions by these methods should be confirmed by DBPCFC, except perhaps in very young infants. In clinical practice, open or single-blind challenges will be all that is necessary. Prior to undertaking DBPCFC, several factors need to be taken into consideration. Suspect foods should be eliminated for 7 to 14 days prior to challenge, longer in some non-IgE-mediated gastrointestinal disorders. Antihistamines should be discontinued long enough to establish a normal histamine skin test, and other medications should be minimized to levels sufficient to prevent breakthrough of acute symptoms. In some asthmatic patients, short bursts of corticosteroids may be necessary to insure adequate pulmonary reserve for testing (FEV_1 > 70% predicted).

The food challenge is administered in the fasting state, starting with a dose unlikely to provoke symptoms (5 mg to 250 mg of lyophilized food) (177). The dose is then doubled every 15 to 60 minutes, depending on the type of reaction suspected. Once the patient has tolerated 10 g of lyophilized food blinded in capsules or liquid, clinical reactivity is generally ruled out. If the blinded challenge is negative, however, it must be confirmed by an open feeding under observation to rule-out the rare false-negative challenge.

To control for a variety of potential confounding factors, an equal number of food antigen and placebo challenges are necessary; the order of administration should be randomized by a noninterested third party (e.g., dietitian) (178). The length of observation is dependent on the type of reaction suspected, e.g., generally up to 2 hours for IgE-mediated reactions, up to 4 to 8 hours for milk-induced enterocolitis and 3 to 4 days for allergic eosinophilic gastroenteritis. Results of blinded challenges for objective signs and symptoms are rarely equivocal, but can be made more objective by monitoring a variety of laboratory parameters, such as plasma histamine, pulmonary function tests, and nasal airway resistance; serum β-tryptase is rarely shown to rise following food allergic reactions (68,179).

In non-IgE-mediated food allergies, e.g., dietary protein-induced enterocolitis, allergen challenges may require up to 0.15 g to 0.3 g of food/kg of body weight given in one or two doses (180,181). In other non-IgE-mediated disorders, e.g., allergic eosinophilic esophagitis or gastroenteritis, the patient may require several feedings over a 1- to 3-day period to elicit symptoms. In most IgE-mediated disorders, challenges to more foods often may be conducted every 1 to 2 days, whereas with non-IgE-mediated disorders, challenges to new foods often need to be at least 3 to 5 days apart.

Oral food challenges should be conducted in a clinic or hospital setting, especially if an IgE-mediated reaction or dietary protein-induced enterocolitis is suspected, and only when trained personnel and equipment for treating systemic anaphylaxis are immediately available (173,182). Patients with histories of life-threatening anaphylaxis should be challenged only when the causative antigen cannot be conclusively determined by history and laboratory testing, or the patient is believed to have "outgrown" his or her sensitivity. The evaluation of many so-called delayed reactions (e.g., most IgE-negative gastrointestinal allergies) can be conducted safely in a physician's office, except perhaps for FPIES where intravenous access is generally required because of the risk of hypotension. In cases where patients' symptoms are largely subjective, three cross-over trials with reactions developing only during the allergen challenge are necessary to conclude that a cause-and-effect relationship exists.

Practical Approach to Diagnosing Food Allergy

The diagnosis of food allergy remains a clinical exercise dependent on a careful history, selective skin tests, or in vitro measurement of food-specific IgE, and when clinically indicated, an appropriate exclusion diet and blinded provocation. At the present time, there are no controlled trials supporting the diagnostic value for food-specific IgG or IgG_4 antibody levels, food antigen-antibody complexes, evidence of lymphocyte activation (^3H uptake, IL-2 production, leukocyte inhibitory factor production), or sublingual or intracutaneous provocation. In gastrointestinal disorders where pre- and post-challenge biopsy studies are required for diagnosis, blinded challenge may not be essential. An exclusion diet eliminating all foods implicated by history and/or skin testing (for IgE-mediated disorders) should be conducted for 1 to 2 weeks in suspected IgE-mediated disorders and food-induced enterocolitis and colitis. Diets may need to be extended for up to 12 weeks in other gastrointestinal disorders, following appropriate biopsies. If no improvement is noted, it is unlikely that food allergy is involved. However, in cases of atopic dermatitis and chronic asthma, other precipitating factors may make it difficult to discriminate the effects of the food allergen from other provocative factors.

Open or single-blind food challenges in a clinic setting may be used to screen suspected food allergens. Multiple food allergies are becoming more common, especially with minor allergens; therefore, physicians must weigh the benefit of accurately identifying clinical reactivity and the risk of challenge. In such cases, the use of open or single-blind challenges is less time consuming, and if positive can be confirmed by DBPCFC. Elimination diets may lead to malnutrition and/or eating disorders, especially if they include a large number of foods and/or utilized for extended periods of time. Presumptive diagnoses of food allergy based on patient history and skin test or in vitro IgE results are unreliable, except in cases where serum food-specific IgE levels exceed decision point values (169) and unequivocal allergic symptoms (i.e., anaphylaxis) occur following an isolated ingestion of a specific food.

■ TREATMENT

Once the diagnosis of food hypersensitivity is established, the only proven therapy is strict *elimination* of the offending allergen. Patients and their families must be educated about how to avoid accidental ingestion of food allergens, teaching them to recognize early symptoms of an allergic reaction, and educating them in the early management of a potential anaphylactic reaction (1). Patients must learn to read all food ingredient labels for the presence of specific food allergens, to become familiar with situations where cross-contamination is likely, and to avoid high-risk situations, such as buffets, ice cream parlors, and unlabeled candies and desserts (183). In addition, considerable educational material is available through organizations such as the Food Allergy and Anaphylaxis Network (FAAN—Fairfax, VA; 1-800-929-4040 or http://www.foodallergy.org) and the American Partnership for Eosinophilic Disorders Web site (http://www.apfed.org).

Patients with multiple food allergies, especially children, are at risk for nutritional deficiencies resulting from their restricted diets; some of these patients may require a hypoallergenic formula to meet their needs. Hypoallergenic formulas for children with milk allergy are either based on extensively hydrolyzed casein-derived from cow's milk (Pregestimil^{TM}, Nutramigen^{TM}, or Alimentum^{TM}) or on a mixture of single amino acids (Neocate^{TM}, Neocate 1+^{TM}, or Elecare^{TM}). Hypoallergenic formulas are well tolerated by children with IgE-mediated and cell-mediated food allergy. If feasible, it is important to utilize the services of a nutritionist for education of the patient and family. Their help in managing the patient's diet is extremely important to ensure that there is adequate nutritional intake while on a restricted diet.

In spite of best efforts at strictly avoiding food allergens, accidental ingestions and exposures can occur; patients must be educated and prepared to recognize symptoms and initiate treatment of food allergic reactions. Individuals with a history of immediate allergic reactions or anaphylaxis, especially those with asthma, and those with allergy to foods typically associated with severe reactions (e.g., peanuts, tree nuts, fish, shellfish) should be prescribed an epinephrine auto-injector (EpiPen^{TM} or EpiPen Jr^{TM} [0.3 mg or 0.15 mg], Dey, Napa, CA; or Twinject^{TM}, Verus Pharmaceuticals, Inc., San Diego, CA). An emergency treatment plan indicating symptoms that require treatment with oral antihistamine (preferably liquid diphenhydramine or cetirizine) or epinephrine or both should be provided to the patient. Templates of anaphylaxis emergency treatment plans may be downloaded from the FAAN Web site (http://www.foodallergy.org), the Food Allergy Initiative Web site (http://www.foodallergyinitiative.org), or the American Academy of Allergy, Asthma and Immunology Web site (http://www.aaaai.org). Use of the autoinjector

should be demonstrated to the patient (and caregivers) and the technique reviewed periodically. At every physician encounter, patients should be reminded about the importance of having their emergency medications with them at all times and to check the expiration dates of their auto-injectors. Patients also must be instructed to seek evaluation at an emergency department or contact emergency services (i.e., contact 911) following the use of an epinephrine, since there is an approximate 20% risk of recurrence of allergic symptoms following initial improvement with or without treatment (so-called *biphasic anaphylaxis*), a minimum 4-hour observation period is recommended. Medic Alert bracelets indicating food allergy and specifying the treatment needed in case of a sudden reaction are helpful for older children and adults.

Studies in both children and adults indicate that symptomatic reactivity to food allergens is often lost over time, including peanuts, nuts, and seafood (99,184–189). Recent studies suggest that about 20% of young infants who experience peanut allergic reactions will outgrow their allergy if they have low levels (less than 2 kU$_A$/L) of peanut-specific serum IgE antibodies (169,188). Therefore, children with low levels of peanut-specific IgE should be re-evaluated to determine whether they have outgrown their allergy. Symptomatic IgE-dependent reactivity to food allergens is generally very specific and uncommonly involves more than one member of a botanical family (190,191) or animal species (58,192). Consequently, institution of an elimination diet totally excluding only foods proven to provoke food allergic reactions will result in symptomatic improvement, may lead to resolution of food allergy within a few years, and is unlikely to induce malnutrition or other eating disorders. Neither medications nor immunotherapy has emerged as useful treatment for most food allergies (193–196).

One approach being investigated is the use of anti-IgE antibody in the treatment of patients with peanut allergy. Using "humanized" monoclonal antibodies specific for the C$_e$3 domain of IgE (portion of the IgE Fc region that binds to the high affinity Fc$_e$ receptor), investigators have shown that anti-IgE therapy leads to a dose-dependent decrease in circulating IgE and respiratory symptoms, as well as a decrease in basophil and mast cell Fc$_e$ receptor numbers (197,198). In a double-blind placebo-controlled dose ranging trial, injections of anti-IgE antibodies (TNX-901) in patients with peanut allergy were shown to increase the average amount of peanut tolerated by peanut-allergic subjects, but 25% of the group showed no improvement (199). A less traditional approach, Chinese herbal medication, also has shown some promise in the murine model of peanut anaphylaxis (200,201).

Specific immunotherapy utilizing "engineered" recombinant food proteins are currently under development for the treatment of peanut allergy. One approach involves the mutation of IgE-binding epitopes on major peanut proteins. Mutational analyses of the immunodominant epitopes on the three major peanut proteins, *Ara h 1–3*, revealed that amino acid substitutions dramatically reduced IgE binding to individual epitopes (202). T-cell epitope mapping with peanut-specific T-cell lines demonstrated four immunodominant T-cell regions on the *Ara h 2* molecule, three of which mapped to different locations than the immunodominant IgE-binding epitopes. In a murine model of peanut anaphylaxis, the mutated recombinant proteins were able to "desensitize" peanut-sensitized mice in a manner similar to standard immunotherapy without the risk of inducing anaphylactic symptoms (201). In human subjects, oral desensitization has had mixed results and remains investigational as long-term oral tolerance has yet to be established (202–207).

■ **PREVENTION**

The role of dietary manipulation in the prevention of atopic disease in infants of allergic parents has been debated for many years. Recently, probiotic and prebiotic infant feedings have been proposed as preventive strategies. In short, conflicting results of various prevention strategies have been reported, and more studies are needed (208–215).

■ **NATURAL HISTORY**

The vast majority of childhood food allergies are lost over time, although certain food allergies tend to persist, such as those to peanuts, tree nuts, fish, and shellfish. Of note, despite clinical tolerance, the presence of IgE, as detected by skin test or RAST, may persist (216–218). The majority of cases of egg allergy resolve within a few years (219,220). Patients with an egg-specific IgE level greater than 50 kU/L are unlikely to develop egg tolerance (221). Cow's milk allergy affects 2.5% of children under 2 years of age (222,223). The potential for persistence of cow's milk allergy along with cow's milk-specific IgE levels effect on prognosis should be taken into consideration when counseling families regarding expected clinical outcomes (224). Non-IgE-mediated cow's milk allergy is typically a transient childhood condition that is almost always outgrown but must be managed carefully as challenge can be hazardous (86). IgE-mediated cow's milk allergy may persist in up to 20% of children. In children with cow's milk or egg IgE-mediated sensitivity, those who became tolerant had antibodies to conformational epitopes, whereas those with persistent hypersensitivity reacted primarily to linear epitopes (37). Peanut and tree nut allergies affect about 0.5% to 1.3% of children and may be increasing over time (50,188,225). It is likely to be a lifelong disorder for most patients, although 20% to 25% outgrow peanut (188,226–228), and up to 9% outgrow tree nut

allergies (184). Immunodominant IgE epitopes of the major peanut allergens *Ara h 1* (recognized by >90% of peanut-allergic individuals) and *Ara h 2* are linear (229,230) and may explain the persistence of peanut allergy. A food allergy rarely recurs once it has resolved, although this has been documented in unusual cases with peanut and tree nut (231). Most allergy experts use a combination of historical information from accidental exposures and periodic *in vitro* or skin testing to assess if oral tolerance has developed. Medically supervised food challenges are required to confirm that a food allergy has resolved, as *in vitro* and skin tests can remain positive in patients who achieve clinical tolerance, and conversely, tests can become negative in patients who still react on ingestion (1).

■ **SUMMARY**

Food allergy is a common medical problem seen particularly early in life. Many of the common food allergies are outgrown in the first few years of life. Ingestion of foods in an allergic individual can quickly provoke cutaneous, respiratory, and gastrointestinal symptoms and in a subset of patients, anaphylaxis can occur. Recent research has continued to characterize the various food hypersensitivity disorders, but our understanding of the basic immunopathologic mechanisms remains incomplete. It is anticipated that new information regarding the pathogenesis of food allergy and new forms of therapy will become available as future studies are completed, analyzed, and reported. Further tables on food allergy are included on the Web site.

■ **REFERENCES**

1. Sampson HA. Update on food allergy. *J Allergy Clin Immunol.* 2004;113(5):805–819.
2. Steinke M, Fiocchi A, Kirchlechner V, et al. Perceived food allergy in children in 10 European nations. A randomised telephone survey. *Int Arch Allergy Immunol.* 2007;143(4):290–295.
3. Bock SA. Prospective appraisal of complaints of adverse reactions to foods in children during the first 3 years of life. *Pediatrics.* 1987;79(5):683–688.
4. Cruz NV, Wilson BG, Fiocchi A, et al. Survey of physicians' approach to food allergy, Part 1: Prevalence and manifestations. *Ann Allergy Asthma Immunol.* 2007;99(4):325–333.
5. Rona RJ, Keil T, Summers C, et al. The prevalence of food allergy: a meta-analysis. *J Allergy Clin Immunol.* 2007;120(3):638–646.
6. Sicherer SH, Sampson HA. Peanut allergy: emerging concepts and approaches for an apparent epidemic. *J Allergy Clin Immunol.* 2007;120(3):491–503.
7. Sicherer SH, Munoz-Furlong A, Sampson HA. Prevalence of seafood allergy in the United States determined by a random telephone survey. *J Allergy Clin Immunol.* 2004;114(1):159–165.
8. Eigenmann PA, Sicherer SH, Borkowski TA, et al. Prevalence of IgE-mediated food allergy among children with atopic dermatitis. *Pediatrics.* 1998;101(3):E8.
9. Hill DJ, Hosking CS. Food allergy and atopic dermatitis in infancy: an epidemiologic study. *Pediatr Allergy Immunol.* 2004; 15(5):421–427.
10. Venter C, Pereira B, Grundy J, et al. Incidence of parentally reported and clinically diagnosed food hypersensitivity in the first year of life. *J Allergy Clin Immunol.* 2006;117(5):1118–1124.
11. Venter C, Pereira B, Voigt K, et al. Prevalence and cumulative incidence of food hypersensitivity in the first 3 years of life. *Allergy.* 2008;63(3):354–359.

12. Chehade M, Mayer L. Oral tolerance and its relation to food hypersensitivities. *J Allergy Clin Immunol.* 2005;115(1):3–12.

13. Mestecky J, McGhee JR, Elson C. Intestinal IgA system. *Immunol Allergy Clin North Am.* 1988;8:349–368.

14. Husby S, Foged N, Host A, et al. Passage of dietary antigens into the blood of children with coeliac disease. Quantification and size distribution of absorbed antigens. *Gut.* 1987;28(9):1062–1072.

15. Wilson SJ, Walzer M. Absorption of undigested proteins in human beings, IV. Absorption of unaltered egg protein in infants. *Am J Dis Child.* 1935;50:49–54.

16. Gray I, Walzer. Studies in mucous membrane hypersensitiveness. III The allergic reaction of the passively sensitized rectal mucous membrane. *Am J Digest Dis.* 1938;4:707–711.

17. Mayer L. Mucosal immunity. *Pediatrics.* 2003;111(6 Pt 3):1595–1600.

18. Sudo N, Sawamura S, Tanaka K, et al. The requirement of intestinal bacterial flora for the development of an IgE production system fully susceptible to oral tolerance induction. *J Immunol.* 1997;159(4):1739–1745.

19. Johansson SG, Dannaeus A, Lilja G. The relevance of anti-food antibodies for the diagnosis of food allergy. *Ann Allergy.* 1984;53(6 Pt 2):665–672.

20. Savilhati E, Salmenpera L, Tainio V, et al. Prolonged exclusive breast-feeding results in low serum concentration of immunoglobulin G, A, and M. *Acta Paediatr Scand.* 1987;76:1–6.

21. Kletter B, Gery I, Freier S, et al. Immune responses of normal infants to cow milk. I. Antibody type and kinetics of production. *Int Arch Allergy Appl Immunol.* 1971;40(4–5):656–666.

22. May CD, Remigio L, Feldman J, et al. A study of serum antibodies to isolated milk proteins and ovalbumin in infants and children. *Clin Allergy.* 1977;7(6):583–595.

23. Breiteneder H, Radauer C. A classification of plant food allergens. *J Allergy Clin Immunol.* 2004;113(5):821–830.

24. Sampson HA. Food allergy. Part 1: immunopathogenesis and clinical disorders. *J Allergy Clin Immunol.* 1999;103(5 Pt 1):717–728.

25. Vadas P, Wai Y, Burks W, et al. Detection of peanut allergens in breast milk of lactating women. *JAMA.* 2001;285(13):1746–1748.

26. Wal JM. Cow's milk allergens. *Allergy.* 1998;53(11):1013–1022.

27. Bleumink E, Young E. Identification of the atopic allergen in cow's milk. *Int Arch Allergy Appl Immunol.* 1968;34(6):521–543.

28. Chatchatee P, Jarvinen KM, Bardina L, et al. Identification of IgE and IgG binding epitopes on beta- and kappa-casein in cow's milk allergic patients. *Clin Exp Allergy.* 2001;31(8):1256–1262.

29. Jarvinen KM, Beyer K, Vila L, et al. B-cell epitopes as a screening instrument for persistent cow's milk allergy. *J Allergy Clin Immunol.* 2002;110(2):293–297.

30. Vila L, Beyer K, Jarvinen KM, et al. Role of conformational and linear epitopes in the achievement of tolerance in cow's milk allergy. *Clin Exp Allergy.* 2001;31(10):1599–1606.

31. Sicherer SH, Sampson HA. Cow's milk protein-specific IgE concentrations in two age groups of milk-allergic children and in children achieving clinical tolerance. *Clin Exp Allergy.* 1999;29(4):507–512.

32. Bellioni-Businco B, Paganelli R, Lucenti P, et al. Allergenicity of goat's milk in children with cow's milk allergy. *J Allergy Clin Immunol.* 1999;103(6):1191–1194.

33. Werfel SJ, Cooke SK, Sampson HA. Clinical reactivity to beef in children allergic to cow's milk. *J Allergy Clin Immunol.* 1997;99(3):293–300.

34. Kulig M, Bergmann R, Klettke U, et al. Natural course of sensitization to food and inhalant allergens during the first 6 years of life. *J Allergy Clin Immunol.* 1999;103(6):1173–1179.

35. Aabin B, Poulsen LK, Ebbehoj K, et al. Identification of IgE-binding egg white proteins: comparison of results obtained by different methods. *Int Arch Allergy Immunol.* 1996;109(1):50–57.

36. Sampson HA. Legumes, eggs, and milk. *Allergy.* 1998;53(46 Suppl):38–43.

37. Cooke SK, Sampson HA. Allergenic properties of ovomucoid in man. *J Immunol.* 1997;159(4):2026–2032.

38. Urisu A, Ando H, Morita Y, et al. Allergenic activity of heated and ovomucoid-depleted egg white. *J Allergy Clin Immunol.* 1997;100(2):171–176.

39. Nowak-Wegrzyn A, Sicherer S, Shreffler W, et al. A trial diet containing baked egg in children with egg allergy. [abstract]. *J Allergy Clin Immun.* 119[1], S194. 2007.

40. Illi S, von Mutius E, Lau S, et al. The pattern of atopic sensitization is associated with the development of asthma in childhood. *J Allergy Clin Immunol.* 2001;108(5):709–714.

41. Burks AW, Williams LW, Helm RM, et al. Identification of a major peanut allergen, Ara h I, in patients with atopic dermatitis and positive peanut challenges. *J Allergy Clin Immunol.* 1991;88(2):172–179.

42. Burks AW, Williams LW, Connaughton C, et al. Identification and characterization of a second major peanut allergen, Ara h II, with use of the sera of patients with atopic dermatitis and positive peanut challenge. *J Allergy Clin Immunol.* 1992;90(6 Pt 1):962–969.

43. Rabjohn P, West C, Helm E, et al. A third major peanut allergen identified by soy-adsorbed serum IgE from peanut sensitive individuals. [abstract] *J Allergy Clin Immun.* 101[S240]. 1998.

44. Kleber-Janke T, Crameri R, Scheurer S, et al. Patient-tailored cloning of allergens by phage display: peanut (Arachis hypogaea) profilin, a food allergen derived from a rare mRNA. *J Chromatogr B Biomed Sci Appl.* 2001;756(1–2):295–305.

45. Mittag D, Akkerdaas J, Ballmer-Weber BK, et al. Ara h 8, a Bet v 1-homologous allergen from peanut, is a major allergen in patients with combined birch pollen and peanut allergy. *J Allergy Clin Immunol.* 2004;114(6):1410–1417.

46. Glaspole IN, de Leon MP, Rolland JM, et al. Characterization of the T-cell epitopes of a major peanut allergen, Ara h 2. *Allergy.* 2005;60(1):35–40.

47. Hourihane JO, Bedwani SJ, Dean TP, et al. Randomised, double blind, crossover challenge study of allergenicity of peanut oils in subjects allergic to peanuts. *BMJ.* 1997;314(7087):1084–1088.

48. Beardslee TA, Zeece MG, Sarath G, et al. Soybean glycinin G1 acidic chain shares IgE epitopes with peanut allergen Ara h 3. *Int Arch Allergy Immunol.* 2000;123(4):299–307.

49. Bush RK, Taylor SL, Nordlee JA, et al. Soybean oil is not allergenic to soybean-sensitive individuals. *J Allergy Clin Immunol.* 1985;76(2 Pt 1):242–245.

50. Sicherer SH, Munoz-Furlong A, Sampson HA. Prevalence of peanut and tree nut allergy in the United States determined by means of a random digit dial telephone survey: a 5-year follow-up study. *J Allergy Clin Immunol.* 2003;112(6):1203–1207.

51. Green TD, LaBelle VS, Steele PH, et al. Clinical characteristics of peanut-allergic children: recent changes. *Pediatrics.* 2007;120(6):1304–1310.

52. Sicherer SH, Furlong TJ, Munoz-Furlong A, et al. A voluntary registry for peanut and tree nut allergy: characteristics of the first 5149 registrants. *J Allergy Clin Immunol.* 2001;108(1):128–132.

53. Hourihane JO, Kilburn SA, Dean P, et al. Clinical characteristics of peanut allergy. *Clin Exp Allergy.* 1997;27(6):634–639.

54. Sicherer SH, Burks AW, Sampson HA. Clinical features of acute allergic reactions to peanut and tree nuts in children. *Pediatrics.* 1998;102(1):e6.

55. O'Neil C, Helbling AA, Lehrer SB. Allergic reactions to fish. *Clin Rev Allergy.* 1993;11(2):183–200.

56. Van Do T, Elsayed S, Florvaag E, et al. Allergy to fish parvalbumins: studies on the cross-reactivity of allergens from 9 commonly consumed fish. *J Allergy Clin Immunol.* 2005;116(6):1314–1320.

57. Elsayed S, Apold J. Immunochemical analysis of cod fish allergen M: locations of the immunoglobulin binding sites as demonstrated by the native and synthetic peptides. *Allergy.* 1983;38(7):449–459.

58. Bernhisel-Broadbent J, Scanlon SM, Sampson HA. Fish hypersensitivity. I. In vitro and oral challenge results in fish-allergic patients. *J Allergy Clin Immunol.* 1992;89(3):730–737.

59. Reese G, Ayuso R, Carle T, et al. IgE-binding epitopes of shrimp tropomyosin, the major allergen Pen a 1. *Int Arch Allergy Immunol.* 1999;118(2–4):300–301.

60. Waring NP, Daul CB, deShazo RD, et al. Hypersensitivity reactions to ingested crustacea: clinical evaluation and diagnostic studies in shrimp-sensitive individuals. *J Allergy Clin Immunol.* 1985;76(3):440–445.

61. Reese G, Ayuso R, Lehrer SB. Tropomyosin: an invertebrate pan-allergen. *Int Arch Allergy Immunol.* 1999;119(4):247–258.

62. Sutton R, Hill DJ, Baldo BA, et al. Immunoglobulin E antibodies to ingested cereal flour components: studies with sera from subjects with asthma and eczema. *Clin Allergy.* 1982;12(1):63–74.

63. Palosuo K, Varjonen E, Kekki OM, et al. Wheat omega-5 gliadin is a major allergen in children with immediate allergy to ingested wheat. *J Allergy Clin Immunol* 2001;108(4):634–638.

64. Palosuo K, Varjonen E, Nurkkala J, et al. Transglutaminase-mediated cross-linking of a peptic fraction of omega-5 gliadin enhances IgE reactivity in wheat-dependent, exercise-induced anaphylaxis. *J Allergy Clin Immunol.* 2003;111(6):1386–1392.

65. Sandiford CP, Tatham AS, Fido R, et al. Identification of the major water/salt insoluble wheat proteins involved in cereal hypersensitivity. *Clin Exp Allergy.* 1997;27(10):1120–1129.

66. Ebner C, Hoffmann-Sommergruber K, Breiteneder H. Plant food allergens homologous to pathogenesis-related proteins. *Allergy.* 2001;56 Suppl 67:43–44.

67. Breiteneder H, Clare Mills EN. Plant food allergens—structural and functional aspects of allergenicity. *Biotechnol Adv.* 2005;23(6):395–399.

68. Sampson HA, Mendelson L, Rosen JP. Fatal and near-fatal anaphylactic reactions to food in children and adolescents. *N Engl J Med.* 1992;327(6):380–384.

69. Greaves M. Chronic urticaria. *J Allergy Clin Immunol.* 2000;105(4):664–672.

70. Bruijnzeel-Koomen C, Ortolani C, Aas K, et al. Adverse reactions to food. European Academy of Allergology and Clinical Immunology Subcommittee. *Allergy.* 1995;50(8):623–635.

71. Chan EF, Mowad C. Contact dermatitis to foods and spices. *Am J Contact Dermat.* 1998;9(2):71–79.

72. Burks AW, James JM, Hiegel A, et al. Atopic dermatitis and food hypersensitivity reactions. *J Pediatr.* 1998;132(1):132–136.

73. Burks AW, Mallory SB, Williams LW, et al. Atopic dermatitis: clinical relevance of food hypersensitivity reactions. *J Pediatr.* 1988;113(3):447–451.

74. Sampson HA. Food hypersensitivity and atopic dermatitis. *Allergy Proc.* 1991;12(5):327–331.

75. Sampson HA, Broadbent KR, Bernhisel-Broadbent J. Spontaneous release of histamine from basophils and histamine-releasing factor in patients with atopic dermatitis and food hypersensitivity. *N Engl J Med.* 1989;321(4):228–232.

76. Stenton GR, Vliagoftis H, Befus AD. Role of intestinal mast cells in modulating gastrointestinal pathophysiology. *Ann Allergy Asthma Immunol.* 1998;81(1):1–11.

77. Gonsalves N. Food allergies and eosinophilic gastrointestinal illness. *Gastroenterol Clin North Am.* 2007;36(1):75–91, vi.

78. Steffen RM, Wyllie R, Petras RE, et al. The spectrum of eosinophilic gastroenteritis. Report of six pediatric cases and review of the literature. *Clin Pediatr (Phila).* 1991;30(7):404–411.

79. Talley NJ, Shorter RG, Phillips SF, et al. Eosinophilic gastroenteritis: a clinicopathological study of patients with disease of the mucosa, muscle layer, and subserosal tissues. *Gut.* 1990;31(1):54–58.

80. Snyder JD, Rosenblum N, Wershil B, et al. Pyloric stenosis and eosinophilic gastroenteritis in infants. *J Pediatr Gastroenterol Nutr.* 1987;6(4):543–547.

81. Spergel JM. Eosinophilic esophagitis in adults and children: evidence for a food allergy component in many patients. *Curr Opin Allergy Clin Immunol.* 2007;7(3):274–278.

82. Brown-Whitehorn T, Liacouras CA. Eosinophilic esophagitis. *Curr Opin Pediatr.* 2007;19(5):575–580.

83. Ferguson DD, Foxx-Orenstein AE. Eosinophilic esophagitis: an update. *Dis Esophagus.* 2007;20(1):2–8.

84. Canani RB, Ruotolo S, Auricchio L, et al. Diagnostic accuracy of the atopy patch test in children with food allergy-related gastrointestinal symptoms. *Allergy.* 2007;62(7):738–743.

85. Sugnanam KK, Collins JT, Smith PK, et al. Dichotomy of food and inhalant allergen sensitization in eosinophilic esophagitis. *Allergy.* 2007;62(11):1257–1260.

86. Maloney J, Nowak-Wegrzyn A. Educational clinical case series for pediatric allergy and immunology: allergic proctocolitis, food protein-induced enterocolitis syndrome and allergic eosinophilic gastroenteritis with protein-losing gastroenteropathy as manifestations of non-IgE-mediated cow's milk allergy. *Pediatr Allergy Immunol.* 2007;18(4):360–367.

87. Egger M, Mutschlechner S, Wopfner N, et al. Pollen-food syndromes associated with weed pollinosis: an update from the molecular point of view. *Allergy.* 2006;61(4):461–476.

88. Mari A, Ballmer-Weber BK, Vieths S. The oral allergy syndrome: improved diagnostic and treatment methods. *Curr Opin Allergy Clin Immunol.* 2005;5(3):267–273.

89. Enberg RN, Leickly FE, McCullough J, et al. Watermelon and ragweed share allergens. *J Allergy Clin Immunol.* 1987;79(6):867–875.

90. Lahti A, Bjorksten F, Hannuksela M. Allergy to birch pollen and apple, and cross-reactivity of the allergens studied with the RAST. *Allergy.* 1980;35(4):297–300.

91. Andersen KE, Lowenstein H. An investigation of the possible immunological relationship between allergen extracts from birch pollen, hazelnut, potato and apple. *Contact Dermatitis.* 1978;4(2):73–79.

92. Halmepuro L, Lowenstein H. Immunological investigation of possible structural similarities between pollen antigens and antigens in apple, carrot and celery tuber. *Allergy.* 1985;40(4):264–272.

93. Ballmer-Weber BK, Vieths S, Luttkopf D, et al. Celery allergy confirmed by double-blind, placebo-controlled food challenge: a clinical study in 32 subjects with a history of adverse reactions to celery root. *J Allergy Clin Immunol.* 2000;106(2):373–378.

94. Gall H, Kalveram KJ, Forck G, et al. Kiwi fruit allergy: a new birch pollen-associated food allergy. *J Allergy Clin Immunol.* 1994;94(1):70–76.

95. Ortolani C, Ispano M, Pastorello EA, et al. Comparison of results of skin-prick tests (with fresh foods and commercial food extracts) and RAST in 100 patients with oral allergy syndrome. *J Allergy Clin Immunol.* 1989;83(3):683–690.

96. Jankiewicz A, Aulepp H, Baltes W, et al. Allergic sensitization to native and heated celery root in pollen-sensitive patients investigated by skin test and IgE binding. *Int Arch Allergy Immunol.* 1996;111(3):268–278.

97. James J. Anaphylactic reactions to foods. *Immunol Allergy Clin North Am.* 2001;21:653–667.

98. Yunginger JW, Sweeney KG, Sturner WQ, et al. Fatal food-induced anaphylaxis. *JAMA.* 1988;260(10):1450–1452.

99. Bock SA, Atkins FM. Patterns of food hypersensitivity during sixteen years of double-blind, placebo-controlled food challenges. *J Pediatr.* 1990;117(4):561–567.

100. Onorato J, Merland N, Terral C, et al. Placebo-controlled double-blind food challenge in asthma. *J Allergy Clin Immunol.* 1986;78(6):1139–1146.

101. Novembre E, de Martino M, Vierucci A. Foods and respiratory allergy. *J Allergy Clin Immunol.* 1988;81(5 Pt 2):1059–1065.

102. Oehling A, Baena Cagnani CE. Food allergy and child asthma. *Allergol Immunopathol (Madr).* 1980;8(1):7–14.

103. Businco L, Falconieri P, Giampietro P, et al. Food allergy and asthma. *Pediatr Pulmonol. Suppl.* 1995;11:59–60.

104. Yazicioglu M, Baspinar I, Ones U, et al. Egg and milk allergy in asthmatic children: assessment by immulite allergy food panel, skin-prick tests and double-blind placebo-controlled food challenges. *Allergol Immunopathol (Madr).* 1999;27(6):287–293.

105. Hill DJ, Firer MA, Shelton MJ, et al. Manifestations of milk allergy in infancy: clinical and immunologic findings. *J Pediatr.* 1986;109(2):270–276.

106. Bock SA. The incidence of severe adverse reactions to food in Colorado. *J Allergy Clin Immunol.* 1992;90(4 Pt 1):683–685.

107. James JM, Bernhisel-Broadbent J, Sampson HA. Respiratory reactions provoked by double-blind food challenges in children. *Am J Respir Crit Care Med.* 1994;149(1):59–64.

108. James JM, Eigenmann PA, Eggleston PA, et al. Airway reactivity changes in asthmatic patients undergoing blinded food challenges. *Am J Respir Crit Care Med.* 1996;153(2):597–603.

109. Zwetchkenbaum JF, Skufca R, Nelson HS. An examination of food hypersensitivity as a cause of increased bronchial responsiveness to inhaled methacholine. *J Allergy Clin Immunol.* 1991;88(3 Pt 1):360–364.

110. Baur X, Posch A. Characterized allergens causing bakers' asthma. *Allergy.* 1998;53(6):562–566.

111. Pavlovic M, Spasojevic M, Tasic Z, et al. Bronchial hyperactivity in bakers and its relation to atopy and skin reactivity. *Sci Total Environ.* 2001;270(1–3):71–75.

112. Bulat P, Myny K, Braeckman L, et al. Exposure to inhalable dust, wheat flour and alpha-amylase allergens in industrial and traditional bakeries. *Ann Occup Hyg.* 2004;48(1):57–63.

113. Quirce S, Polo F, Figueredo E, et al. Occupational asthma caused by soybean flour in bakers—differences with soybean-induced epidemic asthma. *Clin Exp Allergy.* 2000;30(6):839–846.

114. Codina R, Ardusso L, Lockey RF, et al. Identification of the soybean hull allergens involved in sensitization to soybean dust in a rural population from Argentina and N-terminal sequence of a major 50 KD allergen. *Clin Exp Allergy.* 2002;32(7):1059–1063.

115. Rodrigo MJ, Cruz MJ, Garcia MD, et al. Epidemic asthma in Barcelona: an evaluation of new strategies for the control of soybean dust emission. *Int Arch Allergy Immunol.* 2004;134(2):158–164.

116. Rodriguez J, Reano M, Vives R, et al. Occupational asthma caused by fish inhalation. *Allergy.* 1997;52(8):866–869.

117. Douglas JD, McSharry C, Blaikie L, et al. Occupational asthma caused by automated salmon processing. *Lancet.* 1995;346(8977):737–740.

118. Kalogeromitros D, Makris M, Gregoriou S, et al. IgE-mediated sensitization in seafood processing workers. *Allergy Asthma Proc.* 2006;27(4):399–403.

119. Cartier A, Malo JL, Ghezzo H, et al. IgE sensitization in snow crab-processing workers. *J Allergy Clin Immunol.* 1986;78(2):344–348.

120. Malo JL, Cartier A, Ghezzo H, et al. Patterns of improvement in spirometry, bronchial hyperresponsiveness, and specific IgE antibody levels after cessation of exposure to occupational asthma caused by snow-crab processing. *Am Rev Respir Dis.* 1988;138(4):807–812.

121. Malo JL, Chretien P, McCants M, et al. Detection of snow-crab antigens by air sampling of a snow-crab production plant. *Clin Exp Allergy.* 1997;27(1):75–78.

122. Wang J, Sampson HA. Food anaphylaxis. *Clin Exp Allergy.* 2007;37(5):651–660.

123. Beaudouin E, Renaudin JM, Morisset M, et al. Food-dependent exercise-induced anaphylaxis–update and current data. *Allerg Immunol* (Paris). 2006;38(2):45–51.

124. Roberts G. Anaphylaxis to foods. *Pediatr Allergy Immunol.* 2007;18(6):543–548.

125. Derby CJ, Gowland MH, Hourihane JO. Sesame allergy in Britain: a questionnaire survey of members of the Anaphylaxis Campaign. *Pediatr Allergy Immunol.* 2005;16(2):171–175.

126. Gangur V, Kelly C, Navuluri L. Sesame allergy: a growing food allergy of global proportions? *Ann Allergy Asthma Immunol.* 2005;95(1):4–11.

127. Navuluri L, Parvataneni S, Hassan H, et al. Allergic and anaphylactic response to sesame seeds in mice: identification of Ses i 3 and basic subunit of 11s globulins as allergens. *Int Arch Allergy Immunol.* 2006;140(3):270–276.

128. Webb LM, Lieberman P. Anaphylaxis: a review of 601 cases. *Ann Allergy Asthma Immunol.* 2006;97(1):39–43.

129. Cianferoni A, Novembre E, Mugnaini L, et al. Clinical features of acute anaphylaxis in patients admitted to a university hospital: an 11-year retrospective review (1985–1996). *Ann Allergy Asthma Immunol.* 2001;87(1):27–32.

130. Sheffer AL, Tong AK, Murphy GF, et al. Exercise-induced anaphylaxis: a serious form of physical allergy associated with mast cell degranulation. *J Allergy Clin Immunol.* 1985;75(4):479–484.

131. Kidd JM III, Cohen SH, Sosman AJ, et al. Food-dependent exercise-induced anaphylaxis. *J Allergy Clin Immunol.* 1983;71(4):407–411.

132. Novey HS, Fairshter RD, Salness K, et al. Postprandial exercise-induced anaphylaxis. *J Allergy Clin Immunol.* 1983;71(5):498–504.

133. Du TG. Food-dependent exercise-induced anaphylaxis in childhood. *Pediatr Allergy Immunol.* 2007;18(5):455–463.

134. Maulitz RM, Pratt DS, Schocket AL. Exercise-induced anaphylactic reaction to shellfish. *J Allergy Clin Immunol.* 1979;63(6):433–434.

135. Sicherer SH. Food protein-induced enterocolitis syndrome: case presentations and management lessons. *J Allergy Clin Immunol.* 2005;115(1):149–156.

136. Xanthakos SA, Schwimmer JB, Melin-Aldana H, et al. Prevalence and outcome of allergic colitis in healthy infants with rectal bleeding: a prospective cohort study. *J Pediatr Gastroenterol Nutr.* 2005;41(1):16–22.

137. Kagnoff MF. Celiac disease: pathogenesis of a model immunogenetic disease. *J Clin Invest.* 2007;117(1):41–49.

138. Craig D, Robins G, Howdle PD. Advances in celiac disease. *Curr Opin Gastroenterol.* 2007;23(2):142–148.

139. Torres MI, Lopez Casado MA, Rios A. New aspects in celiac disease. *World J Gastroenterol.* 2007;13(8):1156–1161.

140. Rubin CE, Brandborg LL, Phelps PC, et al. Studies of celiac disease. I. The apparent identical and specific nature of the duodenal and proximal jejunal lesion in celiac disease and idiopathic sprue. *Gastroenterology.* 1960; 38:28–49.

141. Yardley JH, Bayless TM, Norton JH, et al. Celiac disease. A study of the jejunal epithelium before and after a gluten-free diet. *N Engl J Med.* 1962; 267:1173–1179.

142. Baklien K, Brandtzaeg P, Fausa O. Immunoglobulins in jejunal mucosa and serum from patients with adult coeliac disease. *Scand J Gastroenterol.* 1977; 12(2):149–159.

143. Kumar V, Lerner A, Valeski JE, et al. Endomysial antibodies in the diagnosis of celiac disease and the effect of gluten on antibody titers. *Immunol Invest.* 1989; 18(1–4):533–544.

144. Levine A, Bujanover Y, Reif S, et al. Comparison of assays for anti-endomysial and anti-transglutaminase antibodies for diagnosis of pediatric celiac disease. *Isr Med Assoc.* J 2000; 2(2):122–125.

145. Sugai E, Selvaggio G, Vazquez H, et al. Tissue transglutaminase antibodies in celiac disease: assessment of a commercial kit. *Am J Gastroenterol.* 2000;95(9):2318–2322.

146. Trier JS. Celiac Sprue. In: Sleisenger M, Fordtran JS, eds. *Gastrointestinal Disease: Pathophysiology, Diagnosis, Management.* Philadelphia: WB Saunders;1993:1078.

147. NIH. *NIH Consensus Development Conference on Celiac Disease.* 21(1), 1–22. 2004.

148. Alonso-Llamazares J, Gibson LE, Rogers RS III. Clinical, pathologic, and immunopathologic features of dermatitis herpetiformis: review of the Mayo Clinic experience. *Int J Dermatol.* 2007;46(9):910–919.

149. Hall RP. The pathogenesis of dermatitis herpetiformis: recent advances. *J Am Acad Dermatol.* 1987;16(6):1129–1144.

150. Katz SI, Hall RP, III, Lawley TJ, et al. Dermatitis herpetiformis: the skin and the gut. *Ann Intern Med.* 1980;93(6):857–874.

151. Taudorf E, Malling HJ, Laursen LC, et al. Reproducibility of histamine skin-prick test. Inter- and intravariation using histamine dihydrochloride 1, 5, and 10 mg/ml. *Allergy.* 1985;40(5):344–349.

152. Bock SA, Lee WY, Remigio L, et al. Appraisal of skin tests with food extracts for diagnosis of food hypersensitivity. *Clin Allergy.* 1978;8(6):559–564.

153. Sporik R, Hill DJ, Hosking CS. Specificity of allergen skin testing in predicting positive open food challenges to milk, egg and peanut in children. *Clin Exp Allergy.* 2000;30(11):1540–1546.

154. Hill DJ, Hosking CS, Reyes-Benito LV. Reducing the need for food allergen challenges in young children: a comparison of in vitro with in vivo tests. *Clin Exp Allergy.* 2001;31(7):1031–1035.

155. Heine RG, Laske N, Hill DJ. The diagnosis and management of egg allergy. *Curr Allergy Asthma Rep.* 2006;6(2):145–152.

156. Sampson HA, Albergo R. Comparison of results of skin tests, RAST, and double-blind, placebo-controlled food challenges in children with atopic dermatitis. *J Allergy Clin Immunol.* 1984;74(1):26–33.

157. Sampson HA. Comparative study of commercial food antigen extracts for the diagnosis of food hypersensitivity. *J Allergy Clin Immunol.* 1988;82(5 Pt 1):718–726.

158. Atkins FM, Steinberg SS, Metcalfe DD. Evaluation of immediate adverse reactions to foods in adult patients. I. Correlation of demographic, laboratory, and skin-prick test data with response to controlled oral food challenge. *J Allergy Clin Immunol.* 1985;75(3):348–355.

159. Sampson HA. Role of immediate food hypersensitivity in the pathogenesis of atopic dermatitis. *J Allergy Clin Immunol.* 1983; 71(5):473–480.

160. Rosen JP, Selcow JE, Mendelson LM, et al. Skin testing with natural foods in patients suspected of having food allergies: is it a necessity? *J Allergy Clin Immunol.* 1994;93(6):1068–1070.

161. Menardo JL, Bousquet J, Rodiere M, et al. Skin test reactivity in infancy. *J Allergy Clin Immunol.* 1985;75(6):646–651.

162. De Boissieu D, Waguet JC, Dupont C. The atopy patch tests for detection of cow's milk allergy with digestive symptoms. *J Pediatr.* 2003;142(2):203–205.

163. Niggemann B, Reibel S, Wahn U. The atopy patch test (APT)—a useful tool for the diagnosis of food allergy in children with atopic dermatitis. *Allergy.* 2000;55(3):281–285.

164. Turjanmaa K. "Atopy patch tests" in the diagnosis of delayed food hypersensitivity. *Allerg Immunol* (Paris). 2002;34(3):95–97.

165. Spergel JM, Andrews T, Brown-Whitehorn TF, et al. Treatment of eosinophilic esophagitis with specific food elimination diet directed by a combination of skin-prick and patch tests. *Ann Allergy Asthma Immunol.* 2005;95(4):336–343.

166. Mehl A, Rolinck-Werninghaus C, Staden U, et al. The atopy patch test in the diagnostic workup of suspected food-related symptoms in children. *J Allergy Clin Immunol.* 2006;118(4):923–929.

167. Sampson HA, Ho DG. Relationship between food-specific IgE concentrations and the risk of positive food challenges in children and adolescents. *J Allergy Clin Immunol.* 1997;100(4):444–451.

168. Sampson HA. Utility of food-specific IgE concentrations in predicting symptomatic food allergy. *J Allergy Clin Immunol.* 2001;107(5):891–896.

169. Perry TT, Matsui EC, Kay Conover-Walker M, et al. The relationship of allergen-specific IgE levels and oral food challenge outcome. *J Allergy Clin Immunol.* 2004;114(1):144–149.

170. Sampson HA. Utility of food-specific IgE concentrations in predicting symptomatic food allergy. *J Allergy Clin Immunol.* 2001;107(5):891–896.

171. Perry TT, Matsui EC, Connover-Walker MK, et al. The relationship of allergen-specific IgE levels and oral food challenge outcome. *J Allergy Clin Immun.* 2004;114(1):127–130.

172. Sampson HA. Food allergy. Part 2: diagnosis and management. *J Allergy Clin Immunol.* 1999;103(6):981–989.

173. Bock SA, Sampson HA, Atkins FM, et al. Double-blind, placebo-controlled food challenge (DBPCFC) as an office procedure: a manual. *J Allergy Clin Immunol.* 1988;82(6):986–997.

174. Sampson H. Diagnosing food allergy. In: Spector S, ed. *Provocation Testing in Clinical Practice.* New York: Marcel Dekker; 1995:623–646.

175. Hansen TK, Bindslev-Jensen C. Codfish allergy in adults. Identification and diagnosis. *Allergy.* 1992;47(6):610–617.

176. Norgaard A, Bindslev-Jensen C. Egg and milk allergy in adults. Diagnosis and characterization. *Allergy.* 1992;47(5):503–509.

177. Sicherer SH, Morrow EH, Sampson HA. Dose-response in double-blind, placebo-controlled oral food challenges in children with atopic dermatitis. *J Allergy Clin Immunol.* 2000;105(3):582–586.

178. Metcalfe D, Sampson H. Workshop on experimental methodology for clinical studies of adverse reactions to foods and food additives. *J Allergy Clin Immunol.* 1990;86:421–442.

179. Schwartz LB, Yunginger JW, Miller J, Bokhari R, Dull D. Time course of appearance and disappearance of human mast cell tryptase in the circulation after anaphylaxis. *J Clin Invest.* 1989;83(5):1551–1555.

180. Sicherer SH, Eigenmann PA, Sampson HA. Clinical features of food protein-induced enterocolitis syndrome. *J Pediatr.* 1998;133(2):214–219.

181. Powell GK. Food protein-induced enterocolitis of infancy: differential diagnosis and management. *Compr Ther.* 1986;12(2):28–37.

182. Executive Committee AAA&I. Personnel and equipment to treat systemic reactions caused by immunotherapy with allergic extracts. *J Allergy Clin Immunol.* 1986;77:271–273.

183. Barnes Koerner C, Sampson H. In: Metcalfe D, Sampson H, Simon R, eds. *Food Allergy: Adverse Reactions to Foods and Food Additives.* Boston: Blackwell Scientific Publications; 1996: 461–484.

184. Fleischer DM, Conover-Walker MK, Matsui EC, et al. The natural history of tree nut allergy. *J Allergy Clin Immunol.* 2005;116(5):1087–1093.

185. Sampson HA, Scanlon SM. Natural history of food hypersensitivity in children with atopic dermatitis. *J Pediatr.* 1989;115(1):23–27.

186. Pastorello EA, Stocchi L, Pravettoni V, et al. Role of the elimination diet in adults with food allergy. *J Allergy Clin Immunol.* 1989;84(4 Pt 1):475–483.

187. Hourihane JO, Roberts SA, Warner JO. Resolution of peanut allergy: case-control study. *BMJ.* 1998;316(7140):1271–1275.

188. Skolnick HS, Conover-Walker MK, Koerner CB, et al. The natural history of peanut allergy. *J Allergy Clin Immunol.* 2001;107(2):367–374.

189. Businco L, Benincori N, Cantani A, et al. Chronic diarrhea due to cow's milk allergy. A 4- to 10-year follow-up study. *Ann Allergy.* 1985;55(6):844–847.

190. Bernhisel-Broadbent J, Taylor S, Sampson HA. Cross-allergenicity in the legume botanical family in children with food hypersensitivity. II. Laboratory correlates. *J Allergy Clin Immunol.* 1989;84(5 Pt 1):701–709.

191. Sicherer SH. Clinical implications of cross-reactive food allergens. *J Allergy Clin Immunol.* 2001;108(6):881–890.

192. Bernhisel-Broadbent J. Allergenic cross-reactivity of foods and characterization of food allergens and extracts. *Ann Allergy Asthma Immunol.* 1995;75(4):295–303.

193. Bindslev-Jensen C, Vibits A, Stahl SP, et al. Oral allergy syndrome: the effect of astemizole. *Allergy.* 1991;46(8):610–613.

194. Sicherer SH, Sampson HA. 9. Food allergy. *J Allergy Clin Immunol.* 2006;117(2 Suppl Mini-Primer):S470–S475.

195. Nelson HS, Lahr J, Rule R, et al. Treatment of anaphylactic sensitivity to peanuts by immunotherapy with injections of aqueous peanut extract. *J Allergy Clin Immunol.* 1997;99(6 Pt 1):744–751.

196. Nowak-Wegrzyn A, Sampson HA. Food allergy therapy. *Immunol Allergy Clin North Am.* 2004;24(4):705–725, viii.

197. MacGlashan DW Jr, Bochner BS, Adelman DC, et al. Down-regulation of Fc (epsilon) RI expression on human basophils during in vivo treatment of atopic patients with anti-IgE antibody. *J Immunol.* 1997;158(3):1438–1445.

198. Beck LA, Marcotte GV, MacGlashan D, et al. Omalizumab-induced reductions in mast cell Fce psilon RI expression and function. *J Allergy Clin Immunol.* 2004;114(3):527–530.

199. Leung DY, Sampson HA, Yunginger JW, et al. Effect of anti-IgE therapy in patients with peanut allergy. *N Engl J Med.* 2003;348(11):986–993.

200. Srivastava KD, Kattan JD, Zou ZM, et al. The Chinese herbal medicine formula FAHF-2 completely blocks anaphylactic reactions in a murine model of peanut allergy. *J Allergy Clin Immunol.* 2005;115(1):171–178.

201. Li XM, Srivastava K, Grishin A, et al. Persistent protective effect of heat-killed Escherichia coli producing "engineered," recombinant peanut proteins in a murine model of peanut allergy. *J Allergy Clin Immunol.* 2003;112(1):159–167.

202. Patriarca G, Nucera E, Roncallo C, et al. Oral desensitizing treatment in food allergy: clinical and immunological results. *Aliment Pharmacol Ther.* 2003;17(3):459–465.

203. Meglio P, Bartone E, Plantamura M, et al. A protocol for oral desensitization in children with IgE-mediated cow's milk allergy. *Allergy.* 2004;59(9):980–987.

204. Rolinck-Werninghaus C, Staden U, Mehl A, et al. Specific oral tolerance induction with food in children: transient or persistent effect on food allergy? *Allergy.* 2005;60(10):1320–1322.

205. Niggemann B, Staden U, Rolinck–Werninghaus C, et al. Specific oral tolerance induction in food allergy. *Allergy.* 2006;61(7):808–811.

206. Buchanan AD, Green TD, Jones SM, et al. Egg oral immunotherapy in nonanaphylactic children with egg allergy. *J Allergy Clin Immunol.* 2007;119(1):199–205.

207. Enrique E, Pineda F, Malek T, et al. Sublingual immunotherapy for hazelnut food allergy: a randomized, double-blind, placebo-controlled study with a standardized hazelnut extract. *J Allergy Clin Immunol.* 2005;116(5):1073–1079.

208. Zeiger RS. Food allergen avoidance in the prevention of food allergy in infants and children. *Pediatrics.* 2003;111(6 Pt 3):1662–1671.

209. Zeiger RS, Heller S, Mellon MH, et al. Effect of combined maternal and infant food-allergen avoidance on development of atopy in early infancy: a randomized study. *J Allergy Clin Immunol.* 1989;84(1):72–89.

210. Zeiger RS, Heller S. The development and prediction of atopy in high-risk children: follow-up at age seven years in a prospective randomized study of combined maternal and infant food allergen avoidance. *J Allergy Clin Immunol.* 1995;95(6):1179–1190.

211. Lilja G, Dannaeus A, Foucard T, et al. Effects of maternal diet during late pregnancy and lactation on the development of atopic diseases in infants up to 18 months of age—in-vivo results. *Clin Exp Allergy.* 1989;19(4):473–479.

212. Muraro A, Dreborg S, Halken S, et al. Dietary prevention of allergic diseases in infants and small children. Part III: Critical review of published peer-reviewed observational and interventional studies and final recommendations. *Pediatr Allergy Immunol.* 2004;15(4):291–307.

213. Greer FR, Sicherer SH, Burks AW. Effects of early nutritional interventions on the development of atopic disease in infants and children: the role of maternal dietary restriction, breastfeeding, timing of introduction of complementary foods, and hydrolyzed formulas. *Pediatrics.* 2008;121(1):183–191.

214. Host A, Halken S, Muraro A, et al. Dietary prevention of allergic diseases in infants and small children. *Pediatr Allergy Immunol.* 2008;19(1):1–4.

215. Osborn DA, Sinn JK. Probiotics in infants for prevention of allergic disease and food hypersensitivity. *Cochrane Database Syst Rev.* 2007;(4):CD006475.

216. Bock SA. The natural history of adverse reactions to foods. *N Engl Reg Allergy Proc.* 1986;7(6):504–510.

217. Bock SA. Natural history of severe reactions to foods in young children. *J Pediatr.* 1985;107(5):676–680.

218. Hill DJ, Firer MA, Ball G, et al. Natural history of cows' milk allergy in children: immunological outcome over 2 years. *Clin Exp Allergy.* 1993;23(2):124–131.

219. Eggesbo M, Botten G, Halvorsen R, et al. The prevalence of allergy to egg: a population-based study in young children. *Allergy.* 2001;56(5):403–411.

220. Ford RP, Taylor B. Natural history of egg hypersensitivity. *Arch Dis Child.* 1982;57(9):649–652.

221. Savage JH, Matsui EC, Skripak JM, et al. The natural history of egg allergy. *J Allergy Clin Immunol.* 2007;120(6):1413–1417.

222. Host A. Frequency of cow's milk allergy in childhood. *Ann Allergy Asthma Immunol.* 2002;89(6 Suppl 1):33–37.

223. Host A, Halken S. A prospective study of cow milk allergy in Danish infants during the first 3 years of life. Clinical course in relation to clinical and immunological type of hypersensitivity reaction. *Allergy.* 1990;45(8):587–596.

224. Skripak JM, Matsui EC, Mudd K, et al. The natural history of IgE-mediated cow's milk allergy. *J Allergy Clin Immunol.* 2007;120(5):1172–1177.

225. Sicherer SH, Munoz-Furlong A, Burks AW, et al. Prevalence of peanut and tree nut allergy in the US determined by a random digit dial telephone survey. *J Allergy Clin Immunol.* 1999;103(4):559–562.

226. Fleischer DM, Conover-Walker MK, Christie L, et al. The natural progression of peanut allergy: resolution and the possibility of recurrence. *J Allergy Clin Immunol.* 2003;112(1):183–189.

227. Bock SA, Atkins FM. The natural history of peanut allergy. *J Allergy Clin Immunol.* 1989;83(5):900–904.

228. Fleischer DM. The natural history of peanut and tree nut allergy. *Curr Allergy Asthma Rep.* 2007;7(3):175–181.

229. Burks AW, Shin D, Cockrell G, et al. Mapping and mutational analysis of the IgE-binding epitopes on Ara h 1, a legume vicilin protein and a major allergen in peanut hypersensitivity. *Eur J Biochem.* 1997;245(2):334–339.

230. Stanley JS, King N, Burks AW, G et al. Identification and mutational analysis of the immunodominant IgE binding epitopes of the major peanut allergen Ara h 2. *Arch Biochem Biophys.* 1997;342(2):244–253.

231. Fleischer DM, Conover-Walker MK, Christie L, et al. Peanut allergy: recurrence and its management. *J Allergy Clin Immunol.* 2004; 114(5):1195–1201.

SECTION ◼V◻

Asthma

CHAPTER **19**

Asthma
PAUL A. GREENBERGER

◼ OVERVIEW

Asthma is a disease characterized by hyperresponsiveness of bronchi to various stimuli as well as changes in airway resistance, lung volumes, and inspiratory and expiratory flow rates, with symptoms of cough, wheezing, dyspnea, or shortness of breath. In 1991, a National Institutes of Health Expert Panel suggested that asthma was a disease characterized by (a) airway obstruction that is reversible—partially or completely, (b) airway inflammation, and (c) airway hyperresponsiveness (1). In 1997, the Expert Panel 2 report described asthma as follows:

"Asthma is a chronic inflammatory disorder of the airways in which many cells and cellular elements play a role, in particular, mast cells, eosinophils, T lymphocytes, macrophages, neutrophils, and epithelial cells. In susceptible individuals, this inflammation causes recurrent episodes of wheezing, breathlessness, chest tightness, and coughing, particularly at night or in the early morning. These episodes are usually associated with widespread but variable airflow obstruction that is often reversible either spontaneously or with treatment. The inflammation also causes an associated increase in the existing bronchial hyperresponsiveness to a variety of stimuli. Reversibility of airflow limitation may be incomplete in some patients with asthma" (2).

The NIH Expert Panel 3 Report of 2007 confirmed this working definition (3). Asthma has been described by other designations, including allergic bronchitis, asthmatic bronchitis, allergic asthma, atopic asthma, nonallergic asthma, cough equivalent asthma (4), and cardiac asthma (5,6). A central feature of asthma from a

physiologic viewpoint is bronchial hyperresponsiveness to stimuli such as histamine or methacholine, a characteristic not shared by patients without asthma. In population screening, such nonspecific hyperresponsiveness has been reported as sensitive but not specific. Surprisingly, in a study of children 7 to 10 years of age, 48% of those with a diagnosis of asthma did not have bronchial hyperresponsiveness (7). Asthma is characterized by wide variations of resistance to airflow on expiration (and inspiration) with remarkable transient increases in certain lung volumes, such as residual volume, functional residual capacity, and total lung capacity.

Asthma is considered, for most patients, a reversible obstructive airway disease as compared with chronic obstructive pulmonary disease (COPD). Many patients with asthma experience symptom-free periods of days, weeks, months, or years in between episodes, whereas chronic symptoms and fixed dyspnea characterize COPD. When daily symptoms of cough, wheezing, and dyspnea have been present for months in a patient with asthma, bronchodilator nonresponsiveness may be present. However, appropriate anti-inflammatory therapy reduces symptoms and improves the quality of life along with improvement in pulmonary function status.

Immunoglobulin E (IgE)-mediated bronchoconstriction can be demonstrated in many patients with asthma, but not all cases of asthma are "allergic." It is thought that about 80% of patients have allergic asthma. In the Inner-City Asthma Study of children ages 5 to 11 years, 94% of children reacted to at least one allergen (8). Some evidence does exist for IgE antibodies to respiratory syncytial virus (RSV) (*9*) and parainfluenza virus (*10*); however, not all studies are consistent with such a mechanistic explanation of antiviral IgE-mediated asthma. Perhaps, RSV infection allows for T_H2 polarization of the immune response and reduced antiviral IFNγ production (11). Serologic tests and nasopharyngeal or sputum cultures were positive for viruses in 23 of 29 (80%) adult patients who reported a recent respiratory tract infection and were hospitalized for asthma (12). Influenza A and rhinovirus were found most often. In children, viral infections (RSV in infants younger than 2 years of age and rhinovirus in children 2 to 16 years of age) were associated with acute wheezing episodes resulting in emergency department treatment or hospitalization (12). It is likely that other viruses or bacteria will be identified as causative of exacerbations of asthma, with use of increasingly sophisticated molecular techniques.

The sudden onset of wheezing dyspnea that occurs within 3 hours of ingestion of aspirin or other nonsteroidal anti-inflammatory drugs (NSAIDs) (13) is not an IgE-mediated reaction but represents alterations of arachidonic acid metabolism, such as blockage of the cyclooxygenase pathway with shunting of arachidonic acid into the lipoxygenase pathway. Potent lipoxygenase pathway products, such as leukotriene D4 (LTD_4), cause acute bronchoconstriction in aspirin- and NSAID-sensitive patients (13–15). Patients with aspirin exacerbated respiratory disease (aspirin intolerant asthma) have a "knock in" condition in that there is increased LTC_4 synthase in bronchial and nasal mucosa and elevated urinary concentrations of LTE_4, a metabolite of LTD_4, even at baseline (13,15). The concentrations of LTE_4 rise significantly after ingestion of aspirin or a NSAID in susceptible patients (13–15).

Many patients with asthma may have symptoms precipitated by nonspecific, non–IgE-mediated triggers, such as cold air, air pollutants including ozone (16) and fine particles (<2.5 μm in diameter) (16), exercise, crying or laughing, and changes in barometric pressure. Fortunately, pharmacologic therapy can minimize the effects of these nonspecific triggers. Psychological stress such as from post traumatic stress disorder (17) and violence and sexual or physical abuse (18) also are associated with asthma.

■ GENETIC AND ENVIRONMENTAL FACTORS

Genetic and environmental factors are important in terms of development of asthma, but the effects of heredity are much greater (19). Heritability of asthma ranges from 30% to 87% (19,20). In a study of 4,910 4-year-old twins, heredity accounted for 68% and the shared environment accounted for 13% (19). Non-shared environmental factors contributed 19% (19). The authors concluded that "rearing environment, family diet, and air pollutants seem to play a minor role" (19). If the approximate population prevalence for an allergic-type disease in a child is 20%, then having 1 parent with allergies increases the prevalence to 50% (*21*). If both parents are allergic, there is a 66% chance of the child developing an allergic condition (*21*). In twin studies, the concordance for asthma in monozygotic twins reared together was similar to that for twins reared apart (*22,23*). In addition, in a study of 5,864 twins who were evaluated from infancy to age 25 years, the cumulative incidence of asthma was 6% in males and 5.4% in females. If one twin developed asthma, the relative risk of the co-twin developing asthma was 17.9 for identical twins, compared with 2.3 for fraternal twins (23). More than 80% of cases of asthma began by 15 years of age, when nearly all of the study subjects lived in the same home environment (23). These data support a strong genetic effect on development of asthma. Methacholine responsiveness, total serum IgE concentration, and immediate skin test reactivity have been found to be more concordant in monozygotic twins than in dizygotic twins (*24*), which supports a genetic influence over an environmental influence. Both factors should be considered as contributory, and production of specific antiallergen IgE appears to be affected by environmental and local allergic exposures in the genetically susceptible subject. In Table 19.1, there are some examples of candidate genes for asthma or immunologic aspects involved with asthma (25). Single nucleotide polymorphisms (SNPs) have been associated with asthma (26), and it is likely that more will be identified and then replicated. Examples of SNPs that are associated with asthma include IL4RR551 and IL13+2044GA as they are associated with "Gain of

TABLE 19.1   EXAMPLES OF CHROMOSOMES ASSOCIATED WITH ASTHMA AND ATOPY

Asthma	1p, 2q, 4q, 5q, 6p, 12q,13q, 14q, 19q, 21q
Atopy	3q, 4q, 6p, 11q, 17q
Total IgE concentration	2q, 3q, 5q, 6p, 7q, 12q
Total blood eosinophil counts	15q

Data was compiled from Blumenthal MN. The role of genetics in the development of asthma and atopy. Curr Opin Allergy Clin Immunol. 2005;5:141–145.

function" or enhanced biologic activity of IL-4 and IL-13, respectively (26).

The onset of early childhood asthma has been associated with smoking *in utero* (27) and parental smoking (28). For development of severe asthma in children, cigarette smoking by grandparents also has been identified (29). However, once asthma begins, evidence exists for increased childhood respiratory symptoms from passive smoking (30,31) and added deficits in lung function when there had been *in utero* smoking (32).

Environmental factors, such as viral infections, have been associated with development of IgE antibodies. Frick et al. (33) demonstrated development of antiallergen IgE in association with increasing antiviral antibodies in a prospective study of high-risk infants whose parents both had allergic diseases. Croup in early childhood has been associated with subsequent development of asthma (34–36), as have RSV, influenza, parainfluenza virus, and metapneumovirus infections (37–39). When infections occur in an at-risk infant, defined when the mother, father, or sibling has asthma, there is a greater incidence of wheezing (35). This association is magnified if there is concomitant parental smoking or sensitization to dust mites (35). These findings demonstrate the overlap between family history, allergic sensitization, and respiratory infections on development of asthma.

Indoor allergen exposures from house dust mites (40), cats (41), and cockroaches (42) have been associated with the development of childhood asthma. New-onset asthma in older men (aged 61 years or older) was associated with detectable serum IgE antibodies to cat allergen but not dust mites, ragweed, or mouse urinary antigen (43). In this study, IgE antibodies to dog dander and cockroach excreta were not measured.

Environmental factors can predispose to development of asthma but also can be associated with a reduced risk of asthma. The concept is that there are beneficial effects of microbes in the home that do not cause any recognizable infection or illness (28,44). The "protective" home environments consist of stables and dairy farms that are part of the family home, which is an L-shape. The home and barn are attached. This observation has been associated with the "hygiene hypothesis" and the purported beneficial effects of certain infections that would shift the T_H1/T_H2 paradigm toward T_H1. Absence of such exposures would permit asthma or atopy. Some specific protective factors have been identified and include small scale pig farming (<10 pigs/farm) but not sheep farming, raw milk consumption, a child's involvement in frequent haying and staying in animal sheds (45). There remains some controversy about the "hygiene hypothesis" and development of asthma or atopy, but the microbe-rich environments seem to be protective against development of asthma by altering the predominant cytokines generated by $CD4^+$ lymphocytes and interactions with innate immunity and its Toll-like receptors (TLRs) (45). A process that favors asthma includes generation of the helper T-cell subset T_H2, which is central to IgE production, as opposed to T_H1, which would diminish an "atopic" pattern and contribute to a classic delayed-type hypersensitivity response (type IVa_1). In a study of 867 children in Japan who had received Bacille Calmette Guérin (BCG) immunization after birth and at 6 and 12 years of age, the presence of and induration of tuberculosis skin tests were studied in relation to the emergence of atopy (asthma, rhinitis, and atopic dermatitis) (46). By age 12 years, 58% of the children had developed positive ($\geq$10 mm in duration) responses to tuberculin testing, and 36% of children had reported atopic symptoms (46). Asthma symptoms and atopy were associated negatively with positive tuberculin responses, and presence of tuberculin reactivity was associated with remission from asthma by years 6 or 12 (46). The data raised the possibility that the T_H1 response produced by BCG immunization resulted in increases in the T_H1 cytokines, interferon-γ (IFN-γ), and interleukin-12 (IL-12) and decreases in incidence of asthma, possibly even inducing remissions of atopy. In addition, there were reduced quantities of the T_H2 cytokines IL-4, IL-13, and IL-10, compared with the BCG nonresponders, who had more atopy and asthma. Alternatively, these data might be interpreted that children likely to become atopic have a reduced ability to develop T_H1 memory lymphocytes after BCG immunization or, by analogy, reduced response to measles vaccination (47). The latter stems from data revealing less atopy when there was a previous episode of measles (47). These studies and the association between RSV and other viral infections and childhood asthma suggest that the critical link may be the predominance of the T_H1 cytokines and protective innate immune responses. The latter may be specific such as for TLR 5 for people exposed to pigs and TLRs 6 and 8 for people working with silage (45). The notion that asthma is "an epidemic in the absence of infection" has been suggested (48) and demonstrates how complex asthma and the identification of its origins are.

The effects of air pollution on the early development of asthma remain under investigation although the effects of air pollution from ozone and small particles have been associated with hospitalizations for acute severe asthma (49).

■ COMPLEXITY OF ASTHMA

The cause of asthma remains unknown, although asthma is considered a very complex, heterogeneous, inflammatory disease (50, 51) or syndrome. Some important pathologic findings include a patchy loss of bronchial epithelium, usually associated with eosinophil infiltration (52–54), neutrophilic infiltration (55), lymphocyte infiltration (52), mast cell degranulation (52), contraction and hypertrophy of bronchial smooth muscles, bronchial mucosa edema and increased blood flow (56), bronchial gland hyperplasia, hypersecretion of thick bronchial mucus, and basement membrane thickening (52,57). Collagen synthesis may result from stimulation or injury to airway epithelial cells (58). A key cell is the myofibroblast, which is a hybrid cell of fibroblast and smooth muscle cell origins. These cells produce types III and I collagen (58). Epithelial cells obtained during bronchoalveolar lavage (BAL) from patients with asthma have been found to be much less viable than in subjects without asthma (59). However, the epithelial cells from patients with asthma produced much more (a) fibronectin, a glycoprotein involved with cell attachment, cell growth, and chemotaxis; and (b) 15- hydroxy-eicosatetraenoic acid (15-HETE), a metabolite of arachidonic acid (59). The increased metabolic activity of epithelial cells appears to contribute to airway damage and remodeling. There is subepithelial "fibrosis" that is composed of collagen types I, II, and V, which contributes to the basement membrane thickening of asthma.

When bronchial biopsy samples were obtained from 14 patients who had asthma for 1 year or less, increases in numbers of mast cells, eosinophils, lymphocytes, and macrophages were found in the epithelium (60). Deeper in the lamina propria, eosinophils, lymphocytes, macrophages, and plasma cells were present, suggesting that patients with mild asthma, who had not received anti-inflammatory therapy, had marked cellular infiltration in the bronchial mucosa (60).

Human bronchial epithelium from patients with asthma express Fas ligand (Fas L) and Fas on eosinophils and T lymphocytes (61). Activation of Fas by Fas L induces apoptosis. Biopsy samples from patients, who had not received inhaled corticosteroids, had reduced numbers of apoptotic eosinophils and reduced expression Fas L and *Bcl-2*, which help regulate apoptosis. Conversely, inhaled corticosteroid–treated patients had fewer eosinophils and increased numbers of apoptotic eosinophils (61). In a study of BAL of 12 newly diagnosed and untreated patients with asthma, reduced expression of messenger RNA (mRNA) for both Fas and the Fas receptor (CD95) on $CD3^+$ T lymphocytes was found (62). These findings are consistent with a persisting inflammatory cell infiltrate that characterizes asthma and offers the possibility of targeted anti-inflammatory therapy.

Some physiologic characteristics of asthma include bronchial hyperresponsiveness to stimuli such as histamine (63), methacholine (64), or LTD_4 (65) and at least a 12% improvement in forced expiratory volume in 1 second (FEV_1) after inhalation of a β_2-adrenergic agonist, unless the patient is experiencing acute severe asthma (status asthmaticus) or has had severe, ineffectively treated airway obstruction. There are large changes in lung compliance, depending on severity of the disease.

On a cellular level, during acute episodes of asthma, there are activated or hypodense eosinophils present in increased numbers (66–68) and hyperadhesive eosinophils in the sense of increased binding to VCAM and ICAM (69). Eosinophil products such as major basic protein (MBP) can be identified in sputum (67) and in areas where bronchial epithelium has been denuded (68). Eosinophil cationic protein has been identified in areas of denuded bronchial epithelium. This cationic protein has been reported to be even more cytotoxic than MBP (70). Mast cells in the bronchial lumen and submucosa are activated, and their many cell products are released, whether preformed or synthesized *de novo*. Mast cells are found to be in close proximity to smooth muscle and their interactions are being investigated regarding the ability of smooth muscle to stretch maximally (71). Indeed, it has been suggested that the mast cells infiltrate smooth muscle causing "mast cell myositis" (71). Macrophages, lymphocytes, and epithelial cells participate as well and when epithelial cells are damaged, the production of the protective PGE_2 is reduced. Epithelial cells are able to produce many different effector molecules.

Evidence supports neuroimmunologic abnormalities in asthma, such as the lack of the bronchodilating nonadrenergic noncholinergic (NANC) vasoactive intestinal peptide (VIP) in lung sections from patients with asthma (72) and reduced concentrations of VIP during acute exacerbations of asthma (73). There are increased concentrations of IgG autoantibodies that catalyze the hydrolysis of VIP in women whose asthma became more difficult to control during pregnancy (73). Substance P concentrations in induced sputum have been reported to be markedly elevated, compared with that in controls (74). The concentrations of the tachykinin, neurokinin A, is elevated in bronchoalveolar lavage fluid from patients with asthma compared to normal (75), and the potent vasodilator, calcitonin gene-related peptide, has been detected during late asthmatic reactions (76).

The free radical nitric oxide is detectable in expired air in patients with asthma, and its concentration increases further after allergen challenge (77). Inhaled corticosteroids, such as fluticasone, result in about a 60% reduction in exhaled nitric oxide (eNO) within 6 weeks (78). It has been hypothesized that management of asthma could be improved by using the biomarker, eNO. Nevertheless, when asthma management compared the use of the National Asthma Education and Prevention Program Expert Panel (NAEPP) guidelines combined with measurement of eNO to the guidelines alone, there was no meaningful difference in control of asthma (79). A free radical generated from arachidonic acid, 8-isoprostane, is increased in asthma and reflects ongoing oxidative stress (80). There are progressively greater amounts in expired air as asthma severity increases from mild-to-severe (80).

In addition to the above-described features of asthma, asthma is heterogeneous in its clinical presentations (phenotypes) and responses to pharmacologic treatment. Patients vary in their responses to β_2 adrenergic agonists (81), inhaled corticosteroids (82), leukotriene antagonists (83), and oral corticosteroids (84).

These findings demonstrate some but not all of the complexities of asthma, which decades ago was considered a psychological condition. Asthma is not a psychological disorder. Nevertheless, the burden of asthma as a chronic disease, especially when the patient has experienced repeated hospitalizations or emergency department visits, may result in psychological disturbances or abnormal coping styles that coexist with asthma (17,18,85–88).

■ INCIDENCE AND SIGNIFICANCE

Asthma affects more than 22 million people in the United States, as of 2005, consisting of 6.5 million children and 15.7 million adults (89). It is estimated that 32.6 million people have at one time been diagnosed with asthma (89). The World Allergy Organization (WAO) has estimated that 300 million people worldwide have asthma, of which half are in developing countries (90). In the United States, using a random digit dialing system, the estimated prevalence of asthma was 8.4% of adults at least 18 years of age (91). The range by various counties across the country was 3% to 13.8% (91). Puerto Rican responders had a prevalence of asthma 80% to 140% higher than non-Hispanic whites (89,91). Native Americans and Alaskan Natives had prevalence rates 40% greater than non-Hispanic whites (89). Acute asthma is the most common childhood medical emergency (92). Disturbingly, the rate of emergency department visits for asthma was 350% higher in black people than in white people (89). Hospitalizations in black people were 240% greater (89). Often, adults and children requiring acute treatment of asthma have not received or are not using optimal anti-inflammatory therapy. In children in the United States, the attack rate (episode in the past 12 months) was 5.9% for boys and 4.5% among girls (89). Morbidity from asthma remains a major issue in that children, ages 5 to 17 years, missed 12.8 million days of school in 2003 and adults, ages 18 years and older, missed 10.1 million work days (89). The rate for hospitalizations for asthma based on the population has remained unchanged during the period from 1980 to 2004 (93) despite vast increments in the knowledge of asthma.

For many countries, the prevalence of "clinical asthma" is greater than the 10.9% reported for the United States (94). For example, Scotland (18.4%), England (15.3), Australia (14.7%), Canada (14.1%), Peru (13.0%), and Brazil (11.4%) had higher rates than the United States (94). "Clinical asthma" in children was reported as 50% of the prevalence data for self-reported wheezing in the past 12 months (94). For adults, the rate for "clinical asthma" was from "breathlessness and wheeze" which was 50% of those reporting current wheeze (94).

Mortality from asthma appears to be decreasing somewhat in that there were 4,055 deaths in 2003, of which 195 were in children (89). There was a disproportionate increase in deaths in Puerto Ricans and black people (89). About 0.5% of hospitalizations for asthma are associated with a death from asthma, ranging from 0.3% in black people to 0.6% in white people more than 5 years of age (95). About one-third of deaths from asthma occur in the hospital (95). In the same study, the typical hospitalization for asthma was 2.7 days with hospital charges of $9,078 in year 2000 (95). Overall, in light of the unchanged per population rate of hospitalizations for asthma from 1980 to 2004 (93), the daunting challenge remains to reduce the number of hospitalizations (and deaths) from asthma.

Intermittent respiratory symptoms may exist for years before the actual diagnosis of asthma is made in patients older than 40 years of age. The diagnosis of asthma may be more likely made in women and non-smokers, whereas men may be labeled as having chronic bronchitis, when in fact they do not have chronic sputum production for 3 months each year for 2 consecutive years. Asthma may have its onset in the geriatric population and medication nonadherence is found frequently (96). Asthma may begin during or after an upper respiratory tract infection. The prevalence of asthma was found to be 7% or greater, and all cause deaths, but not asthma specifically, have been reported to be increased in geriatric patients with asthma as compared to control patients without asthma (97).

Asthma morbidity can be enormous from a personal and family perspective as well as from the societal aspect. The number of hospitalizations in the United States for asthma increased almost fourfold from 1965 to 1983, with absolute numbers growing from 127,000 to 459,000 per year (98). This number has been stable from 1980 to 2004 based on per population calculation (93). The number of days of school missed from asthma is excessive, as is work absenteeism or presenteeism (present but not fully productive).

Asthma was thought to be related to occupational causes in 2% of the 6 million people with asthma in the United States in 1960. As of 2000, it was estimated that 5% to 15% of newly diagnosed asthma in working adults is caused by an occupational exposure (99). The 2008 Consensus Statement of the American College of Chest Physicians reported that 10% to 15% of asthma cases are related to occupational exposures (100). Terminology includes "work-related asthma" which consists of occupational asthma (*de novo* asthma or return of previously quiescent asthma) or work-exacerbated asthma (100).

The asthma death rate is over 4,000 annually in the United States (89) which reflects a decline in absolute numbers despite greater U.S. population. The number of fatalities from asthma increased in the United States from 0.8 deaths per 100,000 general population in 1977 to 2.0 in 1989 and still 2.0 in 1997 (101). By 2003, the rate had declined to 1.4 per 100,000 population (89). The fatality rate among Puerto Ricans (4.4/100,000), black people (3.2/100,000 population), American Indians (1.7/100,000 population), and Alaskan natives (2.0/100,000 population) remains higher than among white people (1.2/100,000 population) (89).

A disturbing finding was reported in a study of asthmatics conducted in the Detroit area. Black patients received or filled fewer prescriptions for inhaled corticosteroids and were less likely to be referred to an asthma specialist than Caucasians in the managed care setting in which the study took place. (102) All the patients in this study were enrolled in the same large health maintenance organization; thus, factors such as insurance type or access to medications would not explain the discrepancy in care for black patients as compared to Caucasians.

The costs of asthma include direct costs of medications, hospitalizations, and physician charges in addition to indirect costs for time lost from work (absenteeism) and loss of worker productivity (presenteeism). Some 20% of the patients used 80% of the resources ($2,584, compared with $140 per patient) (103). Some patients have been labeled as the "$100,000 asthmatic patients" because of repeated hospitalization and emergency department visits (104). Emotional costs of asthma are great for the sufferer and the family if asthma is managed ineffectively or if the patient refuses to adhere to appropriate medical advice.

The death of a family member or friend from asthma is shocking; the person may be young, and the fatal attack may not have been anticipated by others or even the patient. It must be kept in mind that with current understanding and treatment of asthma, nearly all fatalities should be avoidable, and asthma need not be a fatal disease. More than half of the deaths from asthma occur outside of the hospital. This observation has led some physicians to conclude that emergency medical services should be improved or even that every patient with asthma should receive a prescription for an albuterol metered-dose inhaler (MDI). One cannot dispute such an argument about emergency services, but it is advisable for the physician managing the patient with asthma to have an emergency plan (action plan) available for the patient or family so that asthma is not managed from a crisis orientation but rather on a preventive basis. Further, an education program or patient instructions can identify what patients should do when their medications are not effective, such as with a change in the level of control or for an exacerbation of asthma.

■ ANATOMY AND PHYSIOLOGY

The central function of the lungs is gas exchange with delivery into the blood stream of oxygen and removal of carbon dioxide. The lung is an immunologic organ and has endocrine and drug-metabolizing properties that affect respiration. The lung consists of an alveolar network with capillaries passing near and through alveolar walls and progressively larger intrapulmonary airways, including membranous bronchioles (1 mm or smaller noncartilaginous airways) and larger cartilaginous bronchi and upper airways. Inspired air must reach the gas exchange network of alveoli. The first 16 airway divisions of the lung are considered the conducting zone, whereas subsequent divisions from 17 to 23 are considered transitional and respiratory zones. The conducting zone consists of trachea, bronchi, bronchioles, and terminal bronchioles and produces what is measured as airway resistance. The terminal bronchioles as a rule have diameters as small as 0.5 mm. Respiratory bronchioles, alveolar ducts, and sacs comprise the transitional and respiratory zones (*105*) and are the sites of gas exchange.

The structures of bronchi and trachea are similar, with cartilaginous rings surrounding the bronchi completely until the bronchi enter the lungs, at which point there are cartilage plates that surround the bronchi. When bronchioles are about 1 mm in diameter, the cartilage plates are not present. Smooth muscle surrounds bronchi and is present until the end of the respiratory bronchioles.

The lining mucous membrane of the trachea and bronchi is composed of pseudostratified ciliated columnar epithelium (*Fig. 19.1*). Goblet cells are mucin-secreting epithelial cells and are present in airways until their disappearance at the level of terminal bronchioles. In the terminal bronchioles, the epithelium becomes that of cuboidal cells with some cilia, Clara (secretory) cells, and goblet cells until the level of respiratory bronchioles, where the epithelium becomes alveolar in type. Mucus consists of a superficial gel phase composed of glycoproteins and a sol phase consisting of isotonic fluid in contact with the mucous membrane cells. The cilia move in the sol phase proximally to help remove luminal material (debris, cells, mucus) by the ciliary "mucus escalator." Other cells such as mast cells, alveolar macrophages, polymorphonuclear leukocyte lymphocytes, eosinophils, and airway smooth muscle cells contribute to lung pathology in different ways. Epithelial cells may be thought of in a constant state of "injury" and are not able to be "repaired" completely. There is loss of columnar epithelial cells and the tight junctions. Permeability is increased (106). Primary bronchial epithelial cells from subjects with asthma have been shown to replicate rhinovirus *in vitro* to several logs, whereas those of normal control subjects were resistant to infection. This resistance was a result of rapid induction of apoptosis and of interferon (IFN)-β in the normal cells, whereas these responses were deficient in asthmatic cells. These studies were recently extended to a novel family of three related proteins, the IFN-γs 1–3, production of which was also deficient *in vitro* and related to asthma exacerbation severity *in vivo*. (106).

The bronchial wall is characterized by mucosa, lamina propria, smooth muscle, submucosa, submucosal glands, and then cartilaginous plates. Submucosal glands produce either mucous or serous material depending on their functional type. Mast cells can be identified in the bronchial lumen or between the basement membrane and epithelium. They are "microlocalized" to smooth muscle cells and mucosal glands (107). Mast cells have been recovered from BAL samples but are low in number in these samples (*108*). Mast cell heterogeneity has been recognized based on contents and functional properties. Briefly, mucosal mast cells are not recognized in a formalin-fixed specimen, but connective tissue mast cells are. Mucosal mast cells are present in the lung and contain tryptase but not chymase, whereas connective tissue mast cells contain tryptase and chymase (109). Mast cells participate in airway remodeling because they activate fibroblasts (109,110) and infiltrate and interact with smooth muscle cells (109,110) causing a "mast cell myositis" of the smooth muscle. Mast cell–derived tryptase is a mitogen for epithelial cells and stimulates synthesis of collagen (109). The mucosal mast cells are stimulated by IL-3, IL-4, and IL-9 (a growth factor for mast cells) (109). The sub-mucosal (connective tissue) mast cells are present in large and small airways and are thought to participate in localized fibrogenesis (109). These mast cells interact with stem cell factor (c-kit ligand) and smooth muscle cells (109). In addition to mast cell generation of histamine, prostaglandin D_2 (PGD_2), LTD_4, and tryptase, they secrete IL-4, which upregulates vascular cell adhesion molecule (VCAM) on vessel endothelial surfaces. Eosinophil entry into tissues is facilitated by VCAM. IL-4 also favors isotype switching within the nucleus to cause production of IgE antibodies. The mast cell has many effects, from mediator release and cytokine production to fibrogenic activity. Their interactions with smooth muscle cells are intriguing in the context of induced "myositis" of the smooth muscle (109).

Neutrophils have been recovered in induced sputum using 3.5% saline in an ultrasonic nebulizer (111) from patients with asthma. The numbers were increased in patients with severe asthma (53%) compared with moderate (49%) and mild (35%) asthma. Sputum from nonatopic, nonasthmatic subjects had 28% neutrophils (111). The concentrations of IL-8, which is chemoattractant for neutrophils and is an angiogenic cytokine, and of myeloperoxidase were increased in sputum from patients with moderate and severe asthma (111). Neutrophils have been identified in some (112) but not all (113) patients with sudden (<3 hours) death from asthma.

Macrophages serve as antimicrobial and pro-inflammatory cells and are accessory cells for presenting antigens. Macrophages are present in patients with asthma but are found in greater numbers in patients with chronic bronchitis. Macrophages have been detected during both early and late bronchial responses to allergens. These cells are metabolically active in that they can generate prostaglandins, leukotrienes, proinflammatory cytokines, chemokines, free radicals, and mucus secretagogues.

Increased numbers of eosinophils in bronchial biopsy specimens and sputum can be expected in patients with asthma. It has been estimated that for every 1 eosinophil in peripheral blood, there are 100 to 1,000 in the tissue. Patients with mild asthma have eosinophils detected in bronchial biopsy samples, and eosinophils can be found in postmortem histological sections (112,113). Eosinophils produce major basic protein, eosinophil cationic protein, eosinophil derived neurotoxin, eosinophil peroxidase, free radicals, leukotrienes, and T_H2 cytokines. Eosinophils are proinflammatory cells that participate in the pathogenesis of airway remodeling in patients with persistent asthma.

Epithelial cells are shed especially in patients with severe asthma but also in patients with mild asthma. There are a vast number functions and interactions of epithelial cells (114). In addition to being antimicrobial, one of many actions is to produce neutral endopeptidase, which degrades substance P. The loss of functioning epithelium could lead to potentiated effects of this neuropeptide. Similarly, epithelial cells generate smooth muscle–relaxing factors that could be decreased in amount as epithelium is denuded. Epithelial cell fluid obtained during BAL was analyzed for a gelatinase, which is in the family of matrix metalloproteinases (*115*). Mechanically ventilated patients with asthma were found to have very high quantities of a 92-kDa gelatinase, compared with patients with mild asthma and with ventilated, nonasthmatic subjects (115). This enzyme may damage collagen and elastin and the subepithelial basal lamina region (115). Increased permeability could result because of epithelial cell shedding and alterations of types IV and V collagens that are present in this basement membrane region (115). In this study, mechanically ventilated patients had increased numbers of eosinophils and neutrophils, compared with nonventilated patients with mild asthma (115). There was no difference in numbers of epithelial cells in BAL between patients with mild asthma and the mechanically ventilated patients with asthma, but both groups had twice the percentage as the nonasthmatic subjects, emphasizing that epithelial cell denudation occurs in mild as well as severe asthma.

Innervation

The nervous system and various muscle groups participate in respiration. *Table 19.2* lists muscles; their innervation; other respiratory responses, such as smooth muscle cell and bronchial glands; and nonadrenergic, noncholinergic responses. Efferent parasympathetic (vagal) nerves innervate smooth muscle cells and bronchial glands. The vagus nerve also provides for afferent innervation of three types of sensory responses. The irritant (cough) reflex is rapidly adapting and originates in the trachea and main bronchi. Pulmonary stretch or slowly adapting afferents are also located in the trachea and main bronchi, whereas C fibers are located in small airways and alveolar walls. Afferent stimulation occurs through the carotid body (sensing oxygen tension) and nervous system chemoreceptors in the medulla (sensing hypercapnia).

Efferent respiratory responses include cervical and thoracic nervous system innervation of respiratory muscles, such as those listed in *Table 19.2*. Fortunately, not all respiratory muscles are essential for respiration should a spinal cord injury occur. In addition to efferent parasympathetic innervation of smooth muscle cells and bronchial glands, another source of efferent stimulation is through the nonadrenergic, noncholinergic epithelial sensory nerves. Stimulation of these nerves by epithelial cell destruction that occurs in asthma can trigger release of bronchospastic agonists, such as substance P and neurokinins (A and B), through an antidromic axon reflex. The bronchodilating NANC neurotransmitter, VIP, may oppose effects of other bronchoconstricting agonists, such as substance P. Nitric oxide is a mediator of the NANC system and could offset some of the bronchoconstriction induced by histamine and bradykinin (116). The absence of VIP could contribute to bronchoconstriction.

Smooth muscle cells participate in the Hering-Breuer inflation reflex, in which inspiration leading to inflation of the lung causes bronchodilation. This reflex has been described in animals and humans. The clinical significance in human respiratory disease may be minimal. For example, when a patient with asthma experiences bronchoconstriction when inhaling methacholine or histamine, there is increased airway resistance during a deep inspiration (117). In contrast, patients without asthma and those with rhinitis demonstrate bronchodilation and reduced airway resistance at total lung capacity. During a bronchial challenge procedure in a patient with rhinitis, if the patient performs a FVC maneuver by inhaling to total lung capacity after inhaling the bronchoconstricting agonist in question, the resultant bronchodilation may mask any current airway obstruction. To obviate this possibility, the initial forced expiratory maneuver should be a partial flow volume effort, not a maximal one, which requires maximal inspiration. Otherwise, the dose of agonist necessary to achieve finally a 20% decline in FEV$_1$ will be higher than necessary.

■ PATHOPHYSIOLOGIC CHANGES IN ASTHMA

From a pathophysiologic perspective, the changes that occur in asthma are multiple, diverse, and complex.

Further, some of the abnormalities, such as bronchial hyperresponsiveness and mucus obstruction of bronchi, can be present when patients do not have symptoms. Major pathophysiologic abnormalities in asthma are (a) widespread smooth muscle contraction, (b) mucus hypersecretion, (c) mucosal and submucosal edema, (d) bronchial hyperresponsiveness, and (e) inflammation of airways. Obstruction to airflow during expiration and inspiration results in greater limitation during expiration. Hypertrophy and even hyperplasia of smooth muscle have been recognized in asthma. Smooth muscle contraction occurs in large and or small bronchi. The concept of "airway remodeling" includes inflammation, mucus hypersecretion, subepithelial fibrosis, airway smooth muscle hypertrophy and angiogenesis (3).

Bronchial challenge of patients with asthma by inhalation of histamine demonstrated two abnormal responses compared with patients without asthma (*118*). First, the patients with asthma have increased sensitivity to histamine (or methacholine) because a smaller-than-normal dose of agonist is usually necessary to produce a 20% decline in FEV$_1$. Second, the maximal response to the agonist in asthma is increased over that which occurs in nonasthmatic, nonrhinitic subjects. In fact, the maximal bronchoconstrictive response (reduction of FEV$_1$) that occurs in the nonasthmatic, nonrhinitis subject, if one occurs at all, reaches a plateau beyond which increases in agonist produce no further bronchoconstriction. In contrast, were it possible (and safe) to give a patient with asthma increasing amounts of an agonist such as histamine, or methacholine, increasing bronchoconstriction would occur. In an analysis of 146 patients with mild asthma who had undergone bronchial provocation challenge with histamine, two patterns were identified (119). The first was the decline of FEV$_1$ and FEV$_1$/FVC without a change in FVC at the dose of histamine causing a 20% decline in FEV$_1$ (PC$_{20}$). The second pattern, detected at the time of the PC$_{20}$ response, had reductions in FVC and FEV$_1$ but not FEV$_1$/FVC. It was concluded that the latter subjects experienced excessive bronchoconstriction (119). The authors identified a clinical connection in that there was a moderate correlation between the percentage decline in FVC at the PC$_{20}$ and patients necessitating prescriptions for oral corticosteroids (but not β$_2$-adrenergic agonists) (119). In the patients who develop a declining FVC and FEV$_1$ after bronchoprovocation challenge, there is a concurrent increase in residual volume, which is detrimental if it continues. In summary from these findings, the ease of bronchoconstriction (PC$_{20}$) is one parameter, but the extent of bronchoconstriction (drop in FVC), when the patient has reached the PC$_{20}$, correlated with need for oral corticosteroids.

Hypersecretion of bronchial mucus may be limited or extensive in patients with asthma. Autopsy studies of patients who died from asthma after having symptoms for days or weeks classically reveal extensive mucus plugging of airways. Large and small airways are filled with viscid mucus that is so thick that the plugs must be cut for examination (*120*). Reid (120) has described this pattern as consistent with endobronchial mucus suffocation. Other patients have mild amounts of mucus, suggesting that perhaps the fatal asthma episode occurred suddenly (over hours) and that severe bronchial obstruction from smooth muscle contraction contributed to the patient's death. A virtual absence of mucus plugging, called *empty airways* or *sudden asphyxic asthma*, has been reported (120,121). Desquamation of bronchial epithelium can be identified on histological examination (122) or when a patient coughs up clumps of desquamated epithelial cells (creola bodies). Bronchial mucus contains eosinophils, which may be observed in expectorated sputum. Charcot-Leyden crystals (lysophospholipase) are derived from eosinophils and appear as dipyramidal hexagons or needles in sputum. Viscid mucus plugs, when expectorated, can form a cast of the bronchi and are called Curschmann's spirals.

In clinically active asthma, mucus hypersecretion is reduced or eliminated after treatment with systemic and then inhaled corticosteroids. Mucus from patients with asthma has tightly bound glycoprotein and oligosaccharide, compared with mucus from patients with chronic bronchitis (123). It remains unknown why the mucus of patients with asthma is so tenacious compared to patients with cystic fibrosis or chronic bronchitis.

The bronchial mucosa is edematous, as is the submucosa, and both are infiltrated with mast cells, activated eosinophils, and $CD4^+$ T_H2 lymphocytes (3). Neutrophils can be a manifestation of severe asthma (3). Macrophages and epithelium both amplify the inflammatory responses of asthma (3). Venous dilation, plasma leakage and proliferation of new vessels occur along with the cellular infiltration (3). In addition to its presence on mast cells, basophils, and eosinophils, IgE has been identified in bronchial glands, epithelium, and basement membrane. Because plasma cell staining for IgE was not increased in number, it has been thought that IgE is not produced locally. However, because the lung is recognized as an immunologic organ, further work may show that IgE is produced in the lung.

The mechanism of bronchial hyperresponsiveness in asthma is unknown but is perhaps the central abnormality physiologically. Bronchial hyperresponsiveness occurs in patients with asthma to agonists, such as histamine, methacholine, leukotriene D_4, allergens, platelet-activating factor (PAF), PGD_2 (short-lived response), adenosine monophosphate, and mannitol. Bronchial hyperresponsiveness is sensitive for asthma if one considers a maximum dose of methacholine of 8 mg/mL, which is necessary to cause a decline in FEV_1 of 20%. Patients with active symptomatic asthma often experience such a decline in FEV_1 when the dose of

---

TABLE 19.3   CONDITIONS OF PATIENTS THAT MAY DEMONSTRATE BRONCHIAL HYPERRESPONSIVENESS

1. After a viral upper respiratory infection for 6 weeks in nonasthma patients
2. In absence of changes in FEV_1 in patients with asthma
3. In chronic bronchitis
4. In left ventricular failure
5. In allergic rhinitis in absence of asthma
6. In apparently normal subjects
7. In subjects exposed to irritants
8. In smokers
9. In some normal infants
10. In first-degree relatives of asthma patients
11. In sarcoidosis
12. In patients with quadriplegia or high paraplegia (lesions T1 to T6)

FEV_1, forced expiratory volume in 1 second.

---

methacholine is 2 mg/mL or less. However, bronchial hyperresponsiveness is not specific for asthma because it occurs in patients who have disease other than asthma (Table 19.3).

Bronchial hyperresponsiveness is measured physiologically by reductions in expiratory flow rates, FEV_1, or decreases in specific conductance. Nevertheless, hyperresponsiveness consists of bronchoconstriction, hypersecretion, and hyperemia (mucosal edema). It has been easier to measure airway caliber by changes in FEV_1 than to measure changes in bronchial gland secretion, cellular infiltration, or blood vessels (dilation and increased permeability) that also contribute to hyperresponsiveness and cause airways obstruction. Indeed, there has yet to be an "inflammamometer" for asthma. The bronchial responsiveness detected after challenge with histamine or methacholine measures bronchial sensitivity or ease of bronchoconstriction (119). As stated, an additional finding in some patients with asthma is excessive bronchoconstriction, which can be attributable to associated increases in residual volume and possibly more rapid clinical deterioration (119).

Often, on opening the thorax of a patient who has died from status asthmaticus, the lungs are hyperinflated and do not collapse (Fig. 19.2). Mucus plugging and obstruction of bronchi and bronchioles are present. In some cases, complicating factors, such as atelectasis or acute pneumonia, are identified. On histological examination, there is a patchy loss of bronchial epithelium with desquamation and denudation of mucosal epithelium. Eosinophils are present in areas of absent epithelium, and immunologic staining has revealed evidence of eosinophil MBP at sites of bronchial epithelium desquamation. Activated (EG2-positive) eosinophils are

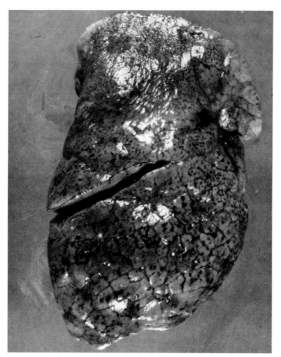

■ **FIGURE 19.2**   Distended lung of patient who died in acute severe asthma (status asthmaticus).

present in the mucosa, submucosa, and connective tissue. Other histological findings include hyperplasia of bronchial mucus glands, bronchial mucosal edema, smooth muscle hypertrophy, and basement membrane thickening (Fig. 19.3). The latter occurs from the remodeling process from collagen deposition (types I, III, and IV), immunoglobulin deposition and cellular infiltrates as evidence of inflammation. The mucus plugs typically contain eosinophils. Occasionally, bronchial epithelium is denuded, but histologic studies do not identify eosinophils. In some cases, neutrophils

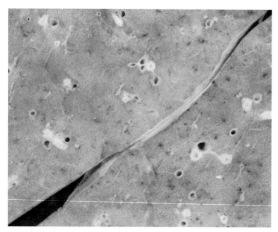

■ **FIGURE 19.3**   Close-up view of pulmonary parenchyma in a case of acute severe asthma. Bronchi are dilated and thickened.

have been present (112). Other mechanisms of lung damage are present but not understood completely. Similarly, although many autopsy examinations reveal the classic pattern of mucus plugging (*Fig. 19.4*) of large and smaller bronchi and bronchioles leading to mucus suffocation or asphyxia as the terminal asthmatic event, some autopsies reveal empty bronchi (113,120,121). Eosinophils have been identified in such cases in airways or in basement membranes, but a gross mechanical explanation, analogous to mucus suffocation, is not present. A third morphologic pattern of patients dying from asthma is that of mild-to-moderate mucus plugging (120).

Some patients dying from asthma have evidence of myocardial contraction band necrosis, which is different from myocardial necrosis associated with infarction. Contraction bands are present in necrotic myocardial smooth muscle cell bands in asthma and curiously the cells are thought to die in tetanic contraction whereas in cases of fatal myocardial infarction, cells die in relaxation.

In patients who experience acute severe asthma but do not die from it, it can be expected that when the patient presents with an FEV_1 of 50% of predicted value, there may be a 10-fold increase in inspiratory muscle work. Pleural pressure becomes more negative, so that as inspiration occurs, the patient is able to apply sufficient radial traction on the airways to maintain their patency. Air can get in more easily than it can be expired, which results in progressively breathing at higher and higher lung volumes. The residual volume (RV) increases several-fold, and functional residual capacity (FRC) expands as well. Expiratory flow rates decrease in large and small airways. The lung hyperinflation is not distributed evenly, and some areas of the lung have a high or low ventilation-perfusion ratio (V/Q). Overall, the hypoxemia that results from acute severe asthma occurs from reduced V/Q, not from shunting of blood. The lung hyperinflation also results in "dynamic autopeep" as the patient attempts to maintain airway caliber by applying some endogenous positive airway pressure.

There is no evidence of chest wall (inspiratory muscle) weakness in patients with asthma. Nevertheless, some patients who have received prolonged courses of daily or twice-daily prednisone or who have been mechanically ventilated with muscle relaxants and corticosteroids can be those who have respiratory muscle fatigue.

After successful treatment of an attack of acute severe asthma, the increases in lung volume may remain present for 6 weeks. The changes are primarily in RV and FRC. Small airways may remain obstructed for weeks or months; in some patients, they do not become normal again. At the same time, it can be expected that the patient has no sensation of dyspnea within 1 week of treatment of acute severe asthma

TABLE 19.4   FACTORS THAT AFFECT THE SENSATION OF DYSPNEA IN ASTHMA

1. Age
2. Gender
3. Temporal adaptation to airway obstruction
4. Severity of asthma
5. Extent of decline in FEV_1*
6. Personality (high anxiety, low anxiousness, etc.)
7. Psychologic profile
8. Medications
9. Concurrent pulmonary, cardiac or neurologic conditions

* For patients who have mild dyspnea at a reduction of 20% of FEV1, the dyspnea would be much more noticeable with a 50% decline in FEV_1. Some "poor perceiver" patients have no appreciation of dyspnea when the FEV_1 has decreased by 50%.

despite increases in RV and reduced small airways caliber. This divergence between symptom recognition in asthma and physiologic measurements has been demonstrated in ambulatory patients who did not have acute severe asthma (status asthmaticus) (124). When patients with an FEV_1 percentage of 60% were studied, 31% overestimated and 17% underestimated the extent of airway obstruction (124). Some patients reported fewer symptoms despite no improvement in FEV_1 or peak expiratory flow rate (PEFR). The reduction in trapped gas in the lung can result in symptom reduction even without improvement in expiratory flow rates.

Asthma pathophysiology includes poor or impaired symptom perception in some patients and in management of asthma, increased symptom perception in others (125,126). There may be poor sensitivity or discrimination (recognizing improvement or worsening status) (125). Dyspnea has been classified into either (a) inspiratory difficulty, (b) chest tightness, (c) unsatisfied inspiration, or (d) work (126). In Table 19.4, factors that alter the perception of dyspnea in asthma are presented. As the exacerbation of asthma becomes worse, the reduction in inspiratory capacity is associated with increases in functional residual capacity (hyperinflation) and increasing dyspnea (126).

■ CONTROL OF AIRWAY TONE

The patency of bronchi and bronchioles is a function of many factors. There is the overriding loss of airway distensibility will less elastic recoil pressures (127). Bronchomotor patency is affected by mediators secreted by mast cells, the autonomic nervous system, the nonadrenergic noncholinergic nervous system, circulating humoral substances, the respiratory epithelium,

smooth muscle cells, and effects of cellular infiltration and glandular secretions (Tables 19.5 and 19.6). Even this list is oversimplified because asthma must be considered a very complex condition in terms of airway caliber and tone.

Mediator release caused by mast cell activation results in acute and late bronchial smooth muscle contraction, cellular infiltration, and mucus production. Autonomic nervous stimulation contributes through vagal stimulation. The neurotransmitter for postganglionic parasympathetic nerves is acetylcholine, which causes smooth muscle contraction. Norepinephrine is the neurotransmitter for postganglionic sympathetic nerves. However, there appears to be little if any significant smooth muscle relaxation through stimulation of postganglionic sympathetic nerves. Exogenously administered epinephrine can produce smooth muscle relaxation. Circulating endogenous epinephrine apparently does not serve to produce relaxation of smooth muscles. Sensory nerves in the respiratory epithelium are stimulated and lead to release of a host of neuropeptides that may be potent bronchoconstrictors or bronchodilators. Respiratory epithelium itself may contain bronchi-relaxing factors that may become unavailable when epithelium is denuded. Tables 19.5 and 19.6 list some chemical mediators derived from mast cells and cytokines and neuropeptides that may contribute to pathogenesis of asthma.

Although much attention has been directed at understanding the contribution of IgE and mast cell activation in asthma, triggering or actual regulation of some of the allergic inflammation of asthma may occur because of other cells in lungs of patients. Low-affinity IgE receptors (FcεR II) are present on macrophages, eosinophils, monocytes, B lymphocytes, and platelets. These cells, as well as mast cells in the bronchial mucosa or lumen, can be activated in the absence of classic IgE-mediated asthma.

Bronchial biopsy specimens from patients with asthma demonstrate mucosal mast cells in various stages of activation in patients with and without symptoms. Mast cell hyperreleasibility may occur in asthma, in that bronchoalveolar mast cells recovered during lavage contain and release greater quantities of histamine when stimulated by allergen or anti-IgE in vitro.

Eosinophils are thought to contribute to proinflammatory effects by secretion of damaging cell products, such as MBP, that can result in bronchial epithelial denudation, exposing sensory nerves, and leading to smooth muscle contraction. Eosinophils are proinflammatory in that they cause eosinophil and neutrophil chemotaxis, which produces positive feedback in terms of leukotriene and PAF production from attracted and newly activated eosinophils. The latter can be demonstrated by activation markers such as EG2 and reduced density on centrifugation, so called hypodense eosinophils.

TABLE 19.5 SELECTED MAST CELL MEDIATORS AND CYTOKINES AND THEIR PROPOSED ACTIONS IN ASTHMA

MEDIATOR	PREFORMED	NEWLY SYNTHESIZED	ACTIONS
Histamine	+		Smooth muscle contraction (H_1 and via vagus); increased vascular permeability; vasodilator; mucus production (H_2)
Tryptase	+		Degrades vasoactive intestinal polypeptide; cleaves kininogen to form bradykinin, complement C3
Eosinophil chemotactic factor	+		Eosinophil chemoattractant
Neutrophil chemotactic factor	+		Neutrophil chemoattractant
Peroxidase	+		Inactivates leukotrienes
Bradykinin		+	Smooth muscle contraction
Leukotriene D_4 (generated from leukotriene C_4)		+	Smooth muscle contraction; increases vascular permeability, mucus secretion
Prostaglandin D_2, $F_{2\alpha}$		+	Smooth muscle contraction; increases vascular permeability, mucus secretion
Platelet-activating factor		+	Smooth muscle contraction; increases vascular permeability, neutrophil and eosinophil chemoattractant; aggregates platelets; sensitizes airways to the agonists
Leukotriene B_4		+	Neutrophil and eosinophil chemoattractant
Interleukin-3 (IL-3)		+	Eosinophil growth factor and chemoattractant, stem cell growth, mast cell growth
IL-5		+	Eosinophil growth factor and chemoattractant
Granulocyte-macrophage colony-stimulating factor		+	Eosinophil growth factor and chemoattractant
IL-1		+	Cytokine production; B-cell differentiation and proliferation
IL-2		+	Proliferation of T cells
IL-4		+	Growth of B cells; class switching from immunoglobulin M (IgM) to IgE production; increases VCAM on endothelium. Favors T_H2 phenotype of CD_4^+ T cells
Tumor necrosis factor-α		+	Activation of macrophages with increased major histocompatibility complex (MHC) molecules (increased antigen presentation)
Interferon-γ		+	Increased MHC molecules on macrophages, antiviral

On a cellular level, the control of airway tone is influenced by even more fundamental factors, including IL-1, IL-2, IL-3, IL-4, IL-6, IL-10, IL-12, IL-16, and IFN-γ, among others, that influence lymphocyte development and proliferation. IL-3 and IL-5 are eosinophil growth factors. IL-8, detected in bronchial epithelium, binds to secretory IgA and serves to chemoattract eosinophils that generate PAF and LTC_4. IL-8 is also a potent chemotactic substance for neutrophils.

During an acute attack of asthma, there is an increase in inspiratory efforts, which apply greater radial traction to airways. Patients with asthma have great ability to generate increases in inspiratory pressures. Unfortunately, patients who have experienced nearly fatal attacks of asthma have blunted perception of dyspnea and impaired ventilatory responses to hypoxia (128).

Patients with persistent severe asthma have been divided into eosinophil-positive (and macrophage-positive) and eosinophil-negative categories based on results on bronchial biopsy findings (129). Both subgroups of patients were prednisone-dependent (average, 28 mg daily) and had asthma for about 20 years

(129). The residual volume measurements were about 200% of predicted and FEV_1 percentage was 56% of predicted in eosinophil-positive and 42% of predicted in eosinophil-negative patients (129). The ratio of the FVC to slow vital capacity was 88%, indicating more airway collapsibility in eosinophil-positive patients, compared with 97% in eosinophil-negative patients. Perhaps the former patients who had somewhat higher FEV_1 percentages had more loss of elastic recoil in their lungs, so that their airways collapsed more easily (129). On biopsy assessments, sub-basement membrane thickening was higher in these eosinophil-predominant patients than in eosinophil-negative patients. These findings were associated with eosinophil-predominant patients with severe asthma having an increased number of $CD3^+$ lymphocytes and activated eosinophils ($EG2^+$) in biopsy samples and an increased quantity of β-tryptase in BAL. It is likely that the cellular inflammation and cell products participate in control or perturbation of airway tone, and continued investigations of the many aspects of allergic inflammation should help clarify this difficult issue.

■ CLINICAL OVERVIEW

Clinical Manifestations

Asthma results in coughing, wheezing, dyspnea, sputum production, and shortness of breath. Symptoms vary from patient to patient and within the individual patient depending on the activity of asthma. Some patients experience mild, nonproductive coughing after exercising or exposure to cold air or odors as examples of transient mild bronchoconstriction. The combination of coughing and wheezing with dyspnea is common in patients who have a sudden moderate to severe episode (such as might occur within 3 hours after aspirin ingestion in an aspirin-intolerant patient). Symptoms of asthma may be sporadic and are often present on a nocturnal basis. Some patients with asthma present with a persistent nonproductive cough as a main symptom of asthma (130). Typically, the cough has occurred on a daily basis and may awaken the patient at night. Repetitive spasms of cough from asthma are refractory to treatment with expectorants, antibiotics, antitussives, and opioids. The patient likely may respond to an inhaled β2-adrenergic agonist; if that is unsuccessful, inhaled corticosteroids or the combination may work. At times, oral corticosteroids are necessary to stop the coughing and are very useful as a diagnostic therapeutic trial (130). Pulmonary physiologic studies usually reveal large airway obstruction, as illustrated by reductions in FEV_1 with preservation of forced expiratory flow, midexpiratory phase ($FEF_{25\%-75\%}$) or small airways function (131). The latter may be reduced in patients with this cough variant form of asthma. Conversely, some patients present with isolated dyspnea as a manifestation of asthma. Some of these patients have small airways obstruction with preservation of function of larger airways. The recognition of variant forms of asthma emphasizes that not all patients with asthma have detectable wheezing on auscultation. The medical history is important, as is a diagnostic-therapeutic trial with antiasthma medications. Pulmonary physiologic abnormalities, such as reduced FEV_1 that responds to therapy, or bronchial hyperresponsiveness to methacholine ($PC_{20} <8$ mg/mL) can provide additional supportive data.

During an acute, moderately severe episode of asthma or in longer-term ineffectively controlled asthma, patients typically produce clear, yellow, or green sputum that can be viscid. The sputum contains eosinophils, which supports the diagnosis of asthma. If measured, expired nitric oxide concentrations will be elevated. Because either polymorphonuclear leukocytes or eosinophils can cause the sputum to be discolored, it is inappropriate to consider such sputum as evidence of a secondary bacterial infection. Patients with nonallergic asthma also produce eosinophil-laden sputum. An occasional patient with asthma presents with cough syncope, a respiratory arrest that is perceived as anaphylaxis, chest pain, pneumomediastinum, or pneumothorax, or with symptoms of chronic bronchitis or bronchiectasis.

The physical examination may consist of no coughing or wheezing if the patient has stable persistent asthma or if there has not been a recent episode of intermittent asthma. Certainly, patients with variant asthma may not have wheezing or other supportive evidence of asthma. Usually, wheezing is present in other patients and can be associated with reduced expiratory flow rates. A smaller number of patients always have wheezing on even tidal breathing, not just with a forced expiratory maneuver. Such patients may not report symptoms and may or may not have expiratory airflow obstruction when FVC and FEV_1 are measured. The physical examination must be interpreted in view of the patient's clinical symptoms and supplemental tests, such as the chest radiograph or pulmonary function tests. There may be a surprising lack of correlation in some ambulatory patients between symptoms and objective evidence of asthma (physical findings and spirometric values) (132). Attempts at using a biomarker such as exhaled nitric oxide have (133) and have not (79,134) been helpful as a noninvasive marker.

An additional physical finding in patients with asthma is repetitive coughing on inspiration. Although not specific for asthma, it is frequently present in unstable patients. In normal patients, maximal inspiration to total lung capacity results in reduced airway resistance, whereas in patients with asthma, increased resistance occurs with a maximal inspiration. Coughing spasms can be precipitated in patients who otherwise may not be heard to wheeze. This finding is transient and, after effective therapy, will not occur. The patient with a very severe episode of asthma may be found to have pulsus paradoxus and use of accessory muscles of respiration. Such findings correlate with an FEV_1 of less than 1.0 L and air trapping as manifested by hyperinflation of the functional residual capacity and residual volume (135). The most critically ill patients have markedly reduced tidal volumes, and their maximal ventilatory efforts are not much higher than their efforts during tidal breathing. A silent chest with absence of or greatly reduced breath sounds indicates likely alveolar hypoventilation (normal or elevated arterial PCO_2) and hypoxemia. Such patients may require intubation or, in most cases, admission to the intensive care unit. Great difficulty in speaking more than a half sentence before needing another inspiration is likely present in such patients.

Persistent asthma may be occurring in patients who have concurrent gastroesophageal reflux disease (GERD), rhinosinusitis, and allergic or nonallergic rhinitis, all of which can cause a cough or worsen ongoing asthma (136).

Radiographic and Laboratory Studies

In about 90% of patients, the presentation chest radiograph is considered within normal limits (137). The most frequently found abnormality is hyperinflation. The diaphragm is flattened, and there may be an increase in the anteroposterior diameter and retrosternal air space. The chest radiograph is indicated because it is necessary to exclude other conditions that mimic asthma and to search for complications of asthma. Congestive heart failure, COPD, pneumonia, sarcoidosis, and neoplasms are just some other explanations for acute wheezing dyspnea that may mimic or coexist with asthma. Asthma complications include atelectasis as a result of mucus obstruction of bronchi, mucoid impaction of bronchi (often indicative of allergic bronchopulmonary aspergillosis), pneumomediastinum, and pneumothorax. Atelectasis often involves the middle lobe, which may collapse. The presence of pneumomediastinum or pneumothorax may have associated subcutaneous emphysema with crepitus on palpation of the neck, supraclavicular areas, or face (Figs. 19.5 and 19.6). Sharp pain in the neck or shoulders should be a clue to the presence of a pneumomediastinum in status asthmaticus.

Depending on the patients examined, abnormal findings on sinus CT examination may be frequent. Some findings may include air-fluid levels, indicative of infection; mucoperiosteal thickening, which is consistent with current or previous infection; and opacification of a sinus or presence of nasal polyps (see Chapters 10 and 12). Clinical research studies of acutely ill patients with asthma have been carried out with V/Q scans. These procedures are not indicated in most cases and, in the markedly hypoxemic patient, may be

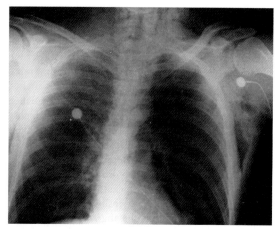

■ **FIGURE 19.5**   Anteroposterior view of the chest of a 41-year-old woman demonstrates hyperinflation of both lungs, with pneumomediastinum and subcutaneous emphysema.

harmful because the technetium-labeled albumin macrospheres injected for the perfusion scan can lower arterial PO_2. Ventilation is extremely uneven (138). Perfusion scans reveal abnormalities such that there may or may not be matched V/Q inequalities. In some patients, the V/Q in the superior portions of the lungs has declined from its relatively high value (138). The explanation for such a finding is increased perfusion of upper lobes presumably from reduced resistance relative to lower lobes that receive most of the pulmonary blood flow. Little evidence for shunting exists (138). Of note, even bronchoprovocation challenge with allergen results in 20% increases in ventilation and perfusion with associated evidence of gas trapping (139).

Pulmonary emboli typically do not complicate episodes of acute asthma, but when a pulmonary embolus is suspected, spiral CT examination of the lung may provide the characteristic findings.

In the assessment of the emergency department patient with acute severe wheezing dyspnea, the measurement of arterial PO_2, PCO_2, and pH can be invaluable. Although hypoxemia is a frequent and expected finding and is identified by measuring the pulse oximetry, the PCO_2 provides information on the effectiveness of alveolar ventilation. This latter status will not be assessed if just oxygen saturation is determined. The PCO_2 should be decreased initially during the hyperventilation stage of acute asthma. A normal or elevated PCO_2 is evidence of alveolar hypoventilation and may be associated with subsequent need for intubation to try to prevent a fatal outcome.

Pulmonary function measurements can help to establish patient status. However, such measurements must be correlated with the physical examination. In the emergency department or ambulatory setting, many physicians determine spirometric values for expiratory flow rates with either PEFR or FEV_1. These tests are effort dependent, and patients with acute symptoms may be unable to perform the maneuver satisfactorily. This finding could be from severe obstruction or patient inability or unwillingness to perform the maneuver appropriately. When properly performed, spirometric measurements can be of significant clinical utility in assessing patient status. For example, as a rule, patients presenting with spirometric determinations of 20% to 25% of predicted value should receive immediate and intensive therapy. Frequent measurements of PEFR or FEV_1 in ambulatory patients can establish a range of baseline values for day and night. Declines of more than 20% from usual low recordings or wide swings in PEFF (such as from a best of 400 L/min to 225 L/min) can alert the patient to the need for more intensive pharmacologic therapy. Nevertheless, such measurements can be insensitive in some patients. Pulmonary physiologic values such as PEFR and FEV_1 have demonstrated value in clinical research studies, such as in documenting a 12% increase in expiratory flow rates after bronchodilator. Such a response (including a 200-mL increase in FEV_1) meets criteria for a bronchodilator response (3). Similarly, in testing for bronchial hyperresponsiveness, a 20% decline in FEV_1 is a goal during incremental administration of methacholine or histamine.

Some patients may benefit from measuring PEFR daily at home (1–3). Unfortunately, some patients do not continue to measure this PEFR or may fabricate results. Other patients manipulate spirometric measurements to make a convincing case for occupational asthma. Thus, the physician must correlate pulmonary physiologic values with the clinical assessment. A complete set of pulmonary function tests should be obtained in other situations, such as in assessing the degree of reversible versus nonreversible obstruction in patients with heavy smoking histories. The diffusing capacity for carbon monoxide (DLCO) is reduced in the COPD patient but normal or elevated in the patient with asthma. Such tests should be obtained after 2 to 4 weeks of intensive therapy to determine what degree of reversibility exists. In acutely ill patients with asthma, the DLCO may be reduced. Thus, its usefulness in differentiating COPD from asthma will be obscured if the wrong time is chosen to obtain this test. Flow-volume loops will demonstrate intrathoracic obstruction in patients with asthma (140) or extrathoracic obstruction in those with vocal cord dysfunction (VCD) (141) (Fig. 19.7).

The complete blood count should be obtained in the emergency setting. First, the hemoglobin and

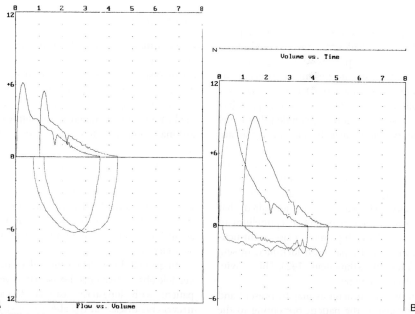

■ **FIGURE 19.7 (A)** A 46-year-old man with persistent asthma since childhood. He had been taking prednisone, 60 mg daily for 6 weeks; salmeterol, 2 puffs twice a day; and budesonide, 800 µg twice a day. He had mild expiratory wheezes on examination. The pattern is that of intrathoracic obstruction from asthma. The forced vital capacity (FVC) was 3.6 L (72%), and the forced expiratory volume in 1 second (FEV_1) was 2.3 L (62%). The FEV_1 percentage was 64%. The forced expiratory flow, midexpiratory phase ($FEF_{25\%-75\%}$) was 1.36 L/sec (36%). The inspiratory loop is not altered. **(B)** A 47-year-old man with adult-onset asthma and intermittent sinusitis, nonallergic rhinitis, and gastroesophageal reflux disease. Medications included prednisone, 35 mg on alternate days; budesonide, 800 µg twice a day; salmeterol, 2 puffs twice a day; omeprazole, 40 mg daily; fexofenadine, 60 mg twice daily; and triamcinolone nasal spray. He had mild end-expiratory wheezes and a hoarse voice. No stridor was present. The FVC was 3.9 L (78%), the FEV_1 was 2.9 L (77%), and the FEV_1 percentage was 74%. The $FEF_{25\%-75\%}$ was 2 L/sec (56%). The inspiratory loop is truncated, consistent with vocal cord dysfunction.

hematocrit provide status regarding anemia, which if associated with hypoxemia can compromise oxygen delivery to tissues. Conversely, an elevated hematocrit is consistent with hemoconcentration such as occurs from dehydration or polycythemia. The latter does not occur in asthma in the absence of other conditions. The white blood count may be elevated from infection or systemic corticosteroids, the mechanism of which includes demargination and release from bone marrow. In the absence of prior systemic corticosteroids, the acutely ill patient with allergic or nonallergic asthma often has peripheral blood eosinophilia. For best accuracy, an absolute eosinophil count is required. However, in the management of most patients with asthma, both those with acute symptoms and long-term sufferers, eosinophil counts are not of value. The presence of eosinophilia in patients receiving long-term systemic corticosteroids should suggest nonadherence or possibly rare conditions, such as Churg-Strauss Syndrome, allergic bronchopulmonary aspergillosis, or chronic eosinophilic pneumonia. Usually, the eosinophilia in asthma does not exceed 10% to 20% of the differential. (Some patients with both asthma and atopic dermatitis have persistently elevated absolute eosinophil counts in the absence of idiopathic hypereosinophilic syndrome or other conditions). Much higher values should suggest an alternative diagnosis (Chapter 35).

Sputum examination reveals eosinophils, eosinophils plus polymorphonuclear leukocytes (asthma and purulent bronchitis or bacterial pneumonia), or absence of eosinophils. In mild asthma, no sputum is produced. In severely ill patients with asthma, the sputum is thick, tenacious, and yellow or green. MBP from eosinophils has been identified in such sputum. Dipyramidal hexagons from eosinophil cytoplasm may be identified and are called Charcot-Leyden crystals. These crystals contain lysophospholipase. Curschmann spirals are expectorated yellow or clear mucus threads that are remnants or casts of small bronchi. Expectorated ciliated and nonciliated bronchial epithelial cells can also be identified that emphasize the patchy loss of bronchial epithelium in asthma. On a related basis, high-molecular-weight neutrophil chemotactic activity has been identified in sera from patients with status asthmaticus (*142*). This activity declined with effective therapy.

Serum electrolyte abnormalities may be present and should be anticipated in the patient presenting to the emergency department. Recent use of oral corticosteroids can lower the potassium concentration (as can β_2-adrenergic agonists) and cause a metabolic alkalosis. Oral corticosteroids may raise the blood glucose in some patients, as can systemic administration of β_2-adrenergic agonists. Elevations of atrial natriuretic peptide and antidiuretic hormone can occur in acute asthma or COPD (*143*). Clinically, few patients have large declines of serum sodium. Because intravenous

fluids will be administered, it is necessary to determine the current status of electrolytes and serum chemistry values. After prolonged high-dose corticosteroids, hypomagnesemia or hypophosphatemia may occur.

Rarely, a patient younger than 30 years of age may be thought to have asthma when the underlying condition is α_1-antitrypsin deficiency. More commonly, patients with wheezing dyspnea have asthma and cystic fibrosis. The sweat chloride should be elevated markedly in such patients. A properly performed sweat chloride test is essential, as is proper performance of genetic analysis and pancreatic function.

In the outpatient management of asthma, determination of the presence or absence of antiallergen IgE is of value. For decades, skin testing for immediate cutaneous reactivity has been the most sensitive and specific method. Some physicians prefer *in vitro* tests. One cannot emphasize enough the need for high quality control for both skin testing and *in vitro* testing. Both tests are subject to misinterpretation. The experienced physician should use either method of demonstration of antiallergen IgE as adjunctive to, rather than a substitute for, the narrative history of asthma. More patients have immediate cutaneous reactivity or detectable *in vitro* IgE than have asthma that correlates with exposure to the specific allergen.

Complications

Complications from asthma include death, adverse effects of hypoxemia or respiratory failure on other organ systems, growth retardation in children, pneumothorax or pneumomediastinum, rib fractures from severe coughing, cough syncope, and adverse effects of medications or therapeutic modalities used to treat asthma. Some patients develop psychological abnormalities because of the burden of a chronic illness such as asthma. Ineffectively treated asthma in children can result in chest wall abnormalities, such as "pigeon chest," because of sustained hyperinflation of the chest. Further, the annual rate of decline of FEV_1 is increased; for example, it may be 38 mL/year in patients with asthma, compared with 22 mL/year in patients without asthma (*144*).

In general, long-term asthma does not result in irreversible obstructive lung disease. However, an occasional patient with long-term asthma develops apparently irreversible disease in the absence of cigarette smoking, α_1-antitrypsin disease, or other obvious cause (*145*). Usually, these patients have childhood-onset asthma and are dependent on oral corticosteroids. Intensive therapy with oral and inhaled corticosteroids does not result in a normal FEV_1 of 80% of the predicted value as the mean FEV_1 was 57% (*145*). In contrast to the few patients with irreversible asthma, patients with asthma do not become "respiratory cripples," as might occur from COPD. Nevertheless, pulmonary physiologic studies do not reveal return of parameters to the expected normal ranges. Asthma patients are not deficient in the antiproteases that can be measured, and they do not have bullous abnormalities on chest radiographs. CT demonstrates gas trapping, especially on expiration, as well as bronchial wall thickening caused by increased smooth muscle mass and elastic and collagenous tissue. Some patients with asthma have evidence of bronchial dilatation on high resolution CT examination (146), but there are few areas of involvement in contrast to that of ABPA (Chapter 24).

Pneumomediastinum or pneumothorax can occur in patients presenting with acute severe asthma. Neck, shoulder, or chest pain is common, and crepitations can be detected in the neck or supraclavicular fossae. Rupture of distal alveoli results in dissection of air proximally through bronchovascular bundles. The air can then travel superiorly in the mediastinum to the supraclavicular or cervical areas. At times, the air dissects to the face or into the subcutaneous areas over the thorax. Treating the patient's asthma with systemic corticosteroids is indicated to reduce the likelihood of hyperinflation and continued air leak. Unless the pneumothorax is very large, conservative treatment is effective. Otherwise, thoracostomy with tube placement is necessary.

Fatalities from asthma are unnecessary because asthma is not an inexorably fatal disease. Fatalities do occur, however, and many factors have been suggested as explanations (1–3,50, 85,86,95,104,121,147–150). While some deaths from asthma are unavoidable despite appropriate medical care, a high percentage of deaths from asthma should be considered preventable. Survivors of major asthma events, such as respiratory failure or arrest, patients with pneumomediastinum or pneumothorax on two occasions, and those with repeated status asthmaticus despite oral corticosteroids have potentially fatal asthma and are at higher risk for fatality than other patients with asthma (50,151,152). The NAEPP refers to high risk patients as near fatal asthma (1–3).

Uncontrolled asthma can lead to mucus plugging of airways and frank collapse of a lobe or whole lung segment. The middle lobe can collapse, especially in children. Repeated mucoid impactions should raise the possibility of ABPA or cystic fibrosis.

Cough syncope or cough-associated cyanosis occurs in patients whose respiratory status has deteriorated and in whom acute severe asthma or need for emergency therapy has occurred. In the setting of severe airway obstruction from asthma, during inspiration, intrathoracic pressure is negative because the patient must generate very high negative pressures to apply radial traction on bronchi in an attempt to maintain their patency. During expiration, the patient must overcome severe airway resistance and premature airways collapse. Increases in intrathoracic pressure during expiration with severe coughing, as compared with intra-abdominal pressure, causes a decline in venous return to the right atrium. There may also be increased blood flow to the lung during a short inspiration, but that is accompanied by pooling in the pulmonary vasculature from the markedly elevated negative inspiratory pressure. There will be reduced blood flow to the left ventricle with temporary decreases in cardiac output and cerebral blood flow.

Pulsus paradoxus is present when there is greater than a 10-mm Hg decline in systolic blood pressure during inspiration. It is associated with severe airway obstruction and hyperinflation (153,154). The most frequent electrocardiographic findings during acute asthma are sinus tachycardia followed by right axis deviation, clockwise rotation, prominent R in lead V_1 and S in lead V_5, and tall peaked P waves consistent with cor pulmonale.

Linear growth retardation can occur from ineffectively controlled asthma and potentially as a complication of high-dosage inhaled corticosteroids. Administration of oral corticosteroids is indicated to prevent repeated hospitalizations and frequent episodes of wheezing dyspnea. The child often responds with a growth spurt. Alternate-day prednisone and recommended doses of inhaled corticosteroids do not result in growth retardation, especially when the prednisone dose is 30 mg on alternate days or less. Even high alternate-day doses in children can be tolerated reasonably well as long as episodes of acute severe asthma are prevented. In contrast, depot corticosteroids given every 2 to 3 weeks in high doses may result in growth retardation. Despite efficacy in asthma, such corticosteroid administration causes hypothalamic-pituitary-adrenal (HPA) suppression (152). The use of depot corticosteroids should be considered only in the most recalcitrant children (or adults) in terms of asthma management. Ineffective parental functioning or poor compliance usually accompanies such cases in which reliable administration of prednisone and inhaled corticosteroids is impossible. The term *malignant, potentially fatal asthma* has been suggested for such patients who are essentially impossible to manage according to guideline based management (151).

The overuse of short acting β_2-adrenergic agonists (>8 inhalations/day and especially 16 inhalations/day) is a risk factor for more severe episodes of asthma and fatalities (148). There has been controversy about scheduled use of long-acting β_2-adrenergic agonists, but the data do not support harmful effects (149,150) when used in combination with inhaled corticosteroids.

Psychological Factors

Asthma has evolved from a disorder considered to be psychological to one recognized as extremely complex and of unknown etiology. Psychological stress can cause modest reductions in expiratory flow rates such as occur while watching a terrifying movie (155). Laughing and crying or frank emotional upheaval, such as an argument with a family member, can result in wheezing. Some patients require additional anti-inflammatory medication to suppress such wheezing. Usually, if the patient has stable baseline respiratory status, acute severe asthma does not result. Nevertheless, some fatal episodes of asthma have been associated with a report of a high level of emotional stress. In an absence of how to quantitate stress and determine whether there is a dose-response effect in asthma, such information must be considered speculative. Specific personality patterns have not been identified in patients with asthma.

The patient with asthma may develop strategies to function with the burden of asthma as a chronic, disruptive, and potentially fatal disease. A variety of behavior patterns have been recognized, including (a) disease denial, with complacency or outright denial of symptoms, wishful thinking, refusal to alert the managing physician about a major change in respiratory symptoms, or personally decreasing medications; (b) using asthma for obvious secondary gain, such as to not attend school or work, or to gain compensation; (c) developing compulsive or manipulative patterns of behavior that restrict the lifestyle of the patient and family members excessively; and (d) resorting to quackery. Some patients display hateful behavior toward physicians and their office staff. Psychiatric care can be of value in some cases (Chapter 43), but patients may refuse appropriate psychiatric referrals. The use of PEFR monitoring devices can be misleading because patients can generate or report truly inaccurate measurements. Obviously, in contrast to theories implying that wheezing dyspnea in patients with asthma was primarily psychologic, the physician must now decide how much of a patient's symptoms and signs are from asthma and how much might be psychologic as a result of asthma. Indeed, a psychologist, psychiatrist, or social worker may help identify what the patient might lose should asthma symptoms be controlled better.

Major management problems occur when asthma patients also have schizophrenia, delusional behavior, neurosis, depression, or manic-depressive disorders (50,85–88). Suicidal attempts are recognized from unjustified cessation of prednisone or theophylline overdosage. Repeated episodes of life-threatening acute severe asthma are difficult to avoid in the setting of untreated major psychiatric conditions (Chapter 43). The presence of post-traumatic stress disorder (17) and a situation of violence and abuse (18) or serious psychiatric disease may make it difficult or impossible to achieve goals of asthma control according to national or international guidelines.

The presence of factitious asthma indicates significant psychiatric disturbance (156). Initially, there must be trust established between the patient and physician. Abrupt referral of the patient to a psychiatrist can result in an unanticipated suicidal attempt. Psychiatric care can be valuable if the patient is willing to participate in

therapy. Abnormal coping styles (88), such as wishful thinking instead of active involvement, impair the quality of life and interfere with optimal control of asthma.

■ CLASSIFICATION

Some types of asthma with an emphasis on etiology are listed in Table 19.7. It is helpful to categorize the type of asthma because treatment programs vary depending on the type of asthma present. Some patients have more than one type of asthma. The NAEPP Report 3 suggests assessing signs and symptoms of asthma in association with spirometry (3). Asthma severity is classified as intermittent (most of the time, implying mild asthma) or persistent (mild, moderate, or severe). In Table 19.8, a version of this classification system is presented. It can be helpful to determine that patients have "moderate persistent allergic asthma" and use the classifications from Tables 19.7 and 19.8 together when applicable.

Asthma in children may be classified by age of onset and persistence of wheezing. (Chapter 20). Designations include "transient early wheeze" (wheezing with lower respiratory tract illnesses before age 3 years but not thereafter), "late-onset wheeze" (wheezing beginning at or after age 6 years), and "persistent wheeze" (wheeze with lower respiratory tract illnesses before age 3 years and wheeze at age 6 years) (157).

In adults, another approach is that of grouping of patients with asthma into clusters using pre-specified variables including induced sputum eosinophil numbers (158). For example, some patients are classified as "concordant disease" because there is a match between symptoms and eosinophilic inflammation, whereas others are either "discordant symptoms" (excessive symptoms with little sputum eosinophilia that could

TABLE 19.7 CLINICAL CLASSIFICATION OF ASTHMA

Allergic asthma
Nonallergic asthma
Potentially fatal asthma
Malignant potentially fatal asthma
Aspirin-intolerant asthma
Occupational asthma
Exercise-induced asthma
Variant asthma
Factitious asthma
Vocal cord dysfunction and asthma
Coexistent asthma and chronic obstructive pulmonary disease
Irreversible asthma

TABLE 19.8   NATIONAL ASTHMA EDUCATION AND PREVENTION PROGRAM ASTHMA CLASSIFICATION SYSTEM: EXPERT PANEL REPORT 3

DESIGNATION	SYMPTOMS/SHORT-ACTING β_2-ADRENERGIC AGONIST USE	NOCTURNAL AWAKENINGS	PULMONARY FUNCTION
Intermittent	$\leq$2 days a week/ $\leq$2 days a week (not counting prophylaxis for exercise-induced bronchoconstriction)	$\leq$2 times a month	FEV_1 >80%; FEV_1/FVC normal; FEV_1 normal between exacerbations
Persistent (mild)	$\geq$2 days a week but not daily/ $\geq$2 days a week but not daily or more than once on a given day	3 to 4 times a month	FEV_1 > 80%; FEV_1/FVC normal
Persistent (moderate)	Daily symptoms/daily use	>1 night/week but not nightly	FEV_1 > 60% but <80%; FEV_1/FVC reduced by 5%
Persistent (severe)	Throughout the day/several times per day	Often 7 times/week	FEV_1 < 60% FEV_1/FVC reduced >5%

FEV_1, forced expiratory volume in 1 second; FVC, forced vital capacity.

RECOMMENDED INITIAL/ALTERNATIVE MEDICATIONS BASED ON ASTHMA SEVERITY

DESIGNATION	INITIAL	ALTERNATIVES
Intermittent	Short-acting β_2-adrenergic agonist prn	
Mild	Low-dose inhaled corticosteroid	Cromolyn, leukotriene receptor antagonist, nedocromil, theophylline
Moderate	Low-dose inhaled corticosteroid + long-acting β_2 adrenergic agonist or medium dose inhaled corticosteroid	Low-dose inhaled corticosteroid + leukotriene receptor antagonist, leukotriene biosynthesis inhibitor, or theophylline
Severe	Medium-dose corticosteroid,* + long-acting β_2 adrenergic agonist	Medium or high-dose inhaled corticosteroid* + Leukotriene receptor antagonist, leukotriene biosynthesis inhibitor, theophylline and consider omalizumab

* May require initial oral corticosteroid course to stabilize

For intermittent asthma or mild, moderate and severe persistent asthma, the components of patient education, environmental control and management of comorbities are recommended.

For patients with mild, moderate or severe persistent allergic asthma, subcutaneous allergen immunotherapy should be considered.

Modified from the National Heart, Lung, and Blood Institute. *Expert Panel Report 3: guidelines for the diagnosis and management of asthma.* National Heart, Lung and Blood Institute, National Institutes of Health, U. S. Department of Health and Human Services. 2007 (http://www.nhlbi.nih.gov/guidelines/asthma/asthgdln.htm)

characterize obese subjects or hypervigilant people) or "discordant inflammation" (few symptoms but high levels of sputum eosinophilia) (158).

Allergic Asthma

Allergic asthma is caused by inhalation of allergen that interacts with IgE present in high-affinity receptors (FcϵRI) on bronchial mucosal mast cells. Twenty-four hours after allergen bronchoprovocation challenge, bone marrow examination demonstrates increased numbers of eosinophil/basophil progenitor cells (159). These cells have been identified in both early responders and dual responders (159). The inflammatory progenitors then can populate the lungs (and nasal mucosa). There are many dimensions of the immunologic basis for allergic asthma (*108*).

Allergic asthma often occurs from ages 2 to 4 to 60+ years and has been recognized in the geriatric population (97). The use of the term *allergic asthma* implies that a temporal relationship exists between respiratory symptoms (clinical reactivity) and allergen exposure and that antiallergen IgE antibodies can be demonstrated or suspected. Approximately 75% to 90% of patients with persistent asthma have clinical reactivity or at least allergic sensitization depending on the study.

Respiratory symptoms may develop within minutes or in an hour after allergen exposure; however, they may not be obvious when there is uninterrupted allergen exposure. Common allergens associated with IgE-mediated asthma include pollens, such as from trees, grasses, and weeds; fungal spores; dust mites; animal dander; and in some settings, animal urine or cockroach excreta. IgE-mediated occupational asthma is considered under the category of occupational asthma. Allergen particle size must be less than 10 μm to penetrate into deeper parts of the lung because larger particles, such as ragweed pollen (19 μm), impact in the oropharynx. However, submicronic, "subpollen" ragweed particles have been described that could reach smaller airways (160). Particles smaller than 1 μm, however, may not be retained in the airways. Fungal spores, such as *Aspergillus* species, are 2 μm to 3 μm in size, and the major cat allergen (*Fel d 1*) has allergenic activity from 0.4 μm to 10 μm in size (*161*). Another study reported that 75% of *Fel d 1* was present in particles of at least 5 μm and that 25% of *Fel d 1* was present in particles of less than 2.5 μm (*162*). Cat dander allergen can be present in indoor air, on clothes, and in schoolrooms where no cats are present (163).

The potential severity of allergic asthma should not be minimized because experimentally, after an antigen-induced early bronchial response, bronchial hyperresponsiveness to an agonist such as methacholine or histamine can be demonstrated. This hyperresponsiveness precedes a late (3- to 11-hour) response (164). In addition, fungus-related (mold-related) asthma may result in a need for intensive antiasthma pharmacotherapy, including inhaled corticosteroids and even alternate-day prednisone in some patients. Exposure to *A. alternata*, a major fungal aeroallergen, was considered an important risk factor for respiratory arrests in 11 patients with asthma (165). The risk of asthma deaths is higher on days with mold spore counts >1000/mm^3 (166). Dust mites and animal danders are important triggers of allergic asthma. Cockroaches are another indoor allergen that can be associated with allergic sensitization and childhood asthma (167).

The diagnosis of allergic asthma should be suspected when symptoms and signs of asthma correlate closely with local patterns of pollinosis and fungal spore recoveries. For example, in the upper midwestern United States after a hard freeze in late November, which reduces (but does not eliminate entirely) fungal spore recoveries from outdoor air, patients suffering from mold-related asthma note a reduction in symptoms and medication requirements. When perennial symptoms of asthma are present, potential causes of asthma include animal dander, dust mites, cockroach excreta, mouse urine, and depending on the local conditions, fungal spores and pollens. Cockroach allergen (*Bla g 1*) is an important cause of asthma in infested buildings, usually in low socioeconomic areas. High indoor concentrations of mouse urine protein (*Mus d 1*) have been identified with volumetric sampling, and monoclonal antibodies directed at specific proteins suggested additional indoor allergens. The physician should correlate symptoms with allergen exposures, support the diagnosis by demonstration of antiallergen IgE antibodies, and institute measures when applicable to decrease allergen exposure.

Some recommendations for environmental control have been made (1–3). There is evidence supporting a multicomponent home-based environmental control program (8). In a study of inner-city children with asthma, where 94% of children had at least one positive skin test to an indoor allergen, the interventions included home visits for teaching; creating a plan of action; allergen-impermeable encasings for the mattress, box spring, and pillows; and a high efficiency particulate air (HEPA) filtered vacuum cleaner (8). If there were mold or animal sensitization or passive smoking, a HEPA air filter was used. For cockroach exposure and sensitization, professional pest control services were obtained. The 20% reduction in symptoms and days of wheeze with intensive environmental control measures was found to be as great as what has been reported in studies of inhaled corticosteroids (8). The beneficial effects of environmental control helps support the notion of allergic asthma being exacerbated by indoor allergens.

Detection of a major cat allergen, *Fel d 1*, in homes or schools never known to have cat exposure is consistent with transport of *Fel d 1* into such premises and sensitivity of immunoassays for cat allergen. The removal of an animal from a home and effectively encasing a mattress and pillow are interventions known to decrease the concentration of allergen below which many patients do not have clinical asthma symptoms.

Although food ingestion can result in anaphylaxis, persistent asthma is not explained by IgE-mediated reactions to ingested food. Food production exposure, such as occurs in bakers (168), egg handlers, flavoring producers, and workers exposed to vegetable gums, dried fruits, teas (169), or enzymes (170), is known to produce occupational asthma mediated by IgE antibodies.

Nonallergic Asthma

In nonallergic asthma, IgE-mediated airway reactions to common allergens are not present. Nonallergic asthma occurs at any age range, as does allergic asthma, but the former is generally more likely to occur in subjects younger than 4 years of age or older than 60 years of age. Episodes of nonallergic asthma are triggered by ongoing inflammation or by upper respiratory tract infections, purulent rhinitis, or exacerbations of chronic rhinosinusitis (CRS). Most patients have no evidence of IgE antibodies to common allergens. In youngsters, "transient early wheezers" have about a 70% likelihood of not having asthma by ages 9 to 11 years (171).

In other patients, skin tests are positive, but despite the presence of IgE antibodies, there is no temporal relationship between exposure and symptoms. Often, but not exclusively, the onset of asthma occurs in the setting of a viral upper respiratory tract infection. Virus infections have been associated with mediator release and bronchial epithelial shedding, which can lead to ongoing inflammation and asthma symptoms. Commonly recovered viruses that are associated with worsening asthma include picornaviruses (rhinoviruses), coronaviruses, RSV, parainfluenza viruses, influenza viruses, and adenovirus. CRS can be identified in some patients with asthma, as can nasal polyps with or without aspirin intolerance (aspirin exacerbated respiratory disease). Indoor air pollution (3) from volatile organic compounds, formaldehyde, wood burning stoves, and cigarette smoking can contribute to asthma of any kind including nonallergic asthma.

Some experimental data exist on the presence of antiviral IgE antibodies and asthma, but the clinical correlation remains to be established. It is important to consider occupation- or hobby-related exposures that may in fact be IgE-mediated in patients with nonallergic asthma. The T_H2 ("hygiene hypothesis") theory of asthma was supported in part by a study finding that protection against developing asthma in children aged 6 to 13 years was associated with day care attendance during the first 6 months of life or with having two or more older siblings at home (172). The "protected" children by age 13 years had a 5% incidence of asthma, compared with 10% in children who had not attended day care or who had one or no sibling (172). Of note is that at 2 years of age, the ultimately protected children had a 24% prevalence of wheezing, compared with 17% in nonprotected children. Overall, the frequent exposure to other children in early childhood, which is presumably associated with more viral infections, could result in a T_H1 predominance as opposed to a T_H2 or allergy profile of $CD4^+$ lymphocytes. Allergen immunotherapy is not indicated and will not be beneficial in patients with nonallergic asthma despite any presence of antiallergen IgE antibodies.

Potentially (Near) Fatal Asthma

The term *potentially (near) fatal asthma* describes the patient who is at high risk for an asthma fatality (86,151,152). The initial series of patients with potentially fatal asthma had one or more of the following criteria: (a) respiratory acidosis or failure from asthma, (b) endotracheal intubation from asthma, (c) two or more episodes of acute severe asthma despite use of oral corticosteroids and other antiasthma medications, or (d) two or more episodes of pneumomediastinum or pneumothorax from asthma. Other factors have been associated with a potentially fatal outcome from asthma, and these criteria may not identify all high-risk patients (2,3). The NAEPP summary lists some additional factors associated with exacerbations or deaths including persistent severe airflow obstruction, acute severe airflow obstruction, and being frightened by one's asthma (3). The physician managing the high-risk patient should be aware of the potential of a fatality and strive to prevent this outcome (151,152). The impossible-to-manage patient who has both severe asthma and noncompliance is referred to as having malignant, potentially fatal asthma (151).

Aspirin-induced Asthma

Selected patients with asthma, often nonallergic, have acute bronchoconstrictive responses to aspirin and or nonselective NSAIDs that inhibit cyclooxygenase-1 (13–15). The onset of acute bronchoconstrictive symptoms after ingestion of such agents can be within minutes (such as after chewing Aspergum) to within 3 hours (13). Some physicians accept a respiratory response that occurs within 8 to 12 hours after aspirin or NSAID ingestion; however, a shorter time interval seems more appropriate, such as up to 3 hours. In persistent asthma, variations in expiratory flow rates occur frequently, so that confirming that aspirin produces a reaction at 8 hours requires careful evaluation. The most severe reactions occur within minutes to 2 hours after ingestion. With indomethacin, 1 mg or 5 mg oral challenges have resulted in acute responses (*173*). Cross-reaction exists, such that certain nonselective NSAIDs that inhibit cyclooxygenase-1 (ibuprofen, indomethacin, flufenamic acid, and mefenamic acid) have a higher likelihood of inducing bronchospastic responses in aspirin-sensitive subjects than other NSAIDs. Because fatalities have occurred in aspirin-sensitive subjects with asthma, challenges should be carried out only with appropriate explanation to the patient, with obvious need for the challenge (such as presence of rheumatoid arthritis), and by experienced physicians. Interestingly, some aspirin-sensitive patients can be desensitized to aspirin after experiencing early bronchospastic responses (13,173). Subsequent regular administration of aspirin does not cause acute bronchospastic responses (13,173).

The term *aspirin exacerbated respiratory disease* (13) has replaced the term *aspirin triad* (*174*) and refers to aspirin-intolerant patients with asthma who also have chronic nasal polyps and CRS. The onset of asthma often precedes the recognition of aspirin intolerance by years. Approximately one-third to two-thirds of patients have immediate skin reactivity to common allergens (13). At one time, tartrazine (FD&C Yellow No. 5) was reported to result in immediate broncho-spastic reactions in 5% of patients with the aspirin triad (174). Contrary results in double-blind studies have been reported in that none of the patients responded to tartrazine (175). The risk for inadvertent exposure to tartrazine by the aspirin-intolerant patient appears to be smaller than initially reported and ranges from nonexistent (175) to 2.3% (176).

The drugs that produce such immediate respiratory responses share the ability to inhibit the enzyme cyclooxygenase-1, which is known to metabolize arachidonic acid into PGD_2, $PGF_{2\alpha}$, and thromboxanes. Structurally, these drugs are different but they have a common pharmacologic effect. Data suggest that the blockade of cyclooxygenase-1 diverts arachidonic acid away from production of PGE_2, with loss of its "braking effects" on the lipoxygenase pathway. This effect results in unrestrained overproduction of LTC_4 and LTD_4 (13,177,178). The latter is a potent bronchoconstrictive agonist. Patients with aspirin-exacerbated respiratory disease have higher baseline $PGF_{2\alpha}$ concentrations and higher urinary LTE_4 concentrations (13,178) than aspirin-tolerant patients with asthma. After aspirin ingestion, intolerant patients have profound increases in urinary LTE_4 compared with aspirin-tolerant subjects (13,178). When bronchial biopsy specimens were obtained from aspirin-intolerant and aspirin-tolerant patients with asthma, there were many more cells (primarily activated eosinophils, but also mast cells and macrophages) that expressed LTC_4 synthase in the aspirin-intolerant patients (13,179). This critical finding supports the urinary LTE_4 results, which are the marker for the bronchoconstrictor LTD_4 that requires LTC_4 synthase for generation. In other words, these data support a "knock in" as opposed to a "knock out" state. It has been demonstrated that after aspirin or NSAID ingestion, there is a decline in the protective PGE_2, whose main effect is the "brake" on synthesis of 5-lipoxygenase (5-LO) and 5-lipoxygenase-activating protein (FLAP) (13). The lack of or reduced inhibition of these two key enzymes in the lipoxygenase pathway, allows for excessive generation of LTC_4 at baseline and after aspirin or nonselective NSAID ingestion (13). The overexpression of LTC_4 synthase primarily by eosinophils results in profound increases in LTD_4 after aspirin or a nonselective cyclooxygenase inhibitor is ingested. Bronchial biopsies have not identified differential staining for cycloxygenase-1, cyclooxygenase-2, 5-lipoxygenase, LTA_4 hydrolase, or FLAP in aspirin-intolerant versus aspirin-tolerant patients (180). The effects of excessive LTD_4 production appear to be amplified by increased numbers of its receptor, specifically cysteinyl leukotriene type 1 receptor as compared to cysteinyl leukotriene type 2 receptor (13,181,182).

Mast cell activation occurs after aspirin challenges as well. There are increases in histamine (and LTC_4) in bronchial lavage and nasal fluid after aspirin challenges (13,183). In some patients, there is an increase in tryptase and PGD_2, a potent bronchoconstrictor, vasodilator and chemoattractant for eosinophils (13,184). For virtually all patients, selective cyclooxygenase-2 inhibitors will be tolerated safely in aspirin-intolerant patients (13,185,186).

Occupational Asthma

Occupational asthma has been estimated to occur in 5% to 15% of all patients with asthma (99,100). Specific industry prevalence may be even higher (e.g., 16%) in snow crab processors in Canada (187). Occupational asthma may or may not be IgE-mediated. When it is IgE-mediated, accumulating longitudinal data support a time of sensitization followed by development of bronchial hyperresponsiveness and then bronchoconstriction (99,100,187). After removal from the workplace exposure, the reverse sequence has been recorded. At the time of removal from exposure, factors associated with persistent asthma include having symptoms for more than 1 year, having abnormal pulmonary function tests, and taking asthma medications. Malo et al. documented that spirometry and bronchial hyperresponsiveness in patients no longer working with snow crabs reached a plateau of improvement by 2 years after cessation of work exposure (187). In workers with occupational asthma attributable to detergent enzymes such as proteases, amylase, and cellulases, some 71% of workers continued to report respiratory symptoms 3 years after removal from the workplace (170). Occupational asthma has been recognized among health care professionals (from 4.2% in physicians to 7.3% in nurses) (188). It is thought that some of the cases are irritant as opposed to allergic (188). The assessment of patients with possible occupational asthma is discussed in detail in Chapter 25. Some workers have early, late, dual, or irritant bronchial responses, such as occur to trimellitic anhydride, which is used in the plastics industry as a curing agent in the manufacture of epoxy resins.

The differential diagnosis of occupational asthma is complex and includes consideration of irritants, smoke, toxic gases, metal exposures, insecticides, organic chemicals and dusts, infectious agents, and occupational chemicals. In addition, one must differentiate true occupational asthma from exposed workers who have coincidental adult-onset asthma not affected by workplace exposure. Some workers have chemical exposure and a compensation syndrome, but no objective asthma despite symptoms and usually a poor response to medications. One must exclude work-related neuroses with fixation on an employer as well as a syndrome of reactive airways dysfunction, which occurs after an accidental exposure to a chemical irritant or toxic gas (*189,190*).

Atopic status and smoking do not predict workers who will become ill to lower-molecular-weight chemicals. Atopic status and smoking are predictors of IgE-mediated occupational asthma to high-molecular-weight chemicals. For example, Western red cedar workers display bronchial hyperresponsiveness during times of exposure, with reductions in hyperresponsiveness during exposure-free periods. It is still undetermined whether antiplicatic acid IgE is necessary for development of Western red cedar asthma because immediate skin tests may be negative while bronchial responses are present.

The complexity of diagnosing occupational asthma cannot be underestimated in some workers. Respiratory symptoms may intensify when a worker returns from a vacation but may not be dramatic when deterioration occurs during successive days at work. In patients with preexisting asthma, fumes at work may cause an aggravation of asthma without having been the cause of asthma initially.

Avoidance measures and temporary pharmacologic therapy can suffice to help confirm a diagnosis in some cases. Resumption of exposure should produce objective bronchial obstruction and clinical changes. The physician must be aware that workers may return serial PEFR measurements that coincide with expected abnormal values during work or shortly thereafter. Such values should be assessed critically because they are effort dependent and may be manipulated. Demonstration of IgE or IgG antibodies to the incriminated workplace allergen or to an occupational chemical bound to a carrier protein has been of value in supporting the diagnosis of occupational asthma and even in prospective use to identify workers who are at risk for occupational asthma (*191*). Such assays are not commonly available but are of discriminatory value when properly performed.

If a bronchial provocation challenge is deemed necessary, it is preferable to have the employee perform a job-related task that exposes him or her to the usual concentration of occupational chemicals. Subsequent blinding may be necessary as well, and successive challenges may be needed. The PC_{20} to histamine can decrease after an uneventful challenge, but the next day, when the employee is exposed to the incriminated agent again, a 30% decline in FEV_1 can occur, which confirms the diagnosis (*192*).

Exercise-induced Asthma/Bronchoconstriction

Exercise-induced asthma occurs in response to either an isolated disorder in patients with intermittent asthma or an inability to complete an exercise program in symptomatic patients with persistent asthma. Control of the latter often permits successful participation in a reasonable degree of exercise. In patients with intermittent asthma, whose only symptoms might be triggered by exercise, the pattern of bronchoconstriction is as follows: during initial exercise, the FEV_1 is slightly increased (about 5%), unchanged, or slightly reduced, but no symptoms occur. This is followed by declines of FEV_1 and onset of symptoms 5 to 15 minutes after cessation of exercise. The decline of FEV_1 is at least 15% (*193–195*). Airway hyperresponsiveness is present in the patients with asthma, and there is an increase in eNO (196). The term *exercise-induced bronchoconstriction* refers to airway closure that occurs only with exercise, especially common in elite athletes (194). Not all of these athletes have hyperresponsive bronchi when challenged with histamine or methacholine as direct agonists; some athletes react only to indirect agonists such as mannitol and hypertonic saline (4.5%) (194). This finding has led to the notion that there may be injury to the airway in elite athletes as opposed to airway inflammation that characterizes asthma (193,194).

Exercise-induced asthma resulting in a decline in FEV_1 of at least 15% is associated with inspiration of cold or dry air. In general, greater declines in spirometry and the presence of respiratory symptoms are directly proportional to the level of hyperventilation and inversely proportional to inspired air temperature and humidity. The mechanism of bronchoconstriction is considered to be related to an increase in osmolarity of the periciliary fluid that accompanies the necessary conditioning of inspired air (197). It has been thought that the loss of water is able to increase the osmolarity of the periciliary fluid to over 900 mOsm so that there is bronchoconstriction (197). Another explanation is that postexertional airway rewarming causes increased bronchial mucosal blood flow as a possible mechanistic explanation (198). Clinically, it has been recognized that running outdoors while inhaling dry, cold air is a far greater stimulus to asthma than swimming or running indoors while breathing warmer humidified air. It has been argued that the hyperventilation of exercise causes a loss of heat from the airway, which is followed by cooling of the bronchial mucosa. The "resupply" of warmth to the mucosa causes hyperemia and edema of the airway wall (198). In addition, there are greater declines in FEV_1 during exercise when there are higher levels of eosinophils in induced sputum. This finding supports an association between eosinophilic inflammation and exercise-induced asthma (199).

Exercise-induced bronchoconstriction (EIB) can occur in any form of asthma on a persistent basis but also can be prevented completely or to a great extent by pharmacologic treatment. In prevention of isolated episodes of EIB, medications such as short-acting inhaled β-adrenergic agonists inspired 10 to 15 minutes before exercise often prevent significant exercise-associated symptoms. Long acting β₂-adrenergic agonists also are bronchoprotective. Cromolyn by inhalation is effective, as to a lesser extent are oral β-adrenergic agonists and theophylline. Leukotriene receptor antagonists have a positive but more modest protective effect and suggest that LTD_4 participates in EIB (200). Histamine$_1$ antagonists may provide bronchoprotection is some subjects. For patients with persistent asthma, overall improvement in respiratory status by avoidance measures and regular pharmacotherapy can minimize exercise symptoms. Pretreatment with short-acting or long-acting β_2-adrenergic agonists in addition to scheduled antiasthma therapy can allow asthma patients to participate in exercise activities successfully. Inhaled corticosteroids can help modify the extent of decline in FEV_1 from exercise (199).

Variant Asthma

Most patients with asthma report symptoms of coughing, chest tightness, and dyspnea, and the physician can auscultate wheezing or rhonchi on examination. *Variant asthma* refers to asthma with the primary symptoms of paroxysmal and repetitive coughing or dyspnea in the absence of wheezing. The coughing often occurs after an upper respiratory infection, exercise, or exposure to odors, fresh paint, or allergens. Sputum is usually not produced, and the cough occurs on a nocturnal basis. Antitussives, expectorants, antibiotics, and use of intranasal corticosteroids do not suppress the coughing. The chest examination is free of wheezing or rhonchi. McFadden (*201*) documented increases in large airways resistance, moderate to severe reductions in FEV_1 (mean, 53%), and bronchodilator responses. The mean RV was 152%, consistent with air trapping. In addition, patients with exertional dyspnea as the prime manifestation of asthma had an FEV_1 value still within normal limits but a RV of 236% (201) and not greatly increased airways resistance. Both phenotypes had reduced small airways flow rates. Some patients can be induced to wheeze after exercise or after performing an FVC maneuver.

Pharmacologic therapy can be successful to suppress the coughing episodes or sensation of dyspnea. When inhaled, β_2-adrenergic agonists have not been effective; the best way to suppress symptoms is with an inhaled corticosteroid. If using an inhaler produces coughing, a 5- to 7-day course of oral corticosteroids often stops the coughing (*130,202*). At times, even longer courses of oral corticosteroids and antiasthma therapy are necessary.

Factitious Asthma

Factitious asthma presents diagnostic and management problems that often require multidisciplinary approaches to treatment (156,*203*). The diagnosis may not be suspected initially because patient history, antecedent triggering symptoms, examination, and even abnormal pulmonary physiologic parameters may appear consistent with asthma. Nevertheless, there may be no response to appropriate treatment or, in fact, worsening of asthma despite what would be considered effective care. Some patients are able to adduct their vocal cords during inspiration and on expiration, emit a rhonchorous sound,

simulating asthma. Other patients have repetitive coughing paroxysms or "seal barking" coughing fits. A number of patients with factitious asthma are physicians, nurses, or paramedical personnel who have an unusual degree of medical knowledge. Psychiatric disease can be severe, yet patients seem appropriate in a given interview. Factitious asthma episodes do not occur during sleep, and the experienced physician can distract the patient with factitious asthma and temporarily cause an absence of wheezing or coughing. Invasive procedures may be associated with conversion reactions or even respiratory "arrests" from breath holding.

Vocal Cord Dysfunction and Asthma

Vocal cord disfunction (VCD) (also called *laryngeal dyskinesia*) may coexist with asthma (140,141,204) (Fig. 19.7B). In a series of 95 patients with VCD, 53 patients had asthma. The level of medication prescriptions can be very high in patients with VCD with or without asthma (140). Of great concern is the prolonged use of oral corticosteroids for dyspnea that is, in fact, due to VCD and not from asthma. Patients with VCD and asthma may or may not have insight into the VCD. Some patients can be taught by a speech therapist to avoid vocal cord adduction during inspiration. The diagnosis can be suspected when there is a truncated inspiratory loop on a flow-volume loop and when direct visualization of the larynx identifies vocal cord adduction on inspiration, on CT examination of the neck (204), or by bedside examination. In the latter case, the patient may have a diagnosis of asthma and be hospitalized. While symptoms are present, the patient has limited wheezing or a quiet chest, relatively normal blood gases or pulse oximetry, and is unwilling to phonate the vowel "e" for more than 3 seconds. Also, when prompted, there is no large inspiratory effort made. In the series of 95 patients, many were health care providers and females who were obese (140). Gastroesophageal reflux disease (GERD) was present in 15 of 40 (37.5%) patients who had both VCD and asthma, compared with 11 of 33 (33%) with VCD without asthma (140). Thirty-eight percent of the 95 patients had a history of abuse, such as physical, sexual, or emotional (140). VCD should be suspected in difficult-to-control patients with asthma, in patients whose symptoms or medical requirements do not concur with the relatively normal spirometric or arterial blood gas findings, and in those who have prolonged hoarseness with dyspnea, wheezing, or coughing, with or without asthma.

Coexistent Asthma and Chronic Obstructive Pulmonary Disease

Usually, in the setting of long-term cigarette smoking (at least 30 to 40 pack-years), asthma may coexist with COPD. Obviously, the patients with asthma or COPD should not smoke. Multiple medications may be administered in patients with asthma and COPD to minimize signs and symptoms. However, some dyspnea likely will be fixed and not transient because of underlying COPD. The component of asthma can be significant, perhaps 25% to 50% initially. However, with continued smoking, the reversible component, using oral and inhaled corticosteroids, β_2-adrenergic agonists, combination inhaled corticosteroid/long-acting β_2-adrenergic agonist, theophylline, tiotropium, and leukotriene antagonists, diminishes or becomes nonexistent. At that point, the fewest medications possible should be used. When there is no benefit from oral corticosteroids, it is advisable to taper and discontinue them.

Initially, such as after hospitalization for asthma, the patient with combined asthma and COPD may benefit from a 2- to 4-week course of oral corticosteroids. The effort to identify the maximal degree of reversibility should be made even when asthma is a modest component of COPD. The lack of bronchodilator responsiveness or peripheral blood eosinophilia does not preclude a response to a 2-week course of prednisone.

Long-term care of patients with coexistent asthma and COPD can be successful in improving quality of life and reducing or eliminating disabling wheezing. A combination of inhaled corticosteroid and long-acting β_2-adrenergic agonist may improve patient outcomes (205). However, eventually, patients may succumb to end-stage COPD or coexisting cardiac failure.

■ NONANTIGENIC PRECIPITATING STIMULI

Hyperresponsiveness of bronchi in patients with asthma is manifested clinically by responses to various nonantigenic triggers. Some airborne triggers include odors such as cigarette smoke, fresh paint, cooking, perfumes, cologne, insecticides, and household cleaning agents (206). In addition, sulfur dioxide, ozone, nitrogen dioxide, carbon monoxide and other combustion products, both indoors and outdoors, can trigger asthma signs and symptoms. Emergency department visits for asthma in adults in New York City peaked 2 days after increases in ambient air ozone levels (207). The effect was most pronounced in patients who had smoked more than 14 pack-years of cigarettes (207). There was no ozone effect for adult nonsmokers or light smokers (<13 pack-years) with asthma. In this study, most patients had persistent severe asthma, and there was no effect of relative humidity on emergency department visits. These data support an effect of ozone on patients with severe asthma who were cigarette smokers. Adverse effects of ozone were not found in light or nonsmokers. Bronchoconstriction likely occurs on an irritant basis. Effective management of patients with asthma may permit patients to tolerate most inadvertent exposures with little troubling effects. Diesel exhaust particles have been shown to stimulate increases in allergen-specific IgE antibodies and increase IL-4 and IL-13 production. Further, these particles were able to induce isotype switching from IgM to IgE antibodies in B cells (208). The public health effects of diesel exhaust particles may be very great on emergence of allergen responses (208,209).

GERD has been a recognized trigger of asthma episodes (3,210). Frank GERD with aspiration into the bronchi has been associated with chronic cough, episodic wheezing, rhonchi, and even cyanosis if aspiration is severe. Reflux of gastric acid into the lower esophagus can precipitate symptoms of asthma or cough without frank aspiration, perhaps by micro aspiration or an esophagobronchial vagal reflex (210). While patients with asthma and GERD who have undergone esophageal acid infusion have demonstrated increases in airways resistance and decreases in PEFR, patients with asthma without GERD can also have these changes. An acute episode of asthma can cause increased negative intrathoracic pressures, which can increase reflux. Medical therapy, such as avoiding meals for 3 hours before recumbency, weight reduction, cessation of cigarette smoking, discontinuation of drugs that decrease gastroesophageal sphincter tone (theophylline), diet manipulation, and raising the head of the bed 6 inches, may be of value. Elevation of the head of the bed and sleeping in the left lateral decubitus position can help reduce the symptoms of reflux (211). Pharmacotherapy with protein-pump inhibitors (PPIs) for 3 months is advisable and then an assessment should be made regarding continued therapy. Some patients will benefit from twice daily PPI (taken 30 minutes before breakfast and dinner) and a histamine$_2$ receptor antagonist at bedtime (212). Surgical intervention is indicated rarely but has been successful in varying degrees with either laparoscopic fundoplication or open procedures in patients with large hiatal hernias, strictures, or previous surgery (213). Nonacid reflux also contributes to cough and may be present when there has been an inadequate response to twice daily, PPI therapy with or without a histamine$_2$ receptor antagonist (214).

Some patients with asthma have "atypical reflux" which is considered a preferable description for supraesophageal reflux disease (SERD) or laryngopharyngeal reflux (LPR), characterized by hoarseness, throat clearing, globus sensation, and persistent cough. Other patients have nonerosive reflux disease (NERD), in which case the endoscopic exam reveals little or no evidence of reflux and there are normal esophageal pH measurements despite symptoms consistent with GERD.

Chronic rhinosinusitis (Chapter 27) and acute exacerbations of rhinosinusitis can cause acute severe asthma or exacerbations of asthma. Patients with intermittent asthma may experience an exacerbation of asthma in the setting of acute rhinosinusitis, upper respiratory tract infection or community acquired pneumonia. Common

variable immunodeficiency or specific antibody deficiency (Chapter 4) may be diagnosed in the patient with
an infectious cause for an exacerbation of asthma or
chronic rhinosinusitis and persistent asthma.

Left-sided congestive heart failure (CHF) has been
associated with exacerbations of asthma. Bronchial
hyperresponsiveness has been recognized in nonasthmatic patients who developed left ventricular failure.
When patients with asthma develop CHF, at times, sudden episodes of wheezing dyspnea can occur in the absence of neck vein distention or peripheral edema,
which would support a diagnosis of left ventricular failure. Differentiating pulmonary edema from acute asthma
may be difficult in brittle cardiac patients who have persistent moderate or severe asthma or asthma, COPD, and
left ventricular failure. B-type natriuretic peptide can be
elevated in the setting of left ventricular failure (215).
Some cases of exacerbations of asthma or asthma and
CHF are precipitated by acute pulmonary emboli. In
patients with CHF and acute asthma or COPD, a non-
elevated concentration of B-type natriuretic peptide
(<100 pg/mL) essentially excludes heart failure and
supports exacerbations of asthma or COPD (215).

■ DIFFERENTIAL DIAGNOSIS OF WHEEZE, DYSPNEA & COUGH

There are many causes of wheezing, dyspnea, and
coughing individually and collectively. A partial listing
follows:

I. Commonly encountered diseases or conditions
  A. Asthma
  B. Upper respiratory tract infection
    1. Bronchiolitis
    2. Croup
    3. Viruses (e.g., RSV, rhinovirus, influenza, par-
ainfluenza, metapneumovirus, etc.)
    4. Acute and chronic bronchitis
    5. Acute community acquired pneumonia
    6. Bronchiectasis
    7. Rhinosinusitis
  C. Congestive heart failure (CHF)
    1. Left ventricular failure
    2. Mitral stenosis
    3. Congenital heart disease
  D. COPD (Chronic Obstructive Pulmonary Disease)
  E. Hyperventilation syndrome
  F. Pulmonary infarction or embolism
  G. Cystic fibrosis
  H. Vocal cord dysfunction
  I. Laryngotracheomalacia
  J. Bronchopulmonary dysplasia
  K. Vascular rings
  L. GERD

II. Less common conditions
  A. Tuberculosis
  B. Hypersensitivity pneumonitis (avian or microor-
ganisms, e.g., fungi and bacteria)
  C. Inhalation of irritant gases, odors, or dusts
  D. Physical obstruction of the upper airways
    1. Neoplasms (benign or malignant)
    2. Foreign bodies
    3. Acute laryngeal or pharyngeal angioedema
    4. Bronchial stenosis
      a. Postintubation
      b. Granulomatous
      c. Postburn
  E. Interstitial lung disease
  F. *Pneumocystis carinii* pneumonia
  G. Sarcoidosis
  H. Bronchomalacia
III. Uncommon conditions
  A. Restrictive lung disease
  B. Churg-Strauss vasculitis
  C. Mediastinal enlargement
  D. Diphtheria
  E. Carcinoid tumor of main-stem bronchi
  F. Thymoma
  G. Tracheoesophageal fistula
  H. Allergic bronchopulmonary aspergillosis (ABPA)
  I. α1-Antitrypsin deficiency
  J. Factitious coughing, wheezing, or stridor

■ TREATMENT

The treatment of an episode of acute asthma varies
according to its clinical severity. Similarly, long-term
treatment regimens depend on the type of asthma by
classification and severity (Tables 19.7 and 19.8). The
basic objective of treatment, as in other chronic illnesses, is to achieve significant control (3) of symptoms
to prevent physical as well as psychological impairment
(Table 19.9). The NAEPP Expert Panel Report 3

TABLE 19.9 GOALS OF THERAPY IN MANAGEMENT OF ASTHMA

Prevent fatalities

Maximize asthma control

Prevent hospitalizations, emergency department visits and unscheduled care visits

Prevent/reduce nocturnal asthma

Prevent/reduce limitations of activities, school/work absenteeism/presenteeism

Maximize respiratory status and pulmonary function

Use appropriate medications

Prepare an action plan for exacerbations (know the patient)

suggests considering three dimensions: the level of severity, control, and responsiveness (ease of treatment) (3).

In addition to clinical improvement, the practical goals of treatment are best measured by avoidance of fatalities, hospitalizations, school or work absenteeism/presenteeism, and the ability of the patient to lead a normal, functional life with little or no impairment of exercise activities and sleep habits. The NAEPP Expert Panel Report 3 suggested specific management protocols for patients categorized with intermittent or persistent mild, moderate, and severe asthma (3) as listed in Table 19.8. The goals should be to maximize control of symptoms of asthma, permit as normal a lifestyle as possible, avoid nocturnal asthma, and achieve the best respiratory status possible. Another goal is preservation of lung function to avoid excessive loss of FEV_1. Finally, it is advisable to avoid untoward effects of medications, if possible, and to provide cost-effective and "personalized" therapies, recognizing differences in responses to therapies.

Principles

The treatment of asthma consists of therapeutic measures to control inflammatory changes and to reverse bronchial mucosal edema, bronchospasm, hypersecretion of mucus, and V/Q imbalance. Depending on the severity of the attack, degree of hypocarbia or hypercarbia and the resultant acid-base changes, individualized specific therapy is often required. Finally, other emergency measures may be necessary to prevent or treat acute respiratory failure.

Preventive measures are very important in the proper management of asthma. In exercise-induced asthma/bronchoconstriction, appropriate premedication can prevent symptoms. In allergic asthma, removing the offending allergen or allergens is of primary importance because it can reduce symptoms, decrease the need for medications, and eventually decrease bronchial hyperresponsiveness. If this is impossible, immunotherapy should be considered (3,216,217). Immunomodulatory treatment (omalizumab) can be instituted for patients with persistent moderate and severe asthma (218). Protective measures must also be included to lessen the deleterious effects of certain aggravating factors, such as dust mites and fungi. In addition, drugs that precipitate asthma should be avoided.

Asthma is a complex disorder! An approach to treatment of asthma consists of determining the clinical classification (Table 19.7), the functional classification (Table 19.8), necessary avoidance measures, drug therapy, allergen immunotherapy, or immunomodulator therapy when indicated, and other conditions that may affect the patient (Tables 19.9, 19.10, and 19.11).

TABLE 19.10 ACUTE ASTHMA TIPS

In the emergency department

1. Establish severity of asthma:
   Cannot speak in a sentence?
   Accessory muscle use?
   Cyanotic?
   Heart rate 120 beats/min or greater?
   Cannot perform spirometry or peak flow is less than 200 L/min?
   β_2-adrenergic agonist overuse?
   Marked nocturnal symptoms?
2. Send the patient who clears after emergency therapy home with a short course of oral corticosteroids. Arrange follow-up care.

In the office

1. Does the patient need hospitalization or emergency therapy?
2. A combination of regular β_2-adrenergic agonist and inhaled corticosteroid may suffice. Otherwise add a short course of an oral corticosteroid.
3. Check inhaler technique.
4. Schedule follow-up care.
5. Consider referral to an allergist-immunologist.

Drug Therapy

β_2-Adrenergic Receptor Antagonists

The effects of an adrenergic agonist depend on its specific (α or β) receptor-stimulating capacity as well as on the type and density of receptor present in the organ or tissue stimulated (*Table 19.12*). The bronchi contain predominantly β_2-adrenergic receptors, which promote bronchodilation. β-Receptors themselves may from organ to organ. Those in the heart are primarily β_1-adrenergic receptors, which increase cardiac contractibility and heart rate. Thus, adrenergic drugs possessing β_2-stimulating activity are most effective in the treatment of asthma (see Chapter 34 and Table 19.13).

Biochemical mechanisms of action of the β-stimulating adrenergic drugs have not been completely clarified, but they are known to increase the rate of formation of 3'5'-cyclic adenosine monophosphate (cAMP) from adenosine triphosphate (ATP) in the presence of adenylyl cyclase (formerly called *adenylate* or *adenyl cyclase*) (Fig. 19.8). The increased cAMP in turn triggers other intermediate processes, which ultimately result in both bronchodilation and inhibition of the mediator release in immediate hypersensitivity reactions. These effects reverse or inhibit some of the pathophysiologic events known to occur in asthma.

β_2-Adrenergic agonists have great value in management of asthma and limitations as well. Although often not considered "anti-inflammatory" therapy, β_2-adrenergic agonists increase the function of cilia in

---

TABLE 19.11   PERSISTENT ASTHMA TIPS

1. Appreciate limitations of inhaled β_2-adrenergic agonists, cromolyn, leukotriene receptor antagonists and biosynthesis inhibitors, and theophylline.
2. Check and improve inhaler technique even in patients using spacer devices.
3. Reassess the patient after initial therapy and change management if satisfactory improvement has not occurred.
4. Emphasize anti-inflammatory therapy as opposed to scheduled β_2-adrenergic agonists (and possibly theophylline).
5. Address allergic factors at home, school, and workplace. Consider referral to an allergist-immunologist.
6. Exclude allergic bronchopulmonary aspergillosis.
7. Many patients are managed successfully with inhaled corticosteroids with or without β_2-adrenergic agonists.
8. Avoid excessively demanding medication regimens.
9. Arrange for emergencies or deteriorations in respiratory status by involving the patient or family, if possible.
10. Use oral corticosteroids early to decrease asthma symptoms in a patient who has deteriorated after an upper respiratory tract infection rather than as a "last resort."
11. Identify patients with potentially (near) fatal asthma.

---

epithelial cells, decrease microvascular permeability, and facilitate the translocation of the glucocorticoid receptor from the cytoplasm into the nucleus of the cell (219). Long-acting β_2-adrenergic agonists also can inhibit both the early and late bronchoprovocation responses to inhaled allergen (*Table 19.14*). Thus, there are at least some actions of long-acting β_2-adrenergic agonists that could be considered as anti-inflammatory. However, there are some limitations to consider; as with inhaled corticosteroids and theophylline, the dose-response curve for β_2-adrenergic agonists becomes flattened as the dose of medication is increased. The combination of an inhaled corticosteroid and 12-hour β_2-adrenergic agonist provides effective asthma control and is indicated for patients with persistent moderate and severe asthma (3). As patients improve, less or no β_2-adrenergic agonist can be used, whether short-acting or long-acting agonist. Alternatively, full control may not be achievable with combination inhaled corticosteroid/β_2-adrenergic agonist therapy (220).

With short-acting β_2-adrenergic agonists, there is concern about their scheduled use potentiating allergic inflammation. In a study of 11 patients with allergic asthma who had dual responses on bronchoprovocation challenges, 1 week's use of albuterol by MDI, 200 µg 4 times daily, was associated with a larger late asthmatic response (*221*). With placebo inhaler, there was a decline in FEV_1 during the early response of 17.9%, and with albuterol 21.1%, a nonsignificant trend was noted (211). However, the late asthmatic response was affected in that the placebo response was a decline in FEV_1 of 13.2%, compared with 23.1% after 1 week of albuterol (221). The conclusion was that regular, scheduled use of albuterol could cause continued airway inflammation. In this study, nonspecific bronchial responsiveness changed modestly from 1.9 mg/mL with

placebo to 2.4 mg/mL with albuterol treatment (221). How much clinical effect these data have on asthma control and management has been controversial. For patients with persistent moderate or severe asthma, however, it has been advisable to use an inhaled corticosteroid and a β_2-adrenergic agonist together, trying not to use additional scheduled short-acting β_2-adrenergic agonists. A medication may be a bronchodilator, and it may or may not have bronchoprotective/anti-inflammatory properties. As regards salmeterol, 24 patients with mild asthma received either salmeterol 50 µg twice daily or placebo for 8 weeks (**222**). Methacholine challenges were performed initially and at the end of the study. Salmeterol caused a steady, almost 10% increase in FEV_1 throughout the 8 weeks (222). There was no evidence for tachyphylaxis. Nevertheless, there was a 10-fold shift (from 1.5 mg/mL to 16 mg/mL) in the PC_{20} to methacholine 1 hour after the initial salmeterol dose, meaning less responsive airways. By 4 weeks, the PC_{20} was 3 mg/mL and remained at that concentration at 8 weeks (222). Thus, although a bronchodilator effect continued, bronchoprotection was temporary and associated with tolerance (222).

In a 16-week study of 255 patients with mild asthma, "as-needed" and "scheduled" albuterol produced similar degrees of bronchodilation and symptom control (223). Patients with moderate or severe persistent asthma may require scheduled salmeterol or formoterol and intermittent albuterol or other short-acting β_2-adrenergic agonist. Responses of FEV_1 to albuterol were preserved for 6 hours despite regular use of salmeterol (224). Such patients should receive inhaled corticosteroid therapy, but even in its absence, in this study, tachyphylaxis to albuterol did not occur (224).

There is significant variability in responses to β_2-adrenergic agonists which has led to studies of single

TABLE 19.13 β_2-ADRENERGIC AGONISTS FOR ASTHMA

NAME	SINGLE ENTITY FORMULATION
Albuterol	Proair HFA inhalation suspension 90 mcg Proventil HFA inhalation suspension 90 mcg Ventolin HFA inhalation suspension 90 mcg Albuterol inhalation solution 0.083%, 0.5% Accuneb inhalation solution 0.21%, 0.42% Ventolin syrup 2 mg/5 mL VoSpire ER extended-release tablets 4 mg, 8 mg
Salmeterol	Serevent inhalation suspension 21 mcg Serevent Diskus 50 mcg
Levalbuterol	Xopenex pediatric inhalation solution 0.31 mg/3mL, Xopenex inhalation solution 0.63 mg/3mL, 1.25 mg/3mL, 1.25 mg/0.5mL Xopenex HFA inhalation suspension 45 mcg
Pirbuterol	Maxair Autohaler 200 mcg
Metaproterenol	Alupent inhalation aerosol 0.65 mg Metaproterenol inhalation aerosol 0.4%, 0.6% Alupent syrup 10 mg/5 mL Albuterol tablets 10mg, 20mg
Terbutaline	Terbutaline solution for injection 1 mg/mL Terbutaline tablets 2.5 mg, 5 mg
Formoterol	Foradil aerolizer inhalation powder 12 mcg Perforomist nebulizer solution 20 mcg/2mL
Fenoterol	Berotec inhalation solution 0.25 mg/mL, 0.625 mg/mL Berotec inhalation aerosol 100 mcg Berotec tablets 2.5 mg
	COMBINATIONS
Albuterol/Ipratropium bromide	Combivent inhalation suspension Duoneb nebulizer solution
Fluticasone/Salmeterol	Advair Diskus inhalation powder 100/50, 250/50, 500/50 Advair HFA inhalation suspension 45/21, 115/21, 230/21
Budesonide/Formoterol	Symbicort 80/4/5, 160/4.5 inhalation aerosol

nucleotide polymorphisms of the gene on chromosome 5 that codes for the β_2-adrenergic receptor. The genotype of the β_2-adrenergic receptor has been explored in the context of control of asthma and bronchodilator responses (225). Most patients with mild asthma have the Glycine/Glycine genotype at the 16th amino acid position of the β_2-adrenergic receptor and such patients have a better response to β_2-adrenergic agonist therapy compared with patients who have the Arginine/Arginine genotype (225). This finding has not been replicated in patients treated with either formoterol/budesonide or salmeterol/fluticasone combinations (226). Thus, although there are differences in responses to short-acting β_2-adrenergic agonists, additional investigations are needed to understand therapeutic differences and how to provide "personalized" pharmacotherapy.

Excessive use of short-acting β_2-adrenergic agonists has been associated with fatalities from asthma (148). Physicians, other health care providers, and pharmacists need to be aware of overuse of MDIs, dry-powder inhalers, or nebulizers by patients. Unlimited or unsupervised prescription refills cannot be recommended because patient self-management when asthma is worsening may result in a fatality. As an asthma attack worsens and continued β_2-adrenergic agonist therapy is used in the absence of inhaled or oral corticosteroids, there may be development of arterial hypoxemia, carbon dioxide retention, and acidosis not recognized by the patient. Data support the use of regularly scheduled

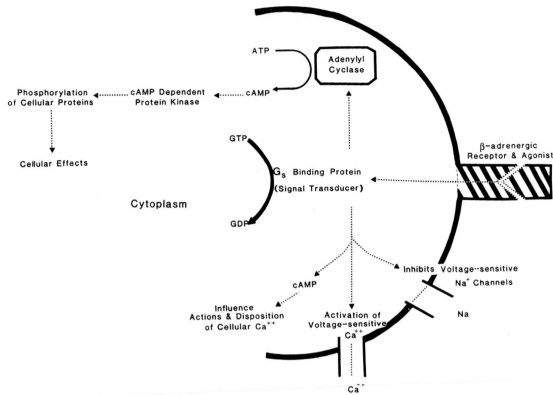

■ **FIGURE 19.8**   A simplified schematic of β_2-adrenergic receptor stimulation. B_2-Adrenergic agonist stimulation of its receptor causes a conformational change in the guanine nucleotide-binding regulatory protein G_S. There is increased guanosine triphosphatase (GTPase) activity and then a transduced signal, resulting in activation of adenylate cyclase. The sequence raises the concentration of cyclic adenosine monophosphate (cAMP). The regulatory protein G_S couples β_2-adrenergic receptors to adenylate cyclase and calcium channels. G_S interacts with the sodium channel, resulting in its inhibition.

long-acting β_2-adrenergic agonists (149,150) with inhaled corticosteroids for moderate and severe persistent asthma.

Various alterations of the molecular structure of the catecholamine nucleus have resulted in a variety of antiasthma drugs (*Fig. 19.9*).

Albuterol

Albuterol is the leading short-acting β_2-adrenergic agonist. Comparable bronchodilation occurs with use of MDIs and nebulizers, although larger doses of albuterol are necessary during nebulization because of the nebulizer's inefficiency (227). In acute asthma, adults may receive three 2.5-mg doses every 30 minutes by nebulization. This protocol was compared with two 5-mg aerosolized treatments given 40 minutes apart (228). Both protocols were effective. The initial PEFR was 35% to 39% in the two groups. Both treatment groups were able to improve the PEFR to about 60%, although the 5-mg doses produced a somewhat faster bronchodilator response. The outcomes from treatment were separated by whether patients were released from the emergency department or whether hospitalization

occurred. Discharged patients whose presentation PEFR was 43% improved their PEFR to 72.5%, whereas hospitalized patients whose initial PEFR was 29% improved to about 40% (228) (*Table 19.15*). These data differentiate the patients with an adequate response to emergency department treatment from those who have acute severe asthma (status asthmaticus), defined by an inadequate response to two or three albuterol treatments or continuous nebulization. Continuously nebulized albuterol solution for treatment of acute episodes of asthma has consisted of preparing 7.7 mL of 0.5% albuterol in 100 mL of saline. A pump infuses the solution initially from 14 mL/h to 26 mL/h while the nebulizer supplies 100% oxygen. Alternatively, 15 mg albuterol can be nebulized in 60 mL of normal saline over 2 hours (229). However, studies have not demonstrated superior results compared with repeated nebulized albuterol administration (230) nor in comparison to the addition of 2 mg to15 mg ipratropium bromide, an anticholinergic agent, to continuously nebulized albuterol (229). For children >12 years of age and adults with episodes of acute asthma, the recommendations of the NAEPP include 2 to 4 inhalations from a metered dose inhaler every 20 minutes up to 3 times (3).

Levalbuterol

Levalbuterol is available as a MDI or nebulized inhalation solution of either a pediatric dosage of 0.31 mg or for older children and adults 0.63 mg or 1.25 mg. It can be administered every 4 to 6 hours. Levalbuterol is about 4 times as potent as albuterol; 0.63 mg of levalbuterol provided comparable bronchodilation to 2.5 mg of albuterol (231). Levalbuterol is indicated for children 4 years of age and older and for adults. For patients who experience tremulousness and palpitations with albuterol, levalbuterol is a useful alternative, but maximal bronchodilation is similar to that achieved with albuterol.

Salmeterol

Salmeterol is a potent β_2-adrenergic agonist with a long half-life, so that administration is 1 to 2 inhalations every 12 hours. It is 50 times more potent experimentally than albuterol but provides similar peak bronchodilation as albuterol. Its onset of action begins in 20 minutes so it is not considered a reliever medication. Anti-inflammatory (bronchoprotective) therapy should be administered concurrently. A combination salmeterol and fluticasone discus or pressurized MDI is available as Advair (Table 19.13).

Formoterol

Formoterol is similar to salmeterol in that the bronchodilator effect is for 12 hours. The drug is administered by inhalation and has its onset of action within 5 minutes. It has an indication for prevention of exercise-induced bronchoconstriction. Its maximum bronchodilator effects are similar to those of salmeterol or albuterol administered every 6 hours. It is available as an inhaler (Foradil) and nebulized solution (Perforomist). For patients with moderate or persistent asthma, formoterol should be used with an inhaled corticosteroid (Table 19.13).While not approved in the United States as a reliever medication, the combination of budesonide/formoterol is used in other countries both as reliever and maintenance therapy (232–234).

Other β_2-Adrenergic Agonists

Pirbuterol, metaproterenol, and terbutaline are older, effective, short-acting β_2-adrenergic agonists (Chapter 34).

Older Medications Once Used for Asthma

Epinephrine

Epinephrine, the drug of choice for anaphylaxis, is administered intramuscularly. Because of its potent bronchodilating effect and rapid onset of action, it was used for initial treatment of acute asthma. It directly stimulates both α- and β-adrenergic receptors. The recommended adult dose is 0.30 mL of a 1:1000 solution administered intramuscularly. In infants and children, the dose is 0.01 mL/kg, with a maximum of 0.25 mL. The dose may be repeated in 15 to 30 minutes if necessary. Intramuscular epinephrine may still have a place for some patients with acute severe asthma who have not responded to albuterol because they are unable to inspire sufficiently or in patients with acute severe wheezing where it is not clear whether the patient with asthma is experiencing anaphylaxis. Nebulized racemic epinephrine is effective but is not used unless a patient has upper airway obstruction (epiglottitis or stridor).

Some side effects of epinephrine include agitation, tremulousness, tachycardia, and palpitation. Hypertension in the presence of acute asthma often resolves with epinephrine administration. This occurs because of a decrease in bronchospasm and as a result of a decrease in peripheral vascular resistance by stimulation of β_2 receptors in smooth muscle of blood vessels in skeletal muscle. Epinephrine must be administered with caution in patients with cardiovascular disease and hypertension but should not be considered contraindicated when bronchoconstriction is significant if albuterol is not being used. The maximum bronchodilator effect of epinephrine given intramuscularly is about equivalent to that of inhaled β_2-adrenergic agonists and occasionally in the severely obstructed patient exceeds what can be gained by aerosol therapy. Although epinephrine is an old drug, it is expedient, effective, and rapidly metabolized.

Ephedrine

Although less potent than isoproterenol, albuterol, and epinephrine, ephedrine, was used for decades because it was effective by oral administration and possessed a longer duration of action (3 to 6 hours). Its onset of action is about 1 hour, with a peak effect of 2 to 3 hours. Ephedrine stimulates α- and β-adrenergic receptors directly and indirectly. Ephedrine is an integral component of some nonprescription combination oral preparations available for treatment of asthma. The adult dose is 25 mg four times daily. Adverse effects of ephedrine include central nervous system (CNS) stimulation. Ephedrine is an outdated drug for treatment of asthma. The 25-mg ephedrine capsule has been shown to have about the same efficacy as 2.5 mg of terbutaline. Currently, in the United States, 50 mg of ephedrine is marketed to motor vehicle drivers as a CNS stimulant, not a bronchodilator. Cardiovascular toxicity is well recognized (235).

Adverse Effects of β_2-Adrenergic Therapy

The immediate relief of short-acting β_2-adrenergic agonists has made it widely acceptable to both patients and physicians. Unfortunately, some patients develop an almost addictive relationship with their inhalers, which results in excessive use and risk of arrhythmias and death. The most common side effects are related to β_1 stimulation, resulting in cardiac symptoms as listed previously with epinephrine. Potential adverse effects from β_2-adrenergic agonists include overuse, systemic absorption across bronchial mucosa, delay in receiving anti-inflammatory therapy, and fatality.

Although subjective and objective improvement of airway obstruction is produced by inhaled short-acting β_2-adrenergic agonists, the associated hypoxemia of asthma is not improved and may be increased. This phenomenon results from enhancing the already existing V/Q imbalance by either increasing aeration of those alveoli already overventilated in relation to their perfusion or by reestablishing ventilation to nonperfused alveoli. Absorption of β_2-adrenergic agonists from bronchial mucosa may result in systemic effects, such as increased cardiac output. The resultant hypoxemia is usually clinically insignificant, unless the initial PO_2 is on the steep portion of the oxygen–hemoglobin dissociation curve (i.e., less than 60 mm Hg). In moderately severe acute asthma, oxygen should be administered to correct the hypoxemia.

Of concern is the paradoxical response of increased bronchial obstruction seen in occasional patients using β_2-adrenergic agonists by inhalation. With an exacerbation of asthmatic symptoms, these patients may overuse inhalation therapy because of a decreasing response to preceding inhalations. A cycle begins of increasing obstruction with increasing use of the aerosol. This pattern may progress to acute severe asthma or respiratory/cardiac arrest. Patients identified as using β_2-adrenergic agonist inhalation or nebulizers excessively should have this therapy terminated or monitored more aggressively. The physician should begin a short course of prednisone to control underlying bronchoconstriction and airway inflammation. There remains a public health concern of asthma fatalities that occur in patients with persistent asthma, who rely on short- or long-acting β_2-adrenergic agonists in the absence of inhaled corticosteroids or other controller therapy.

Long-acting β_2-adrenergic agonists appear to have an appropriate safety profile when used with inhaled corticosteroids (149,150) although there have been differences of opinion in the literature. The long-acting β_2-adrenergic agonists are not intended for monotherapy for management of persistent asthma.

Practical Considerations in Using β_2-Adrenergic Receptor Agonists

Proper technique is essential. Patients may fail to expire fully to FRC before actuating their MDI or dry-powder inhaler (DPI). Other patients may inhale too rapidly to TLC, take a submaximal inspiration, flex the neck during inspiration, forget to shake the canister before

actuation, or not hold their breath for 10 seconds after a full inspiration. Some patients activate the inhaler twice during one inhalation. Others may not have washed the mouthpiece at least once a week or may not have primed the hydrofluroalkane (HFA) MDI after absence of use for 7 to 14 days, depending on the manufacturer's instructions. All of these variables may decrease drug delivery to the lung periphery and explain poor therapeutic responses. Rarely, the inhaler cap can be inhaled inadvertently, or coins, paper clips, or capsules stored inside the MDI cap may be inhaled. When effective synchronization of inhalation with actuation of the air inhaler cannot be corrected, improvement in patient care may be achieved by replacing the MDI with a DPI or adding spacer devices.

A number of devices have been developed in an effort to improve the dynamics of aerosol administration by a pressurized inhaler (see Chapter 37). These devices attempt to minimize aerosol deposition in the oropharynx and increase delivery to the airways. Further, by necessitating a slower inspiration, more drug may be distributed to obstructed peripheral airways than with a rapid inspiration, which favors central airway deposition at the expense of the peripheral airways.

Motor-driven nebulizers do not result in greater bronchodilation than that achieved with pressurized metered-dose aerosol canisters. Drug delivery by motor-driven nebulizers has been considered more efficacious because the patient inhales a relatively large concentration of drug from the nebulizer. For example, the dose of albuterol added to the nebulizer is 5 mg, which is 56 times the dose generated by the metered dose inhaler (90 μg). However, it has been demonstrated that perhaps 15% to 20% of the drug is actually nebulized during inspiration, and only 10% of the nebulized dose would reach the bronchi. Thus, the dose delivered to the lung from the nebulizer may be approximately similar to that given by a pressurized aerosol canister. The delivery system can also cause nosocomial infections. On the other hand, it has been suggested that nebulizers formalize the process of drug administration and do not require the patient to learn correct inhalation technique as for the MDIs.

In summary, the physician and other health care providers should become familiar with β_2-adrenergic agonists and emphasize proper inhalation technique. In some patients, spacer devices or breath-activated units improve drug delivery. It is advisable to recheck the patient's inhaler technique periodically because errors are made frequently that impede drug delivery and because some patients use delivery devices improperly. The goal should be to have the patient use β_2-adrenergic agonists intermittently rather than on a scheduled basis.

It must be recognized that, useful as the β_2-adrenergic agonists are, even combined with inhaled corticosteroids, leukotriene receptor antagonists, leukotriene biosynthesis inhibitor (zileuton), cromolyn, theophylline, and nedocromil, they are not capable of controlling some cases of severe, persistent asthma. This limitation must be kept in mind, and oral corticosteroids should be used when appropriate.

Corticosteroids

Overview

Corticosteroids are the most effective drugs in the treatment of asthma (Chapter 35). Parenteral corticosteroids are prescribed for the treatment of acute severe asthma with a minimum dosage of methylprednisolone 80 mg/day being as effective as higher dosages (236). It may be possible to administer the equivalent as prednisone 100 mg/day as well as oral treatment instead of intravenous methylprednisolone. Objective evidence of improvement in flow rates and FEV_1 requires about 12 hours of therapy (237). In some patients, beneficial effects occur by 6 hours (238). The administration of systemic corticosteroids within the first hour of presentation to the emergency department reduces the number of hospitalizations (239). Short-term outpatient administration decreases the incidence of return visits to emergency medical facilities (240,241). High-dose budesonide (1,600 μg daily) resulted in almost a 50% reduction in relapses (12.8% versus 24.5%) over a 21-day follow-up period in a study in which all patients received prednisone, 50 mg daily for the first 7 days after treatment in the emergency department (242). Very high and frequent doses of inhaled corticosteroids appear to be beneficial in emergency department treatment (243) and can be combined with systemic corticosteroids.

Chronic (scheduled) administration of inhaled and oral corticosteroids prevents work and school absenteeism, disabling wheezing, and episodes of acute severe asthma or respiratory failure in patients with persistent severe asthma. Because of the potentially serious side effects of oral corticosteroids, their use is advised only when other measures have not provided sufficient control of acute or persistent symptoms. Their indiscriminate employment in mild asthma is not indicated unless as a diagnostic-therapeutic trial for cough variant asthma. Failure to use them when indicated, however, may result in unwarranted morbidity and mortality. In life-threatening asthma, corticosteroids are essential, but because of their delayed onset of action, they cannot replace other necessary emergency measures, including β_2-adrenergic agonists, patent airway, and oxygen. Patients who are still wheezing after initial emergency treatment with β_2-adrenergic agonists are in acute severe asthma (status asthmaticus) and should receive systemic corticosteroids. Patients who must be hospitalized for exacerbations of asthma should receive systemic corticosteroids immediately without attempting to determine whether continued β_2-adrenergic agonists (and possibly ipratropium bromide or theophylline) will work without systemic corticosteroids.

Oral corticosteroids are of value in prevention of repeated emergency department visits or office visits in acutely ill patients who respond to β_2-adrenergic agonists and do not require hospitalization. A prednisone dosage regimen of 30 mg to 60 mg each morning for 5 to 7 days is often effective in adults, and in children 1 mg/kg to 2 mg/kg prednisone is necessary, often the latter dosage for the first few days. On an ambulatory basis, doubling of inhaled corticosteroids, when the patient already is receiving recommended doses, does not appear to be helpful to avoid administration of oral corticosteroids (244). In some adult patients whose asthma is controlled with 200 mcg to 400 mcg of budesonide or equivalent corticosteroid, then doubling the dose may be sufficient during a mild exacerbation.

Inhaled corticosteroids are recommended for persistent mild, moderate and severe asthma (3) (Table 19.8) and are associated with improved control of asthma (245). Unfortunately, inhaled corticosteroids administered to high-risk toddlers and young children have not been associated with prevention or suppression of the emergence of asthma (246–248).

There is significant variability with inhaled corticosteroids as some patients have >15% improvements in FEV_1 and others have poor responses (<5% improvement in FEV_1) (249). In a study of patients with mild asthma and in which bronchodilator reversibility was not used as an inclusion criterion, the response to inhaled corticosteroid over 6 weeks was split into responders (54%) and nonresponders (46%) (250). In the best responders, the FEV_1 improved by as much as 60% whereas the FEV_1 decreased by 20% in others. The mode was a 0 to 5% increase in FEV_1 (250). The nonresponse to the inhaled corticosteroid, beclomethasone dipropionate, was associated with a nonresponse to inhaled albuterol (250).

The exact mode of action of corticosteroids is complex (see Chapter 35 and references 251,252), but they have many anti-inflammatory effects (Table 19.16). As valuable as inhaled corticosteroids are, they cannot "do everything." For example, after allergen bronchoprovocation challenges, there are increases in bone marrow $CD34^+$ (mast cell) progenitor cells and eosinophil and basophil colony-forming units (254). These findings suggest that asthma is truly a systemic disorder. While budesonide, 400 μg inhaled daily for 8 days could not prevent this activation of the bone marrow, budesonide did inhibit the early and late bronchial responses to allergen challenge and the number of eosinophils in sputum. Not to minimize their important effects in the treatment of asthma, in a study of 16,941 subjects enrolled in a health maintenance organization, inhaled corticosteroids and cromolyn in children were associated with about a 50% reduction in risk for hospitalization, compared with patients who did not receive inhaled corticosteroids (255). There was no dose-response relationship noted for inhaled corticosteroids

---

TABLE 19.16   CLINICAL AND ANTI-INFLAMMATORY EFFECTS OF CORTICOSTEROIDS IN ASTHMA

- Reduction of symptoms (cough, wheezing, dyspnea) from asthma
- Improvement in morning expiratory flow rates and intraday variation
- Reduces need for β_2-adrenergic agonists in persistent asthma
- Increases the β_2-adrenergic receptor density
- Can prevent deterioration leading to acute severe asthma (status asthmaticus)
- Improves oxygenation and time to discharge after acute severe asthma (status asthmaticus)
- Reduces recidivism to emergency department after acute therapy
- Decreases mucus production and sputum eosinophilia
- Reduction of expired NO
- Regeneration of bronchial epithelium
- Increases the ratio of ciliated columnar cells to goblet cells in the bronchial epithelium
- Causes a modest lessening of nonspecific bronchial hypersensitivity
- Increases numbers of intraepithelial nerves
- Partial inhibition of the late bronchoconstrictive responses to aerosol allergen provocation after one dose of inhaled corticosteroid
- Partial inhibition of the early and late bronchoconstrictive responses to aerosol allergen provocation after 1 week of inhaled corticosteroids and early response after 1 week of prednisone
- Reduction in recovery of eosinophils and mast cells in bronchoalveolar lavage
- Reduction of eosinophils, mast cells in the respiratory epithelium and lamina propria
- Reduction of production of superoxide anions by eosinophils
- Reduction of numbers of activated lymphocytes in bronchoalveolar lavage and mucosa
- Reduction of *ex vivo* bronchoalveolar (macrophage) cell synthesis of leukotriene B_4 and thromboxane B_2
- Reduction in bronchoalveolar lavage cells expressing mRNA for interleukin-4 (IL-4) and IL-5 with an increase in interferon-γ–positive cells
- Activation of the glucocorticoid receptor in the cytoplasm causing translocation into the nucleus
- Reduces histone acetyltransferase activity which reduces unwinding of chromatin (DNA-histone) and transcription
- Increases histone deacetylation causing transcriptional repression of inflammatory gene expression
- Increases FOXP3 mRNA expression in CD4$^+$CD25$^+$T $_{reg}$ cells
- Reduction in the stability of mRNA transcripts

---

regarding avoidance of hospitalizations from asthma (255).

In addition to their therapeutic importance, corticosteroids may be useful as a diagnostic tool. Often, it is helpful to document the extent of reversibility of a patient's signs and symptoms to establish whether the basic underlying process is asthma or irreversible obstructive airways disease. Therapeutic doses of corticosteroids for 7 to 14 days should significantly reverse the airway obstruction of asthma in almost all patients but would result in little or no reversal in most patients with chronic bronchitis or emphysema. The initial therapeutic dose of prednisone in children is 1 mg/kg/day to 2 mg/kg/day and in adults is 40 mg to 80 mg per day.

To minimize side effects, it is important to use these drugs for the shortest time necessary to achieve the clinical goal. A 3- to 5-day course of prednisone in therapeutic doses may be sufficient to reverse an occasional acute episode of asthma that has not responded adequately to the common modes of therapy, such as inhaled corticosteroids and β_2-adrenergic agonists. If oral corticosteroids are required for longer periods, abrupt discontinuation may be followed by the return of acute symptoms. Until significant clearing of signs and symptoms of asthma occur, prednisone or the equivalent should be administered at a steady dosage rate over the first 1 to 2 weeks. In a small group of patients who have abruptly discontinued corticosteroids after prolonged use, a withdrawal syndrome may occur, consisting of malaise, emotional lability, myalgia, and low-grade fever.

In patients requiring maintenance oral therapy, the lowest possible dose (preferably, alternate-day dosing) compatible with adequate control of symptoms should be used, and there should be use of inhaled corticosteroids as well. There is a relatively flat dose-response curve for inhaled corticosteroids, especially when increases in FEV$_1$ are used as an end point (249). Perhaps it is not surprising that adding a long-acting β_2-adrenergic agonist to a moderate dose of inhaled steroid achieved greater increases in FEV$_1$ and PEFR than did doubling the inhaled corticosteroid dose (256–258). Some patients have better control of asthma on moderate- to high-dose inhaled corticosteroids and can have prednisone tapered or discontinued. These patients should have little need for β_2-adrenergic agonists over time as the airway inflammation recedes.

In patients who are managed with inhaled corticosteroids and other medications for asthma and require single-morning prednisone for adequate control, the attempt to use alternate-day prednisone requires tripling the dose of prednisone. Simply doubling the prednisone for use on alternate days often will be unsuccessful.

Measures to prevent or correct abnormalities in bone mineral metabolism induced by oral corticosteroids or high-dose inhaled corticosteroids require cooperative patients and physician expertise. Estrogen/progestin replacement therapy has proven value in prevention of bone loss and fractures in postmenopausal women, but its risk profile includes cardiovascular disease and breast cancer (259). It should be administered only if truly indicated. Regular gynecologic examinations are necessary. Prevention of osteopenia is of paramount importance and should begin early because bone mass increases until about 25 to 45 years of age and then declines over years. Exercise, sedentary lifestyle, cigarette smoking, excessive alcohol consumption, and overuse of thyroxine in euthyroid or possibly hypothyroid patients are some additional factors to address in terms of bone health. Adequate calcium intake of 1,200 mg or more for women (1,000 mg for men) and of vitamin D, 800 IU for women, is advisable. Bisphosphonates often are indicated for patients with osteopenia. Patients with established osteopenia or osteoporotic fractures may require combinations of medications in different categories including bisphosphonates, calcitonin, parathyroid hormone (teriparatide), fluorides, selective estrogen receptor modulators (raloxifene), vitamin D, and calcium supplementation.

If necessary on a long-term basis, oral corticosteroids should be administered as alternate-day therapy with short-acting agents such as prednisone or methylprednisolone. Split daily doses should be avoided in stable ambulatory patients. Effective dosages of inhaled corticosteroids should be used, but with a flat dose-response effect, large doses may produce little additional benefit and cause adrenal suppression or osteopenia.

A potentially serious side effect from corticosteroids is suppression of the HPA axis. This results in an impaired ability to tolerate stress, and for this reason, patients must receive increased doses of corticosteroids during stressful situations such as surgery, infectious illness, and even exacerbations of asthma. The extent of suppression, however, is variable from patient to patient. The time required for a return to normal HPA activity after discontinuation of oral corticosteroids also varies and is unpredictable. In a rare patient, inability of the HPA axis to respond to stress may continue for up to 1 year after the cessation of therapy; in other patients, normal HPA reactivity may persist despite their taking corticosteroids for as long as 10 years. Fortunately, surgery with modern anesthesia techniques rarely results in maximal adrenal output of about 300 mg cortisol; output is more likely 100 mg (260).

Some patients with severe persistent asthma cannot be controlled effectively without oral corticosteroids. To minimize the occurrence of adverse side effects from oral corticosteroids, the use of alternate-day prednisone therapy is recommended. The total daily dose of a short-acting corticosteroid preparation (prednisone, prednisolone, methylprednisolone) should be taken in the morning every 48 hours, as long as underlying airways obstruction is controlled adequately. Daily prednisone is indicated in the acutely ill patient. Often, a short course (5 to 7 days) of daily prednisone is required to control asthma. Alternate-day prednisone therapy should be considered for patients who still require corticosteroids after 3 weeks of daily medication for severe asthma. Most patients obtain adequate control of symptoms by this form of therapy, with little, if any, deterioration in pulmonary function on the alternate-day schedule (261).

Although major side effects are not usually observed in patients receiving less than 20 mg of prednisone daily (administered as a single-morning dose), the physician should attempt to convert to an alternate-day regimen. One common mistake is to try to accomplish the conversion too rapidly. If a patient has been receiving split doses of prednisone on a daily basis, the first step should be to establish control of the severe asthma with a single-morning dose of prednisone. Once the patient is stable, tripling the daily dose on alternate days may be adequate for control of the disease. Close patient supervision is essential during this critical changeover period. Some patients will not tolerate alternate-day steroid therapy even with very large doses of prednisone and should be managed on daily steroids using a single-morning prednisone dose. The half-life of prednisolone is about 200 minutes in patients requiring daily prednisone or alternate-day prednisone, and other pharmacokinetic parameters are similar (262).

Parenteral Corticosteroids

Intravenous corticosteroids usually are administered for acute severe asthma (status asthmaticus). Hydrocortisone (400 mg/day), prednisone (100 mg/day), methylprednisolone (80 mg/day), and dexamethasone (12 mg/day) are the minimum effective dosages and are often as effective as higher dosages (236). It is possible to manage status asthmaticus with oral corticosteroids if access is difficult or if there are shortages of parenteral agents. The minimum equivalent dose is prednisone 100 mg/day. For malignant, potentially fatal asthma, intramuscular methylprednisolone can be a short-term consideration. It is available in 20-mg/mL, 40 mg/mL, and 80-mg/mL preparations for injection into the gluteus maximus. For adults who can be considered nonadherent and unreliable, a dose of 40 mg to 120 mg can be given to try to prevent a hospitalization or potential fatality from asthma. Regular administration should be avoided unless there is no other alternative.

Inhaled Corticosteroids

Bronchial mucosa atrophy has not been described in patients who have used topical corticosteroids in recommended doses, even for decades. Because of the absence of serious side effects and with the impressive array of anti-inflammatory effects (Table 19.16), primary monotherapy of asthma with inhaled corticosteroids continues to be recommended for mild and moderate persistent asthma (3) (see Chapter 35 and Table 19.8). The benefits of treatment have been confirmed in many investigations (3) (Chapters 22 and 35). In an important early study of newly diagnosed patients with mild asthma, budesonide, 600 µg twice daily, was considered superior to inhaled terbutaline, 375 µg twice daily (263). Patients were treated for 2 years with this moderately high dose of budesonide and then received budesonide, 400 µg/day or placebo (264). Not surprisingly, patients who received budesonide had better asthma control (FEV_1, peak flow, and bronchial responsiveness) than patients who received the placebo. Further, patients who initially had received terbutaline improved after therapy with 1,200 µg/day of budesonide (264). The physician or other health care provider should individualize the therapeutic options for patients with persistent asthma and verify that IgE-mediated triggering allergens are avoided. In patients who truly have persistent mild asthma, it is possible to utilize an inhaled corticosteroid on an as needed basis (134).

Leukotriene Antagonists and Biosynthesis Inhibitors

Montelukast (Singulair) and zafirlukast (Accolate) are leukotriene receptor antagonists, and zileuton (Zyflo) is an inhibitor of the 5-lipoxygenase enzyme that catalyzes synthesis of leukotrienes. All these medications can block declines in FEV_1 from exercise, allergen challenge, and aspirin administration (265–267) (see Chapter 36). Administration of montelukast or zafirlukast to adults with persistent mild-to-moderate asthma results in reduced symptoms and increased FEV_1 up to 13%, compared with a placebo response of 4.2% (268). Comparable results were reported in children 6 to 14 years of age (269). These findings support the concept that leukotrienes contribute to airway tone. In adult patients "incompletely controlled" with inhaled beclomethasone dipropionate, 200 µg twice daily, montelukast 10 mg or placebo was added. The combination drugs produced 6% increases in FEV_1, compared with no change with continued beclomethasone dipropionate (270). However, days with asthma symptoms decreased by 25%, and asthma attacks decreased by 50% (270). These findings demonstrate that control of asthma extends beyond bronchodilator responses and have been replicated in other studies (266,271). The leukotriene recep-

tor antagonists can help some patients with persistent asthma lower their dosage of inhaled corticosteroids.

There is variation of improvement in FEV_1 after administration of montelukast. About 15% of patients bronchodilate by 18% to 25%, which is greater than 8% to 10% that occurs in other patients (83). Polymorphisms in the cysteinyl leukotriene receptor 2 gene explain some of the differences. It has been hypothesized that genetic polymorphisms in the loci that participate in biosynthesis of leukotrienes may result in increased concentrations of leukotrienes and more potential for effects of inhibition (83).

Zileuton inhibits from 26% to 86% of production of leukotrienes (266) and also results in bronchodilation (14.6% versus 0% for placebo using FEV_1 after 60 minutes) (272). In a 12-week study of controlled release zileuton, 1,200 mg twice daily, the improvement in FEV_1 was 20.8% with active treatment and 12.7% with placebo (273). Reversible elevations of alanine aminotransferase, over three times the normal limits, occurred in less than 2.5% of patients and 0.5% of controls (273). Next-generation leukotriene receptor antagonists or 5-lipoxygenase inhibitors presumably will be even more effective than the currently available products.

Cromolyn

Cromolyn sodium (Intal) was shown to be effective in preventing bronchospasm from inhaled allergens and exercise 35 years ago (see Chapter 36). It has been used in the United States since 1973 and has a very high therapeutic index. It is available as a MDI containing 112 or 200 actuations or by nebulized aerosol inhalation. Ampules contain 20 mg of cromolyn in 2 mL of diluent. Intal can be added to a nebulizer containing a β_2-adrenergic agonist such as albuterol for inhalation. With an HFA formulation of the MDI, patients had a 28% to 33% reduction in asthma symptoms after cromolyn administration, compared with placebo (274). However, a Cochrane Analysis found little to no improvement over placebo for maintenance therapy in children (275).

Cromolyn has been of value for prevention or minimization of exercise-induced bronchoconstriction when inhaled up to 2 hours pre-exercise (276). Cromolyn has value for pre-treatment before allergen, cold air, or odor exposure.

Nedocromil

Nedocromil (Tilade) is a pyranoquinoline that blocks release of mediators from several cell types in the airway, including mast cells. Experimentally, it inhibits both early and late bronchial responses to allergen (see Chapter 36). It is of value in prevention or minimization of exercise-induced bronchoconstriction when inhaled up to 2 hours pre-exercise (276). Nedocromil was used in comparison with budesonide in the Childhood Asthma Management Program but, as with budesonide, does not appear to protect against loss of FEV_1/FVC in mild-to-moderate asthma (277). The magnitude of response is similar to cromolyn (277). Nedocromil inhibits afferent nerve transmission from respiratory nerves, so that substance P may be limited in its effect as a bronchoconstrictor or trigger of cough. It can also decrease nonspecific bronchial hyperresponsiveness. Nedocromil is administered by MDI, with each actuation delivering 1.75 mg. The canister contains 112 inhalations, and the initial dosage for children aged 12 years and older and adults is 2 inhalations four times daily. The dosage may be reduced as improvement (cessation of coughing) occurs. Some adverse effects include unpleasant (bitter) taste and slight temporary yellowing of teeth; use of a spacer device is helpful.

Nedocromil is efficacious in patients with mild-to-moderate asthma and in patients with difficult to control nonproductive cough. If nedocromil does not help reduce the dose of inhaled corticosteroids or reduce symptoms after 1 to 2 months of use, it should be discontinued.

Theophylline

Theophylline, a drug with a very narrow therapeutic index, is not essential in the management of asthma for the ambulatory patient or for the hospitalized patient (see Chapter 36). It is listed as an alternative medication for persistent moderate and severe asthma (Table 19.8). The most important pharmacologic action of theophylline (1,3-dimethylxanthine) is bronchodilation. Other properties of the drug include central respiratory stimulation, inotropic and chronotropic cardiac effects, diuresis, relaxation of vascular smooth muscles, improvement in ciliary action, and reduction of diaphragmatic muscle fatigue.

Theophylline has been shown *in vitro* to increase cAMP concentrations by inhibiting phosphodiesterase, the enzyme that converts $3'5'$-cAMP to $5'$-AMP. However, the inhibition of phosphodiesterase by theophylline was accomplished with concentrations that would be toxic *in vivo*; thus, theophylline's mechanism of action is unlikely attributable to phosphodiesterase inhibition. Possible explanations for theophylline-induced bronchodilation are adenosine antagonism and induction of histone deacetylase, which would lead to repression of pro-inflammatory cytokines (278). Indeed, the latter effect would be consistent with theophylline being an anti-inflammatory medication.

Optimal bronchodilation from theophylline is a function of the serum concentration. Maximal bronchodilation is usually achieved with concentrations between 8 and 15 μg/mL. Some patients achieve adequate clinical improvement with serum theophylline levels at 5 μg/mL

or even lower. The explanation for this phenomenon is that the bronchodilator effect of theophylline, as measured by percentage increase in FEV_1, is related to and fairly dependent on the logarithm of the serum level concentration (279). A dose-related improvement in pulmonary function was reported in six patients. The mean improvement in FEV_1 was 19.7% with theophylline concentration 5 μg/mL, 30.9% at 10 μg/mL, and 42.2% at 20 μg/mL. Two methods of graphic presentation of these data are shown in *Figure 19.10*. At these concentrations, improvement in pulmonary function occurs in linear fashion with the log of the theophylline concentration. However, using an arithmetic scale on the abscissa, improvement in pulmonary function occurs in a hyperbolic manner. Thus, although continued improvement occurs with increasing serum concentrations, the incremental increase with each larger dose decreases. About half of the improvement in FEV_1 that is achievable with a theophylline concentration of 20 μg/mL is reached with concentration of 5 μg/mL and 75% of the improvement is reached with a concentration of 10 μg/mL.

Theophylline is an alternative medication for use in patients with persistent moderate and severe asthma (3) or COPD. Theophylline may be tolerated if peak concentrations are 8 μg/mL to 15 μg/mL. When added to inhaled corticosteroid and/or β_2-adrenergic agonist combinations, theophylline may add no additional benefit. The indications for theophylline remains problem-patients with persistent severe asthma, COPD, steroid-phobic patients, and perhaps patients who cannot afford inhaled corticosteroid and/or β_2-adrenergic agonists.

Anticholinergic Agents

Anticholinergic agents diminish cyclic guanosine monophosphate concentrations and inhibit vagal efferent pathways. Bronchodilation then could occur in a multiplicative fashion when ipratropium bromide is administered with albuterol (Combivent inhalation aerosol). Monotherapy with anticholinergic bronchodilators will not replace β_2-adrenergic agonists in acute asthma, in that the onset of action is slower and effect smaller than with β_2-adrenergic agonists. Combination therapy in acute asthma possibly is superior to albuterol alone, but whether this approach is clinically important is not clear. Combivent is useful for patients with persistent asthma and COPD, perhaps because of the greater relative contribution of cholinergic tone in COPD as compared with asthma.

Although the anticholinergic agent, tiotropium bromide, is not approved for use for asthma, it may have a role in some patients who do not benefit from short- or possibly long-acting β_2-adrenergic agonists. A case report has described the use of both anticholinergics, tiotropium bromide and ipratropium bromide, in an African-American patient whose polymorphism for the β_2-adrenergic receptor was Arg-Arg instead of Gly-Gly (280).

Immunomodulatory Therapy

Omalizumab

Omalizumab, a recombinant IgG_1 monoclonal antibody to IgE, marketed under the name Xolair in the United States, is approved for adolescents (age 12+) and adults with moderate to severe persistent asthma\ (Chapter 38). Patients must have at least one positive immediate skin test reaction to a perennial allergen, be inadequately controlled on inhaled steroids, and have a total serum IgE from 30 KU/L to 700 KU/L. Omalizumab reduces the free total IgE by 95% and both the early and late reactions on bronchoprovocation challenge with allergen (281). It decreases the numbers of Fcε RI receptors on mast cells (282), basophils, and dendritic cells (283). Omalizumab interferes with antigen presentation by reducing the binding of complexes of allergen-IgE to B lymphocytes, decreasing their "facilitated antigen presentation" to T lymphocytes (284).

Nonspecific Measures

Meteorologic Factors

Increasing air pollution is a known worldwide health hazard. It is considered to be a major causative factor in certain conditions such as bronchitis, emphysema, and lung cancer. Urban surveys have demonstrated the deleterious effect of pollution on patients with chronic cardiopulmonary disease. In industrialized cities, the alarming morbidity and mortality rates resulting from thermal inversions have dramatized the seriousness of stagnating pollution. Because of inherent bronchial hyperreactivity, the patient with asthma may be more vulnerable to air pollution. However, asthma death rates increased to about 5,000/year in the United States and then plateaued and decreased, while air quality has improved. It is possible that coarse (2.5 μm to 10 μm) or ultrafine (<0.1 μm) particle air pollution (209) will be associated with untoward effects on asthma.

Industrial smog results from incomplete combustion of fossil fuels, and consists of sulfuric acid, sulfur dioxide, nitrogen dioxide, carbon monoxide, and particulate material. Photochemical smog occurs from the action of ultraviolet radiation on nitrogen oxides or hydrocarbons from automobile exhaust. Ozone is the major constituent of photochemical smog. Clinical and immunologic effects of excessive diesel fumes are under investigation but data suggest an association with asthma.

Other meteorologic factors, such as sudden changes in temperature, increases in relative humidity, and increasing or decreasing barometric pressure, also may aggravate asthmatic symptoms in some patients. It is impossible to protect patients from these changes entirely. Why weather changes should aggravate asthma remains completely understood. The breathing of cold, dry air is a potent stimulus that precipitates symptoms in many patients. The use of scarves or facemasks may be beneficial in these patients.

"Thunderstorm asthma" is attributable to fungal spore fragments (285), grasses (286), or the Mediterranean weed, *Parietaria* (287).

Home Environment

Certain interventions for the internal environment of the home are beneficial (8). Extremes of humidity can adversely affect the patient with asthma; the optimal humidity should range from 40% to 50%. Low humidity dries the mucous membranes and can be an irritative factor, although it helps to desiccate house dust mites.

Most patients benefit from air conditioning, but in a few patients, the cold air may increase symptoms. The reduction in spore counts in air-conditioned homes in part results from simply having the windows closed to reduce the influx of outdoor spores. Heating ventilation air conditioning system cleaning does improve indoor air quality (288) and reduces fungal recoveries (289). Removal of visible molds has been associated with reduced symptoms from asthma and rhinitis (290).

Mechanical devices that purify circulating air may be helpful in reducing animal danders (291). Older (fiberglass type) furnace air filters vary in their effectiveness but in general remove only particles larger than 5 μm (e.g., pollens). Many inhalant particles, such as dust mites, fumes, smoke, some fungal spores, some rat urinary proteins, some cat allergen, bacteria, and viruses, are smaller than 5 μm. Efficient air-cleaning devices include the following: the electrostatic precipitator, which attracts particles of any size by high-voltage plates; nonelectronic precipitators in forced air systems; electrostatic filters that remove particles as small as 1 μm; and air cleaners that use a high-efficiency particulate accumulator (HEPA) filtering system. Sensitive immunoassays have documented presence of mouse urinary protein (*Mus d 1*) in indoor environment air samples. Similar findings occur with cockroach fecal particles or saliva (*Bla g 1*) (8). Control measures can be difficult in such conditions but should be encouraged with involvement of those living in that environment (8). It is not possible to reduce indoor concentrations of house dust mite (*Derp 1*) to a mite-free level. A clinical benefit to dust mite–sensitive patients, however, occurs if some avoidance measures are instituted. It is advisable that the mattress, box spring, and pillow be covered with special zippered encasings. Window blinds should be cleaned regularly or not installed, and attention to other dust collection sites should be given. Rugs should be vacuumed each week, and dust mite–trapping vacuum sweeper bags should be used. In that *Der p 1* is heat labile (but *Der p 2* is not), some benefit has been reported of steam-cleaning carpets and upholstery along with applying dry heat (>100°C) to mattresses and blinds (292). Concentrations of both *Der p 1* and *Der p 2* were reduced for 1 year with that intensive treatment (292).

The presence of moist basements and crawl spaces may provoke acute or chronic symptoms in certain patients allergic to fungal spores. Dehumidification and more effective drainage are advised. Patients with mold-induced asthma should not sleep or work in moldy basements. As stated, removal of visible molds has some benefit (290).

Smoking

Cigarette smoking must be discouraged in all patients and their family members. Its deleterious effects probably result from bronchial irritation, impairment of antibacterial defense mechanisms, and mildly reduced responses to inhaled corticosteroids (293). Cigarette smoke has been shown to impair mucociliary transport and to inhibit alveolar macrophage phagocytosis. Patients with asthma who continue to smoke often require progressive increments in medication. Keeping a patient with asthma controlled with medication while the patient continues to smoke is not good medical practice. When COPD occurs, episodes of asthma may be tolerated poorly and may result in frequent hospitalizations or in respiratory failure.

Passive smoking by nonasthmatic subjects has been associated with statistically significant reductions in expiratory flow rates. This finding provides support for the often reported comment that patients with asthma experience increased symptoms in smoke-filled office rooms or homes.

Exercise

As an indicator of control of asthma (3), it is advisable to inquire about the patient's current exercise tolerance and participation in sports. The subjective and psychological value of physical conditioning can be a helpful adjunct in treatment. An important feature of asthma is the occurrence of exercised-induced bronchoconstriction. Many children or adults may be discouraged by their inability to participate in sports or to withstand other normal exertional activities. These feelings of inferiority or anger promote additional physical and psychological incapacitation. Once asthma has been stabilized with appropriate therapy, there should be a noticeable increase in physical capacities and hopefully self-image and self-confidence. Inhaled β_2-adrenergic agonists, inhaled cromolyn, or inhaled nedocromil taken 15 to 30 minutes before exercise will decrease postexercise bronchoconstriction. Some patients require two medications such as β_2-adrenergic agonists and cromolyn to suppress symptoms. Although formoterol has an indication for exercise-induced bronchoconstriction, this author favors a short-acting β_2-adrenergic agonist instead for prophylaxis.

Some patients find that use of an inhaled corticosteroid (199) or leukotriene antagonist such as montelukast (200) as scheduled therapy allows full exercise or sports activities without need for other medications.

Drugs to Use Cautiously or to Avoid

Monotherapy of persistent mild, moderate, or severe asthma with short- or long-acting β_2-adrenergic agonists is not recommended (3) and should not be done.

β_2-Adrenergic blocking drugs have gained wide clinical use in the treatment of cardiac arrhythmias, acute myocardial infarction, congestive heart failure, angina, hypertension, asymmetric septal hypertrophy, thyrotoxicosis, tremor, and migraine. These drugs exert blocking properties on both cardiac and pulmonary β receptors. As a result of the effect on the latter, β blockers may enhance or trigger wheezing in overt and latent asthmatic patients. The adrenergic receptors of the lung are predominantly β_2 in type, and they subserve bronchodilation. When these receptors are blocked, bronchoconstriction may result. Should selective or nonselective β_2-adrenergic antagonists be required in a patient with asthma, cautious increase in dose with close supervision is recommended. Both cardioselective (atenolol, metoprolol) and nonselective (propranolol, carvedilol, lebatalol, timolol, etc.) blockers have been associated with increased numbers of emergency department visits and hospitalizations in patients with asthma (294). Acute bronchospasm has been associated with conjunctival instillation of timolol for glaucoma (*295*).

Bronchoconstriction has been described even for betaxolol, a β_1-adrenergic antagonist, which is less likely to cause declines in FEV_1 than timolol (*296*). Occasionally, parasympathomimetic agents, such as pilocarpine, administered in the conjunctival sac can cause bronchospasm (295). It is advisable to make certain that the patient with persistent asthma is first achieving adequate control of asthma, such as with inhaled corticosteroids or β_2-adrenergic agonist and/or inhaled corticosteroid or other medications, so that any possible effects from necessary ophthalmic drugs are minimized.

Angiotensin-converting enzyme (ACE) inhibitors have been associated with cough and asthma (or pharyngeal or laryngeal angioedema), even after the first dose (*297,298*). Discontinuation of the ACE inhibitor is associated with resolution of cough over several days or up to a month. ACE inhibitors and angiotensin receptor blocker antagonists are not contraindicated in patients with asthma in the absence of prior adverse reactions such as cough or acute angioedema.

Narcotics analgesics, such as morphine, oxycodone, hydromorphone, and fentanyl, are at least relatively (or absolutely) contraindicated during exacerbations of asthma. Moreover, morphine can activate mast cells to release histamine. Nocturnal reductions in PO_2 occur regularly in normal subjects and in patients with asthma. Acute severe asthma (status asthmaticus) is a contraindication for the use of soporific medications.

Antidepressants of the tricyclic or serotonin reuptake inhibitor classes can be continued with asthma medications. Antidepressants of the monoamine oxidase inhibitor class can be utilized but are not recommended in a patient who might receive epinephrine as there could be a severe hypertensive crisis.

Drugs possessing anticholinesterase properties may potentiate wheezing. This results from their parasympathomimetic-enhancing effect due to the inhibition of acetylcholine catabolism. These drugs represent the primary drug treatment of myasthenia gravis; if asthma coexists, a therapeutic problem arises. When anticholinesterases are necessary, maximal doses of β_2-adrenergic agonists and inhaled corticosteroids may be necessary. The addition of oral corticosteroids may be indicated for more adequate control of asthma, but it must be remembered that, in some patients, myasthenic symptoms may initially worsen with addition of oral corticosteroids (299).

Specific Measures

Allergic Asthma

Specific allergy management must be included in the treatment regimen of allergic asthma. Many, but not all, studies suggest that there is a dose response relationship between allergen exposure and development of asthma. Moreover, there are suggestions that there are threshold levels of allergen exposure, below which sensitization and therefore, allergic asthma are unlikely to occur. For a major dust mite allergen Der p 1 it is 2 µg/g dust and for a major cockroach allergen Bla g 1, it is 1 unit/g dust.

When one allergen is the primary cause (e.g., animal dander) and can be removed from the environment, symptomatic relief is achieved, often within 1 to 2 months if there is thorough cleaning. Cat dander (Fel d 1) antigen may require 16 weeks or more to reach threshold levels (<8 µg Fed d 1/g dust); in some cases, it may take longer if additional cleaning is not performed. Most allergic patients, however, are sensitive to more than one allergen, and many allergens cannot be removed completely. In adults, inhalant allergens are the most frequent causative agents.

Certain basic environmental controls in the house are advisable. Hypoallergenic pillows are preferred and should be enclosed in impermeable encasings. Box springs and mattresses should be enclosed similarly. In some situations, additional cleaning of blankets or removal of rugs (especially old ones) is beneficial. Measures to reduce exposure to rodent urine and cockroaches should be implemented and likely require continued effort (8).

Other aspects may be considered with regard to the environmental control in the home. Basement apartments, because of increased moisture, are most likely to have higher levels of airborne fungi and mite antigens. Visible molds should be removed and depending on the severity of asthma or difficulty in achieving adequate control, cleaning of the heating-ventilation-air conditioning ducts should be performed. For the highly dust-allergic patient, appropriate furnace filters and air cleaners should be used and maintained properly. In patients with perennial symptoms, it is generally advisable that pets (e.g., cats, dogs, and birds) be removed from the house if there are symptoms from contact or if there is a positive skin test. Nevertheless, most patients do not remove the pet as advised. The physician and patient must then rely on pharmacologic therapies.

Ingestion of foods essentially is never the cause of asthma; an exception occurs when the cause is acute severe bronchoconstriction from anaphylaxis. Patients may attribute their respiratory symptoms to aspartame or monosodium glutamate when such associations are not justified. Exposure to sulfur dioxide from sodium or potassium metabisulfite used as an antioxidant in foods can cause acute respiratory symptoms in patients with asthma. However, patients with stable asthma who are managed by anti-inflammatory medications will not be affected significantly by metabisulfite.

When environmental control is either impossible or insufficient to control symptoms, subcutaneous allergen immunotherapy should be considered (Chapter 13). Efficacy in asthma has been documented for pollens, dust mites, and Cladosporium species (216,217), and allergen immunotherapy should be considered in patients with persistent asthma, who also are being treated with pharmacotherapy (3,13) (Table 19.8). Other than very modest effects, subcutaneous immunotherapy with cat dander extracts has not been impressive in reducing symptoms when the cat remains in the home environment.

Johnstone and Dutton (301), in a 14-year prospective study of subcutaneous allergen immunotherapy for asthmatic children, reported that 72% of the treated group were free of symptoms at 16 years of age, as compared with only 22% of the placebo group. This publication occurred in 1968 and for decades was treated with healthy skepticism. In 2007, somewhat similar data were reported again, in that rhinitis patients who received allergen immunotherapy had less emergence of asthma than rhinitis patients who did not receive allergen immunotherapy (302).

In the United States, currently, there are no approved extracts for use for sublingual immunotherapy, and this issue is quite controversial (303).

Omalizumab is indicated and should be considered for patients with persistent moderate or severe asthma and at least one positive immediate skin test reaction to a perennial allergen. The total IgE concentration should be between 30 kU/L to 700 kU/L (Chapter 38). Based on data from studies of patients who were not controlled effectively with a combination β_2-adrenergic agonist/high-dosage inhaled corticosteroid, treatment with omalizumab resulted in fewer severe exacerbations and emergency department visits (304). Nevertheless, some have argued that it is not cost-effective therapy (305).

Nonallergic Asthma

Treatment of nonallergic asthma primarily involves the judicious use of pharmacologic therapy as avoidance measures; immunotherapy and immunomodulator treatments are not indicated. The next three paragraphs apply to allergic asthma as well.

Convincing evidence is available that virus-induced upper respiratory infections initiate exacerbations of asthma. Important agents for children 1 to 5 years of age include RSV, parainfluenza virus, and rhinovirus; for older children and adults, influenza virus, parainfluenza virus, and rhinovirus are important. Adenovirus infection rarely acts to initiate asthma attacks. Additional viruses will be understood better (metapneumoviruses) or identified that are associated with episodes of asthma.

Mycoplasma pneumoniae infections may be associated with new onset asthma (306) or likely exacerbations of established asthma (307). In patients with acute exacerbations of asthma, in which serologic evidence of infection with *Mycoplasma pneumoniae* or *Chlamydophilia* (formerly *Chlamydia*) *pneumoniae* was present, the macrolide, telithromycin, reduced symptoms (40% versus 27%) but did not improve PEFR significantly more than placebo (78 L/min versus 67 L/min) (307). It remains to be established whether there will be an indication for macrolides for treatment of asthma, e.g., whether there is an anti-inflammatory or anti-infective role.

Annual influenza vaccination should be administered according to the Centers for Disease Control and Prevention recommendations for children and adults. Treatment of secondary bacterial infections, such as acute (purulent) bronchitis and rhinosinusitis, is desirable. Pneumococcal vaccine can be administered to adults over the age of 65 years with persistent asthma, although pneumococcal pneumonia is an infrequent occurrence.

Aspirin-Exacerbated Respiratory Disease (Aspirin-Intolerant Asthma)

Treatment of aspirin-exacerbated respiratory disease (aspirin-intolerant asthma) includes avoidance measures for patients with IgE-mediated triggers of asthma and anti-inflammatory therapy. It is important to avoid aspirin and nonselective NSAIDs, which may also produce serious acute bronchoconstriction. Patients must be informed that numerous proprietary mixtures contain aspirin, and they must be certain to take no proprietary medication that contains acetylsalicylic acid. Acetaminophen may be used as a safe substitute for aspirin in nearly all patients, and other salicylates, such as sodium salicylate, choline magnesium trisalicylate, or salsalate, can be taken safely. Other patients respond with urticaria, angioedema, or anaphylaxis. The mechanisms of acute bronchoconstriction include the blockade of cyclooxygenase-1, reduced production of PGE_2, and generation of LTC_4 and LTD_4. Patients with aspirin-exacerbated respiratory disease have increased baseline urinary concentrations of LTE_4, a marker of 5-lipoxygenase products. After aspirin ingestion, there is even greater increase in urinary LTE_4 concentrations, consistent with synthesis of the potent agonist LTD_4 (13). Although PGE_2 can be thought of as a bronchodilator, it has a major role in "braking" the production of leukotrienes via inhibitory effects on 5-LO and FLAP. PGE_2 also stabilizes mast cells, but this protective effect also is reduced after aspirin ingestion. The cyclooxygenase-2 inhibitors are tolerated uneventfully (13,185,186). There are very few patients who experience acute bronchoconstriction from both cyclooxygenase-1 and cyclooxygenase-2 antagonists.

In some situations, provocative dose testing with either aspirin or NSAIDs may be carried out to confirm the diagnosis or to treat underlying aspirin-exacerbated respiratory disease (308,309). Because the mean provoking dose of aspirin was 62 mg during oral challenges (308), the physician should be in attendance at all times because of the explosiveness and severity of these reactions, primarily when the initial dosage is the full dose. The FEV_1 should be at least 70% before the challenge. Pulmonary function parameters and vital signs should be measured prospectively. Aspirin should be administered in serial doubling doses, beginning with 30 mg (308). (It may be advisable to begin with 3 mg in some patients.) The dosage is advanced to 60 mg, 100 mg, 150 mg, 325 mg, and 650 mg every 3 hours if there is <20% decrease in FEV_1 with each dosage. If 650 mg of aspirin has been given and there is not a 20% decrease in FEV_1, it is unlikely that aspirin is significant in the patient's condition. When a decrease in FEV_1 of 20% occurs, the provoking dose is repeated every 3 to 24 hours until no bronchospastic response occurs. There may be long-term benefit in patients who undergo successful "aspirin desensitization" followed by daily aspirin treatment, acknowledging that some patients will experience gastritis or gastric bleeding (309).

Conversion ratios between aspirin and NSAIDs are as follows: aspirin 325 mg = ibuprofen 200 mg = naproxen 220 mg = indomethacin 25 mg (308). It has been suggested that in this context acetaminophen of 1,000 mg may be equivalent, but this author believes that a higher dosage of acetaminophen should be used in this comparison.

Formerly, there was a notion that tartrazine intolerance/sensitivity might co-exist with aspirin-exacerbated respiratory disease. However, this issue appears to be nonexistent. Should a challenge have to be perfomed to exclude tartrazine intolerance/sensitivity, begin test dosing FD&C Yellow No. 5, begin 1 mg, 5 mg, 15 mg, and 29 mg every hour and monitor respiratory status and FEV_1.

Potentially (Near) Fatal Asthma

The diagnosis of potentially (near) fatal asthma is helpful because it identifies high-risk patients who are more likely to die from asthma (50,86,151,152). Despite aggressive intervention, such as early and intensive pharmacotherapy, allergen avoidance, and psychological evaluation, the death rate was found to be 7.1%, which is much greater than the asthma death rate overall of 0.0017% (86). Potentially (near) fatal asthma patients do not have an inexorably fatal condition, in that stabilization and clinical improvement can occur if patients are managed effectively and are compliant with office appointments and other factors. Some patient factors that complicate care of potentially (near) fatal asthma and result in noncompliance include psychologic or psychiatric conditions (schizophrenia, bipolar disorder, personality disorders), chaotic dysfunctional family, denial, anger, lack of insight, ignorance, and child abuse by proxy. In the latter situation, some parents refuse to permit essential medications such as prednisone to be administered to their children despite previous episodes of respiratory arrest or repeated status asthmaticus. Some physician- or health care provider-related factors that can contribute to ineffectively managed patients and potential fatalities include (a) lack of appreciation for limitations in effectiveness of β_2-adrenergic agonists, leukotriene modifiers, theophylline, and combinations in increasingly severe asthma; (b) fear of prednisone; (c) failure to increase the dosage of prednisone or to administer prednisone when asthma exacerbations occur, such as during an upper respiratory tract infection; (d) lack of availability; (e) excessively demanding regimens; and (f) limited understanding of importance of a quiet chest on auscultation in severely dyspneic patients.

In survivors of episodes of nearly fatal asthma, defined as acute respiratory arrest, presentation with PCO_2 of at least 50 mm Hg, or impaired level of consciousness, blunted perception of dyspnea has been demonstrated when patients were hospitalized, but these abnormalities normalized or improved considerably. Similarly, the ventilatory response to inhalation of carbon dioxide was not different from that of other patients with less severe asthma or nonasthmatic subjects. However, abnormal respiratory responses to decreases in inspired oxygen have been identified. This group of patients with potentially fatal asthma does not demonstrate persistent physiologic abnormalities that identify them as having intrinsically precarious asthma.

Potentially fatal asthma can be treated with inhaled corticosteroids, inhaled β_2-adrenergic agonists, and usually alternate-day or rarely daily prednisone in compliant patients. It is advisable to institute the nonspecific general areas of care discussed previously. In contrast, in patients with malignant, potentially fatal asthma, depot corticosteroids (Depo-Medrol) can be administered after appropriate documentation is made in the medical record and the patient is informed. As for other types of asthma, prevention of fatalities and acute severe asthma (Chapter 21) involves understanding asthma, knowing the patient, instituting stepwise but effective therapy, establishing a physician–patient relationship, and emphasizing early therapy for increasingly severe asthma.

Personal peak flow monitoring will not help the unreliable, noncompliant patient. A personal peak flow monitor possibly will improve asthma if it can formalize antiasthma therapy in the otherwise noncompliant patient.

Some patients with very severe asthma will have steroid-resistant asthma, defined by a <12% increase in FEV_1 after 1 week of prednisone administered as 20 mg twice daily (84). Steroid-sensitive patients have a >15% increase in FEV_1 (84). The best treatments for steroid-resistant patients are under investigation, but continued moderate to high dosages of prednisone on a daily basis may cause more side effects than therapeutic benefit.

Treatment of the Acute Attack of Asthma

In mild attacks, the use of inhaled (or oral depending on age) short-acting β_2-adrenergic agonists every 4 to 6 hours may suffice. Inhaled β_2-adrenergic agonists can be administered by metered β_2-adrenergic dose inhaler with or without a spacer device, depending on patient technique, or by nebulizer. Patients must be advised about their proper use and warned against overuse. Alternatively, in patients with persistent mild asthma, as needed inhaled corticosteroids may be sufficient therapy (134).

In patients with persistent moderate and severe asthma, it is necessary to continue the currently prescribed inhaled corticosteroids and add a β_2-adrenergic agonist or, depending on severity of the attack and the ease of control of the patient's asthma, and add a short course of oral corticosteroid (e.g., prednisone, 1 mg/kg to 2 mg/kg for children and 40 mg to 60 mg for adults). When signs and symptoms of asthma are refractory to 2 to 3 treatments with inhaled short-acting β_2-adrenergic agonists or nebulized albuterol, acute severe asthma exists, a medical emergency requiring corticosteroids and intensified monitoring. Its treatment is presented in Chapter 21 and Table 19.17. For patients who are not that ill acutely and can initiate therapy at home, doubling of the dosage of inhaled corticosteroid from a therapeutic, controlling dosage has not been found to be effective (204). It may be possible to triple the inhaled corticosteroid dose and achieve control of the acute attack, but this issue remains under investigation.

TABLE 19.17   INITIAL TREATMENT OF ACUTE SEVERE ASTHMA

1. Corticosteroid therapy (give immediately in the office or emergency department). Methylprednisolone (Solu-Medrol), 0.5 mg/kg to 1.0 mg/kg intravenously every 6 hours; or hydrocortisone (Solu-Cortef), 4 mg/kg intravenously every 6 hours; or prednisone, 1 mg/kg orally every 6 hours (minimum is 80 mg methylprednisolone equivalent/24 hours)
2. β-Adrenergic agonists
   Choice of approaches available:
   a. Aerosolized therapy; albuterol, levalbuterol, metaproterenol, pirbuterol.
      Repeat twice at 20-minute intervals, then at reduced frequency. May use continuous nebulization of albuterol.
   b. Epinephrine, 0.01 mL/kg of 1:1000 solution, intramuscularly not to exceed 0.3 mL to 0.4 mL in adults. May repeat twice at 20-minute intervals, then at reduced frequency.
   c. If a patient does not respond to (a), try (b).
3. Hospitalize
4. Laboratory studies
   White blood cell count with differential
   Chest radiograph
   Pulse oximetry or arterial blood gas
   Serum electrolytes and chemistries
   Sputum Gram stain, culture, and sensitivities (some cases)
   Bedside spirometer may be useful, but not essential
   Electrocardiogram (some cases)
5. Oxygen therapy; 2 L/min to 3 L/min nasal cannula (best guided by arterial blood gas determination)
6. Correct dehydration
7. Aminophylline therapy (controversial). Check theophylline concentration if chronic therapy. Administration is discouraged because efficacy has been questioned during emergency use.
8. Antibiotic therapy. When indicated for bronchitis or exacerbations of rhinosinusitis.
9. Impending or acute respiratory failure. Repeat β$_2$-adrenergic agonists; endotracheal intubation with assisted or controlled ventilation.

Because tachyphylaxis to short-acting β$_2$-adrenergic agonists has been demonstrated *in vivo* and *in vitro* in some studies, concern has been expressed that prior administration of β$_2$-adrenergic agonists may abrogate clinical response from current emergency treatment of asthma. Failure of a patient to improve suggests increasingly severe asthma (bronchoconstriction, hyperinflation, mucus plugging of airways, etc.), not tachyphylaxis to short-acting β$_2$-adrenergic agonists. In patients using salmeterol regularly but for whom emergency department care for asthma was required, nebulized albuterol at 2.5 mg or 5.0 mg produced similar improvement in PEFR, compared with patients who had not been using salmeterol (310). The responses to albuterol were not impaired. Typically, the PEFR improved from about 200 L/min (40% predicted) to 300 L/min (60% predicted) (310). The patients who were hospitalized (32%) did not respond to albuterol, which is the definition of acute severe asthma. As stated earlier, scheduled use of salmeterol should include concurrently administered inhaled corticosteroid (Table 19.8).

There may be a modest benefit of combining ipratropium bromide with nebulized albuterol (3, 311–313), but other studies have found no advantage (314,315). Although ipratropium bromide is safe, its bronchodilating effect is small. In a study of children, when asthma was stratified into severe asthma and moderate asthma, fewer hospitalizations occurred in the former patients (52.6% versus 37.5%) when ipratropium bromide, 500 μg, was included with albuterol and prednisone or prednisolone, 2 mg/kg (312).

Treatment of Persistent Asthma

The management of persistent asthma entails a continuous broad control that should be tailored to each patient. Features of general management, as discussed previously, must be included in the treatment regimen. Significant allergic factors are treated by environmental control combined with appropriately administered allergen immunotherapy. Immunomodulator treatment (omalizumab) should be considered for persistent moderate and severe asthma in patients with at least one positive skin test response to a perennial allergen and high medication requirements (Table 19.8). In each patient, secondary contributing factors or comorbidities should be evaluated and controlled as best as possible. Some of these factors include cessation of smoking or illicit drug use, adherence with medications, effective inhaler technique, and treatment of concurrent medical conditions, such as allergic rhinitis or rhinosinusitis, GERD (SERD or NERD), COPD, and congestive heart failure. Medication intolerance and variations in responses to pharmacotherapy should be identified.

Patients with persistent asthma require anti-inflammatory therapy (preferably inhaled corticosteroids, but cromolyn, nedocromil, and leukotriene receptor antagonists or inhibitors are acceptable in some situations) (Table 19.8) (3). In patients with intermittent asthma, inhaled (or oral) short-acting β_2-adrenergic agonists taken only when or before symptoms occur may suffice. A patient who has asthma only with upper respiratory infections should be instructed to begin either an inhaled corticosteroid or inhaled corticosteroid/β_2-adrenergic agonist at the first sign of coryza. Children or some adults, who wheeze only with upper respiratory infections, may need to use inhaled corticosteroids (or inhaled corticosteroid/β_2-adrenergic agonist combination) as scheduled therapy because of the persistence of silent pulmonary function abnormalities and airway inflammation. This point needs to be explained clearly to obtain sufficient control of asthma. At a minimum, patients with persistent moderate or severe asthma clearly require scheduled daily inhaled corticosteroids (3) used properly (with or without a spacer device). An action plan for regular or intensified therapy is indicated, especially for times when symptoms are not controlled by ongoing medications.

If the patient has prednisone-dependent asthma with nocturnal symptoms, effective control of these symptoms may be achieved either by increasing the morning prednisone dose or by increasing the use of inhaled corticosteroids. Because of the tradeoff between severe allergic asthma from a pet and incomplete control of asthma with polypharmacy, it is advisable to revisit the recommendation for removal of the pet.

A patient being treated with scheduled, noncorticosteroid therapy using β_2-adrenergic agonists, leukotriene modifier, theophylline, ipratropium bromide, or a combination of these agents may have an exacerbation of asthma. For these patients, additional β_2-adrenergic agonists may result in side effects. Additional theophylline may result in toxicity without clinical improvement. Short-term oral corticosteroid or perhaps inhaled corticosteroid therapy or both, is the most appropriate therapy. If longer use of oral corticosteroids or more frequent courses are required, inhaled corticosteroid/β_2-adrenergic agonist combination therapy or high-dosage inhaled-corticosteroid steroid and alternate-day prednisone should be considered after the patient has improved (Table 19.16). Such patients should undergo allergy-immunology consultation and receive appropriate anti-inflammatory medications.

When persistent asthma is not controlled effectively with inhaled corticosteroids or an inhaled corticosteroid/β_2-adrenergic agonist combination, other medications may be tried. Cromolyn, nedocromil, leukotriene receptor antagonists or biosynthesis inhibitors, or a combination of these should be tried in some patients. Cromolyn can be used prophylactically for intermittent but unavoidable animal exposure. However, if added to scheduled inhaled corticosteroid therapy, the additional benefit of cromolyn may or may not occur. However, a 1- to 2-month trial of cromolyn, nedocromil, or leukotriene receptor antagonist or biosynthesis inhibitor should be attempted (Chapter 36).

Because of their frequent recurrence, it is generally advisable that surgical removal of nasal polyps be considered only after local corticosteroid aerosol treatment, coupled with good medical and allergy-immunology management, have not been effective in decreasing obstruction and repeated infections. Sinus surgery should also be considered when more conservative treatment (medical and allergic-immunologic) has resulted in little or no success in preventing recurrent sinusitis. Some patients with recurrent exacerbations of chronic rhinosinusitis have common variable immunodeficiency or specific antibody deficiency (Chapter 4). Referral for surgery typically occurs when patients have four episodes of rhinosinusitis per year, asthma episodes repeatedly triggered by acute rhinosinusitis, chronic rhinosinusitis resistant to medical therapy, and in patients in whom allergic fungal rhinosinusitis is suspected (Chapter 12).

Anxiety or depression or other psychologic or psychiatric conditions may aggravate asthma. When these conditions are present, antidepressants may be necessary. Psychologic or psychiatric evaluation should be obtained. Often, it has been assumed by the lay public as well as by some members of the medical profession that asthma is primarily an expression of an underlying psychological disturbance. This attitude has inappropriately prevented proper medical and allergy-immunologic management in some patients. In most patients, psychiatric factors are of little to no significance in the cause of the disease. Nevertheless, psychological factors may be a contributory aggravating factor for asthma. Asthma is a chronic disease that also may be associated with significant impairment of physical and social activity. These factors in themselves may lead to the development of psychologic dysfunction with reduced quality of life. Often, when symptoms of asthma are brought under control, concomitant improvement of psychologic dynamics occurs. When schizophrenia and corticosteroid-dependent asthma coexist, the physician may become frustrated because of the patient's prednisone phobia, medication or appointment nonaderence, and abuse of emergency medical facilities. Depot methylprednisolone (Depo-Medrol) may be beneficial or lifesaving in patients if they keep their medical appointments.

The decision to use a peak flow meter should be kept in perspective. In adherent patients, measurements can be an early warning system that leads to implementation of the action plan. If the patient is under effective control of asthma such that exercise tolerance is satisfactory, nocturnal wheezing is absent or infrequent, emergency department visits are not happening, and symptoms of asthma are uncommon or mild, little benefit from a peak flow meter will occur. If the peak flow meter can help emphasize patient adherence with antiasthma measures and medication, its addition to a regimen will be valuable. Some patients submit peak flow diaries consistent with their expectations or perceptions of asthma. Other patients do not contact their physicians or intensify therapy for peak flow rates of 30% of predicted, nullifying any value to the patient or physician. There may be discrepancies between measurements of PEFR and FEV_1, resulting in overestimation or underestimation of the FEV_1.

Treatment of Intractable, Difficult to Treat or Refractory Asthma

Intractable asthma refers to persistent, incapacitating symptoms that have become unresponsive to the usual therapy, including moderate to large doses of oral corticosteroids and high-dose inhaled corticosteroids. These cases fortunately are few. Their constant medical and nonmedical requirements are heavy social and financial burdens on their families. Further, these patients may have cushingoid features from daily prednisone use. Most patients with intractable asthma are not deficient in antiproteases. Some will meet criteria for steroid-resistant asthma. Their asthma may represent an intense inflammatory process with marked bronchial mucosal edema, mucus plugging of airway, and decreased lung compliance and more easily collapsible airways. In cases of intractable asthma, a home visit may be beneficial for the patient as well as for the physician or other health care provider. For example, the finding that an animal resides in the home of a patient with intractable asthma may explain the apparent failure of oral and high-dosage inhaled corticosteroids to improve the control of asthma. Also, when speaking to the patient by telephone, a physician's overhearing of a barking dog may provide the explanation for the difficulty controlling the asthma. Thus, intractable asthma is not always intractable.

Some cases of intractable asthma include those patients with severe, corticosteroid-dependent asthma in whom adequate doses of corticosteroids have not been used, either by physician or patient avoidance. After initiation of appropriate doses of prednisone and clearing of asthma, many cases can be controlled with alternate-day prednisone and inhaled corticosteroids or with inhaled corticosteroid/β_2-adrenergic agonist alone. Leukotriene receptor antagonists or biosynthesis inhibitors should be tried. Other patients require moderate to even high doses of daily prednisone for functional control. Fortunately, this latter group is small. Occasionally, it includes patients with severe lung damage from allergic bronchopulmonary aspergillosis or with irreversible asthma (145). Other patients may have asthma and COPD, with most of their disease being COPD. Pharmacologic improvement of asthma can be achieved, but the irreversible obstructive component cannot be altered significantly.

In an attempt to reduce the prednisone dosage in patients with intractable asthma (severe corticosteroid-dependent asthma), some physicians have recommended using methylprednisolone (Medrol) and the macrolide antibiotic, troleandomycin, in an effort to decrease the prednisone requirement. Although prednisone dosage can be reduced, the decreased clearance of methylprednisolone by the effect of troleandomycin on the liver still may result in cushingoid obesity or corticosteroid side effects, at times exceeding prednisone alone. Therefore, methylprednisolone and troleandomycin are reduced as the patient improves. This approach has little to offer. The antifungal drug itraconazole also decreases metabolism of methylprednisolone. It remains unclear if empiric use of clarithromycin has any role in management of intractable or very severe asthma.

High doses of intramuscular triamcinolone have been recommended and are effective therapy. However, they were associated with expected adverse effects, such as cushingoid facies, acne, hyperglycemia, hirsutism, and myalgias. In patients with severe asthma who were receiving high dosage of beclomethasone dipropionate and oral corticosteroids but still had elevated eosinophils in sputum, intramuscular triamcinolone resulted in reduced sputum eosinophils and increased FEV_1 (316). These findings questioned the notion that patients with severe asthma and sputum eosinophilia, despite oral and inhaled corticosteroid treatment, actually are refractory to corticosteroids.

In adults, methotrexate (15 mg/week) was reported to be steroid sparing in a group of patients whose daily prednisone dosage was reduced by 36.5% (317). A double-blind placebo-controlled trial over a shorter period, 13 weeks, did not confirm a benefit of methotrexate, in that both methotrexate and placebo-treated patients had prednisone reductions of about 40% (318). Such a finding is consistent with the Hawthorne effect, improvement that occurs simply as a result of participant observation; in other words, entry into a study itself can have a beneficial effect. The use of methotrexate (and drugs like azathioprine) remains experimental and unproved for treatment of persistent severe asthma. Cyclosporine also has been disappointing and appears to provide only prednisone-sparing effects that are not sustainable after cyclosporine is discontinued (319, 320). The administration of gold therapy for asthma has been described but is associated with recognized toxicity (321).

It is possible to reduce the elevated levels of $TNF\alpha$ in sputum from patients with severe asthma and $TNF\alpha$ participates in airway hyperreactivity (322). This observation suggests that antagonizing $TNF\alpha$ might be of benefit in treatment of asthma (323). In patients with persistent moderate asthma, infliximab, a recombinant antibody to soluble TNFα reduced peak expiratory flow rate variability, reduced number of exacerbations and delayed time until exacerbation (323). The role of anti-TNFα therapy in severe or intractable asthma remains a possibility for future study. Omalizumab and other recombinant antibodies may provide a role in persistent severe asthma, but it remains to be established whether these antibodies will be effective for difficult to treat asthma.

Studies with dapsone, hydroxychloroquine, and intravenous gammaglobulin (324–326) are not convincing in the management of difficult cases of asthma. Nebulized lidocaine (40 mg to 160 mg, 4 times daily) has been investigated in adults (327) and children (328). Its role remains to be established. In steroid-dependent patients, a confounding factor is unrecognized respiratory or skeletal muscle weakness. Although this finding may result from use of intravenous corticosteroids and muscle relaxants, it can have residual effects. Every attempt must be made to reduce the prednisone dose and eventually to use alternate-day prednisone if possible. Furthermore, very high dosages of inhaled corticosteroids such as >2,000 µg/day may cause adrenal suppression or adverse effects on bone health and still not improve asthma.

Another approach for moderate and severe asthma is bronchial thermoplasty (329,330). With bronchoscopy and the patient receiving either general anesthesia or conscious sedation, there is "controlled thermal energy" delivered to bronchi (330). It is hoped that there is a reduction in the smooth muscle mass. Some therapeutic effectiveness has been described (330). Additional data are required to determine if this approach will provide the proper risk/benefit outcomes.

Asthma is a long-term condition with fluctuations. In a study of the natural history of severe asthma in patients who required at least 1 year of prednisone in addition to other pharmacotherapy (β2-adrenergic agonists, theophylline, and high-dose inhaled corticosteroids), avoidance measures, and possibly immunotherapy, prednisone-free intervals occurred, even lasting several years, before prednisone was required again (331). It was uncommon to have greater prednisone requirements, although usually, in these cases of persistent severe asthma, prednisone dosages were stable over time, or reductions occurred. The conclusion is that in assessment of novel treatments for persistent moderate, severe, or refractory asthma, adequate "wash-in" periods are needed in studies of such patients; otherwise, credit may be given to a new therapy inappropriately.

The term *glucocorticoid-resistant* has been applied to patients with asthma who did not increase the FEV_1 after 2 weeks of prednisone or prednisolone administration (40 mg daily for week 1, 20 mg daily for week 2) (332,333). The evaluation period of prednisone administration also has been suggested as 1 week of prednisone 40 mg daily (84). Experimentally, glucocorticoid receptor downregulation on T lymphocytes has been identified, suggesting that such patients may have impaired inhibition of activated T lymphocytes in asthma. For example, in cells from corticosteroid-resistant patients, dexamethasone *in vitro* did not *inhibit* T-lymphocyte proliferation to the mitogen phytohemagglutinin (334). Excessive and harmful allergic inflammation characterizes this form of difficult to treat asthma.

In summarizing the discussion of intractable or difficult to treat or refractory asthma, it is worth reconsidering the differential diagnosis of asthma. Some patients will have unrecognized vocal cord dysfunction and asthma. Other patients may misrepresent their dosages and use of prednisone.

■ ACUTE SEVERE ASTHMA (STATUS ASTHMATICUS)

Acute severe asthma (status asthmaticus) is defined as severe asthma unresponsive to emergency therapy with β2-adrenergic agonists (Chapter 21). It is a medical emergency for which immediate recognition and treatment are necessary to avoid a fatal outcome. For practical purposes, acute severe asthma is present in the absence of meaningful response to two aerosol treatments with β2-adrenergic agonists or 1 hour of nebulized albuterol.

A number of factors have been shown to be important in inducing acute severe asthma and contributing to the mortality of asthma. About half of patients have an associated respiratory tract infection. Some have overused short acting β2-adrenergic agonists before developing refractoriness. In the aspirin-exacerbated respiratory disease asthmatic patient, ingestion of aspirin or related cyclooxygenase-1 inhibitors may precipitate acute severe asthma. Exposure to animal dander (especially cat dander) in the highly atopic patient may contribute to development of acute severe asthma, particularly when this is associated with an upper respiratory infection. Withdrawal or too sudden reduction of oral or inhaled corticosteroids may be associated with the development of acute severe asthma. In many situations, both the patient and physician or health care provider are unaware of the severity of progression of symptoms, and often earlier and more aggressive medical management would have prevented the need for emergency department visit or hospitalization. The inappropriate use of soporific medications in the treatment of acute severe asthma has contributed to the development of respiratory failure. A problem of the past in the United States, overdose of theophylline has been cited as a cause of death or cardiac arrest in some patients.

Acute severe asthma requires immediate treatment with high-dose corticosteroids either parenterally or orally. Patients with acute severe asthma must be hospitalized where close observation and ancillary treatment by experienced personnel are available. If respiratory failure occurs, optimal treatment often involves the combined efforts of the pulmonary disease critical care specialist and/or anesthesiologist.

Initial laboratory studies should include a complete blood count, Gram stain with culture and sensitivity of the sputum, chest radiograph, serum electrolytes, and chemistries, pulse oximetry, and perhaps arterial blood gas studies (Tables 19.17 and 19.18). There may be considerable improvement during treatment of acute severe asthma without improvement in peak expiratory flow rate, FEV_1, or forced vital capacity. This apparent lack of spirometric improvement occurs even though the hyperinflation of lung volumes is diminishing in association with a reduction in the elastic work of breathing.

The severity of acute asthma is organized into four stages (Table 19.18). Stage I signifies the presence of airway obstruction only. Because of the associated hyperventilation, the PCO_2 is low, and the pH is therefore slightly alkalotic (respiratory alkalosis). The PO_2 in stage I is normal. Spirometric study shows only a decrease in FEV_1, with a normal vital capacity. As symptoms progress, obstruction of the airway increases, compliance decreases, and air trapping and hyperinflation develop. As a result of the latter changes, the FRC increases, and the vital capacity is decreased. In stage II, V/Q imbalance with hypoxemia occurs. These changes, however, are not enough to impair net alveolar ventilation; thus, although PO_2 is lowered, PCO_2 remains low, and an alkalotic pH persists. With progressive severity, net alveolar ventilation decreases, and a transitional period exists (stage III), in which the PCO_2 increases and the pH decreases, so that now both values appear to be normal. When the blood gas study shows hypoxemia in the presence of a normal PCO_2 and pH, close supervision and frequent determinations of pH and PCO_2 are essential to evaluate the adequacy of treatment and the possible progression to respiratory failure characterized by hypoxemia and elevated PCO_2

(stage IV). Clinical observation alone is inadequate in determining the seriousness of acute severe asthma.

Patients who experience a single episode of acute severe asthma can be at increased risk of future episodes of acute severe asthma or fatalities from asthma. It is important to consider what factors contributed to the acute episode and what approaches may be taken to prevent future emergency department visits, hospitalizations, or fatality from asthma. A virtual "discharge conference," performed during the allergy-immunology or asthma specialist consultation, for example, should focus on prevention of future episodes requiring emergency treatment.

Treatment

Although many patients with acute severe asthma manifest signs of restlessness and anxiety, the use of anxiolytic drugs is contraindicated. The inability to achieve adequate ventilation may cause the patient to appear excessively anxious. Such patients likely are in stage III or IV (Table 19.18) and may require emergent intubation. Some patients in acute severe asthma are dehydrated. The hyperventilation and increased work of breathing cause water loss through the lungs and skin.

In patients with a compromised cardiovascular system, sodium and water overload must be avoided. Because a high dose of parenteral corticosteroids is used in these patients, adequate potassium supplementation must be included in the intravenous therapy. In some adults, 80 mEq of potassium chloride per 24 hours (not to exceed 20 mEq/hour) is indicated. Frequent serum electrolyte determinations provide the best guide for continued electrolyte therapy.

It is no longer considered that aminophylline should be administered. However, if it is used, aminophylline should be given intravenously using constant infusion and being cognizant of serum theophylline concentrations and drug interactions.

TABLE 19.18 SPIROMETRY AND BLOOD GASES IN ASTHMA AS RELATED TO THE STAGE OR SEVERITY

	FEV_1	VITAL CAPACITY	PO_2 (NORMAL, 90 MM HG–100 MM HG)	PCO_2 (NORMAL, 35 MM HG–40 MM HG)	PH (NORMAL, 7.35 MM HG–7.43 MM HG)
Stage I (respiratory alkalosis)	↓	Normal	Normal	↓	>7.43
Stage II (respiratory alkalosis)	↓↓	↓	↓	↓↓	>7.43
Stage III	↓↓↓	↓↓	↓↓	35–40	7.35–7.43
Stage IV (respiratory acidosis)	↓↓↓↓	↓↓↓	↓↓↓	↑↑↑	<7.35

FEV_1, forced expiratory volume in 1 second; ↑, increased; ↓, reduced.

Because nearly all patients are hypoxemic, oxygen therapy is required. Ideally, blood gas determinations should guide proper therapy. Therapeutically, a PO_2 of 60 mm Hg or slightly higher is sufficient. This often can be accomplished with low flow rates of 2 L/min to 3 L/min by nasal cannula. Ventimasks calibrated to deliver 24%, 28%, and 35% oxygen may also be used. The necessity for higher concentration of oxygen to maintain a PO_2 of 60 mm Hg usually signifies the presence of thick tracheobronchial secretions and of V/Q mismatch. Also, β_2-adrenergic agonists initially may cause a mild decrease in PO_2 by increasing pulmonary blood flow to poorly ventilated alveoli, increasing V/Q mismatch. Oxygen helps protect against this effect. It is cautioned that, in patients with asthma complicated by COPD, chronic hypercapnia may be present, and hypoxemia remains the only respiratory stimulus. Oxygen therapy during an acute respiratory insult in these patients may enhance progression to respiratory failure. Close clinical observation and frequent blood gas monitoring are important in preventing this complication.

With evidence of infection (i.e., purulent sputum containing polymorphonuclear leukocytes, fever, acute rhinosinusitis, or radiographic evidence of pneumonia), antibiotics should be administered. In some instances, infection may be present in the absence of these suggestive findings; conversely, eosinophils may result in sputum that appears purulent but contains no bacteria or neutrophils. Thus, antibiotics should not be prescribed routinely. Results of sputum culture should dictate change in antibiotic therapy. If rhinosinusitis is present, other antibiotics, such as amoxicillin-clavulanate, azithromycin, clarithromycin, or trimethoprim-sulfamethoxazole, can be administered.

Large doses of corticosteroids are essential immediately in acute severe asthma with a minimum of 80 mg/day of methylprednisolone in adolescents and adults (236). With improvement, oral doses of prednisone can be substituted at 60 mg/day to 80 mg/day in an adult and 2 mg/kg/day in children. There is no additional benefit of 1,000-mg doses/day of methylprednisolone. It is possible to manage acute severe asthma without giving intravenous corticosteroids. For example, when prednisone, 2 mg/kg twice daily, was compared in children with methylprednisolone, 1 mg/kg four times daily given intravenously, equal efficacy was found for hospital length of stay and respiratory parameters (335). For adults, prednisone, 60 mg immediately and every 6 hours, can be administered. Chemistries, including glucose and potassium, should be determined. Magnesium rarely can be decreased in ambulatory patients and may contribute to respiratory muscle dysfunction but should be considered in some situations, especially after mechanical ventilation.

For acute dyspnea, nebulized or aerosolized β_2-adrenergic agonists may be administered every 4 hours or continuously (a fad that does not produce superior results); however, little or no effect may be seen in the first 24 hours. Treatment of acute severe asthma is summarized in Tables 19.10, 19.17, 19.18, and Chapter 21. There remains no defined role for magnesium (unless the patient has hypomagnesemia) or heliox.

■ RESPIRATORY FAILURE

Most patients with acute severe asthma respond favorably to the management described previously and in Chapter 21. In those patients who continue to deteriorate, other aggressive measures must be included to prevent respiratory failure, which may be defined as a PCO_2 of greater than 50 mm Hg or a PO_2 of less than 50 mm Hg. The important features of treatment at this stage include measures to maintain adequate alveolar ventilation and to protect from the severe acid-base disturbances that may arise.

Signs of impending respiratory failure result from the combined effects of hypercapnia, hypoxia, and acidosis. Clinically, because of fatigue, inability to talk, and exhaustion, thoracic excursion is decreased, and auscultation of the chest may show decreased respiratory sounds because there is a decrease in air flow. Because of accompanying stupor, the patient may appear to be struggling less to breathe. These two features may give a false impression of improvement. Signs and symptoms of hypoxia include restlessness, confusion or delirium, and central cyanosis, which is present when arterial saturation is less than 70% and arterial PO_2 is less than 40 mm Hg. Hypercapnia is associated with headache or dizziness, confusion, unconsciousness, asterixis, miosis, papilledema, hypertension, and diaphoresis. Other danger signs in the patient with acute severe asthma include the presence of pulsus paradoxus, marked inspiratory retractions, inability to speak in full sentences, and cardiac arrhythmias that may lead to cardiac arrest. It has been suggested that retractions (154) are equivalent to pulsus paradoxus and certainly easier to detect.

Acute chest pain is consistent with myocardial ischemia or infarction, pulmonary infarction (emboli usually cause dyspnea without chest wall pain), or rib fractures. When subcutaneous emphysema is present, chest pain suggests pneumomediastinum or pneumothorax. Acidosis and hypoxemia contribute to pulmonary vasoconstriction, with resultant pulmonary hypertension and right ventricular strain. The acidosis is primarily respiratory in origin, but with severe hypoxemia, aerobic metabolism is impaired, and there is an accumulation of pyruvic and lactic acid (end products of anaerobic metabolism). These result in a superimposed metabolic acidosis. The presence of these signs and symptoms associated with development of acidosis and hypercapnia usually demands the institution of mechanical ventilation.

Patients who survive an episode of acute severe asthma who have required mechanical ventilation should be considered to have potentially (near) fatal asthma (50,86,151,152). Attempts should be made to identify reasons for the episode of acute severe asthma. Some examples include allergic asthma from animal exposure, such as cats, dogs, gerbils, or hamsters; molds (fungi); upper respiratory infections; acute rhinosinusitis; nonadherence with outpatient advice; undertreatment on an ambulatory basis (failure to receive a short course of prednisone when the deterioration began); use of aspirin or cyclooxygenase-1 inhibitor within 3 hours of onset of severe asthma symptoms; or substance abuse, such as cocaine or heroin use (336). Some patients have unanticipated severe attacks, but these patients should undergo allergy-immunology or asthma specialist evaluation and receive more intensive pharmacotherapy. Acute respiratory failure may occur seemingly without apparent explanation and can be fatal. Furthermore, not all patients with acute respiratory failure report moderate to severe persistent symptoms of asthma. However, some of these patients are poor perceivers of dyspnea and decreases in FEV_1 and are not recognized as having more than mild (persistent) symptoms.

■ PREPARATION OF THE ASTHMATIC PATIENT FOR SURGERY

For elective surgery, the patient with asthma ideally should be evaluated 1 to 3 weeks in advance as an ambulatory patient so that adequate treatment can be instituted to ensure optimal bronchopulmonary status. If the patient is a corticosteroid-dependent asthmatic patient currently requiring a maintenance dose of prednisone, increase the dose of prednisone instead of relying on increased use of β_2-adrenergic agonists or inhaled corticosteroids to ensure complete control of asthma. If the patient is receiving scheduled inhaled corticosteroids, a short course (4 to 5 days) of prednisone (20 mg/day to 40 mg/day) before surgery is recommended to maximize pulmonary function (337,338). Pulmonary function testing should be obtained, at least FVC and FEV_1. The main need for oral corticosteroids, however, is prevention of intraoperative or postoperative asthma rather than adrenal crisis.

Hydrocortisone, 100 mg intravenously, should be started before surgery and continued every 8 hours until the patient can tolerate oral or inhaled medications (337,338). Often, just one dose of hydrocortisone is necessary. If no postoperative asthma occurs, the hydrocortisone dose can be discontinued. The doses of prednisone and hydrocortisone needed to control asthma do not increase postoperative complications, such as wound infection or dehiscence (337,338).

In patients with asthma, optimal respiratory status should be achieved before surgery occurs. Manipulation of the upper airway (e.g., suction, oropharyngeal airway) may cause bronchoconstriction during conscious sedation or anesthesia.

After surgery, the patient should be evaluated carefully. β_2-adrenergic agonists, deep-breathing exercises, adequate hydration, and gentle coughing should be instituted to avoid accumulation of secretions and atelectasis. Use of epidural or spinal anesthesia is not necessarily safer than general anesthesia.

■ COMPLICATIONS OF ASTHMA

Although they are rare, pneumothorax, pneumomediastinum, and subcutaneous emphysema can occur during an attack of severe asthma. These complications are thought to result from the rupture of overdistended peripheral alveoli. The escaping air then follows and dissects through bronchovascular sheaths of the lung parenchyma. Often, the amount of air is minimal, and no chest tube insertion is required. When severe tension symptoms occur, insertion of a chest tube under a water seal for pneumothorax may be needed. Tracheostomy may be required for severe tension complications of pneumomediastinum. A common feature of these conditions is chest pain; this is not expected with uncomplicated asthma, and when present should suggest the possibility of the extravasation of air. On auscultation of the heart, a crunching sound synchronous with the heartbeat may be present in a patient with pneumomediastinum (Hamman sign).

Minimal areas of atelectasis may occur in asthma. Atelectasis of the middle lobe is a common complication of asthma in children. It is often reversible with prednisone or parenteral corticosteroids and β_2-adrenergic agonists. It results from mucus plugging and edema of the middle lobe bronchus. When the atelectasis does not respond to the above treatment within a few days, bronchoscopy is indicated for both therapeutic and diagnostic reasons. Occasionally, children may develop atelectasis of other lobes or of an entire lung. Allergic bronchopulmonary aspergillosis (see Chapter 24) and cystic fibrosis must be excluded in these patients, as in any patient with asthma.

Rib fracture and costochondritis may occur as a result of coughing during attacks of asthma. In a few patients, severe coughing from asthma may result in cough syncope. In women, severe coughing results in urinary incontinence. Men or women may experience fecal incontinence in rare cases.

Chronic bronchitis and emphysema are not complications of asthma. These conditions occur with irreversible destruction of lung tissue, whereas asthma is at least a partially to completely reversible inflammatory condition. In some patients, asthma and emphysema or chronic bronchitis may coexist. The identification of bronchiectasis in a patient with asthma should raise the possibility of allergic bronchopulmonary aspergillosis, undiagnosed cystic fibrosis, or hypogammaglobulinemia or specific antibody deficiency. Hypoxemia from uncontrolled asthma has been associated with adverse effects on other organs, such as myocardial ischemia or infarction.

Another complication of asthma is excessive loss of FEV_1 compared with patients without asthma (145). Although this effect typically produces no clinical ramifications, in the exceptional patient, "irreversible asthma" occurs (145). Most of these adults could be considered as persistent wheezers since childhood (145). These patients do not have COPD, ABPA, cystic fibrosis, occupational asthma, or other lung disease, and α_1-antitrypsin concentrations are not reduced. High-resolution CT scanning of the lungs does not demonstrate fibrosis or other explanations. Most of these patients do not have steroid-resistant asthma because they have more than 15% bronchodilator response to 2 weeks of daily prednisone. However, their ultimate FEV_1 after prednisone and other pharmacotherapy is markedly impaired, with a mean FEV_1 percentage of 57 (145).

Treatment of asthma can help avoid the excessive loss of FEV_1 and preserve lung function (339,340) in patients with mild-to-severe asthma. For example, in a study over a period of 10 years in adults, the group of nonsmokers receiving inhaled corticosteroid therapy had an annualized loss of FEV_1 of 22.8 mL/yr compared with 46.1 mL/yr in those patients who did not use inhaled corticosteroids (339). There are advantages of initiating inhaled corticosteroid therapy within the first 2 years of the diagnosis of asthma (340). In children, loss of lung function occurs in the first 3 years of life and can persist (341). In a study of 16-year-old adolescents who had been evaluated since birth, when there was a history of transient wheezing with lower respiratory tract infections in the first 3 years of life or persistent wheezing (wheezing before age 3 years and wheezing at age 6 years), there was a loss of FEV_1 of 75 mL and 87 mL respectively compared with 23 mL in late onset wheeze patients (wheeze by age 6 years but not earlier) (341). These data support the finding that transient wheezers and persistent wheezers by age 6 years *already* have reductions in lung function that persist, whereas, the onset of asthma from ages 6 years and greater did not result in excessive loss of FEV_1 by age 16 (341).

Complications of treatment of asthma include adverse effects of inhaled corticosteroids and oral corticosteroids, such as the possibility of bone loss (osteopenia), osteoporosis, or even fracture. Complications of long acting β_2-adrenergic agonists have been a source of dispute, but their benefits when combined with an inhaled corticosteroid are far greater than risks.

■ MORTALITY

Death from asthma commonly occurs either as a result of acute severe asthma progressing to respiratory failure or suddenly and unexpectedly from severe bronchoconstriction and hypoxia, perhaps with a terminal cardiac arrhythmia. The increase in mortality rate from asthma that occurred in the 1980s in the United States appeared to stabilize by 1996 and peaked at over 5,000 cases/year before declining to 4,055 cases as of 2003 (86). The use of repeated doses of β_2-adrenergic aerosols has been suspected to be a contributing factor in some of these deaths. This interpretation alone is unlikely to be a satisfactory explanation as the quality of care, or lack of it, in the antecedent days (or weeks) before the fatal event is insufficient or misguided. In some cases, the death is seemingly unavoidable.

Undue reliance on inhaled β_2-adrenergic agonists by patients and physicians may contribute to fatalities in patients with severe exacerbations of asthma because essential corticosteroid therapy is not being administered. For historical purposes, the surge in deaths in the 1980s in New Zealand associated with the availability of albuterol inhalers without prescription and physician guidance has been considered possibly analogous to the earlier epidemics of the 1960s with potent short-acting β_2-adrenergic agonists. In addition, excessive deaths associated with the potent longer-acting, β_2-adrenergic agonist, femoterol, have been reported. This observation has led to the recommendation that, in persistent asthma, inhaled corticosteroids should be used in conjunction with β_2-adrenergic agonists.

Some factors that have been implicated in contributing to asthma deaths include the use of sedation in the hospital, illicit drugs and substance abuse outside of the hospital, the failure to use adequate doses of oral corticosteroids, theophylline toxicity, excessive use of β_2-adrenergic agonists, nonadherence with physician or other health care provider instructions, failure to initiate oral corticosteroids for exacerbations of asthma, and ineffective (lack of aggressive) outpatient management of asthma (50,101,336,342). One example of the latter phenomenon may be exemplified by the use of inhaled corticosteroids or β_2-adrenergic agonists, which will not substitute for oral corticosteroids given acutely as the attack of asthma intensifies. Although there are data supporting the combination product as reliever and maintenance therapy (232–234), it is not certain that this approach will be of value for patients experiencing a severe and potentially fatal episode of asthma. High-risk patients include those who have persistent moderate or severe asthma with frequent episodes of hospitalizations or chronic oral corticosteroid use, chest deformities such as pectus carinatum (pigeon breast), significant wheezing in-between exacerbations of asthma, or gross pulmonary function abnormalities when asymptomatic (poor perceivers) and patients previously requiring mechanical ventilation (343) during respiratory failure, such as those with potentially fatal asthma (150). After an episode of intubation for asthma, as many as 10% of patients may succumb from their asthma (343). Because of the reduction in functional residual capacity and less ability to apply negative radial traction on bronchi during acute asthma, patients with underlying restrictive lung disease tolerate episodes of acute severe asthma poorly.

■ FUTURE CONSIDERATIONS

Asthma management will be improved by continued improvements in therapy, implementation of these advances, health care system improvement, and stability of the family. Specific curative therapy can be realized only when basic pathophysiologic mechanisms are understood. Then, therapeutic modalities can be devised rationally to reverse the underlying pathogenesis.

Many patients with persistent asthma can be managed successfully with an inhaled corticosteroid and intermittent but not excessive use of β_2-adrenergic agonists. Additional anti-inflammatory therapies include cromolyn, nedocromil, and LTD_4-antagonists or biosynthesis inhibitors. None of the medications can substitute for prednisone in patients with oral corticosteroid–dependent asthma. Future therapies can be assessed for their ability to (a) decrease symptoms, (b) allow for withdrawal for prednisone or inhaled corticosteroids, (c) preserve lung function or limit the loss of FEV_1, and (d) permit improved quality of life without unacceptable adverse effects. Physicians managing patients with asthma should consider allergic triggers in all patients with persistent asthma because about 80% of patients have IgE antibodies by skin testing. Subcutaneous allergen vaccine therapy (immunotherapy), especially with trees, grasses, ragweed, and dust mites, remains effective as an immunomodulatory therapy. Some patients respond to injection of molds (fungi).

Humanized monoclonal antibody therapy, such as the anti-IgE antibody, omalizumab, is of value in some patients with persistent asthma (304). The antibody is primarily human IgG_1 and does form small immune complexes, but does not activate complement. Immediate and late bronchial responses to inhaled allergen challenge can be reduced by intravenous anti-IgE infusions (281). In a study using a soluble IL-4 receptor to inactivate IL-4, apparent benefit was reported initially (*344*). The requirement for β_2-adrenergic agonists and asthma symptom scores were reduced. Theoretically, such a "decoy" therapy, which binds free IL-4, would be of value in asthma therapy. The true measure of an agonist in asthma such as TNFα (322,323) is the effect when antagonists interact with the agonist and disease severity is reduced. There is an increasing array of targets in the pulmonary immune system that can be assessed for clinical benefit (Chapter 38).

Fundamental principles of asthma management include (a) preventing death, disability, and school or work absenteeism/presenteeism, (b) trying to minimize or overcome the effects of airway remodeling and allergic inflammation, mast cell activation, smooth muscle contraction, and pulmonary physiologic abnormalities; and (c) using medications effectively and as safely as possible. It is expected that our treatment modalities will continue to improve and that more specific therapies, whether pharmacologic, allergen immunotherapy, immunologically targeted treatments or other innovative approaches, will be of help to patients. It is hoped that we can take advantage of pharmacogenomic patterns to provide optimal "personalized medicine" for patients with asthma and allergic-immunologic conditions.

■ REFERENCES

1. National Institutes of Health, National Heart, Lung, and Blood Institute, Expert Panel Report, National Asthma Education Program, Executive Summary. *Guidelines for the Diagnosis and Management of Asthma.* Bethesda, MD: Public Health Service, U.S. Department of Health and Human Services, 1991; NIH Publication No. 91-3042A.

2. National Heart, Lung, and Blood Institute, Expert Panel Report 2. *Guidelines for the Diagnosis and Management of Asthma.* Bethesda, MD: U.S. Department of Health and Human Services, 1997; NIH publication No. 97-4051.

3. National Heart, Lung, and Blood Institute, National Asthma Education and Prevention Program. Expert Panel Report 3. *Guidelines for the Diagnosis and Management of Asthma.* Full report 2007. Bethesda, MD: U.S. Department of Health and Human Services, 2007; NIH publication no.07-0451.

4. Dicpinigaitis PV. Chronic cough due to asthma: ACCP evidence-based clinical practice guidelines. *Chest.* 2006;129:75S–79S.

5. Quesenberry PJ. Cardiac asthma: a fresh look at an old wheeze. *N Engl J Med.* 1989;320:1346–1348.

8. Morgan WJ, Crain EF, Gruchalla RS, et al. Results of a home-based environmental intervention among urban children with asthma. *N Engl J Med.* 2004;351:1068–1080.

11. Becker Y. Respiratory syncytial virus (RSV) evades the human adaptive immune system by skewing the Th1/Th2 cytokine balance toward increased levels of Th2 cytokines and IgE, markers of allergy—a review. *Virus Genes.* 2006;33:235–252.

12. Rakes GP, Arruda E, Ingram JM, et al. Rhinovirus and respiratory syncytial virus in wheezing children requiring emergency care. *Am J Respir Crit Care Med.* 1999;159:785–790.

13. Stevenson DD, Szczeklik K. Clinical and pathologic perspectives on aspirin sensitivity and asthma. *J Allergy Clin Immunol.* 2006;118:773–786.

14. Israel E, Fischer AR, Rosenberg MA, et al. The pivotal role of 5-lipoxygenase products in the reaction of aspirin-sensitive asthmatic subjects to aspirin. *Am Rev Respir Dis.* 1993;148:1447–1451.

15. Nasser SM, Patel M, Bell GS, et al. The effect of aspirin desensitization on urinary leukotriene E_4 concentrations in aspirin-sensitive asthma. *Am J Respir Crit Care Med.* 1995;151:1326–1330.

16. Gent JF, Triche WE, Holford TR, et al. Association of low-level ozone and fine particles with respiratory symptoms in children with asthma. *JAMA.* 2003;290:1859–1867.

17. Goodwin RD, Fischer ME, Goldberg J. A twin study of post-traumatic stress disorder symptoms and asthma. *Am J Respir Crit Care Med.* 2007;176:983–987.

18. Cohen RT, Canino GJ, Bird HR, et al. Violence, abuse, and asthma in Puerto Rican children. *Am J Resp Crit Care Med.* 2008;178:453–459.

19. Koeppen-Schomerus G, Stevenson J, Plomin R. Genes and environment in asthma: a study of 4 year old twins. *Arch Dis Child.* 2001;85:398–400.

20. Raby BA, Van Steen K, Caledon J, et al. Paternal history of asthma and airway responsiveness in children with asthma. *Am J Respir Crit Care Med.* 2005;172:552–558.

23. Harris JR, Magnus P, Samuelson SO, et al. No evidence for effects of family environment on asthma: a retrospective study of Norwegian twins. *Am J Respir Crit Care Med.* 1997;156:43–49.

25. Blumenthal MN. The role of genetics in the development of asthma and atopy. *Curr Opin Allergy Clin Immunol.* 2005;5:141–145.

26. Vercelli D. Advances in asthma and allergy genetics in 2007. *J Allergy Clin Immunol.* 2008;122:267–271.

27. Metsala J, Kilkkinen A, Kaila M, et al. Perinatal factors and the risk of asthma in childhood—a population-based register study in Finland. *Am J Epidemiol.* 2008:168:170–78.

28. Eder W, Ege MJ, von Mutius E. The asthma epidemic. *N Engl J Med.* 2006;355:2226–235.

29. Ratageri VH, Kabra SK, Dwivedi SN, et al. Factors associated with severe asthma. *Indian Pediatr.* 2000;37:1072–1082.

31. Withers NJ, Low L, Holgate ST, et al. The natural history of respiratory symptoms in a cohort of adolescents. *Am J Respir Crit Care Med.* 1998;158:352–357.

32. Gilliland FD, Berhane K, Li Y-F, et al. Effects of early onset asthma and *in utero* exposure to maternal smoking on childhood lung function. *Am J Respir Crit Care Med.* 2003;167:917–924.

34. Nicolai T, von Mutius E. Risk of asthma in children with a history of croup. *Acta Paediatr.* 1996;85:1295–1299.

35. Kuiper S, Muris JWM, Dompeling E, et al. Interactive effect of family history and environmental factors on respiratory tract-related morbidity in infancy. *J Allergy Clin Immunol.* 2007;120:388–395.

36. Alper Z, Sapan N, Ercan I, et al. Risk factors for wheezing in primary school children in Bursa, Turkey. *Am J Rhinol.* 2006;20:53–56.

37. Martinez FD, Wright AL, Taussig LM, et al. Asthma and wheezing in the first six years of life. *N Engl J Med.* 1995;332:133–138.

38. Martinez FD. Respiratory syncytial virus bronchiolitis and the pathogenesis of childhood asthma. *Pediatr Infect Dis J.* 2003;22:S76–S82.

39. Williams JV, Harris PA, Tollefson SJ, et al. Human metapneumovirus and lower respiratory tract disease in otherwise healthy infants and children. *N Engl J Med.* 2004;350:443–450.

41. von Mutius E. The environmental predictors of allergic disease. *J Allergy Clin Immunol.* 2000;105:9–19.

42. Rosenstreich DL, Eggleston P, Kattan M, et al. The role of cockroach allergy and exposure to cockroach allergen in causing morbidity among inner-city children with asthma. *N Engl J Med.* 1997;336:1356–1363.

43. Litonjua AA, Sparrow D, Weiss ST, et al. Sensitization to cat allergen is associated with asthma in older men and predicts new-onset airway hyperresponsiveness. *Am J Respir Crit Care Med.* 1997;156: 23–27.

44. Braun-Fahrlander C, Lauener R. Farming and protective agents against allergy and asthma. *Clin Exp Allergy.* 2003;33:409–411.

45. Ege MJ, Frei R, Bieli C, et al. Not all farming environments protect against the development of asthma and wheeze in children. *J Allergy Clin Immunol.* 2007;119:1140–1147.

46. Shirakawa T, Enomoto T, Shimazu S, et al. The inverse association between tuberculin responses and atopic disorder. *Science.* 1997; 275:77–79.

47. Shaheen SO, Aaby P, Hall AJ, et al. Measles and atopy in Guinea-Bissau. *Lancet.* 1996;347:1792–1796.

48. Cookson WOCM, Moffat MF. Asthma: an epidemic in the absence of infection? *Science.* 1997;275:41–42.

49. Tatum AJ, Shapiro GG. The effects of outdoor air pollution and tobacco smoke on asthma. *Immunol Allergy Clin North.* 2005;25:15–30.

50. Greenberger PA, Patterson R. Potentially fatal asthma and asthma deaths: knowledge is greater but implementation appears problematic. *Ann Allergy Asthma Immunol.* 2000;84:563–564.

51. Greenberger PA. Allergic rhinitis and asthma connection: Treatment implications. *Allergy Asthma Proc.* 2008;29:557–564.

52. Busse WW, Lemanske RF. Asthma. *N Engl J Med.* 2001;344:350–362.

53. Gleich GJ, Motojima S, Frigas E, et al. The eosinophilic leukocyte and the pathology of fatal bronchial asthma: evidence for pathologic heterogeneity. *J Allergy Clin Immunol.* 1987;80:412–415.

55. Shaw DE, Berry MA, Hargadon B, et al. Association between neutrophilic airway inflammation and airflow limitation in adults with asthma. *Chest.* 2007;132:1871–1875.

56. Kuman SD, Emery MJ, Atkins ND, et al. Airway mucosal blood flow in bronchial asthma. *Am J Respir Crit Care Med.* 1998;158:153–156.

58. Morishima Y, Nomura A, Uchida Y, et al. Triggering the induction of myofibroblast and fibrogenesis by airway epithelial shedding. *Am J Respir Cell Mol Biol.* 2001;24:1–11.

59. Campbell AM, Chanez P, Bignola AM, et al. Functional characteristics of bronchial epithelium obtained by brushing from asthmatic and normal subjects. *Am Rev Respir Dis.* 1993;147:529–534.

60. Laitinen LA, Laitinin A, Haahtela A. Airway mucosal inflammation even in patients with newly diagnosed asthma. *Am Rev Respir Dis.* 1993;147:697–704.

61. Druilhe A, Wallaert B, Tsicopoulos A, et al. Apoptosis, proliferation, and expression of Bcl-2, Fas, and Fas ligand in bronchial biopsies from asthmatics. *Am J Respir Cell Mol Biol.* 1998;19:747–757.

62. Spinozzi F, Fizzotti M, Agea E, et al. Defective expression of Fas messenger RNA and Fas receptor on pulmonary T cells from patients with asthma. *Ann Intern Med.* 1998;128:363–369.

64. Cookson WOCM, Musk AW, Ryan G. Associations between asthma history, atopy and non-specific bronchial responsiveness in young adults. *Clin Allergy.* 1986;16:425–432.

66. Frick WE, Sedgwick JB, Busse WW. The appearance of hypodense eosinophils in antigen-dependent late phase asthma. *Am Rev Respir Dis.* 1989;139:1401–1406.

67. Frigas E, Loegering DA, Solley GO, et al. Elevated levels of eosinophil granule major basic protein in the sputum of patients with bronchial asthma. *Mayo Clin Proc.* 1981;56:345–353.

69. Barthel SR, Jarjour NM, Mosher DF, et al. Dissection of the hyperadhesive phenotype of airway eosinophils in asthma. *Am J Respir Cell Mol Biol.* 2006;35:378–386.

71. Bradding P, Walls AF, Holgate ST. The role of the mast cell in the pathophysiology of asthma. *J Allergy Clin Immunol.* 2006;117: 1277–1284.

73. Olopade CO, Yu J, Abubacher J, et al. Catalytic hydrolysis of VIP in pregnant women with asthma. *J Asthma.* 2006;43:429–437.

74. Tomaki M, Ichinose N, Miura M, et al. Elevated substance P content in induced sputum from patients with asthma and patients with chronic bronchitis. *Am J Respir Crit Care Med.* 1995;151:613–617.

75. Heaney LG, Cross LJM, McGarvey LPA, et al. Neurokinin A is the predominant tachykinin in human bronchoalveolar lavage fluid in normal and asthmatic subjects. *Thorax.* 1998;53:357–362.

76. Kay AB, Ali FR, Heaney LG, et al. Calcitonin gene-related peptide-induced late asthmatic reactions in atopics. *Allergy.* 2007;62:495–503.

77. Sanders SP. Nitric oxide in asthma: pathogenic, therapeutic or diagnostic? *Am J Respir Cell Mol Biol.* 1999;21:147–149.

78. Sorkness CA, Lemanske RF Jr, Mauger DT, et al. Comparison of 3 controller regimens for mild-moderate persistent childhood asthma: the Pediatric Asthma Controller Trial. *J Allergy Clin Immunol.* 2007;119:64–72.

79. Szefler SJ, Mitchell H, Sorkness CA, et al. Management of asthma based on exhaled nitric oxide in addition to guideline-based treatment for inner-city adolescents and young adults: a randomized controlled trial. *Lancet.* 2008;372:1065–1072.

80. Montuschi P, Corradi M, Ciabattoni G, et al. Increased 8-isoprostane, a marker of oxidative stress, in exhaled condensate of asthma patients. *Am J Respir Crit Care Med.* 1999;160:216–220.

81. Hawkins GA, Weiss ST, Bleecker ER. Clinical consequences of ADRbeta2 polymorphisms. *Pharmacogenomics.* 2008;9:349–358.

82. Martin RJ, Szefler SJ, King TS, et al. The Predicting Response to Inhaled Corticosteroid Efficacy (PRICE) trial. *J Allergy Clin Immunol.* 2007;119:73–80.

83. Klotsman M, York TP, Pillai SG, et al. Pharmacogenetics of the 5-lipoxygenase biosynthetic pathway and variable clinical response to montelukast. *Pharmacogenet Genomics.* 2007;17:189–196.

84. Golena E, Hauk PJ, Hall CF, et al. Corticosteroid-resistant asthma is associated with classical antimicrobial activation of airway macrophages. *J Allergy Clin Immunol.* 2008;122:550–559.

86. Walker CL, Greenberger PA, Patterson R. Potentially fatal asthma. *Ann Allergy.* 1990;64:487–493.

88. Adams RJ, Wilson D, Smith BJ, et al. Impact of coping and socioeconomic factors on quality of life in adults with asthma. *Respirology.* 2004;9:87–95.

89. Akinbami L. *Asthma prevalence, health care use and mortality: United States, 2003–05.* National Center for Health Statistics. November 2006.

90. Pawankar R, Baena-Cagnani CE, Bousquet J, et al. State of world allergy report 2008: allergy and chronic respiratory diseases. *WAO Journal.* 2008:Supplement: S4–S17.

91. Kilmer G, Roberts H, Hughes E, et al. Surveillance of certain health behaviors and conditions among states and selected local areas—Behavioral Risk Factor Surveillance System (BRFSS), United States, 2006. *MMWR Surveillance Summaries.* August 15, 2008/ 57(SS07);1–188.

92. Measuring childhood asthma prevalence before and after the 1997 redesign of the national health interview survey–United States. *MMWR Morb Mortal Wkly Rep.* 2000;49:908–911.

93. Moorman JE, Rudd RA, Johnson CA, et al. National surveillance for asthma—United States, 1980–2004. *MMWR Surveillance Summaries.* October 19, 2007/56(SS08):1–14;18–54.

94. Masoli M, Fabian D, Hold S, et al. The global burden of asthma: executive summary of the GINA Dissemination Committee Report. *Allergy.* 2004;59:469–478.

95. Krishnan V, Diette GB, Rand CS, et al. Mortality in patients hospitalized for asthma exacerbations in the United States. *Am J Respir Crit Care Med.* 2006;174:633–638.

96. Malik A, Saltoun CA, Yarnold PR, et al. Prevalence of obstructive airways disease in disadvantaged elderly of Chicago. *Allergy Asthma Proc.* 2004;25:169–173.

97. Bellia V, Pedone C, Catalano F, et al. Asthma in the elderly: mortality rate and associated risk factors for mortality. *Chest.* 2007; 132:1175–1182.

99. Beckett WS. Occupational respiratory diseases. *N Engl J.* 2000; 342:406–413.

100. Tarlo SM, Balmes J, Balkissoon R, et al. Diagnosis and management of work-related asthma. American College of Chest Physicans Consensus Statement. *Chest.* 2008;134:(3 Suppl)1S–41S.

101. Sly RM. Decreases in asthma mortality in the United States. *Ann Allergy Asthma Immunol.* 2000;85:121–127.

102. Zoratti EM, Havstad S, Rodriguez J, et al. Health service use by African Americans and Caucasians with asthma in a managed care setting. *Am J Respir Crit Care Med.* 1998;158:371–377.

103. Smith DH, Malone DC, Lawson KA, et al. A national estimate of the economic costs of asthma. *Am J Respir Crit Care Med.* 1997;156:787–793.

104. Greenberger PA. Preventing the emergence of the $100,000 asthmatic. *Medscape Respir Care.* 1998;2(1).

106. Johnston SL. Innate immunity in the pathogenesis of virus induced asthma exacerbations. *Pro Am Thorac Soc.* 2007;4:267–270.

107. Woodman L, Sutcliffe A, Kaur D, et al. Chemokine concentrations and mast cell chemotactic activity in BAL fluid in patients with eosinophilic bronchitis and asthma, and in normal control subjects. *Chest.* 2006;130:371–378.

109. Holgate ST. Pathogenesis of asthma. *Clin Exper Allergy* 2008; 38:872–897.

110. Bousquet J, Jeffery PK, Busse WW, et al. Asthma: from bronchoconstriction to airways inflammation and remodeling. *Am J Respir Crit Care Med.* 2000;161:1720–1745.

111. Jatakanon A, Uasuf C, Maziak W, et al. Neutrophilic inflammation in severe persistent asthma. *Am J Respir Crit Care Med.* 1999;160:1532–1539.

112. Sur S, Crotty TB, Kephart GM, et al. Sudden-onset fatal asthma: a distinct clinical entity with few eosinophils and relatively more neutrophils in the airway submucosa? *Am Rev Respir Dis.* 1993;148: 713–719.

113. Jerath Tatum A, Greenberger PA, Mileusnic D, et al. Clinical, pathologic, and toxicologic findings in asthma deaths in Cook County, Illinois. *Allergy Asthma Proc.* 2001;22:285–291.

114. Schleimer RP, Kato A, Kern R, et al. Epithelium: at the interface of innate and adaptive immune responses. *J Allergy Clin Immunol.* 2007;120:1279–1284

116. Di Maria GU, Spicuzza L, Mistretta A, et al. Role of endogenous nitric oxide in asthma. *Allergy.* 2000;55:Suppl 61:31–35.

117. Burns GP, Gibson GJ. Airway hyperresponsiveness in asthma: not just a problem of smooth muscle relaxation with inspiration. *Am J Respir Crit Care Med.* 1998;158:203–206.

119. Gibbons WJ, Sharma A, Lougheed D, et al. Detection of excessive bronchoconstriction in asthma. *Am J Respir Crit Care Med.* 1996;153:582–589.

121. Robin ED, Lewiston N. Unexpected, unexplained sudden death in young asthmatic subjects. *Chest.* 1989;96:790–93.

122. Hamid QA, Minshall EM. Molecular pathology of allergic disease I. Lower airway disease. *J Allergy Clin Immunol.* 2000;105:20–36.

123. Jeffery PK. Differences and similarities between chronic obstructive pulmonary disease and asthma. *Clin Exp Allergy.* 1999;29:Suppl 2:14–26.

124. Teeter JG, Bleecker ER. Relationship between airway obstruction and respiratory symptoms in adult asthmatics. *Chest.* 1998;113:272–277.

125. Banzett RB, Dempsey JA, O'Donnell DE, et al. Symptom perception and respiratory sensation in asthma. *Am J Respir Crit Care Med.* 2000;162:1178–1182.

126. Lougheed MD. Variability in asthma: symptom perception, care, and outcomes. *Can J Physiol Pharmacol.* 2007;85: 149–154.

127. Brown NJ, Salome CM, Berend N, et al. Airways distensibility in adults with asthma and healthy adults, measured by forced oscillation technique. *Am J Respir Crit Care Med.* 2007;176:129–37.

128. Banzett RB, Dempsey JA, O'Donnell DE, et al. Symptom perception and respiratory sensation in asthma. *Am J Respir Crit Care Med.* 2000;162:1178–1182.

129. Wenzel SE, Schwartz LB, Langmack EL, et al. Evidence that severe asthma can be divided pathologically into two inflammatory subtypes with distinct physiologic and clinical characteristics. *Am J Respir Crit Care Med.* 1999;160:1001–1008.

132. Teeter JG, Bleecker ER. Relationship between airway obstruction and respiratory symptoms in adult asthmatics. *Chest.* 1998;113:272–277.

133. Smith AD, Cowan JO, Brasset KP, et al. Use of exhaled nitric oxide measurements to guide treatment in chronic asthma. *N Engl J Med.* 2005;352:2163–2173.

134. Boushey HA, Sorkness CA, King TS, et al. Daily versus as-needed corticosteroids for mild persistent asthma. *N Engl J Med.* 2005;352: 1519–1528.

136. Greenberger PA. Preventing hospitalizations for asthma by improving ambulatory management. *Am J Med.* 1996;100:381–382.

139. Parameswaran K, Knight AC, Keaney NP, et al. Ventilation and perfusion lung scintigraphy of allergen-induced airway responses in atopic asthmatic subjects. *Can Respir J.* 2007;14:285–291.

140. Newman KB, Mason UG III, Schmaling KB. Clinical features of vocal cord dysfunction. *Am J Respir Crit Care Med.* 1995:152:1382–1386.

141. Bacharier LB, Strunk RC. Vocal cord dysfunction: a practical approach to diagnosis. *J Respir Dis.* 2001;22:93–103.

144. Lange P, Perner J, Vestbo J, et al. A 15-year follow-up study of ventilatory function in adults with asthma. *N Engl J Med.* 1998; 339:1194–1200.

145. Backman KS, Greenberger PA, Patterson RP. Airways obstruction in patients with long-term asthma consistent with 'irreversible asthma.' *Chest.* 1997;112:1234–1240.

146. Takemura M, Niimi A, Minakuchi M, et al. Bronchial dilatation in asthma: relation to clinical and sputum indices. *Chest.* 2004;125:1352–1358.

147. Sly RM. Decreases in asthma mortality in the United States. *Ann Allergy Asthma Immunol.* 2000;85:121–127.

148. Suissa S, Ernst P, Boivin J-F, et al. A cohort analysis of excess mortality in asthma and the use of inhaled B-agonists. *Am J Respir Crit Care Med.* 1994;149:604–610.

149. Anderson HR, Ayres JG, Sturdy PM, et al. Bronchodilator treatment and deaths from asthma: case-control study. *BMJ.* 2005;330:117: Epub 2004 Dec 23.

150. Bateman E, Nelson H, Bousquet J, et al. Meta-analysis: effects of adding salmeterol to inhaled corticosteroids on serious asthma-related events. *Ann Intern Med.* 2008;149:33–42.

152. Miller TP, Greenberger PA, Patterson R. The diagnosis of potentially fatal asthma in hospitalized adults: patient characteristics and increased severity of asthma. *Chest.* 1992; 102:515–518.

154. Arnold DA, Gebretsadik T, Minton PA, et al. Clinical measures associated with FEV$_1$ in persons with asthma requiring hospital admission. *Am J Emerg Med.* 2007;25:425–429.

157. Morgan WJ, Stern DA, Sherrill DL, et al. Outcome of asthma and wheezing in the first 6 years of life: follow-up through adolescence. *Am J Respir Crit Care Med.* 2005;172:1253–1258.

158. Haldar P, Pavord ID, Shaw DE, et al. Cluster analysis and clinical asthma phenotypes. *Am J Respir Crit Care Med.* 2008;178:218–224.

159. Wood LJ, Inman MD, Watson RM, et al. Changes in bone marrow inflammatory cell progenitors after inhaled allergen in asthmatic subjects. *Am J Respir Crit Care Med.* 1998;157:99–105.

160. Bacsi A, Choudhury BK, Dharajiya N, et al. Subpollen particles: carriers of allergenic proteins and oxidases. *J Allergy Clin Immunol.* 2006;118:844–850.

163. Perry TT, Vargas PA, Buford J, et al. Classroom aeroallergen exposure in Arkansas head start centers. *Ann Allergy Asthma Immunol.* 2008;100:358–363.

164. Cockcroft DW, Hargreave FE, O'Byrne PM, et al. Understanding allergic asthma from allergen inhalation tests. *Can Respir J.* 2007;14:414–418.

165. O'Hollaren MT, Yunginger JW, Offord KP, et al. Exposure to an aeroallergen as a possible precipitating factor in respiratory arrest in young patients with asthma. *N Engl J Med.* 1991;321:359–363.

166. Targonski PV, Persky VW, Ramekrishnan V. Effect of environmental molds on risk of death from asthma during the pollen season. *J Allergy Clin Immunol.* 1995;95:955–961.

167. Canfield SM, Jacobson JS, Perzanowski MS, et al. Total and specific IgE associations between New York City Head Start children and their parents. *J Allergy Clin Immunol.* 2008;121:1422–427.

168. Van Kampen V, Rabstein S, Sander I, et al. Prediction of challenge test results by flour-specific IgE and skin prick test in symptomatic bakers. *Allergy.* 2008;63:897–902.

169. Zuskin E, Kanceljak B, Schacter EN, et al. Respiratory function and immunologic status in workers processing dried fruits and teas. *Ann Allergy Asthma Immunol.* 1996;77:417–422.

170. Brant A, Zekveld C, Welch J, et al. The prognosis of occupational asthma due to detergent enzymes: clinical, immunological and employment outcomes. *Clin Exp Allergy.* 2006;36:483–488.

171. De Sario M, Di Domenicantonio R, Corbo G, et al. Characteristics of early transient, persistent, and late onset wheezers at 9 to 11 years of age. *J Asthma.* 2006;43:633–638.

172. Ball TM, Castro-Rodriguez JA, Griffith KA, et al. Sibling, day-care attendance, and the risk of asthma and wheezing during childhood. *N Engl J Med.* 2000;343:538–543.

175. Mathison DA, Stevenson DD, Simon RA. Precipitating factors in asthma: aspirin, sulfites, and other drugs and chemicals. *Chest.* 1985;87:50S–54S.

176. Szczeklik A, Gryglewski RJ, Czerniawska-Mysik G, et al. Aspirin sensitive asthma and arachidonic acid transportation. *N Engl Reg Allergy Proc.* 1986;7:21–25.

177. Israel E, Fischer AR, Rosenberg MA, et al. The pivotal role of 5-lipoxygenase products in the reaction of aspirin-sensitive asthmatic subjects to aspirin. *Am Rev Respir Dis.* 1993;148:1447–1451.

178. Nasser SM, Patel M, Bell GS, et al. The effect of aspirin desensitization on urinary leukotriene E_4 concentrations in aspirin-sensitive asthma. *Am J Respir Crit Care Med.* 1995;151:1326–1330.

179. Cowburn AS, Sladek K, Soja J, et al. Overexpresssion of leukotriene C_4 synthase in bronchial biopsies from patients with aspirin-intolerant asthma. *J Clin Invest.* 1998;101:834–846.

180. Szczeklik A, Sanak M, Nizankowska-Mogilnicka E, et al. Aspirin intolerance and the cyclooxygenase-leukotriene pathways. *Curr Opin Pul Med.* 2004;10:51–56.

181. Corrigan C, Mallett K, Ying S, et al. Expression of the cysteinyl leukotriene receptors $cysLT_1$ and $cysLT_2$ in aspirin-sensitive and aspirin-tolerant chronic rhinosinusitis. *J Allergy Clin Immunol.* 2005;115:316–322.

182. Zhu J, Qiu Y-S, Figueroa DJ, et al. Localization and upregulation of cysteinyl leukotriene-1 receptor in asthmatic bronchial mucosa. *Am J Respir Crit Care Med.* 2005;33:531–540.

183. Szczelik A, Sladek K, Dworski R, et al. Bronchial aspirin challenge causes specific eicosanoid response in aspirin-sensitive asthmatics. *Am J Respir Crit Care Med.* 1996;154:1608–1614.

184. Bochenek G, Nagraba K, Nizankowska E, et al. A controlled study of $9\alpha,11\beta$-PGF2 (a prostaglandin D2 metabolite) in plasma and urine of patients with bronchial asthma and healthy controls after aspirin challenge. *J Allergy Clin Immunol.* 2003;111:743–749.

185. Woessner KM, Simon RA, Stevenson DD. Safety of high-dose rofecoxib with aspirin-exacerbated respiratory disease. *Ann Allergy Asthma Immunol.* 2004;93:339–344.

186. Dahlén B, Szczeklik A, Murray JJ. Celecoxib in patients with asthma and aspirin intolerance. *N Engl J Med.* 2001;344:142.

187. Malo J-L, Cartier A, Ghezzo H, et al. Patterns of improvement in spirometry, bronchial hyperresponsiveness and specific IgE antibody levels after cessation of exposure in occupational asthma caused by snow-crab processing. *Am Rev Respir Dis.* 1988;138:807–812.

188. Delclos GL, Gimeno D, Arif AA, et al. Occupational risk factors and asthma among health care professionals. *Am J Respir Crit Care Med.* 2007;175:667–675.

194. Fitch KD, Sue-Chu M, Anderson SD, et al. Asthma and the elite athlete: Summary of the International Olympic Committee's Consensus Conference, Lausanne, Switzerland, January 22–24, 2008. *J Allergy Clin Immunol.* 2008;122:254–260.

196. Kotaru C, Coreno A, Skowronski M, et al. Exhaled nitric oxide and thermally induced asthma. *Am J Respir Crit Care Med.* 2001;163:383–388.

197. Rundell KW, Slee JB. Exercise and other indirect challenges to demonstrate asthma or exercise-induced bronchoconstriction in athletes. *J Allergy Clin Immunol.* 2008;122:238–246.

198. McFadden ER, Nelson JA, Skowronski ME, et al. Thermally induced asthma and airway drying. *Am J Respir Crit Care Med.* 1999;160:221–226.

199. Duong M, Subbarao P, Adelroth E, et al. Sputum eosinophils and the response of exercise-induced bronchoconstriction to corticosteroid in asthma. *Chest.* 2008;133:404–411.

200. Leff JA, Busse WW, Pearlman D, et al. Montelukast, a leukotriene-receptor antagonist, for the treatment of mild asthma and exercise-induced bronchoconstriction. *N Engl J Med.* 1998;339:147–152.

204. Beckman DB, Greenberger DA. Diagnostic dilemma. Vocal cord dysfunction. *Am J Med.* 2001;101:731, 741.

205. Calverley PM, Anderson JA, Celli B, et al. Salmeterol and fluticasone propionate and survival in chronic obstructive pulmonary disease. *N Engl J Med.* 2007;356:775–89.

206. Mohammed F, Bootoor S, Panday A, et al. Predictors of repeat visits to the emergency room by asthmatic children in primary care. *J Natl Med Assoc.* 2006;98:1278–185.

207. Cassino C, Ito K, Bader I, et al. Cigarette smoking and ozone-associated emergency department use for asthma by adults in New York City. *Am J Respir Crit Care Med.* 1999;159:1773–1779.

208. Fujieda S, Diaz-Sanchez D, Saxon A. Combined nasal challenge with diesel exhaust particles and allergen induces *in vivo* IgE isotype switching. *Am J Respir Cell Mol Biol.* 1998;19:507–512.

209. McCreanor M, Cullinan P, Nieuwenhuijsen MJ, et al. Respiratory effects of exposure to diesel traffic in persons with asthma. *N Engl J Med.* 2007;357:2348–2358.

210. Nordenstedt H, Nilsson M, Johansson S, et al. The relation between gastroesophageal reflux and respiratory symptoms in a population-based study: the Nord-Trondelag health survey. *Chest.* 2006;129:1051–1056.

211. Kaltenback T, Crockett S, Gerson LB. Are lifestyle measures effective in patients with gastroesophageal reflux disease? An evidence-based approach. *Arch Intern Med.* 2006;166:965–971.

212. Mainie I, Tutuian R, Castell DO. Addition of a H2 receptor antagonist to PPI improves acid control and decreases nocturnal acid breakthrough. *J Clin Gastroenterol.* 2008;42:676–679.

213. Vakil N. Review article: the role of surgery in gastro-oesophageal reflux disease. *Aliment Pharmacol Ther.* 2007;25:1365–1372.

214. Tutuian R, Mainie I, Agrawal A, et al. Nonacid reflux in patients with chronic cough on acid-suppressive therapy. *Chest.* 2006;130:386–391.

215. Mueller C, Laule-Kilian K, Frana B, et al. Use of B-type naturietic peptide in the management of acute dyspnea in patients with pulmonary disease. *Am Heart J.* 2006;151:471–477

216. Abramson MJ, Puy RM, Weiner JM. Allergen immunotherapy for asthma. *Cochrane Database Syst Rev.* 2003;(4):CD001186.

217. Joint Task Force on Practice Parameters: American Academy of Allergy, Asthma and Immunology, American College of Allergy, Asthma and Immunology, and the Joint Council of Allergy, Asthma and Immunology. Allergen immunotherapy: a practice parameter second update. *J Allergy Clin Immunol.* 2007;120:S25–S85.

218. Casale TB, Stokes JR. Immunomodulators for allergic respiratory disorders. *J Allergy Clin Immunol.* 2008;121:288–296.

219. Usmani OS, Ito K, Maneechotesuwan K, et al. Glucocorticoid receptor nuclear translocation in airway cells after inhaled combination therapy. *Am J Respir Crit Care Med.* 2005:172: 704–712.

220. Bateman ED, Boushey HA, Boushey J, et al. Can guideline-defined asthma control be achieved? The Gaining Optimal Asthma Control Study. *Am J Respir Crit Care Med.* 2004;170:836–844.

223. Drazen JM, Israel E, Boushey HA, et al. Comparison of regularly scheduled with as-needed use of albuterol in mild asthma. *N Engl J Med.* 1996;335:841–847.

224. Nelson HS, Berkowitz RB, Tinkelman DA, et al. Lack of subsensitivity to albuterol after treatment with salmeterol in patients with asthma. *Am J Respir Crit Care Med.* 1999;159:1556–1561.

225. Israel E, Chinchilli VM, Ford JG, et al. Use of regularly scheduled albuterol treatment in asthma: genotype-stratified, randomized, placebo-controlled cross-over trial. *Lancet.* 2004;364:1505–1512.

226. Bleecker ER, Postma DS, Lawrance RM, et al. Effect of ADRB2 polymorphisms on response to longacting β-agonist therapy: a pharmacogenetic analysis of two randomised studies. *Lancet.* 2007;370:2118–2125.

229. Salo D, Tuel M, Lavery RF, et al. A randomized, clinical trial comparing the efficacy of continuous nebulized albuterol (15 mg) versus continuous nebulized albuterol (15 mg) plus ipratropium bromide (2 mg) for the treatment of acute asthma. *J Emerg Med.* 2006;31:371–376.

230. Peters SG. Continuous bronchodilator therapy. *Chest.* 2007;131:286–289.

231. Handley DA, Tinkelman D, Noonan M, et al. Dose-response evaluation of levalbuterol versus racemic albuterol in patients with asthma. *J Asthma.* 2000;37:319–327.

232. Kuna P, Peters MJ, Manjra AI, et al. Effect of budesonide/formoterol maintenance and reliever therapy on asthma exacerbations. *Int J Clin Pract.* 2007;61:725–736.

233. O'Byrne PM, Bisgaard H, Godard PP, et al. Budesonide/formoterol combination therapy as both maintenance and reliever medication in asthma. *Am J Respir Crit Care Med.* 2005;171:129–136.

234. Rabe KF, Pizzichini E, Stallberg B, et al. Budesonide/formoterol in a single inhaler for maintenance and relief in mild-to-moderate asthma: a randomized, double-blind trial. *Chest.* 2006; 129:246–256.

235. Enders JM, Dobesh PP, Ellison JN. Acute myocardial infarction induced by ephedrine alkaloids. *Phamacology.* 2003;23:1645–1651.

236. Manser R, Reid D, Abramson M. Corticosteroids for acute severe asthma in hospitalized patients. *Cochrane Database Syst Rev.* 2001;(1):CD001740.

238. Rodrigo G, Rodrigo C. Corticosteroids in the emergency department therapy of acute adult asthma: an evidence-based evaluation. *Chest.* 1999;116:285–295.

239. Rowe BH, Spooner C, Ducharme FM, et al. Early emergency department treatment of acute asthma with systemic corticosteroids. *Cochrane Database Syst Rev.* 2001;(1):CD002178.

241. Chapman KR, Verbeek PR, White JG, et al. Effect of a short course of prednisone in the prevention of early relapse after the emergency room treatment of acute asthma. *N Engl J Med.* 1991;324: 788–794.

242. Rowe BH, Bota GW, Fabris L, et al. Inhaled budesonide in addition to oral corticosteroids to prevent asthma relapse following discharge from the emergency department: a random controlled trial. *JAMA.* 1999;281:2119–2126.

243. Rodrigo GJ. Rapid effects of inhaled corticosteroids in acute asthma: an evidence-based evaluation. *Chest.* 2006;130:1301–1311.

244. Harrison TW, Osborne J, Newton S, et al. Doubling the dose of inhaled corticosteroid to prevent asthma exacerbations: randomised controlled trial. *Lancet.* 2004;363:271–275.

245. Busse WW, Pedersen S, Pauwels RA, et al. The Inhaled Steroid Treatment As Regular Therapy in Early Asthma (START) study 5-year follow-up: effectiveness of early intervention with budesonide in mild persistent asthma. *J Allergy Clin Immunol.* 2008;121:1167–1174.

246. Guillbert TW, Morgan WJ, Zeiger RS, et al. Long-term inhaled corticosteroids in preschool children at high risk of asthma. *N Engl J Med.* 2006;354:1985–1997.

247. Bisgaard H, Hermansen MN, Loland L, et al. Intermittent inhaled corticosteroids in infants with episodic wheezing. *N Engl J Med.* 2006;354:1998–2005.

248. Murray CS, Woodcock A, Langley SJ, et al. Secondary prevention of asthma by the use of Inhaled Fluticasone propionate in Wheezy Infants (IFWIN): double-blind, randomised, controlled study. *Lancet.* 2006;368:754–762.

249. Szefler SJ, Martin RJ, King TS, et al. Significant variability in response to inhaled corticosteroids for persistent asthma. *J Allergy Clin Immunol.* 2002;109:410–418.

250. Martin RJ, Szefler SJ, King TS, et al. The Predicting Response to Inhaled Corticosteroid Efficacy (PRICE) trial. *J Allergy Clin Immunol.* 2007;119:73–80.

251. Rhen T, Cidlowski JA. Antiinflammatory action of glucocorticoids—new mechanisms for old drugs. *N Engl J Med.* 2005;353:1711–1723.

252. Giembycz MA, Kaur M, Leigh R, et al. A Holy Grail of asthma management: toward understanding how long-acting β2-adrenoceptor agonists enhance the clinical efficacy of inhaled corticosteroids. *Brit J Pharmacol.* 2008 153:1090–1104.

253. Adcock IM, Barnes PJ. Molecular mechanisms of corticosteroid resistance. *Chest.* 2008;134:394–401.

254. Wood LJ, Sehmi R, Gauvreau GM, et al. An inhaled corticosteroid, budesonide, reduces baseline but not allergen-induced increases in bone marrow inflammatory cell progenitors in asthmatic subjects. *Am J Respir Crit Care Med.* 1999;159:1457–1463.

255. Donahue JG, Weiss ST, Livingston JM, et al. Inhaled steroids and the risk of hospitalization for asthma. *JAMA.* 1997;277:887–891.

256. Pauwels RA, Löfdahl C-G, Postma DS, et al. Effect of inhaled formoterol and budesonide on exacerbations of asthma. *N Engl J Med.* 1997;337:1405–1411.

257. Verberne AAPH, Frost C, Duiverman EJ, et al. Addition of salmeterol versus doubling the dose of beclomethasone in children with asthma. *Am J Respir Crit Care Med.* 1998;158:213–229.

258. Shrewsbury S, Pyke S, Britton M. Meta-analysis of increased dose of inhaled steroid or addition of salmeterol in symptomatic asthma (MIASMA). *Br Med J.* 2000;320:1368–1373.

259. Cauley JA, Robbins J, Chen Z, et al. Effects of estrogen plus progestin on risk of fractures and bone mineral density: The Women's Health Initiative Randomized Trial. *JAMA.* 2003;290:1729–1738.

265. Leff JA, Busse WW, Pearlman D, et al. Montelukast, a leukotriene-receptor antagonist, for the treatment of mild asthma and exercise-induced bronchoconstriction. *N Engl J Med.* 1998;339:147–152.

266. Peters–Golden M, Henderson WR. Leukotrienes. *N Engl J Med.* 2007;357;1841–1854.

267. Edelman JM, Turpin JA, Bronsky EA, et al. Oral montelukast compared with inhaled salmeterol to prevent exercise-induced bronchoconstriction. *Ann Intern Med.* 2000;132:97–104.

268. Reiss TF, Chervinsky P, Dockhorn RJ, et al. Montelukast, a once-daily leukotriene receptor antagonist, in the treatment of chronic asthma: a multicenter, randomized, double-blind trial. *Arch Intern Med.* 1998;158:1213–1220.

269. Knorr B, Matz J, Bernstein JA, et al. Montelukast for chronic asthma in 6- to 14-year-old children: a randomized double-blind trial. *JAMA.* 1998;279:1181–1186.

270. Laviolette M, Malmstrom K, Lu S, et al. Montelukast added to inhaled beclomethasone in treatment of asthma. *Am J Respir Crit Care Med.* 1999;160:1862–1868.

271. Zeiger RS, Bird SR, Kaplan MS, et al. Short-term and long-term asthma control in patients with mild persistent asthma receiving montelukast or fluticasone: a randomized controlled trial. *Am J Med.* 2005;118:649–646.

273. Nelson H, Kemp J, Berger W, et al. Efficacy of zileuton controlled-release tablets administered twice daily in the treatment of moderate persistent asthma: a 3-month randomized controlled study. *Ann Allergy Asthma Immunol.* 2007;99:78–84.

274. Furukawa C, Atkinson D, Forster TJ, et al. Controlled trial of two formulations of cromolyn sodium in the treatment of asthmatic patients 12 years of age. *Chest.* 1999;116:65–72.

275. van der Wouden JC, Uijen JHM, Bernsen RMD, et al. Inhaled sodium cromoglycate for asthma in children. *Cochrane Database Syst Rev.* 2008. DOI:10.1002/14651858.CD002173.pub2.

276. Kelly KD, Spooner C, Rowe BH. Nedocromil sodium versus sodium cromoglycate for prevention of exercise-induced bronchoconstriction. *Cochrane Database Syst Rev.* 2008. DOI:10.1002/14651858.CD002731.

277. Strunk RC, Weiss ST, Yates KP, et al. Mild to moderate asthma affects lung growth in children and adolescents. *J Allergy Clin Immunol.* 2006;118:1040–1047.

278. Boswell-Smith V, Cazzola M, Page CP. Are phosphodiesterase 4 inhibitors just more theophylline? *J Allergy Clin Immunol.* 2006;117:1237–1243.

280. Metzger NL, Knockler DR, Gravatt LA. Confirmed beta16 Arg/Arg polymorphism in a patient with uncontrolled asthma. *Ann Pharmacother.* 2008;42:874–881.

281. Fahy JV, Fleming HE, Wong HH, et al. The effect on an anti-IgE monoclonal antibody on the early- and late-phase responses to allergen inhalation in asthmatic subjects. *Am J Respir Crit Care Med.* 1997;155:1828–1834.

282. Beck LA, Marcotte GV, MacGlashan D, et al. Omalizumab-induced reductions in mast cell FcεRI expression and function. *J Allergy Clin Immunol.* 2004;114:527–30.

283. Prussin C, Griffith DT, Boesel KM, et al. Omalizumab treatment downregulates dendritic cell FcεRI expression. *J Allergy Clin Immunol.* 2003;112:1147–1154.

284. Klunker S, Saggar LR, Seyfert-Margolis V, et al. Combination treatment with omalizumab and rush immunotherapy for ragweed-induced allergic rhinitis; Inhibition of IgE-facilitated allergen binding. *J Allergy Clin Immunol.* 2007;120:688–695.

285. Pulimood TB, Corden JM, Bryden C, et al. Epidemic asthma and the role of fungal mold Alternaria alternate. *J Allergy Clin Immunol.* 2007;120:610–617.

286. Marks GB, Colquhoun JR, Girgis ST, et al. Thunderstorm outflows preceding epidemics of asthma during spring and summer. *Thorax.* 2001;56:468–471.

287. D'Amato G, Cecchi L, Liccardi G. Thunderstorm-related asthma: not only grass pollen and spores. *J Allergy Clin Immunol.* 2008; 121:537–538.

288. Ahmad I, Tansel B, Mitrani JD. Effectiveness of HVAC dust cleaning procedures in improving air quality. *Environ Monit Assess.* 2001;72:265–276.

289. Garrison RA, Robertson LD, Koehn RD, et al. Effect of heating-ventilation-air conditioning system sanitation on airborne fungal populations in residential environments. *Ann Allergy.* 1993;71: 548–556.

290. Burr ML, Matthews IP, Arthur RA, et al. Effects on patients with asthma of eradicating visible indoor mould: a randomized controlled trial. *Thorax.* 2007;62:767–772.

291. Francis H, Gletcher G, Anthony C, et al. Clinical effects of air filters in homes of asthmatic adults sensitized and exposed to pet allergens. *Clin Exp Allergy.* 2003;33:101–105.

292. Htut T, Higenbottam TW, Gill GW, et al. Eradication of house dust mite from homes of atopic asthmatic subjects: a double-blind trial. *J Allergy Clin Immunol.* 2001;107:55–60.

293. Lazarus SC, Chinchilli VM, Rollings, NJ, et al. Smoking affects response to inhaled corticosteroids or leukotriene receptor antagonists in asthma. *Am J Respir Crit Care Med.* 2007;175:783–790.

294. Brooks TWA, Creekmore FM, Young DC, et al. Rates of hospitalizations and emergency department visits in patients with asthma and chronic obstructive pulmonary disease taking β-blockers. *Pharmacotherapy.* 2007;27:684–690.

298. Dicpinigaitis PV. Angiotensin-converting enzyme inhibitor-induced cough: ACCP evidence-based clinical practice guidelines. *Chest.* 2006;129:169S–173S.

300. Wood RA, Chapman MD, Atkinson NF Jr, et al. The effect of cat removal on allergen content in household-dust samples. *J Allergy Clin Immunol.* 1989;83:730–734.

301. Johnstone DE, Dutton A. The value of hyposensitization therapy for bronchial asthma in children: a 14 year study. *Pediatrics.* 1968;42:793–802.

302. Jacobsen L, Niggemann B, Dreborg S, et al. Specific immunotherapy has long-term preventive effect of seasonal and perennial asthma: 10-year follow-up on the PAT study. *Allergy.* 2007; 62:943–948.

303. Greenberger PA, Ballow M, Casale TB, et al. Sublingual immunotherapy and subcutaneous immunotherapy: issues in the United States. *J Allergy Clin Immunol.* 2007;120:1466–1468.

304. Humbert M, Beasley R, Ayres J, et al. Benefits of omalizumab as add-on therapy in patients with severe persistent asthma who are inadequately controlled despite best available therapy (GINA 2002 step 4 treatment): INNOVATE. *Allergy.* 2005;60:309–316.

305. Wu AC, Paltiel AD, Kuntz KM, et al. Cost-effectiveness of omalizumab in adults with severe asthma: results from the Asthma Policy Model. *J Allergy Clin Immunol.* 2007;120:1146–1152.

306. Ou CY, Tseng YF, Chiou YH, et al. The role of Mycoplasma pneumoniae in acute exacerbation of asthma in children. *Acta Paediatr Taiwan.* 2008;49:14–18.

307. Sutherland ER, Martin RJ. Asthma and atypical bacterial infection. *Chest.* 2007;132:1962–1966.

308. Williams AN, Simon RA, Woessner KM, et al. The relationship between historical aspirin-induced asthma and severity of asthma induced during oral aspirin challenges. *J Allergy Clin Immunol.* 2007;120:273–277.

309. Berges-Gimeno MP, Simon RA, Stevenson DD. Long-term treatment with aspirin desensitization in asthmatic patients with aspirin-exacerbated respiratory disease. *J Allergy Clin Immunol.* 2003;111:180–186.

311. Rodrigo GJ, Rodrigo C. First-line therapy for adult patients with acute asthma receiving a multiple-dose protocol of ipratropium bromide plus albuterol in the emergency department. *Am J Respir Crit Care Med.* 2000;161:1862–1868.

314. Fitzgerald JM, Grunfeld A, Pare PD, et al. The clinical efficacy of combination nebulized anticholinergic and adrenergic bronchodilators vs. nebulized adrenergic bronchodilator alone in acute asthma. *Chest.* 1997;111:311–315.

316. ten Brinke A, Zwinderman AH, Sterk PJ, et al. "Refractory" eosinophilic airway inflammation in severe asthma: effect of parenteral corticosteroids. *Am J Respir Crit Care Med.* 2004;170:601–605.

320. Evans DJ, Cullinan P, Geddes DM. Cyclosporine as an oral corticosteroid sparing agent in stable asthma. *Cochrane Database Syst Rev.* 2001;(2):CD002993.

322. Li Y-F, Gauderman J, Avol A, et al. Associations of tumor necrosis factor G-308A with childhood asthma and wheezing. *Am J Respir Crit Care Med.* 2006;173:970–976.

323. Erin EM, Leaker BR, Nicholson GC, et al. The effects of monoclonal antibody directed against tumor necrosis factor-α in asthma. *Am J Respir Crit Care Med.* 2006;174:753–762.

325. Salmun LM, Barlan I, Wolf HM, et al. Effect of intravenous immunoglobulin on steroid consumption in patients with severe asthma: a double-blind, placebo-controlled, randomized trial. *J Allergy Clin Immunol.* 1999;103:810–815.

326. Landwehr LP, Jeppson JD, Katlan MG, et al. Benefits of high-dose IV immunoglobulin in patients with severe steroid-dependent asthma. *Chest.* 1998;114: 1349–1356.

327. Hunt LW, Swedlund HA, Gleich GJ. Effect of nebulized lidocaine on severe glucocorticoid-dependent asthma. *Mayo Clin Proc.* 1996;71:361–368.

328. Decco ML, Neeno TA, Hunt LW, et al. Nebulized lidocaine in the treatment of severe asthma in children: a pilot study. *Ann Allergy Asthma Immunol.* 1999;82:29–32.

329. Miller JD, Cox G, Vincic L, et al. A prospective feasibility study of bronchial thermoplasty in the human airway. *Chest.* 2005;127: 1999–2006.

330. Cox G, Thomson NC, Rubin AS, et al. Asthma control during the year after bronchial thermoplasty. *N Engl J Med.* 2007;356:1327–37.

334. Borish L, Culp JA. Asthma: a syndrome comprised of heterogeneous diseases. *Ann Allergy Asthma Immunol.* 2008;101:1–8.

336. Levenson T, Greenberger PA, Donoghue ER, et al. Asthma deaths confounded by substance abuse: an assessment of fatal asthma. *Chest.* 1996;110:604–610.

337. Su FW, Beckman DB, Yarnold PA, et al. Low incidence of complications in asthmatic patients treated with preoperative corticosteroids. *Allergy Asthma Proc.* 2004;25:327–333.

338. Tirumalasetty J, Grammer LC. Asthma, surgery, and general anesthesia: a review. *J Asthma.* 2006;43:251–254.

339. Lange P, Scharling H, Ulrik CS, et al. Inhaled corticosteroids and decline of lung function in community residents with asthma. *Thorax.* 2006;61:100–104.

340. O'Byrne PM, Pedersen S, Busse WW, et al. Effects of early intervention with inhaled budesonide on lung function in newly diagnosed asthma. *Chest.* 2006; 129:1478–1485.

341. Morgan WJ, Stern DA, Sherrill DL, et al. Outcome of asthma and wheezing in the first 6 years of life: follow-up through adolescence. *Am J Respir Crit Care Med.* 2005;1721:1253–1258.

342. Jerath Tatum A, Greenberger PA, Mileusnic D, et al. Clinical, pathologic, and toxicologic findings in asthma deaths in Cook County, Illinois. *Allergy Asthma Proc.* 2001;22:285–291.

343. McFadden ER Jr. Acute severe asthma. *Am J Respir Crit Care Med.* 2003;168:740–759.

CHAPTER 20

The Infant and Toddler with Asthma

MARY BETH HOGAN AND NEVIN W. WILSON

Recurrent wheezing is a common problem among infants, toddlers, and young children. The 2007 National Heart, Lung, and Blood Institute (NHLBI) Guidelines for the treatment of asthma attempt to address the significant problems of asthma in the very young. Despite recent scientific advances, the pathogenesis of recurrent wheezing, its relationship to the development of asthma, and ultimately its treatment options continue to be poorly defined. The purpose of this chapter is to review the factors important in the development of asthma in infants and very young children. The current difficulties of evaluation and management of wheezing in very young children also are discussed. In this chapter, infantile asthma refers to asthma in children less than 3 years of age with four or more episodes of wheezing. These episodes improve with bronchodilators or anti-inflammatory medications and may or may not be associated with viral infections. In many of these young asthmatics, environmental allergy is already playing an underappreciated role.

■ EPIDEMIOLOGY

The prevalence rate for asthma in infants and young children is increasing, particularly in westernized countries (1). An increase in atopy may be a contributing factor (2). Hospital admission rates are climbing for infants with asthma (3). Asthmatic children under 24 months of age are four times more likely to be admitted to the hospital than teenagers with asthma (4). In Norway, 75% of all children hospitalized for asthma are under 4 years of age (5). Although the number of days in the hospital is declining in older children, hospital length of stay for asthmatic infants is not changing (6). In addition, infants are more likely to require emergency department assistance for asthma exacerbations (7). Ten percent of all childhood mortality from asthma occurs in children under 4 years of age (8). Overall, it appears that hospitalization rates may be improving for older children, but no substantial progress has been made in improving the quality of life of asthmatic infants.

■ NATURAL HISTORY

Wheezing in infants and young children can be divided into three specific phenotypes: early transient wheezers; late-onset nonatopic wheezers; persistent atopic wheeze/asthma (9). The early transient wheezers have symptoms primarily with viral infections, do not wheeze in between infectious episodes, and are no longer wheezing by the time they are 6 years of age. They often respond poorly to bronchodilators and asthma-controller medications. The late-onset, nonatopic wheezers will wheeze with viral infections and also under other conditions such as exercise. Their prevalence peaks between 3 and 6 years of age and then gradually declines and frequently becomes asymptomatic early in the second decade of life. The third phenotype combines wheezing with evidence of IgE-mediated disease. This atopic phenotype is the group most likely to have persistent wheezing. This phenotype gradually increases until it becomes the most common cause of wheezing by 6 years of age.

Based on these observations, an Asthma Predictive Index (API) (10) was developed to predict which infants were more likely to go on to develop asthma when they were older. It was subsequently modified to include allergic sensitization to at least one aeroallergen as a major criteria and allergic sensitization to milk, egg, or peanut as minor criteria (11) (Table 20.1). In the API, recurrent wheezing episodes in the first 3 years of life was combined with at least one major risk factor consisting of a parental history of asthma or child atopic dermatitis. Two of three minor criteria are required; they include wheezing unrelated to colds, blood eosinophil counts of ≥4%, and physician diagnosed allergic rhinitis. The API was modified and used as the mAPI in the Prevention of Early Asthma in Kids (PEAK) study (12) to characterize the atopic profile of toddler-aged children with recurrent wheezing at high risk of developing persistent asthma.

TABLE 20.1 MODIFIED ASTHMA PREDICTIVE INDEX

1. A history of 4 or more wheezing episodes with at least one physician-diagnosed
2. In addition, the child must meet at least one of the following major criteria or at least two of the following minor criteria:

Major Criteria
Parental history of asthma
Physician-diagnosed atopic dermatitis
Allergic sensitization to at least one aeroallergen

Minor Criteria
Allergic sensitization to milk, egg, or peanut
Wheezing unrelated to colds
Blood eosinophilia above 4%

Adapted from Guilbert TW, Morgan WJ, Zeiger RS, et al. Atopic characteristics of children with recurrent wheezing at high risk for the development of childhood asthma. *J Allergy Clin Immunol.* 2004;114:1282–1287.

They found that more than 60% of young children were already sensitized to either food or aeroallergens. Male toddlers were significantly more likely to be sensitized to aeroallergens, to have a blood eosinophil level of more than 4% and elevated serum IgE levels. Eosinophilia and total serum IgE concentration were strongly correlated with aeroallergen sensitization. The presence of allergen sensitization is considered significant criteria for the diagnosis of allergic rhinitis and indicative of increased risk of developing asthma. On the other hand a negative mAPI in the first 3 years of life has been shown to accurately predict 95% of those without persistent asthma between the ages of 6 and 13 years.

The PEAK trial was initiated to determine if young children at high risk of developing asthma could be treated with inhaled corticosteroids to modify the natural history of the disease. Guilbert et al. (12) randomly assigned 2-year-old to 3-year-old children with a positive mAPI to treatment with fluticasone propionate (88 µg twice daily) or placebo for 2 years. Patients then were followed for a subsequent 1-year period without study medication. During the treatment period, fluticasone use was associated with more episode-free days, less asthma exacerbations, and decreased supplementary use of rescue medication. However, after the treatment period ended, there was no difference between the treatment group and placebo for episode-free days, the number of exacerbations, or pulmonary function (12). Guilbert et al. concluded that in preschool children at high risk for asthma, 2 years of inhaled-corticosteroid therapy did not provide a subsequent long-term disease-modifying effect after treatment discontinuation.

Care for the asthmatic infant is predicated on the correct identification of asthma versus other conditions that cause wheezing. It is critical to identify triggers such as allergies or gastroesophageal reflux that cause asthma exacerbations. Once any triggers are identified, correct therapy, and ultimately long-term disease-modifying treatments can be delivered.

■ TRIGGERS OF ASTHMA IN INFANTS

Gastroesophageal Reflux

Gastroesophageal reflux (GER) is a common cause of wheezing in infants under 1 year of age. The clinical difficulty of GER in small children is that it is a trigger for both wheezing and asthma (13). In nonatopic infants with wheezing but without asthma, BAL samples were noted to contain increased neutrophils, lipid laden macrophages, IL-8, and myeloperoxidase. These findings suggest that aspiration associated with GER is characterized by a neutrophilic inflammatory response (13). Sheikh et al. noted that, in a population of infants, silent GER was related to wheezing and that treatment with acid suppression and prokinetics decreased the need for daily asthma medications (14). In fact, 64% of infants with silent GER were able to discontinue all daily asthma medications. However, 73% of infants without GER were unable to discontinue inhaled steroids. In a study of adequately treated, nonatopic wheezing in 1- to 16-year-olds, clinical improvement occurred with acid suppression therapy as compared to a control group (15). These studies illustrate the difficulty in ascertaining which infants and young children have asthma versus which have GER-induced wheezing.

Few studies describe the effect of GER on asthma symptoms or exacerbations in infants. In a population of 5-month-old to 6-year-old asthmatics, Condino et al. noted that equal numbers of acid and nonacid reflux events occurred after a meal. There did not appear to be a direct link of reflux events to symptoms (16). In a controlled study of older asthmatic children, anti-GER therapy did result in a significant reduction in asthma medication (17). A Cochrane analysis has been performed inclusive of adults and children to determine whether GER treatment affects asthma. Broadly, no treatment effect was noted while subgroups did respond to treatment, it was not possible to predict which patients were in the responding subgroup (18).

■ PASSIVE SMOKE INHALATION

Parental smoking is a profound trigger for infantile asthma. Passive smoking increases airway responsiveness in normal 4 1/2-week-old infants (19). Overall, as much as 13% of asthma in children under 4 years of age is estimated to be secondary to maternal smoking (20). In lower socioeconomic households, children of mothers who smoke 10 cigarettes or more per day are at increased risk of asthma (21). Lower socioeconomic children of smoking parents have more emergency department visits for asthma than nonsmoking parents (22). The likelihood of infantile asthma increases with increasing exposure to smoke by-products (23). Parents of asthmatics often underestimate how much smoke their children are actually exposed to when urinary nicotine metabolites are compared with parental history (24). It is believed that children with glutathione-S-transferase deficiency may be at increased risk for asthma symptoms (25).

Fetal smoke exposure during pregnancy is linked to childhood asthma (26) and may play a larger role in the development of childhood asthma than postnatal exposure (26,27). Prenatal exposure to smoke is associated with decreased peak expiratory flow, mid-expiratory flow, and forced expiratory flow rates by the time children become school-aged (28). In fact, this decrease in pulmonary function is noted shortly after birth in apparently normal infants. This increase in risk of asthma due to prenatal and post-natal asthma is linked to increased risk of adult asthma (29). The most discouraging aspect to this public health problem is that maternal smoking during pregnancy is an entirely preventable cause of asthma.

Outdoor and Indoor Air Pollution

Outdoor air pollution exacerbates asthma. Increased emergency department visits, hospitalizations, and asthma severity among children with asthma are associated with elevated pollution levels (30,31). Increases in hospitalization risk for young children in Hong Kong are reported for every 10 $\mu g/m^3$ increase in NO_2 (32). Infants with asthma also are affected by outdoor air pollution; in fact, the number of emergency department related visits was the highest in this age group (33).

Indoor air pollution is an additional important trigger for asthma in this age group. Prevalence of asthma symptoms is highest in children whose households have open wood burning stoves (34). Wood burning stoves are linked to increased respiratory symptoms in infants due to increased airborne particulate matter (35).

Allergy

Until recently, allergy was not considered a risk factor for the development of wheezing in infants and very young children. Bernton and Brown (36) skin-tested allergic children in 1970 to cockroach allergen and found no child under 4 years of age with a positive skin test. Other early studies also suggested that immunoglobulin E (IgE)-mediated allergy did not act as a trigger for infantile asthma (37). These studies have formed the groundwork for the case that allergy is unimportant to infantile asthma.

The Case for Indoor Atopic Sensitization Affecting Asthma in Infants and Toddlers

In more recent studies, allergy has been commonly found in infants. Delacourt et al. (38) reported that 25% of infants with recurrent wheezing had positive skin test results to either dust mites or cat allergen. The prevalence rate for reactivity to one inhalant in a general population of 1-year-olds and 6-year-olds was 11%, and 30% respectively (39). Wilson et al. evaluated 196 rural children less than 3 years of age with infantile asthma for allergy (40). Forty-five percent of the infants who were tested to indoor inhalant allergens had at least one positive skin test result. For the 49 children who were under 1 year of age, 28.5% had a positive skin test to cockroach and 10.2% to dust mite. Welch et al. subsequently demonstrated that mouse allergy is present in 12% of asthmatic children (41). Cockroach sensitization is linked to previous episodes of wheezing in young children (42). Increased cockroach allergen in family rooms is associated with wheezing in the first year of life (43). In addition, 30% of asthmatic children may have sensitization to flying insects such as mayfly, housefly, caddis fly, moth, and ant (44).

These sensitizations have significant clinical implications. Frequent use of humidifiers is associated with increased wheezing. Damp housing increases the likelihood of a diagnosis of asthma in infants and increases the hospitalization rate (45). Visible moisture damage, particularly in the bedroom or main living quarters, was linked to new asthma cases in infants and young children (46). Sensitization to mouse, presumably from indoor exposure has been linked to increased asthma symptoms and hospitalization in very young asthmatic children (47).

The Case for Aeroallergen Sensitization Affecting Asthma in Infants and Toddlers

Many allergists have been reluctant to test very young children and infants to aeroallergens. However, recent studies suggest that aeroallergen sensitization in very young children may in fact occur despite "common wisdom." In a birth cohort study, aeroallergen sensitized 4-year-old children had significant allergic diseases such as asthma (48). Forty-two percent of children sensitized to grass had asthma. In addition, a majority of children were already sensitized to more than one allergen and this increased sensitization was associated with an increased risk of asthma (48). Ogershok et al. found that while no children under 12 months of age had aeroallergen sensitization, an astonishing 29% of 12- to 24-month-olds with asthma were pollen sensitized (49). In this study, equal numbers of 3-year-old asthmatic infants and toddlers were sensitized to pollen as to indoor allergens. Overall, 40% of asthmatic children between 12 months to 36 months of age were noted to be pollen sensitized. In another study, up to 52% of children less than 3 years of age with asthma were sensitized to pollen (50). This early sensitization to pollen in wheezing infants predicted subsequent asthma through adolescence (51). As of yet, there have not been studies of the effect of pollen sensitization on rates of infantile asthmatic symptoms or hospitalization. However, it is well documented in older individuals that aeroallergen sensitization is linked to increased pediatric hospitalizations, and emergency department visits for asthma exacerbations during the concurrent pollen season (52–54).

Viral Infections

In infants, viral respiratory illnesses are a major trigger for asthma. A viral trigger for status asthmaticus is reported in 86% of hospitalized infants (55). Respiratory syncytial virus (RSV) is the predominant viral organism causing wheezing in infants who present to an emergency department for care (56). In younger children, RSV is responsible for longer duration of illness prior to hospitalization for asthma (57). In fact, the presence of asthma was related to increased risk of hospitalization during RSV infection in children less than 18 months of age (58). Metapneumovirus is a newly identified virus which causes febrile winter-time asthma exacerbations in children (59). Children presenting with status asthmaticus had prolonged hospitalizations when infected with metapneumovirus (60). In asthmatic children under the age of 3 years, Manoha et al. found that metapneumovirus and rhinovirus were more significant viral triggers of asthma exacerbations than RSV (61).

■ EVALUATION OF THE PERSISTENTLY WHEEZING INFANT

Infants and young children with repeated episodes of wheezing require a complete history and physical examination. The frequency of hospitalizations and emergency department visits helps indicate the severity of the problem. Response to bronchodilators or steroids may provide clues supportive of a diagnosis of asthma. Coughing and wheezing associated with triggers other than viral infections strongly suggests asthma. A history of wheezing with exposure to pets, foods, or indoor or outdoor allergens is an indication for skin testing. Factors important in the history of the wheezing infant are listed in Table 20.2. In taking an environmental history, one should remember that many infants spend significant amounts of time in more than one household.

The differential diagnosis of infantile wheezing may be complex (Table 20.3). Asthma in a child under 1 year of age is a diagnosis of exclusion because congenital defects are more prevalent in this age group. The height and weight should be compared with standard norms to determine the growth pattern. On auscultation, the presence of inspiratory wheezing may indicate extra-thoracic obstruction. Wheezing due to asthma occurs throughout the entire expiratory phase. Specifically, expiratory stridor mimicking wheezing will not carry

through to the end of expiration. Rales or rhonchi may indicate atelectasis or pneumonia.

■ ALLERGY EVALUATION AND OTHER TESTS

Allergy appears to be a more significant trigger in infants and toddlers than previously appreciated. Skin testing using the prick-puncture technique to relevant indoor and outdoor (≥1 year of age) should be considered in infants and young children with asthma. Appropriate environmental control measures can then be instituted for those who are found to have evidence of atopy. Identification of outdoor aeroallergen sensitization can assist in determining issues of concomitant allergy therapy with asthma therapy and designing a maintenance asthma plan which accounts for peak pollen season.

Infants under 1 year of age with persistent wheezing and older children with a suggestive history should be evaluated for GER, anatomic abnormalities, and feeding disorders. An upper gastrointestinal series performed after consultation with a radiologist will provide information about anatomic abnormalities such as tracheoesophageal fistulas and vascular rings and may provide evidence of GER if it occurs during the examination. Feeding disorders may be diagnosed with a modified barium swallow. The most helpful and accurate study for the evaluation of GER in infants and small children is 24-hour esophageal pH monitoring. Bronchoscopy may be necessary if the presence of a foreign body or ciliary dyskinesia is suspected.

Standard pulmonary function testing such as spirometry or peak flow monitoring is not applicable to this population because they are not capable of performing the required maneuvers. Involuntary methods of assessing pulmonary function in small infants have been used for experimental purposes but are not generally available to clinicians. Methacholine provocation tests in very young children also have been studied experimentally, but are not routinely performed.

A chest film should be performed the first time an infant has an acute episode of wheezing. Repeated radiographs for each subsequent episode of wheezing are not necessary. A sweat chloride test to exclude cystic fibrosis should be considered in any infant under 1 year of age with repeated episodes of wheezing or respiratory distress. Wheezing associated with increased numbers of severe or unusual infections should lead to evaluation for an immune deficiency.

■ TREATMENT

The treatment of asthmatic infants is similar to that in older children and consists of avoiding identified triggers of wheezing, regular use of an anti-inflammatory

TABLE 20.2   IMPORTANT FACTORS IN THE HISTORY OF THE WHEEZING INFANT

HISTORY	POTENTIAL ETIOLOGY
Sudden onset	Foreign object
Intubation at birth	Subglottic stenosis, chronic lung disease of prematurity
Maternal papillomatosis	Laryngeal papilloma
Forceps delivery	Vocal cord injury
Difficulty feeding	Congenital heart defect Neurogenic defect
Irritability, regurgitation, torticollis	Sandifer syndrome (gastroesophageal reflux)
Recurrent pneumonia	Aspiration Tracheoesophageal fistula Cystic fibrosis Ciliary dyskinesia Immunodeficiency Human immunodeficiency virus infection
Formula changes	Milk or soy allergy
Isolated episode	Tuberculosis Respiratory syncytial virus Adenovirus Histoplasmosis Parainfluenza virus Metapneumovirus
Eczema, urticaria	Atopic diseases associated with asthma
Severe or recurrent infections	Immunodeficiencies
Recurrent wheezing ≥4 episodes	Asthma

medication, and a bronchodilator for symptomatic relief. However, treatment of this age group poses certain challenges. Many medications and delivery systems for asthma have been inadequately tested in this population or there is conflicting data concerning their use. Monitoring the effectiveness of treatment in infants is more difficult due to a lack of clinical availability of pulmonary function testing. Compliance with daily treatment is difficult due to the poor cooperation inherent in this age group as well as the reluctance of parents to have their children on medications when they are asymptomatic. Fortunately, the newer medications for asthma in infants promise better control of wheezing with improved safety and convenience. A summary of current asthma medications for infants is listed in Table 20.4.

The recent 2007 NHLBI guidelines (62) emphasize the need for assessment of both impairment and risk. Impairment includes both functional limitations experienced by the patient or frequent or intense exacerbations. Functional limitations in infants can include coughing/wheezing/breathlessness during daytime, nighttime, or with play; feeding difficulties or post-tussive emesis *or*

use of short-acting β agonist >2 times/week. Possible risks to be prevented include limited lung growth *or* recurrent exacerbations of asthma with emergency department and hospital visits. The most difficult group to determine maintenance medication for is the infants with severe exacerbations; but no perceivable daily symptoms between episodes. The NHBLI guidelines note that children with ≥4 episodes/year which last longer than a day *and* affect sleep *and* have a positive asthma risk profile (API) should have daily long-term control therapy. Other groups of infants requiring long-term controller therapy include 2 oral corticosteroid bursts for exacerbations in 6 months *or* children who require β-agonist treatment for >2 days/week for >4 weeks. If at any point a notable clinical response is not observed with asthma specific medications, alternative diagnoses should be considered.

β Agonists

β Agonists are clearly effective in infants and young asthmatic children for acute wheezing. Side effects of these medications may include tremors, irritability,

TABLE 20.3   DIFFERENTIAL DIAGNOSIS OF WHEEZING IN INFANTS

Congenital Disorders	Infectious/Post-Infectious
Cystic fibrosis	Epiglottitis
Tracheoesophageal fistula	Croup
Primary ciliary dyskinesia	Tracheitis
Immunodeficiency	Bronchiolitis
Sickle cell disease (acute chest syndrome)	Diphtheria
Diaphragmatic hernia	Chlamydia
Chronic lung disease of prematurity	Pneumocytisis carnii
α_1-antitrypsin deficiency	Histoplasmosis
Pulmonary lymphangiectasia	Bronchiectasis
Carnitine deficiency	Pertussis
Congenital Heart Disease	Retropharyngeal abscess
Aberrant left coronary artery	Bronchiolitis obliterans
Chronic heart failure	**Compression Syndromes**
Upper Airway Disorders	Tuberculosis
Foreign body	Lymphadenopathy
Laryngotracheomalacia	Vascular ring
Vocal cord dysfunction/paralysis	Pulmonary sling
Laryngeal web, papillomatosis, cleft	Mediastinal masses
Subglottic or tracheal stenosis	Congenital goiter
Hemangioma	Thyroglossal duct cyst
Laryngeal paralysis	Teratoma
Lower Airway Disorders	Aspiration syndromes
Bronchial stenosis	Neurogenic
Foreign object	**Other**
Bronchial casts	Munchausen syndrome by proxy
Asthma	Neurofibroma
Bronchomalacia	Gastroesophageal reflux
Lobar emphysema	Pulmonary langerhans cell histiocytosis

sleep disturbances, and behavioral problems. At higher doses, tachycardia, agitation, hypokalemia, and hyperglycemia may also be seen. Oral preparations are more likely to produce side effects than inhaled ones. Continuous nebulized albuterol has been successfully administered to infants with severe wheezing (63).

An initial clinical study did not demonstrate clinical efficacy of β agonists in infants under 18 months of age (64). However this study used a mixed population of infants with asthma and bronchiolitis. It has been subsequently determined that infants do have functioning β receptors (65), and recent studies in infants specifically diagnosed with asthma suggest that β agonists decrease wheezing as well as improve pulmonary functions. This improvement is noted both for nebulized

medications and metered-dose inhalers (MDIs) with face mask spacer devices (67,68). It is prudent to administer a trial of inhaled β agonists to all wheezing infants regardless of the underlying etiology to determine whether there is any improvement. Infants with true asthma should be given inhaled β agonists as needed for wheezing during acute exacerbations of their disease.

Anticholinergics

Ipratropium bromide is a quaternary isopropyl derivative of atropine available as a nebulizer solution. A pediatric asthma consensus group suggests that ipratropium may be useful as a second- or third-line

TABLE 20.4 OUTPATIENT- OR OFFICE-BASED MEDICATIONS FOR THE TREATMENT OF INFANTILE ASTHMA

MEDICATION	DOSAGE
Short-course Systemic Steroids	
Prednisolone (5 mg/5 mL or 15 mg/5 mL)	1 mg/kg/day to 2 mg/kg/day orally; maximum 60 mg/day
Methylprednisolone acetate (40 mg/mL; 80 mg/mL)	7.5 mg/kg intramuscularly × 1
Dexamethasone acetate	1.7 mg/kg intramuscularly
*Rescue Medications**	
Albuterol ampules* (0.63 mg/3mL; 1.25 mg/3mL; 2.5 mg/3mL)	0.63 mg/3ml to 2.5 mg/3ml saline every 4 to 6 hours as needed (may be dosed 2.5 mg every 20 minutes × 3 doses *or* 0.15 mg/kg to 0.3 mg/kg up to 10 mg every 1 to 4 hours as needed *or* up to 0.5 mg/kg/hr continuous nebulization for acute exacerbations)
Levalbuterol (R-albuterol)* (0.63 mg/3 mL; 1.25 mg/3mL)	0.63 mg/3 ml to 1.25 mg/3 ml saline every 4 to 6 hours as needed (may be dosed 1.25 mg every 20 minutes for 3 doses then 0.075 mg/kg to 0.15 mg/kg up to 5 mg every 1 to 4 hours as needed)
Ipratroprium (0.25 mg/mL saline*) (severe exacerbation only, is not to be used as first-line therapy)	0.25 mg to 0.5 mg every 20 minutes × 3 then as needed (may mix with albuterol in nebulizer)
Ipratroprium with albuterol nebulizer solution: (0.5 mg ipratroprium bromide and 2.5 mg albuterol)	1.5 mL every 20 minutes × 3 doses then as needed for up to 3 hours
Epinephrine 1:1000 (1mg/mL)	0.01 mg/kg subcutaneously up to 0.3 mg to 0.5 mg every 20 minutes up to 3 doses
Terbutaline (1 mg/mL)	0.01 mg/kg every 20 minutes for 3 doses then every 2 to 6 hours as needed subcutaneously
Maintenance Medications	
Cromolyn sodium	1 ampule 3 to 4 times per day
Montelukast	4 mg orally daily
Budesonide ampules*,#	0.25 mg, 0.5 mg, 1 ampule daily
Fluticasone HFA (44 µg, 110 µg, or 220 µg/puff) with antistatic valved holding chamber and mask*,§	*Low dose:* 88 µg/day to 176 µg/day *Medium dose:* 176 µg/day to 352 µg/day *High dose:* >352 µg/day

* 2007 NHBLI guidelines specifically note that blow by technique for nebulized aerosol delivery is inadequate.

2007 NHBLI guidelines specifically note doubling the dose of inhaled steroid during exacerbations is not effective.

§ 2007 NHBLI guidelines note that HFA use with spacer and face mask may reduce lung delivery by 50%.

medication in severe infantile asthma exacerbations. A recent meta-analysis of clinical trials of ipratropium for wheezing in children under the age of 2 years concluded that there is not enough evidence to support the routine use of anticholinergic therapy for wheezing infants (69). A current NHLBI consensus statement notes that data suggest that ipratropium is appropriate to use during severe exacerbations in infants as add-on therapy in the emergency department. Further benefit of ipratropium treatment during the remainder of the hospitalization has not been noted.

Cromolyn Sodium

Cromolyn sodium (sodium cromoglycate) is an anti-inflammatory medication that inhibits the degranulation of mast cells and inhibits early- and late-phase asthmatic reactions to allergen. It is not a bronchodilator, but a prophylactic medication that must be used on a regular basis to have an effect. In the past, its safety and lack of toxicity made it particularly attractive as a first-line therapy for the prevention of wheezing in this age group (70). However, it is clearly not as efficacious as low-dose inhaled corticosteroids in controlling symptoms.

A study reported that cromolyn is no more effective than placebo in children under 1 year of age or in children 1 to 4 years of age using MDIs with a face mask spacer device (71). However, nebulized cromolyn in infants over 12 months of age is effective for treating asthma (72). Cromolyn is no longer recommended by the NIH Expert Panel Report (62) as the first-line anti-inflammatory medication for infants and small children with chronic asthma symptoms. In addition, daily treatment for any length of time in an uncooperative infant or toddler may become tedious for parents, adversely affecting compliance. Nevertheless, due to its high safety profile, cromolyn remains one of the prophylactic medications currently available for the prevention of wheezing in this age group, particularly in parents wishing to avoid daily inhaled corticosteroids.

Leukotriene Antagonists

Leukotrienes are chemical mediators that produce bronchospasm, eosinophilia, stimulate mucus secretion, and increase vascular permeability, all critical features of asthma. Leukotriene antagonists block these inflammatory effects. Montelukast is approved for children as young as age 1 by the U.S. Food and Drug Administration. So far, these medications appear to have a good safety profile and are well tolerated (73). Montelukast has been reported to decrease asthma exacerbations in 2- to 5-year-olds with intermittent asthma (74). In 10- to 26-month-old children with asthma, treatment with montelukast significantly improved infantile FEV 0.5 nitric oxide and symptom score measurements (75). This study reflects that montelukast can have a positive effect on airway inflammation measured in these patients with early childhood asthma. In head-to-head comparisons to inhaled steroids in children with mild persistent asthma, both montelukast and inhaled steroids improved symptom control, but those patients on inhaled steroids utilized less oral corticosteroid rescue (76). NHLBI asthma treatment guidelines list inhaled corticosteroids as preferred first-line treatment for asthma as a result of these studies. Montelukast is noted by the NIHBI guidelines (62) to be alternative therapy or add-on therapy for mild persistent to more severe asthma. These recommendations do not reflect that parents of mild infantile asthmatics perceive montelukast as a particularly attractive long-term controller medication because it can be taken as a tablet once daily, it has a high safety profile, and it is not a corticosteroid.

Theophylline

Despite its long use and previous popularity in this age group, few data are available on theophylline effectiveness in infants. Concern about theophylline side effects ranging from mild nausea, insomnia, and agitation to life-threatening cardiac arrhythmias and encephalopathic seizures has limited its use now that safer medications are available (77). Checking serum concentrations of theophylline is necessary to achieve maximal benefits without significant side effects, and minor symptoms are not predictive of elevated levels (78). Most serious side effects occur when the serum concentration of theophylline exceeds 20 mg/dL. Age, diet, fever, viral infections, and drug interactions may affect the metabolism of this medication particularly in children less than 1 year old. Drugs that increase serum theophylline concentrations include certain antibiotics such as ciprofloxacin, clarithromycin, and erythromycin, as well as cimetidine, verapamil, propranolol, and thiabendazole (79). Nevertheless, NHLBI treatment guidelines list theophylline as an acceptable alternative or add-on therapy for children under 4 years of age due to proven efficacy.

Corticosteroids

Corticosteroids are potent anti-inflammatory medications that have profound effects on asthma. They decrease inflammatory mediators, reduce mucus production, decrease mucosal edema, and increase β-adrenergic responsiveness. Clinically, corticosterids improve lung function, reduce airway hyperreactivity, and modify the late-phase asthmatic response. The efficacy of steroids in treating true infantile asthma is well known. For acute exacerbations, asthmatic infants treated with steroids have a significantly reduced need for hospitalization, reduced length of stay once hospitalized, and reduced asthma medications (80,81). Intramuscular dexamethasone may be used in those infants who do not tolerate oral steroids (82).

Maintenance inhaled steroids provide many of the beneficial anti-inflammatory properties of corticosteroids without numerous unwanted side effects. Young children with severe asthma treated with inhaled nebulized corticosteroids have markedly decreased symptoms and days of oral corticosteroid use (83). This study was replicated in children less than 4 years of age utilizing fluticasone HFA with valved holding chamber and face mask (84) for asthma symptom scores. Studies have also reported that inhaled corticosteroids for asthmatic 1- to 3-year-old children are more efficacious than cromolyn (85). Lastly, inhaled glucocorticosteroids have been demonstrated to improve pulmonary function tests, decrease β-agonist use, and improve symptoms in the youngest children with asthma (<2 years old) (86,87). Due to the significant anti-inflammatory effect of inhaled corticosteroids, NHLBI guidelines indicate that inhaled steroids are the initial drug of choice in asthmatic children under 4 years of age.

Some studies demonstrate short-term linear growth in children on inhaled steroids may be decreased, and that these effects may be dose dependent. Other studies demonstrate that short-term (6- to 12-month) exposure has no effect on growth (88). These issues are difficult to assess due to the nature of growth, which is intermittent in children. However, the long-term effects on adult height remain unknown because catch-up growth may occur during puberty (89). Other theoretical concerns include adrenal suppression. Current studies have determined that there is no evidence of altered adrenal function due to inhaled steroids in infants or small children, albeit this may be susceptible to a dose effect (83,88). Currently being studied is a new inhaled steroid, ciclesonide, which is only bioavailable through esterification in the respiratory tree. Lack of bioavailable drug deposited in the GI tract virtually eliminates systemic corticosteroid effects. Awaiting further study, ciclesonide holds promise to end concerns of systemic growth or adrenal effects in asthmatic children (89).

Allergen Avoidance

Dust mite avoidance measures have been noted to have a modest treatment effect in infants (90). In older asthmatic children, mattress encasing has been linked to lower inhaled steroid doses (91). However, some studies indicate that utilizing prophylactic encasements at birth does not affect the dust mite sensitization rate at 4 years of age (92). In addition, the allergen reducing effects of dust mite covers may decrease over time (92). Reduced levels of cockroach allergen have been associated with decreasing number of cockroaches by utilizing better eradication efforts (93). However, a study linking decreased cockroach levels in the dwelling with improved asthma symptoms in infants has not been reported. Clearly more studies are required to determine best treatment options including allergen avoidance.

Allergy Immunotherapy

Potential deleterious outcomes of childhood asthma have been convincingly shown to develop despite the use of inhaled steroids (12). The increasingly apparent role of aeroallergens in the progression of infant wheezing to clinical long-term asthma has suggested that allergen immunotherapy might provide a more permanent disease-modifying outcome after the treatment is discontinued. In older children, a 3-year course of subcutaneous immunotherapy with standardized allergen extracts has shown long-term clinical effects (94). In addition, subcutaneous immunotherapy has shown potential to prevent development of asthma in children with allergic rhinoconjunctivitis. This clinical effect was noted up to 7 years after treatment (94). However, subcutaneous immunotherapy in very young children is very problematic due to their immaturity and inability to verbalize or cooperate. Sublingual immunotherapy might be better tolerated in young children, and there are data in children as young as age 3, that sublingual immunotherapy with standardized extracts might reduce symptom scores and rescue medication use in allergic asthma compared with placebo (95). Further studies are needed to determine the role of immunotherapy in altering the natural history of asthma in young children.

■ REFERENCES

1. Beasley R, Crane J, Lai CKW, et al. Prevalence and etiology of asthma. *J Allergy Clin Immunol.* 2000;105 (Part 2; suppl):466–472.
2. Shamssain MH, Shamsian N. Prevalence and severity of asthma, rhinitis, and atopic eczema: the north east study. *Arch Dis Child.* 1999;81:313–317.
3. Lin S, Fitzgerald E, Hwang SA, et al. Asthma hospitalization rates and socioeconomic status in New York State (1987–1993). *J Asthma.* 1999;36:239–251.
4. Goodman DC, Stukel TA, Chang CH. Trends in pediatric asthma hospitalization rates: regional and socioeconomic differences. *Pediatrics.* 1998;101:208–213.
5. Jonasson G, Lodrup Carlsen KC, Leegard J, et al. Trends in hospital admissions for childhood asthma in Oslo, Norway, 1980–1995. *Allergy.* 2000;55:232–239.
6. Wennergren G, Krisjansson S, Strannegard IL. Decrease in hospitalization for the treatment of asthma with increased use of anti-inflammatory treatment, despite an increase in prevalence of asthma. *J Allergy Clin Immunol.* 1996;97:742–748.
7. Schaubel D, Johansen H, Mao Y, et al. Risk of preschool asthma: incidence, hospitalization, recurrence, and readmission probability. *J Asthma.* 1996;33:97–103.
8. Weitzman JB, Kanarek NF, Smialek JE. Medical examiner asthma death autopsies: a distinct subgroup of asthma deaths with implications for public health preventive strategies. *Arch Pathol Lab Med.* 1998;122:691–699.
9. Martinez, FD, Wright AL, Taussig LM, et al. Asthma and wheezing in the first six years of life. *N Engl J Med.* 1995;332;133–138.
10. Castro-Rodriguez JA, Holberg CJ, Wright AL, et al. A clinical index to define risk of asthma in young children with recurrent wheezing. *Am J Respir Crit Care Med.* 2000;25:1403–1406.
11. Guilbert TW, Morgan WJ, Zeiger RS, et al. Atopic characteristics of children with recurrent wheezing at high risk for the development of childhood asthma. *J Allergy Clin Immunol.* 2004;114:1282–1287.
12. Guilbert TW, Morgan WJ, Zeiger RS, et al. Long-term inhaled corticosteroids in preschool children at high risk for asthma. *N Engl J Med.* 2006;354:1985–1996.
13. Sacco O, Silvestri M, Sabatini F, et al. IL-8 and airway neutrophilia in children with gastroespophageal reflux and asthma-like symptoms. *Respir Med.* 2006;100:307–315.
14. Sheikh S, Stephen T, Howell L, et al. Gastroesophageal reflux in infants with wheezing. *Pediatr Pulmonol.* 1999;28:181–186.
15. Yuksel H, Yilmaz O, Kirmaz C, et al. Frequency of gastroesophageal reflux disease in nonatopic children with asthma-like airway disease. *Respir Med.* 2006;100:393–398.
16. Condino AA, Sondheimer J, Pan Z, et al. Evaluation of gastroesophageal reflux in pediatric patients with asthma using impedance-pH monitoring. *J Pediatr.* 2006;149:216–219.
17. Khoshoo V, Le T, Haydell RM Jr, et al. Role of gastroesophageal reflux in older children with persistent asthma. *Chest.* 2003;123:1008–1013.
18. Gibson PG, Henry RL, Coughland L. Gastroesophageal reflux treatment for asthma in adults and children. *Cochrane Database Syst Rev.* 2003;(2):CD001496.
19. Young S, Le Souef PN, Geelhoed GC, et al. The influence of a family history of asthma and parental smoking on airway responsiveness in early infancy. *N Engl J Med.* 1991;324:1168–1173.
20. Lister SM, Jorm LR. Parental smoking and respiratory illness in Australian children aged 0–4 years: ABS 1989–90 National Health Survey results. *Aust N Z J Public Health.* 1998;22:781–786.
21. Martinez FD, Cline M, Burrows B. Increased incidence of asthma in children of smoking mothers. *Pediatrics.* 1992;89:21–26.
22. Wang HC, McGeady SJ, Yousef E. Patient, home residence and neighborhood characteristics in pediatric emergency department visits for asthma. *J Asthma.* 2007;44:95–98.
23. Ehrlich RI, Du Toit D, Jordaan E, et al. Risk factors for childhood asthma and wheezing. Importance of maternal and household smoking. *Am J Respir Crit Care Med.* 1996;154:681–688.

24. Kohler E, Sollich V, Schuster R, et al. Passive smoke exposure in infants and children with respiratory tract diseases. *Hum Exp Toxicol.* 1999;18:212–217.

25. Kabesch M, Hoefler C, Carr D, et al. Glutathione S transferase deficiency and passive smoking increase childhood asthma. *Thorax.* 2004;59:569–573.

26. Moshammer H, Hoek G, Luttmann-Gibson H, et al. Parental smoking and lung function in children: an international study. *Am J Respir Crit Care Med.* 2006;173:1255–1263.

27. Stein RT, Holberg CJ, Sherrill D, et al. Influence of parental smoking on respiratory symptoms during the first decade of life: the Tucson Children's Respiratory Study. *Am J Epidemiol.* 1999;149:1030–1037.

28. Gilliland FD, Berhane K, McConnell R, et al. Maternal smoking during pregnancy, environmental tobacco smoke exposure, and childhood lung function. *Thorax.* 2000;55:271–276.

29. Skorge TD, Eagan TM, Eide GE, et al. The adult incidence of asthma and respiratory symptoms by passive smoking in utero or in childhood. *Am J Respir Crit Care Med.* 2005;172:61–66.

30. Tseng RY, Li CK, Spinks JA. Particulate air pollution and hospitalization for asthma. *Ann Allergy.* 1992;68:425–432.

31. Su HL, Chou MC, Lue KH. The relationship of air pollution to ED visits for asthma differ between children and adults. *Am J Emerg Med.* 2006;24:709–713.

32. Ko FW, Tam W, Wong TW, et al. Effects of air pollution on asthma hospitalization rates in different age groups in Hong Kong. *Clin Exp Allergy.* 2007;37:1312–1319.

33. Babin SM, Burkom HS, Holtry RS, et al. Pediatric patient asthma-related emergency department visits and admissions in Washington, DC, from 2001–2004, and associations with air quality, socioeconomic status and age group. *Environ Health.* 2007;21:6–9.

34. Schei MA, Hessen JO, Smith KR, et al. Childhood asthma and indoor woodsmoke from cooking in Guatemala. *J Expo Anal Environ Epidemiol.* 2004;14(Suppl1):S110–117.

35. Honicky RE, Osborn JS, Akpom CA. Symptoms of respiratory illness in young children and the use of wood-burning stoves for indoor heating. *Pediatrics.* 1985;75:587–593.

36. Bernton HS, Brown H. Cockroach allergy: age of onset of skin reactivity. *Ann Allergy.* 1970;28:420–422.

37. Rowntree S, Cogswell JJ, Platts-Mills TAE, et al. Development of IgE and IgG antibodies to food and inhalant allergies in children at risk of allergic disease. *Arch Dis Child.* 1985;75:633–637.

38. Delacourt C, Labbe D, Vassault A, et al. Sensitization to inhalant allergens in wheezing infants is predictive of the development of infantile asthma. *Allergy.* 1994;49:843–847.

39. Kulig M, Bergmann R, Klettke U, et al. Natural course of sensitization to food and inhalant allergens during the first 6 years of life. *J Allergy Clin Immunol.* 1999; 103:1173–1179.

40. Wilson NW, Robinson NP, Hogan MB. Cockroach and other inhalant allergies in infantile asthma. *Ann Allergy Asthma Immunol.* 1999;83:27–30.

41. Welch JE, Hogan MB, Wilson NW. Mouse allergy among asthmatic children from rural Appalachia. *Ann Allergy Asthma Immunol.* 2003;90:223–225.

42. De Vera MJ, Drapkin S, Moy JN. Association of recurrent wheezing with sensitivity to cockroach allergen in inner-city children. *Ann Allergy Asthma Immunol.* 2003;91:455–459.

43. Gold DR, Burge HA, Carey V, et al. Predictors of repeated wheeze in the first year of life. The relative roles of cockroach, birth weight, acute lower respiratory illness, and maternal smoking. *Am J Respir Crit Care Med.* 1999;160:227–236.

44. Smith TS, Hogan MB, Welch JE, et al. Modern prevalence of insect sensitization in rural asthma and allergic rhinitis patients. *Allergy Asthma Proc.* 2005;26:356–360.

45. Pekkanen J, Hyvarinen A, Haverinen-Shaughnessy U, et al. Moisture damage and childhood asthma: a population-based incident case-control study. *Eur Respir J.* 2007;29:509–515.

46. Wever-Hess J, Kowenberg JM, Duiverman EJ, et al. Risk factors for exacerbations and hospital admissions in asthma of early childhood. *Pediatr Pulmonol.* 2000;29:250–256.

47. Matsui EC, Eggleston PA, Buckley TJ, et al. Household mouse allergen exposure and asthma morbidity in inner-city preschool children. *Ann Allergy Asthma Immunol.* 2006;97:514–520.

48. Arshad SH, Tariq SM, Matthews S, et al. Sensitization to common allergens and its association with allergic disorders at age 4 years: a whole population birth cohort study. *Pediatrics.* 2001;108:E33.

49. Ogershok PR, Warner DJ, Hogan MB, et al. Prevalence of pollen sensitization in younger children who have asthma. *Allergy Asthma Proc.* 2007;28:654–658.

50. Emin O, Nermin G, Ulker O, et al. Skin sensitization to common allergens in Turkish wheezy children less than 3 years of age. *Asian Pac J Allergy Immunol.* 2004:22:97–101.

51. Piippo-Savolainen E, Remes S, Korppi M. Does early exposure or sensitization to inhalant allergens predict asthma in wheezing infants? A 20 year follow-up. *Allergy Asthma Proc.* 207;28:454–461.

52. Wang HC, Yousef E. Air quality and pediatric asthma-related emergencies. *J Asthma.* 2007;44:839–841.

53. Im W, Schneider D. Effect of weed pollen on children's hospital admissions for asthma during the fall season. *Arch Environ Occup Health.* 2005;60:257–265.

54. Heguy L, Garneau M, Goldberg MS, et al. Associations between grass and weed pollen and emergency department visits for asthma among children in Montreal. *Envrion Res.* 2008;106:203–211.

55. Freymuth F, Vabret A, Brouard J, et al. Detection of viral, *Chlamydia pneumoniae,* and *Mycoplasma pneumoniae* infections in exacerbations of asthma in children. *J Clin Virol.* 1999;13:131–139.

56. Rakes GP, Arruda E, Ingram JM, et al. Rhinovirus and respiratory syncytial virus in wheezing children requiring emergency care. IgE and eosinophil analyses. *Am J Respir Crit Care Med.* 1999;159:785–790.

57. Lazzaro T, Hogg G, Barnett P. Respiratory syncytial virus infection and recurrent wheeze/asthma in children under five years: an epidemiological survey. *J Paediatr Child Health.* 2007:43:29–33.

58. Stensballe LG, Kristensen K, Simoes EA, et al. Atopic disposition, wheezing, and subsequent respiratory syncytial virus hospitalization in Danish children younger than 18 months: a nested case-control study. *Pediatrics.* 2006;118:1360–1368.

59. Bosis S, Esposito S, Niesters HG, et al. Impact of human metapneumovirus in childhood: comparison with respiratory syncytial virus and influenza viruses. *J Med Virol.* 2005;75:101–104.

60. Estrada B, Carter M, Barik S, et al. Severe human metapneumovirus infection in hospitalized children. *Clin Pediatr (Phila).* 2007:46:258–262.

61. Manoha C, Espinosa S, Aho SL, et al. Epidemiological and clinical features of hMPV, RSV, and RVs infections in young children. *J Clin Virol.* 2007;28:221–226.

62. National Heart, Lung, and Blood Institute, National Asthma Education and Prevention Program Expert Panel Report 3. *Guidelines for the Diagnosis and Management of Asthma.* Full Report 2007, National Institutes of Health, 2007. Available at http://www.nhlbi.nih.gov/guidelines/asthma/asthmafullrpt.pdf.

63. Katz RW, Kelly HW, Crowley MR, et al. Safety of continuous nebulized albuterol for bronchospasm in infants and children. *Pediatrics.* 1993;92:666–669.

64. Prendiville A, Green S, Silverman M. Paradoxical response to nebulized salbutamol in wheezy infants, assessed by partial expiratory flow-volume curves. *Thorax.* 1987;42:86–91.

65. Prendiville A, Green S, Silverman M. Airway responsiveness in wheezy infants: evidence for functional beta adrenergic receptors. *Thorax.* 1987;42:100–104.

66. Lenney W, Milner AD. Alpha and beta adrenergic stimulants in bronchiolitis and wheezy bronchitis in children under 18 months of age. *Arch Dis Child.* 1978;53:707–709.

67. Bentur L, Canny GJ, Shields MD, et al. Controlled trial of nebulized albuterol in children younger than 2 years of age with acute asthma. *Pediatrics.* 1992;89:133–137.

68. Kraemer R, Frey U, Sommer CW, et al. Short-term effect of albuterol, delivered via a new auxiliary device, in wheezy infants. *Am Rev Respir Dis.* 1991;144:347–351.

69. Everard ML, Bara A, Kurian M. Anti-cholinergic drugs for wheeze in children under the age of two years. *Cochrane Database Syst Rev.* 2005(3)CD001279.

70. Brugman SM, Larson GL. Asthma in infants and small children. *Clin Chest Med.* 1995;16:637–656.

71. Tasche MJ, van der Wouden JC, Uijen JH, et al. Randomised placebo-controlled trial of inhaled sodium cromoglycate in 1–4-year-old children with moderate asthma. *Lancet.* 1997;350:1060–1064.

72. O'Callahan C, Milner AD, Swarbrick A. Nebulized sodium cromoglycate in infancy: airway protection after deterioration. *Arch Dis Child.* 1990;65:404–406.

73. van Adelsberg J, Moy J, Wei LX, et al. Safety, tolerability and exploratory efficacy of montelukast in 6- to 24-month-old patients with asthma. *Curr Med Res Opin.* 2005;21:971–979.

74. Bisgaard H, Zielen S, Garcia-Garcia ML, et al. Montelukast reduces asthma exacerbations in 2- to 5-year-old children with intermittent asthma. *Am J Respir Crit Care Med.* 2005;171:315–322.

75. Straub DA, Moeller A, Minocchieri S, et al. The effect of montelukast on lung function and exhaled nitric oxide in infants with early childhood asthma. *Eur Respir J.* 2005;25:289–294.

76. Szefler SJ, Baker JW, Uryniak T, et al. Comparative study of budesonide inhalation suspension and montelukast in young children with mild persistent asthma. *J Allergy Clin Immunol.* 2007;120:1043–1050.

77. Hendeles L, Weinberger M, Szefler S, et al. Safety and efficacy of theophylline in children with asthma. *J Pediatr.* 1992;120:177–183.

78. Melamed J, Beaucher WN. Minor symptoms are not predictive of elevated theophylline levels in adults on chronic therapy. *Ann Allergy Asthma Immunol.* 1995;75:516–520.

79. Weinberger M, Hendeles L. Theophylline in asthma. *N Engl J Med.* 1996;334:1380–1388.

80. Fox GF, Marsh MJ, Milner AD. Treatment of recurrent acute wheezing episodes in infancy with oral salbutamol and prednisolone. *Eur J Pediatr.* 1996;155:512–516.

81. Csonka P, Kaila M, Laippala P, et al. Oral prednisolone in the acute management of children age 6 to 35 months with viral respiratory infection-induced lower airway disease: a randomized, placebo-controlled trial. *J Pediatr.* 2003;143:725–730.

82. Gries DM, Moffitt DR, Pulos E, et al. A single dose of intramuscularly administered dexamethasone acetate is as effective as oral prednisone to treat asthma exacerbations in young children. *J Pediatr.* 2000;136: 298–303.

83. Delacourt C, Dutau G, Lefrancios G, et al. Beclospin Clinical Development Group. Comparison of the efficacy and safety of nebulized beclometasone dipropionate and budesonide in severe persistent childhood asthma. *Respir Med.* 2003;97(Suppl B):S27–S33.

84. Qaqundah PY, Sugerman RW, Ceruti E, et al. Efficacy and safety of fluticasone propionate hydrofluoroalkane inhalation aerosol in preschool-age children with asthma; a randomized, double-blind, placebo-controlled study. *J Pediatr.* 2006;149:663–670.

85. Bisgaard H, Allen D, Milanowski J, et al. Twelve-month safety and efficacy of inhaled fluticasone propionate in children aged 1 to 3 years with recurrent wheezing. *Pediatrics.* 2004;113:e87–94.

86. Teper AM, Kofman CD, Szulman GA, et al. Fluticasone improves pulmonary function in children under 2 years old with risk factors for asthma. *Am J Respir Crit Care Med.* 2005;171:587–590.

87. Mellon M. Efficacy of budesonide inhalation suspension in infants and young children with persistent asthma. Budesonide Inhalation Suspension Study Group. *J Allergy Clin Immunol.* 1999;104(Part 2):191–199.

88. Berger WE, Qaundah PY, Blake K, et al. Safety of budesonide inhalation suspension in infants ages six to twelve months with mild to moderate persistent asthma or recurrent wheeze. *J Pediatr.* 2005;146:91–95.

89. Skoner DP, Maspero J, Banerji D; Ciclesonide Pediatric Growth Study Group. Assessment of the long-term safety of inhaled ciclesonide on growth in children with asthma. *Pediatrics.* 2008;121:179–180.

90. van Strien RT, Koopman LP, Kerkhof M, et al. Mattress encasings and mite allergen levels in the prevention and incidence of asthma and mite allergy study. *Clin Exp Allergy.* 2003;33(4):490–495.

91. Halken S, Host A, Niklassen U, et al. Effect of mattress and pillow casings on children with asthma and house dust mite allergy. *J Allergy Clin Immunol.* 2003;111(1):169–176.

92. Corver K, Kerkhof M, Brussee JE, at al. House dust mite allergen reduction and allergy at 4 yr: follow-up of the PIAMA study. *Pediatr Allergy Immunol.* 2006;17(5):329–336.

93. Sever ML, Arbes SJ, Gore JC, et al. Cockroach allergen reduction by cockroach control in low-income urban homes: a randomized control trial. *J Allergy Clin Immunol.* 2007;120:849–855.

94. Jacobsen L, Niggemann B, Dreborg S, et al. (The PAT investigator group). Specific immunotherapy has long-term preventive effect of seasonal and perennial asthma: 10-year follow-up on the PAT study. *Allergy.* 2007;62 (8):943–948.

95. Penagos M, Passalacqua G, Compalati E, et al. Meta-analysis of the efficacy of sublingual immunotherapy in the treatment of allergic asthma in pediatric patients, 3 to 18 years of age. *Chest.* 2008; 133(3):599–609.

CHAPTER 21

Management of Acute Severe Asthma

THOMAS CORBRIDGE AND SUSAN CORBRIDGE

Acute severe asthma (ASA) all too commonly results from inadequately controlled asthma—particularly in the subgroup of patients that depends on emergency-oriented management and under uses inhaled corticosteroids (1). Each year in the United States, acute asthma accounts for approximately 1.8 million emergency department (ED) visits, 480,000 hospitalizations, and 4,000 deaths, most of which occur in the outpatient setting (2,3). While these statistics have improved recently, a gender and racial gap exists with women and African Americans at greatest risk for hospitalization and death (4).

It follows that management of an acutely ill asthmatic involves not only treatment of the exacerbation but also prevention of future attacks by educational efforts, initiation of controller therapy, and scheduling follow-up appointments with an asthma specialist (5). The focus of this chapter, however, is on the more immediate concern of improving airflow rates through the appropriate use of pharmacologic therapy, and, when required, the use of nonpharmacologic means to support ventilation. Fortunately, β-agonist bronchodilators with or without anticholinergics and systemic corticosteroids are sufficient in most cases. For patients with acute respiratory failure requiring intubation, a strategy that minimizes lung hyperinflation improves outcome (6,7).

■ PATHOPHYSIOLOGY OF ACUTE AIRFLOW OBSTRUCTION

The speed with which ASA develops varies (8). In sudden asphyxic asthma, severe obstruction develops in less than 3 hours from a more pure form of smooth muscle-mediated bronchospasm. Patients have fewer airway secretions and may respond quickly to bronchodilators alone (9,10). Triggers of sudden attacks include medications such as nonsteroidal anti-inflammatory agents and β blockers in susceptible patients, allergen

or irritant exposure, sulphites, and inhalation of illicit drugs (11). Respiratory tract infection is not common; often no cause is identified (12).

Most attacks evolve over 24 hours with progressive airway wall inflammation, accumulations of thick intraluminal mucus, and bronchospasm. Mucus obstructs large and small airways and consists of sloughed epithelial cells, eosinophils, fibrin, and other serum components that have leaked through the denuded airway epithelium. These types of exacerbations are triggered by a variety of infectious, allergic, and nonspecific irritant exposures and take longer to resolve. Importantly, they epitomize clear and missed opportunities to increase anti-inflammatory medications in the outpatient setting.

The critical endpoint of ASA, regardless of tempo, is expiratory airflow obstruction. It takes longer to exhale through bronchospastic, inflamed, and mucus-filled airways. Indeed it may take as long as 60 seconds for termination of expiratory flow during tidal breathing, but, of course, with respiratory rates in the 20s or 30s, there are only 1 to 2 seconds available for expiration. The result is incomplete emptying of gas and dynamic lung hyperinflation (DHI). Fortunately, DHI may be self-limiting because hyperinflation increases lung elastic recoil pressure and airway diameter, which improves expiratory flow.

At the end of exhalation, incomplete gas emptying elevates alveolar volume and pressure, a state referred to as auto–positive end-expiratory pressure (auto-PEEP). Auto-PEEP is a threshold pressure that must be overcome during inhalation which increases inspiratory work of breathing. At the same time diaphragm force generation is diminished by the adverse effects of DHI and possible respiratory acidosis to create an imbalance between strength and load that predisposes to hypercapneic respiratory failure (13).

Airway obstruction further decreases ventilation (V) relative to perfusion (Q) in alveolar-capillary units, resulting in hypoxemia (14). Because this is not shunt physiology as is seen in alveolar filling processes, supplemental oxygen typically corrects hypoxemia, even in severely affected patients. Refractory hypoxemia is rare and suggests other problems such as pneumonia, aspiration, atelectasis, or pneumothorax.

There is a rough correlation between severity of airflow obstruction as measured by spirometry and hypoxemia. However, there are no cut-off values that accurately predict hypoxemia. Furthermore, hypoxemia may occur sooner and/or resolve later than spirometric measures of airflow (15).

Cardiovascular complications of ASA include accentuation of the normal inspiratory reduction in stroke volume and blood pressure termed the *pulsus paradoxus* (PP). Wide swings in pleural pressure during labored breathing are responsible for this phenomenon. During vigorous inspiration to overcome the effects of auto-PEEP, intra-thoracic pressure falls and blood flow increases to the right heart. The right ventricle fills early in inspiration and shifts the intra-ventricular septum leftward causing diastolic dysfunction of the left ventricle (LV) and incomplete LV filling. Large negative pleural pressures further impair LV emptying by increasing LV afterload (16). Rarely, these effects cause pulmonary edema. During forced exhalation, however, positive intra-thoracic pressure decreases venous return to the right heart setting up the cyclical changes in venous return that underlie the development of PP. Further complicating the cardiovascular response to asthma is the potential for lung hyperinflation to increase pulmonary vascular resistance and pulmonary artery pressures (17). A widened PP can be a valuable sign indicating asthma severity. However, the absence of a widened PP does not ensure a mild attack because PP decreases in the fatiguing patient unable to generate large swings in pleural pressure.

■ CLINICAL PRESENTATION, DIFFERENTIAL DIAGNOSIS, AND SEVERITY ASSESSMENT

Analysis of multiple factors, including the medical history, physical examination, objective measures of airflow obstruction, initial response to therapy, arterial blood gases, and chest radiography is all important in the assessment of acutely ill patients (18). Risk factors for asthma-related death including prior intubation should be identified. (Table 21.1) (11,19,20).

Differential Diagnosis

"All that wheezes is not asthma" is a fitting clinical saw worth considering during the initial evaluation. An extensive smoking history suggests chronic obstructive pulmonary disease and a more fixed form of expiratory airflow obstruction. Congestive heart failure may

TABLE 21.1   RISK FACTORS FOR FATAL OR NEAR-FATAL SEVERE ASTHMA
Frequent emergency department visits
Frequent hospitalization
Intensive care unit admission
Intubation
Hypercapnia
Barotrauma
Psychiatric illness
Medical noncompliance
Illicit drug abuse
Low socioeconomic status
Inadequate access to medical care
Use of more than two canisters per month of inhaled β agonist
Difficulty perceiving airflow obstruction
Comorbidities such as coronary artery disease
Sensitivity to *Alternaria* species

present with wheezing (termed *cardiac asthma*) that responds to bronchodilators (21). However, heart failure is typically associated with an enlarged cardiac silhouette, vascular redistribution, interstitial or pulmonary edema, and small lung volumes. Regardless of concerns regarding heart failure, myocardial ischemia should be considered in patients at risk for coronary artery disease, particularly those receiving high-dose bronchodilators. Moreover, ASA alone can trigger an imbalance between myocardial oxygen supply and demand (22).

Foreign body obstruction occasionally mimics asthma. It should be considered in the very young and old, in patients with altered mental status or neuromuscular disease, and when symptoms occur after eating or dental work. Localized wheeze and, rarely, asymmetric hyperinflation on chest radiography are clues to foreign body aspiration.

Upper airway obstruction including vocal cord dysfunction (VCD) should also be considered in the differential diagnosis of ASA. In contrast to asthma, classic upper airway (extra-thoracic) obstruction flattens the inspiratory portion of the flow-volume loop. Fiberoptic laryngoscopy should be considered when VCD is suspected because of normal oxygenation, lack of response to bronchodilators, normal airway pressures after prior intubation, or stridor to confirm paradoxical vocal cord movement (23). Significant response to helium-oxygen mixtures (heliox) also suggests upper airway obstruction, although heliox response likely occurs in some asthmatics and should not be used to distinguish upper from lower airway obstruction. In cases of suspected tracheal stenosis (e.g., from prior intubation), fiberoptic bronchoscopy, or spiral computed tomography (CT) are the tests of choice.

Pneumonia complicating asthma is unusual, but it should be considered in patients with fever, localizing signs, and refractory hypoxemia. Antibiotics are frequently prescribed for asthmatics with increased sputum production alone. Antibiotics have not been shown to improve outcome and should be reserved for treatment of concurrent sinusitis or pneumonia (19,24).

Wheezing occurs rarely in pulmonary embolism (25). When dyspnea is out of proportion to objective findings, particularly the peak expiratory flow rate (PEFR), consider evaluation with chest CT angiography, ventilation-perfusion imaging, d-dimer analysis, or lower extremity Doppler ultrasonography.

Physical Examination

The general appearance of the patient (posture, speech, positioning, and alertness) provides a quick guide to severity, response to therapy, and need for intubation. Patients assuming the upright position have a higher heart rate, respiratory rate, and pulsus paradoxus, and a significantly lower partial pressure of arterial oxygen (PaO_2) and PEFR than patients who are able to lie supine (26). Diaphoresis is associated with an even lower PEFR. Accessory muscle use and a widened PP indicate severe asthma; however, their absence does not exclude a severe attack (27). Depressed mental status suggests impending arrest and is an indication for intubation (19).

Examination of the head and neck helps identify barotrauma (crepitus) and upper airway obstruction (prolongation of inspiration and stridor). Tracheal deviation, asymmetric breath sounds, mediastinal crunch, and subcutaneous emphysema variably suggest pneumomediastinum, pneumothorax, or atelectasis. The mouth and neck should be inspected quickly for mass lesions, signs of previous surgery, and angioedema.

Chest auscultation typically reveals expiratory phase prolongation and wheeze. However, wheeze is not a reliable indicator of the severity of airflow obstruction (28). A silent chest indicates severe obstruction and impending respiratory arrest. (In this situation emerging wheeze signals improvement.) Localized wheeze or crackles may represent mucus plugging and atelectasis, but should prompt consideration of pneumonia, pneumothorax, endobronchial lesions, or foreign body.

Tachycardia is common (29). Heart rate generally decreases in improving patients, but some patients remain tachycardic despite clinical improvement because of medications. The usual rhythm is sinus tachycardia but supraventricular and ventricular arrhythmias occur; bradycardia is an ominous sign of imminent arrest (19).

Measurement of Airflow Obstruction

Measuring PEFR or forced expiratory volume in 1 second (FEV_1) helps assess the severity of airflow obstruction. Objective measures are important because physician estimates of severity are often wrong—with errors equally distributed between over- and underestimates of the actual PEFR. However, PEFRs are not always obtainable in severely dyspneic patients. Indeed it is wiser to defer measurements in the sickest subgroup because they rarely alter initial management and performing a PEFR maneuver may worsen bronchospasm even to the point of respiratory arrest (30).

According to the Expert Panel Report 3 of the National Institutes of Health, mild attacks are characterized by PEFR >70% of predicted or personal best, moderate attacks by PEFRs between 40% to 69%, severe attacks by PEFR <40%, and life-threatening attacks by PEFR <25% (19). Measuring the change in PEFR or FEV_1 is one of the best ways to predict the need for hospitalization. Several studies have demonstrated that inconsequential changes or deterioration after 30 to 60 minutes of therapy predicts a more severe course and need for hospitalization (31).

Arterial Blood Gases

In patients with severe or life-threatening ASA, arterial blood gas analysis demonstrates the degree of hypoxemia and allows for acid-base analysis. In the early stages of ASA, mild hypoxemia and respiratory alkalosis are common. As the severity of airflow obstruction increases, $PaCO_2$ generally increases so that eucapnia and hypercapnia are worrisome findings; however, hypercapnia alone is not an indication for intubation as many of these patients respond adequately to pharmacotherapy (32). Conversely, the absence of hypercapnia does not rule out a life-threatening attack (33).

Patients with persistent respiratory alkalosis compensate by wasting serum bicarbonate which manifests later as a normal anion gap metabolic acidosis (referred to as post hypocapneic metabolic acidosis). Metabolic acidosis with an elevated anion gap may stem from lactic acidosis secondary to increased work of breathing, tissue hypoxia, or intracellular alkalosis. Lactic acidosis indicates a severe exacerbation and occurs more commonly in men and in patients receiving parenteral β agonists (34).

Serial blood gases are not necessary to determine clinical course. In most cases, valid judgments follow serial examinations with attention to patient posture, accessory muscle use, diaphoresis, chest auscultation, pulse oximetry, and PEFR measurements. Patients who deteriorate on these grounds are candidates for intubation regardless of $PaCO_2$. Conversely, patients improving by multifactorial assessment should not be intubated despite hypercapnia. Serial blood gases are required in mechanically ventilated patients to guide ventilator management.

Chest Radiography

In classic cases of ASA, chest X-rays rarely alter management (35). In one study (36) reporting radiographic abnormalities in 34% of cases, the majority of findings were likely attributable to common asthma features of airway wall thickening and intraluminal mucus. Chest radiography is thus best reserved for cases with localizing signs or symptoms and when the diagnosis is in question. In mechanically ventilated patients, chest radiography further confirms proper endotracheal tube position.

■ EMERGENCY DEPARTMENT MANAGEMENT

Patients with mild to moderate attacks responding well to initial therapy may be considered for discharge. Observation in the ED for at least 60 minutes after the last β-agonist treatment helps ensure suitability for discharge. Patients should receive written medication instructions, a written asthma action plan, and instructions for follow-up. Invariably patients should be discharged on inhaled and/or oral steroids. Patients presenting with a mild exacerbation that completely resolves after bronchodilators may be discharged on inhaled steroids or the combination of a long-acting β agonist and inhaled steroid, particularly if they were not previously on controller therapy. Patients with incomplete responses or attacks of greater severity should receive a course of oral steroids such as subcutaneously an 8-day course of 40 mg/day prednisone (37). Alternatively, a single dose of triamcinolone diacetate 40 mg intramuscularly also has been reported to be as effective as prednisone 40 mg/day for 5 days (38). When considering hospitalization, health care providers should err on the side of admission when there is a risky home environment or directly observed therapy is needed in the case of noncompliance.

Clearly patients with more severe attacks, or who demonstrate a lackluster response or a deteriorating response to initial therapy require hospital admission. Indications for intensive care unit admission include frank or impending respiratory arrest, progressive hypercapnia, mechanical ventilation, altered mental status, cardiac arrhythmias, myocardial injury, and need for frequent bronchodilator treatments (19).

■ PHARMACOLOGIC THERAPY

Oxygen

Supplemental oxygen by nasal cannula is titrated to maintain arterial oxygen saturations greater than 92%

(>95% with pregnancy and ischemic heart disease). Adequate oxygenation is generally not difficult to achieve with low-flow supplementation (see above) and is important in maintaining oxygen delivery to tissue beds and minimizing hypoxic pulmonary vasoconstriction. Supplemental oxygen further protects against hypoxemia resulting from β agonist–induced pulmonary vasodilation and increased blood flow to low V/Q units (39).

ββ Agonists

Inhaled short-acting β agonists such as albuterol and levalbuterol are used to treat the smooth muscle–mediated bronchoconstriction of ASA. Approximately two-thirds of patients respond convincingly to initial inhaled therapy in the ED, leaving one-third of patients with a lackluster response. This latter group invariably requires prolonged treatment in the ED or admission to hospital. In the study by Rodrigo and Rodrigo, 67% of patients improved significantly and were discharged from the ED after 2.4 mg albuterol (Fig. 21.1) (40). Half of the responders in this study met discharge criteria

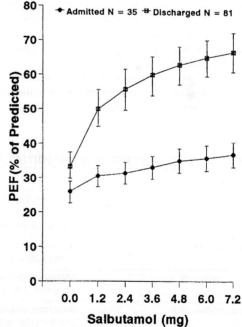

■ **FIGURE 21.1** Dose–response relationship to 4 puffs albuterol (400 μg) every 10 minutes in 116 acute asthmatics. Sixty-seven percent of patients achieved discharge criteria after administration of 2.4 mg albuterol within 1 hour; half of the responders met discharge criteria after 12 puffs. Patients with a blunted cumulative dose-response relationship were hospitalized. (Reprinted with permission from Rodrigo C, Rodrigo G. Therapeutic response patterns to high and cumulative doses of salbutamol in acute severe asthma. *Chest* 1998;113:593.)

after receiving only 12 puffs of albuterol. Similarly, Strauss and co-workers found that two-thirds of patients with acute asthma could be discharged after three 2.5-mg doses of albuterol by nebulization every 20 minutes (41).

The optimal dose of albuterol in ASA has yet to be established. McFadden and colleagues compared two 5.0-mg nebulized treatments of albuterol over 40 minutes with three 2.5-mg albuterol every 20 minutes in 160 ED patients (42), demonstrating a dose–response relationship between albuterol and PEFR. One 5 mg albuterol dose achieved the same effect as two doses of 2.5 mg, and 10 mg albuterol resulted in higher PEFRs than 7.5 mg. The 5-mg regimen increased peak flows more rapidly and to a greater extent than the standard 2.5-mg approach. Patients receiving 5-mg doses reached discharge criteria quicker and left the ED with higher PEFRs. There was also a trend toward fewer hospitalizations in the high-dose group (25 of 80 patients, 31%) than in the lower dose group (37 of 80 patients, 46%) ($p = 0.06$). However, Emerman and colleagues compared the effects of three doses of 2.5 or 7.5 mg albuterol every 20 minutes in 160 acutely ill asthmatics, finding no differences in spirometry or admission rates (43). In sum, these data support the standard recommendation of administering albuterol 2.5 mg by nebulization every 20 minutes during the first hour of treatment (i.e., 3 doses); for more severe exacerbations 10 mg to 15 mg of albuterol by continuous nebulization may be used (19).

Albuterol should be used in a continuous or repetitive manner until there is convincing improvement or side effects limit further administration (Table 21.2)

(44). Fortunately, high-doses of inhaled β agonists are generally well tolerated. Tremor and tachycardia are common, but significant cardiovascular morbidity is rare (45).

Racemic albuterol consists of equal amounts of R- and S-albuterol. The R isomer confers bronchodilator effects whereas the S isomer has been viewed as either inert or pro-inflammatory. These observations provide the rationale for using just the R-isomer or levalbuterol. Emerging data suggest that levalbuterol is at least as effective as albuterol in children and adults. A large, multicenter and prospective trial enrolled acutely ill asthmatics with an FEV_1 between 20% and 55% of predicted (46). Patients received prednisone and either 1.25 mg levalbuterol or 2.5 mg of racemic albuterol every 20 minutes over the first hour, then every 40 minutes for 3 additional doses, and finally as needed for up to 24 hours. There was no difference between groups for the primary endpoint of time to meeting discharge criteria. However, levalbuterol improved FEV_1 more than albuterol after the first dose (0.5 L versus 0.43 L, P = 0.02), particularly in patients not recently on inhaled or oral steroids. In this same subgroup of steroid naïve patients, fewer patients were admitted in the levalbuterol group (3.8% versus 9.3%, P = 0.03).

Inhaled β agonists can be delivered well by metered-dose inhaler (MDI) or hand-held nebulizer. Four to 12 puffs by MDI with spacer achieves the same degree of bronchodilation as one 2.5-mg nebulized treatment of albuterol (47). MDIs with spacers carry the advantage of lesser cost and faster drug delivery times; hand-held nebulizers require fewer instructions, less supervision, and less coordination.

TABLE 21.2 DRUGS USED IN THE INITIAL TREATMENT OF ACUTE ASTHMA IN ADULTS

Standard Therapies	
Albuterol	2.5 mg in 2.5 mL normal saline by nebulization every 20 minutes three times over the first hour or 4 to 8 puffs by MDI with spacer every 20 minutes three times; for intubated patients, titrate to physiologic effect and side effects.
Epinephrine	0.3 mL of a 1:1,000 solution subcutaneously every 20 min three times. Use with caution in older patients.
Corticosteroids	Methylprednisolone 40 mg to 60 mg intravenously every 6 to 12 hours or prednisone 40 mg orally every 12 hours.
Anticholinergics	Ipratropium bromide 0.5 mg by nebulization every 20 min three times in combination with albuterol, or 4 to 8 puffs by MDI with spacer every 20 min for 3 doses.
Adjunctive Therapies	
Magnesium sulfate	2 g intravenously over 20 min, repeat in 20 min (total dose 4 g unless hypomagnesemic).
Heliox	80:20 or 70:30 helium:oxygen mix by tight-fitting, non-rebreathing face mask. Higher helium concentrations are needed for maximal effect.

MDI, metered-dose inhaler

Long-acting β agonists are not indicated in the initial treatment of ASA, although formoterol (which has acute onset of action) may prove effective. However, the addition of a long-acting β agonist to albuterol in hospitalized asthmatics appears to be safe and results in greater improvements in FEV_1 after 48 hours compared with placebo (48).

There is no advantage to parenteral administration of β agonists in the initial management of ASA unless the patient is unable to comply with inhaled therapy (such as those with altered mental status and impending cardiopulmonary arrest) (49). However, lack of response to several hours of inhaled β-agonist therapy may be an indication for subcutaneous epinephrine in patients at low risk for complications (50). Intravenous β agonists are not recommended, with the possible exception of patients in cardiac arrest, because they are less effective and more toxic than their inhaled counterparts. (51).

Ipratropium Bromide

Bronchodilating properties of ipratropium bromide are modest, precluding its use as a sole drug in asthma. However, data support adding ipratropium to albuterol in the initial management of severe cases of ASA, decreasing time in the ED, albuterol dose requirements and hospitalization rates (52,53).

To the contrary, Weber and colleagues conducted a prospective, randomized, double-blind, placebo-controlled trial of 67 patients receiving either a combination of albuterol plus ipratropium bromide or albuterol alone by continuous nebulization for a maximum of 3 hours (54). Primary outcome measures were improvement in PEFR, hospital admission rates, and length of stay in the ED. Although trends favored combination therapy, differences did not reach statistical significance. Fitzgerald et al. have reported similar results (55); in children, Ducharme and Davis did not demonstrate benefit from combination therapy in their study of nearly 300 asthmatics with mild to moderate acute asthma (56).

To study high and cumulative doses of ipratropium bromide plus albuterol, Rodrigo and Rodrigo conducted a double-blind, randomized, prospective trial of albuterol plus ipratropium bromide versus albuterol plus placebo in 180 patients with acute asthma (57). Four puffs of combination therapy by MDI with spacer totaling 480 μg albuterol and 84 μg ipratropium bromide were administered every 10 minutes for 3 hours compared to 4 puffs of albuterol with placebo every 10 minutes for the same duration. Combination therapy improved spirometric measures more than albuterol alone and decreased the rate of hospitalization. Subgroup analysis showed that patients with more severe obstruction and symptoms for more than 24 hours prior to presentation were most likely to benefit from the addition of ipratropium bromide.

The current recommendation is to mix ipratropium bromide 0.5 mg (0.25 mg to 0.5 mg in children) with albuterol in the same nebulizer and deliver 3 treatments over the first hour to patients in severe exacerbation (19). Once the patient is admitted, however, there are no data to support continued combination therapy in adults; in hospitalized children, two controlled trials failed to demonstrate benefit (58,59).

Corticosteroids

Systemic corticosteroids should be quickly prescribed to most patients unless there has been an immediate and marked response to β agonists alone. Because corticosteroids treat airway wall inflammation by promoting new protein synthesis, their effects may not be apparent for several hours. This delay may explain the results of some studies demonstrating that corticosteroid use in the ED does not improve lung function acutely or decrease hospitalization rates (60). However, two controlled trials have shown benefit to the early use of methylprednisolone. Littenberg and Gluck showed intravenous (IV) methylprednisolone 125 mg given on presentation reduced the number of hospitalizations. Lin et al. studied the effects of methylprednisolone 125 mg IV in ED patients with PEFRs <50% of predicted after initial albuterol therapy. In their study methylprednisolone treated patients had improved PEFRs at 1 and 2 hours and a trend toward decreased rates of hospitalization compared to controls. Early benefit to the use of systemic steroids was further demonstrated by recent meta-analysis (61). Corticosteroids have also been shown to improve the speed of acute asthma resolution, the number of relapses in the first week or two after treatment, and the risk of asthma-related mortality (62,63).

Whether there is a dose-response relationship to systemic steroids in acute asthma is not clear. Manser et al. found low doses (<80 mg/day of methylprednisolone) were adequate in the management of hospitalized adults (64). Emerman and Cydulka compared 100-mg and 500-mg doses of methylprednisolone administered in the ED, finding no benefit to higher dose therapy (65).

The recommendation of the Expert Panel 3 report is to administer 40 mg to 80 mg/day of prednisone, methylprednisolone, or prednisolone in one or two divided doses until the PEFR reaches 70% of predicted or personal best (19). Orally administered therapy is as effective as parenteral therapy but should be avoided in patients at risk for intubation (66).

There is a limited role for inhaled corticosteroids in the management of acute asthma. Rodrigo and Rodrigo conducted a randomized, double-blind trial of flunisolide 1 mg or placebo added to 400 μg salbutamol delivered by MDI every 10 minutes for 3 hours in 94 ED patients not on systemic steroids (67). PEFRs and FEV_1 were approximately 20% higher in the flunisolide group beginning at 90 minutes. On the other hand, other investigators using different inhaled steroids and different protocols have not demonstrated efficacy in this setting (68,69).

Inhaled corticosteroids play a pivotal role in achieving outpatient asthma control. Patients discharged from an ED or hospital after successful treatment of acute asthma should receive an inhaled steroid or the combination of an inhaled steroid with a long-acting β agonist to help achieve control and prevent future attacks.

Theophylline and Aminophylline

On the whole, the data do not support the use of theophylline in acute asthma. Parameswaran et al. conducted a meta-analysis for the *Cochrane Review* and concluded that the use of intravenous aminophylline does not result in additional bronchodilation in adults compared to standard therapy with inhaled short-acting β-adrenergic agonists and that the frequency of adverse effects was higher with aminophylline use (70). The Expert Panel Report 3 does not recommend use of theophylline for adults or children in the ED or hospital setting (19).

In patients taking theophylline, serum concentrations should be checked on arrival to the ED before additional theophylline is prescribed. If the serum level is therapeutic and adverse effects have not been identified, then a continuous infusion may be started (or the oral preparation continued).

Magnesium Sulfate

Prospective trials have yielded conflicting results regarding the efficacy of magnesium sulfate ($MgSO_4$) in acute asthma. Several studies have failed to show a benefit to adding $MgSO_4$ to standard therapies (71); others have demonstrated improved lung function and/or decreased hospitalization rates (72). Published meta-analyses have also reached different conclusions (73). In their meta-analysis for the *Cochrane Review*, Rowe et al. concluded that routine use of IV $MgSO_4$ was not indicated in adults with acute asthma (74). However, these authors further concluded that $MgSO_4$ was safe and improved spirometry in the subgroup of patients with severe exacerbations. Further data support the use of inhaled $MgSO_4$ as a vehicle for nebulized albuterol in acute asthma (75).

Leukotriene Modifiers

Limited data support the use of leukotriene receptor antagonists in ASA. The most compelling study is a randomized, double-blinded, parallel group trial by Camargo et al. in 201 acutely ill asthmatics (76). When added to standard therapy, IV montelukast improved FEV_1 over the first 20 minutes compared to placebo (14.8% versus 3.6%, P = 0.007). Effects were seen within 10 minutes and lasted for 2 hours. Of note, montelukast

is not currently available for IV administration in the United States.

Heliox

Heliox consists of 20% oxygen and 80% helium (30:70% mixtures are also available). This low-density gas can be delivered by tight-fitting face mask in an attempt to lower work of breathing; alternatively it has been used as the driving gas for albuterol nebulization. Data regarding efficacy in ASA are mixed. Several studies have failed to demonstrate that heliox is beneficial in nonintubated patients, including a recent meta-analysis of six randomized controlled trials involving a total of 369 adults and children (77). A recent study further failed to demonstrate a benefit to heliox as a driving gas for albuterol nebulization (78). To the contrary, there are data supporting a benefit to heliox-driven over oxygen-driven albuterol nebulization in children and adults (79). Methodological differences between studies, small patient numbers, and failure to control for upper airway obstruction preclude strong conclusions at this time; however, it is reasonable to consider heliox-driven albuterol nebulization in patients with life-threatening acute asthma.

Antibiotics

In their 2007 update, the Expert Panel did not recommend antibiotics for most patients with acute asthma unless necessary to treat comorbid conditions such as pneumonia or bacterial sinusitis (19). However, this recommendation is based more on consensus than data as there are very few well designed studies available for review.

■ MECHANICAL VENTILATION

Noninvasive Positive Pressure Ventilation

Soroksky et al. have reported their prospective, randomized, controlled trial of Noninvasive positive pressure ventilation (NPPV in 15 adult asthmatics compared to 15 asthmatic control patients receiving sham NPPV for 3 hours (80). NPPV improved lung function (mean rise in FEV_1 was 53.5 ± 23.4% in NPPV- treated patients compared to 28.5 ± 22.6% in the control group, P = 0.006) and decreased hospitalization rates (17.6% in the NPPV group versus 62.5% in the control group, P = 0.013). Ram et al. analyzed the literature to determine the efficacy of NPPV in adults with ASA compared to standard therapy (81). Ten of 11 identified trials were excluded for analysis leaving only the above study by Soroksky for analysis. Ram concluded that Soroksky's data are promising but that larger controlled trials are required.

Thill et al. conducted a prospective, randomized, crossover study of NPPV in children with acute lower airway obstruction (82). Twenty children were randomized to receive either 2 hours of NPPV followed by 2 hours of standard therapy (group 1) or 2 hours of standard therapy followed by 2 hours of NPPV (group 2). Results demonstrated that NPPV was associated with lower clinical asthma score (CAS) and improvements in respiratory rate, accessory muscle use, wheezing, and dyspnea. Discontinuation of NPPV in group 1 at the 2-hour crossover point resulted in an increase in respiratory rate and CAS score. NPPV did not improve oxygen saturation or transcutaneous CO_2 measurements but NPPV-treated patients required less supplemental oxygen to maintain adequate oxygen saturations.

Although the data are limited, use of NPPV is sensible in patients with life-threatening exacerbations who are alert, cooperative, and hemodynamically stable and not in need of endotracheal intubation to protect the airway or clear secretions. Reasonable initial settings are IPAP 10 cmH_2O and EPAP 0 cmH_2O. After the mask is secured and the patient is breathing synchronously, IPAP can be increased quickly to 12 cmH_2O to 15 cmH_2O and EPAP to 5 cmH_2O to decrease respiratory rate, work of breathing, and dyspnea.

Intubation

Respiratory arrest and impending respiratory arrest (e.g., extreme exhaustion, a quiet chest, or altered mental status) are clear indications for intubation. Oral intubation is preferred because it allows for a larger endotracheal tube which decreases airway resistance and facilitates removal of intraluminal mucus. Nasal intubation may be considered in an awake patient anticipated to be difficult to intubate and mask ventilate in the supine position (e.g., a short, obese patient), but this approach mandates a smaller endotracheal tube and increases the risk of sinusitis.

Post-intubation Hypotension

The immediate post-intubation period can be extremely challenging and considerable care must be taken to stabilize the patient through the thoughtful use of sedatives, bronchodilators, fluids, and positive pressure ventilation. One pressing concern is post-intubation hypotension. Hypotension occurs for several reasons including sedation, loss of sympathetic activity, and hypovolemia from increased insensible losses and decreased oral fluid intake. Overzealous Ambu-bag ventilation can also result in dangerous levels of DHI and elevated airway pressures. This decreases venous return on to hypotension and tachycardia. When this occurs a 30 to 60 second trial of hypopnea (2 to 3 breaths/min) or apnea in a pre-oxygenated patient is both diagnostic and therapeutic. This maneuver deflates the lung by prolonging expiratory time and helps restore hemodynamic parameters.

Failure of a deflation trail to improve cardiopulmonary stability mandates immediate consideration of unilateral or bilateral tension pneumothorax. (Note that hemodynamic improvement with deflation does not completely exclude tension pneumothorax.) Management of pneumothorax consists of urgent tube thoracostomy and volume resuscitation.

Initial Ventilator Settings and Dynamic Hyperinflation

During mechanical ventilation, the expiratory time, tidal volume, and severity of airway obstruction determine the level of DHI. Because airway obstruction is generally refractory in this subgroup of patients, expiratory time and tidal volume are the key manipulable variables during ventilator management. Expiratory time is determined by minute ventilation (respiratory rate tidal volume) and inspiratory flow rate (83,84). When minute ventilation is increased, expiratory time is shortened and there is more DHI. To avoid dangerous levels of DHI, the initial minute ventilation should not exceed 115 mL/kg/min or approximately 8 L/min in a 70-kg patient (85). To this end, we recommend a respiratory rate of 12 to 14 breaths/min and a tidal volume of 7 mL/kg to 8 mL/kg. The use of relatively low tidal volumes avoids excessive peak lung inflation.

High inspiratory flow rates further prolong expiratory time, but also may result in tachypnea and unduly elevated peak airway pressures. We favor an inspiratory flow rate of 60 L/min, using a square flow pattern (i.e., a constant flow rate). This strategy often results in high peak airway pressures, but high peak airway pressures per se do not correlate with morbidity or mortality. Rather it is the state of lung hyperinflation that appears to predict outcome (85).

There is no consensus as to which ventilator mode should be used in asthmatic patients. In paralyzed patients, synchronized intermittent mandatory ventilation (SIMV) and assist-controlled ventilation are equivalent. In patients triggering the ventilator, assist-controlled ventilation may increase minute ventilation more than SIMV, but SIMV may increase work of breathing. Volume-controlled ventilation is recommended over pressure-controlled ventilation (PC) for several reasons, including staff familiarity with its use. PC offers the advantage of limiting peak airway pressure to a predetermined set value. However, during PC, tidal volume is inversely related to auto-PEEP and minute ventilation is not guaranteed.

Ventilator-applied PEEP is not recommended in sedated and paralyzed patients because it may increase lung volume if used excessively (86). In spontaneously breathing patients, small amounts of ventilator-applied PEEP (e.g., 5 cm H_2O) decrease inspiratory work of breathing by decreasing the pressure gradient required to overcome auto-PEEP.

Assessing Lung Inflation

Determination of the severity of DHI is central to risk assessment and adjustment of ventilator settings. Numerous methods have been proposed to measure DHI. The volume at end-inspiration, termed Vei, is determined by collecting expired gas from total lung capacity to functional residual capacity during 40 to 60 seconds of apnea. A Vei of greater than 20 mL/kg has been correlated with barotrauma (85). Indeed, Vei is the only measure of DHI that has been shown to predict barotrauma (even though it may underestimate the degree of air trapping with very slowly emptying air spaces). The utility of this measure is limited by the need for paralysis and the fact that most clinicians and respiratory therapists are unfamiliar with expiratory gas collection.

Surrogate measures of lung inflation include the single-breath plateau pressure (Pplat) and auto-PEEP. Pplat is an estimate of average end-inspiratory alveolar pressures determined by stopping flow at end-inspiration. Auto-PEEP is the lowest average alveolar pressure achieved during the respiratory cycle. It is obtained by measuring airway opening pressure during an end-expiratory hold maneuver. In the presence of auto-PEEP, airway opening pressure increases by the amount of auto-PEEP present. Persistence of expiratory gas flow at the beginning of inspiration (which can be detected by auscultation or monitoring of flow tracings) also suggests auto-PEEP.

Accurate measurement of Pplat and auto-PEEP requires patient–ventilator synchrony and absence of patient effort. Unfortunately, both measures are problematic and neither has been proved to predict complications. Pplat is affected by the entire respiratory system, including lung tissue and chest wall; thus, significant variations in DHI may occur from patient to patient at the same pressure. For example, an obese patient will likely have a higher Pplat than a thin patient for the same degree of DHI. Despite these limitations, experience suggests that a Pplat <30 cm H_2O is generally associated with good outcomes.

Auto-PEEP may underestimate the severity of DHI (87). This occurs when severe airway narrowing limits the communication between the alveolus and mouth so that during an end-exhalation hold maneuver airway opening pressure fails to increase. In most cases, however, auto-PEEP of less than 15 cm H_2O appears to be acceptable.

Ventilator Adjustments

With the above considerations in mind, we offer the following algorithm for ventilator adjustment. This algorithm relies on Pplat as the measure of DHI and arterial pH as a marker of ventilation. If initial ventilator settings result in Pplat of more than 30 cm H_2O,

respiratory rate should be decreased until this goal is achieved. Hypercapnia may ensue, but fortunately this is generally well tolerated (88). Anoxic brain injury and myocardial dysfunction are contraindications to permissive hypercapnia because it causes cerebral vasodilation, decreased myocardial contractility, and pulmonary vasoconstriction (89). If hypercapnia results in a blood pH of less than 7.15 (and respiratory rate cannot be increased because of the Pplat limit), we consider a slow infusion of sodium bicarbonate, although this has not been shown to improve outcome. If Pplat is less than 30 cm H_2O and pH is less than 7.20, respiratory rate can be safely increased to lower $PaCO_2$ and elevate arterial pH until Pplat nears the threshold pressure. Commonly, patients can be ventilated to a pH of more than 7.20 with a Pplat of less than 30 cm H_2O, particularly as they improve and near extubation.

Sedation and Paralysis

Sedation is indicated to improve comfort, safety, and patient–ventilator synchrony. This is particularly true when hypercapnia serves as a potent stimulus to respiratory drive. Some patients (such as those with sudden asphyxic asthma) may be extubated within hours. In these patients, propofol is attractive because it can be rapidly titrated to a deep level of sedation and still allow for quick awakening after discontinuation (90). Benzodiazepines, such as lorazepam and midazolam, are alternatives, but time to awakening after discontinuation of these drugs is longer and less predictable than with propofol.

To provide the best combination of amnesia, sedation, analgesia, and suppression of respiratory drive, we recommend the addition of a narcotic (best given by continuous infusion) to either propofol or a benzodiazepine. Regardless of strategy, sedative and analgesic agents should be held daily to assess mental status (91).

Ketamine, an intravenous anesthetic with sedative, analgesic, and bronchodilating properties, is generally reserved for intubated patients with severe bronchospasm precluding safe mechanical ventilation (92). Ketamine must be used with caution because of its sympathomimetic effects and ability to cause delirium.

When safe and effective mechanical ventilation cannot be achieved by sedation alone, consider short-term muscle paralysis. Short- to intermediate-acting agents include atracurium, cis-atracurium, and vecuronium. Pancuronium is a longer acting drug that may cause untoward tachycardia. Pancuronium and atracurium both release histamine, but the clinical significance of this property is doubtful (93). We prefer cis-atracurium because it is essentially free of cardiovascular effects, does not release histamine, and does not require hepatic and renal function for clearance.

Paralytics may be given intermittently by bolus or continuous intravenous infusion. Continuous infusions require a nerve stimulator or withholding the drug every 4 to 6 hours to avoid accumulation and prolonged paralysis. Paralytic agents should be minimized whenever possible because of the risk of post-paralytic myopathy (94).

Administration of Bronchodilators during Mechanical Ventilation

Many questions remain regarding the optimal administration of inhaled bronchodilators during mechanical ventilation, with the common problem being inadequate drug delivery. Manthous et al. compared the efficacy of albuterol delivered by MDI via a simple inspiratory adapter (no spacer) to nebulized albuterol in mechanically ventilated patients (95). Using the peak-to-pause pressure gradient at a constant inspiratory flow to measure airway resistance, they found no effect (and no side effects) from the administration of 100 puffs (9.0 mg) of albuterol; whereas albuterol delivered by nebulizer to a total dose of 2.5 mg reduced inspiratory flow-resistive pressure by 18%. Increasing the nebulized dose to a total of 7.5 mg reduced airway resistance further in 8 of 10 patients, but caused side effects in half of these patients. When MDIs are used during mechanical ventilation, they must be delivered by a spacing device on the inspiratory limb of the ventilator (96). In general, nebulizers should be placed close to the ventilator, and in-line humidifiers stopped during treatments. Inspiratory flow should be reduced to approximately 40 L/min during treatments to minimize turbulence, although this strategy has the potential to worsen lung hyperinflation and must be time-limited. Patient–ventilator synchrony is crucial to optimize drug delivery. In either case (MDI with spacer or nebulizer), higher drug dosages are required and dosage should be titrated to achieve a decrease in the peak-to-pause airway pressure gradient. If no measurable decrease in airway resistance occurs, other causes of elevated airway resistance such as a kinked or plugged endotracheal tube should be excluded.

Other Considerations

Rarely, the above strategies are unable to stabilize the ventilated patient and consideration should be given to the use of other strategies. Halothane and enflurane are general anesthetic bronchodilators that can reduce Ppk and $PaCO_2$ (97). These agents cause myocardial depression, arterial vasodilation, and arrhythmias, and their benefits do not last after drug discontinuation. Heliox delivered through the ventilator circuit may decrease Ppk and $PaCO_2$ (98). However, safe use of heliox requires significant institutional expertise and careful planning. Ventilator flow meters that are gas-density dependent must be recalibrated to low-density gas, and a spirometer should be placed on the expiratory port of the ventilator during heliox administration to measure tidal volume. Strategies to mobilize mucus, such as chest physiotherapy and mucolytics are not recommended because they are of unproven value and may worsen bronchospasm.

Extubation

Although some patients with labile asthma respond to therapy within hours, more typically patients require 24 to 48 hours of bronchodilator and/or anti-inflammatory therapy before they are ready for extubation. Patients should be considered for a spontaneous breathing trial once they are alert or easily arousable, have minimal oxygen requirements and normalized their PCO_2, require infrequent suctioning, and are hemodynamically stable. If pneumonia, central nervous system injury, or muscle weakness has not complicated the patient's course, progression to spontaneous breathing should be prompt. Patients successfully completing a 30- to 120-minute spontaneous breathing trial are evaluated for extubation. After extubation, observation in the intensive care unit is recommended for an additional 12 to 24 hours.

■ REFERENCES

1. Chapman KR, Boulet LP, Rea RM, et al. Suboptimal asthma control: prevalence, detection and consequences in general practice. *Eur Respir J.* 2008;31:320–325.
2. Mannino DM, Homa DM, Akinbami LJ, et al. Surveillance for Asthma—United States, 1980–1999. *MMWR.* March 29, 2002/51(SS01); 1–13.
3. Krishnan V, Diette GB, Rand CS, et al. Mortality in patients hospitalized for asthma exacerbations in the United States. *Am J Respir Crit Care Med.* 2006;174:633–638.
4. Getahun D, Demissie K, Rhoads GG. Recent trends in asthma hospitalization and mortality in the United States. *J Asthma.* 2005;42:373–378.
5. Lugogo NL, Macintyre NR. Life-threatening asthma: pathophysiology and management. *Respir Care.* 2008;53(6):726–739.
6. Corbridge T, Hall JB. The assessment and management of status asthmaticus in adults. *Am J Respir Crit Care Med.* 1995;151:1296–1316.
7. McFadden ER Jr. Acute severe asthma: state of the art. *Am J Respir Crit Care Med.* 2003;168:740–759.
8. Barr RG, Woodruff PG, Clark S, et al. Sudden-onset asthma exacerbations: clinical features, response to therapy, and 2-week follow-up. Multicenter Airway Research Collaboration (MARC) investigators. *Eur Respir J.* 2000;15;266–273.
9. Wasserfallen JB, Schaller MD, Feihl F, et al. Sudden asphyxic asthma: a distinct entity? *Am Rev Respir Dis.* 1990;142:108–111.
10. Sur S, Crotty TB, Kephart GM, et al. Sudden-onset fatal asthma: a distinct clinical entity with few eosinophils and relatively more neutrophils in the airway submucosa. *Am Rev Respir Dis.* 1993;148:713–729.
11. Cygan J, Trunsky M, Corbridge T. Inhaled heroin-induced status asthmaticus. *Chest.* 2000;117:272–275.
12. Rodrigo G, Rodrigo C. Rapid-onset asthma attack: a prospective cohort study about characteristics and response to emergency department treatment. *Chest.* 2000;118:1547–1552.
13. Yanos J, Wood LDH, Davis K, et al. The effect of respiratory and lactic acidosis on diaphragm function. *Am Rev Respir Dis.* 1993; 147:616–729.
14. Rodriguez-Roisin R, Ballester E, Roca J, et al. Mechanisms of hypoxemia in patients with status asthmaticus requiring mechanical ventilation. *Am Rev Respir Dis.* 1989;139:732–739.
15. Ferrer A, Roca J, Wagner PD, et al. Airway obstruction and ventilation–perfusion relationships in acute severe asthma. *Am Rev Respir Dis.* 1993;147:579–584.
16. Scharf S, Brown R, Saunders N, et al. Effects of normal and loaded spontaneous inspiration on cardiovascular function. *J Appl Physiol.* 1979;47:582–590.

17. Corbridge T, Hall JB. Pulmonary hypertension in status asthmaticus. In: Cosentino AM, Martin RJ, eds. *Cardiothoracic Interrelationships in Clinical Practice.* Armonk, NY: Futura;1997:137–156.

18. Rodrigo G, Rodrigo C. Assessment of the patient with acute asthma in the emergency department: a factor analytic study. *Chest.* 1993; 104:1325–1328.

19. National Heart, Lung and Blood Institute. *Expert Panel Report 3: Guidelines for the diagnosis and management of asthma (EPR-3 2007).* NIH Item No. 08-4051. Bethesda, MD: National Institutes of Health, 2007. http://www.nhlbi.nih.gov/guidelines/asthma/asthgdln.pdf.

20. Levenson T, Greenberger PA, Donoghue ER, et al. Asthma deaths confounded by substance abuse: an assessment of fatal asthma. *Chest.* 1996;110:604–610.

21. Fishman AP. Cardiac asthma—a fresh look at an old wheeze. *N Engl J Med.* 1989;320:1346–1348.

22. Scharf S. Mechanical cardiopulmonary interactions with asthma. *Clin Rev Allergy.* 1985;3:487–500.

23. Baughman RP, Loudon RC. Stridor: differentiation from wheezing or upper airway noise. *Am Rev Respir Dis.* 1989;139:1407–1419.

24. Graham VAL, Knowles GK, Milton AF, et al. Routine antibiotics in hospital management of acute asthma. *Lancet* 1982;1:418–420.

25. Hall JB, Wood LDH. Management of the critically ill asthmatic patient. *Med Clin North Am.* 1990;74:779–796.

26. Brenner BE, Abraham E, Simon RR. Position and diaphoresis in acute asthma. *Am J Med.* 1983;74:1005–1009.

27. Kelsen SG, Kelsen DP, Fleegler BF, et al. Emergency room assessment and treatment of patients with acute asthma. *Am J Med.* 1978;64:622–628.

28. Shim CS, Williams MH. Relationship of wheezing to the severity of obstruction in asthma. *Arch Intern Med.* 1983;143:890–892.

29. Josephson GW, Kennedy HL, MacKenzie EJ. Cardiac dysrhythmias during the treatment of acute asthma: a comparison of two treatment regimens by a double blind protocol. *Chest.* 1980;78:429–435.

30. Lemarchand P, Labrune S, Herer B, et al. Cardiorespiratory arrest following peak expiratory flow measurement during attack of asthma. *Chest.* 1991;100:1168–1169.

31. Rodrigo G, Rodrigo C. Early prediction of poor response in acute asthma patients in the emergency department. *Chest.* 1998;114:1016–1021.

32. Mountain RD, Sahn S. Clinical features and outcome in patients with acute asthma presenting with hypercapnia. *Am Rev Respir Dis.* 1988;138:535–539.

33. McFadden ER Jr, Lyons HA. Arterial-blood gas tension in asthma. *N Engl J Med.* 1968;278:1027–1032.

34. Mountain RD, Heffner JE, Brackett NC. Acid-base disturbances in acute asthma. *Chest.* 1990;98:651–655.

35. Sherman S, Skoney JA, Ravikrishnan KP. Routine chest radiographs in exacerbations of acute obstructive pulmonary disease. *Arch Intern Med.* 1989;149:2493–2496.

36. White CS, Cole RP, Lubetsky HW, et al. Acute asthma: admission chest radiography in hospitalized adult patients. *Chest.* 1991;100:14–16.

37. Cydulka RK, Emerman CL. A pilot study of steroid therapy after emergency department treatment of acute asthma: is a taper needed? *J Emerg Med.* 1998;16:15–19.

38. Schuckman H, DeJulius DP, Blanda M, et al. Comparison of intramuscular triamcinolone and oral prednisone in the outpatient treatment of acute asthma: a randomized controlled trial. *Ann Emerg Med.* 1998;31:333–338.

39. Ballester E, Reyes A, Roca J, et al. Ventilation–perfusion mismatching in acute severe asthma: effects of salbutamol and 100% oxygen. *Thorax.* 1989;44:258–267.

40. Rodrigo C, Rodrigo G. Therapeutic response patterns to high and cumulative doses of salbutamol in acute severe asthma. *Chest.* 1998;113:593–598.

41. Strauss L, Hejal R, Galan G, et al. Observations of the effects of aerosolized albuterol in acute asthma. *Am J Respir Crit Care Med.* 1997;155:454–458.

42. McFadden ER Jr, Strauss L, Hejal R, et al. Comparison of two dosage regimens of albuterol in acute asthma. *Am J Med.* 1998;105:12–17.

43. Emerman CL, Cydulka RK, McFadden ER. Comparison of 2.5 mg vs 7.5 mg of inhaled albuterol in the treatment of acute asthma. *Chest.* 1999;115:92–96.

44. Besbes-Ouanes L, Nouira S, Elatrous S, et al. Continuous versus intermittent nebulization of salbutamol in acute severe asthma: a randomized, controlled trial. *Ann Emerg Med.* 2000;36:198–203.

45. Newhouse MT, Chapman KR, McCallum AL, et al. Cardiovascular safety of high doses of inhaled fenoterol and albuterol in acute severe asthma. *Chest.* 1996;110:595–603.

46. Nowak R, Emerman C, Hanrahan JP, et al. A comparison of levalbuterol with racemic albuterol in the treatment of acute severe asthma exacerbations in adults. *Am J Emerg Med.* 2006;24:259–267.

47. Rodrigo C, Rodrigo G. Salbutamol treatment of acute severe asthma in the ED: MDI vs hand-held nebulizer. *Am J Med.* 1998;16:637–642.

48. Peters JI, Shelledy DC, Jones AP, et al. A randomized, placebo-controlled study to evaluate the role of salmeterol in the in-hospital management of asthma. *Chest.* 2000;118:313–320.

49. Fanta CH, Rossing TH, McFadden ER Jr. Treatment of acute asthma: is combination therapy with sympathomimetics and methylxanthines indicated? *Am J Med.* 1986;80:5–10.

50. Cydulka R, Davison R, Grammer L, et al. The use of epinephrine in the treatment of older adult asthmatics. *Ann Emerg Med.* 1990;17:322–326.

51. Salmeron S, Brochard L, Mal H, et al. Nebulized versus intravenous albuterol in hypercapnic acute asthma: a multicenter, double-blind, randomized study. *Am J Respir Crit Care Med.* 1994;149:1466–1470.

52. Zorc JJ, Pusic MV, Ogborn CJ, et al. Ipratropium bromide added to asthma treatment in the pediatric emergency department. *Pediatrics.* 1999;103:748–752.

53. Qureshi F, Pestian J, Davis P, et al. Effect of nebulized ipratropium on hospitalization rates of children with asthma. *N Engl J Med.* 1998;339:1030–1035.

54. Weber EJ, Levitt A, Covington JK, et al. Effect of continuously nebulized ipratropium bromide plus albuterol on emergency department length of stay and hospital admission rates in patients with acute bronchospasm. *Chest.* 1999;115:937–944.

55. Fitzgerald JM, Grunfeld A, Pare PD, et al., and the Canadian Combivent Study Group. The clinical efficacy of combination nebulized anticholinergic and adrenergic bronchodilators vs nebulized adrenergic bronchodilator alone in acute asthma. *Chest.* 1997;111:311–315.

56. Ducharme FM, Davis GM. Randomized controlled trial of ipratropium bromide and frequent low doses of salbutamol in the management of mild and moderate acute pediatric asthma. *J Pediatr.* 1998;133:479–485.

57. Rodrigo GJ, Rodrigo C. First-line therapy for adult patients with acute severe asthma receiving a multiple-dose protocol of ipratropium bromide plus albuterol in the emergency department. *Am J Respir Crit Care Med.* 2000;161:1862–1868.

58. Craven D, Kercsmar CM, Myers TR, et al. Ipratropium bromide plus nebulized albuterol for treatment of hospitalized children with acute asthma. *J Pediatr.* 2001;138:51–58.

59. Goggin N, Macarthur C, Parkin PC. Randomized trial of the addition of ipratropium bromide to albuterol and corticosteroid therapy in children hospitalized because of an acute asthma exacerbation. *Arch Pediatr Adolesc Med.* 2001; 115: 1329–1334.

60. Rodrigo G, Rodrigo C. Corticosteroids in the emergency department therapy of acute asthma: an evidence-based evaluation. *Chest.* 1999;116:285–295.

61. Rowe BH, Spooner C, Ducharme FM, et al. Early emergency department treatment of acute asthma with systemic corticosteroids. *Cochrane Database Syst Rev.* 2000;2:CD002178. DOI: 10.1002/14651858. CD002178.

62. Connett GJ, Warde C, Wooler E, et al. Prednisolone and salbutamol in the hospital treatment of acute asthma. *Arch Dis Child.* 1994;70:170–173.

63. Scarfone RJ, Fuchs SM, Nager AL, et al. Controlled trial of oral prednisone in the emergency room treatment of children with acute asthma. *Pediatrics.* 1993;2:513–518.

64. Manser R, Reid D, Abramson M. Corticosteroids for acute severe asthma in hospitalised patients. *Cochrane Database Syst Rev.* 1999;3:CD001740. DOI: 10.1002/14651858.CD001740.

65. Emerman CL, Cydulka RK. A randomized comparison of 100-mg vs 500-mg dose of methylprednisolone in the treatment of acute asthma. *Chest.* 1995;107:1559–1563.

66. Engel T, Dirksen A, Frolund L. Methylprednisolone pulse therapy in acute severe asthma. A randomized, double-blind study. *Allergy.* 1990;45:224–230.

67. Rodrigo G, Rodrigo C. Inhaled flunisolide for acute severe asthma. *Am J Respir Crit Care Med.* 1998;157:698–703.

68. Guttman A, Afilalo M, Colacone A, et al. The effects of combined intravenous and inhaled steroids (beclomethasone dipropionate) for the emergency treatment of acute asthma. The Asthma ED Study Group. *Acad Emerg Med.* 1997;4:100–106.

69. Afilalo M, Guttman A, Colacone A, et al. Efficacy of inhaled steroids (beclomethasone dipropionate) for treatment of mild to moderately severe asthma in the emergency department: a randomized clinical trial. *Ann Emerg Med.* 1999;33:304–309.

70. Parameswaran K, Belda J, Rowe BH. Addition of intravenous aminophylline to beta2-agonists in adults with acute asthma. *Cochrane Database Syst Rev.* 2000;4: CD002742. DOI: 10.1002/14651858. CD002742.

71. Scarfone RJ, Loiselle JM, Joffe MD, et al. A randomized trial of magnesium in the emergency department treatment of children with asthma. *Ann Emerg Med.* 2000;36:572–578.

72. Ciarallo L, Brousseau D, Reinert S. Higher-dose intravenous magnesium therapy for children with moderate to severe acute asthma. *Arch Pediatr Adolesc Med.* 2000;154:979–983.

73. Alters HJ, Koepsell TD, Hilty WM. Intravenous magnesium as an adjuvant in acute bronchospasm: a meta-analysis. *Ann Emerg Med.* 2000;36:191–197.

74. Rowe BH, Bretzlaff JA, Bourdon C, et al. Magnesium sulfate for treating exacerbations of acute asthma in the emergency department. *Cochrane Database Syst Rev.* 1999;2: CD001490. DOI: 10.1002/14651858.CD001490.

75. Nannini LJ, Pendino JC, Corna RA, et al. Magnesium sulfate as a vehicle for nebulized salbutamol in acute asthma. *Am J Med.* 2000;108:193–197.

76. Camargo CA, Jr, Smithline HA, Malice MP, et al. A randomized controlled trial of intravenous montelukast in acute asthma. *Am J Resp Crit Care Med.* 2003;167:528–533.

77. Rodrigo G, Pollack C, Rodrigo C, et al. Heliox for nonintubated actue asthma patients. *Cochrane Database Syst Rev.* 2001;1: CD002884. DOI: 10.1002/14651858.CD002884.pub 2.

78. Rivera ML, Kim TY, Stewart GM, et al. Albuterol nebulized in heliox in the initial ED treatment of pediatric asthma: a blinded, randomized controlled trial. *Am J Emerg Med.* 2006;24:38–42.

79. Kim IK, Phrampus E, Venkataraman S, et al. Helium/oxygen-driven albuterol nebulization in the treatment of children with moderate to severe asthma exacerbations: a randomized, controlled trial. *Pediatrics.* 2005;116(5):1127–1133.

80. Soroksky A, Stav D, Shpirer I. A pilot prospective, randomized, placebo-controlled trial of bilevel positive pressure airway pressure in acute asthma attack. *Chest.* 2003;123:1018–1025.

81. Ram FSF, Wellington SR, Rowe B, et al. Non-invasive positive pressure ventilation for treatment of respiratory failure due to severe acute exacerbations of asthma. *Cochrane Database Syst Rev.* 2005;1: CD004360. DOI: 10.1002/14651858.CD004360.pub3.

82. Thill PJ, McGuire JK, Baden HP, et al. Noninvasive positive-pressure ventilation in children with lower airway obstruction. *Pediatr Crit Care Med.* 2004;5:337–342.

83. Tuxen DV, Lane S. The effects of ventilatory pattern on hyperinflation, airway pressures, and circulation in mechanical ventilation of patients with severe air-flow obstruction. *Am Rev Respir Dis.* 1987;136:872–879.

84. Tuxen DV, Williams TJ, Scheinkestel CD, et al. Use of a measurement of pulmonary hyperinflation to control the level of mechanical ventilation in patients with acute severe asthma. *Am Rev Respir Dis.* 1992;146:1136–1142.

85. Williams TJ, Tuxen DV, Scheinkestel CD, et al. Risk factors for morbidity in mechanically ventilated patients with acute severe asthma. *Am Rev Respir Dis.* 1992;146:607–615.

86. Tuxen DV. Detrimental effects of positive end-expiratory pressure during controlled mechanical ventilation of patients with severe airflow obstruction. *Am Rev Respir Dis.* 1989;140:5–9.

87. Leatherman JW, Ravenscraft SA. Low measured auto-positive end-expiratory pressure during mechanical ventilation of patients with severe asthma: hidden auto-positive end-expiratory pressure. *Crit Care Med.* 1996;24:541–546.

88. Feihl F, Perret C. State of the art: permissive hypercapnia: how permissive should we be? *Am J Respir Crit Care Med.* 1994;150:1722–1737.

89. Tuxen DV. Permissive hypercapnic ventilation. *Am J Respir Crit Care Med.* 1994;150:870–874.

90. Kress JP, O'Connor MF, Pohlman AS, et al. Sedation of critically ill patients during mechanical ventilation: a comparison of propofol and midazolam. *Am J Respir Crit Care Med.* 1996;153:1012–1018.

91. Kress JP, Pohleman A, O'Connor MF, et al. Daily interruption of sedative infusions in critically ill patients undergoing mechanical ventilation. *N Eng J Med.* 2000;342:1471–1477.

92. Sarma VJ. Use of ketamine in acute severe asthma. *Acta Anaesthesiol Scand.* 1992;36:106–107.

93. Caldwell JE, Lau M, Fisher DM. Atracurium versus vecuronium in asthmatic patients. A blinded, randomized comparison of adverse events. *Anesthesiology.* 1995;83:986–991.

94. Behbehani NA, Al-Mane F, D'yachkova Y, et al. Myopathy following mechanical ventilation for acute severe asthma: the role of muscle relaxants and corticosteroids. *Chest.* 1999;115:1627–1631.

95. Manthous CA, Hall JB, Schmidt GA, et al. Metered-dose inhaler versus nebulized albuterol in mechanically ventilated patients. *Am Rev Respir Dis.* 1993;148:1567–1570.

96. Manthous CA, Hall JB. Update on using therapeutic aerosols in mechanically ventilated patients. *J Crit Illness.* 1996;11:457–468.

97. Saulnier FF, Durocher AV, Deturck RA, et al. Respiratory and hemodynamic effects of halothane in status asthmaticus. *Intensive Care Med.* 1990;16:104–107.

98. Gluck EH, Onorato DJ, Castriotta R. Helium-oxygen mixtures in intubated patients with status asthmaticus and respiratory acidosis. *Chest.* 1990;98:693–698.

CHAPTER 22

Asthma Clinical Trials

PEDRO C. AVILA

Clinical trials are the gold standard to prove efficacy of new therapies and management approaches for any disease. These trials take place after preclinical development of new drugs usually based on our understanding of disease pathogenesis. Drugs vary widely from low-molecular-weight molecules to large recombinant compounds such as monoclonal antibodies. Once a candidate drug is selected for development, it is submitted to several toxicology tests before the U.S. Food and Drug Administration (FDA) approves it for investigational studies in humans. Under FDA supervision, clinical development takes place with phases I, II, and III studies to learn the pharmacokinetics, pharmacodynamics, and clinical efficacy of the new drug. Several drugs have been developed for asthma, targeting airway inflammation and relaxation of airway smooth muscle. As our understanding of asthma pathogenesis evolves, new drugs are being developed to manage a disease that affects 20 million Americans and 300 million worldwide.

■ DEVELOPMENT OF A DRUG

A drug undergoes several phases of development until it is marketed (Fig.22.1) (1). A drug is initially developed from the understanding of the essential biological processes in disease pathogenesis based on human studies and animal models of human disease. One approach to developing a drug is to model a critical step of a pathway in an *in vitro* system (e.g., biological response to a cytokine receptor) and test several compounds to identify which ones affect the pathway. Pharmaceutical industries have libraries with thousands of natural and synthetic chemicals, peptides, nucleic acids, and other organic molecules which can be screened in high throughput assay systems to test their biological activity. Another approach is to design new compounds based on crystallography three-dimensional structure and computer drug design. In this case, scientists use crystallography to discover the three-dimensional structure of the target molecules and how they spatially interact (e.g., ligand-receptor binding). Using this information, they

use computer programs to design drugs, atom by atom, creating a three-dimensional molecule that can potentially disturb the spatial interaction between the target molecules. These designed drugs are then synthesized and tested in biological systems for their activities. A third approach is to use biotechnology to produce recombinant molecules that are agonists (e.g., a cytokine) or antagonists (e.g., monoclonal antibodies, soluble receptors) in the target pathway. In the case of monoclonal antibodies, they were initially produced in mouse cell systems, but the latest biotechnology allows humanization of these antibodies by changing murine IgG antibody protein sequences to human IgG sequences except for the principal amino acids responsible for binding to the target epitope. This humanization of the antibody minimizes immunogenicity while sparing specificity and biological activity. For example, omalizumab and mepolizumab were originally murine monoclonal antibodies—against IgE and interleukin 5, respectively—that were humanized by changing most of their amino acids to human IgG sequences (2,3). Besides antibodies, biotechnology has produced recombinant human molecules for asthma trials such as interleukin-4 soluble receptor (4), interferon gamma (5), and interleukin 12 (6). Still newer approaches are under development such as using human cell systems to produce human monoclonal antibodies, genetic alteration of animals to produce human molecules (e.g., making goats secrete human growth hormone in the milk), DNA vaccines, virus vectors for human gene therapy, and epigenetic tools (e.g., small interfering RNAs).

A drug is usually developed together with several chemically similar counterparts. These similar compounds are tested in biological systems *in vitro* and in animal models of human disease for their biological activities to eventually identify a single or a few compound(s) for further development. These compounds may undergo chemical modifications to improve their eventual clinical application because a lot is known about organic chemical characteristics necessary for resistance to gastrointestinal digestion and successful oral absorption (bioavailability), to prolong half-life by affecting distribution and metabolism, and to avoid

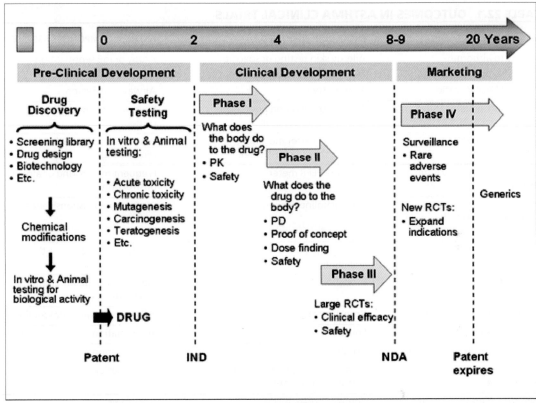

■ **FIGURE 22.1**   Phases of drug development. IND, Investigational New Drug approval; NDA, New Drug Application approval; PD, pharmacodynamics; PK, pharmacokinetics; RCTs, randomized clinical trials.

toxicity. After *in vitro* testing, the drug is tested in animals for bioavailability, biological activity, specificity of action, and toxicity. After a lead compound is selected, the pharmaceutical company files for a patent to obtain exclusive rights to market it for 20 years. Next, the drug enters the pre-clinical phase of development to establish an extensive safety profile of the drug in standard animal and cell culture systems. This phase includes *in vitro* and animal experiments to assess dose range, lethal dose 50% (dose that kills 50% of the exposed animals) acute and chronic toxicity, teratogenesis, mutagenesis, carcinogenesis, effects on pregnancy, etc. During this phase the pharmaceutical company discusses with the FDA what safety data in animals will be required to start human studies. Once the pharmaceutical company and the FDA discuss the design of the first human study with the new drug, the company submits an Investigational New Drug (IND) application. Only after the FDA approves the IND can the first clinical trial begin, initiating the clinical phase of drug development.

The clinical development of a drug involves three phases of clinical studies before a drug is approved for marketing. All studies in this phase are designed by the pharmaceutical company with continuous discussions and oversight of the FDA. In Phase I studies, the drug is administered to few humans (e.g., n=10) for the first time after completion of extensive animal studies. Phase I helps us to understand drug pharmacokinetics (PK) and begin to assess safety in humans. In addition, biomarkers of drug activity can be measured, although this is a secondary objective. At the end of phase I studies, researchers have the first data on adverse effects in humans, determine the maximum tolerated dose, and define the drug's PK characteristics such as time to peak serum level, bioavailability, half-life, metabolism, volume distribution, and route of elimination.

Based on the dose that worked in animal studies and on PK data in humans, Phase II studies are designed to assess pharmacodynamics (PD), that is, to determine whether the drug causes the expected biological effects for the targeted human disease. Two kinds of studies are usually conducted in this phase: proof-of-concept and dose-finding studies. In proof-of-concept studies, the biological effect of the drug on the disease of interest is assessed in small randomized clinical trials where usually maximal dose is administered to determine if the new drug really works. In asthma, a common proof-of-concept study is to assess the inhibitory effect of the drug on the early and late airway responses to inhaled allergen challenge. Often pharmaceutical companies conduct a couple of proof-of-concept studies that are considered "go" or "no-go" trials; that is, if the drug

TABLE 22.1   OUTCOMES IN ASTHMA CLINICAL TRIALS

MEASUREMENT	PROCEDURE REQUIRED	ASTHMA COMPONENT ASSESSED
Allergy to airborne allergens	Allergy skin testing or specific serum IgE	Atopy or IgE sensitization
FEV_1 or FEV_1/FVC ratio	Spirometry	Airway obstruction
Post-bronchodilator FEV_1	Spirometry pre- and post-short-acting bronchodilator	Reversible bronchospasm component
Best achievable FEV_1 or FEV_1/FVC ratio	Spirometry after maximum asthma therapy for 1 week	Possibly a measure of remodeling
Peak Expiratory Flow Rate (PEFR)	Portable PEFR meter	Frequent monitoring of airway obstruction
Provocative concentration to decline FEV_1 by 20% (PC20)	Methacholine challenge	Airway hyperresponsiveness
Early and late airway responses to allergen	Whole lung inhalation allergen challenge	IgE-mediated response to allergen in lower airways
Segmental allergen challenge	Bronchoscopy	Induction of T_H2-inflammation in a segment of lower airways
Bronchial mucosal biopsy	Bronchoscopy	Inflammation and remodeling
Sputum eosinophils	Sputum induction	Inflammation
Exhaled nitric oxide (eNO)	Exhaling into NO analyzer	Inflammation
Exhaled breath condensate	Measure small molecular inflammatory markers and pH	Inflammation
Symptom diary	Complete diary forms	Symptoms
Asthma Quality of Life Questionnaire	Complete questionnaire	Impact of asthma on own life (patient's perspective)
Asthma Control Questionnaire	Complete questionnaire	Ongoing severity of asthma (physician's perspective)

Abbreviations: FEV_1: Forced expiratory volume in 1 second. FVC: Forced vital capacity.

shows no signs of efficacy in these trials, clinical development is stopped. In a dose-finding trial, a few hundred subjects are randomized to placebo or 2 or more different dose regimens in a double-blind fashion to determine what doses improve disease-related outcomes (e.g., forced expiratory volume in 1 second [FEV_1] in asthma). Surrogate biological markers of efficacy are often used to enable these trials to be short and thus less costly. Such secondary outcomes may include assays in patients' samples to determine whether the drug had the expected biological effects in the targeted pathway. For example, in trials of omalizumab, a neutralizing anti-IgE antibody, besides asthma clinical outcomes, serum-free IgE concentration was also measured as a surrogate marker to titrate dose to drive free IgE to undetectable levels. At the end of phase II trials, researchers know the dose that affects important disease physiological outcomes and have additional safety data in hundreds of individuals. This information is then used to plan and design phase III clinical trials to assess efficacy aiming at obtaining the necessary data

on efficacy in clinically important outcomes and safety data to apply for FDA approval to market the drug.

Phase III studies are large double-blind, placebo-controlled, randomized clinical trials to determine whether the drug improves clinically relevant outcomes. For asthma some of the main outcomes to establish efficacy are airway obstruction, symptoms, quality of life, and frequency of exacerbations (see Table 22.1). When phase III studies are conducted, the pharmaceutical company and the FDA have a clear idea of what efficacy and safety data will be needed for drug approval. The FDA usually requires more than one phase III trial demonstrating efficacy. If phase III trials are successful, the pharmaceutical company submits to the FDA a new drug application to obtain approval for marketing. This application contains all data available on the drug since its preclinical development, and therefore contains several thousands of pages, including data on drug administration to 3,000 to 5,000 subjects. The FDA takes on average 6 months to approve or deny a new drug application (range: 3 months to years) and may seek input from outside experts. Once approved, the pharmaceutical company can market the drug with exclusivity until the patent expires, at which point other companies can start producing and marketing the drug without having to pay a fee to the patent holder. After approval, new phase III studies can be undertaken to expand indications to different age groups (e.g., pediatrics) and new diseases, which can help extend duration of patents.

After FDA approval, phase IV studies are designed to monitor safety aiming at identifying severe and rare side effects such as those occurring at a rate of 1:10,000 or rarer. Examples of rare adverse events discovered in this phase include liver toxicity caused by telithromycin, cardiovascular events caused by rofecoxib, progressive multifocal leukoencephalopathy caused by JC virus in those receiving rituxan (anti-CD20), tendon rupture in patients taking quinolones, and possibly, increased risk of asthma-related death in patients taking long-acting bronchodilators, particularly in African Americans. Besides phase IV trials, these rare serious events can be captured through the FDA surveillance system for medications' adverse events called MedWatch (http://www.fda.gov/medwatch/), which allows health care professionals to report adverse events directly to the FDA online. Rare serious adverse events proven to be related to a drug lead to "black box warnings" in the drug's package insert, limitations of FDA-approved indications based on new risk:benefit ratio assessments, and even drug withdrawal from the market.

The costly development of new drugs is a risky business. It is estimated that the cost to bring a new drug to market is about $900 million. Many drugs fail during clinical development and only 30% of marketed drugs return the costs for their development. New drugs can fail even after marketing in phase IV studies because of rare life-threatening adverse events leading to restrictions in use or withdrawal from the market. Although patents protect marketing of new drugs for 20 years, it usually takes 8 to 10 years to obtain FDA approval to market a drug, leaving 10 or fewer years for the pharmaceutical company to profit from the drug. This profit not only should cover the expenses incurred to develop the drug itself, but also fund research and development of new drugs to keep the pharmaceutical company in business. Successful drugs can be highly profitable such as atorvastatin (Lipitor) with over $10 billion dollars in sales in 2004, or fluticasone-salmeterol inhaler (Advair) with almost $8 billion dollars in sales in 2008.

■ OUTCOMES IN ASTHMA TRIALS

Outcomes measured in asthma trials have evolved as did our knowledge of asthma pathogenesis, clinical trials science, and biomedical research technology. In the early 1900s, pathological and clinical evidence

already indicated that asthma pathogenesis involved bronchoconstriction, eosinophilic bronchitis, and exposure to external allergen triggers, which also caused hay fever. With the advent of pulmonary function testing in the 1940s to 1950s, it was noticed that patients with asthma had reversible airway obstruction and airway hyperresponsiveness. In the 1970s, it was documented that inhalation allergen challenges caused early and late airway bronchoconstriction associated with increased blood eosinophilia. In the 1980s, bronchoscopic biopsies of bronchial mucosa revealed chronic airway inflammation even in the mild cases, which is characterized mainly by eosinophilic bronchitis, and increase in $CD4^+$ T cells. In the 1990s, remodeling was described, which entails alterations in the resident cells resulting from chronic inflammation driven by infiltrating leukocytes. Remodeling includes goblet-cell hyperplasia, smooth-muscle-cell hyperplasia, collagen deposition in the subepithelial reticular membrane, and increased vasculature, among other changes (7). Currently, research continues to focus on mechanisms of inflammation, particularly inflammatory mediators produced by resident cells, innate response, and interactions between resident cells and leukocytes.

The number and variety of clinical outcomes measured in asthma trials expanded based on our understanding of pathogenesis of airway disease as aforementioned. Initial trials measured spirometric outcomes such as FEV_1 to assess changes in airway caliber. Later, portable peak expiratory flow (PEF) meters allowed patients to monitor airway flow at home. More recently, electronic portable devices can measure and record PEF, FEV_1 and forced vital capacity (FVC) of 6 seconds, greatly expanding our ability to monitor variability in airway obstruction, a hallmark of asthma.

Airway hyperresponsiveness to nonspecific stimuli is also measured in asthma trials because it is an important feature of asthma (8,9) and because it correlates with airway inflammation. It is commonly measured as the provocative concentration of methacholine or histamine to cause a 20% decline in FEV_1 (PC20). Airways of asthmatic subjects undergo excessive bronchoconstriction upon inhalation of methacholine or histamine, which acts directly on smooth muscles causing contraction. Airway hyperactivity is defined as a PC20 less than 8 mg/mL for direct agents (10). Inhaled corticosteroid therapy simultaneously improves both hyperresponsiveness and airway inflammation. Indirect agents are also used to assess PC20. They cause bronchoconstriction indirectly by stimulating mast cells to release bronchospastic mediators including histamine, cysteinyl leukotrienes, and prostaglandin D2. Examples of indirect agents to assess airway responsiveness include exercise, inhalation of adenosine, or inhalation of osmotic stimulants such as cold dry air, distilled water, hypertonic saline, or mannitol (11). PC20 using indirect agents can correlate more closely with airway

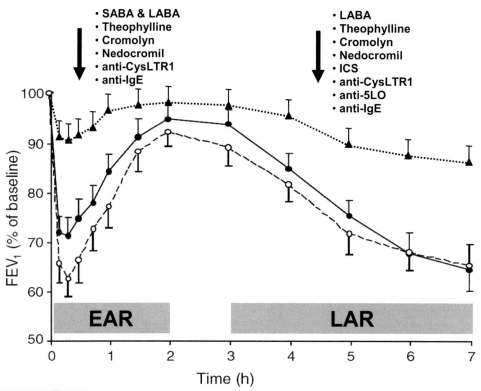

FIGURE 22.2 Inhalation allergen challenge causing biphasic airway response in asthmatic patients. Graph shows percentage changes in mean FEV_1 and SEM from baseline to 7 hours post-challenge. Changes are reproducible between inhalation challenges performed 4 weeks apart (traced and continuous lines). Bronchoconstriction occurs within minutes and improves in 2 hours (early airway response—EAR) mostly as a consequence of smooth cell contraction. Then, 3-8 hours after challenge bronchoconstriction recurs as a consequence of increased influx of leukocytes, particularly eosinophils, T_H2 lymphocytes and basophils (late airway response—LAR). Listed are medications that inhibit EAR and LAR (dotted line) when administered before the challenge.

Anti-CysLTR1, antagonists of cysteinyl leukotriene receptor 1 (e.g. montelukast, zafirlukast); Anti-5LO, antagonist of 5-lipoxygenase (e.g. zileuton); Anti-IgE, antibody anti-IgE (e.g. omalizumab); ICS, Inhaled corticosteroids; LABA, long-acting beta-2 receptor agonist bronchodilators (e.g. salmeterol, formoterol); SABA, short-acting beta-2 receptor agonist bronchodilators (e.g. albuterol, terbutaline).

inflammation than PC20 using direct agents (e.g., methacholine and histamine). Airway hyperresponsiveness can also occur in medical conditions other than asthma, including allergic rhinitis without asthma, up to 6 weeks after respiratory virus infections, and in smokers with chronic obstructive pulmonary disease (10).

The realization that IgE-sensitization and inhalation of a relevant allergen caused reproducible **early and late airway responses (EAR and LAR)** led to the development of a widely used proof-of-concept asthma study model. In this model, subjects inhaled increasing amounts of allergen to which they reacted in allergy skin testing to determine the concentration of allergen that causes a 20% decline in FEV_1. Then, the subject receives placebo and/or drug therapy for a period of time and returns for a repeat allergen challenge using the same allergen and dose as the initial challenge to determine whether the drug attenuated airway responses to the allergen. Because EAR and LAR are very reproducible, only 10 to 12 patients are needed per group to assess whether a drug attenuates any response by 30% or more. Almost all currently available asthma drugs attenuate EAR, LAR, or both (2,12–25), making this study model a common phase II trial to determine whether a new drug works for asthma (Fig. 22.2). Drugs that inhibit mast cell activation and bronchoconstriction should attenuate EAR, whereas drugs that inhibit delayed production of mediators or airway influx of leukocytes (e.g., eosinophils, dendritic cells, and lymphocytes) can inhibit LAR. This model of inhalation allergen challenge to induce 20% decline in FEV_1 also increases airway hyperresponsiveness and sputum eosinophilia 24 hours after the challenge, allowing researchers to assess the effects of new drugs in these outcomes as well. Presence of LAR seems to be driven by T cells because studies of peptide immunotherapy revealed late phase reactions to injections (26). BB Peptides are too small to cross-link IgE and stimulate mast cells, but they do bind to human leukocyte antigens and stimulate T cells. Lastly, EAR and LAR responses in the lower airways are not unique to asthmatic patients. They can also be present in nonasthmatic allergic rhinitic patients after rhinovirus colds (27) raising the hypothesis that a spectrum of disease progression in the lower airways may occur such as IgE-sensitization, bronchial hyperresponsiveness, bronchial EAR and LAR to allergen challenge, and finally full-blown asthma.

Another common proof-of-concept study design used in phase II trials to assess efficacy of new drugs that aim at chronic asthma control rather than acute relief of bronchospasm is the **corticosteroid withdrawal model**. In this model, subjects with moderate-to-severe asthma enter a run-in period on inhaled plus or minus oral corticosteroid therapy that is titrated to the minimum corticosteroid dose necessary to control symptoms, at which point subjects are randomized to placebo or the new drug as an add-on therapy. Then, after a period on corticosteroid therapy and study medication (either active drug or placebo), corticosteroid therapy is tapered to determine whether the new drug is more efficacious than placebo in maintaining asthma control. In this type of study, patients need to be monitored very closely and protocols for action plan need to be in place to rescue patients when their asthma deteriorates. The corticosteroid withdrawal model is sometimes mistakenly called *asthma exacerbation* model. This is incorrect because exacerbations are caused by common colds in up to 80% of the episodes (28,29). Exacerbations occur when virus-induced inflammation superimposes to chronic allergen-driven inflammation. Studies evaluating exacerbations recruit patients who have exacerbated in the previous year and follow them for a long period (e.g., 12 or more months) to capture new episodes of acute asthma deterioration requiring a short course of systemic corticosteroid therapy. The corticosteroid withdrawal model is a model of loss of asthma control of chronic allergen-driven inflammation for lack of sufficient controller therapy.

The recognition that asthma is a chronic inflammatory airway condition led to implementation of **measurements of inflammation** in clinical trials (see Table 22.1). Blood eosinophilia was an initial marker. Bronchoalveolar lavage and bronchial mucosal biopsy reliably assess luminal and tissue inflammatory infiltrates, but necessitate bronchoscopy precluding their use in large clinical trials. In the 1990s, **sputum induction** using hypertonic saline solution started to be used in asthma studies as a noninvasive technique to assess airway inflammation. Sputum eosinophilia (more than 2% of nonsquamous cells) is characteristic of asthma, increases after allergen challenge (30), and decreases with therapy, including systemic (31) or inhaled corticosteroids (32), leukotriene antagonists (33), and anti-IgE (omalizumab) (34). Mast cell stabilizers (cromolyn and nedocromil) improve symptoms of asthma and airway function, but have mild and inconsistent anti-inflammatory effects as measured by eosinophil count or products in airways and blood (35–38). However, sputum eosinophilia is not pathognomonic of asthma and can also occur in patients with eosinophilic bronchitis or chronic eosinophilic pneumonia. In addition, sputum neutrophilia, not eosinophilia, can be found in some asthmatic patients, particularly those with nonatopic or more severe disease (39–41).

Because of the risk of severe bronchospasm with inhalation allergen challenge, other models have been developed to study the effects of drugs in airway inflammation. In one model, allergen is infused into a bronchial tree segment to induce localized airway allergic inflammation, the so-called **segmental allergen challenge model** (42). In this model, a small amount of allergen is delivered to a segmental bronchus of one lung whereas another segmental bronchus in the contralateral lung is challenged with saline. Repeated bronchoscopies for bronchoalveolar lavages of the same segments evaluate local EARs and LARs. Yet another model to induce mild airway inflammation of lower airways is the **repeated low-dose inhalation allergen challenge model** (43), in which subjects inhale the allergen dose calculated to cause only 5% decline in FEV_1, based on a baseline allergen challenge. The same dose is inhaled daily for 5 or more days to induce airway eosinophilia, worsen hyperresponsiveness, and cause none-to-mild short-living asthma symptoms, thus reproducing many features of asthma while avoiding the risk of severe bronchoconstriction associated with high-dose inhalation allergen challenges to induce EAR and LAR. Both the segmental and the repeated low-dose allergen challenge models are not widely used due to the need for bronchoscopy and labor. Bronchoscopy with mucosal biopsy, however, has been used in clinical trials to assess the effect of therapy on airway inflammation (34) and remodeling (e.g., subepithelial collagen deposition [44,45]).

An approach to indirectly **measure remodeling** is to administer a short course of maximal therapy. Because it is not practical to perform bronchoscopy for mucosal biopsy to histologically measure remodeling, researchers have used a short course of maximal therapy to obtain "the best achievable" FEV_1. This measure can be applied to large clinical trials (46). In this study model, before and after an intervention, patients undergo a week of oral corticosteroid, maximum-dose of inhaled corticosteroid-long-acting bronchodilator (ICS+LABA) combination, and a leukotriene antagonist treatment.

At the end of the week of maximal asthma therapy, FEV_1 is measured before and after maximal broncho-dilation with administration of a short-acting bron-chodilator (SABA). This best achievable FEV_1 may be considered a practical measurement of remodeling, which is assumed to be the irreversible component of airway obstruction after maximal therapy to improve any reversible component of bronchial inflammation and to reverse bronchospasm. However, this assumption has not been validated by comparing best-achievable FEV_1 (or FEV_1/FVC ratio) with bronchial biopsy measures of remodeling (e.g., goblet and gland cell volume, smooth muscle volume, and subepithelial reticular membrane thickening).

Noninvasive measurements of airway inflammation were developed in the 1990s and 2000s and include **exhaled nitric oxide (eNO) and exhaled breath condensate (EBC)**. Nitric oxide (NO) can be measured as a gas in exhaled air. It is produced by the action of nitric oxide synthases (NOS) on L-arginine. In the lungs, NOS are found in airway epithelial and endothelial cells. Airway epithelial cells express inducible NOS (a.k.a. iNOS or NOS2) on stimulation by several inflammatory pathways including interferons (via signal transducer and activator of transcription [STAT]-1), toll-like receptors (via nuclear factor kappa B), and interleukin 4 (via STAT-6). NO has several roles including vasodilation, bronchodilation, and innate defense by inflicting nitrosative distress via nitration, nitrosation, and nitrosylation of molecules. Guidelines have been devised on how to measure eNO because several factors can alter its concentration such as food intake, contamination with upper airway NO, air flow, and other diseases besides asthma (47). Normal levels are less than 10 parts per billion and untreated atopic asthmatic patients usually have levels more than 35 parts per billion. Intermediary levels are not indicative of asthma. As with sputum eosinophilia, eNO correlates with more severe disease and airway inflammation, and decreases promptly with inhaled corticosteroid therapy. eNO can be elevated in other conditions such as bronchiectasis, alveolitis, chronic bronchitis, cystic fibrosis exacerbation, atopic individuals (e.g., allergic rhinitis), chronic cough, and pneumonia. It can be decreased in systemic or pulmonary hypertension, heart failure, smokers, and after caffeine intake. eNO can be helpful, particularly in atopic asthmatic patients, to monitor the need to increase inhaled corticosteroid therapy or to improve patient compliance (48), although this is still controversial (49,50). At present, two companies have NO analyzers approved by the FDA for clinical use: Aerocrine manufactures the NIOX analyzer and Apieron produces the Insight Monitor.

Another noninvasive measure of airway inflammation is EBC, which is collected by the patient breathing out through a cooled tube where water vapor from exhaled breath condensates and accumulates. Guidelines have been established for its collection as well (51). An example of a research collection device is the Aeriflux, a three-way valve connected to a disposable plastic collection tube not yet FDA approved for clinical use. A three-way valve directs air flow so that the patient breathes in via an intake opening and out into a tube surrounded by a removable and reusable metal sheath that is kept in the -20°C freezer until used. After breathing through the device for 10 minutes, the tube contains 1 mL to 2 mL of breath condensate. This condensate (EBC) contains low-molecular-weight inflammatory mediators including chemokines, cytokines (e.g., IL-8, IL-6), prostaglandins, thromboxanes, leukotrienes, 8-isoprostane, and markers of oxidative and nitrosative stress. EBC pH can also be measured and it lowers during asthma exacerbations (52). Analysis of EBC is currently a research tool, but has the future potential to aid in diagnosing asthma, asthma exacerbation, gastroesophageal reflux (53), and in monitoring airway inflammation.

Besides new measurements to assess disease pathogenesis, new tools have also been developed to assess clinical improvement in trials, namely **quality of life (QOL)** and asthma control questionnaires. QOL questionnaires are patient-centered and aim at assessing how disease severity affects the patient from the patient's perspective. They are developed by asking patients with the disease of interest how the disease affects them in terms of the most bothersome symptoms, limitations on daily activities specifically caused by the disease, and emotions resulting from disease severity. Several QOL questionnaires specifically developed to assess the impact of asthma in patients' lives have been validated; that is, changes in QOL scores correlated well with changes in traditional outcome variables (54,55). These asthma-specific QOL tools have between 12 to 30 or more questions asking how asthma has affected patients' lives in the previous few weeks regarding different domains such as symptoms, ability to perform daily activities, emotions elicited by asthma severity, and environmental exposures that trigger symptoms. Often, studies report the scores for each domain. This tool, therefore, assesses changes in disease severity from the patient's standpoint.

A similar approach was employed to develop the **asthma control questionnaires** to assess disease severity from the physician's perspective. Experts in asthma were asked which variables were the most important to ensure that asthma was well controlled and minimally impacting the patients' lives. A few variables that the majority of the experts considered the most important to assess control were included in the tool and validated. There are a few validated asthma control tools that usually contain questions about frequency of daytime and nocturnal symptoms, limitation of activities because of asthma, and use of rescue bronchodilators. Asthma QOL tools and asthma control tools have joined the traditional symptom diary as measures of

TABLE 22.2   SOURCES OF INFORMATION ON ASTHMA CLINICAL TRIALS

DATABASE	TYPES OF TRIALS	INTERNET URL
MEDLINE / PubMed EMBASE	Published articles describing clinical trials.	http://www.ncbi.nlm.nih.gov/sites/entrez http://www.embase.com/
Cochrane Library Clinical Evidence	Meta-analyses and systematic reviews of published and unpublished asthma trials.	http://www.cochrane.org/ http://clinicalevidence.bmj.com/
ClinicalTrials.gov Current Controlled Trials	Registries of governmental and privately supported clinical trials, both completed and ongoing trials.	http://www.clinicaltrials.gov http://www.controlled-trials.com
FDA EMEA	Regulatory agencies that approve marketing of drugs. Industry's filing documents may be posted online.	http://www.fda.gov/ http://www.emea.europa.eu/

Abbreviations: EMBASE, Excerpta Medica Database of publisher Elsevier; EMEA, European Medicines Agency. FDA, U.S.Food and Drug Administration; MEDLINE, Medical Literature Analysis and Retrieval System online database of the National Library of Medicine.

clinical severity of asthma in trials. Additional variables used in clinical trials are asthma-free days and exacerbations. An **asthma-free day** is defined as a day in which symptoms, asthma impact on patient's life, and use of rescue medication were minimal or nonexistent. **Asthma exacerbations** have been defined as aggravation of symptoms associated with moderate worsening in airway obstruction, but nowadays it is more commonly defined as deterioration of asthma necessitating systemic steroid therapy or unscheduled physician's visit, a more clinically relevant definition and rarer event.

Current clinical trials assess several outcomes to ensure that the drug or intervention benefits the hallmark components of asthma: symptoms, airway obstruction, airway hyperresponsiveness, and airway inflammation. Symptoms are appraised with symptom diary, and periodic assessments of asthma quality of life and asthma control. Airway obstruction is monitored twice daily via peak expiratory flow measurements and at study visits with spirometry. Airway hyperresponsiveness is assessed through methacholine inhalation challenges and airway inflammation monitored with eNO and/or sputum eosinophil measurements. No single measurement can assess all components of asthma. It is reassuring when a therapy consistently improves all of these measurements in clinical trials.

■ ASTHMA CLINICAL TRIALS

Thousands of clinical trials have been conducted in asthma. Using the National Library of Medicine's PubMed's "Clinical Queries" search mode (http://www.ncbi.nlm.nih.gov/entrez/query/static/clinical.shtml) for "asthma" and "therapy" together with the "Limits" option for "randomized controlled trial," PubMed displays more than 6,440 articles reporting results of trials

in asthma from 1965 to 2008. Sources for information on ongoing clinical trials and on published and unpublished completed trials are listed in Table 22.2. Table 22.3 lists the results of important clinical trials conducted in asthmatic patients. These clinical trials and many others have shaped the recommendations in national and international asthma guidelines (56,57).

Asthma clinical trials have assessed many medications for asthma treatment over the years. Some of the first clinical trials in asthmatic patients evaluated the efficacy of inhaled short-acting bronchodilators (beta-2 receptor agonists [SABA] and anticholinergic drug) and oral corticosteroids for acute deterioration of asthma. For chronic control, the drugs developed for asthma included methylxanthines (e.g., theophylline, aminophylline), inhaled cromolyn, inhaled corticosteroids (ICS), inhaled nedocromil, inhaled long-acting beta-2 receptor agonists (LABA), oral leukotriene antagonists, and subcutaneous antibody anti-IgE. For asthma exacerbations, SABA and systemic corticosteroids have been the mainstay of therapy for over 30 years. Addition of inhaled anticholinergic drug can reduce admissions from the emergency department, and high-dose ICS decreases risk of relapse of exacerbation symptoms within a few weeks. For chronic asthma control, ICS is the most efficacious therapy and reduces asthma mortality (56,58). If it is insufficient to control asthma, addition of LABA improves control and is preferable than increasing ICS dose. The next step for refractory asthma not controlled on maximal dose of ICS+LABA combination is not very clear based on the evidence. Options include daily oral corticosteroid, leukotriene antagonists, theophylline, and/or anti-IgE antibody (omalizumab) which are all efficacious as monotherapy in steroid-naïve asthmatic patients, but as an add-on therapy only provide a small degree of additional

TABLE 22.3 IMPORTANT ASTHMA CLINICAL TRIALS

TRIAL (REF.)	AIM	POPULATION	INTERVENTIONS	RESULTS	CONCLUSION
Haahtela T, et al. (61) 1991	To evaluate the effect of terbutaline (Ter) versus budesonide (Bud) in recently diagnosed asthma.	N=103. 15–64 years old. Mild asthma diagnosed within 1 year.	• 600 mcg Bud versus 375 mcg Ter bid. Duration: 2 years.	Bud improved AHR, symptoms, and AM PEF to a greater extent than Ter. These results were present at the third month of therapy.	ICS is better than SABA for long-term treatment of recently diagnosed asthma.
Haahtela T, et al. (62) 1994	To evaluate the effect of delayed Bud therapy in recently diagnosed asthma.	Follow up of the above study. N=74. 15–64 years old. Mild asthma diagnosed within 3 years.	In the third year: • Bud group above was randomized to Bud 200 mcg bid or switched to Ter. • Ter group was started on Bud 600 mcg bid. Duration: 1 year.	• Bud group: Lower Bud dose was 2x more effective than Ter. But lowering Bud dose worsened AHR, symptom, and AM PEF. • Ter group improved on Bud, but to a lesser extent than original Bud group (see study above).	Delayed start of ICS in recent onset of mild asthma may reduce overall efficacy of ICS therapy.
Drazen JM, et al. (63). BAGS (Beta AGoniSt for mild asthma) 1996	To evaluate whether regular albuterol (Alb) is deleterious to asthma.	N=255. 12–55 years old. • $FEV_1 \geq 70\%$. • $PC20 \leq 16$ mg/mL. • SABA prn only. • No ICS.	Alb 180 mcg qid + prn versus prn only. Duration: 16 weeks.	AM PEF was similar in both groups as was FEV_1, rescue use of Alb, symptoms, QOL, and PC20.	Regular SABA qid provided neither deleterious, nor beneficial effects. It should be used prn.
Pauwels RA, et al. (64). FACET (Formoterol And Corticosteroids Establishing Therapy) 1997	To evaluate the effect of adding formoterol (For) to low and high doses of budesonide (Bud).	N=852. 18–72 years old. • $FEV_1 \geq 50\%$. • $\geq 15\%$ FEV_1 reversibility. • ICS $\leq 1,600$ mcg/day of Bud equivalent.	Randomized to 4 arms: • Bud 100 mcg bid. • Bud 100 mcg + For 12 mcg bid. • Bud 400 mcg bid. • Bud 400 mcg + For 12 mcg bid. Duration: 12 months.	Adding For better controlled symptoms and improved FEV_1 and AM PEF than 4X Bud. Higher dose of Bud better protected against exacerbations than adding For.	Adding LABA to ICS better controls symptoms and improves airway obstruction than increasing ICS 4X. ICS best prevents exacerbations.
Rowe BH, et al. (65) 1999	To evaluate whether high dose inhaled Bud reduces relapse of asthma exacerbations within 3 weeks after ED discharge.	N=188. 16–60 years old. • Severe exacerbation presenting to ED. • Peak flow < 80%.	Usual ED care for exacerbation. At discharge, Prednisone 50 mg/day x 7 days and: Bud 800 mcg or Pbo bid x 3 weeks. Duration: 3 weeks	Bud reduced in 48% the relapse of exacerbation. QOL and symptoms were better and use of rescue Alb lessened in Bud group. PEF was similar.	High dose ICS (e.g., Bud) given at ED discharge reduces relapse of exacerbations.

Study / Year	Objective	Population	Design	Results	Conclusions
Milgrom H, et al. (66) 1999	To evaluate the effect of anti-IgE monoclonal antibody (omalizumab) in moderate-to-severe asthma.	N=317. 11–50 years old. • On ICS ≥ 400 mcg/day. • Daily need for rescue Alb therapy. • Allergy to indoor allergens and IgE. Serum IgE for dosing.	Randomized to 3 arms: • Pbo. • Anti-IgE, low dose. • Anti-IgE, high dose. All given intravenously. Duration: 5 months.	Compared with Pbo, anti-IgE allowed more reduction in oral and ICS, improved symptoms, AM PEF, QOL, and reduced frequency of exacerbations.	This phase II trial showed that anti-IgE can be efficacious in asthmatic subjects not well controlled on ICS therapy.
Malmstrom K, et al. (67) 1999	To compare efficacy of ICS beclometasone (Bec) versus LTA (Montelukast [Mon]) in asthma.	N=895. 15–85 years old. • FEV$_1$ 50%–85%.	Randomized to 3 arms: • Pbo. • Mon 10 mg qd. • Bec 200 mcg bid. Duration: 12 weeks.	Bec > Mon > Pbo in improving FEV$_1$, symptoms, QOL, and reducing exacerbations.	Bec is superior to Mon, which is better than Pbo to treat moderate-to-severe asthma.
CAMP (68). Childhood Asthma Management Program research group 2000	To compare long-term efficacy and safety of nedocromil (Ned) versus ICS therapy in childhood asthma.	N=1,041. 5–12 years old. • Mild-to-moderate asthma.	Randomized to 3 arms: • Pbo bid. • Ned 8 mg bid. • Bud 200 mcg bid. Duration: 4–6 years.	No significant change in postbronchodilator FEV$_1$. Bud > Ned > Pbo in providing greater benefits in symptoms, AHR, exacerbation rate, and rescue Alb use.	Bud is superior to Ned which is better than Pbo for chronic therapy of childhood asthma. Bud caused a decrease in growth of 1.1 cm in the first year only.
Lazarus SC, et al. (69). SOCS (Salmeterol Or CorticoSteroids trial) 2001	To examine whether salmeterol (Sal) can control mild persistent asthma as well as inhaled triamcinolone (Tri).	N=164. 12–65 years old. • FEV$_1$ 50%–85%. • 12% FEV$_1$ reversibility. or PC20 < 8 mg/mL.	After 6 weeks run-in on Tri 400 mcg bid, if FEV$_1$ ≥ 80%, randomized to: • Pbo. • Tri 400 mcg bid. • Sal 42 mcg bid. Duration: 16 weeks. Run out: Pbo for 6 weeks.	During the 16-week treatment phase Tri and Sal kept control of asthma symptoms, QOL, lung function, and rescue SABA use. But on Sal alone inflammation worsened, exacerbation and treatment failure rates were greater. In the run-out phase all groups became similar.	Patients with persistent asthma well controlled on ICS can not be switched to LABA monotherapy, because airway inflammation worsens and risk of treatment failure and exacerbations increase.
Lemanske RF, et al. (70). SLIC (SaLmeterol ± Inhaled Corticosteroids trial) 2001	To examine whether inhaled Tri can be tapered off in patients with asthma well controlled on Tri + Sal.	N=175. 12–65 years old. • FEV$_1$ 50%–85% • 12% FEV$_1$ reversibility or PC20 < 8 mg/mL. • After 6 weeks run-in on Tri 400 mcg bid, if FEV$_1$ < 80%. Then, all	Randomized to 3 arms: • Switch Sal to Pbo (n=21). • Continue Sal (n=74). • Continue Sal and reduce Tri 50% for 8	• Pbo subjects worsened. • 50% reduction in Tri increased treatment failure from 2.8% to 8.3%. • Elimination of Tri increased treatment	In patients with moderate asthma taking combination inhalers ICS+LABA, ICS cannot be completely eliminated because of

(continued)

TABLE 22.3 IMPORTANT ASTHMA CLINICAL TRIALS (CONTINUED)

TRIAL (REF.)	AIM	POPULATION	INTERVENTIONS	RESULTS	CONCLUSION
		subjects received added Sal 42 mcg bid for 2 weeks.	weeks, then stopped it (n=74). Duration: 16 weeks.	failure from 13.7% to 46.3%. Elimination of Tri caused nonsignificant worsening of symptoms, FEV$_1$, AM PEF, and PC20.	increased risk of exacerbations.
Hughes R, et al. (71) 2003	To evaluate the effect of nebulized magnesium in asthma exacerbation.	N=52. 16–65 years old. • Severe exacerbation presenting to ED. • FEV$_1$ ≤ 70%.	• Saline versus MgSO4 250 mM nebulized with Alb every 30 min X 3 together via face mask.	Nebulized MgSO4 improved twice as much FEV$_1$ and reduced admission by 40% compared with saline.	MgSO4 nebulized with alb improves airway obstruction to a greater extent than Alb alone.
Pauwels RA et al. (72). START (Inhaled Steroid Treatment as Regular Therapy in early asthma study) 2003	To determine long-term benefit of early start of ICS therapy for asthma.	N=7,241. 5–66 years old. • Asthma diagnosed within 1 year. • Reversibility of airway obstruction. • FEV$_1$ ≥ 60%.	• Bud 400 mcg/day (200 mcg/day if < 11 years old) versus Pbo. Duration: 3 years.	Bud reduced in 46% risk of severe exacerbations. Bud slightly increased postbronchodilator FEV$_1$ by 0.88%. Bud reduced growth in children by 1.3 cm.	Bud reduces the risk for severe need of systemic corticosteroids and improved asthma control in patients with asthma of recent onset.
Israel E, et al. (73). BARGE (Beta-Adrenergic Response byGenotype) 2004	To determine whether asthmatic subjects homozygous for arginine (Arg) or glycine (Gly) in the 16th amino acid of the B2AR respond differently to Alb.	N=76. 11–50 years old. • FEV$_1$ ≥ 70% • Daily need for rescue Alb therapy, but <56 puffs/week. • Treated with SABA only.	Cross-over design: • 16 weeks of Alb 180 mcg or pbo qid Duration: 16 weeks for each treatment phase. Wash out of 8 weeks. Ipratropium prn.	Arg/Arg patients improved AM PEF, FEV$_1$, symptoms and reducedrescue ipratropium use while off of Alb. Gly/Gly patients did better on Alb than on Pbo.	Patients homozygous for Arg in the 16th amino acid of the B2AR have worse asthma while taking Alb regularly qid.
Morgan WJ, et al. (74) 2004	To determine if tailored allergen avoidance improves asthma in inner city pediatric population.	N=937. 5–11 years old. • Allergen skin test showing allergy to aeroallergens (dust, rat, mouse, cockroach, mold, pets).	Randomized to real versus mock intervention tailored to decrease allergen and tobacco exposure. Education and implementation. Duration: 2 years.	Real intervention successfully reduced amount of allergens in home dust samples. It also reduced symptoms, missed school days, and unscheduled doctor's visits for asthma.	Tailored environmental intervention to reduce exposure to allergens and tobacco in children with asthma improves symptoms and reduces exacerbations.

Study	Objective	Population	Methods	Results	Conclusions
Bateman ED, et al. (75). GOAL (Gaining Optimal Asthma control) 2004	To determine whether complete asthma control is achievable in practice with either fluticasone (Flu) or combination Flu + salmeterol (Sal), namely (Flu/Sal).	N=3,421. 12–83 years old. • $FEV_1 \geq 70\%$. • $\geq 15\%$ FEV_1 reversibility.	Randomized to Flu versus Flu/Sal. Every 12 weeks assessed for totally, or well, or not controlled asthma and dose adjusted per guidelines. Duration: 1 year.	Total control was achieved in 43% of Flu/Sal and in 31% of Flu alone groups ($p=0.001$). The worse the severity, the more efficacious was Flu/Sal. Flu/Sal was also better at preventing exacerbations.	Total control is achievable in a good proportion of patients following Asthma Guidelines. Flu/Sal is more successful than Flu in this endeavor.
O'Byrne PM, et al. (76). SMART (Symbicort MAintenance and Reliever Therapy) 2005	To determine whether Bud/For can be used as maintenance and rescue medications for asthma.	N=2,760. 4–80 years old. • $FEV_1 = 60\%$–100%. • Receiving 200 mcg–1,000 mcg ICS. • $\geq 12\%$ reversibility. • Using SABA prn almost daily.	Randomized to 3 arms: • Bud/For 80 mcg/4.5 mcg bid + Ter prn. • Bud 320 mcg bid + Ter prn. • Bud/For 80 mcg/4.5 mcg bid + prn. Duration: 2 years.	Bud/For bid + prn reduced exacerbation risk by 45% and symptoms, and improved lung function compared with the other 2 groups.	Bud/For can be used as maintenance and rescue medication. For is a fast-acting LABA, improving lung function within 5 min.
Boushey HA, et al. (46). IMPACT (IMProving Asthma Control Trial) 2005	To evaluate daily versus as-needed ICS for mild persistent asthma.	N=225. 18–65 years old. • $FEV_1 \geq 70\%$. • $\geq 12\%$ reversibility or PC20 < 16 mg/mL. • Mild persistent asthma in run-in phase.	Randomized to 3 arms: • Pbo bid (intermittent Bud). • Bud 200 mcg bid. • Zafirlukast 20 mg bid. All received as needed Bud 800 mcg bid x 10–14 days, or Prednisone x 5 days if asthma worsened. Duration: 12 months.	Daily Bud better improved baseline FEV_1, sputum eosinophils, PC20, and eNO than the other 2 treatments. QOL, symptoms, and FEV_1 after 1 week of maximal therapy did not differ among groups, suggesting no deterioration of remodeling.	It may be possible to treat mild persistent asthma with as needed ICS. Although intermittent ICS controlled well QOL and symptoms, its ability to prevent severe exacerbations and deaths is unknown.
Guilbert TW, et al. (77). PEAK (Prevention of Early Asthma inKids) 2006	To determine whether ICS prevents asthma in high-risk young children.	N=285. 2–3 years old. • Positive asthma predictive index (≥ 4 wheezing episodes + atopy markers).	Fluticasone (Flu) 88 mcg or Pbo bid for 2 years, then 1 year of follow-up off study medication.	During the 2 years of treatment Flu improved symptoms, reduced exacerbations, and need for rescue medications. In the third year, there were no differences between groups.	Two years of ICS in young children at high risk to develop asthma did not prevent asthma. But ICS controlled well asthma-like symptoms.

(continued)

TABLE 22.3 IMPORTANT ASTHMA CLINICAL TRIALS (CONTINUED)

TRIAL (REF.)	AIM	POPULATION	INTERVENTIONS	RESULTS	CONCLUSION
Rabe KF, et al (78) 2006	To determine whether Bud/For is safe when used as maintenance and rescue therapy for asthma.	N=3,394. ≥ 12 years old. • FEV_1 = 50%–100%. • ED or hospitalization for asthma within 12 months. • ≥ 12% reversibility. • Using SABA prn almost daily.	Daily Bud/For 160 mcg/ 4.5 mcg bid for all. Randomized to 3 arms of prn therapy: • Ter 400 mcg. • For 4.5 mcg. • Bud/For 160 mcg/4.5 mcg. Duration: 1 year.	Bud/For prn reduced number of exacerbations (ED or hospitalization) by 33%–50% compared with Ter or For, which were similar. Likewise, symptoms and lung function were better with Bud/For prn.	Bud/For used as maintenance and rescue therapy provided superior daily control of asthma symptoms, improved lung function, and reduced exacerbations.
Nelson HS, et al (79). SMART (Salmeterol Multicenter AsthmaResearch Trial) 2006	To examine the safety of Sal added to usual asthma therapy.	N=26,355. • ≥ 12 years old. • Physician-diagnosed asthma.	Inhaled Sal 42 mcg bid versus pbo. Duration: 28 weeks.	Death rate 1:1,000. Trial was stopped early due to nonsignificant higher death rate in the Sal group. Sal group also had increase in asthma-related deaths (RR=4.3; 95% CI=1.3–15.3), largely due to events in African Americans.	LABA may increase risk of death, asthma-related (or respiratory) deaths, particularly in African Americans. Decision to add LABA therapy needs to carefully weigh benefits and risks.
Papi A, et al. (80). BEST (BEclomethasone plus Salbutamol [albuterol] Treatment) 2007	To determine whether rescue therapy with combined Alb + Bec (Bec/Alb) is better than Alb alone in mild persistent asthma.	N=455, 18–65 years old. • FEV_1 ≥ 75%. • ≥ 12% reversibility or PC20 < 8 mg/mL.	Randomized to 4 arms: • A: Pbo bid + rescue prn Bec/Alb 250 mcg/ 100 mcg. • B: Pbo bid + rescue Alb 100 mcg prn. • C: Bec 250 mcg bid + rescue Alb 100 mcg prn. • D: Bec/Alb 250 mcg/ 100 mcg bid + rescue Alb 100 mcg prn. Duration: 6 months.	Exacerbation rate was lower in group A than B, but similar among A, C, and D. Group A received the lowest cumulative ICS dose over the 6 months. Group A was consistently better in improving lung function, symptoms, and use of rescue inhaler.	Patients with mild persistent asthma can be treated with symptomdriven ICS/SABA therapy as needed instead of regular ICS daily therapy.

AHR, airway hyperresponsiveness; Alb, albuterol; AM PEF, morning peak flow rate; B2AR, Beta-2 adrenergic receptor; Bec, beclomethasone; bid, 2x per day; Bud, budesonide; ED, emergencydepartment; eNO, exhaled nitric oxide; FEV_1, forced expiratory volume in 1 second; For, formoterol; ICS, Inhaled corticosteroids; LABA,Long-acting beta agonist (e.g., salmeterol, formoterol); LTA, leukotriene antagonist; Mg, magnesium; $MgSO_4$, magnesiumsulfate; Pbo, placebo; PC20, provocation concentration ofmethacholine to cause a decline of ≥ 20% in FEV_1; prn, as needed; qid, 4x per day; QOL, quality of life; SABA, short-acting beta agonist (e.g., terbutaline, albuterol); Alb, albuterol; Sal, salmeterol; Ter, terbutaline; Tri, triamcinolone.

symptomatic relief. Mast cell stabilizers such as inhaled cromolyn and nedocromil are no longer widely used because they are less efficacious than ICS as monotherapy and provide minimal benefit when added to ICS for refractory cases. New treatments continue to be explored for asthma, particularly biotechnology-derived drugs targeting cytokines, adhesion molecules, and other mediators of T_H2-inflammatory pathway.

The asthma clinical trials conducted so far have defined appropriate and effective therapies for most asthmatic patients. As a result, clinical research is now focusing on specific phenotypes of asthma and on exacerbations. Among the specific phenotypes are refractory asthma (59), asthma with accelerated loss of lung function (60), nonatopic asthma, asthma with sputum neutrophilia (39,40), and frequent exacerbators. New therapies are also needed to reverse airway remodeling and to treat acute asthma exacerbations, especially those precipitated by common colds, because exacerbations cause the most severe and costly asthma outcomes including unscheduled visits to doctors, missed school or work days, emergency department visits, hospitalizations, intubations, and death. Current clinical trials are now investigating these remaining issues in asthma management.

■ REFERENCES

1. Berkowitz BA. Development & regulation of drugs. In: Katzung BG, ed. *Basic & Clinical Pharmacology*. 10th ed. New York: McGraw-Hill Companies; 2007:64–74.

2. Fahy JV, Fleming HE, Wong HH, et al. The effect of an anti-IgE monoclonal antibody on the early- and late-phase responses to allergen inhalation in asthmatic subjects. *Am J Respir Crit Care Med*. 1997;155:1828–1834.

3. Leckie MJ, ten Brinke A, Khan J, et al. Effects of an interleukin-5 blocking monoclonal antibody on eosinophils, airway hyper-responsiveness, and the late asthmatic response. *Lancet*. 2000;356:2144–2148.

4. Borish LC, Nelson HS, Corren J, et al. Efficacy of soluble IL-4 receptor for the treatment of adults with asthma. *J Allergy Clin Immunol*. 2001;107:963–970.

5. Boguniewicz M, Schneider LC, Milgrom H, et al. Treatment of steroid-dependent asthma with recombinant interferon-gamma. *Clin Exp Allergy*. 1993;23:785–790.

6. Bryan SA, O'Connor BJ, Matti S, et al. Effects of recombinant human interleukin-12 on eosinophils, airway hyper-responsiveness, and the late asthmatic response. *Lancet*. 2000;356:2149–2153.

7. Bosse Y, Pare PD, Seow CY. Airway wall remodeling in asthma: from the epithelial layer to the adventitia. *Curr Allergy Asthma Rep*. 2008;8:357–366.

8. Rosi E, Ronchi MC, Grazzini M, et al. Sputum analysis, bronchial hyperresponsiveness, and airway function in asthma: results of a factor analysis. *J Allergy Clin Immunol*. 1999;103:232–237.

9. Oddera S, Silvestri M, Penna R, et al. Airway eosinophilic inflammation and bronchial hyperresponsiveness after allergen inhalation challenge in asthma. *Lung*. 1998;176:237–247.

10. Crapo RO, Casaburi R, Coates AL, et al. Guidelines for methacholine and exercise challenge testing-1999. This official statement of the American Thoracic Society was adopted by the ATS Board of Directors, July 1999. *Am J Respir Crit Care Med*. 2000;161:309–329.

11. Joos GF, O'Connor B, Anderson SD, et al. Indirect airway challenges. *Eur Respir J*. 2003;21:1050–1068.

12. Cockcroft DW, Murdock KY. Comparative effects of inhaled salbutamol, sodium cromoglycate, and beclomethasone dipropionate on allergen-induced early asthmatic responses, late asthmatic responses, and increased bronchial responsiveness to histamine. *J Allergy Clin Immunol*. 1987;79:734–740.

13. Hutson PA, Holgate ST, Church MK. The effect of cromolyn sodium and albuterol on early and late phase bronchoconstriction and airway leukocyte infiltration after allergen challenge of nonanesthetized guinea pigs. *Am Rev Respir Dis*. 1988;138:1157–1163.

14. Siergiejko Z. [The effect of salmeterol on specific and non-specific bronchial response in allergic asthma patients]. *Pneumonol Alergol Pol*. 1998;66:440–449.

15. Duong M, Gauvreau G, Watson R, et al. The effects of inhaled budesonide and formoterol in combination and alone when given directly after allergen challenge. *J Allergy Clin Immunol*. 2007;119:322–327.

16. Palmqvist M, Balder B, Lowhagen O, et al. Late asthmatic reaction decreased after pretreatment with salbutamol and formoterol, a new long-acting beta 2-agonist. *J Allergy Clin Immunol*. 1992;89:844–849.

17. Pauwels R, Van Renterghem D, Van der Straeten M, et al. The effect of theophylline and enprofylline on allergen-induced bronchoconstriction. *J Allergy Clin Immunol*. 1985;76:583–590.

18. Crescioli S, Spinazzi A, Plebani M, et al. Theophylline inhibits early and late asthmatic reactions induced by allergens in asthmatic subjects. *Ann Allergy*. 1991;66:245–251.

19. Taylor IK, O'Shaughnessy KM, Choudry NB, et al. A comparative study in atopic subjects with asthma of the effects of salmeterol and salbutamol on allergen-induced bronchoconstriction, increase in airway reactivity, and increase in urinary leukotriene E4 excretion. *J Allergy Clin Immunol*. 1992;89:575–583.

20. Twentyman OP, Finnerty JP, Harris A, et al. Protection against allergen-induced asthma by salmeterol. *Lancet*. 1990;336:1338–1342.

21. Diamant Z, Grootendorst DC, Veselic-Charvat M, et al. The effect of montelukast (MK-0476), a cysteinyl leukotriene receptor antagonist, on allergen-induced airway responses and sputum cell counts in asthma. *Clin Exp Allergy*. 1999;29:42–51.

22. Aalbers R, Kauffman HF, Groen H, et al. The effect of nedocromil sodium on the early and late reaction and allergen-induced bronchial hyperresponsiveness. *J Allergy Clin Immunol*. 1991;87:993–1001.

23. Howarth PH, Durham SR, Lee TH, et al. Influence of albuterol, cromolyn sodium and ipratropium bromide on the airway and circulating mediator responses to allergen bronchial provocation in asthma. *Am Rev Respir Dis*. 1985;132:986–992.

24. Hui KP, Taylor IK, Taylor GW, et al. Effect of a 5-lipoxygenase inhibitor on leukotriene generation and airway responses after allergen challenge in asthmatic patients. *Thorax*. 1991;46:184–189.

25. Roquet A, Dahlen B, Kumlin M, et al. Combined antagonism of leukotrienes and histamine produces predominant inhibition of allergen-induced early and late phase airway obstruction in asthmatics. *Am J Respir Crit Care Med*. 1997;155:1856–1863.

26. Haselden BM, Larche M, Meng Q, et al. Late asthmatic reactions provoked by intradermal injection of T-cell peptide epitopes are not associated with bronchial mucosal infiltration of eosinophils or T(H)2-type cells or with elevated concentrations of histamine or eicosanoids in bronchoalveolar fluid. *J Allergy Clin Immunol*. 2001;108:394–401.

27. Lemanske RF Jr, Dick EC, Swenson CA, et al. Rhinovirus upper respiratory infection increases airway hyperreactivity and late asthmatic reactions. *J Clin Invest*. 1989;83:1–10.

28. Nicholson KG, Kent J, Ireland DC. Respiratory viruses and exacerbations of asthma in adults. *BMJ*. 1993;307:982–986.

29. Johnston SL, Pattemore PK, Sanderson G, et al. Community study of role of viral infections in exacerbations of asthma in 9-11 year old children. *BMJ*.1995;310:1225–1229.

30. Avila PC, Boushey HA, Wong H, et al. Effect of a single dose of the selectin inhibitor TBC1269 on early and late asthmatic responses. *Clin Exp Allergy*. 2004;34:77–84.

31. Claman DM, Boushey HA, Liu J, et al. Analysis of induced sputum to examine the effects of prednisone on airway inflammation in asthmatic subjects. *J Allergy Clin Immunol*. 1994;94:861–869.

32. van Rensen EL, Straathof KC, Veselic-Charvat MA, et al. Effect of inhaled steroids on airway hyperresponsiveness, sputum eosinophils, and exhaled nitric oxide levels in patients with asthma. *Thorax*. 1999;54:403–408.

33. Pizzichini E, Leff JA, Reiss TF, et al. Montelukast reduces airway eosinophilic inflammation in asthma: a randomized, controlled trial. *Eur Respir J*. 1999;14:12–18.

34. Djukanovic R, Wilson SJ, Kraft M, et al. Effects of treatment with anti-immunoglobulin E antibody omalizumab on airway inflammation in allergic asthma. *Am J Respir Crit Care Med*. 2004;170:583–593.

35. Devalia JL, Rusznak C, Abdelaziz MM, et al. Nedocromil sodium and airway inflammation in vivo and in vitro. *J Allergy Clin Immunol*. 1996;98:S51–S57; discussion S64–S56.

36. Rytila P, Pelkonen AS, Metso T, et al. Induced sputum in children with newly diagnosed mild asthma: the effect of 6 months of treatment with budesonide or disodium cromoglycate. *Allergy*. 2004;59:839–844.

37. Stelmach I, Jerzynska J, Brzozowska A, et al. Double-blind, randomized, placebo-controlled trial of effect of nedocromil sodium on clinical and inflammatory parameters of asthma in children allergic to dust mite. *Allergy*. 2001;56:518–524.

38. Stelmach I, Majak P, Jerzynska J, et al. Comparative effect of triamcinolone, nedocromil and montelukast on asthma control in children: A randomized pragmatic study. *Pediatr Allergy Immunol*. 2004;15:359–364.

39. Jatakanon A, Uasuf C, Maziak W, et al. Neutrophilic inflammation in severe persistent asthma. *Am J Respir Crit Care Med*. 1999;160:1532–1539.

40. Woodruff PG, Khashayar R, Lazarus SC, et al. Relationship between airway inflammation, hyperresponsiveness, and obstruction in asthma. *J Allergy Clin Immunol*. 2001;108:753–758.

41. Green RH, Brightling CE, Woltmann G, et al. Analysis of induced sputum in adults with asthma: identification of subgroup with isolated sputum neutrophilia and poor response to inhaled corticosteroids. *Thorax*. 2002;57:875–879.

42. Liu MC, Proud D, Lichtenstein LM, et al. Effects of prednisone on the cellular responses and release of cytokines and mediators after segmental allergen challenge of asthmatic subjects. *J Allergy Clin Immunol*. 2001;108:29–38.

43. Sulakvelidze I, Inman MD, Rerecich T, et al. Increases in airway eosinophils and interleukin-5 with minimal bronchoconstriction during repeated low-dose allergen challenge in atopic asthmatics. *Eur Respir J*. 1998;11:821–827.

44. Hoshino M, Nakamura Y, Sim JJ, et al. Inhaled corticosteroid reduced lamina reticularis of the basement membrane by modulation of insulin-like growth factor (IGF)-I expression in bronchial asthma. *Clin Exp Allergy*. 1998;28:568–577.

45. Sont JK, Willems LN, Bel EH, et al. Clinical control and histopathologic outcome of asthma when using airway hyperresponsiveness as an additional guide to long-term treatment. The AMPUL Study Group. *Am J Respir Crit Care Med*. 1999;159:1043–1051.

46. Boushey HA, Sorkness CA, King TS, et al. Daily versus as-needed corticosteroids for mild persistent asthma. *N Engl J Med*. 2005; 352:1519–1528.

47. ATS, ERS. ATS/ERS recommendations for standardized procedures for the online and offline measurement of exhaled lower respiratory nitric oxide and nasal nitric oxide, 2005. *Am J Respir Crit Care Med*. 2005;171:912–930.

48. Smith AD, Cowan JO, Brassett KP, et al. Use of exhaled nitric oxide measurements to guide treatment in chronic asthma. *N Engl J Med*. 2005;352:2163–2173.

49. Szefler SJ, Mitchell H, Sorkness CA, et al. Management of asthma based on exhaled nitric oxide in addition to guideline-based treatment for inner-city adolescents and young adults: a randomised controlled trial. *Lancet*. 2008;372:1065–1072.

50. Petsky HL, Cates CJ, Li AM, et al. Tailored interventions based on exhaled nitric oxide versus clinical symptoms for asthma in children and adults. *Cochrane Database Syst Rev*. 2008:CD006340.

51. Horvath I, Hunt J, Barnes PJ, et al. Exhaled breath condensate: methodological recommendations and unresolved questions. *Eur Respir J*. 2005;26:523–548.

52. Hunt JF, Fang K, Malik R, et al. Endogenous airway acidification. Implications for asthma pathophysiology. *Am J Respir Crit Care Med*. 2000;161:694–699.

53. Shimizu Y, Dobashi K, Mori M. Exhaled breath marker in asthma patients with gastroesophageal reflux disease. *J Clin Biochem Nutr*. 2007;41:147–153.

54. Juniper EF, Buist AS, Cox FM, et al. Validation of a standardized version of the Asthma Quality of Life Questionnaire. *Chest*. 1999;115:1265–1270.

55. Juniper EF. Health-related quality of life in asthma. *Curr Opin Pulm Med*. 1999;5:105–110.

56. Expert Panel Report 3. *NHLBI Guidelines for the Diagnosis and Management of Asthma*. 2007 11/26/2008]. Available from: http://www.nhlbi.nih.gov/guidelines/asthma/.

57. Global Initiative for Asthma. *GINA Report, Global Strategy for Asthma Management and Prevention*. 2007 11/26/2008]. Available from: http://www.ginasthma.com/.

58. Suissa S, Ernst P, Benayoun S, et al. Low-dose inhaled corticosteroids and the prevention of death from asthma. *N Engl J Med*. 2000;343:332–336.

59. ATS. Proceedings of the ATS workshop on refractory asthma: current understanding, recommendations, and unanswered questions.

American Thoracic Society. *Am J Respir Crit Care Med*. 2000;162:2341–2351.

60. Lange P, Parner J, Vestbo J, et al. A 15-year follow-up study of ventilatory function in adults with asthma. *N Engl J Med*. 1998;339:1194–1200.

61. Haahtela T, Jarvinen M, Kava T, et al. Comparison of a beta 2-agonist, terbutaline, with an inhaled corticosteroid, budesonide, in newly detected asthma. *N Engl J Med*. 1991;325:388–392.

62. Haahtela T, Jarvinen M, Kava T, et al. Effects of reducing or discontinuing inhaled budesonide in patients with mild asthma. *N Engl J Med*. 1994;331:700–705.

63. Drazen JM, Israel E, Boushey HA, et al. Comparison of regularly scheduled with as-needed use of albuterol in mild asthma. Asthma Clinical Research Network. *N Engl J Med*. 1996;335:841–847.

64. Pauwels RA, Lofdahl CG, Postma DS, et al. Effect of inhaled formoterol and budesonide on exacerbations of asthma. Formoterol and Corticosteroids Establishing Therapy (FACET) International Study Group. *N Engl J Med*. 1997;337:1405–1411.

65. Rowe BH, Bota GW, Fabris L, et al. Inhaled budesonide in addition to oral corticosteroids to prevent asthma relapse following discharge from the emergency department: a randomized controlled trial. *JAMA*. 1999;281:2119–2126.

66. Milgrom H, Fick RB Jr, Su JQ, et al. Treatment of allergic asthma with monoclonal anti-IgE antibody. rhuMAb-E25 Study Group. *N Engl J Med*. 1999;341:1966–1973.

67. Malmstrom K, Rodriguez-Gomez G, Guerra J, et al. Oral montelukast, inhaled beclomethasone, and placebo for chronic asthma. A randomized, controlled trial. Montelukast/Beclomethasone Study Group. *Ann Intern Med*. 1999;130:487–495.

68. CAMP. Long-term effects of budesonide or nedocromil in children with asthma. The Childhood Asthma Management Program Research Group. *N Engl J Med*. 2000;343:1054–1063.

69. Lazarus SC, Boushey HA, Fahy JV, et al. Long-acting beta2-agonist monotherapy vs continued therapy with inhaled corticosteroids in patients with persistent asthma: a randomized controlled trial. *JAMA*. 2001;285:2583–2593.

70. Lemanske RF Jr, Sorkness CA, Mauger EA, et al. Inhaled corticosteroid reduction and elimination in patients with persistent asthma receiving salmeterol: a randomized controlled trial. *JAMA*. 2001; 285:2594–2603.

71. Hughes R, Goldkorn A, Masoli M, et al. Use of isotonic nebulised magnesium sulphate as an adjuvant to salbutamol in treatment of severe asthma in adults: randomised placebo-controlled trial. *Lancet*. 2003;361:2114–2117.

72. Pauwels RA, Pedersen S, Busse WW, et al. Early intervention with budesonide in mild persistent asthma: a randomised, double-blind trial. *Lancet*. 2003;361:1071–1076.

73. Israel E, Chinchilli VM, Ford JG, et al. Use of regularly scheduled albuterol treatment in asthma: genotype-stratified, randomised, placebo-controlled cross-over trial. *Lancet*. 2004;364:1505–1512.

74. Morgan WJ, Crain EF, Gruchalla RS, et al. Results of a home-based environmental intervention among urban children with asthma. *N Engl J Med*. 2004;351:1068–1080.

75. Bateman ED, Boushey HA, Bousquet J, et al. Can guideline-defined asthma control be achieved? The Gaining Optimal Asthma ControL study. *Am J Respir Crit Care Med*. 2004;170:836–844.

76. O'Byrne PM, Bisgaard H, Godard PP, et al. Budesonide/formoterol combination therapy as both maintenance and reliever medication in asthma. *Am J Respir Crit Care Med*. 2005;171:129–136.

77. Guilbert TW, Morgan WJ, Zeiger RS, et al. Long-term inhaled corticosteroids in preschool children at high risk for asthma. *N Engl J Med*. 2006;354:1985–1997.

78. Rabe KF, Atienza T, Magyar P, et al. Effect of budesonide in combination with formoterol for reliever therapy in asthma exacerbations: a randomised controlled, double-blind study. *Lancet*. 2006; 368:744–753.

79. Nelson HS, Weiss ST, Bleecker ER, et al. The Salmeterol Multicenter Asthma Research Trial: a comparison of usual pharmacotherapy for asthma or usual pharmacotherapy plus salmeterol. *Chest*. 2006; 129:15–26.

80. Papi A, Canonica GW, Maestrelli P, et al. Rescue use of beclomethasone and albuterol in a single inhaler for mild asthma. *N Engl J Med*. 2007;356:2040–2052.

SECTION VI

Other Immunologic Pulmonary Disease

CHAPTER 23

Hypersensitivity Pneumonitis

MICHAEL C. ZACHARISEN AND JORDAN N. FINK

Hypersensitivity pneumonitis, also known as extrinsic allergic alveolitis, is a multifaceted immunologically mediated pulmonary disease with associated constitutional symptoms due to sensitization and then repeated inhalation of a wide variety of inhaled organic dusts. It is characterized by nonimmunoglobulin E (IgE)-mediated inflammation of the pulmonary interstitium, terminal airways, and alveoli. This syndrome occurs in both atopic and nonatopic individuals and may present in several clinical forms depending on the duration, frequency, and intensity of antigen exposure, the antigenicity of the offending agent, and the patient's age and immunologic responsiveness. The preponderance of cases occurs in occupational and agricultural settings. However, various hobbies and medications are also associated with hypersensitivity pneumonitis. Despite the many antigens recognized to cause hypersensitivity pneumonitis, the clinical, immunologic, and pathophysiologic findings are generally comparable.

■ ALLERGENS OF HYPERSENSITIVITY PNEUMONITIS

Hypersensitivity pneumonitis was recognized by Ramazzini in 1713 in grain workers (1). As awareness of this pulmonary disease has increased, there has been identi-fication of new antigens implicated in the disease currently encompassing over 200 different agents (2). Although the immunopathophysiology of the disease is becoming clarified, there continue to be cases of hypersensitivity pneumonitis in which the specific antigen has not been defined. The primary exposures for the development of hypersensitivity pneumonitis are occupational, agricultural, and those related to hobbies. To reach the terminal airways and alveoli, the allergenic particles must be smaller than 3 μm to 5 μm. The variety of causative antigens includes airborne microbial antigens, animal or plant products, and low-molecular-weight chemicals (Table 23.1). Many of these same antigens, such as diisocyanates, mammalian and insect proteins, and wood dusts, also can induce IgE-mast cell mediated allergic responses including asthma.

Thermophilic actinomycetes were recognized as the causative agent in farmer's lung in 1932 in England (3). These bacteria thrive at temperatures of 70°C and can be found in high concentrations in compost piles or in silos where animal fodder is stored and becomes a culture medium for the organism. Identification and clarification of the responsible antigens have been described by a number of investigators (4,5). Increased awareness of the environmental factors favoring disease and changes in farming techniques have reduced the incidence of this disorder (6).

TABLE 23.1   SOME ANTIGENS OF HYPERSENSITIVITY PNEUMONITIS

ANTIGENS	SOURCE OF ANTIGEN	DISEASE NAME
Bacteria		
Thermophilic actinomycetes (Saccharopolyspora rectivirgula, Thermoactinomyces vulgaris)	Moldy hay, compost, silage, grain, moldy sugarcane	Farmer's lung, mushroom picker's lung, bagassosis
Bacillus, Klebsiella, Cytophaga	Air conditioner, humidifier	Ventilation pneumonitis, humidifier lung
Pseudomonas, Acinetobacter	Contaminated metal-working fluids	Machine operator's lung
Bacillus subtilis	Enzyme dust	Enzyme/detergent worker's lung
Mycobacterium	Hot tub, metal-working fluids	Hot tub lung
Fungi		
Aspergillus	Moldy brewing malt, stucco, compost, soy sauce, home contamination	Malt worker's lung, stipatosis, compost lung
Alternaria, Pullaria	Moldy redwood, wood dust	Wood worker's lung, sequoiosis
Cephalosporium	Moldy wood floors or basement, sewer water	Floor finisher's lung
Epicoccum, Rhodotorula	Cellar, bathroom and shower walls	
Penicillium	Moldy cheese, cork dust, hay, wood dust, salami seasoning, compost	Cheese worker's/washer's lung, suberosis, residential composter's lung
Penicillium, Monocillium	Moldy peat moss	Peat moss processor's lung
Cryptostroma corticale	Moldy maple bark	Maple bark disease
Trichosporum	Moldy homes in Japan	Summer pneumonitis
Pleurotus, Hypsizigus, Lyphyllum, Cortinus shiitake, Pholiota	Indoor mushroom cultivation	Mushroom picker's/worker's lung
Candida	Moldy reed	Saxophonist's lung
Pezizia, Penicillium, Fusarium	Moldy home	El Niño lung
Cladosporium	Contaminated water, moldy home	Hot tub lung/sauna taker's lung
Rhizopus, Mucor	Moldy wood trimmings	Wood trimmer's disease
Amebae		
Naegleria, Acanthamoeba	Contaminated humidifier/ventilation	Ventilation pneumonitis
Animal protein		
Avian proteins (pigeon, duck, goose, turkey, chicken, dove, parakeet, parrot, lovebird, owl, canary, pheasant)	Droppings, feather bloom	Bird/pigeon breeder's lung/disease, bird fancier's disease, budgerigar disease, plucker's lung, duck fever
Rodent urine/serum protein	Rat or gerbil urine or serum	Lab worker's lung, gerbil keeper's lung
Pearl oyster/mollusk shell protein	Shell dust	Oyster shell lung/sericulturist lung
Animal fur dust (e.g., cat)	Animal pelts, fur	Furrier's lung
Insect (grain weevil, silk worm)	Sitophilus granarius, silk worm larvae	Wheat weevil disease

(continued)

TABLE 23.1   SOME ANTIGENS OF HYPERSENSITIVITY PNEUMONITIS (*CONTINUED*)

ANTIGENS	SOURCE OF ANTIGEN	DISEASE NAME
Drugs/Medications		
Amiodarone, chlorambucil, cloza-pine, cyclosporin, gold, β blocker, sulfonamide, nitrofurantoin, mino-cycline, procarbazine, leflunomide, methotrexate	HMG-CoA reductase inhibitor, fluoxetine, roxithromycin, lenali-domide, loxoprofen, mesal-amine, sirolimus, tocainamide, trofosfamide, hydroxyurea, nasal heroin	Drug-induced hypersensitivity pneumonitis
Chemicals		
Isocyanates (TDI, HDI, MDI)	Paint/chemical catalyst, varnish, lacquer, polyurethane foam plasticizer, spandex fibers, poly-urethane elastomers	Bathtub refinisher's disease, paint refinisher's disease, plastic worker's lung, chemical worker's lung
Phthalic anhydride	Heated epoxy resin, dyes, insecticides	Epoxy resin lung
Dimethyl phthalate or styrene	Chemicals used in manufacture of yachts	Yacht-maker's lung
Methylmethacrylate	Dental prosthesis making	
Others	Tobacco leaves	Tobacco grower's lung
	Insecticide	Pyrethrum lung
	Coffee bean and tea leaf dust	Coffee worker's lung, tea grower's lung
	Sawdust (pine, Cabreuva wood)	Wood worker's lung
	Fish meal extract	Fish meal worker's lung
	Veterinary feed containing soybean hulls	

HMG-CoA, 3-hydroxy-3-methyl-glutaryl–coenzyme A; TDI, toluene diisocyanate; HDI, hexamethylene diisocyanate; MDI, methylene diphenyl diisocyanate.

Both commercial and residential exposures to mold-contaminated materials have been implicated in a number of cases of hypersensitivity pneumonitis with the descriptive names of many of these diseases reflecting the source of exposure. For example, ventilation pneumonitis, caused by contaminated heating or cooling units, is probably the most common building-related form of hypersensitivity pneumonitis (7,8). This syndrome may occur as a result of the inhalation of aerosols containing antigens found in small home ultrasonic humidifiers to large industrial air handling units (9). Over the past decade, respiratory illness related to inhalation of metal-working fluids containing gram-negative bacteria has been reported; this finding has far-reaching consequences for industry (10–12). While fungal exposure is ubiquitous outdoors, indoor exposure in water-damaged environments is less well characterized, but many case reports incriminate fungi as the cause of the disease in both adults and children (13). The role of fungal fragments in initiating human disease has yet to be clarified, but it provides a new par-adigm for fungal exposure (14). Workers cultivating mushrooms in indoor facilities have been identified as another occupation with many affected individuals (15,16). Pigeon breeders and bird fanciers have long been recognized to develop hypersensitivity pneumonitis to inhaled antigens in dried avian droppings and feather bloom (17,18). A variety of exotic, wild, and domestic birds have also been identified as causing bird breeder's disease (19–21).

As new cases of hypersensitivity pneumonitis are recognized, measures to identify the antigen and decrease antigen exposure can be implemented. This recognition, as well as changes in exposure, has resulted in some hypersensitivity diseases such as smallpox handler's lung and pituitary snuff taker's lung (porcine and bovine allergens) being of historical interest only (22). Occupational exposures recently recognized include the manufacture of yacht hulls where inhalation of fumes from heated chemicals in rolling fiberglass has been implicated (23). Kiln-dried wood heavily contaminated with Paecilomyces has affected workers in a hardwood floor processing plant (24). Inhalation of the coolant HFC134a used during laser removal of body hair has been reported to trigger HP symptoms with peripheral blood and bronchial biopsy eosinophilia (25).

Medications are also an important cause of pulmonary disease that resembles hypersensitivity pneumonitis. Among the implicated medications are nitrofurantoin, amiodarone, minocycline, roxithromycin, lenalidomide, nadolol, and sulphasalazine (26–31). Intranasal heroin has also been reported to cause the syndrome (32).

Specific syndromes of hypersensitivity pneumonitis occur in different parts of the world. For example, esparto grass is used in the production of rope, matting, paper pulp, and plaster in Mediterranean countries. Individuals such as stucco workers have developed hypersensitivity pneumonitis to *Aspergillus fumigates*-contaminated esparto fiber dust in their workplace environments (33). Workers in Eastern Canada who are employed in peat moss processing plants are frequently exposed to loose dry material which may contain many microorganisms, of which molds have been implicated in causing hypersensitivity pneumonitis (34). Summer-type hypersensitivity pneumonitis due to Trichosporon is an important example of a disease not found in the United States, but is the most prevalent form of hypersensitivity pneumonitis in Japan (35). In the Midwest United States, of 85 patients with hypersensitivity pneumonitis identified from 1997 to 2002, the most common causes were avian-related (34%), hot tub lung (21%), farmer's lung (11%), household mold exposure (9%), and unidentified antigen (25%) (36). Controversy surrounds the classification of "hot tub lung" as hypersensitivity pneumonitis versus infection with nontuberculous mycobacteria.

EPIDEMIOLOGY

The exact incidence of hypersensitivity pneumonitis is unknown, but it has been identified in 2% to 8% of farmers (37) and in 6% to 21% of pigeon breeders (38). Of 36 cases of chronic hypersensitivity pneumonitis identified by a hospital survey in Japan, reported etiologies were summer-type hypersensitivity pneumonitis (10 cases), other home-related causes (5 cases), bird fancier's disease (7 cases), isocyanate (5 cases), farmer's lung (4 cases), and five miscellaneous cases (39). In Ireland, haymaking methods were revolutionized in the 1980s and between 1997 and 2002, a marked decline in hypersensitivity pneumonitis was observed (40). In the United Kingdom, however, the overall incidence of hypersensitivity pneumonitis is stable at 600 new cases per year (1 per 100,000 general population) (41). In the United States, the "healthy worker effect" and high employee turnover may be partly responsible for the underreporting or underrecognition of work-related cases of hypersensitivity pneumonitis.

DIAGNOSTIC CRITERIA AND CLINICAL FEATURES

The criteria for the diagnosis of hypersensitivity pneumonitis consist of recognizing the clinical features with supporting exposure history, laboratory, pulmonary function, and radiographic characteristics (Fig. 23.1.) (42). While there is no single confirmatory test for hypersensitivity pneumonitis, not even lung biopsy, six significant predictors were identified that provide a 95% confidence interval. These include: (a) exposure to a known offending allergen; (b) positive precipitating antibodies to the offending antigen; (c) recurrent episodes of symptoms; (d) inspiratory crackles on lung auscultation; (e) symptoms occurring 4 to 8 hours after exposure, and (f) weight loss (43). The clinical presentation follows repeated exposure and can vary from sudden and explosive systemic and respiratory symptoms to an insidious, progressive course of dyspnea, fatigue, and weight loss. Based on these clinical presentations, hypersensitivity pneumonitis has been divided into acute, subacute, and chronic forms (44).

The patient with the acute form presents with nonproductive cough, dyspnea, sweating, myalgia, and malaise occurring 4 to 12 hours after intense exposure to the inciting allergen. Acute viral or bacterial infections may mimic this presentation, leading to treatment with antibiotics. With avoidance of the allergen, the symptoms spontaneously resolve over 18 to 24 hours, with complete resolution within days. This is in contrast to viral infections. On repeat exposure, the symptoms recur with either more severe and progressive symptoms or less intense and nonprogressive symptoms. The patient may recognize this pattern and try to minimize their exposure. The chronic form is characterized by the insidious onset of dyspnea that especially occurs with exertion. Other symptoms include productive cough, fatigue, and anorexia with weight loss. Fever is not typical unless there is a high-dose allergen exposure superimposed on the chronic symptoms. This form is usually related to continuous low-level antigen exposure and is not often recognized resulting in a delay in the correct diagnosis. An antigen exposure history could be the only clue to the diagnosis. The subacute form is characterized by symptoms intermediate to the acute and chronic form with progressive lower respiratory symptoms. The acute and subacute forms may overlap clinically, just as the subacute and chronic forms may.

PHYSICAL EXAMINATION

The physical examination may be normal in the asymptomatic patient between widely spaced episodes of acute hypersensitivity pneumonitis. Fine, dry rales may be present, depending on the degree of lung disease present and the timing following the most recent exposure. Wheezing is not a prominent symptom. An

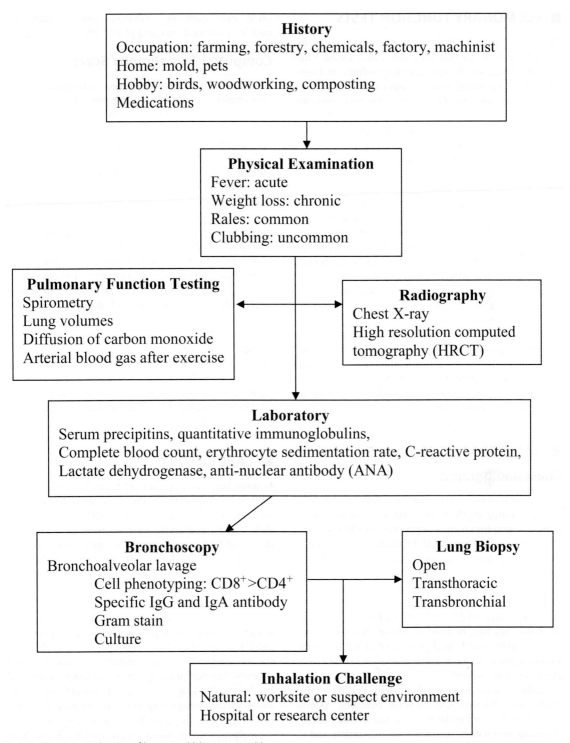

History
Occupation: farming, forestry, chemicals, factory, machinist
Home: mold, pets
Hobby: birds, woodworking, composting
Medications

Physical Examination
Fever: acute
Weight loss: chronic
Rales: common
Clubbing: uncommon

Pulmonary Function Testing
Spirometry
Lung volumes
Diffusion of carbon monoxide
Arterial blood gas after exercise

Radiography
Chest X-ray
High resolution computed tomography (HRCT)

Laboratory
Serum precipitins, quantitative immunoglobulins,
Complete blood count, erythrocyte sedimentation rate, C-reactive protein,
Lactate dehydrogenase, anti-nuclear antibody (ANA)

Bronchoscopy
Bronchoalveolar lavage
    Cell phenotyping: $CD8^+ > CD4^+$
    Specific IgG and IgA antibody
    Gram stain
    Culture

Lung Biopsy
Open
Transthoracic
Transbronchial

Inhalation Challenge
Natural: worksite or suspect environment
Hospital or research center

■ **FIGURE 23.1** Evaluation of hypersensitivity pneumonitis.

acute flare-up of hypersensitivity pneumonitis is associated with an ill-appearing patient in respiratory distress with temperature elevation up to 40°C 6 to 12 hours after antigen exposure. Rash, lymphadenopathy, or rhinitis should prompt investigation for causes other than hypersensitivity pneumonitis. With extensive fibrosis that occurs in the chronic form of the disease, dry rales and decreased breath sounds predominate. Some patients with end-stage disease may have digital clubbing (45).

■ PULMONARY FUNCTION TESTS

The classic pulmonary function abnormality in the acute form is restriction with decreased forced vital capacity (FVC) and forced expiratory volume in 1 second (FEV_1) occurring 6 to 12 hours after exposure to the offending antigen (*Fig. 23.2*). A biphasic obstructive response similar to that seen in the early and late phases of asthma has been observed in patients who develop both asthma and hypersensitivity pneumonitis as a result of sensitization to the same antigen. Peripheral airways obstruction as determined by decreased FEV_1 and/or forced midrange flow measurements ($FEF_{25-75\%}$) has frequently been reported. Decreased gas transfer across the alveolar wall as measured by the diffusion capacity of carbon monoxide (DLCO) is often detected. This is in contrast to asthma, a disease in which an elevated DLCO commonly occurs. Although hypoxemia at rest may be observed with severe lung damage, hypoxemia with exercise is common and can be documented by pre- and postexercise arterial blood gas measurements. Bronchial hyperresponsiveness as determined by methacholine challenge is present in a majority of patients with hypersensitivity pneumonitis and is likely due to the inflammatory response of the airways. In subacute and chronic hypersensitivity pneumonitis, there is usually a demonstrable combination of obstruction and restriction.

■ RADIOGRAPHIC FEATURES

Chest Radiographs

Radiographic abnormalities may be transient or permanent depending on the form or stage of disease. Transient radiographic changes occur primarily in the acute form with patchy, peripheral, bilateral interstitial infiltrates with a fine, reticulonodular pattern similar to acute pulmonary edema (46) as seen in *Figure 23.3*. There may be bilateral ground-glass opacities in the middle to lower lung fields that are indistinguishable from other interstitial lung disorders. Central lymphadenopathy also may be present. These changes usually resolve spontaneously with avoidance or with corticosteroid therapy. Between acute attacks, the chest radiograph is usually normal.

In the subacute form, nodular, patchy, or diffuse infiltrates with bilateral ground-glass opacities; poorly defined small centrilobular nodules; and lobular areas of decreased attenuation, vascularity on inspiration, and of air-trapping on expiration have been observed (47).

In the chronic form, fibrotic changes with patchy or random reticulation, traction bronchiectasis, and areas of emphysema may be seen superimposed on acute or subacute changes, typically sparing the lung bases. Less commonly, subpleural honeycombing is found (47). Findings not characteristic of hypersensitivity pneumonitis include calcification, cavitation, atelectasis, solitary pulmonary nodules, pneumothorax, and pleural effusions.

Computed Tomography Scans

High-resolution chest computed tomography (CT) scans may be helpful when vague parenchymal changes are present on plain chest radiographs. Findings include ground-glass opacification and diffuse consolidation suggestive of alveolar disease. A normal chest CT scan does not rule out acute hypersensitivity pneumonitis because the sensitivity of this technique may be only 55% (48). In subacute disease, 1- to 3-mm ill-defined centrilobular nodules with superimposed areas of ground-glass opacity may be seen (49). The CT findings of the chronic form are honeycombing, pulmonary fibrosis, and traction bronchiectasis. CT features to suggest hypersensitivity pneumonitis are predominantly middle lung involvement, extensive ground-glass opacities, and small nodules often in the central and peripheral compartments. The role of magnetic resonance imaging has been limited due to respiratory and cardiac motion artifact. Similarly, gallium lung scan and the clearance rate from the alveolar epithelium using a technetium-label are being investigated in the early detection of inflammation or damage to the alveolar-capillary unit, respectively, in infiltrative lung diseases, but studies specifically in hypersensitivity pneumonitis are lacking (50).

■ LABORATORY

Routine laboratory studies are typically normal in the asymptomatic patient. In the acute form, leukocytosis with a white blood cell count to 25,000 mm^3 and a left shift, an elevated erythrocyte sedimentation rate, and decreased DLCO are common. Eosinophilia is uncommon. Total serum IgE levels are normal unless the patient has coexisting atopic disease (51). Quantitative immunoglobulin measurements are normal, or at times serum IgG may be elevated.

The characteristic immunologic feature of hypersensitivity pneumonitis is the presence of high titers of precipitating IgG and other classes of antibodies directed against the offending antigen demonstrated in the sera of affected patients (52). Serum precipitating antibodies, as detected by the Ouchterlony double-gel immunodiffusion technique, indicate antigen exposure, but not necessarily disease (*Fig. 23.4*). In pigeon breeders, as many as 50% of similarly exposed but asymptomatic individuals may have detectable precipitins (53). False negative precipitin panels could result from omission of the responsible antigen from the test panel. Enzyme-linked immunosorbent assays and complement fixation techniques for antibody measurements may be too sensitive. However, a small study using an automated solid-phase indirect enzyme-assay with fluorimetry was shown to be more sensitive in detecting symptomatic bird fanciers using antibody level of 10 mg/L in contrast to precipitin formation which detects antibody at over 40 mg/L. The assay was rapid and may be able to differentiate between pigeon breeders who have subacute or insidious onset of chronic avian hypersensitivity pneumonitis (54). Compared to double diffusion, electrosyneresis (electrophoresis on cellulose acetate sheets) demonstrated value to detect mold antigens in symptomatic patients, but only if the appropriate antigens were selected (55). If these tests are negative despite a suggestive history, additional testing with antigens specifically prepared from the suspect environment may be necessary. Depending on the exposure, an airborne mist, fluid, dust, or soil sample may be obtained and cultured for contaminating microorganisms. This cultured material can then be used as an antigen in gel diffusion reactions.

■ SKIN TESTING

In contrast to asthma and other IgE-mast cell mediated diseases, immediate wheal-and-flare skin reactivity to allergens is not useful because the immunopathogenesis of hypersensitivity pneumonitis does not involve IgE. Skin testing with antigens that cause hypersensitivity pneumonitis has been associated with late-onset skin reactions that histologically resemble Arthus-type reactions with mild vasculitis. On occasion, necrosis also has been observed. When differentiating IgE-mast cell mediated occupational asthma from hypersensitivity pneumonitis, skin testing can aid in the diagnosis. Both asthma and hypersensitivity pneumonitis may occur in the same individual; in that case, both immediate and late reactions to antigens used in cutaneous testing may occur.

■ BRONCHOALVEOLAR LAVAGE

Pulmonary consultation to conduct bronchoscopy and bronchoalveolar lavage may be indicated when other studies are normal or other diagnoses such as tuberculosis, pulmonary sarcoidosis, alveolar proteinosis, or idiopathic pulmonary fibrosis are entertained. Bronchoalveolar lavage fluid (BALF) is helpful in the diagnosis of hypersensitivity pneumonitis as there is a lymphocytosis with preponderance of CD8$^+$ T lymphocytes over CD4$^+$ T cells (56). An elevated lymphocyte count may not always be demonstrated in the chronic form. In contrast to the subacute and chronic forms of HP, increased alveolar macrophages are observed in the acute form. Lymphocytosis with a normal CD4/CD8 ratio correlated with more severe interstitial disease on HRCT (57). Recently, elevated levels of albumin in BALF using eriochrome cyanine R in fluorimetric determination was found in patients with HP (58). Cultures of BALF can help exclude infectious disorders.

■ PATHOLOGIC FEATURES

If a biopsy is deemed necessary, open lung biopsy is recommended to obtain an adequate tissue sample. Studies of transbronchial biopsy results suggest that the sample may not be adequate. Lung biopsy findings depend on the form of the disease and extent of lung damage that has occurred. The cells specifically are activated "foamy" macrophages, and have a marked predominance of lymphocytes, plasma cells, and neutrophils (59). The acute form has a marked neutrophilic infiltration in the alveoli and respiratory bronchioles with diffuse alveolar damage. Specimens of the subacute form classically reveal a triad of cellular bronchiolitis, patchy chronic interstitial lymphocytic pneumonitis, and scattered small alveolar noncaseating granulomas (47) *Fig. 23.5*. The granulomas differ from pulmonary sarcoidosis in that they appear smaller, dispersed in interstitial fibrosis, loosely arranged, poorly formed, and are distributed away from bronchioles and vessels. Immunoglobulin or complement has only rarely been demonstrated in pulmonary biopsies. In the later stages of chronic HP, interstitial fibrosis with collagen-thickened bronchiolar walls and less prominent lymphocytic alveolitis is common. In chronic bird fancier's lung, nonspecific interstitial pneumonia or usual interstitial pneumonia patterns may be seen (47).

■ SPECIFIC INHALATION CHALLENGE

Although purposeful inhalation challenge is not required for diagnosis, it can be helpful in situations in which the history is convincing but other data are lacking and the diagnosis is unclear. An allergen challenge can be performed in two ways. First, the patient can return to the workplace or the suspect environment where the antigen is present. In conjunction with pulmonary function and laboratory studies, this approach can implicate the suspect environment, but it will not necessarily identify the allergen. In evaluating these individuals, vital signs, including temperature, spirometry, diffusing capacity, and white blood cell counts with differentials, should be monitored before exposure and at intervals up to 12 hours later.

An inhalation challenge also can be performed in the hospital pulmonary function laboratory. In this situation, vital signs, including temperature, spirometry, and complete blood count should be monitored before, during, and after a controlled antigen exposure. Unfortunately, there generally is no specified concentration of allergen or commercially available allergen preparations for this use. The concentration of antigen used can be determined by using air sampling data, which reflects usual exposure. Nonspecific antigen should also be used as a control challenge. This inhalation test requires careful observation by trained personnel because severe systemic febrile and respiratory reactions requiring intervention with corticosteroids may occur.

■ DIFFERENTIAL DIAGNOSIS

Hypersensitivity pneumonitis should be considered in any patient with acute or chronic respiratory distress with or without systemic symptoms or interstitial pneumonia (*Table 23.2*). Like other occupational respiratory diseases, a detailed knowledge of the work and home environment is required. Documentation of cross-shift lung function changes can be detected in some individuals. It should be noted that hypersensitivity pneumonitis is limited to the lung and involvement of extra-pulmonary tissues has not been described.

The acute form of hypersensitivity pneumonitis is commonly confused with atypical, community-acquired pneumonia. A group of conditions referred to as organic dust toxic syndrome (ODTS) is also often confused with hypersensitivity pneumonitis (60). ODTS occurs in the agricultural setting, presents in individuals exposed to grain, silage, or swine materials, and primarily affects younger age groups and those without prior sensitization to offending agents. In contrast to hypersensitivity pneumonitis, ODTS is thought to be due to inhalation of endotoxin and other phlogistic agents. Diseases such as humidifier fever also can occur in outbreaks and may be related to inhalation of endotoxin from Gram-negative bacteria that contaminate ventilation and humidification systems (61).

The differential diagnosis of the subacute form of hypersensitivity pneumonitis includes chronic bronchitis, recurrent episodes of influenza, and idiopathic pulmonary fibrosis. "Hot tub lung" refers to a noncaseating granulomatous lung disease with nontuberculous mycobacteria (usually MAC) from exposure to hot water aerosols from hot tubs or spas, showers, and indoor swimming pools. Features of both infectious and immunologic pathogenesis have resulted in treatment with both corticosteroids and antituberculous agents although mere abstinence from hot tubs has been successful in some cases. While the chest CT scan findings are similar to HP, the histopathologic features are distinct (62,63).

The chronic form of hypersensitivity pneumonitis must be differentiated from many chronic interstitial lung diseases, including idiopathic pulmonary fibrosis, chronic eosinophilic pneumonia, collagen vascular disorders (dermatomyositis), emphysema, lymphogenous spread of carcinoma, sarcoid, desquamative interstitial pneumonia, and Hamman-Rich syndrome Table 23.3. Extrapulmonary findings of liver or spleen enlargement, generalized or local lymphadenopathy, severe sinusitis, or myositis are not consistent with hypersensitivity pneumonitis.

■ PATHOGENESIS

Although the mechanisms of inflammation are complex and still not fully clarified, the Gell and Coombs type III immune complex and IV cell-mediated reactions are the best paradigm for explaining the immunologic mechanisms that result in hypersensitivity pneumonitis. Several animal models and many animal studies have been conducted to elucidate the complexity of the immune inflammation-inducing disease (64–67). Unfortunately, the findings do not appear to directly parallel the inflammatory process seen in human disease. Also, there is difficulty evaluating exposed but asymptomatic animals, as can be done in human studies. Animal models suggest that hypersensitivity pneumonitis is facilitated by the overproduction of interferon-γ (IFN-γ), a helper T-cell type 1 (T_H1) response (68). This is supported by observations that interleukin-10 (IL-10), a T_H1 suppressor molecule, ameliorates the severity of the disease.

Human studies are more difficult to perform, relying on patients who have already experienced symptoms and therefore not truly evaluating the course of inflammation from the onset. The relative contributions of cellular versus humoral immunity in the pathogenesis are not entirely defined. A case report of a patient with hypogammaglobulinemia and hypersensitivity pneumonitis supports the central role of cellular immunity in mediating the disease (69).

The study data are frequently based on bronchoalveolar lavage findings compared with biopsy or peripheral blood. The data suggest that the most important elements in the inflammatory process are the activation of alveolar macrophages, $CD8^+$ cells and T_H1 lymphocytes. The hypothesized mechanism for hypersensitivity pneumonitis is depicted in *Fig. 23.6*. When antigens 2 μm to 10 μm in size are inhaled, they are engulfed and processed by activated alveolar macrophages that can be detected by an increase in surface IL-2R (CD25). The activated macrophages release proinflammatory cytokines such as IL-1 and tumor necrosis factor α (TNF-α) (70). This in turn activates endothelial cells to increase adhesion molecules by upregulating intracellular adhesion molecule type 1 (ICAM-1) and e-selectin (71).

Antigens also may combine with antibodies, forming immune complexes that directly activate complement releasing C3a and C5a, which promote chemotaxis of neutrophils. The neutrophils release superoxide anions, hydroxyl radicals, and toxic oxygen radicals, which contribute to the inflammation.

Alveolar macrophages have cognate interaction with regulatory $CD8^+$ T lymphocytes through the T-cell receptor in the presence of B7 costimulatory molecules CD80 and CD86 on macrophages, which act as an accessory signal (72). In healthy subjects, alveolar macrophages have a normal suppressive activity. In contrast, the activated alveolar macrophages in hypersensitivity pneumonitis increase the antigen-presenting capacity through the increased expression of CD80 and CD86, thus enhancing the lymphocytic alveolitis. Cigarette smoking may provide a protective effect from hypersensitivity pneumonitis by decreasing the expression of B7 costimulatory molecules, whereas viral infections could enhance hypersensitivity pneumonitis by increasing B7 expression. BALF CD8$^+$ T lymphocytes release multiple T_H1 cell type cytokines, including IL-2, IL-8, IL-12, IL-16, and IFN-γ. These cytokines are associated with an intense inflammatory process. In direct contrast to asthma, there is an imbalance of IL-10 and IL-12. Stimulated by TNF-α, IL-10 normally functions to inhibit ICAM-1 and B7 molecule expression to prevent the alveolar macrophage from interacting with the T cell, thus preventing activation. In hypersensitivity pneumonitis there is a decreased production of IL-10, leading to activated macrophages and ongoing inflammation. Gene polymorphisms for TNF-α, IL-10, and TGF-β examined by restriction fragment length polymorphism analysis did not support an association between genetic control of cytokine production and disease susceptibility in 61 patients with hypersensitivity pneumonitis compared to 101 healthy controls (73).

BALF T cells from patients with hypersensitivity pneumonitis have high levels of functioning IL-12R compared with peripheral blood T cells. When stimulated with recombinant IL-12, lung T cells significantly increased IFN-γ production (74). T lymphocytes along with mast cells can both produce and respond to nerve growth factor (NGF). This neurotrophic cytokine not only contributes to the development and survival of sympathetic and sensory neurons, but is associated with cough and found in higher levels in asthmatics and correlates with IgE levels. In asymptomatic pigeon fanciers, serum concentrations of NGF were normal, but increased in parallel with serum CRP as a marker of inflammation. *In vitro* studies using mitogen-induced production of NGF by lymphocytes was higher than normal (75).

NKT cells are a distinct subset of $\alpha\beta$ T cells and are characterized by the coexpression of surface markers of both these cell types and release large amounts of IL-4 and IFN-γ regulating the innate and adaptive immune response by modulating the T_H1/T_H2 balance. In mice, these cells can attenuate hypersensitivity pneumonitis by suppressing the IFN-γ producing neutrophils (76).

Increased expression of the integrin $\alpha^E\beta_7$ on the surface of T cells function as mucosal homing receptors for the selective retention of T lymphocytes in lung mucosa (77). The chemokines IL-8 and monocyte chemoattractant protein-1/monocyte chemotactic and activating factor (MCP-1/MCAF) are significantly increased in BALF, suggesting a role in the accumulation of cells such as neutrophils, lymphocytes, and monocyte/macrophages into the alveoli of patients with hypersensitivity pneumonitis (78). Arachidonic acid metabolites are released from many cell types. Along with hydrolytic enzymes, these further contribute to inflammation.

Surfactant is responsible for the regulatory activities of lung lymphocytes and alveolar macrophages. Alveolar macrophages from patients with hypersensitivity pneumonitis enhance PHA-induced peripheral blood mononuclear cell (PBMC) proliferation, whereas normal alveolar macrophages suppress this proliferation. Surfactant from normal individuals decreases mitogen-induced proliferation of PBMC greater than surfactant from patients with hypersensitivity pneumonitis in the presence of alveolar macrophages (79). Thus, the alveolitis in hypersensitivity pneumonitis also may be due in part to alteration in the surfactant immunosuppressive effect.

Viruses including influenza A have been demonstrated by polymerase chain reaction in the lower airways of patients with acute hypersensitivity pneumonitis. In experimental murine models infected with respiratory syncytial virus, both the early and late inflammatory responses are augmented in hypersensitivity pneumonitis. Avian circoviruses can be detected in the T lymphocytes of respiratory organs of free-ranging and captive birds worldwide. These viruses may be potential triggers in avian-induced-hypersensitivity pneumonitis (80). Further studies are required to clarify the nature of this relationship between viral infection and the modulation of pulmonary immune response (81,82).

■ MANAGEMENT

Avoidance

The most important element of management, as in any allergic lung disease, is avoidance of the offending antigen. This can occur in two ways: removal of the individual from the antigen or removal of the antigen exposure from the individual's environment. Workplace reassignment is a reasonable means of managing affected employees. Although this straightforward approach is simple to recommend, adherence by patients can be more difficult. For example, farmers afflicted with farmer's lung may be unable to change careers. Machinists with metal-working fluid–induced lung disease may be unable to work in other capacities. Pigeon breeders frequently continue intermittent pigeon exposure. Although elimination of the antigen seems essential for a long-term solution to the problem, continued antigen exposure may not lead to clinical deterioration for some persons (83). Depending on the source of the antigen and the conditions surrounding its generation, various industrial hygiene measures have been proposed. For instance, reducing the humidity in silos has resulted in a decline in the prevalence and incidence of farmer's lung. Other measures include alterations in plant management, increased automation, improved exhaust ventilation, and personal protective face masks. Frequently, assays for the presence of the material in the environment are lacking, or the minimum concentration to provoke symptoms or initiate sensitization is not known.

Pharmacologic Treatment

Few data exist on the various pharmacologic treatments for hypersensitivity pneumonitis. Corticosteroid therapy should be instituted in the acute and subacute forms because this has been reported to reduce symptoms and detectable inflammation and improve pulmonary function. Oral corticosteroids are recommended for acute disease starting at prednisone doses of 40 mg to 80 mg daily until clinical and laboratory improvements are observed, then decreased stepwise to 5 mg to 10 mg every other day for 6 weeks. Although indefinite corticosteroid therapy is not necessary, individualized treatment is recommended. Unfortunately, the long-term outcome of patients treated with a course of prednisone for acute farmer's lung has not always been complete recovery (84). Ongoing follow-up visits should include pulmonary function studies, not peak flow measurements, because they are not sensitive enough. Inhaled corticosteroid therapy is not as effective as oral drug therapy. If obstructive pulmonary function changes are present, then treatment with bronchodilators can be attempted. Steroid-sparing agents in the treatment of chronic progressive hypersensitivity pneumonitis are unproven. Drugs that have shown potential *in vitro* include thalidomide as it reduces IL-18, IL-8, and TNF-α release from alveolar macrophages in interstitial lung disease. However, unfavorable side effect profiles limit current use (85).

■ PREVENTION AND SCREENING

The presence of occupational lung disease in a worker usually represents a sentinel event. As in other occupational lung diseases, a systematic evaluation and investigation of the work environment and exposed cohort is recommended, although not mandated by law or always conducted (86). The investigation for additional cases may include a screening questionnaire survey with positive responses undergoing chest radiographs, serum precipitins, and lung function testing. Questionnaire surveys can be used to screen for further cases of disease, and to compare rates of symptoms between different locations in the same plant. If possible, the numbers of workers on medical leave should be reviewed. Survey questions should include demographics, risk factors, and protective factors in the home and workplace, including tobacco use and the presence of a humidifier and/or dehumidifier. Industrial hygiene surveys should include reviewing building maintenance records, visual inspection for standing water, mold growth, stained ceiling tile or carpet, roof drainage patterns, measurement of temperature and humidity, and measurement and culture of

airborne, soil, or water microorganisms. In 1998, the National Institute for Occupational Safety and Health published recommended exposure limits for metal working fluids (0.4 mg/m^3 as a time-weighted average for up to 10 hours) designed to prevent respiratory disorders (87). Unfortunately, companies may not strictly enforce this exposure limit or provide specific medical surveillance programs for employees exposed to higher levels. Changes in agricultural processes such as haymaking can reduce the microbiological concentrations including fungus (88).

■ PROGNOSIS

There have been limited studies on the factors determining prognosis of hypersensitivity pneumonitis. Factors identified as having predictive value in the likelihood of recovery from pigeon breeder's disease and farmer's lung include age at diagnosis, duration of antigen exposure after onset of symptoms, and total years of exposure before diagnosis. The effect of other factors including the nature of the allergen, especially its inflammatory potential, host susceptibility, severity of lung function at diagnosis, and form of the disease are not well clarified. Although most cases of acute disease improve, those patients with ongoing exposure continue to experience symptoms, and have abnormal lung function and abnormal chest radiographs. The mortality rates from hypersensitivity pneumonitis range from 1% to 29% with agricultural industries closely associated with mortality. Farmer's lung deaths accounted for 40% of all hypersensitivity pneumonitis deaths. A population-based study of 26 states using data from the National Institute for Occupational Safety and Health found Wisconsin to have the highest mortality rate at 1.04 per million and the death rate increasing over the period 1980 to 2002 (89). It is unclear what factors account for this increase, making additional epidemiological and surveillance research a priority in an effort to implement regional prevention and control strategies. The presence of pulmonary fibrosis is an important predictor of mortality (90). Deaths from pigeon breeder's disease have also been reported (91).

■ CONCLUSION

The diagnosis of hypersensitivity pneumonitis requires a high index of suspicion, because the primary focus of treatment is avoidance of the offending allergen even if the specific allergen is not identified. Efforts are needed to prevent recurrent and progressive disease in individuals already sensitized and prevent potential epidemics in occupational settings. Because the diagnosis is difficult and occupational evaluation complex, a team approach including the collaborative efforts of allergists, pulmonologists, occupational physicians, industrial hygienists, and microbiologists is important.

■ REFERENCES

1. Ramazzini B. *De morbus artificum diatriba* (originally published 1713). Chicago: University of Chicago Press, 1940.

2. Mohr LC. Hypersensitivity pneumonitis. *Current Opinion Pulm Med.* 2004;10:401–411.

3. Campbell JM. Acute symptoms following work with hay. *BMJ.* 1932;2:1143–1144.

4. Dickie HA, Rankin J. Farmer's lung: an acute granulomatous interstitial pneumonitis occurring in agricultural workers. *JAMA.* 1958;167:1069–1076.

5. Emanuel DA, Wenzel FJ, Bowerman CI, et al. Farmer's lung: clinical, pathologic and immunologic study of twenty-four patients. *Am J Med.* 1964;37:392–401.

6. Ranalli G, Grazia L, Roggeri A. The influence of hay-packing techniques on the presence of saccharopolyspora rectivirgula. *J Appl Microbiol.* 1999;87:359–365.

7. Fink JN, Banaszak EF, Thiede WH, et al. Interstitial pneumonitis due to hypersensitivity to an organism contaminating a heating system. *Ann Intern Med.* 1971;74:80–83.

8. Banaszak EF, Thiede WH, Fink JN. Hypersensitivity pneumonitis due to contamination of an air conditioner. *N Engl J Med.* 1970;283:271–276.

9. Volpe BT, Sulavik SB, Tran P, et al. Hypersensitivity pneumonitis associated with a portable home humidifier. *Conn Med.* 1991;55:571–573.

10. Bernstein D, Lummus Z, Santilli G, et al. Machine operator's lung, hypersensitivity pneumonitis disorder associated with exposure to metalworking fluid aerosols. *Chest.* 1995;108:636–641.

11. Fox J, Anderson H, Moen T, et al. Metal working fluid-associated hypersensitivity pneumonitis: an outbreak investigation and case-control study. *Am J Industrial Med.* 1999;35:58–67.

12. Dawkins P, Robertson A, Robertson W, et al. An outbreak of extrinsic alveolitis at a car engine plant. *Occup Med.* 2006;56:559–565.

13. Temprano J, Becker B, Hutcheson PS, et al. Hypersensitivity pneumonitis secondary to residential exposure to *Aureobasidium pullulans* in 2 siblings. *Ann Allergy Asthma Immunol.* 2007;99:562–566.

14. Green BJ, Tovey ER, Sercombe JK, et al. Airborne fungal fragments and allergenicity. *Med Mycology.* 2006;44:S245–S255.

15. Tsushima K, Furuya S, Yoshikawa S, et al. Therapeutic effects for hypersensitivity pneumonitis induced by Japanese mushroom (Buna-shimeji). *Amer J Indust Med.* 2006;49:826–835.

16. Hoy RF, Pretto JJ, van Gelderen D, et al. Mushroom worker's lung: organic dust exposure in the spawning shed. *Med J of Australia.* 2007;186:472–474.

17. Reed CE, Sosman AJ, Barbee RA. Pigeon breeder's lung. *JAMA.* 1965;193:261–265.

18. Tebo T, Moore V, Fink JN. Antigens in pigeon breeder's disease. *Clin Allergy.* 1977;7:103–108.

19. Cunningham A, Fink JN, Schlueter D. Hypersensitivity pneumonitis due to doves. *Pediatrics.* 1976;58:436–442.

20. Saltoun CA, Harris KE, Mathisen TL, et al. Hypersensitivity pneumonitis resulting from community exposure to Canada goose droppings: when an external environmental antigen becomes an indoor environmental antigen. *Ann Allergy Asthma Immunol.* 2000:84:84–86.

21. Boyer RS, Klock LE, Schmidt CD, et al. Hypersensitivity lung disease in the turkey-raising industry. *Am Rev Respir Dis.* 1974;109:630–635.

22. Mahon WE, Scott DJ, Ansell G, et al. Hypersensitivity to pituitary snuff with miliary shadowing in the lungs. *Thorax.* 1967;22:13–20.

23. Volkman K, Merrick J, Zacharisen MC. Yacht-maker's lung: a case of hypersensitivity pneumonitis in yacht manufacturing. *Wisc Med J.* 2006;105:47–50.

24. Veillette M, Cormier Y, Israel-Assayaq E, et al. Hypersensitivity pneumonitis in a hardwood processing plant related to heavy mold exposure. *J Occup Environ Hygiene.* 2006;3:301–307.

25. Ishiguro T, Yasui M, Nakade Y, et al. Extrinsic allergic alveolitis with eosinophil infiltration induced by 1,1,1,2-tetrafluoroethane (HFC-134a): a case report. *Int Med.* 2007;46:1455–1457.

26. Akoun GM, Cadranel JL, Blanchette G, et al. Bronchoalveolar lavage cell data in amiodarone associated pneumonitis. *Chest.* 1991;99:1177–1182.

27. Leino R, Liipo K, Ekfors T. Sulphasalazine-induced reversible hypersensitivity pneumonitis and fatal fibrosing alveolitis: report of two cases. *J Intern Med.* 1991;229:553–556.

28. Guillon JM, Joly P, Autran B, et al. Minocycline-induced cell mediated hypersensitivity pneumonitis. *Ann Intern Med.* 1992;117:476–481.

29. Ridley MG, Wolfe CS, Mathews JA. Life threatening acute pneumonitis during low dose methotrexate treatment for rheumatoid arthritis: a case report and review of the literature. *Ann Rheum Dis.* 1988;47:784–788.

30. Thornburg A, Abonour R, Smith P, et al. Hypersensitivity pneumonitis-like syndrome associated with the use of lenalidomide. *Chest.* 2007;131:1572–1574.

31. Chew GYJ, Hawkins CA, Cherian M, et al. *Pathology.* 2006;38:475–477.

32. Suresh K, D'Ambrosio C, Einarsson O, et al. Hypersensitivity pneumonitis induced by intranasal heroin use. *Am J Med.* 1999;107:392–395.

33. Quirce S, Hinojosa M, Blanco R, et al. *Aspergillus fumigatus* is the causative agent of hypersensitivity pneumonitis caused by esparto dust. *J Allergy Clin Immunol.* 1998;102:147–148.

34. Cormier Y, Israil-Assayag E, Bedard G, et al. Hypersensitivity pneumonitis in peat moss processing plant workers. *Am J Respir Crit Care Med.* 1998;158:412–417.

35. Kawai T, Tamura M, Murao M. Summer type hypersensitivity pneumonitis: a unique disease in Japan. *Chest.* 1984; 85:311–317.

36. Hanak V, Golbin JM, Ryu JH. Causes and presenting features in 85 consecutive patients with hypersensitivity pneumonitis. *Mayo Clinic Proc.* 2007;82:812–816.

37. Madsen D, Kloch LE, Wenzel FJ, et al. The prevalence of farmer's lung in an agricultural population. *Am Rev Respir Dis.* 1976;113:171–174.

38. Lopez M, Salvaggio JE. Epidemiology of hypersensitivity pneumonitis/allergic alveolitis. *Monogr Allergy.* 1987;21:70–86.

39. Yoshizawa Y, Ohtani Y, Hayakawa H, et al. Chronic hypersensitivity pneumonitis in Japan: a nationwide epidemiologic survey. *J Allergy Clin Immunol.* 1999; 103:315–320.

40. Arya A, Roychoudhury K, Bredin C. Farmer's lung is now in decline. *Irish Med J.* 2006;99:203–205.

41. Solaymani-Dodaran M, West J, Smith C, et al. Extrinsic allergic alveolitis: incidence and mortality in the general population. *QJ Med.* 2007;100:233–237.

42. Richerson H, Berstein IL, Fink JN, et al. Guidelines for the clinical evaluation of hypersensitivity pneumonitis. *J Allergy Clin Immunol.* 1989;84:839–844.

43. Lacasse Y, Selman M, Costabel U, et al. Clinical diagnosis of hypersensitivity pneumonitis. *Am J Respir Crit Care Med.* 2003;168:952–958.

44. Fink JN, Sosman AJ, Barboriak JJ, et al. Pigeon breeder's disease: a clinical study of a hypersensitivity pneumonitis. *Ann Intern Med.* 1968;68:1205–1219.

45. Sansores R, Salas J, Chapela R et al. Clubbing in hypersensitivity pneumonitis. *Arch Intern Med.* 1990;150: 1849–1851.

46. Unger JD, Fink JN, Unger GF. Pigeon breeder's disease: roentgenographic lung findings in a hypersensitivity pneumonitis. *Radiology.* 1968;90:683–687.

47. Silva CIS, Churg A, Muller NL. Hypersensitivity pneumonitis: spectrum of high-resolution CT and pathologic findings. *Am J Radiol.* 2007;188:334–344.

48. Lynch DA, Rose CS, Way D, et al. Hypersensitivity pneumonitis: sensitivity of ARCT in a population based study. *Am J Radiol.* 1992;159:469–472.

49. Buschman DL, Gamsu G, Waldron JA, et al. Chronic hypersensitivity pneumonitis: use of CT in diagnosis. *Am J Radiol.* 1992;159:957–960.

50. Uh S, Lee SM, Kim HT, et al. The clearance rate of alveolar epithelium using 99mTc-DTPA in patients with diffuse infiltrative lung diseases. *Chest.* 1994;106:161–165.

51. Patterson R, Fink JN, Pruzansky JJ, et al. Serum immunoglobulin levels in pulmonary allergic aspergillosis and certain other lung diseases, with special reference to immunoglobulin E. *Am J Med.* 1973;54:16–22.

52. Moore VL, Fink JN, Barboriak JJ, et al. Immunologic events in pigeon breeder's disease. *J Allergy Clin Immunol.* 1974:53:319–328.

53. Fink JN, Schlueter DP, Sosman AJ, et al. Clinical survey of pigeon breeder's. *Chest.* 1972; 62:277–281.

54. McSharry C, Dye GM, Ismail T, et al. Quantifying serum antibody in bird fanciers' hypersensitivity pneumonitis. *BMC Pulmonary Med.* 2006;6:16.

55. Fenoglio CM, Reboux G, Sudre B, et al. Diagnostic value of serum precipitins to mould antigens in active hypersensitivity pneumonitis. *Eur Respir J.* 2007;29:706–712.

56. Leatherman JW, Michael AF, Schwartz BA, et al. Lung T-cells in hypersensitivity pneumonitis. *Ann Intern Med.* 1984;100:390–392.

57. Sterclova M, Vasakova M, Dutka J, et al. Extrinsic allergic alveolitis: comparative study of the bronchoalveolar lavage profiles and radiological presentation. *Postgrad Med J.* 2006;82:598–601.

58. Sato T, Saito Y, Chikuma M, et al. Fluorimetric determination of trace amounts of albumin in bronchoalveolar lavage fluid with eriochrome cyanine R. *Biological Pharmaceutical Bulletin.* 2007;30:1187–1190.

59. Kawanami O, Basset F, Barrios R, et al. Hypersensitivity pneumonitis in man. Light and electron microscope studies of 18 lung biopsies. *Am J Pathol.* 1983;110:275–289.

60. Parker JE, Petsonk LE, Weber SL. Hypersensitivity pneumonitis and organic dust toxic syndrome. *Immunol Allergy Clin North Am.* 1992;12:279–290.

61. Rylander R, Haglind P. Airborne endotoxins and humidifier disease. *Clin Allergy.* 1984;14:109–112.

62. Sood A, Sreedhar R, Kulkarni P, et al. Hypersensitivity pneumonitis-like granulomatous lung disease with nontuberculous mycobacteria from exposure to hot water aerosols. *Environ Health Perspect.* 2007; 115:262–266.

63. Hartman TE, Jensen E, Tazelaar H, et al. CT findings of granulomatous pneumonitis secondary to Mycobacterium avium-intracellulare inhalation: "hot tub lung." *Am J Radiol.* 2007;188:1050–1053.

64. Fink JN, Hensley GT, Barboriak JJ. An animal model of hypersensitivity pneumonitis. *J Allergy.* 1970;46:156–161.

65. Moore VL, Hensley GT, Fink JN. An animal model of hypersensitivity pneumonitis in the rabbit. *J Clin Invest.* 1975;56:937–944.

66. Takizawa H, Ohta K, Horiuchi T, et al. Hypersensitivity pneumonitis in athymic nude mice. *Am Rev Respir Dis.* 1992;146:479–484.

67. Bice D, Salvaggio J, Hoffman E. Passive transfer of experimental hypersensitivity pneumonitis with lymphoid cells in the rabbit. *J Allergy Clin Immunol.* 1976;58:250–262.

68. Denis M, Ghadirian E. Murine hypersensitivity pneumonitis: bidirectional role of interferon-gamma. *Clin Exp Allergy.* 1992;22: 783–792.

69. Schkade PA, Routes JM. Hypersensitivity pneumonitis in a patient with hypogamma-globulinemia. *J Allergy Clin Immunol.* 1996;98: 710–712.

70. Denis M. Interleukin-1 (IL-1) is an important cytokine in granulomatous alveolitis. *Cell Immunol.* 1994;157:70–80.

71. Pforte A, Schiessler A, Gais P, et al. Expression of the adhesion molecule ICAM-1 on alveolar macrophages and in serum in extrinsic allergic alveolitis. *Respiration.* 1993;60:221–226.

72. Israil-Assayag E, Dakhama A, Lavigne S, et al. Expression of costimulatory molecules on alveolar macrophages in hypersensitivity pneumonitis. *Am J Respir Crit Care Med.* 1999;159:1830–1834.

73. Kondoh K, Usui Y, Ohtani Y, et al. Proinflammatory and anti-inflammatory cytokine gene polymorphisms in hypersensitivity pneumonitis. *J Med Dental Sci.* 2006;53:75–83.

74. Yamasaki H, Ando M, Brazer W, et al. Polarized type 1 cytokine profile in bronchoalveolar lavage T cells of patients with hypersensitivity pneumonitis. *J Immunol.* 1999;163:3516–3523.

75. McSharry CP, Fraser I, Chaudhuri R, et al. Nerve growth factor in serum and lymphocyte culture in pigeon fanciers' acute hypersensitivity pneumonitis. *Chest.* 2006;130:37–42.

76. Hwang SJ, Kim S, Park WS, et al. IL-4 secreting NKT cells prevent hypersensitivity pneumonitis by suppressing IFN-γ producing neutrophils. *J Immunol.* 2006;177:5258–5268.

77. Lohmeyer J, Friedrich J, Grimminger F, et al. Expression of mucosa-related integrin $\alpha^E\beta_7$ on alveolar T cells in interstitial lung diseases. *Clin Exp Immunol.* 1999;116:340–346.

78. Sugiyama Y, Kasahara T, Mukaida N, et al. Chemokines in bronchoalveolar lavage fluid in summer-type hypersensitivity pneumonitis. *Eur Respir J.* 1995;8:1084–1090.

79. Israel-Assayag E, Cormier Y. Surfactant modifies the lymphoproliferative activity of macrophages in hypersensitivity pneumonitis. *Am J Physiol.* 1997;273:L1258–L1264.

80. Bougiouklis PA. Avian circoviruses of the genus Circovirus: a potential trigger in pigeon breeder's lung (PBL)/bird fancier's lung (BFL). *Medical Hypothesis.* 2007;68:320–323.

81. Dakhama A, Hegele RG, Laflamme G, et al. Common respiratory viruses in lower airways of patients with acute hypersensitivity pneumonitis. *Am J Respir Crit Care Med.* 1999;159:1316–1322.

82. Gudmundsson G, Monick M, Hunninghake G. Viral infection modulates expression of hypersensitivity pneumonitis. *J Immunol.* 1999;162:7397–7401.

83. Cuthbert OD, Gordon MF. Ten year follow-up of farmers with farmer's lung. *Br J Industrial Med.* 1983;40:173–176.

84. Kokkarinen JI, Tukiainen HO, Terho EO. Effect of corticosteroid treatment on the recovery of pulmonary function in farmer's lung. *Am Rev Respir Dis.* 1992;145: 3–5.

85. Ye Q, Chen B, Tong Z, et al. Thalidomide reduces IL-18, IL-8 and TNF-α release from alveolar macrophages in interstitial lung disease. *Eur Respir J.* 2006;28:824–831.

86. Weltermann BM, Hodgson M, Storey E, et al. Hypersensitivity pneumonitis: a sentinel event investigation in a wet building. *Am J Industrial Med.* 1998;34:499–505.

87. Cohen H, White EM. Metalworking fluid mist occupational exposure limits: a discussion of alternative methods. *J Occup Environ Hygiene.* 2006;3:501–507.

88. Reboux G, Reiman M, Roussel S, et al. Impact of agricultural practices on microbiology of hay, silage, and flour on Finnish and French farms. *Annal Agricult Environ Med.* 2006;13:267–273.

89. Bang KM, Weissman DN, Pinheiro GA, et al. Twenty-three years of hypersensitivity pneumonitis mortality surveillance in the United States. *Amer J Indust Med.* 2006;49:997–1004.

90. Vourlekis JS, Schwarz MI, Cherniack RM, et al. The effect of pulmonary fibrosis on survival in patients with hypersensitivity pneumonitis. *Am J Med.* 2004;116:662–668.

91. Greenberger PA, Pien LC, Patterson R, et al. End-stage lung and ultimately fatal disease in a bird fancier. *Am J Med.* 1989;86: 119–122.

CHAPTER 24

Allergic Bronchopulmonary Aspergillosis

PAUL A. GREENBERGER

Allergic bronchopulmonary aspergillosis (ABPA) is characterized by immunologic reactions to antigens of *Aspergillus fumigatus* that are present in the bronchial tree and result in pulmonary infiltrates, mucus plugging and proximal bronchiectasis. Allergic bronchopulmonary aspergillosis was first described in England in 1952 in patients with asthma who had recurrent episodes of fever, roentgenographic infiltrates, peripheral blood and sputum eosinophilia, and sputum production containing *A. fumigatus* hyphae (1). The first adult with ABPA in the United States was described in 1968 (2), and the first childhood case was reported in 1970 (3). Since then, the increasing recognition of ABPA in children (4–10), adults (10–12), corticosteroid-dependent asthmatic patients (13), patients with cystic fibrosis (CF) (11–25), and patients with allergic fungal rhinosinusitis (26–29) is probably the result of the increasing awareness by physicians of this complication of asthma or CF. Diagnosis has been helped by serologic aids such as total serum immunoglobulin E (IgE) (30), serum IgE and IgG antibodies to *A. fumigatus* (31–33), precipitating antibodies (34), and familiarity with chest radiography and high-resolution computed tomography (CT) findings. Some atypical patients seemingly have no documented history of asthma and present with chest roentgenographic infiltrates, lobar collapse, and peripheral blood eosinophilia (35).

Allergic bronchopulmonary aspergillosis was identified in 6.0% of 531 patients in Chicago with asthma and immediate cutaneous reactivity to an *Aspergillus* mix (36), whereas 28% of such patients in Cleveland had ABPA (37). These surprisingly high prevalence figures were generated from the ambulatory setting of the allergist-immunologist practice and suggest that the overall prevalence of ABPA in patients with persistent asthma is 1% to 2% (36). Allergic bronchopulmonary aspergillosis has been identified on an international basis (1,10,27,28,34,38), and because of its destructive potential should be confirmed or excluded in all patients with persistent asthma.

Aspergillus species are ubiquitous, thermotolerant, and can be recovered on a perennial basis (39,40). Spores (conidia) measure 2 μm to 3.5 μm and can be cultured on Sabouraud's agar slants incubated at 37° to 40°C. Growth at this warm temperature is a somewhat unique property of *Aspergillus fumigatus*. *Aspergillus* hyphae may be identified in tissue by hematoxylin and eosin staining, but identification and morphology are better appreciated with silver methenamine or periodic acid-Schiff stains. Hyphae are 7 μm to 10 μm in diameter, septate, and classically branch at 45-degree angles. *Aspergillus* spores, which often are green, are inhaled from outdoor and indoor air and can reach terminal airways. They then could grow as hyphae. Airway epithelial cells phagocytose spores (41), but it is the alveolar macrophages that ingest and kill the spores (conidia) (41–43). Polymorphonuclear leukocytes do not ingest hyphae but bind to them and kill the hyphae by damaging their cell walls with a powerful, oxidative burst (41,44). Protection against invasive aspergillosis occurs due to multiple factors, but most crucial is the presence of functioning polymorphonuclear leukocytes because prolonged neutropenia (<500 cells/mm^3) and possibly thrombocytopenia (as platelets bind to hyphae and become activated), injured pulmonary epithelium (from chemotherapy), insufficient local complement to facilitate opsonization and the oxidative burst by polymorphonuclear leukocytes, and overwhelmed innate immunity contribute to invasive disease.

Aspergillus species, particularly *A. flavus* and *A. fumigatus*, produce some toxic metabolites, of which aflatoxin is the most widely known. The measurement of aflatoxin is used to verify that foods, such as coffee beans and corn, are not contaminated. On a cellular level, a toxic and immunosuppressive metabolite, gliotoxin, inhibits macrophage phagocytosis and lymphocyte activation (41,45,46). *A. fumigatus* produces proteolytic enzymes and ribosome toxins (RNAses)

(41) that are thought to contribute to bronchial wall damage when *A. fumigatus* hyphae are present in bronchial mucus. Epithelial cells could be damaged by proteases from *A. fumigatus* that also would decrease ciliary function (40). Virulence factors generated by *A. fumigatus* include elastase, phospholipase, and acid phosphatase (47). In that cell membranes are composed of proteins and lipids, these enzymes could destroy the cell membranes and allow for unrestrained growth of spores and resultant damage to the bronchial wall (47). Also, surfactant is approximately 80% phospholipid, so that the phospholipases could interfere with normal lining fluid and immune responses to *Aspergillus* species (47).

A. flavus and *A. fumigatus* have been incriminated in avian aspergillosis, a major economic concern in the poultry industry. For example, aspergillosis is common in turkey poults and can cause 5% to 10% mortality rates in production flocks (48). *Aspergillus* infections as a cause of abortions and mammary gland infections in sheep are recognized, as are infections in horses (pneumonia), cattle (pneumonia), camels (ulcerative tracheobronchitis), and dolphins (pneumonias including a condition resembling ABPA with cough, weight loss, and pulmonary infiltrates).

Aspergillus terreus is used in the pharmaceutical industry for synthesis of the cholesterol-lowering drug, levostatin. *Aspergillus oryzae* is invaluable in the production of soy products. *Aspergillus niger* is critical for production of citric acid. For use in the baking industry, *Aspergillus* species produce α-amylase, cellulase, and hemicellulase. Because these enzymes are powdered, some bakery workers may develop IgE-mediated rhinitis and asthma (49,50).

The genus *Aspergillus* may produce different types of disease, depending on the immunologic status of the patient. In nonatopic patients, *Aspergillus* hyphae may grow in damaged lung and cause a fungus ball (aspergilloma). Morphologically, an aspergilloma contains thousands of tangled *Aspergillus* hyphae in pulmonary cavities, and can complicate sarcoidosis, tuberculosis, old histoplasmosis, carcinoma, CF, or ABPA (51). Hypersensitivity pneumonitis may result from inhalation of large numbers of *A. fumigatus* or *A. clavatus* spores by malt workers. These spores also may produce farmer's lung disease. *Aspergillus* species may invade tissue in the immunologically compromised (neutropenic and thrombocytopenic) host, causing sepsis and death. A rare patient, who seemingly is immunocompetent, may develop acute respiratory failure from bilateral "community acquired" pneumonia due to *A. fumigatus* infection. *Aspergillus* species have been associated with emphysema, colonization of cysts, pulmonary suppurative reactions, and necrotizing pneumonia in other patients (52,53). In the atopic patient, fungal spore–induced asthma may occur from IgE-mediated processes in response to inhalation of *Aspergillus* spores. About 25% of patients with persistent asthma

have immediate cutaneous reactivity to *A. fumigatus* or a mix of *Aspergillus* species. Why some of these patients with asthma develop ABPA remains unclear. Genetic susceptibility includes HLA-DR2+, DRB*1501, and HLA-DQ2- as well as gain of function polymorphisms for IL-4 (54–56). In patients without asthma, *Aspergillus* hyphae have been identified in mucoid impactions of sinuses, a condition that morphologically resembles mucoid impaction of bronchi in ABPA (57–64). Such allergic *Aspergillus* rhinosinusitis may occur in patients with ABPA (26,27,65) (see Chapters 10 and 12).

There are over 185 *Aspergillus* species and additional variants. When *A. fumigatus* is grown in culture, changing media components and conditions alter the characteristics of the resultant strains of *A. fumigatus*. The International Union of Immunological Societies has recognized 22 allergens of *A. fumigatus*, which are listed as *Asp f* 1, 2, 3–18, 22w, 23, 27, 28, and 29 (see Chapter 6).

■ DIAGNOSTIC CRITERIA AND CLINICAL FEATURES

The criteria used for diagnosis of classic ABPA consist of five essential criteria and other criteria that may or may not be present, depending on the classification and stage of disease. The minimal essential criteria are (a) asthma, even cough-variant asthma or exercise-induced asthma; (b) central (proximal) bronchiectasis; (c) elevated total serum IgE ($\geq$417 kU/L or 1,000 ng/mL); (d) immediate cutaneous reactivity to *Aspergillus*; and (e) elevated serum IgE and/or IgG antibodies to *A. fumigatus*. (66–68). Central (proximal) bronchiectasis in the absence of distal bronchiectasis, as occurs in CF or chronic obstructive pulmonary disease, is virtually pathognomonic for ABPA. Such patients are labeled ABPA-CB, for central bronchiectasis. Other features of ABPA are often present. For example, the expected diagnostic criteria (Table 24.1) of ABPA-CB include (a) asthma; (b) immediate cutaneous reactivity to *A. fumigatus*; (c) precipitating antibodies to *A. fumigatus*; (d) elevated total serum IgE concentration; (e) peripheral blood eosinophilia ($\geq$1,000/mm^3); (f) a history of either transient or fixed roentgenographic infiltrates; (g) proximal bronchiectasis; and (h) elevated serum IgE–*A. fumigatus* and IgG–*A. fumigatus* (66–68). These diagnostic criteria may not apply to ABPA-S (seropositive), where bronchiectasis cannot be detected by high-resolution chest tomography (12). Patients, who have all the criteria for ABPA but in whom proximal bronchiectasis is not present, have ABPA-S (12). The minimal essential criteria for ABPA-S include (a) asthma; (b) immediate cutaneous reactivity to *Aspergillus*; (c) elevated total serum IgE concentration; and (d) elevated serum IgE and IgG antibodies to *A. fumigatus* compared with sera from skin test positive patients with asthma without ABPA (12,67).

TABLE 24.1 DIAGNOSTIC CRITERIA FOR ALLERGIC BRONCHOPULMONARY ASPERGILLOSIS

Asthma
Chest roentgenographic infiltrates
Immediate cutaneous reactivity to *Aspergillus*
Elevated total serum IgE concentration (>417 kU/mL)
Elevated serum IgE-Af and/or IgG-Af antibodies
Serum precipitating antibodies to Af
Proximal bronchiectasis
Peripheral blood eosinophilia ($\geq$1,000/mm^3)
Minimal essential criteria for ABPA-CB^a
Asthma
Immediate cutaneous reactivity to *Aspergillus*
Elevated total IgE concentration
Elevated serum IgE-Af and or IgG-Af antibodies
Proximal bronchiectasis

^{a}Suitable for diagnosis of ABPA in cystic fibrosis.

Af, *Aspergillus fumigatus*; ABPA, allergic bronchopulmonary aspergillosis; CB, central bronchiectasis.

Other features of ABPA may include positive sputum cultures for *A. fumigatus* and a history of expectoration of golden brown plugs containing *A. fumigatus* hyphae. Patients with asthma without ABPA may have positive cutaneous tests for *A. fumigatus*, peripheral blood eosinophilia, and a history of roentgenographic infiltrates (due to atelectasis from inadequately controlled asthma). *Aspergillus* precipitins are not diagnostic of ABPA, and sputum cultures may be negative for *A. fumigatus* or even unobtainable if the patient has little bronchiectasis. In ABPA-S, bronchiectasis cannot be detected by high-resolution CT. Serologic measurements have proven useful in making the diagnosis of ABPA. A marked elevation in total serum IgE concentration and IgE and IgG antibodies to *A. fumigatus* is of value in making the diagnosis (32,67–69). Furthermore, the decline in total serum IgE concentration by at least 35% by 6 weeks after institution of prednisone has been shown to occur in ABPA (70).

Allergic bronchopulmonary aspergillosis initially should be suspected in all patients with asthma who have immediate cutaneous reactivity to *A. fumigatus* (36,67). The absence of a documented chest roentgenographic infiltrate or mucoid infiltrates demonstrable by CT does not exclude ABPA-CB. Familial ABPA has been described occasionally, which emphasizes the need for screening family members for evidence of ABPA if they have asthma. Clearly, ABPA should be suspected in patients with a history of roentgenographic infiltrates,

pneumonia, or abnormal chest films and in patients with allergic fungal rhinosinusitis. Increasing severity of asthma without other causes may indicate evolving ABPA, but some patients present solely with asymptomatic pulmonary infiltrates. Consolidation on the chest roentgenogram caused by ABPA often is not associated with the rigors, chills, as high a fever, and overall malaise as with a bacterial pneumonia causing the same degree of roentgenographic consolidation. The time of onset of ABPA may precede recognition by many years (72–74), or there may be early diagnosis of ABPA before significant lung destruction and roentgenographic infiltrates have occurred (12). Allergic bronchopulmonary aspergillosis must be considered in the patient over 40 years of age with chronic bronchitis, idiopathic bronchiectasis, or interstitial fibrosis. Further lung damage may be prevented by prednisone treatment of ABPA exacerbations. The dose of prednisone necessary for controlling persistent asthma may be inadequate to prevent the emergence of ABPA, although the total serum IgE concentration may be elevated only moderately because of suppression by prednisone.

Patients with ABPA manifest multiple allergic conditions. For example, only one of the initial 50 patients diagnosed and managed at Northwestern University Feinberg School of Medicine had isolated cutaneous reactivity to *A. fumigatus* (72). Other atopic disorders (rhinitis, urticaria, atopic dermatitis, drug allergy) may be present in patients with ABPA (72). The severity of asthma ranges from intermittent asthma to mildly persistent, to severe prednisone-dependent persistent asthma. Occasionally, patients deny developing wheezing or dyspnea on exposure to raked leaves, moldy hay, or damp basements, but they noted nonimmunologic triggering factors such as cold air, infection, or weather changes. The findings in these patients emphasize that ABPA may be present in patients who appear to have no obvious IgE-mediated asthma. Such patients can present with mucoid impactions and tenacious sputum and then have the diagnosis of ABPA made.

The number of diagnostic criteria vary depending on the classification (ABPA-CB or ABPA-S) and stage of ABPA. Furthermore, prednisone therapy causes clearing of the chest roentgenographic infiltrates, decline of the total serum IgE concentration, disappearance of precipitating antibodies, peripheral blood or sputum eosinophilia, and absence or reduction of sputum production.

■ PHYSICAL EXAMINATION

The physical examination in ABPA may be completely unremarkable in the asymptomatic patient, or the patient may have crackles, bronchial breathing, or wheezing, depending on the degree and quality of lung disease present. An acute exacerbation of ABPA may be associated with temperature elevation to 103°F (although this is most uncommon), with malaise, dyspnea, wheezing, and sputum production. In some cases of ABPA, extensive pulmonary consolidation on roentgenography may be accompanied by few or no clinical symptoms, in contrast to the usual manifestations of a patient with a bacterial pneumonia and the same degree of consolidation. When extensive pulmonary fibrosis has occurred from ABPA, posttussive crackles will be present. Allergic bronchopulmonary aspergillosis has been associated with collapse of a lung from a mucoid impaction, and it was associated with a spontaneous pneumothorax (72). The physical examination yields evidence for these diagnoses. When ABPA infiltrates affect the periphery of the lung, pleuritis may occur and it may be associated with restriction of chest wall movement on inspiration and a pleural friction rub. Some patients with end-stage ABPA (fibrotic stage V) have digital clubbing and cyanosis (73,74). The latter findings should suggest concomitant CF as well.

■ RADIOLOGY

Chest roentgenographic changes may be transient or permanent (Figs. 24.1 to 24.6) (75,76). Transient roentgenographic changes, which may clear with or without oral corticosteroid therapy, appear to be the result of parenchymal infiltrates, mucoid impactions, or secretions in damaged bronchi (9,10,75–81). These nonpermanent findings include (a) perihilar infiltrates simulating adenopathy; (b) air-fluid levels from dilated central bronchi filled with fluid and debris; (c) massive consolidation that may be unilateral or bilateral; (d) roentgenographic infiltrates; (e) "toothpaste" shadows that result from mucoid impactions in damaged bronchi; (f) "gloved-finger" shadows from distally occluded bronchi filled with secretions; and (g) "tramline" shadows, which are two parallel hairline shadows extending out from the hilum. The width of the transradiant zone between the lines is that of a normal bronchus at that level (75). Tramline shadows, which represent edema of the bronchial wall, may be seen in asthma without ABPA, in CF, and in left ventricular failure with elevated pulmonary venous pressure. Permanent roentgenographic findings related to proximal bronchiectasis have been shown to occur in sites of previous infiltrates, which are often, but not exclusively, in the upper lobes. This is in contrast to postinfectious bronchiectasis, which is associated with distal abnormalities and normal proximal bronchi. When permanent lung damage occurs to large bronchi, parallel line shadows and ring shadows are seen. These do not change with oral corticosteroids. Parallel line shadows

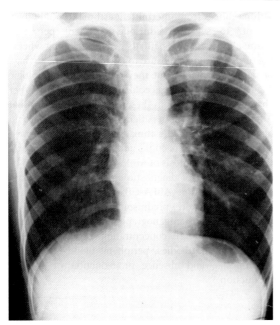

■ **FIGURE 24.1** An 11-year-old boy with far-advanced allergic bronchopulmonary aspergillosis. Presentation chest radiograph shows massive homogeneous consolidation in left upper lobe. (Reprinted from Mintzer RA, Rogers LF, Kruglick GD, et al. The spectrum of radiologic findings in allergic bronchopulmonary aspergillosis. *Radiology* 1978;127:301; with permission.)

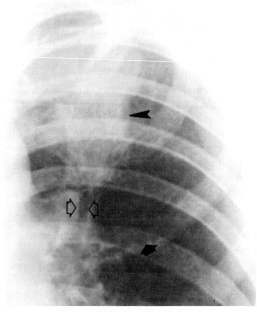

■ **FIGURE 24.2** Magnified view of the left upper lobe shows massive homogenous consolidation (*narrow arrowhead*), parallel lines (*open broad arrowheads*), and ring shadows (*closed broad arrowhead*). (Reprinted from Mintzer RA, Rogers LF, Kruglick GD, et al. The spectrum of radiologic findings in allergic bronchopulmonary aspergillosis. *Radiology* 1978;127:301; with permission.)

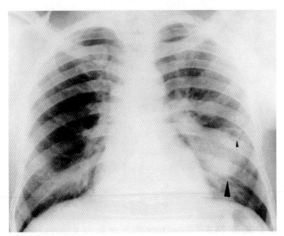

■ **FIGURE 24.3** A 31-year-old man with far-advanced allergic bronchopulmonary aspergillosis. Presentation chest radiograph. Note massive homogeneous consolidation (*large arrowhead*) and air-fluid level (*small arrowhead*). (Reprinted from Mintzer RA, Rogers LF, Kruglick GD, et al. The spectrum of radiologic findings in allergic bronchopulmonary aspergillosis. *Radiology* 1978;127:301; with permission.)

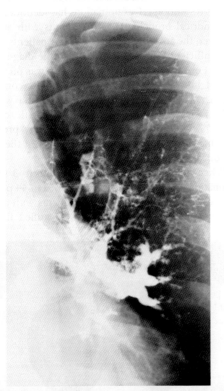

■ **FIGURE 24.4** Bronchogram showing classic proximal bronchiectasis with normal peripheral airways in a 25-year-old woman with allergic bronchopulmonary aspergillosis. (Reprinted from Mintzer RA, Rogers LF, Kruglick GD, et al. The spectrum of radiologic findings in allergic bronchopulmonary aspergillosis. *Radiology* 1978;127:301; with permission.)

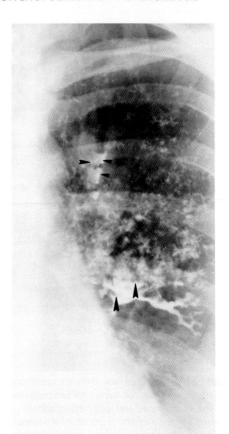

■ **FIGURE 24.5** Posttussive films after bronchography. Air-fluid levels (*large arrowheads*) are present in several partially filled ectatic bronchi. A bronchus in the left upper lobe is filled after the tussive effort, confirming that a portion of the density seen in this area is in fact a filled ectatic proximal bronchus (*small arrowheads*). (Reprinted from Mintzer RA, Rogers LF, Kruglick GD, et al. The spectrum of radiologic findings in allergic bronchopulmonary aspergillosis. *Radiology* 1978;127:301; with permission.)

are dilated tramline shadows that result from bronchiectasis; the transradiant zone between the lines is wider than that of a normal bronchus. These shadows are believed to be permanent, representing bronchial dilation. The ring shadows, 1 cm to 2 cm in diameter, are dilated bronchi *en face*. Pulmonary fibrosis may occur and might be irreversible. Late findings in ABPA include cavitation, contracted upper lobes, fibrosis, and localized emphysema. When bullous changes are present, a spontaneous pneumothorax may occur (72).

With high clinical suspicion of ABPA (bronchial asthma, high total serum IgE concentration, immediate cutaneous reactivity to *A. fumigatus*, precipitating antibody against *A. fumigatus*) and a negative chest roentgenogram, central bronchiectasis may be demonstrated by high-resolution computed tomography (CT) (77–81). This examination should be performed as an initial radiologic test beyond the chest roentgenogram (Figs. 24.7

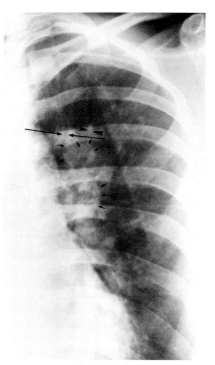

■ **FIGURE 24.6** Magnified view of the left upper lung of the patient shown in Figs. 24.4 and 24.5 demonstrates parallel lines (*long arrows*) and toothpaste shadows (*arrowheads*). Perihilar infiltrates (pseudohilar adenopathy) and a gloved-finger shadow also are seen (*small arrows*). (Reprinted from Mintzer RA, Rogers LF, Kruglick GD, et al. The spectrum of radiologic findings in allergic bronchopulmonary aspergillosis. *Radiology* 1978;127:301; with permission.)

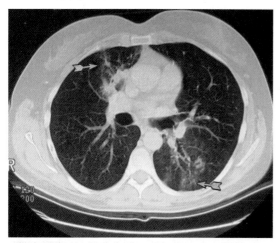

■ **FIGURE 24.7** Computed tomography scan of a 42-year-old woman demonstrating right upper lobe and left lower lobe infiltrates, the latter not seen on the posteroanterior and lateral radiographs. Dilated bronchioles are present in areas of infiltrates (*arrows*).

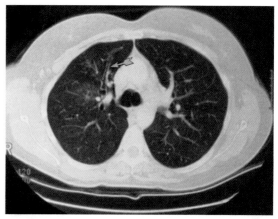

■ **FIGURE 24.8** Dilated bronchi from an axial longitudinal orientation (*arrow*) consistent with bronchiectasis (same patient as in Fig. 24.7).

through 24.9). If findings are normal, studies should be repeated in 1 to 2 years for highly suspicious cases.

High-resolution CT using 1.5-mm section cuts has proved valuable in detecting bronchiectasis in ABPA (77–81). The thin-section cuts were obtained every 1 cm to 2 cm from the apex to the diaphragm. The use of high-resolution CT examinations has identified areas of cylindrical bronchiectasis in patients with asthma. However, the areas are localized and the patients do not have sufficient other criteria to make the diagnosis of ABPA. For example, bronchial dilatation was present in 41% of lung *lobes* in eight ABPA patients compared with 15% of *lobes* in patients with asthma without ABPA. Bronchiectasis may be cylindrical, cystic, or varicose (77–79). From the axial perspective, proximal bronchiectasis is present when it occurrs in the inner two-thirds of the lung.

When high-resolution CT using 1 mm to 3 mm of collimation (thin sections) was performed in 44 patients with ABPA and compared with 38 patients with asthma without ABPA, bronchiectasis was identified in both

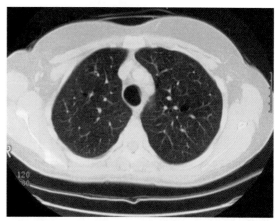

■ **FIGURE 24.9** Cystic (dilated) bronchi and bronchioles (same patient as in Fig. 24.7).

patient groups (79). Bronchiectasis was present in 42 (95%) ABPA patients compared with 11 (29%) patients with asthma. The CT scans revealed bronchiectasis in 70% of *lobes* examined in ABPA versus 9% of *lobes* from patients with asthma (79). Some 86% of ABPA patients had three or more bronchiectatic *lobes*, whereas 91% of the patients with asthma had bronchiectasis in one or two *lobes*. In the ABPA patients, bronchiectasis was varicose in 41% of patients, cystic in 34% of patients, and cylindrical in 23% of patients. Consolidation was identified in 59% of ABPA patients, primarily being located peripherally, whereas consolidation was present in 9% of patients with asthma (79).

■ STAGING

Five stages of ABPA have been identified (11). These stages are acute, remission, exacerbation, corticosteroid-dependent asthma, and fibrotic. The acute stage (stage I) is present when all the major criteria of ABPA can be documented. These criteria are asthma, immediate cutaneous reactivity to A. fumigatus, precipitating antibody to A. fumigatus, elevated serum IgE concentration, which is over the upper limit of normal adults (>417 kU/L), peripheral blood eosinophilia, history of or presence of roentgenographic infiltrates, and proximal bronchiectasis, unless the patient has ABPA-S. If measured, sera from stage I patients have elevated serum IgE and IgG antibodies to A. fumigatus compared with sera from patients with asthma and immediate cutaneous reactivity to *Aspergillus* but not sufficient criteria for ABPA. After therapy with prednisone, the chest roentgenogram clears and the total serum IgE concentration declines substantially (66,70). Remission (stage II) is defined as clearing of the roentgenographic lesions and decline in total serum IgE for at least 6 months. Exacerbation (stage III) of ABPA is present when, after the remission that follows prednisone therapy, the patient develops a new roentgenographic infiltrate, total IgE concentration rises over baseline, and the other criteria of stage I appear. Corticosteroid-dependent asthma (stage IV) includes patients whose prednisone cannot be terminated without occurrence of persistent moderate-to-severe allergic asthma requiring oral corticosteroids for control or new roentgenographic infiltrates. Despite prednisone administration, most patients have elevated total serum IgE concentrations, precipitating antibody, and elevated serum IgE and IgG antibodies to A. fumigatus. Roentgenographic infiltrates may or may not occur. Stage V ABPA is present when extensive cystic or fibrotic changes are demonstrated on the chest roentgenogram (73,74). Patients in the fibrotic stage have some degree of irreversible obstructive flow rates on pulmonary function testing. A reversible obstructive component requires prednisone therapy, but high-dose prednisone does not reverse the roentgenographic lesions of irreversible obstructive disease. At the time of the initial diagnosis, the stage of ABPA may not be defined, but it becomes clear after several months of observation and treatment.

Patients with ABPA-S can be in stages I through IV, but not stage V (12). Patients with ABPA and CF often are in stage III (recurrent exacerbation) but may be in any stage.

■ LABORATORY FINDINGS

All patients exhibit immediate cutaneous reactivity (wheal and flare) to A. fumigatus antigen. Because of the lack of standardized A. fumigatus antigens for clinical testing, differences in skin reactivity have been reported by different researchers (Table 24.2) (66,82–84). Approximately 25% of patients with asthma without ABPA demonstrate immediate skin reactivity to A. fumigatus, and about 10% show precipitating antibodies against A. fumigatus (85,86). Conversely a nonreactive skin test (prick and intradermal) to reactive extracts of A. fumigatus essentially excludes the diagnosis of ABPA. Some commercial mixes of *Aspergillus* species contain little or no A. fumigatus; it is advised to skin test with a reactive extract of A. fumigatus.

Some ABPA patients display a diphasic skin response to the intradermal injection of *Aspergillus* antigen. This consists of a typical immediate wheal and flare seen within 20 minutes, which subsides, to be followed in 4 to 8 hours by erythema and induration that resolves in 24 hours. IgG, IgM, IgA, and C3 have been reported on biopsies of these late reactions, suggesting an Arthus (type III) immune response (87). IgE antibodies also likely participate in the late reactions. Few ABPA patients treated at Northwestern University Feinberg School of Medicine have biphasic skin reactivity despite the presence of anti-A. fumigatus IgE antibodies and precipitating antibodies. Conversely, few patients are tested by intradermal injection, because skin-prick test results are positive in most patients. As shown in Table 24.2, precipitating antibody to A. fumigatus is not uncommon in patients without ABPA and likely represents previous exposure to A. fumigatus antigens. In ABPA, however, these antibodies may be important in the pathogenesis of the disease, or at least a manifestation of very high levels of anti-A. fumigatus IgG antibody production.

A. fumigatus extracts are mixtures containing well over 200 proteins, glycoproteins, and polysaccharides (88,89). This has led to utilization of recombinant allergens for diagnosis (90). In addition, there are hundreds of secondary metabolites of A. fumigatus (91). There is marked heterogeneity of immunoglobulin and lymphocyte binding or stimulation with A. fumigatus allergens (88,89). Initially, it was demonstrated that after rocket immunoelectrophoresis of A. fumigatus mycelia and addition of A. fumigatus antisera raised in rabbits, 35 different bands could be detected by that methodology. Immunoblotting has resulted in identification of 100 proteins (glycoproteins) that bind to immunoglobulins (89). It is

TABLE 24.2 INCIDENCE OF IMMUNOLOGIC REACTIONS TO *ASPERGILLUS FUMIGATUS*

PATIENTS STUDIED	IMMEDIATE SKIN REACTIVITY (%)	PRECIPITINS (%)
Normal population	1–4	0–3
Hospitalized patients		2.5–6
Asthma without aspergillosis	12–38	9–25
Asthma without aspergillosis[a]		
London	23	10.5
Cleveland	28	7.5
Allergic bronchopulmonary aspergillosis	100	100[b]
Aspergilloma	25	100
Cystic fibrosis	39	31

[a]Similar antigenic material used for both groups.

[b]May be negative at times.

Data from Hoehne JH, Reed CE, Dickie HA. Allergic bronchopulmonary aspergillosis is not rare. *Chest.* 1973;63:177; Longbottom JL, Pepys J. Pulmonary aspergillosis: diagnostic and immunologic significance of antigens and C-substance in *Aspergillus fumigatus. J Pathol Bacteriol.* 1964;88:141; Reed C. Variability of antigenicity of *Aspergillus fumigatus. J Allergy Clin Immunol.* 1978;61:227; Rosenberg M, Patterson R, Mintzer R, et al. Clinical and immunologic criteria for the diagnosis of allergic bronchopulmonary aspergillosis. *Ann Intern Med.* 1977;86:405; and Schwartz HJ, Citron KM, Chester EH, et al. A comparison of the prevalence of sensitization to *Aspergillus* antigens among asthmatics in Cleveland and London. *J Allergy Clin Immunol,* 1978;62:9.

now thought that there are over 30,000 proteins that are produced by *A. fumigatus* (92), which is a testament to the challenges of identifying critical immunodominant peptides and allergens that would be useful in diagnosis.

One characterized polypeptide is called *Asp f* 1 and has a molecular weight of 18,000 daltons. It is generated from a culture filtrate that was found to react with IgE and IgG antibodies and was toxic to lymphocytes (93,94). *Asp f* 1 is a member of the mitogillin family, which demonstrates ribonuclease (ribotoxic) activity. Sera from ABPA patients react with several ribotoxins, and far greater quantities of IgE and IgG antibodies to ribotoxins from *Aspergillus* are present in patients with ABPA as compared with nonatopic patients with asthma (41). As stated, recombinant *A. fumigatus* allergens have been identified and labeled up to *Asp f* 29. Some peptides (12 to 16 amino acids from *Asp f* 1) induce TH_1, and others produce TH_2 cytokine responses. Peptides that are three to seven amino acids long have been obtained from the IgE binding region of *Asp f* 2 and evaluated for IgE binding with sera from ABPA patients. Overall, just a few amino acids of *Asp f* 2 provide the conformation to react with IgE, whereas these short IgE-specific peptides did not react with IgG antibodies (92,95,96). These results emphasize the complexities to be addressed in the future (88,90,92,95,96). Reactive epitopes of *A. fumigatus* are under investigation for use in skin testing and *in vitro* assays. It is hoped that more precise skin testing and

in vitro test results using recombinant allergens will lead to more accurate diagnoses. However, such an approach, at least with ragweed proteins, was unsuccessful in that a particular "immunologic fingerprint" did not occur as proposed. The genotypes were different for the "hay fever" phenotype.

In the double-gel diffusion technique, most patients' sera have at least one to three precipitin bands to *A. fumigatus.* Some sera must be concentrated five times to demonstrate precipitating antibody. A precipitin band with no immunologic significance may be seen, caused by the presence of C-reactive protein in human sera that cross-reacts with a polysaccharide antigen in *Aspergillus.* This false-positive band can be avoided by adding citric acid to the agar gel.

Because of the high incidence of cutaneous reactivity and precipitating antibodies to *A. fumigatus* in patients with CF and transient roentgenographic infiltrates attributed to *Aspergillus,* there is concern that *A. fumigatus* bronchial colonization or ABPA could contribute to the ongoing lung damage of CF. Nevertheless, this notion may not be true (23). Use of high-dose tobramycin by nebulization might favor the growth of *A. fumigatus* in the bronchial mucus of CF patients. The question also has been raised whether ABPA might be a variant form of the latter. Genetic testing has identified the ΔF508 mutation in one allele of some ABPA patients or other variant patterns (24,97). Eleven patients with ABPA who had normal sweat electrolytes ($\leq$40 mM) had extensive genetic analysis of the coding region for the cystic fibrosis transmembrane regulator (CFTR). Five patients had one CF mutation (ΔF508 in four and R117H in one), whereas another patient had two CF mutations (ΔF508/R347H). In comparison were 53 patients with chronic bronchitis who did not have any with the ΔF508 mutation, demonstrating clear-cut differences and suggesting that ABPA in some patients includes CF heterozygosity. In a study of 16 patients with ABPA, 6 (37.5%) patients were homozygous for ΔF508 and 6 were heterozygous with other mutations in 4 patients (23). In our patient population, all but one patient tested had normal sweat chloride concentrations in the absence of CF. Nevertheless, there is increasing evidence that ABPA can complicate CF, and it must be considered in that population because 1% to 10% of patients with CF have ABPA (16–25).

Serum IgE concentrations in patients with ABPA are elevated, but the degree of elevation varies markedly. In most patients, the total serum IgE concentration is greater than 417 kU/L (1,000 ng/mL) (1 IU/mL = 2.4 ng/mL). It has been demonstrated that *A. fumigatus* growing in the respiratory tract without tissue invasion, as in ABPA, can provide a potent stimulus for production of total "nonspecific" serum IgE (98). When serum IgE or serum IgG antibodies, or both, against *A. fumigatus* are elevated compared with sera from skin-prick–positive asthmatic patients without evidence for ABPA, ABPA is highly probable or definitely present (67). With prednisone therapy and clinical improvement, the total IgE concentration and IgE–*A. fumigatus* decrease, although at different rates. Seemingly, this decrease is associated with a decrease in the number of *A. fumigatus* organisms in the bronchi and suppression of $CD4T_H2$ allergic inflammation. It is possible, but unlikely, that the reduction in IgE concentration is due directly to prednisone without an effect on *A. fumigatus* in the lung, because in other conditions, such as atopic dermatitis and asthma, corticosteroids did not lower total serum IgE concentrations significantly (99,100).

Because of the wide variation of total serum IgE concentrations in atopic patients with asthma, some difficulty exists in differentiating the patient with ABPA from the patient with asthma and cutaneous reactivity to *A. fumigatus*, with or without precipitating antibody to *A. fumigatus* and a history of an abnormal chest roentgenogram. Detection of elevated serum IgE and IgG antibodies to *A. fumigatus* has proved useful to identify patients with ABPA (67). Sera from patients with ABPA have at least twice the level of antibody to *A. fumigatus* than do sera from patients with asthma with skin-prick–positive reactions to *A. fumigatus*. During other stages of ABPA, the indices have diagnostic value if results are elevated, but are not consistently positive in all patients. In patients with suspected ABPA, serodiagnosis should be attempted before prednisone therapy is started so that the total IgE concentration is at its

peak. Hyperimmunoglobulinemia E should raise the possibility of ABPA in any patient with asthma, although other causes besides asthma include atopic dermatitis, hyper-IgE syndrome, immune deficiency, Churg-Strauss syndrome, allergic bronchopulmonary mycosis, parasitism, and, remotely, IgE myeloma.

Lymphocyte transformation is present in some cases but is not a diagnostic feature of ABPA (66). Delayed hypersensitivity (type IV) reactions occurring 48 hours after administration of intradermal *Aspergillus* antigens typically are not seen (101).

T- and B-cell analysis of selected patients with ABPA has not shown abnormal numbers of B cells, CD4 (helper), or CD8 (suppressor) cells. However, some patients have evidence for B-cell activation ($CD19^+$ $CD23^+$) or T-cell activation ($CD3+$ $CD25^+$). T-cell clones from peripheral blood from three ABPA patients, two of whom had been in remission, were generated and analyzed (102). The clones were specific for *Asp f* 1 and were reported to be HLA class II molecules restricted to HLA-DR2 or HLA-DR5 alleles. Furthermore, the T-cell clones produced high quantities of interleukin 4 (IL-4) and little interferon-γ, consistent with helper T cell type 2 (T_H2 subtype of $CD4^+$ cells). Additional experiments explored major histocompatibility complex (MHC) class II restriction in 15 additional ABPA patients to determine whether specific HLA class II molecules were likely associated with *A. fumigatus* presentation (103). Sixteen of 18 (88.8%) patients overall were either HLA-DR2 or HLA-DR5 compared with 42.1% frequency in normal individuals (103). Using polymerase chain reaction techniques to investigate HLA-DR subtypes, it was determined that three HLA-DR2 alleles (identified as subtypes DRB1 1501, 1503, and 1601) and three HLA-DR5 alleles (identified as subtypes DRB1 1101, 1104, and 1202) were recognized by T cells in their activation (103). In other words, T-cell activation after binding to *Asp f* 1 was restricted to certain subtypes of class II molecules HLA-DR2 or HLA-DR5, raising the possibility that selective HLA-DR alleles might provide the genetic disadvantage that permits T-cell activation and possibly ABPA to evolve. Because not all patients with these genotypes have ABPA, additional insight is attributable to gain of function polymorphisms for IL-4 in ABPA (55). Using CD20 (B cells), incubation with IL-4 increases the number of CD23 molecules on the CD20 cells greater in ABPA than non-ABPA cell populations (55).

Circulating immune complexes have been described during an acute flare-up of ABPA with activation of the classic pathway (104). Although Clq precipitins were present in patient sera, it was not proven that *Aspergillus* antigen was present in these complexes. ABPA is not considered to be characterized by circulating immune complexes as in serum sickness. But it has been demonstrated that *A. fumigatus* can convert C3 proactivator to C3 activator, a component of the alternate pathway

(105). It is known that secretory IgA can activate the alternate pathway, and that *Aspergillus* in the bronchial tract can stimulate IgA production (106).

In vitro basophil histamine release resulted from exposure to an *Aspergillus* mix, anti-IgE, and other fungi in patients with ABPA and fungi-sensitive asthma (with immediate cutaneous reactivity to *A. fumigatus*) (107). There was much greater histamine release to *Aspergillus* and anti-IgE from basophils of patients with ABPA than there was from fungi-sensitive asthmatic patients without ABPA. Furthermore, patients with stage IV and stage V ABPA demonstrated greater histamine release to *Aspergillus* than did patients in stages I, II, or III. There was greater histamine release to other fungi from cells taken from ABPA patients than there was from other patients with asthma. These data document a cellular difference in ABPA patients when compared with fungi-sensitive asthmatic patients. There was no difference between ABPA patients and patients with asthma in terms of cutaneous end-point titration using a commercially available *Aspergillus* mix.

A positive sputum culture for *A. fumigatus* is a helpful, but not pathognomonic, feature of ABPA. Repeated positive cultures may be significant. Whereas some patients produce golden brown plugs or "pearls" of mucus containing *Aspergillus* mycelia, others produce no sputum at all, even in the presence of roentgenographic infiltrates. Sputum eosinophilia usually is found in patients with significant sputum production, but is not essential for diagnosis and clearly is not specific.

Peripheral blood eosinophilia is common in untreated patients, but need not be extremely high, and often is about 10% to 25% of the differential in patients who have not received oral corticosteroids. Bronchial inhalational challenges with *Aspergillus* are not required to confirm the diagnosis, and are not without risk. Nevertheless, a dual reaction usually occurs after bronchoprovocation. An immediate reduction in flow that resolves, to be followed in some cases by a recurrence of obstruction after 4 to 10 hours, has been described (87). Pretreatment with β adrenergic agonists prevents the immediate reaction; pretreatment with corticosteroids prevents the late reaction; and cromolyn sodium has been reported to prevent both. Inhalational challenge with *A. fumigatus* in a patient with asthma sensitive to *Aspergillus* produces the immediate response only. Aspergilloma patients may respond only with a late pattern.

■ LUNG BIOPSY

Because of the increasing recognition of ABPA and the availability of serologic tests, the need for lung biopsy in confirming the diagnosis appears unnecessary unless other diseases must be excluded. Bronchiectasis in the affected lobes in segmental and subsegmental bronchi,

with sparing of distal branches, characterizes the pattern of proximal or central bronchiectasis (108–110). Bronchi are tortuous and very dilated. Histologically, bronchi contain tenacious mucus, fibrin, Curschmann spirals, Charcot-Leyden crystals, and inflammatory cells (mononuclear cells and eosinophils). Fungal hyphae can be identified in the bronchial lumen, and *Aspergillus* can be isolated in culture. Except for a few unusual case reports, no evidence exists for invasion of the bronchial wall, despite numerous hyphae in the lumen. Bronchial wall damage is associated with the presence of mononuclear cells and eosinophils, and in some cases with granulomata. Organisms of *Aspergillus* may be surrounded by necrosis, or acute or chronic inflammation. In other areas, there is replacement of submucosa with fibrous tissue. It is not known why bronchial wall destruction is focal with uninvolved adjacent areas.

A variety of morphologic lesions have been described in patients meeting criteria of ABPA (108–110). These include *Aspergillus* hyphae in granulomatous bronchiolitis, exudative bronchiolitis, *Aspergillus* hyphae in microabscess, eosinophilic pneumonia, lipid pneumonia, lymphocytic interstitial pneumonia, desquamative interstitial pneumonia, pulmonary vasculitis, and pulmonary fibrosis. Some patients with ABPA may show pathology consistent with bronchocentric granulomatosis. Mucoid impaction related to ABPA may cause proximal bronchial obstruction with distal areas of bronchiolitis obliterans. Examples of microscopic sections from ABPA patients are shown in Figures 24.10 through 24.13.

■ PATHOGENESIS

On a historical basis, in some asthma patients who had a normal bronchogram before they developed ABPA, bronchiectasis has been found to occur at the sites of roentgenographic infiltrates. This phenomenon has

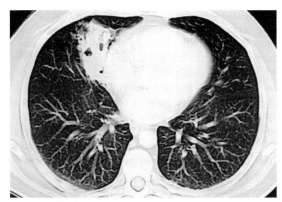

■ **FIGURE 24.10** Computed tomography scan demonstrating a cavitary mass in the right lower lobe in a 56-year-old man. The total serum IgE was 4,440 ng/mL. His only symptom was a mild nonproductive cough.

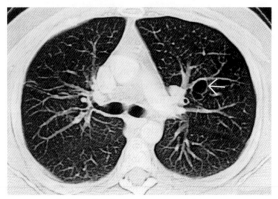

■ **FIGURE 24.11** The same patient as in Fig. 24.10. The computed tomography scan at the level of the carina demonstrates cystic bronchiectasis (*arrow*).

been confirmed by repeated CT examinations as well. It is thought that inhaled *Aspergillus* spores grow in the patient's tenacious mucus and release antigenic glyco-proteins and perhaps other reactants that activate bronchial mast cells, lymphocytes, macrophages, and eosinophils, and generate antibodies, cytokines and chemokines, followed by tissue damage that is associated with subsequent bronchiectasis or roentgenographic infiltrates. *Aspergillus* spores are thermophilic; therefore, growth is feasible in bronchi. It is unclear whether *Aspergillus* spores are trapped in the viscid mucus, or whether they have a special ability (virulence) to colonize the bronchial tree and result in development of tenacious

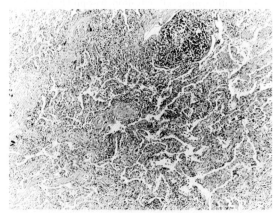

■ **FIGURE 24.12** Typical microscopic appearance representing eosinophilic pneumonia. The collapsed alveolus contains a predominance of large mononuclear cells, few lymphocytes, plasma cells, and clumps of eosinophils; similar cells infiltrate the alveolar walls. Superior segment of the upper lobe was resected for a cavitary and infiltrative lesion. (Reprinted from Imbeau SA, Nichols D, Flaherty D, et al. Allergic bronchopulmonary aspergillosis. *J Allergy Clin Immunol* 1978;62:243; with permission. Photographs from the specimen collection of Enrique Valdivia; magnification ×120, hematoxylin and eosin stain.)

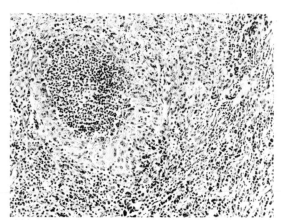

■ **FIGURE 24.13** Right lower lobectomy. The lung has prominent cellular infiltration and an area of early bronchocentric granulomatosis, with leukocytes and a crown of epithelioid cells. *Aspergillus* was demonstrated in the center of the lesions with special stains. (Reprinted from Imbeau SA, Nichols D, Flaherty D, et al. Allergic bronchopulmonary aspergillosis. *J Allergy Clin Immunol* 1978;62:243; with permission. Photographs from the specimen collection of Enrique Valdivia; magnification ×240, hematoxylin and eosin stain.)

mucus. The latter is such that during bronchoscopy, the mucoid material may remain impacted after 30 minutes of attempted removal. In contrast, in patients with CF without ABPA, such difficulty is not encountered. Pro-teolytic enzymes and possibly gliotoxins and ribotoxins produced by *A. fumigatus* growing in the bronchial tree may contribute to lung damage on a nonimmunologic or immunologic basis. Immunologic injury could occur because the release of antigenic material is associated with production of IgE, IgA, and IgG antibodies and acti-vation of the pulmonary immune response with a pano-ply of harmful proinflammatory effects.

Although peripheral blood lymphocytes from stable ABPA patients have not been reported to form excess IgE *in vitro* compared with nonatopic patients at the time of an ABPA flare-up, these cells produced signifi-cantly increased amounts of IgE (111). This suggests that during an ABPA flare-up IgE-forming cells are released into the systemic circulation, presumably from the lung. The biphasic skin reaction requires IgE and possibly IgG, and it has been suggested that a similar reaction occurs in the lung. Nevertheless, the lack of immunofluorescence in vascular deposits is evidence against an immune complex vasculitis as a cause of bronchial wall damage.

The passive transfer of serum containing IgG and IgE antibodies from a patient with ABPA to a monkey, followed by bronchial challenge with *Aspergillus*, has been associated with pulmonary lesions in the monkey. When monkeys were immunized with *A. fumigatus* and generated IgG antibodies, normal human serum was infused into both immunized and nonimmunized monkeys, and allergic human serum from a patient with ABPA (currently without any precipitating antibody) was infused into other monkeys, immunized and nonimmunized (112). All animals were challenged with aerosolized *A. fumigatus*, and lung biopsy samples were obtained on the fifth day. Only the monkey with precipitating antibody (IgG) to *Aspergillus* who received human allergic serum (IgE) showed biopsy changes consistent with ABPA (112). Mononuclear and eosinophilic infiltrates were present, with thickening of alveolar septa, but without evidence of vasculitis. These findings confirm that IgE and IgG directed against *Aspergillus* are necessary for the development of pulmonary lesions.

Similarly, a murine model of ABPA was developed that resulted in blood and pulmonary eosinophilia (113) using *A. fumigatus* particulates simulating spores that were inoculated by the intranasal route. However, if *A. fumigatus* in alum was injected into the peritoneal cavity, anti–*A. fumigatus*-IgG1 and total IgE concentrations increased, but pulmonary and peripheral blood eosinophilia did not occur. In contrast, intranasal inoculation of *A. fumigatus* resulted in perivascular eosinophilia, as well as pulmonary lymphocytes, plasma cells, histocytes, and eosinophils consistent with ABPA. A true model of ABPA where animals develop spontaneously occurring pulmonary infiltrates has yet to be described.

It is known that lymphocytes produce IL-4 (or IL-13) and IL-5 to support IgE synthesis and eosinophilia, respectively. Elevated soluble IL-2 receptors suggest $CD4^+$ lymphocyte activation (114), and $CD4^+$-T_H2 type clones have been produced from ABPA patients (56). It appears as if presentation of *Asp f* 1 is restricted to certain class II MHC molecules, HLA-DR2 and HLA-DR5 (54,56). The demonstration of hyperreleasability of mediators from basophils of patients with stage IV and V ABPA (107) is consistent with the hypothesis that a subgroup of patients may be most susceptible to immunologic injury if peripheral blood basophils are representative bronchial mast cells. The fact that basophils from patients with any stage of ABPA have increased *in vitro* histamine release as compared with basophils from *A. fumigatus* skin-prick–positive patients with asthma suggests that mast cell mediator release to various antigens (fungi) may contribute to lung damage in ABPA if these findings can be applied to bronchial mast cells.

Analysis of bronchoalveolar lavage from stages II and IV ABPA patients who had no current chest roentgenographic infiltrates revealed evidence for local antibody production of IgA–*A. fumigatus* and IgE–*A. fumigatus* compared with peripheral blood (115). Bronchial lavage IgA–*A. fumigatus* was 96 times that of peripheral blood, and IgE–*A. fumigatus* in lavage was 48 times that found in peripheral blood. Although total serum IgE was elevated, there was no increase in bronchial lavage total IgE corrected for albumin. These results suggest that the bronchoalveolar space is not the source of the markedly elevated total IgE in ABPA. Perhaps pulmonary interstitium or nonpulmonary sources (tonsils or bone marrow) serve as sites of total IgE production in ABPA.

In a serial analysis of serum IgA–*A. fumigatus* in 10 patients, there were sharp elevations over baseline before (five cases) or during (five cases) roentgenographic exacerbations of ABPA for IgA1–*A. fumigatus* (116). Serum IgA2–*A. fumigatus* was elevated before the exacerbation in two cases and during the exacerbation in five cases. Heterogeneous polyclonal antibody responses to seven different molecular weight bands of *A. fumigatus* were present on immunoblot analysis of sera (116). Band intensity increased during ABPA exacerbations, and patient's sera often had broader reactivity with *A. fumigatus* bands from 24-kDa to 90-kDa molecular weights during disease flare-ups. Some patients had immunoblot patterns consistent with increases in IgE, IgG, or IgA antibodies binding to different *A. fumigatus* antigens but no consistent binding to a particular *A. fumigatus* band.

A summary of immunopathogenesis includes virulence factors, including proteases from *A. fumigatus*, that can damage epithelium and interfere with surfactant, generation of tenacious eosinophil-rich mucoid impactions, a brisk CD4 T_H2 response with its characteristic cytokines and chemokines, activation of CD20 B cells and upregulation of CD23 (the low affinity IgE receptor that binds allergen-IgE complexes) by IL-4, remarkable amounts of isotypic antibody production in the bronchoalveolar space and presumably interstitium, genetic restriction of HLA-DR2 and HLA-DR5 and gain of function polymorphisms for IL-4, eosinophil upregulation and activation, mast cell activation, basophil hyperreleasability, and chemokines such as thymus- and activation-regulated chemokine (34,117). The immunopathogenesis also includes allergic inflammation that is responsive to systemic but not inhaled corticosteroids and poorly responsive to intensive antifungal therapies.

■ DIFFERENTIAL DIAGNOSIS

The differential diagnosis of ABPA includes disease states associated primarily with transient or permanent roentgenographic lesions, asthma, and peripheral blood or sputum eosinophilia. The asthma patient with a roentgenographic infiltrate may have atelectasis from inadequately controlled asthma. Bacterial, viral, or fungal pneumonias must be excluded in addition to tuberculosis and the many other causes of roentgenographic infiltrates. Eosinophilia may occur with parasitism, tuberculosis, Churg-Strauss syndrome, pulmonary infiltrates from drug allergies, neoplasm, eosinophilic pneumonia, and, rarely, avian-hypersensitivity pneumonitis. Mucoid impaction of bronchi may occur without ABPA. All patients with a history of mucoid impaction syndrome or with collapse of a lobe or lung, however, should have ABPA excluded. Similarly, although the morphologic diagnosis of bronchocentric granulomatosis is considered by some to represent an entity distinct from ABPA, ABPA must be excluded in such patients. Although the sweat test for CF is within normal limits in ABPA patients, unless concomitant CF is present, the patient with CF and asthma or changing roentgenographic infiltrates should have ABPA excluded or confirmed. Genetic testing and assessment of pancreatic function for CF may be indicated. The genetics of ABPA are beginning to be studied to determine similarities with CF. Some patients with asthma who develop pulmonary infiltrates with eosinophilia are likely to have ABPA. Some patients will have mucus plugging (tree-in-bud) from atypical Mycobacteria (118).

In the patient without a history of roentgenographic infiltrates, ABPA should be suspected on the basis of (a) a positive, immediate cutaneous reaction to *Aspergillus*; (b) elevated total serum IgE (>417 kU/L); (c) increasing severity of asthma; (d) abnormalities on chest roentgenogram or CT; (e) repeatedly positive sputum cultures for *Aspergillus* species; or (f) bronchiectasis.

A rare patient with asthma, roentgenographic infiltrates, and bronchiectasis or a history of surgical resection for such may present with peripheral eosinophilia, elevated total serum IgE concentration, but other negative serologic results for ABPA. Some other species of *Aspergillus* may be responsible, such as *A. oryzae*, *A. ochraceus*, or *A. niger*. Perhaps a different allergic bronchopulmonary mycosis may be present. For example, illnesses consistent with allergic bronchopulmonary candidiasis, curvulariosis, dreschleriosis, stemphyliosis, fusariosis, and pseudallescheriasis have been described (119–121). Positive sputum cultures, precipitating antibodies, or *in vitro* assays for a fungus other than *Aspergillus* or for different *Aspergillus* species could suggest a causative source of the allergic bronchopulmonary fungosis.

The presence of bronchiectasis from ABPA has been associated with colonization of bronchi by atypical Mycobacteria (118). It appears that the identification of atypical Mycobacteria in the sputum should at least raise the possibility of ABPA in patients with asthma who do not have acquired immunodeficiency syndrome. Similarly, bronchiectatic airways may become colonized by *Pseudomonas aeruginosa* in ABPA patients who do not have CF.

■ NATURAL HISTORY

Although most patients are diagnosed before the age of 40 years, and an increasing number are diagnosed before the age of 20 years, one must not overlook the diagnosis of ABPA in older patients previously characterized as having chronic asthma or chronic bronchiectasis. Some patients as old as 80 have had the diagnosis of ABPA made. Late sequelae of ABPA include irreversible pulmonary function abnormalities, symptoms of chronic bronchitis, and pulmonary fibrosis. Death

results from respiratory failure and cor pulmonale. Allergic bronchopulmonary aspergillosis has been associated with respiratory failure in the second or third decade of life. Most patients who have ABPA do not progress to the end-stage disease, especially if there is early diagnosis and appropriate treatment. Patients who present in the acute stage (stage I) of ABPA may enter remission (stage II), recurrent exacerbation (stage III), or may develop corticosteroid-dependent asthma (stage IV). One patient who had a single roentgenographic infiltrate when her ABPA was diagnosed entered a remission stage that lasted for 8 years until an exacerbation occurred (122). Thus, a remission does not imply permanent cessation of disease activity. This patient may be the exception, but serves to emphasize the need for longer term observation of patients with ABPA. Patients who have corticosteroid-dependent asthma (stage IV) at the time of diagnosis may evolve into having pulmonary fibrosis (stage V). Because prednisone does not reverse bronchiectasis or the pulmonary fibrotic changes in the lung, every effort should be made by physicians managing patients with asthma to suspect and confirm cases of ABPA before significant structural damage to the lung has developed.

In managing patients with ABPA, there is a lack of correlation between clinical symptoms and chest roentgenographic lesions. Irreversible lung damage including bronchiectasis may occur without the patient seeking medical attention. In Great Britain, ABPA exacerbations were reported to occur between October and February during elevations of fungal spore counts (34). In Chicago, 38 of 49 (77.5%) ABPA exacerbations (new roentgenographic infiltrate with elevation of total serum IgE concentration) occurred from June through November in association with increased outdoor fungal spore counts (123).

Acute and chronic pulmonary function changes have been studied in a series of ABPA cases, during which time all patients received corticosteroids and bronchodilators (124). There appeared to be no significant correlation between duration of ABPA (mean follow-up period, 44 months), duration of asthma, and diffusing capacity of the lungs for carbon monoxide, total lung capacity (TLC), vital capacity (VC), forced expiratory volume in 1 second (FEV_1), and FEV_1%. In six patients with acute exacerbations of ABPA, a significant reduction in total lung capacity, vital capacity, FEV_1, and diffusing capacity of the lungs for carbon monoxide occurred, which returned to baseline during steroid treatment. Thus, early recognition and prompt effective treatment of flare-ups appear to reduce the likelihood of irreversible lung damage. Other patients may have reductions in FEV_1 and FEV_1% consistent with an obstructive process during an ABPA exacerbation.

The prognosis for stage V patients is less favorable than for patients classified into stages I through IV (74). Although prednisone has proven useful in patients with end-stage lung disease, 6 of 17 stage V patients, observed for a mean 4.9 years, died. When the FEV_1 was 0.8 L or less after aggressive initial corticosteroid administration, the outcome was poor (53). In contrast, when stage IV patients are managed effectively, deterioration of respiratory function parameters or status asthmaticus has not occurred.

Prednisone is the most effective treatment. In a 5-year follow-up of ABPA cases, it was reported that a daily prednisone dose of 7.5 mg was required to maintain clinical improvement and roentgenographic clearing in 80% of patients, compared with 40% of those treated with either cromolyn or bronchodilators alone (125). In a study of patients from Northwestern University Feinberg School of Medicine, who had periodic blood sampling, both immunologic and clinical improvement occurred with prednisone therapy. Individuals with ABPA have high presentation (stages I and III) total serum IgE concentrations, and those patients previously never requiring oral steroids for control of asthma have the highest concentrations. Treatment with prednisone causes roentgenographic and clinical improvement, as well as decreases in total serum IgE. Total serum IgE and IgE–*A. fumigatus* may increase before and during a flare-up, but the serum IgE–*A. fumigatus* does not fluctuate to the extent that total serum IgE concentration does.

Prognostic factors remain to be established that may identify patients at risk for developing stage IV or V ABPA. The roentgenographic lesion at the time of diagnosis does not appear to provide prognostic data about long-term outcome unless the patient is stage V. The effect of untreated ABPA exacerbations has produced stage V ABPA. In addition, at least some patients with CF who develop ABPA have a worse prognosis. Lastly, the effect of allergic fungal rhinosinusitis (Table 24.3) on the natural history of ABPA is unknown.

■ TREATMENT

Prednisone is the drug of choice but need not be administered indefinitely (Table 24.4). Multiple agents have been tried, including intrabronchial instillation of amphotericin B, oral nystatin, itraconazole, ketoconazole, high-dose inhaled corticosteroids, and omalizumab (126–128). Itraconazole (129–132) or voriconazole or newer antifungals may have an adjunctive role, but prednisone therapy typically eliminates or diminishes sputum plug production. Although the exact pathogenesis of ABPA is unknown, oral corticosteroids have been demonstrated to reduce the clinical symptoms, incidence of positive sputum cultures, and roentgenographic infiltrates. Oral corticosteroids may be effective by decreasing sputum volume, by making the bronchi a less suitable culture media for *Aspergillus* species, and by inhibiting many of the *Aspergillus*–pulmonary immune system interactions. The total serum IgE concentration

TABLE 24.3   CRITERIA FOR DIAGNOSIS OF ALLERGIC FUNGAL SINUSITIS

Chronic sinusitis—at least 6 months duration with nasal polyposis
Allergic mucin (histologic examination with eosinophils and fungal hyphae and "putty" material by rhinoscopy)
Computed tomography of sinuses shows opacification and magnetic resonance imaging shows fungal findings[a]
Absence of invasive fungal disease, diabetes mellitus, HIV

[a]T_1-weighted imaging reveals isointense or hypointense findings of mucin in sinuses; T_2-weighted imaging demonstrates a "signal void" where there is inspissated mucin.

declines by at least 35% within 2 months of initiating prednisone therapy. Failure to observe this reduction suggests noncompliance of patients or a continuing exacerbation of ABPA.

Our current treatment regimen is to clear the roentgenographic infiltrates with daily prednisone, usually at 0.5 mg/kg. Most infiltrates clear within 2 weeks, at which time the same dose, given on a single alternate-day regimen, is begun and maintained for 2 months until the total serum IgE, which should be followed up every 4 to 8 weeks for the first year, has reached a baseline concentration. The baseline total serum IgE concentration can remain elevated despite clinical and radiographic improvement. Slow reductions in prednisone, at no faster than 10 mg/month, can be initiated once a stable baseline of total IgE has been achieved. Acute exacerbations of ABPA often are preceded by a 100% increase in total serum IgE and must be treated promptly with increases in prednisone and reinstitution of daily steroids. Certainly, the physician must exclude other causes for roentgenographic infiltrates. Pulmonary functions should be measured yearly or as necessary for stages IV and V and as required for asthma.

If prednisone can be discontinued, the patient is in remission (stage II), and perhaps only an inhaled corticosteroid will be needed for management of asthma. Alternatively, if the patient has asthma that cannot be managed without prednisone despite avoidance measures and maximal anti-inflammatory medications, alternate-day prednisone will be necessary. The dose of prednisone required to control asthma and to prevent ABPA radiologic exacerbations is usually less than 0.5 mg/kg on alternate days. For corticosteroid-dependent patients (stages IV or V) with ABPA, an explanation of prednisone risks and benefits is indicated, as is the discussion that untreated ABPA infiltrates result in bronchiectasis and irreversible fibrosis. Specific additional recommendations regarding estrogen supplementation

TABLE 24.4   TREATMENT OF ALLERGIC BRONCHOPULMONARY ASPERGILLOSIS

1. Prednisone is drug of choice; 0.5 mg/kg daily for 2 weeks, then on alternate days for 6 to 8 weeks, then attempt tapering by 5 mg on alternate days every 2 weeks.
2. Repeat chest roentgenogram and/or high-resolution computed tomography of lung at 2 to 4 weeks to document clearing of infiltrates.
3. Serum IgE concentration at baseline and at 4 and 8 weeks, then every 8 weeks for first year to establish range of total IgE concentrations (a 100% increase can identify a silent exacerbation).
4. Baseline spirometry or full pulmonary function tests depending on the clinical setting.
5. Environmental control for fungi and other allergens at home or work.
6. Determine if prednisone-dependent asthma (stage IV ABPA) is present; if not, manage asthma with anti-inflammatory medications and other medications as indicated.
7. Future ABPA exacerbations may be identified by

   a. Asymptomatic sharp increases in the total serum IgE concentration
   b. Increasing asthma symptoms or signs
   c. Deteriorations in FVC and/or FEV_1
   d. Cough, chest pain, new production of sputum plugs, dyspnea not explained by other causes
   e. Chest roentgenographic or high-resolution computed tomography findings (patient may be asymptomatic)

8. Document in chart that prednisone side effects were discussed and address bone density issues (e.g., adequate calcium, exercise, hormone replacement and antiosteopenia medication if indicated).
9. Persistent sputum expectoration should be cultured to identify *Aspergillus fumigatus, Staphylococcus aureus, Pseudomonas aeruginosa,* atypical Mycobacteria, etc.
10. If new ABPA exacerbations occur, repeat step 1.

ABPA, Allergic bronchopulmonary aspersillosis; FVC, forced vital capacity; FEV_1, forced expiratory volume in 1 second.

for women, adequate calcium ingestion, bronchial hygiene, and physical fitness and bone density measurements should be considered.

In ABPA patients receiving prednisone, itraconazole, 200 mg twice daily or placebo, was administered for 16 weeks (129). A response was defined as (a) at least a 50% reduction in oral corticosteroid dose, and (b) a decrease of 25% or more of the total serum IgE concentration and at least one of three additional parameters: a 25% improvement in exercise tolerance or similar 25% improvement in pulmonary function tests or resolution of chest roentgenographic infiltrates if initially present with no subsequent new infiltrates, or if no initial chest roentgenographic infiltrates were present, no emergence of new infiltrates. Oral corticosteroids were tapered during the study, although it was not certain that all patients had an attempt at steroid tapering. With that consideration, itraconazole administration was associated with a response as defined. Unfortunately, less than 25% of patients had chest roentgenographic infiltrates at the beginning of the study. More responders (60%) occurred in patients without bronchiectasis (ABPA-S) versus ABPA-CB (31%), compared with 8% in placebo-treated patients (129). Eleven isolates from sputum cultures were analyzed for antifungal susceptibility, and five were susceptible to intraconazole (129). None of the patients whose isolates of *A. fumigatus* were resistant or tolerant *in vitro* to itraconazole had responses to treatment. The conclusions from this study were that patients with ABPA "generally benefit from concurrent itraconazole" (129). The difficulties and complexities in such studies are apparent, and ideally the drug would be of value in patients with ABPA-CB, who are the patients more frequently seen in the office. Itraconazole has anti-inflammatory effects and reduces eosinophils in induced sputum and lowers the total IgE concentration (132).

Itraconazole's absorption is reduced if there is gastric hypochlorhydria, so it should be ingested 1 hour before or 2 hours after meals. It slows hepatic metabolism of drugs that use the CYP 3A4 pathway, including methylprednisolone, inhaled budesonide, statins, coumadin, oral hypoglycemics, tacrolimus, cyclosporines, and benzodiazepines, as examples. Itraconazole itself is potentiated by clarithromycin and some protease inhibitors used for human immunodeficiency virus infection.

Antifungal agents have been administered for 40 years to ABPA patients and are not a substitute for oral corticosteroids. They remain adjunctive at best. The primary pharmacologic therapy remains prednisone, which, if the patient is in stage IV or V, often can be administered on an alternate-day basis. Perhaps itraconazole has anti-inflammatory effects or a delaying effect on corticosteroid elimination. If so, then its effects might resemble those of the macrolide troleandomycin, delaying the metabolism of methylprednisolone. I have seen failures of itraconazole and voriconazole and excessive reliance on it without clearing of chest roentgenographic infiltrates.

Nevertheless, as adjunctive therapy in patients who have susceptible strains of *A. fumigatus*, itraconazole or other antifungal agent could be considered in ABPA. Some studies have reported reductions in daily prednisone use and clearance of *A. fumigatus* from sputum.

In CF patients with ABPA, itraconazole was reported to result in a 47% reduction in oral steroid dose and a 55% reduction in ABPA exacerbations (23). The study group was composed of 16 (9%) patients from a pool of 122 CF patients. Itraconazole was administered to 12 of the 16 patients, who also received inhaled corticosteroids and prednisone and treatment for CF. Elevated serum aspartate aminotransferase or alanine aminotransferase results of greater than three times the upper limit of normal were contraindications to the use of itraconazole. Although there were reductions in acute ABPA exacerbations and oral steroid doses, there were no differences in total cumulative prednisone doses (23). Nepomuceno et al. suggested trying intraconazole in "properly selected" patients with CF, especially because ABPA seems to cause a faster deterioration of FEV_1 per year in CF patients compared with CF without ABPA (23). Whether this antifungal therapy will be effective on a longer term basis remains uncertain. Indeed, just as it is possible that the increasing frequency of ABPA occurring in CF may be a consequence of high-dose nebulized tobramycin allowing for emergence of *A. fumigatus* in bronchial mucus, perhaps resistance to antifungals will occur and create additional issues that complicate the clinical care of patients with CF who have ABPA.

Immunotherapy with *Aspergillus* species probably should not be administered in patients with ABPA, but examples of adverse effects aside from injection reactions have not been reported. It is not expected that immunotherapy with *Aspergillus* extracts would result in immune complex formation. Immunotherapy can be administered with pollens and mites and possibly fungi, but not those in the *Aspergillus* genus.

Inhaled corticosteroids should be used in an effort to control asthma but one should not depend on them to prevent exacerbations of ABPA. Similarly, the leukotriene D_4 antagonists have antieosinophil actions *in vitro* and theoretically might be of value for use in ABPA patients. They can be administered for a trial of 1 to 3 months.

The exact role of environmental exposure of *Aspergillus* spores in the pathogenesis of ABPA remains unknown. *Aspergillus* spores are found regularly in crawl spaces, "unfinished" basements, compost piles, manure, and fertile soil. Some patients have developed acute wheezing dyspnea and recognized ABPA exacerbations after inhalation of heavy spore burdens such as moldy wood chips or after exposure to closed up cottage homes. Attempts should be made to repair leaky basement walls and floors to minimize moldy basements. Because spores of *Aspergillus* species, including *A. fumigatus*, are detected regularly both indoors and outside, a common sense approach seems advisable.

■ REFERENCES

1. Hinson KFW, Moon AJ, Plummer NS. Bronchopulmonary aspergillosis: a review and report of eight new cases. *Thorax*. 1952;73: 317–333.
2. Patterson R, Golbert T. Hypersensitivity disease of the lung. *Univ Michigan Med Center J*. 1968;34:8–11.
3. Slavin RG, Laird TS, Cherry JD. Allergic bronchopulmonary aspergillosis in a child. *J Pediatr*. 1970;76:416–421.
4. Chetty A, Bhargava S, Jain RK. Allergic bronchopulmonary aspergillosis in Indian children with bronchial asthma. *Ann Allergy*. 1985;54:46–49.
5. Turner ES, Greenberger PA, Sider L. Complexities of establishing an early diagnosis of allergic bronchopulmonary aspergillosis in children. *Allergy Proc*. 1989;10:63–69.
6. Kiefer TA, Kesarwala HH, Greenberger PA, et al. Allergic bronchopulmonary aspergillosis in a young child: diagnostic confirmation by serum IgE and IgG indices. *Ann Allergy*. 1986;56:233–236.
7. Greenberger PA, Liotta JL, Roberts M. The effects of age on isotypic antibody responses to *Aspergillus fumigatus*: implications regarding *in vitro* measurements. *J Lab Clin Med*. 1989;114:278–284.
8. Imbeau SA, Cohen M, Reed CE. Allergic bronchopulmonary aspergillosis in infants. *Am J Dis Child*. 1977;131:1127–1130.
9. Huppmann MV, Monson M. Allergic bronchopulmonary aspergillosis: a unique presentation in a pediatric patient. *Pediatr Radiol*. 2008;38:879–883.
10. Agawal R, Gupta D, Aggarwal AN, et al. Allergic bronchopulmonary aspergillosis: lessons from 126 patients attending a chest clinic in North India. *Chest*. 2006;130:442–448.
11. Patterson R, Greenberger PA, Radin RC, et al. Allergic bronchopulmonary aspergillosis: staging as an aid to management. *Ann Intern Med*. 1982;96:286–291.
12. Greenberger PA, Miller TP, Roberts M, et al. Allergic bronchopulmonary aspergillosis in patients with and without evidence of bronchiectasis. *Ann Allergy*. 1993;70:333–338.
13. Basich JE, Graves TS, Baz MN, et al. Allergic bronchopulmonary aspergillosis in steroid dependent asthmatics. *J Allergy Clin Immunol*. 1981;68:98–102.
14. Laufer P, Fink JN, Bruns W, et al. Allergic bronchopulmonary aspergillosis in cystic fibrosis. *J Allergy Clin Immunol*. 1984;73:44–48.
15. Maguire S, Moriarty P, Tempany E, et al. Unusual clustering of allergic bronchopulmonary aspergillosis in children with cystic fibrosis. *Pediatrics*. 1988;82:835–839.
16. Nelson LA, Callerame ML, Schwartz RH. Aspergillosis and atopy in cystic fibrosis. *Am Rev Respir Dis*. 1979;120:863–873.
17. Zeaske R, Bruns WT, Fink JN, et al. Immune responses to *Aspergillus* in cystic fibrosis. *J Allergy Clin Immunol*. 1988;82:73–77.
18. Knutsen AP, Hutchinson PS, Mueller KR, et al. Serum immunoglobulins E and G anti–*Aspergillus fumigatus* antibody in patients with cystic fibrosis who have allergic bronchopulmonary aspergillosis. *J Lab Clin Med*. 1990;116:724–727.
19. Hutcheson PS, Knutsen AP, Rejent AJ, et al. A 12-year old longitudinal study of *Aspergillus* sensitivity in patients with cystic fibrosis. *Chest*. 1996;110:363–366.
20. Geller DE, Kaplowitz H, Light MJ, et al. Allergic bronchopulmonary aspergillosis: reported prevalence, regional distribution, and patient characteristics. *Chest*. 1999;116:639–646.
21. Becker JW, Burke W, McDonald G, et al. Prevalence of allergic bronchopulmonary aspergillosis and atopy in adult patients with cystic fibrosis. *Chest*. 1996;109:1536–1540.
22. Chotirmall SH, Branagan P, Gunaratnam C, et al. Aspergillus/allergic bronchopulmonary aspergillosis in an Irish cystic fibrosis population: a diagnostically challenging entity. *Respir Care*. 2008;53:1035–1041.
23. Skov M, Koch C, Reinert CM, et al. Diagnosis of allergic bronchopulmonary aspergillosis (ABPA) in cystic fibrosis. *Allergy*. 2000;55:50–58.
23a. Nepomuceno IB, Esrig S, Moss BB. Allergic bronchopulmonary aspergillosis in cystic fibrosis: role of atopy and response to itraconazole. *Chest*. 1999;115:364–370.
24. Stevens DA, Moss RB, Kurup VP, et al. Allergic bronchopulmonary aspergillosis in cystic fibrosis—state of the art: Cystic Fibrosis Foundation Consensus Conference. *Clin Infect Dis*. 2003;37 (Suppl 3): S225–S264.
25. Simmonds NJ, Cullinan P, Hodson ME. Growing old with cystic fibrosis—The characteristics of long-term survivors of cystic fibrosis. *Resp Med*. 2008;doi:10.1016/j.rmed.2008.10.011.
26. Bhagat R, Shah A, Jaggi OP, et al. Concomitant allergic bronchopulmonary aspergillosis and allergic *Aspergillus* sinusitis with an operated aspergilloma. *J Allergy Clin Immunol*. 1993;91:1094–1096.

27. Shah A, Bhagat R, Panchal N, et al. Allergic bronchopulmonary aspergillosis with middle lobe syndrome and allergic *Aspergillus* sinusitis. *Eur Respir J.* 1993;6:917–918.

28. Shah A, Panjabi C. Contemporaneous occurrence of allergic bronchopulmonary aspergillosis, allergic *Aspergillus* sinusitis, and aspergilloma. *Ann Allergy Asthma Immunol.* 2006;96:874–888.

29. Slavin RG, Spector SL, Bernstein IL. The diagnosis and management of sinusitis: a practice parameter update. *J Allergy Clin Immunol.* 2005;116:S13–S47.

30. Rosenberg M, Patterson R, Roberts M, et al. The assessment of immunologic and clinical changes occurring during corticosteroid therapy for allergic bronchopulmonary aspergillosis. *Am J Med.* 1978;64:599–606.

31. Wang JLF, Patterson R, Rosenberg M, et al. Serum IgE and IgG antibody activity against *Aspergillus fumigatus* as a diagnostic aid in allergic bronchopulmonary aspergillosis. *Am Rev Respir Dis.* 1978;117:917–927.

32. Greenberger PA, Patterson R. Application of enzyme linked immunosorbent assay (ELISA) in diagnosis of allergic bronchopulmonary aspergillosis. *J Lab Clin Med.* 1982;99:288–293.

33. Barton RC, Hobson RP, Denton M, et al. Serologic diagnosis of allergic bronchopulmonary aspergillosis in patients with cystic fibrosis through the detection of immunoglobulin G to *Aspergillus fumigates.* *Diag Micro Infect Dis.* 2008;62:287–291.

34. Pepys J. Hypersensitivity disease of the lungs due to fungi and organic dusts. In: *Karger Monographs in Allergy.* Vol. 4. Basel: Karger; 1969: 63–68.

35. Glancy JJ, Elder JL, McAleer R. Allergic bronchopulmonary fungal disease without clinical asthma. *Thorax.* 1981;36:345–349.

36. Greenberger PA, Patterson R. Allergic bronchopulmonary aspergillosis and the evaluation of the patient with asthma. *J Allergy Clin Immunol.* 1988;81:646–650.

37. Schwartz HJ, Greenberger PA. The prevalence of allergic bronchopulmonary aspergillosis in patients with asthma, determined by serologic and radiologic criteria in patients at risk. *J Lab Clin Med.* 1991; 117:138–142.

38. Geller M. Allergic Bronchopulmonary Aspergillosis does exist in Brazil. *Ann Allergy.* 1989;63:325–326.

39. Solomon WR, Burge HP, Boise JR. Airborne *Aspergillus fumigatus* levels outside and within a large clinical center. *J Allergy Clin Immunol.* 1978;62:56–60.

40. Latge J-P. *Aspergillus fumigatus* and aspergillosis. *Clin Microbiol Rev.* 1999;12:310–350.

41. Kurup VP, Kumar A, Kenealy WR, et al. *Aspergillus* ribotoxins react with IgE and IgG antibodies of patients with allergic bronchopulmonary aspergillosis. *J Lab Clin Med.* 1994;123:749–756.

42. Berkova N, Lair-Fulleringer S, Femenia F, et al. *Aspergillus fumigatus* conidia tumour necrosis factor- and staurosporine-induced apoptosis in epithelial cells. *Internat Immunol.* 2005;18:139–150.

43. Dubourdeau M, Athman R, Balloy V, et al. *Aspergillus fumigates* induces immune responses in alveolar macrophages through the MAPK pathway independently of TLR2 and TLR4. *J Immunol.* 2006;177:3994–4001.

44. Rambach G, Hadleitner M, Mohsenipour I, et al. Antifungal activity of local complement system in cerebral aspergillosis. *Microbes Infect.* 2005;7:1285–1295.

45. Spikes S, Xu R, Nguyen CK, et al. Gliotoxin production in Aspergillus fumigates contributes to host-specific differences in virulence. *J Infect Dis.* 2008;197:479–486.

46. Stanzani M, Orciuolo E, Lewis R, et al. Aspergillus fumigates suppresses the human cellular immune response via gliotoxin-mediated apoptosis of monocytes. *Blood.* 2005;105:2258–2265.

47. Alp S, Arikan S. Investigation of extracellular elastase, acid proteinase and phospholipase activities as putative virulence factors in clinical isolates of Aspergillus species. *J Basic Micro.* 2008;48:331–337.

48. Morris MP, Fletcher OJ. Disease prevalence in Georgia turkey flocks in 1986. *Avian Dis.* 1988;32:404–406.

49. Quirce S, Cuevas M, Diez-Gomez ML, et al. Respiratory allergy to *Aspergillus*-derived enzymes in bakers' asthma. *J Allergy Clin Immunol.* 1992;90:970–978.

50. Houba R, Heederik DJ, Doekes G, et al. Exposure-sensitization relationship for alpha-amylase allergens in the baking industry. *Am J Respir Crit Care Med.* 1996;154:130–136.

51. Rosenberg IL, Greenberger PA. Allergic bronchopulmonary aspergillosis and aspergilloma: long-term followup without enlargement of a large multiloculated cavity. *Chest.* 1984;85:123–125.

52. Binder RE, Faling LJ, Pugatch RE, et al. Chronic necrotizing pulmonary aspergillosis: a discreet clinical entity. *Medicine.* 1982;151: 109–124.

53. Barth PJ, Rossberg C, Kock S, et al. Pulmonary aspergillosis in an unselected autopsy series. *Pathol Res Pract.* 2000;196:73–80.

54. Knutsen AP, Noyes B, Warrier MR, et al. Allergic bronchopulmonary aspergillosis in a patient with cystic fibrosis: diagnostic criteria when the IgE level is less than 500 IU/mL. *Ann Allergy Asthma Immunol.* 2005;95:488–493.

55. Knutsen AP, Kariuki B, Consolino JD, et al. IL-4 alpha chain receptor (IL-4Ralpha) polymorphisms in allergic bronchopulmonary aspergillosis. *Clin Mol Allergy.* 2006;17:4:3.

56. Chauhan B, Santiago L, Hutcheson PS, et al. Evidence for the involvement of two different MHC class II regions in susceptibility or protection in allergic bronchopulmonary aspergillosis. *J Allergy Clin Immunol.* 2000;106:723–729.

57. Katzenstein AL, Sale SR, Greenberger PA. Allergic *Aspergillus* sinusitis: a newly recognized form of sinusitis. *J Allergy Clin Immunol.* 1983;72:89–93.

58. Goldstein MF, Atkins PC, Cogan FC, et al. Allergic *Aspergillus* sinusitis. *J Allergy Clin Immunol.* 1985;76: 515–524.

59. DeShazo RD, Chapin K, Swain RE. Fungal sinusitis. *N Engl J Med.* 1997;337:254–259.

60. Kohn FA, Javer AR. Allergic fungal sinusitis: a four-year followup. *Am J Rhinol.* 2000;14:149–156.

61. Marple BF. Surgical fungal sinusitis: surgical management. *Otolaryngol Clin North Am.* 2000;33:409–418.

62. Marple B, Newcomer M, Schwade N, et al. Natural history of allergic fungal rhinosinusitis: a 4- to 10-year follow-up. *Otolaryngol Head Neck Surg.* 2002;127:361–366.

63. Campbell JM, Graham M, Gray HC, et al. Allergic fungal sinusitis in children. *Ann Allergy Asthma Immunol.* 2006;96:286–290.

64. Bassichis BA, Marple BF, Mabry RL, et al. Use of immunotherapy in previously treated patients with allergic fungal sinusitis. *Otolaryngol Head Neck Surg.* 2001;125:487–490.

65. Sher TH, Schwartz HJ. Allergic *Aspergillus* sinusitis with concurrent allergic bronchopulmonary *Aspergillus*: report of a case. *J Allergy Clin Immunol.* 1988;81:844–846.

66. Rosenberg M, Patterson R, Mintzer R, et al. Clinical and immunologic criteria for the diagnosis of allergic bronchopulmonary aspergillosis. *Ann Intern Med.* 1977;86:405–414.

67. Greenberger PA. Allergic bronchopulmonary aspergillosis. *J Allergy Clin Immunol.* 2002;110:685–692.

68. Greenberger PA, Yucha CB, Janson S, et al. Using rare diseases as models for biobehavioral research: allergic bronchopulmonary aspergillosis. *Allergy Asthma Proc.* 2007;28:489–496.

69. Patterson R, Greenberger PA, Halwig JM, et al. Allergic bronchopulmonary aspergillosis: natural history and classification of early disease by serologic and roentgenographic studies. *Arch Intern Med.* 1986;146:916–918.

70. Ricketti AJ, Greenberger PA, Patterson R. Serum IgE as an important aid in management of allergic bronchopulmonary aspergillosis. *J Allergy Clin Immunol.* 1984;74:68–71.

71. Ricketti AJ, Greenberger PA, Patterson R. Immediate type reactions in patients with allergic bronchopulmonary aspergillosis. *J Allergy Clin Immunol.* 1983;71:541–545.

72. Ricketti AJ, Greenberger PA, Glassroth J. Spontaneous pneumothorax in allergic bronchopulmonary aspergillosis. *Arch Intern Med.* 1984;144:181–182.

73. Greenberger PA, Patterson R, Ghory AC, et al. Late sequelae of allergic bronchopulmonary aspergillosis. *J Allergy Clin Immunol.* 1980;66:327–335.

74. Lee TM, Greenberger PA, Patterson R, et al. Stage V (fibrotic) allergic bronchopulmonary aspergillosis: a review of 17 cases followed from diagnosis. *Arch Intern Med.* 1987;147:319–323.

75. Mintzer RA, Rogers LF, Kruglick GD, et al. The spectrum of radiologic findings in allergic bronchopulmonary aspergillosis. *Radiology.* 1978;127:301–307.

76. Mendelson EB, Fisher MR, Mintzer RA, et al. Roentgenographic and clinical staging of allergic bronchopulmonary aspergillosis. *Chest.* 1985;87:334–339.

77. Neeld DA, Goodman LR, Gurney JW, et al. Computerized tomography in the evaluation of allergic bronchopulmonary aspergillosis. *Am Rev Respir Dis.* 1990;142:1200–1205.

78. Goyal R, White CS, Templeton PA, et al. High attenuation mucous plugs in allergic bronchopulmonary aspergillosis: CT appearance. *J Comput Assist Tomogr.* 1992;16:649–650.

79. Ward S, Heyneman L, Lee MJ, et al. Accuracy of CT in the diagnosis of allergic bronchopulmonary aspergillosis in asthmatic patients. *AJR.* 1999;173:937–942.

80. Mitchell TAM, Hamilos DL, Lynch DA, et al. Distribution and severity of bronchiectasis in allergic bronchopulmonary aspergillosis (ABPA). *J Asthma.* 2000;37:65–72.

81. Martinez S, Heyneman LE, McAdams HP, et al. Mucoid impactions: finger-in-glove sign and other CT and radiographic features. *Radiographics.* 2008;28:1369–1382.

82. Hoehne JH, Reed CE, Dickie HA. Allergic bronchopulmonary aspergillosis is not rare. *Chest.* 1973;63:177–181.

83. Kurup VP, Fink JN. Immunologic tests for evaluation of hypersensitivity pneumonitis and allergic bronchopulmonary aspergillosis. In: Rose NR, Conway de Macario E, Folds JD, et al., eds. *Manual of Clinical Laboratory Immunology.* 5th ed. Washington, DC: ASM Press; 1997:908–915.

84. Reed C. Variability of antigenicity of *Aspergillus fumigatus. J Allergy Clin Immunol.* 1978;61:227–229.

85. Schwartz HJ, Citron KM, Chester EH, et al. A comparison of the prevalence of sensitization to *Aspergillus* antigens among asthmatics in Cleveland and London. *J Allergy Clin Immunol.* 1978;62:9–14.

86. Novey HS. Epidemiology of allergic bronchopulmonary aspergillosis. *Immunol Allergy Clin North Am.* 1998;18:641–653.

87. McCarthy DS, Pepys J. Allergic bronchopulmonary aspergillosis: clinical immunology: II. Skin, nasal, and bronchial tests. *Clin Allergy.* 1971;1:415–432.

88. Sarma PU, Banerjee B, Bir N, et al. Immunodiagnosis of allergic bronchopulmonary aspergillosis. *Immunol Allergy Clin North Am.* 1998;18:525–547.

89. Kurup VP, Banerjee B, Greenberger PA, et al. Allergic bronchopulmonary aspergillosis: challenges in diagnosis. *Medscape Respir Care.* 1999;3(6).

90. Sarfati J, Monod M, Recco P, et al. Recombinant antigens as diagnostic markers for aspergillosis. *Diagn Microbiol Infect Dis.* 2006;552:279–291.

91. Frisvad JC, Rank C, Nielsen KF. Metabolomics of Aspergillus fumigatus. *Med Mycol.* 2008;Sept 2, 1–19.

92. Gautam P, Sundaram CS, Madan T, et al. Identification of novel allergens of Aspergillus fumigatus using immunoproteomics approach. *Clin Exp Allergy.* 2007;37:1239–1249.

93. Longbottom JL, Austwick PKC. Antigens and allergens of *Aspergillus fumigatus:* I. Characterization by quantitative immunoelectrophoretic techniques. *J Allergy Clin Immunol.* 1986;78:9–17.

94. Arruda LK, Mann BJ, Chapman MD. Selective expression of a major allergen and cytotoxin, Asp f I, in *Aspergillus fumigatus.* Implications for the immunopathogenesis of *Aspergillus*-related diseases. *J Immunol.* 1992;149:3354–3359.

95. Banerjee B, Kurup VP, Phadnis S, et al. Molecular cloning and expression of a recombinant Aspergillus fumigatus protein Asp f II with significant immunoglobulin E reactivity in allergic bronchopulmonary aspergillosis. *J Lab Clin Med.* 1996;127:253–262.

96. Banerjee B, Greenberger PA, Fink JN, et al. Immunologic characterization of Asp f 2, a major allergen from *Aspergillus fumigatus* associated with allergic bronchopulmonary aspergillosis. *Infect Immun.* 1998;66:5175–5182.

97. Weiner Miller P, Hamosh A, Macek M Jr, et al. Cystic fibrosis transmembrane conductance regulator (CFTR) gene mutations in allergic bronchopulmonary aspergillosis. *Am J Hum Genet.* 1996;59:45–51.

98. Patterson R, Rosenberg M, Roberts M. Evidence that *Aspergillus fumigatus* growing in the airway of man can be a potent stimulus of specific and nonspecific IgE formation. *Am J Med.* 1977;63:257–262.

99. Gunnar S, Johansson O, Juhlin L. Immunoglobulin E in "healed" atopic dermatitis and after treatment with corticosteroids and azathioprine. *Br J Dermatol.* 1970;82:10–13.

100. Settipane GA, Pudupakkam RK, McGowan JH. Corticosteroid effect on immunoglobulins. *J Allergy Clin Immunol.* 1978;62:162–166.

101. Slavin RG, Hutcheson PS, Knutsen AP. Participation of cell-mediated immunity in allergic bronchopulmonary aspergillosis. *Int Arch Allergy Appl Immunol.* 1987;83:337–340.

102. Knutsen AP, Mueller KR, Levine AD, et al. Characterization of Asp f1 CD4+ T cell lines in allergic bronchopulmonary aspergillosis. *J Allergy Clin Immunol.* 1994;94:215–221.

103. Chauhan B, Santiago L, Kirschmann DA, et al. The association of HLA-DR alleles and T cell activation with allergic bronchopulmonary aspergillosis. *J Immunol.* 1997;159:4072–4076.

104. Geha RS. Circulating immune complexes and activation of the complement sequence in acute allergic bronchopulmonary aspergillosis. *J Allergy Clin Immunol.* 1977;60:357–359.

105. Marx JJ, Flaherty DK. Activation of the complement sequence by extracts of bacteria and fungi associated with hypersensitivity pneumonitis. *J Allergy Clin Immunol.* 1976;57:328–334.

106. Apter AJ, Greenberger PA, Liotta JL, et al. Fluctuations of serum IgA and its subclasses in allergic bronchopulmonary aspergillosis. *J Allergy Clin Immunol.* 1989;84:367–372.

107. Ricketti AJ, Greenberger PA, Pruzansky JJ, et al. Hyperreactivity of mediator releasing cells from patients with allergic bronchopulmonary

aspergillosis as evidenced by basophil histamine release. *J Allergy Clin Immunol.* 1983;72:386–392.

108. Chan-Yeung M, Chase WH, Trapp W, et al. Allergic bronchopulmonary aspergillosis. *Chest.* 1971;59:33–39.

109. Imbeau SA, Nichols D, Flaherty D, et al. Allergic bronchopulmonary aspergillosis. *J Allergy Clin Immunol.* 1978;62:243–255.

110. Bosken CH, Myers JL, Greenberger PA, et al. Pathologic features of allergic bronchopulmonary aspergillosis. *Am J Surg Pathol.* 1988;12:216–222.

111. Ghory AC, Patterson R, Roberts M, et al. In vitro IgE formation by peripheral blood lymphocytes from normal individuals and patients with allergic bronchopulmonary aspergillosis. *Clin Exp Immunol.* 1980;40:581–585.

112. Slavin RG, Fischer VW, Levin EA, et al. A primate model of allergic bronchopulmonary aspergillosis. *Int Arch Allergy Appl Immunol.* 1978;56:325–333.

113. Kurup VP, Mauze S, Choi H, et al. A murine model of allergic bronchopulmonary aspergillosis with elevated eosinophils and IgE. *J Immunol.* 1992;148:3783–3788.

114. Brown JE, Greenberger PA, Yarnold PR. Soluble serum interleukin 2 receptors in patients with asthma and allergic bronchopulmonary aspergillosis. *Ann Allergy Asthma Immunol.* 1995;74:484–488.

115. Greenberger PA, Smith LJ, Hsu CCS, et al. Analysis of bronchoalveolar lavage in allergic bronchopulmonary aspergillosis: divergent responses in antigen-specific antibodies and total IgE. *J Allergy Clin Immunol.* 1988;82:164–170.

116. Bernstein JA, Zeiss CR, Greenberger PA, et al. Immunoblot analysis of sera from patients with allergic bronchopulmonary aspergillosis: correlation with disease activity. *J Allergy Clin Immunol.* 1990;86: 532–539.

117. Hartl D, Latzin P, Zissel G, et al. Chemokines indicate allergic bronchopulmonary aspergillosis in patients with cystic fibrosis. *Am J Respir Crit Care Med.* 2006;173: 1370–1376.

118. Greenberger PA, Katzenstein A-LA. Lipoid pneumonia with atypical mycobacterial colonization in allergic bronchopulmonary aspergillosis: a complication of bronchography and a therapeutic dilemma. *Arch Intern Med.* 1983;143:2003–2005.

119. Greenberger PA. Allergic bronchopulmonary aspergillosis and funguses. *Clin Chest Med.* 1988;9:599–608.

120. Miller MA, Greenberger PA, Palmer J, et al. Allergic bronchopulmonary pseudallescheriasis in a child with cystic fibrosis. *Am J Asthma Allergy Pediatr.* 1993;6:177–179.

121. Miller MA, Greenberger PA, Amerian R, et al. Allergic bronchopulmonary mycosis caused by *Pseudoallescheria boydii. Am J Respir Crit Care Med.* 1993;148:810–812.

122. Halwig JM, Greenberger PA, Levin M, et al. Recurrence of allergic bronchopulmonary aspergillosis after seven years of remission. *J Allergy Clin Immunol.* 1984;74:738–740.

123. Radin R, Greenberger PA, Patterson R, et al. Mold counts and exacerbations of allergic bronchopulmonary aspergillosis. *Clin Allergy.* 1983;13:271–275.

124. Nichols D, Dopico GA, Braun S, et al. Acute and chronic pulmonary function changes in allergic bronchopulmonary aspergillosis. *Am J Med.* 1979;67:631–637.

125. Safirstein BH, D'Souza MF, Simon G, et al. Five-year follow-up of allergic bronchopulmonary aspergillosis. *Am Rev Respir Dis.* 1973;108:450–459.

126. Zirbes JM, Milla CE. Steroid-sparing effect of omalizumab for allergic bronchopulmonary aspergillosis and cystic fibrosis. *Pediatr Pulmonol.* 2008;43:607–610.

127. van der Ent CK, Hoekstra H, Rijkers GT. Successful treatment of allergic bronchopulmonary aspergillosis with recombinant anti-IgE antibody. *Thorax.* 2007;62:276–277.

128. Kanu A, Patel K. Treatment of allergic bronchopulmonary aspergillosis (ABPA) in CF with anti-IgE antibody (omalizumab). *Pediatr Pulmonol.* 2008;43:1249–1251.

129. Stevens DA, Schwartz HJ, Lee JY, et al. A randomized trial of itraconazole in allergic bronchopulmonary aspergillosis. *N Engl J Med.* 2000;342:756–762.

130. Denning DW, Van Wye JE, Lewiston NJ, et al. Adjunctive therapy of allergic bronchopulmonary aspergillosis with itraconazole. *Chest.* 1991;100:813–819.

131. Leon EE, Craig TJ. Antifungals in the treatment of allergic bronchopulmonary aspergillosis. *Ann Allergy Asthma Immunol.* 1999;82: 511–517.

132. Wark PAB, Hensley MJ, Saltos N, et al. Anti-inflammatory effect of itraconazole in stable allergic bronchopulmonary aspergillosis: a randomized controlled trial. *J Allergy Clin Immunol.* 2003;111:952–957.

CHAPTER 25

Occupational Immunologic Lung Disease

LESLIE C. GRAMMER AND KATHLEEN E. HARRIS

Occupational asthma (OA) is the most common form of occupational pulmonary disease in developed countries, including the United States (1). Increasing industrialization has led and will likely continue to lead to the production of numerous materials capable of inducing immunologically mediated lung disease in the working population. This is of concern to physicians who diagnose and treat these diseases and to labor, management, and a variety of governmental agencies.

There are two major subdivisions of diseases that constitute occupational immunologic lung disease (OILD): (a) immunologically mediated asthma which is often accompanied by allergic rhinitis and allergic conjunctivitis and (b) hypersensitivity pneumonitis. In addition, there is an asthma syndrome that can occur after high level irritant exposure; this is called *reactive airways dysfunction syndrome* (RADS) (1). There is also a category of OA entitled "work exacerbated asthma" which has been defined as pre-existing or concurrent asthma that is exacerbated by workplace exposures to such things as cold air, fumes, dusts, or exercise (2). According to the 2007 National Asthma Education and Prevention Program Expert Panel Report 3, asthma should be controlled so that patients can exercise, tolerate cold air, and have normal attendance at school or work, in addition to other activities (3). Therefore, some would assert that work-exacerbated asthma is simply asthma that is not being managed in accordance with Expert Panel Guidelines.

This chapter organizes the various exposures into the most relevant disease category. Various overlaps and uncertainties exist generally in OILD, and in OA, in particular. First, some exposures can cause more than one disease. For instance, some antigens, such as trimellitic anhydride (TMA) and various fungal antigens, can cause more than one immunologic pulmonary disease, including asthma or hypersensitivity pneumonitis (4). Second, many reactive chemicals, such as toluene diisocyanate (TDI), can cause disease by inducing either RADS or immunologic asthma (1). Finally, pulmonary

responses to some antigens have not been definitely established as immunologically or nonimmunologically mediated; an example would be Western red cedar.

■ EPIDEMIOLOGY

Incidence and prevalence figures for OILD are difficult to obtain for several reasons. First, there is often a high turnover rate in jobs associated with OILD, thus selecting workers who have not become sensitized. For instance, there is a high turnover rate among platinum workers. In a study of an electronics industry, a substantial proportion of workers who left reported respiratory disease as the reason (5). Second, occupationally related diseases generally are underreported (6). For instance, although the incidence of work-related illness is thought to be upward of 20 per 100, only 2% of these illnesses were recorded in employers' logs, as required by the Occupational Safety and Health Administration (OSHA) (7). Finally, the incidence of disease varies with the antigen exposure involved. For example, the incidence of occupational lung disease among animal handlers is estimated at 8% (8), whereas that of workers exposed to proteolytic enzymes can be up to 45% which is significantly higher (9).

It has been estimated that 2% of all cases of asthma in industrialized nations are occupationally related. In U.S. surveys, 9% to 15% of adult asthma cases were classified as occupational in origin (10,11). The European Community Respiratory Health Survey Study Group reported the highest risk for asthma was in farmers (odds ratio, 2.62), painters (2.34), plastic workers (2.20), cleaners (1.97), and spray painters (1.96) (12). In an American study of work-related asthma in California, Massachusetts, Michigan, and New Jersey, the most common industries where OA occurred were transportation manufacturing equipment (19.3%), health services (14.2%), and educational services (8.7%) (13). In other reported studies, health care workers have been noted to have an increased risk for OA (14,15).

■ MEDICOLEGAL ASPECTS

Most sensitizing agents that have been reported to cause occupational asthma are proteins of plant, animal, or microbial derivation and are, therefore, not specifically regulated by OSHA. Some of the low-molecular-weight sensitizers, such as isocyanates, anhydrides, and platinum, are regulated by OSHA; published standards for airborne exposure can be found in the Code of Federal Regulations (CFR 29.1910.1000) (16). OSHA, a division of the U.S. Department of Labor, is responsible for determining and enforcing these legal standards. The National Institute of Occupational Health and Safety (NIOSH), a division of the U.S. Department of Health and Human Services, is responsible for reviewing available research data on exposure to hazardous agents and providing recommendations to OSHA relative to airborne exposure limits. However, NIOSH has no regulatory or enforcement authority in this regard. More than 200 different substances have been reported to act as respiratory sensitizers and causes of occupational asthma (1). In only a few European countries are such occupational respiratory illnesses recognized by law with rights of compensation. In France, such etiologic agents as isocyanates, biologic enzymes, and tropical wood dusts are recognized. In the United Kingdom, such agents as platinum salts, isocyanates, colophony, and epoxy resins are recognized. It has been reported that in countries where legislation involving compensation exists, implementation may still be difficult because of the lack of explicit criteria for the diagnosis of a given occupational disease (17).

The Hazard Communication Standard, also called "worker right-to-know" legislation at the federal, state, and local levels, was passed in the United States about three decades ago (18). Substances that are capable of inducing respiratory sensitization are generally considered hazardous, and thus workers exposed to such substances are covered in most legislation. The common elements that exist in most hazard communication legislation are (a) that the employer apprise a governmental agency relative to its use of hazardous substances; (b) that the employer inform the employee of the availability of information on hazardous substances to which the employee is exposed; (c) that there be available to the employee alphabetized material safety data sheets for hazardous substances in the workplace; (d) that there be labeling of containers of hazardous substances; and (e) that training be provided to employees relative to health hazards, methods of detection, and protective measures to be used in handling hazardous substances. This sort of hazard communication legislation may make workers more aware of the potential that exists to develop respiratory sensitization and OILD syndromes due to certain exposures. Whether this awareness will have an effect on the incidence of OILD remains to be seen.

Legal and ethical aspects of management of individuals with occupational asthma are major problems (17). Guidelines for assessing impairment and disability from occupational asthma continue to evolve (19,20). The ATS has proposed criteria based on a possible 4 points for each of the following: forced expiratory volume in 1 second (FEV_1), methacholine challenge, and medication. After totaling the points, degree of impairment can be determined (20). Depending on the occupation, disability can then be assessed.

■ ASTHMA

Pathophysiology

The pathophysiology of asthma is reviewed in Chapter 19. The major pathophysiologic abnormalities of asthma, occupational or otherwise, are bronchoconstriction, excess mucus production, and bronchial wall inflammatory infiltration, including activated T cells, mast cells, and eosinophils (21,22). Neutrophilic occupational asthma has also been described (23). There is evidence that these abnormalities may be at least in part explained by neurogenic mechanisms and release of inflammatory mediators and cytokines such as interleukins and interferons. Type I hypersensitivity involving cross-linking immunoglobulin E (IgE) on the surface of mast cells and basophils, resulting in release of mediators such as histamine and leukotrienes and of cytokines such as interleukin-3 (IL-3), IL-4, and IL-5, is believed to be the triggering mechanism in most types of immediate-onset asthma. There is increasing evidence that cellular mechanisms are very important in asthma (23). An updated paradigm of the Gell and Coombs classification is improving our understanding of some of those cellular mechanisms (24). There are now four types of type IV, or cellular, mechanisms. Type IV_{a2} involves T_H2 cells and is probably responsible for late asthmatic responses.

There are also nonsensitizing causes of occupational asthma (25). RADS was originally described two decades ago by Brooks and Lockey. The criteria for RADS are listed in Table 25.1. Several aspects of RADS are very characteristic (26). First, it results from a very high level of exposure to a toxic substance. Second, the asthma-like condition starts with that exposure. Third, the patient has symptoms that persist for at least 3 months. Finally, because of airway hyperreactivity, the patient develops bronchospasm from a variety of stimuli, including exercise, cold air, fumes, and irritant chemicals such as bleach or ammonia.

Reaction Patterns

A number of patterns of asthma may occur after a single inhalation challenge, as shown in Table 25.2 (22). The immediate reaction is mediated by IgE, occurs within

TABLE 25.1   CRITERIA FOR REACTIVE AIRWAYS DYSFUNCTION SYNDROME (RADS)

1. No history of bronchospastic respiratory disease
2. Onset of symptoms follows a high-level exposure to a respiratory irritant
3. Onset of symptoms is abrupt, within minutes to hours
4. Symptoms must persist for at least 3 months
5. Methacholine challenge is positive
6. The symptoms are asthmalike, such as cough and wheeze
7. Other respiratory disorders have been excluded

minutes of challenge, presents as large airway obstruction, and is preventable with cromolyn and reversible by bronchodilators. The late response occurs several hours after inhalation challenge, presents as small airway obstruction in which wheezing may be mild and cough and dyspnea may predominate, lasts for several hours, is usually preventable with steroids (27) or cromolyn, and is only partly reversed by most bronchodilators. It may well result from a type IV_{a2} reaction.

The dual response is a combination of the immediate and late asthmatic responses. It is partially prevented by steroids or bronchodilators. After a single challenge study with certain antigens like Western red cedar, the patient may have repetitive asthmatic responses occurring over several days. This repetitive asthmatic response can be reversed with bronchodilators. Other atypical patterns—square wave, progressive, and progressive and prolonged immediate—have been described after diisocyanate challenges; the mechanisms resulting in these patterns have not been elucidated (28).

Etiologic Agents

Most of the 200 agents that have been described to cause occupational asthma are high-molecular-weight (>1 kDa) heterologous proteins of plant, animal, or microbial origin. Low-molecular-weight chemicals can act as irritants and aggravate preexisting asthma. They may also act as allergens if they are capable of haptenizing autologous proteins in the respiratory tract. Numerous reviews of occupational asthma have information on etiologic agents (1,29,30). A representative list of agents and industries associated with OILD can be found in Table 25.3.

Etiologic Agents of Animal Origin

Proteolytic enzymes are known to cause asthmatic symptoms on the basis of type I immediate hypersensitivity. Examples are pancreatic enzymes, hog trypsin (31) used in the manufacture of plastic polymer resins, *Bacillus subtilis* enzymes (32) incorporated into laundry detergents, and subtilisin. Papain, which is a proteolytic enzyme of vegetable origin used in brewing beer and manufacturing meat tenderizer, has been noted to cause similar symptoms by IgE-mediated mechanisms (33). Lactase is another enzyme reported to cause respiratory hypersensitivity; in the same publication, contact dermatitis is also reported (34).

Animal dander can cause asthma in a variety of workers, including veterinarians, laboratory workers, grooms, shepherds, breeders, pet shop owners, farmers, and jockeys (35). This can be a problem even for people whose work takes them to homes of clients who have pets, such as real estate salespeople, interior designers, and domestic workers.

Immediate asthmatic reactions and late interstitial responses have been reported after inhalation challenge with avian proteins in people who raise poultry and in workers exposed to egg products in egg processing facilities (36). Positive skin test results and *in vitro* IgE have been demonstrated, as well.

A variety of insect scales have been associated with asthma. Occupational exposure to insect scales occurs in numerous circumstances (1,29,30,36). Bait handlers can become sensitized to mealworms used as fishing bait. Positive skin test results, *in vitro* IgE antibody, and

TABLE 25.2   TYPES OF RESPIRATORY RESPONSE TO INHALATION CHALLENGE

ASTHMA	IMMEDIATE	LATE	REPETITIVE
Onset	10 to 20 minutes	4 to 6 hours	Periodic after initial attack
Duration	1 to 2 hours	2 to 6 hours	Days
Abnormality	FEV_1	FEV_1	FEV_1
Immune mechanism	Type I (IgE)	Type IV_{a2}	Type IVb CD8?
Symptoms	Wheezing	Wheezing, dyspnea	Recurrent wheezing
Therapy	Bronchodilators	Bronchodilators, corticosteroids	Bronchodilators

FEV_1, forced expiratory volume in 1 second; IgE, immunoglobulin E; IgG, immunoglobulin G.

TABLE 25.3   EXAMPLES OF OCCUPATIONAL ALLERGENS

AGENT	INDUSTRIES AND OCCUPATIONS
Animal Proteins	
Proteolytic enzymes	Plastic polymer resin manufacturing; detergent industry; pharmaceutical industry; meat tenderizer manufacturing; beer clearing
Animal dander, saliva, urine	Lab researchers; veterinarians; grooms; breeders; pet shop owners; farmers
Avian protein	Poultry breeders; bird fanciers; egg processors
Insect scales	Beekeepers; insect control workers; bait handlers; mushroom workers; entomologists
Vegetable Proteins	
Latex	Health care workers
Flour or contaminants (insects, molds)	Bakers
Green coffee beans, tea, garlic, other spices, soybeans	Workers in processing plants
Grain dust	Farmers; workers in processing plants
Castor beans	Fertilizer workers
Guar gum	Carpet manufacturing
Wood dusts: boxwood, mahogany, oak, redwood, Western red cedar	Carpenters; sawyers, wood pulp workers; foresters; cabinet makers
Penicillium caseii	Cheese workers
Orris root, rice flour	Hairdressers
Thermophilic molds	Mushroom workers
Chemicals	
Antibiotics	Hospital and pharmaceutical personnel
Other drugs; piperazine hydrochloride, α-methyldopa, amprolium hydrochloride	Hospital and pharmaceutical personnel
Platinum	Workers in processing plants
Nickel chromium, cobalt, zinc	Workers using those metals
Anhydrides (TMA, PA, TCPA)	Workers in manufacture of curing agents, plasticizers, anticorrosive coatings
Azo dyes	Dye manufacturers
Ethylenediamine	Shellac and lacquer industry workers
Isocyanates	Production of paints, surface coatings, insulation polyurethane foam
Soldering fluxes, colophony	Welders
Chloramine-T	Sterilization
Acrylates	Surgical or dental personnel

TMA, trimellitic anhydride; PA, phthalic anhydride; TCPA, tetrachlorophthalic anhydride.

inhalation challenges have been demonstrated to mealworms. Positive skin test results have been shown in various workers who have asthma on insect exposure: to screw worm flies in insect control personnel, to moths in fish bait workers, and to weevils in grain dust workers.

Asthma has been reported in workers who crush oyster shells to remove the meat. On the basis of skin tests to various allergens, the authors determined that the allergen was actually the primitive organisms that attached to the oyster shell surface. Similarly, asthma may occur from sea squirt body fluids in workers who gather pearls and oysters and in snow crab workers (37).

Etiologic Agents of Vegetable Origin

In terms of plant protein antigens, exposure to latex antigens, particularly those dispersed by powder in gloves, has become an important cause of occupational asthma in the health care setting (14,15). People working in a number of other occupations, including seamstresses, may develop latex hypersensitivity (38). In the baking industry, flour proteins are well recognized to cause occupational asthma (39). A new occupational allergen, xylanase, has been reported to be the antigen in some cases of baker's asthma (40). Numerous other plant foodstuff proteins have been described to cause occupational asthma with inhalational exposure. These include tea, garlic, coffee beans, spices, soybeans, vegetable gums, castor bean, guar gum, grain dust, wood dust, and dried flowers (1,29,30,36). In addition to the plant-derived proteins enumerated above, a variety of microbial proteins have been reported to be sensitizing agents in OA, including those from *Alternaria, Aspergillus,* and *Cladosporium* species (1,29,30,36). Wood dust from Western red cedar is a well-recognized cause of occupational asthma, but the antigen appears to be the low-molecular-weight chemical, plicatic acid, not a high-molecular-weight plant protein (41).

Chemicals

Asthma has been described in pharmaceutical workers and hospital personnel exposed to pharmacologic products. Numerous antibiotics, including ampicillin, penicillin, spiramycin, and sulfas (1,29,30,36), are known to cause asthma, positive skin test results, and/or specific IgE. Other pharmaceuticals, including amprolium hydrochloride, α-methyldopa, and piperazine hydrochloride, have been reported to cause asthma on an immunologic basis (1,29,30,36).

Workers in platinum-processing plants may have rhinitis, conjunctivitis, and asthma (42). Positive bronchial challenges and specific IgE have been demonstrated in affected workers. Another metal, nickel sulfate, has also been reported to cause IgE-mediated asthma (43). Other metals reported to cause OA include chromium, cobalt, vanadium, and zinc (1,29,30,36).

The manufacture of epoxy resins requires a curing agent, usually an acid anhydride or a polyamine compound. Workers may thus be exposed to acid anhydrides in the manufacture of curing agents, plasticizers, and anticorrosive coating materials. Studies have reported that three different patterns of immunologic respiratory response may occur (4) (Table 25.4).

Initially, it was presumed that the antibody in affected workers was directed only against the trimellityl (TM) haptenic determinant. However, studies of antibody specificity have demonstrated that there is antibody directed against both hapten and TM-protein determinants that are considered new antigen determinants. Other acid anhydrides that have been described to cause similar respiratory hypersensitivity reactions include phthalic anhydride, hexahydrophthalic anhydride, and pyromellitic anhydride (4).

Isocyanates are required catalysts in the production of polyurethane foam, vehicle spray paint, and protective surface coatings. It is estimated that about 5% to 10% of isocyanate workers develop asthma from exposure to subtoxic levels after a variable period of latency (44). The isocyanates that have been described to cause occupational asthma include TDI, hexamethylene diisocyanate, diphenylmethyl diisocyanate, and isopherone diisocyanate (44). The histology of bronchial biopsy specimens from workers with isocyanate asthma appears very similar to that from patients with immunologic asthma and thus is suggestive of an immunologic mechanism. Compared with those isocyanate workers with negative bronchial challenges, workers with positive challenges have a higher incidence and level of antibody against isocyanate–protein conjugates. However, in most studies, isocyanate workers with positive challenges did

TABLE 25.4 TRIMELLITIC ANHYDRIDE–INDUCED RESPIRATORY DISEASES AND IMMUNOLOGIC CORRELATES

DISEASE	MECHANISM	IMMUNOLOGIC TESTS
Asthma or rhinitis	Immunoglobulin E (IgE)	Immediate skin test IgG against TM-protein conjugate
Late respiratory systemic syndrome	IgG and IgA	IgG, IgA, or total antibody against TM-protein conjugate
Pulmonary disease, anemia syndrome	Complement-fixing antibodies	Complement-fixing antibodies against TM cells

TM, trimellityl.

not have detectable specific IgE in their serum. In a more recent study, it is speculated that some isocyanate asthma is mediated by IgE, but more than half is not (45). Hypersensitivity pneumonitis (46) and hemorrhagic pneumonitis (47) due to isocyanates have been reported to be caused by immunologic mechanisms. Human leukocyte antigen (HLA) class II alleles have been studied in isocyanate asthma; a positive association was reported in one study and negative in another (48,49). Formaldehyde, a respiratory irritant at ambient concentrations of 1 ppm or more, is often cited as a cause of occupational asthma; however, documented instances of formaldehyde-induced IgE-mediated asthma are almost nonexistent (50). A bifunctional aldehyde, glutaraldehyde, has been reported to cause occupational asthma (51). Ethylenediamine, a chemical used in shellac and photographic developing industries, has been reported to cause occupational asthma (52). Chloramine T (53), reactive azo dyes (54), methacrylates (55), and dimethyl ethanolamine are other chemicals that also have been reported to be causes of occupational asthma (56).

■ HYPERSENSITIVITY PNEUMONITIS

The signs, symptoms, immunologic features, pulmonary function abnormalities, pathology, and laboratory findings of hypersensitivity pneumonitis are reviewed in Chapter 23. No matter what the etiologic agent, the presentation follows one of three patterns. In the acute form, patients have fever, chills, chest tightness, dyspnea without wheezing, and nonproductive cough 4 to 8 hours after exposure. The acute form resolves within 24 hours. In the chronic form, which results from prolonged low-level exposure, patients have mild coughing, dyspnea, fatigue, pulmonary fibrosis, and weight loss. There is also a subacute form, which presents as a clinical syndrome of productive cough, malaise, myalgias, dyspnea, and nodular infiltrates on chest film. Any form can lead to severe pulmonary fibrosis with irreversible change; thus, it is important to recognize this disease early so that significant irreversible lung damage does not occur.

A variety of organic dusts from fungal, bacterial, or serum protein sources in occupational settings have been identified as etiologic agents of hypersensitivity pneumonitis (57) (Table 25.5). Several chemicals, including anhydrides and isocyanates, as discussed previously, have been reported to cause hypersensitivity pneumonitis; others include organochlorine and carbamate pesticides (58).

■ DIAGNOSIS

The diagnosis of OILD is not complex in the individual worker if symptoms appear at the workplace shortly after exposure to a well-recognized antigen. However, the diagnosis can be very difficult in patients whose symptoms occur many hours after exposure, for instance,

TABLE 25.5 OCCUPATIONAL HYPERSENSITIVITY PNEUMONITIDES

DISEASE	EXPOSURE	SPECIFIC INHALANT
Farmer's lung	Moldy hay	Saccharopolyspora rectivirgula (Formerly Micropolyspora faeni) Thermoactinomyces vulgaris
Malt worker's disease	Fungal spores	Aspergillus clavatus Aspergillus fumigatus
Maple-bark stripper's disease	Moldy logs	Cryptostroma corticale
Wood-pulp worker's disease	Moldy logs	Alternaria species
Sequoiosis	Moldy redwood sawdust	Graphium species; Aureobasidium pullulans
Humidifier/air conditioner disease	Fungal spores	Thermophilic actinomycetes Naegleria gruberi
Bird breeder's disease	Avian dust	Avian serum
Bagassosis	Moldy sugarcane	Thermoactinomyces vulgaris
Mushroom worker's disease	Mushroom compost	Saccharopolyspora rectivirgula (Formerly Micropolyspora faeni) Thermoactinomyces vulgaris
Suberosis	Moldy cork dust	Penicillium frequetans
Isocyanate disease	Isocyanates	Toluene diisocyanate (TDI) Diphenylmethane diisocyanate (MDI)

late asthma from TMA. Because of the increasing importance of OILD, it has now become essential to evaluate patients with respiratory syndromes for a possible association between their present disease states, their pulmonary function test results, and their immunologic exposure in the work environment (59). It is being increasingly reported that rhinoconjunctivitis precedes occupational asthma in many cases (60,61).

In the case of the well-established OILD syndrome, a careful history and physical examination with corroborative immunology and spirometry will suffice (59). The history and physical examination findings in asthma and hypersensitivity pneumonitis are discussed in Chapters 22 and 23. A negative methacholine test can almost exclude occupational asthma (59). Immunologic evaluations may provide important information about the cause of the respiratory disease. Skin tests, with antigens determined to be present in the environment, may detect IgE antibodies and suggest a causal relationship (62). Haptens may be coupled to carrier proteins, such as human serum albumin, and used in skin tests (56) or radioimmunoassays. In cases of interstitial lung disease, double gel immunodiffusion techniques may be used to determine the presence of precipitating antibody, which would indicate antibody production against antigens known to cause disease (57).

It may be necessary to attempt to reproduce the clinical features of asthma or interstitial lung disease by bronchial challenge, followed by careful observation of the worker. Challenge may be conducted by natural exposure of the patient to the work environment with preexposure and postexposure pulmonary functions, compared with similar studies on nonwork days. Another technique used for diagnosis of OILD is controlled bronchoprovocation in the laboratory with preexposure and postexposure pulmonary function measurements (27,62). It is important that the intensity of exposure not exceed that ordinarily encountered on the job and that appropriate personnel and equipment be available to treat respiratory abnormalities that may occur. Some advocate the use of peak flow monitoring, whereas others find it unreliable (59). Evaluating induced sputum eosinophils has been reported to be a potentially useful technique to diagnose occupational asthma (63).

If the analysis of OILD is not for an individual patient but rather for a group of workers afflicted with a respiratory illness, the approach is somewhat different. The initial approach to an epidemiologic evaluation of OILD is usually a cross-sectional survey using a well-designed questionnaire (63). The questionnaire should include a chronologic description of all past job exposures, symptoms, chemical exposures and levels, length of employment, and protective respiratory equipment used. Analysis of the survey can establish possible sources of exposure. All known information about the sources of exposure should be sought in the form of previously reported toxic or immunologic reactions. Ultimately, immunologic tests and challenges may be done selectively.

■ PROGNOSIS

Unfortunately, many workers with occupational asthma do not completely recover, even though they have been removed from exposure to a sensitizing agent (64–66). Prognostic factors that been examined include specific IgE, duration of symptoms, pulmonary function testing, and nonspecific bronchial hyperreactivity (BHR). An unfavorable prognosis has been reported to be associated with a persistent high level of specific IgE, long duration of symptoms (>1 to 2 years), abnormal pulmonary function test results, and a high degree of BHR (67). The obvious conclusion from these studies is that early diagnosis and removal from exposure are requisites for the goal of complete recovery. In workers who remain exposed after a diagnosis of occupational asthma is made, further deterioration of lung function and increase in BHR have been reported (68). It must be appreciated that life-threatening attacks and even deaths have been reported when exposure continued after diagnosis (1).

■ TREATMENT

The management of OILD consists of controlling the worker's exposure to the offending agent. This can be accomplished in various ways. Sometimes, the worker can be moved to another station; efficient dust and vapor extraction can be instituted; or the ventilation can be improved in other ways, so that a total job change is not required (69). Consultation with an industrial hygienist familiar with exposure levels may be helpful in this regard. It is important to remember that levels of exposure below the legal limits that are based on toxicity may still cause immunologic reactions. Facemasks of the filtering type are not especially efficient or well-tolerated. Ideally, the working environment should be designed to limit concentration of potential sensitizers to safe levels. Unfortunately, this is impractical in many manufacturing processes, and even in a carefully monitored facility, recommended thresholds may be exceeded (70). Thus, avoidance may well entail retraining and reassigning an employee to another job.

Pharmacologic management of OILD is rarely helpful in the presence of continued exposure on a chronic basis. Certainly, in acute hypersensitivity pneumonitis, a short course of corticosteroids (as discussed in Chapter 23) is useful in conjunction with avoidance. However, chronic administration of steroids for occupational hypersensitivity pneumonitis is not recommended. Asthma resulting from contact with occupational exposures responds to therapeutic agents such as β-adrenergic receptor agonists, cromolyn, and steroids, as discussed in Chapter 22. As exposure continues, sensitivity may increase, making medication requirements prohibitive.

Immunotherapy has been used with various occupational allergens causing asthma, including treatment of laboratory animal workers, bakers, and oyster gatherers, with reported success. However, there are no double-blind placebo-controlled trials. Immunotherapy may be feasible in a limited number of patients, with certain occupational allergens of the same nature as the common inhalant allergens; however, it is difficult and hazardous with many agents that cause occupational immunologic asthma.

■ PREVENTION

The key principle in OILD is that prevention, rather than treatment, must be the goal. Such preventative measures as improved ventilation and adhering to threshold limits, as discussed under the Treatment section, would be helpful to this end. There should be efforts to educate individual workers and managers in high-risk industries so that affected workers can be recognized early. Right-to-know legislation should increase awareness of occupational asthma.

Currently, there are no preemployment screening criteria that have been shown to be useful in predicting the eventual appearance of OILD. There is conflicting evidence as to whether HLA studies are useful in predicting isocyanate asthma or anhydride asthma. It has been reported that atopy is a predisposing factor for a worker to develop IgE-mediated disease (60), but there is at least one conflicting study (73). Whether or not cigarette smoking is a risk factor for OILD is unclear.

Prospective studies of acid anhydride workers, such as those of Zeiss (74), Baur (62), and Newman-Taylor et al. (75), have reported that serial immunologic studies are useful in predicting which workers are likely to develop immunologically mediated diseases. At the first sign of occupational asthma, those workers then could be removed from the offending exposure and retrained before permanent illness develops. This approach has been studied in TMA-exposed employees. Another prospective study of TMA workers has reported that decreasing the airborne levels will reduce disease prevalence (76). This may prove to be the best approach to preventing OILD from other agents. Already, medical surveillance studies with cost-benefit analyses have been reported to reduce cases of permanent occupational asthma (77).

■ REFERENCES

1. Mapp CE, Boschetto P, Maestraloli P, et al. Occupational asthma. *Am J Resp Crit Care Med.* 2005;172:280–305.
2. Henneberger PK. Work-exacerbated asthma. *Curr Opin in All & Clin Immunol.* 2007;7:146–151.
3. National Heart, Lung, and Blood Institute, NIH, USDHHS. *National Asthma Education and Prevention Program Expert Panel Report 3: Guidelines for the Diagnosis and Management of Asthma.* NIH Pub No 08-5846, 2007.
4. Grammer LC, Harris KE. Trimellitic anhydride and other acid anhydrides. In: Rom WN, Markowitz SB, eds. *Environmental and Occupational Medicine.* 4th ed. Philadelphia: Wolters Kluwer/Lippincott Williams & Wilkins; 2007:1213–1218.
5. Perks WH, Burge PS, Rehahn M, et al. Work-related respiratory disease in employees leaving an electronic factory. *Thorax.* 1979;34:19–22.
6. Markowitz SB. The role of surveillance in occupational health. In: Rom WN, Markowitz SB, eds. *Environmental and Occupational Medicine.* 4th ed. Philadelphia: Wolters Kluwer/Lippincott Williams & Wilkins; 2007:9–21.
7. NIOSH, USDHHS, PHS, CDC. *Work-related Lung Disease Surveillance Report 2002.* NIOSH Pub No. 2003-111; 2003.
8. Cullinan P, Lowson D, Nieuwenshuijsen MJ, et al. Work related symptoms, sensitization, and estimated exposure in workers not previously exposed to laboratory rats. *Occup Environ Med.* 1994;51:589–592.
9. Schweigert MK, Mackenzie DP, Sarlo K. Occupational asthma and allergy associated with the use of enzymes in the detergent industry—a review of the epidemiology, toxicology, and methods of prevention. *Clin Exp Immunol.* 2000; 30:1511–1518.
10. Blanc PD, Toren K. How much asthma can be attributed to occupational factors? *Am J Med.* 1999; 107:580–587.
11. Balmes J, Becklake M, Blanc P, et al. American Thoracic Society statement: occupational contribution to the burden of airway disease. *Am J Resp Crit Care Med.* 2003;167:787–797.
12. Kogevinas M, Anto JM, Sunyer J, et al. Occupational asthma in Europe and other industrialized areas: a population-based study. *Lancet.* 1999;353:1750–1754.
13. Jajosky RA, Harrison R, Reinisch F, et al. Surveillance of work-related asthma in selected U.S. states using surveillance guidelines for state health departments—California, Massachusetts, Michigan, and New Jersey, 1993–1995. *MMWR Suveill Summ.* 1999;48(3):1–20.
14. Mirabelli MC, Zock JP, Plana E, et al. Occupational risk factors for asthma among nurses and related health care professionals in an international study. *Occup Environ Med.* 2007;64:474–479.
15. Delclos GL, Gimeno D, Arif AA, et al. Occupational risk factors and asthma among health care professionals. *Am J Resp Crit Care Med.* 2007;175:667–675.
16. Office of the Federal Register National Archives and Records Administration. *Code of Federal Regulations OSHA Title 29, Labor Parts 1900–1910.* Washington, DC: Federal Register, 2007.
17. Richman SI. Legal treatment of the asthmatic worker: a major problem for the nineties. *J Occup Med.* 1990;32:1027–1031.
18. Howard J. OSHA and the regulatory agencies. In: Rom WN, ed. *Environmental and Occupational Medicine.* 3rd ed. Philadelphia: Lippincott-Raven; 1998:1671–1679.
19. Engleberg AL, ed. *Guides to the Evaluation of Permanent Impairment.* 3rd ed. Chicago: American Medical Association, 1988.
20. Miller A. Guidelines for the evaluation of impairment/disability in patients with asthma. *Am J Resp Crit Care Med.* 1994;149:834–835.
21. Mamessier E, Milhe F, Guillot C, et al. T-cell activation in occupational asthma and rhinitis. *Allergy.* 2007;62:162–169.
22. Hamid QA, Minshall EM. Molecular pathology of allergic disease I: lower airway. *J Allergy Clin Immunol.* 2000;105:20–36.
23. Leigh R, Hargreave FE. Occupational neutrophilic asthma. *Can Respir J.* 1999;6:194–196.
24. Kay AB. Concepts of allergy and hypersensitivity. In: Kay AB, ed. *Allergy and Allergic Diseases.* Oxford: Blackwell Science; 1997:23–35.
25. Lemiere C, Malo J-L, Gautrin D. Nonsensitizing causes of occupational asthma. *Med Clin North Am.* 1996;80:749–774.
26. Alberts WM, do Pico GA. Reactive airways dysfunction syndrome. *Chest.* 1996;109:1618–1626.
27. Boschetto P, Fabbri LM, Zocca E, et al. Prednisone inhibits late asthmatic reactions and airway inflammation induced by toluene diisocyanate in sensitized subjects. *J Allergy Clin Immunol.* 1987;80:261–267.
28. Cartier A, Malo J-L. Occupational challenge tests. In: Bernstein IL, Chan-Yeung M, Malo J-L, et al., eds. *Asthma in the Workplace.* 2nd ed. New York: Marcel Dekker; 1998:211–234.
29. Maol J-L, Chan-Yeung M. Occupational asthma. In: Adkinson NF Jr, Yunginger JW, Busse WW, et al., eds. *Middleton's Allergy: Principles and Practice.* 6th ed. Philadelphia: Mosby; 2003:1333–1352.
30. Brooks SM, Truncale T, McCluskey J. In: Rom WN, Markowitz SB, eds. *Environmental and Occupational Medicine.* 4th ed. Philadelphia: Wolters Kluwer/Lippincott Williams & Wilkins; 2007:418–465.
31. Colten HR, Polakoff PL, Weinstein SF, et al. Immediate hypersensitivity to hog trypsin resulting from industrial exposure. *N Engl J Med.* 1975;292:1050–1053.

32. Lemiere C, Cartier A, Dolovich J, et al. Isolated late asthmatic reaction after exposure to a high-molecular-weight occupational agent, subtilisin. *Chest.* 1996;110:823–824.

33. Novey HS, Keenan WJ, Fairshter RD, et al. Pulmonary disease in workers exposed to papain: clinicophysiological and immunological studies. *Clin Allergy.* 1980;10:721–731.

34. Laukkanen A, Ruoppi P, Remes S, et al. Lactase-induced occupational protein contact dermatitis and allergic rhinoconjunctivitis. *Contact Derm.* 2007;57:89–93.

35. Chapman MD, Wood RA. The role and remediation of animal allergens in allergic disease. *J Allergy Clin Immunol.* 2001;107: S414–21.

36. Boeniger MF, Lummus ZL, Biagini RE et al. Exposure to aeroallergens in egg processing facilities. *Appl Occup Environ Hyg* 2001;16: 660–70.

37. Weytjens K, Cartier A, Malo J-L, et al. Aerosolized snow-crab allergens in a processing facility. *Allergy.* 1999;54:892–893.

38. Weytjens K, Labrecque M, Malo J-L, et al. Asthma to latex in a seamstress. *Allergy.* 1999;54:290–291.

39. Blanco Carmona JG, Juste Picon S, Garces Sotillos M. Occupational asthma in bakeries caused by sensitivity to alpha-amylase. *Allergy.* 1991;46:274–276.

40. Baur X, Sander I, Posch A, et al. Baker's asthma due to the enzyme xylanase—a new occupational allergen. *Clin Exp Allergy.* 1998; 28:1591–1593.

41. Frew A, Chang JH, Chan H, et al. T lymphocyte responses to plicatic acid-human serum albumin conjugates in occupational asthma caused by Western red cedar. *J Allergy Clin Immunol.* 1998;101:841–847.

42. Cromwell O, Pepys J, Parish WE, et al. Specific IgE antibodies to platinum salts in sensitized workers. *Clin Allergy.* 1979;9:109–117.

43. Malo J-L, Cartier A, Doepner M, et al. Occupational asthma caused by nickel sulfate. *J Allergy Clin Immunol.* 1982;69:55–59.

44. Banks DE. The respiratory effects of isocyanates. In: Rom WN, ed. *Environmental and Occupational Medicine.* 3rd ed. Boston: Little, Brown; 1998:537–564.

45. Redlich CA, Bello D, Wisnewski AV. Isocyanate exposures and health effects. In: Rom WN, Markowitz SB, eds. *Environmental and Occupational Medicine.* 4th ed. Philadelphia: Wolters Kluwer/Lippincott Williams & Wilkins; 2007:502–516.

46. Walker CL, Grammer LC, Shaughnessy MA, et al. Diphenylmethan diisocyanate hypersensitivity pneumonitis: a serologic evaluation. *J Occup Med.* 1989;31:315–319.

47. Patterson R, Nugent KM, Harris KE, et al. Case reports: immunologic hemorrhagic pneumonia caused by isocyanates. *Am Rev Respir Dis.* 1990;141:225–230.

48. Mapp CE, Balboni A, Baricordi R, et al. Human leukocyte antigen associations in occupational asthma induced by isocyanates. *Am J Respir Crit Care Med.* 1997;156:S139–S143.

49. Rihs HP, Barbalho-Krolls T, Huber H, et al. No evidence for the influence of HLA class II in alleles in isocyanate-induced asthma. *Am J Ind Med.* 1997;32:522–527.

50. Dykewicz MS, Patterson R, Cugell DW, et al. Serum IgE and IgG to formaldehyde-human serum albumin: lack of relation to gaseous formaldehyde exposure and symptoms. *J Allergy Clin Immunol.* 1991;87:48–57.

51. Chan-Yeung M, McMurren T, Catonio-Begley F, et al. Clinical aspects of allergic disease: occupational asthma in a technologist exposed to glutaraldehyde. *J Allergy Clin Immunol.* 1993;91:974–978.

52. Lam S, Chan-Yeung M. Ethylenediamine-induced asthma. *Am Rev Respir Dis.* 1980;121:151–155.

53. Blasco A, Joral A, Fuente R, et al. Bronchial asthma due to sensitization to chloramine T. *J Invest Allergol Clin Immunol.* 1992;2:167–170.

54. Nilsson R, Nordlinder R, Wass U, et al. Asthma, rhinitis, and dermatitis in workers exposed to reactive dyes. *Br J Ind Med.* 1993;50:65–70.

55. Jaakola MS, Leino T, Tammilehto L, et al. Respiratory effects of exposure to methacrylates among dental assistants. *Allergy.* 2007;62:648–654.

56. Vallieres M, Cockcroft DW, Taylor DM, et al. Dimethyl ethanolamine-induced asthma. *Am Rev Respir Dis.* 1977;115:867–871.

57. Grammer LC, Story RE. Hypersensitivity pneumonitis. In: Rakel RE, Bope ET, eds. *Conn's Current Therapy.* Philadelphia: Saunders; 2004:282–284.

58. Hoppin JA, Umbach DM, Kullman GJ, et al. Pesticides and other agricultural factors associated with self-reported farmer's lung among farm residents in the Agricultural Health Study. *Occup Environ Med.* 2006;64:334–341.

59. Nicholson PJ, Cullinan P, Newman Taylor AJ, et al. Evidence based guidelines for the presention, identification, and management of occupational asthma. *Occup. Environ Med.* 2005;62:290–299.

60. Grammer LC, Ditto AM, Tripathi A, et al. Prevalence and onset of rhinitis and conjunctivitis in subjects with occupational asthma caused by trimellitic anhydride (TMA). *J Occup Environ Med.* 2002;44(12): 1179–1181.

61. Piirilä P, Estlander T, Hytönen M, et al. Rhinitis caused by ninhydrin develops into occupational asthma. *Eur Respir J.* 1997;10:1918–1921.

62. Baur X, Stahlkopf H, Merget R. Prevention of occupational asthma including medical surveillance. *Am J Ind Med.* 1998;34:632–639.

63. Vandenplas O, Ghezzo H, Munoz X, et al. What are the questionnaire items most useful in identifying subjects with occupational asthma? *Eur Resp J.* 2005;26:1056–1063.

64. Barker RD, Harris JM, Welch JA, et al. Occupational asthma caused by tetrachlorophthalic anhydride: a 12-year follow-up. *J Allergy Clin Immunol.* 1998;101:717–719.

65. Park HS, Nahm DH. Prognostic factors for toluene diisocyanate-induced occupational asthma after removal from exposure. *Clin Exp Allergy.* 1997;27:1145–1150.

66. Perfetti L, Cartier A, Ghezzo H. Follow-up of occupational asthma after removal from or diminution of exposure to the responsible agent: relevance of the length of the interval from cessation of exposure. *Chest.* 1998;114:398–403.

67. Marabini A, Siracusa A, Stopponi R, et al. Outcome of occupational asthma in patients: a 3-year study. *Chest.* 2003;124:2372–2376.

68. Marabini A, Dimich-Ward H, Kwan SY, et al. Clinical and socioeconomic features of subjects with red cedar asthma: a follow-up study. *Chest.* 1993;104:821–824.

69. Merget R, Schulte A, Gebler A, et al. Outcome of occupational asthma due to platinum salts after transferral to low-exposure areas. *Int Arch Occup Environ Health.* 1999;72:33–39.

70. Diem JE, Jones RN, Hendrick DJ, et al. Five year longitudinal study of workers employed in a new toluene diisocyanate manufacturing plant. *Am Rev Respir Dis.* 1982;126:420–428.

71. Young RP, Barker RD, Pile KD, et al. The association of HLA-DR3 with specific IgE to inhaled acid anhydrides. *Am J Respir Crit Care Med.* 1995;151:219–221.

72. Nielsen J, Johnson U, Welinder H, et al. HLA and immune nonresponsiveness in workers exposed to organic acid anhydrides. *J Occup Environ Med.* 1996;38:1087–1090.

73. Calverley AE, Rees D, Dowdeswell RJ. Allergy to complex salts of platinum in refinery workers: Prospective evaluations of IgE and Phadiatop[SC] status. *Clin Exp Allergy.* 1999;29:703–711.

74. Zeiss CR, Wolkonsky P, Pruzansky JJ, et al. Clinical and immunologic evaluation of trimellitic anhydride workers in multiple industrial settings. *J Allergy Clin Immunol.* 1982;70:15–18.

75. Barker RD, van Tongeren MJ, Harris JM, et al. Risk factors for sensitization and respiratory symptoms among workers exposed to acid anhydrides: a cohort study. *Occup Environ Med.* 1998;55:684–691.

76. Grammer LC, Harris KE, Sonenthal KR, et al. A cross-sectional survey of 46 employees exposed to trimellitic anhydride. *Allergy Proc.* 1992;13:139–142.

77. Phillips VL, Goodrich MA, Sullivan TJ. Health care worker disability due to latex allergy and asthma: a cost analysis. *Am J Public Health.* 1999;89:1024–1028.

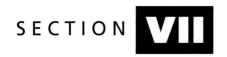

SECTION VII

Upper Respiratory Tract Diseases

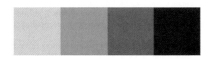

CHAPTER 26

Allergic Rhinitis

ANTHONY J. RICKETTI AND DENNIS J. CLERI

■ INTRODUCTION AND DEFINITIONS

The clinical definition of allergic rhinitis is a symptomatic disorder of the nose induced by an immunoglobulin E (IgE)-mediated inflammatory reaction after allergen exposure of the membranes lining the nose (1). The symptoms that characterize the disorder are rhinorrhea, nasal congestion, sneezing, nasal pruritus, post-nasal drainage, and at times, pruritus of the eyes, ears, and throat.

Previously, allergic rhinitis was subdivided, based on the time of exposure into either a seasonal or a perennial disorder. Perennial allergic rhinitis is most frequently caused by indoor allergens such as dust mites, mold spores, animal danders, and cockroaches. Seasonal allergic rhinitis is related to a wide variety of pollens and molds. However, it became evident that a new classification system was required because of several clinical observations (2):

- In many areas of the world, pollens and molds are perennial allergens (e.g., the weed *Parietaria* pollen allergy in the Mediterranean area [3]; and grass pollen allergy in southern California and Florida) (4).
- Symptoms of perennial allergic rhinitis may not always be present throughout the year.
- Many patients who are sensitive to pollen and also allergic to mold may have difficulty defining a pollen season (5).

- The majority of patients are sensitized to several allergens and therefore manifest symptoms not only seasonally but throughout the year (6).
- The priming effect on the nasal mucosa induced by low levels of pollen allergens (7) and persistent inflammation of the nose in asymptomatic allergic rhinitis patients may result in rhinitis symptoms not confined to the specific allergy season (8).

The 2001 Allergic Rhinitis and its Impact on Asthma (ARIA) workshop guidelines for the classification and treatment of allergic rhinitis (8) have led to the definitions of allergic nasal disease as intermittent or persistent, and mild or moderate-severe (2). Intermittent rhinitis is defined on the basis of symptoms that are present for fewer than 4 days per week or fewer than 4 weeks (2). When symptoms are present for more than 4 days per week and are present for more than 4 weeks, it is defined as persistent rhinitis. Mild symptoms do not affect sleep, impair participation in daily activities, sports, and leisure, or interfere with work or school and are not considered bothersome (2). Conversely, moderate-severe symptoms result in abnormal sleep, interfere with daily activities, sports, and leisure, impair work and school activities, and are considered troublesome. Any one of the designators classifies allergic rhinitis into the moderate-severe category (2).

■ EPIDEMIOLOGY

Although allergic rhinitis may have its onset at any age, the incidence of onset is greatest in children at adolescence, with a decrease in incidence seen in advancing age. The prevalence of allergic rhinitis has been estimated to be between 15% and 20% (9), but physician-diagnosed allergic rhinitis in the pediatric age group has been reported in as many as 42% (10). Although it has been reported in infants (11), in most cases, an individual requires two or more seasons of exposure to a new antigen before exhibiting the clinical manifestations of allergic rhinitis. Older children have a higher prevalence of allergic rhinitis than younger ones, with a peak occurring in children aged 13 to 14 years. Approximately 80% of individuals diagnosed with allergic rhinitis will develop symptoms before the age of 20 years (12). Boys tend to have an increased incidence of allergic rhinitis in childhood, but the sex ratio becomes equal in adulthood.

Epidemiology studies suggest that the prevalence of allergic rhinitis in the United States and around the world is increasing (13). However, accurate estimates of allergic rhinitis are difficult to obtain secondary to variability of geographic pollen counts, misinterpretation of symptoms by patients, and inability of the patient and physician to recognize the disorder. Although there is an increased prevalence of allergic rhinitis, the cause for this increase is unknown. Risk factors associated with development of allergic rhinitis include family history (14), higher socioeconomic status (15), atmospheric pollution (16), ethnicity other than white (17), late entry into daycare (18), lack of other siblings (19), birth during a pollen season (20), heavy maternal smoking during the first year of life (21), exposure to high concentrations of indoor allergens, such as mold spores, dust mites, and animal dander (22), higher serum IgE (>100 IU/mL before age 6 years) (21), presence of positive allergen skin-prick tests (23), early introduction of foods or formula (21), and a trend toward sedentary life styles (24).

Burden of Disease

According to 1997 survey data from primary care physicians, there were 16.9 million office visits for symptoms suggestive of allergic rhinitis (25). In 2000, more than $6 billion was spent on prescription medications for this condition and over-the-counter medications were at least twice that amount (26). In addition to the characteristic nasal and ocular symptoms of allergic rhinitis, patients can also experience fatigue; headache; disrupted sleep patterns; and declines in cognitive processing, psychomotor speed, verbal learning, and memory (27). Hidden direct costs include the treatment of asthma, upper respiratory infection, chronic sinusitis, otitis media, nasal polyposis, and obstructive sleep apnea (28). Surveys report that 38% of patients with allergic rhinitis have coexisting asthma, and as many as 78% of patients with asthma also have allergic rhinitis (29). Asthma and allergic rhinitis are often thought of as conditions that characterize different points on a continuum of inflammation within one common airway (30). Evidence suggests a common pathophysiology for these allergen-induced disorders and supports the observation that treatment of allergic rhinitis reduces the incidence and severity of asthma (31). Allergy has been linked as a contributing factor in 40% to 80% of cases of chronic sinusitis (32). Approximately 21% of children with nasal allergies experience otitis media with effusion (OME). Children with an OME have a 35% to 50% incidence of allergy (33,34). In patients with allergic rhinitis, an allergen challenge induces expression of intercellular adhesion molecule-1 (ICAM-1), the receptor for 90% of human rhinoviruses (32), increasing the susceptibility for an upper respiratory infection. In turn, rhinovirus can accentuate the pattern of airway reactivity in patients with allergic rhinitis (35). Although the link between allergic rhinitis and nasal polyps is considered controversial, the recurrence rate of nasal polyps in patients with allergic rhinitis is higher than for patients who are nonallergic (36). The indirect costs of allergic rhinitis such as absenteeism and presenteeism (decreased productivity while at work) are also substantial. Allergic rhinitis results in impaired productivity and/or missed work in 52% of patients (37). In a survey of 8,267 U.S. employees, 55% experienced allergic rhinitis symptoms for an average of 52.5 days, were absent from work for 3.6 days/year because of their condition, and were unproductive 2.3 hours/workday when experiencing symptoms. The mean total productivity (absenteeism and presenteeism) losses were $593/employee per year (38). In total, allergic rhinitis results in an estimated 3.5 million lost work days and 2 million lost school days (39). Approximately 10,000 children are absent from school on any given day secondary to allergic rhinitis (39). Depending on a child's age, absence from school also may affect parents' productivity or absence from work.

Quality-of-life surveys have evaluated the impairment secondary to allergic rhinitis. In the Medical Outcomes Study Short-Form Health Survey, of 36 items (SF-36) administered to patients with allergic rhinitis and asthma (40), patients with allergic rhinitis had similar impairment with asthma when evaluating energy/fatigue, general health perception, physical role limitations as well as emotional role limitations—mental health, pain, and change in health. Patients with allergic rhinitis actually had significantly lower scores than asthma patients in the area of social functioning. These surveys clearly demonstrate the overall morbidity of the disorder and, therefore, the symptoms of these patients should not be trivialized.

■ GENETICS

The hereditary character of allergic rhinitis and other atopic diseases has been frequently demonstrated in families and twins (41). In a series of 8,633 5-year-old twins in which the prevalence of rhinitis was 4.4%, there was a 93% correlation in full-term monozygotic twins having rhinitis (41). The correlation was 53% in dizygotic twins (41). The influence of environmental factors therefore is small.

Atopy has been linked to multiple genetic loci, including those on chromosomes 2, 5, 6, 7, 11, 13, 16, and 20 (42). A family history, therefore, represents a major risk factor for allergic rhinitis. In one study, development of atopic disease in the absence of parental family history was only present in 17%, whereas when one parent or sibling was atopic, the risk increased to 29%. When both parents were atopic, the risk for developing an atopic disorder was 47% in the next generation (43).

■ ETIOLOGY

Pollen and mold spores are the allergens responsible for intermittent or seasonal allergic rhinitis (Table 26.1). The pollens important in causing allergic rhinitis are from plants that depend on the wind (anemophilous pollens). Many grasses, trees, and weeds produce light-weight pollen in sufficient quantities to sensitize genetically susceptibile individuals. Plants that produce

TABLE 26.1   MAJOR AEROALLERGENS IN ALLERGIC RHINITIS

Outdoor (generally seasonal)
- Pollens
- Weeds (ragweed)
- Grasses (rye, timothy, orchard)
- Trees (oak, elm, birch, alder, hazel)
- Molds (*Alternaria* spp., *Cladosporium* spp.) March, April, May

Indoor (generally perennial)
- House dust mites
- *Dermatophagoides farinae*
- *Dermatophagoides pteronyssinus*
- Warm-blooded pets
- Pests
- Mice
- Cockroaches
- Rats
- Molds
- *Aspergillus* spp.
- *Penicillium* spp.
- Occupational allergens
- Laboratory animals

entomophilous pollens depend on insect pollination, and include golden rod, dandelions, and most other plants with obvious flowers, that do not cause allergic rhinitis symptoms. The pollination season of various plants depends on the individual plant and on the various geographic locations. For a particular plant in a given locale, however, the relative amount of night and day determines the pollinating season and it is constant from year to year. Weather conditions, such as temperature and rainfall, influence the amount of pollen produced but not the actual onset or termination of a specific season. Some of the effects of global warming appear to be lengthening some pollen seasons and increasing concentration of CO_2, which can result in greater recoveries of ragweed pollen.

Ragweed pollen, a significant cause of allergic rhinitis, produces the most severe and longest seasonal rhinitis in the eastern and midwestern portions of the United States and Ontario, Canada. In those areas, ragweed pollen appears in significant amounts from the second or third week of August through September. Occasionally, sensitive patients may exhibit symptoms as early as the first few days of August, when smaller quantities of pollen first appear. Although ragweed is the dominant airborne allergen in North America during the late summer and early fall, there are also other important weed pollens, such as sheep sorrell in the spring and plantain in the summer months. Western ragweed and marsh elder in the western states, sagebrush and franseria in the Pacific areas, and careless weed, pigweed, and franseria in the southwestern United States are important allergens in the late summer and early fall. In the northern and eastern United States, the earliest pollens to appear are tree pollens, usually in March, April, or May. Grass pollens, which appear from May to late June or early July, cause allergic rhinitis in this locale. About 25% of pollinosis patients have both grass and ragweed allergic rhinitis, and about 5% have tree, grass, and ragweed allergies. In other geographic regions, these generalizations are not accurate, because of the particular climate and because some less common plants may predominate. For example, grass pollinates from early spring through late fall in the southwestern regions and accounts for allergic rhinitis that is almost perennial. In Southern California, grass pollen can be detected in all months except January, although the specific "grass" season is from April to September.

Airborne mold spores, the most important of which throughout the United States are *Alternaria* and *Cladosporium* species, also cause seasonal allergic rhinitis. Warm, damp weather favors the growth of molds and thereby influences the severity of the season. Generally, molds first appear in the air in the spring, become most significant during the warmer months, and usually disappear with the first frost. Thus, patients with marked hypersensitivity to molds may exhibit symptoms from early spring through the first frost, whereas those with a lesser degree of hypersensitivity only may have symptoms from early summer through late fall.

Inhalant allergens are the most important cause of perennial allergic rhinitis. The major perennial allergens are house dust mites, mold antigens (i.e., *Aspergillus* and *Penicillium* species), animal danders, cockroaches, and feather pillows which harbor dust mites. Occasionally, perennial allergic rhinitis may be the result of exposure to an occupational allergen. Symptoms tend to be perennial but not constant because there is a clear, temporal association with workplace exposure. Some causes of occupational rhinitis include laboratory animals (rats, mice, guinea pigs, etc.), grains (bakers and agricultural workers), medications such as psyllium or penicillin, wood dust, particularly hard woods (mahogany, Western red cedar, etc.), latex, and chemicals (acid anhydrides, platinum salts, glues, and solvents) (44).

Although some clinicians believe that food allergens may be significant factors in the cause of persistent allergic rhinitis, a direct immunologic relationship between ingested foods and persistent rhinitis symptoms has been difficult to establish. Rarely, hypersensitivity to dietary proteins may induce the symptoms of nonseasonal allergic rhinitis. Double-blind food challenges usually confirm such reactions (45). Cow's milk has been the food often suspected of precipitating or aggravating upper respiratory symptoms. Usually, however, the overwhelming majority of patients with proven food allergies exhibit other symptoms, including gastrointestinal disturbances, urticaria, angioedema, asthma, and anaphylaxis, in addition to rhinitis, after ingestion of the specific food.

Cross-reactive allergens between food and inhalant allergens are common. Patients with allergic rhinitis due to birch and, to a lesser extent, other *Betulaceae* (hazel, alder) pollen frequently develop oral allergic symptoms to tree nuts, fruits, and vegetables, including apples, carrots, celery, and potatoes (46). Most patients develop mild symptoms but anaphylaxis may occur very rarely from these cross-reacting foods. Some birch or hazel pollen allergens cross-react with those of fresh apples, especially those located just beneath the skin. Baked apples are tolerated as is apple sauce (47). Ragweed-sensitive individuals may experience symptoms when eating banana or melon. Latex-sensitive individuals may develop symptoms when ingesting avocado, banana, chestnut, kiwi fruit, or other foods (48).

Nonspecific irritants and infections may influence the course of persistent (perennial) allergic rhinitis. Children with this condition appear to have a higher incidence of respiratory infections that tend to aggravate the condition and may lead to the development of complications. Irritants such as tobacco smoke, and air pollutants (sulfur dioxide, volatile organic compounds (49), particulate matter, ozone, diesel exhaust particles,

nitrogen dioxide) can aggravate the symptoms. Drafts, chilling, and sudden changes in temperature also tend to do so. These features indicate that the patient has concurrent nonallergic rhinitis.

■ CLINICAL FEATURES

The major symptoms of allergic rhinitis are sneezing, rhinorrhea, nasal pruritus, and nasal congestion, although patients may not have the entire symptom complex. When taking a history, one should record the specific characteristics of the symptoms, as follows:

- Define the onset and duration of symptoms and emphasize any relationship to seasons or life events, such as changing residence or occupation, or acquiring a new pet.
- Define the current symptoms including secretions, degree of congestion, sneezing, and nasal itching, or sinus pressure and pain. Obtain a history regarding ocular symptoms, such as itching, lacrimation, puffiness, and chemosis; pharyngeal symptoms of a mild sore throat, throat clearing, and itching of the palate and throat; and associated systemic symptoms of malaise, fatigue, or sleep disturbances.
- Identify exacerbating factors, such as seasonal or perennial allergens and nonspecific irritants (e.g., cigarette smoke, chemical fumes, cold air, etc.).
- Identify other associated allergic diseases, such as asthma or atopic dermatitis, or a family history of allergic diathesis.
- Obtain a complete medication history, including both prescription and over-the-counter medications.

Sneezing is the most characteristic symptom, and occasionally one may have paroxysms of 10 to 20 sneezes in rapid succession. Sneezing episodes may arise without warning, or they may be preceded by an uncomfortable itching or irritated feeling in the nose. Sneezing attacks result in tearing of the eyes because of activation of the nasal-lacrimal reflex. During the pollen season, nonspecific factors, such as dust exposure, sudden drafts, air pollutants, or noxious irritants, may also trigger violent sneezing episodes.

The rhinorrhea is typically a thin discharge, which may be quite profuse and continuous. Because of the copious nature of the rhinorrhea, the skin covering the external nose and the upper lip may become irritated and tender. Purulent discharge is never seen in uncomplicated allergic rhinitis, and its presence usually indicates secondary infection. Nasal congestion resulting from swollen turbinates is a frequent complaint. Early in the season, the nasal obstruction may be more troublesome in the evening and at night, only to become almost continuous as the season progresses. If the nasal obstruction is severe, interference with aeration and drainage of the paranasal sinuses or the eustachian tube may occur, resulting in complaints of headache or earache. The headache is of the so-called vacuum type, presumably caused by the development of negative pressure when air is absorbed from the obstructive sinus or middle ear. Patients also complain that their hearing is decreased and that sounds seem muffled. Patients may also notice a crackling sensation in the ears, especially when swallowing. Nasal congestion alone, particularly in children, occasionally may be the major or sole complaint. With continuous severe nasal congestion, the senses of smell and taste may be lost. Itching of the nose may also be a prominent feature, inducing frequent rubbing of the nose, particularly in children. Eye symptoms (pruritus, erythema, and lacrimation) often accompany the nasal symptoms. Patients with severe eye symptoms often complain of photophobia, inability to wear contact lenses, and sore, "tired" eyes. Conjunctival injection and chemosis often occur. There is marked itching of the ears, palate, throat, or face, which may be extremely annoying. Because of irritating sensations in the throat and the posterior drainage of the nasal secretions, a hacking, nonproductive cough may be present. A constricted feeling of the chest with associated dyspnea may occur suggesting coexistent asthma. Some patients have systemic symptoms of seasonal allergic rhinitis. Complaints may include weakness, malaise, irritability, fatigue, and anorexia. Certain patients relate that nausea, abdominal discomfort, and poor appetite appear to occur with swallowing excess mucous.

A characteristic feature of the symptom complex is the periodicity of its appearance. Symptoms usually recur each year for many years in relation to the duration of the pollinating season of the causative plant. The most sensitive patients exhibit symptoms early in the season, almost as soon as the pollen appears in the air. The intensity of the symptoms tends to follow the course of pollination, becoming more severe when the pollen concentration is highest and waning as the season ends, when the amount of pollen in the air decreases. In some patients, symptoms disappear suddenly when the pollination season is over, whereas in others, symptoms may disappear gradually over a period of 2 to 3 weeks after the pollination season is completed. There may be an increased reactivity of the nasal mucosa after repeated exposure to the pollen. This local and nonspecific increased reactivity has been termed the *priming effect* (50). Under experimental conditions a patient may respond to an allergen not otherwise considered clinically significant if he or she had been exposed or primed to a clinically significant allergen. The nonspecificity of this effect may account for the presence of symptoms in some patients beyond the termination of the pollinating season because an allergen not clinically important by itself may induce symptoms in the "primed" nose. For example, a patient with positive skin tests to mold antigens and ragweed, and no symptoms until August may have symptoms until late October, after the ragweed-pollinating season is over. The symptoms persist because of the presence of molds in the air, which affect the primed mucous membrane. In most patients, however, this does not appear to occur (51). The presence of a secondary infection, or the effects of nonspecific irritants on inflamed nasal membranes, may also prolong and influence the degree of rhinitis symptoms beyond the specific pollinating season. Some nonspecific irritants include tobacco smoke, paints, newspaper ink, and soap powders. Rapid atmospheric changes may aggravate symptoms in predisposed patients. Nonspecific air pollutants may also potentiate the symptoms of allergic rhinitis, such as sulfur dioxide, ozone, carbon monoxide, and nitrogen dioxide.

These symptoms of allergic rhinitis may exhibit periodicity within the season. Many patients tend to have more intense symptoms in the morning because most windborne pollen is released in greatest numbers between sunrise and 9:00 AM. Some specific factors such as rain may decrease symptoms of rhinitis because rain can clear pollen from the air. Also, dry windy days may increase symptoms because higher concentrations of pollen may be distributed over larger areas.

The symptoms of perennial allergic rhinitis are similar to seasonal rhinitis. The decreased severity of symptoms seen in some patients may lead them to interpret their symptoms as resulting from "sinus trouble" or "frequent colds." Nasal congestion may be the dominant symptom, particularly in children, in whom the passageways are relatively small. Sneezing; clear rhinorrhea; itching of the nose, eyes, ears, and throat; and lacrimation may also occur. The presence of itching in the nasopharyngeal and ocular areas is consistent with an allergic cause of the chronic rhinitis. The chronic nasal obstruction may cause mouth breathing, snoring, almost constant sniffing, and a nasal twang to the voice. The obstruction may worsen or be responsible for the development of obstructive sleep apnea. Because of the constant mouth breathing, patients may complain of a dry, irritated, or sore throat. Loss of the sense of smell may occur in patients with marked chronic nasal obstruction. Sneezing episodes on awakening or in the early morning hours are a complaint. Because the chronic edema involves the opening of the eustachian tube and the paranasal sinuses, dull frontal headaches and ear complaints, such as decreased hearing, fullness and popping of the ears, are common. In children, there may be recurrent episodes of serous otitis media. Chronic nasal obstruction may lead to eustachian tube dysfunction. Persistent, low-grade nasal pruritus leads to almost constant rubbing of the nose and nasal twitching. In children, recurrent epistaxis may occur because of the friability of the mucous membranes, sneezing episodes, forceful nose blowing, or nose picking. After exposure to significant levels of an allergen, such as close contact with a pet or when dusting the house, the symptoms may be as severe as in the acute stages of seasonal allergic rhinitis. Constant, excessive postnasal drainage of secretions may be associated with a chronic cough or a continual clearing of the throat.

Physical Examination

Most abnormal physical findings are present during the acute stages of seasonal allergic rhinitis. The physical findings commonly recognized include:

- Nasal obstruction and associated mouth breathing
- Pale to bluish nasal mucosa and enlarged (boggy) inferior tubinates
- Clear nasal secretions (whitish secretions may be seen in patients experiencing severe allergic rhinitis)
- Clear or white secretions along the posterior wall of the nasopharynx
- Conjunctival erythema, lacrimation, and puffiness of the eyes

The physical findings, which are usually confined to the nose, ears, and eyes, aid in the diagnosis. Rubbing of the nose and mouth breathing are common findings. Some children will rub the nose in an upward and outward fashion, which has been termed the *allergic salute*. The eyes may exhibit excessive lacrimation. The sclera and conjunctivae may be reddened, and chemosis is often present. The conjunctivae may be swollen and may appear granular, and the eyelids are often swollen. The skin above the nose may be reddened and irritated because of the continuous rubbing and blowing. Examination of the nasal cavity discloses a pale, wet, edematous mucosa, frequently bluish in color. A clear, thin nasal secretion may be seen within the nasal cavity. Swollen turbinates may completely occlude the nasal passageway and severely affect the patient. Nasal polyps may be present in individuals with allergic rhinitis. Occasionally, there is fluid in the middle ear, resulting in decreased hearing. The pharynx is usually normal. The nose and eye examination are normal during asymptomatic intervals.

In patients with perennial allergic rhinitis, the physical examination may aid in the diagnosis, particularly in a child, who may constantly rub his nose or eyes. These include a gaping appearance due to the constant mouth breathing, and a broadening of the midsection of the nose. There may be a transverse nasal crease across the lower third of the nose where the soft cartilagenous portion meets the rigid bony bridge. This is the result of the continual rubbing and pushing of the nose to relieve itching. The mucous membranes are pale, moist, and boggy, and may have a bluish tinge. Polyps may be present in cases of chronic perennial allergic rhinitis of long duration. Their characteristic appearance is smooth, glistening, and white. They may take the form of grapelike masses. However, polyps may also occur in patients without allergic rhinitis, and thus causality cannot be inferred. The nasal secretions are usually clear and watery, but may be more mucoid and microscopically

may show large numbers of eosinophils. Dark circles under the eyes, known as *allergic shiners*, appear in some children. These are presumed to be due to venous stasis secondary to constant nasal congestion. The conjunctiva may be injected or may appear granular. In children affected with perennial allergic rhinitis early in life, narrowing of the arch of the palate may occur, leading to the Gothic arch. These children may develop facial deformities, such as dental malocclusion or gingival hypertrophy. The throat is usually normal on examination, although the posterior pharyngeal wall may exhibit prominent lymphoid follicles.

■ PATHOPHYSIOLOGY

The nose has the following six major functions:

1. An olfactory organ
2. A resonator for phonation
3. A passageway for airflow in and out of the lungs
4. A means of humidifying and warming inspired air
5. A filter of noxious particles from inspired air
6. A part of the immunologic responses of the nose and sinuses (52)

Allergic reactions occurring in the nasal mucous membranes markedly affect the nose's major functions. The nose can initiate immune mechanisms, and the significance of mediator release from nasal mast cells and basophils in the immediate-type allergic reaction is well established. Patients with allergic rhinitis have IgE antibodies that bind to high-affinity receptors ($F_{C\epsilon}RI$) on mast cells and basophils, and to low-affinity receptors ($F_{C\epsilon}RII$ or CD_{23}) on other cells, such as monocytes, eosinophils, B cells, and platelets. Sensitization to an allergen is necessary to elicit an IgE response. After inhalation, the allergen must first be internalized by antigen-presenting cells, which include macrophages, $CD1^+$ dendritic cells, B-lymphocytes, and epithelial cells (53). After allergen processing, peptide fragments of the allergen are exteriorized and presented with class II (MHC) molecules of host antigen presenting cells to $CD4^+$ T-lymphocytes. Nasal provocation with allergen has been associated with increases of such HLA-DR and HLA-DQ positive cells in the lamina propria and epithelium in allergic subjects (54). These lymphocytes have receptors specific for the particular MHC peptide complex. This interaction results in the release of cytokines by the $CD4^+$ cell. The switch from the T_H1 phenotype to the T_H2 phenotype is the crucial early event in allergic sensitization and is key to the development of allergic inflammation. Allergic inflammation involves two major T_H2-mediated pathways:

1. The secretion of interleukin-4 (IL-4) and IL-13 that results in isotypic switching of B lymphocytes to secrete IgE (55)
2. The secretion of eosinophil growth factor, IL-5 (72)

B-lymphocytes require two signals for isotypic switch to IgE (56). In the first signal, Il-4 or Il-13 stimulate transcription at the Ce locus, the site of exons that encode the constant region of the IgE heavy chain. Interaction of CD40 on the B-cell membrane with CD40 ligand on the surface of T-lymphocytes provides the second signal that activates genetic recombination in the functional IgE heavy chain. IL-4 and IL-13 also upregulate vascular cell adhesion molecule-1 (VCAM-1) on endothelial cells promoting adhesion of inflammatory cell populations and facilitate their migration into areas of allergic inflammation.

After IgE antibodies specific for a certain allergen are synthesized and secreted, they bind to high-affinity receptors on mast cells. On nasal re-exposure to allergen, the allergen cross links the specific cell-bound IgE antibodies on the mast cell surface in a calcium-dependent process resulting in the release of a number of mediators of inflammation. Mediators released include histamine, leukotrienes, prostaglandins, platelet-activating factor, and bradykinin. These mediators are responsible for vasodilatation, increased vascular permeability, increased glandular secretion, and stimulation of afferent nerves, which culminate in the immediate-type rhinitis symptoms (57). Chemokines and cytokines are generated as well.

Mast cells are present in concentrations of $7,000/mm^3$ in the normal nasal submucosa but only $50/mm^3$ in the nasal epithelium. Some studies report increased mast cells in the nasal epithelium in allergic rhinitis. Nasal mast cells are predominantly located in the nasal lamina propria as connective tissue mast cells, although 15% are epithelial and are called mucosal mast cells. Mucosal mast cells express tryptase without chymase. They proliferate in allergic rhinitis under the influence of T_H2 cytokines. The superficial nasal epithelium in patients with allergic rhinitis has 50-fold more mast cell and basophils when compared to the epithelium of nonallergic patients (58).

Mast cells and their mediators are central to the pathogenesis of the early response, as indicated by the demonstration of mast cell degranulation in the nasal mucosa and the detection of mast cell-derived mediators, including histamine, leukotriene C4 (LTC-4), and prostaglandin D_2 (PGD_2) in nasal washings. In addition to mast cell mediators, the early response is associated with an increase in neuropeptides, such as calcitonin gene-related peptide, substance P, vasoactive intestinal peptide, and increasing numbers of cytokines (IL-1, IL-3, IL-4, IL-5, IL-6, granulocyte macrophage colony-stimulating factor [GM-CSF]), and tumor necrosis factor-á (TNF-á) (59–63). The mast cell derived cytokines promote further IgE production, mast cell and eosinophil growth, chemotaxis, and survival. IL-5, TNF-á, and IL-1 promote eosinophil movement by increasing the expression of adhesion molecules on endothelium. In turn, eosinophils secrete a plethora of cytokines including IL-3, IL-4, IL-5, IL-10, and GM-CSF resulting in mast cell growth and T_H2 proliferation. Eosinophils may also function in an autocrine manner by producing cytokines IL-3, IL-5, and GM-CSF, which are important in hematopoiesis, differentiation, and survival of eosinophils. With continuation of allergic inflammation, one sees an accumulation of CD4+ lymphocytes, eosinophils, neutrophils, and basophils (64). Eosinophils release oxygen radicals and proteins including eosinophil major basic protein, eosinophil cationic protein, and eosinophil peroxidases. These proteins may disrupt the respiratory epithelium and promote further mast cell mediator release and hyper-responsiveness (65,66). There are strong correlations between the number of basophils and the level of histamine in the late reaction, and between the number of eosinophils and the amount of eosinophil major basic protein. These findings suggest that these cells may participate in allergic inflammation by not only entering the nose, but also degranulating (67,68). Eosinophils increase during seasonal exposure, and the number of eosinophil progenitors in the nasal scrapings increases after exposure to allergens, and correlates with the severity of seasonal disease (69).

The infiltration of the nasal cavity with basophils, lymphocytes, eosinophils, and neutrophils characterizes the late-phase reaction of allergic rhinitis. The late-phase reaction will occur in approximately 50% of patients with allergic rhinitis who undergo nasal challenge. This reaction is associated with elevated levels of mediators similar to the immediate allergic reaction, except PGD_2 and tryptase are not detected. The absence of the mast cell-derived mediators PGD_2 and tryptase during the late-phase reaction is consistent with basophil-derived histamine release rather than mast cell involvement. Basophils are noted to be significantly increased in nasal lavage fluids 3 to 11 hours after allergen challenge, correlating their role in the late-phase reaction (68). CD4+ CD25 T-cells, in addition to neutrophils, eosinophils, and basophils, are increased during the late-phase response. These CD4 T-lymphocytes help promote the late-phase allergic reaction because they express messenger RNA for IL-3, IL-4, IL-5, and GM-CSF (70).

The heating and humidification of inspired air is an important function of the nasal mucosa. The highly vascularized mucosa of the turbinates in the septum provides an effective structure to heat and humidify air as it passes over them. The blood vessels are under the direction of the autonomic nervous system, which controls reflex adjustments for efficient performance of this function. The sympathetic nervous system provides for vascular constriction with a reduction of secretions. The parasympathetic nervous system enables vascular dilatation and an increase in secretions. This high degree of vascularization in the nasal cavity and the changes in the vasculature may lead to severe nasal obstruction (71). In most individuals under normal conditions, there is a rhythmic alternating congestion and decongestion of the mucosa, referred to as the nasal cycle.

The protecting and cleansing role of the nasal mucosa is also an important function. Relatively large particles are filtered out of the inspired air by the hairs within the nostrils. The nasal secretions contain an enzyme, lysozyme, which is bacteriostatic. The pH of the nasal secretions remains relatively constant at 7. Lysozyme activity and ciliary action are optimal at this pH. Ciliated cells line the major portions of the nose, septum, and paranasal sinuses. The cilia beat at a frequency of 1,000 beats/min, producing a streaming mucus blanket at an approximate rate of 3 mm/min to 25 mm/min. The mucus is produced by mucus and serous glands, and epithelial goblet cells in the mucosa. The density of goblet cells in the nose and in the large airways is approximately 10,000/mm^3 (72). The number of goblet cells and mucus glands does not appear to increase in chronic rhinitis (73). The mucus blanket containing the filtered materials moves toward the pharynx to be expectorated or swallowed.

■ LABORATORY FINDINGS

A characteristic laboratory finding in allergic rhinitis, also termed *intermittent rhinitis* (2), is the presence of large numbers of eosinophils in a Hansel-stained smear of the nasal secretions obtained during a period of symptoms. In classic seasonal allergic rhinitis, this test is usually not necessary to make a diagnosis. Its use is limited to questionable cases and more often in defining chronic allergic rhinitis.

In chronic rhinitis, the presence of large numbers of eosinophils suggests an allergic cause, although nonallergic rhinitis with eosinophilia syndrome (NARES) certainly occurs. The absence of nasal eosinophilia does not exclude an allergic cause, especially if the test is performed during a relatively quiescent period of the disease, or in the presence of bacterial infection when large numbers of polymorphonuclear neutrophils obscure the eosinophils.

Peripheral blood eosinophilia of <12% may or may not be present in active seasonal allergic rhinitis. A significantly elevated concentration of serum IgE may occur in some patients with allergic rhinitis, but many other conditions (including racial factors) may increase the serum levels of total IgE such as concomitant atopic dermatitis. Thus, the measurement of total serum IgE is barely predictive for allergy screening in rhinitis and should not be used as a diagnostic tool (1).

■ DIAGNOSIS

The diagnosis of seasonal (intermittent) allergic rhinitis usually presents no difficulty by the time the patient has had symptoms severe enough to seek medical attention. The seasonal nature of the condition, the characteristic symptom complex, and the physical findings should establish a diagnosis in almost all cases. If the patient is first seen during the initial or second season, or if the major symptom is conjunctivitis, there may be a delay in making the diagnosis from the history alone. Additional supporting evidence is a positive history of allergic disorders in the immediate family and a collateral history of other allergic disorders in the patient. After the history is taken and the physical examination is performed, skin tests should be performed to determine the reactivity of the patient against the suspected allergens. For the proper interpretation of the meaning of a positive skin test, it is important to remember that patients with allergic rhinitis may exhibit positive skin tests to allergens other than those that are clinically important. In seasonal allergic rhinitis, it has been demonstrated that prick puncture testing with standardized extracts is adequate for diagnostic purposes in many patients if standardized extracts are used. Intradermal testing when positive may not always correlate with allergic disease (74,75). Skin testing should be performed and interpreted by trained personnel because results may be altered by the distance placed between allergens (76), the application site (back versus arm), the type of device used for testing (77), the season of the year tested (78), and the quality of extracts used for testing (79).

The first technique used to accurately measure serum specific IgE was the RAST (radioallergosorbent test) (80–82). Newer techniques use enzyme-labeled anti-IgE. The *in vitro* tests have been employed as a diagnostic aid in some allergic diseases. RAST or enzyme-labeled anti-IgE assays of circulating IgE antibody can be used instead of skin testing when high-quality extracts are not available, when a control skin test with a diluent is consistently positive, when antihistamine therapy cannot be discontinued, or widespread skin disease is present.

Initially, RAST, then enzyme-based anti-IgE assays appear to correlate fairly well with other measures of sensitivity, such as skin tests, end-point titration, histamine release, and provocation tests. The frequency of positive reactions obtained by skin testing is usually greater than that found with serum or nasal RAST or enzyme assay (ImmunoCAP, Phadia). In view of these findings, the serum assays may be used as a supplement to skin testing. Skin testing is the diagnostic method of choice to demonstrate IgE antibodies. When the skin test is positive, there is little need for other tests. When the skin test is dubiously positive, the *in vitro* diagnostic test will, as a rule, be negative. Therefore, the information obtained by examining serum IgE antibody by *in vitro* test usually adds little to that gleaned from critical evaluation of skin testing with high-quality extracts.

Another procedure, nasal provocation, is a useful tool (83) but not as a generally recognized diagnostic procedure. Skin testing should be performed because, in contrast to the nasal test, the skin test is quick, inexpensive, safe, and without discomfort. It has the additional advantage of possessing better reproducibility.

■ DIFFERENTIAL DIAGNOSIS

The diagnosis of allergic rhinitis must be established carefully since an incorrect diagnosis could result in expensive treatments and major alterations in a patient's lifestyle and environment. Several medical conditions may be confused with persistent allergic rhinitis (Table 26.2). The main causes of persistent nasal congestion and discharge include rhinitis medicamentosa, drugs, pregnancy, nasal foreign bodies, other bony abnormalities of the lateral nasal wall, concha bullosa (air cell within the middle turbinate), enlarged adenoids, nasal polyps, cerebrospinal fluid rhinorrhea, tumors, hypo-

thyroidism, ciliary dyskinesia from cystic fibrosis, primary ciliary dyskinesia, Kartagener syndrome, granulomatous diseases (i.e., sarcoidosis, Wegener granulomatosis, midline granuloma), nasal mastocytosis, congenital syphilis, gustatory rhinitis, gastroesophageal reflux, atrophic rhinitis, Churg-Strauss vasculitis, allergic fungal sinusitis, nonallergic rhinitis, or NARES.

Rhinitis Medicamentosa

A condition that may enter into the differential diagnosis is rhinitis medicamentosa, which results from the overuse of decongestant (vasoconstricting) nose drops. Every patient who presents with the complaint of chronic nasal congestion should be carefully questioned as to the amount and frequency of the use of nose drops.

Drugs

Patients taking antihypertensive medications such as β-adrenergic blockers, α-adrenergic blockers, hydralazine, alpha methyldopa, erectile dysfunction medications, and certain psychoactive drugs may complain of marked nasal congestion, which is a common side effect of these agents. Discontinuation of these drugs for a few days results in marked symptomatic improvement.

Cyclic changes in rhinitis intensity may be related to the changes in relative concentrations of the complex mix of hormones during the menstrual cycle. In nasal provocation experiments, allergic patients on oral contraceptives having grass challenges had less nasal congestion at day 14 of the menstrual cycle and more sneezing at the end of the cycle (84). Thus, oral contraceptives affect nasal reactivity in complex ways and usually can be continued in patients with allergic rhinitis.

Cocaine sniffing is often associated with frequent sniffing, rhinorrhea, diminished olfaction, and septal perforation (85).

Aspirin and other nonsteroidal anti-inflammatory drugs commonly induce rhinitis. In a population-based random sample, aspirin intolerance was more frequent among subjects with allergic rhinitis than among those without (86). In about 10% of adult patients with asthma, aspirin and other nonsteroidal anti-inflammatory agents that inhibit cyclooxygenase enzymes precipitate asthmatic attacks and nonocular reactions (87). This distinct clinical syndrome, called *aspirin-induced asthma* is characterized by an atypical sequence of symptoms, intense eosinophilic inflammation of the nasal and bronchial tissues, combined with an overproduction of cysteinyl-leukotrienes. After ingestion of aspirin or other NSAIDs, an acute asthma attack occurs within 3 hours, usually accompanied by profuse rhinorrhea, conjunctival injection, periorbital edema, and sometimes a scarlet flushing of the head and neck.

The inflammatory cell populations in the nasal mucosa of aspirin-sensitive rhinitis patients have been

---

TABLE 26.2 DIFFERENTIAL DIAGNOSIS OF NONALLERGIC RHINITIS

Associated drugs
- Topical α-adrenergic agonists
- Oral estrogens
- Ophthalmic and oral β-blockers

Infections
- Chronic sinusitis
- Tuberculosis
- Syphilis
- Fungal infection

Systemic conditions
- Cystic fibrosis
- Immunodeficiencies
- Immotile cilia syndrome
- Hypothyroidism
- Rhinitis of pregnancy

Structural abnormalities
- Marked septal deviation
- Concha bullosa
- Nasal polyps
- Adenoidal hypertrophy
- Foreign body

Neoplasms
- Squamous cell carcinoma
- Nasopharyngeal carcinoma

Granulomatous diseases
- Wegener granulomatosis
- Sarcoidosis
- Midline granuloma
- Churg-Strauss vasculitis

Other
- Atrophic rhinitis
- Gustatory rhinitis
- Allergic fungal sinusitis
- Gastroesophageal reflux disease
- Nonallergic rhinitis with eosinophilia syndrome (NARES)

studied. In comparison to normal subjects, there is an increase in eosinophils, mast cells, and activated T-cells. Marked increases in the numbers of IL-5 mRNA+ cells and lower numbers of IL-4 mRNA+cells are observed in aspirin-sensitive patients. No differences are recognized for either IL-2 or IFN-γ. The predominance of macrophages and the disproportionate increase in IL-5 compared to IL-4 mRNA expression suggest that factors other than "allergic mechanisms" may be important in this disease (63,88). A similar increase in IL-5, an over expression of LTC_4 synthetase, and increase in cysteinyl leukotriene 1 receptor numbers have been noted in the bronchi or cells of patients with aspirin-induced asthma or rhinosinusitis (88,89).

Pregnancy

Rhinitis of pregnancy has been attributed to increasing concentrations of female hormones during pregnancy, and the need for swollen mucosae with mucous hypersecretion for protection of the vagina and cervix (90). The rhinitis characteristically begins at the end of the first trimester and then disappears immediately after delivery (91). It has been reported that increased nasal congestion occurs in from 22% to 72% of gravidas with asthma (92). The course of allergic rhinitis in pregnancy is variable and although many patients remain unchanged, approximately one-third may actually have a worsening of their condition during pregnancy (93).

Foreign Body

On rare occasions, a patient with a foreign body in the nose may be thought to have chronic allergic rhinitis. Foreign bodies usually present as unilateral nasal obstruction accompanied by a foul, purulent nasal discharge. Children may place foreign bodies into the nose, most commonly peas, beans, buttons, and erasers. Sinusitis is often diagnosed if the nose is not examined properly. Examination is best done after secretions are removed so that the foreign body may be visualized.

Physical Obstruction

Careful physical examination of the nasal cavity should be performed to exclude septal deviation, enlarged adenoids, choanal atresia, choncha bullosa, and nasal polyps as a cause of nasal congestion.

Cerebrospinal Fluid Rhinorrhea

Cerebrospinal fluid (CSF) rhinorrhea may at times mimic allergic rhinitis (94). The majority of CSF rhinorrhea cases are the result of trauma (95). Cases of spontaneous (nontraumatic) CSF rhinorrhea may be a high or a normal pressure leak, and can persist for months to years. There are reports of meningitis in 19% of patients with persistent CSF leak (96). The CSF is clear and watery in appearance, and may be either unilateral or bilateral (97). Obtaining Beta 2 transferrin levels from the nasal discharge establishes the diagnosis. The beta 2 transferrin is only present in the CSF, perilymph, and aqueous humor. When present in nasal discharge, it is highly specific for CSF rhinorrhea (98). After localization of the leak with magnetic resonance CT cisternography or high resolution CT examination, surgical repair is required to prevent meningitis (98).

Tumor

Several neoplasms may occur in the nasopharyngeal area. The most important are encephalocele, inverting papilloma, squamous cell carcinoma, sarcoma, and angiofibroma. Encephaloceles are generally unilateral. They usually occur high in the nose and occasionally within the nasopharynx. They increase in size with straining, lifting, or crying. Some have a pulsating quality. CSF rhinorrhea or even meningitis may develop as a complication of biopsy of these lesions.

Inverting papillomas have a somewhat papillary appearance. They are friable and more vascular than nasal polyps, and bleed more readily. They occur either unilaterally or bilaterally, and frequently involve the nasal septum as well as the lateral wall of the nose. A biopsy is necessary to confirm the diagnosis.

Angiofibromas are the most common tumors in preadolescent boys (99). They arise in the posterior choana (*choanae osseae*) of the nasopharynx. They have a polypoid appearance but are usually reddish-blue in color. They do not pit on palpation. Angiofibromas are highly vascular tumors that bleed excessively when injured or when a biopsy is done. Larger tumors may invade bone and extend into adjacent structures (99).

Carcinomas and sarcoma may simulate nasal polyps. They are generally unilateral, may occur at any site within the nasal chamber, are firm, and usually bleed with manipulation. As the disease progresses, adjacent structures become involved.

Hypothyroidism

A careful review of systems and indicated thyroid stimulating hormone level are important to exclude hypothyroidism as a cause of nasal congestion.

Syphilis

Congenital syphilis can cause rhinitis in infancy. The nasal symptom is referred to as *snuffles*.

Ciliary Disorders

With the dyskinetic cilia syndrome, patients may experience rhinitis symptoms secondary to abnormalities of mucociliary transport. The criteria for diagnosis include: (a) absence or near absence of tracheobronchial or nasal mucociliary transport, and (b) total or nearly total absence of dynein arms of the cilia in the nasal or bronchial mucosa. On electron microscopy, one may see defective radial spokes or transposition of a peripheral microtubular doublet to the center of the axoneme. The last criterion is (c) clinical manifestations of chronic upper and lower respiratory tract infections (i.e., sinusitis, bronchitis, and bronchiectasis) (*100*). Rare patients may have the triad of bronchiectasis, sinusitis, and situs inversus (Kartagener syndrome) (101). In some patients, cilia, although abnormal in structure, may be motile. The cilia in patients with this syndrome can be distinguished from those in patients with asthma, sinusitis, chronic bronchitis, and emphysema, who may have nonspecific abnormalities in cilia structure.

Perennial Nonallergic Rhinitis

Perennial nonallergic rhinitis comprises a heterogenous group of at least two subgroups. One subgroup, NARES, was defined in the early 1980s (*102,103*). NARES is characterized by the presence of nasal eosinophilia and perennial symptoms of sneezing, itching, rhinorrhea, nasal obstruction, and occasionally a loss of the sense of smell. The condition may occur in children and adults. NARES appears to evolve in three stages: (a) migration of eosinophils from vessels to secretions,(b) retention of eosinophils in the mucosa, and (c) development of nasal polyps (*104*). NARES usually has a favorable response to intranasal corticosteroids.

Another subgroup of perennial nonallergic rhinitis has been termed *vasomotor rhinitis* (note that this term is no longer used.) In these patients, nasal symptoms, although similar to that of allergic rhinitis, are usually precipitated by nonspecific stimuli such as smoke, perfumes, alcoholic beverages, cold air, hot spicy foods, strong odors, and barometric pressure changes. Treatment of this condition is variable and usually directed to the most prominent nasal symptom. Nerve fiber numbers are increased in nonallergic and allergic rhinitis when biopsies of inferior turbinates are studied (105). Nerve fibers "sprout" under the influence of nerve growth factor and contribute to sensory neurons being hyperexcitable (*142*).

Atrophic Rhinitis

Primary atrophic rhinitis is characterized by progressive atrophy of the nasal mucosa and underlying bone, resulting in a nasal cavity that is widely patent but full of copious foul-smelling crusts (106). The infection may be attributed to *Klebsiella pneumoniae* sp. *ozaenae*, although its role as a primary pathogen is not fully documented. Patients' complaints usually consist of severe nasal congestion, hyposmia, and a constant smell. It must be distinguished from secondary atrophic rhinitis associated with radiation, trauma, excessive nasal surgery, and chronic granulomatous conditions.

Gastroesophageal Reflux

Gastroesophageal reflux can be associated with rhinitis and recurrent otitis media, especially in children (107–109).

Allergic Fungal Rhinosinusitis

The fungi responsible for allergic fungal rhinosinusitis (AFS) are predominantly of the Dematiaceae family (*Aspergillus* spp., *Rhizopus* spp., *Alternaria* spp., *Curvularia* spp., and *Bipolaris specifera*) (110). AFS primarily occurs in atopic patients who develop an IgE-mediated response to the fungus resulting in nasal polyps (111). The sinus mucosa shows a characteristic eosinophilic inflammation, with allergic mucin filling the sinuses. Elevated total IgE and fungal-specific IgG and IgE antibodies are commonly found (112). AFS is unilateral in more than 50% of patients but may involve several sinuses with associated bone erosion. Treatment usually includes surgical intervention with polypectomy and marsupialization of the involved sinuses. Medical management involoves long-term intranasal glucocorticosteroids with use of systemic corticosteroids for more difficult cases (113).

■ COURSE AND COMPLICATIONS

Allergic rhinitis accounts for the largest number of patients with respiratory allergy. Most patients develop symptoms before the age of 20 years, with the highest rate of increase of onset of symptoms occurring between the ages of 12 and 15 years (*114*). Because of a variety of factors (geographic location, allergen load, weather conditions), the course and prognosis for any single patient cannot be predicted. The age of onset of atopy may be an important confounding factor for the development of asthma and rhinitis or rhinitis alone. An Australian study found that atopy acquired before the age of 6 years was a predictive factor for asthma continuing into late childhood and adulthood as well (*115*,116).

Several surveys in children and adults have shown significantly lower prevalence of asthma and allergic diseases in Eastern Europe than in western countries. With unification, there were tremendous changes toward western lifestyle in the former German Democratic Republic (Deutsche Demokratische Republik, a.k.a., East Germany) (117). In 1995 to 1996, a cross-sectional study of 2,334 school children in Leipzig utilized the same methodology of the previous study performed after the fall of communism in 1991 to 1992

(*118*). The prevalence of seasonal allergic rhinitis and atopic sensitization increased significantly between 1991 to 1992 and 1995 to 1996 (*119*). However, there was no significant change in the prevalence of asthma or bronchial hyperresponsiveness (*118*). These findings suggested important differences in the development of atopic disorders. Factors operating very early in life may be particularly important for the acquisition of childhood asthma and rhinitis, whereas environmental factors occurring beyond infancy may also affect the development of atopic sensitization and seasonal rhinitis.

The course of patients with allergic rhinitis is variable (*120*). One study suggested 39% improved, 39% remained unchanged, and in 21%, the symptoms became worse (117). In another study, 8% of those with allergic rhinitis had remissions for at least 2 years' duration (*120*). In a study published in the 1970s, a chance for remission was better in those with seasonal allergic rhinitis and if the disease was present for less than 5 years (*121*).

The possibility of developing asthma as a sequelae to allergic rhinitis may worry the patient or the parents. Allergic rhinitis and positive allergy skin tests are significant risk factors for developing new asthma (*122*). A 10-year prognosis study for childhood allergic rhinitis found that asthma or wheezing developed in 19% of cases and was more common among those with perennial allergic rhinitis than among those with seasonal allergic rhinitis (*123*). Individuals with either of these diagnoses are about three times more likely to develop asthma than negative controls. However, upper and lower airway symptoms may develop simultaneously in about 25% of patients.

Patients with allergic rhinitis may develop complications because of chronic nasal inflammation including recurrent otitis media with hearing loss, impaired speech development, acute and chronic sinusitis, recurrence of nasal polyps, abnormal craniofacial development, sleep apnea with its related complications (123,124), aggravation of asthma, and increased propensity to develop asthma. In patients with allergic rhinitis, a continuous allergen exposure results in persistent inflammation that upregulates expression of ICAM-1 and VCAM-1 in the inflamed epithelium (125). Because ICAM-1 is the ligand for almost 90% of rhinoviruses, its upregulation may be responsible for the increased viral respiratory infections in these patients. Poorly controlled symptoms of allergic rhinitis may contribute to sleep loss, secondary daytime fatigue, learning impairment, decreased overall cognitive functioning, decreased long-term productivity, and decreased quality of life.

The symptoms of allergic rhinitis and skin test reactivity tend to wane with increasing age. In most patients, however, skin tests remain positive despite symptomatic improvement; therefore, symptomatic improvement does not necessarily correlate with skin test conversion to negative.

■ TREATMENT

There are three types of management of seasonal allergic or perennial allergic rhinitis. These methods are (a) avoidance therapy, (b) symptomatic therapy (pharmacologic treatment), and (c) immunotherapy.

Avoidance Therapy

Complete avoidance of an allergen results in a cure when there is only a single allergen of limited and clearly defined distribution. For this reason, attempts should be made to minimize contact with any important allergen, regardless of what other mode of treatment is instituted (Table 26.3). Perennial allergic rhinitis secondary to household pets can be adequately controlled by removing the pet from the home. The allergens of cats and dogs are not the dander itself, but are contained in the saliva and in sebaceous secretions, which can flake off in small particles and remain airborne for considerable periods. This results in an ubiquitous allergen that can be found in many environments outside the home (126), especially schools (127,128). This makes complete avoidance much more difficult, though there is little doubt that removal of the pets from the home will achieve improvement.

In most cases of allergic rhinitis, complete avoidance therapy is difficult, if not impossible, because aeroallergens are so widely distributed. Attempts to eradicate sources of pollen or molds have not proved to be significantly effective. Most mold-sensitive patients should avoid damp, musty basements, raked or burning leaves, barns, moldy hay, and straw. They should disinfect or destroy moldy articles. Some mold-sensitive patients occasionally note a precipitation or aggravation of symptoms after ingestion of certain foods having a high mold content. In these patients, an avoidance of beer, wine, cantaloupe, melons, mushrooms, and various cheeses may be helpful.

In patients with house dust mite allergy, complete avoidance is nearly impossible in most climates, but a comprehensive program for dust mite control may result in a decreased exposure to the allergen. There should be at least one room in the house that is relatively dust-free. The most practical program is to make the bedroom as dust-free as possible, so that the patient may have the sleeping area as a controlled environment. Certain measures to decrease house dust exposure are relatively easy to perform. The patient should wear a mask when house cleaning if such activity precipitates significant symptoms. Recommendations include washing bed linens in very hot water (140°F) and encasing both the mattress and box spring in mite-proof casings. Eliminating upholstered furniture, wall-to-wall carpeting,

TABLE 26.3   TIPS FOR PATIENTS WITH ALLERGIC RHINITIS

1. Keep pets out of the bedroom and preferably outside of the house.
2. Avoid smoking and secondhand smoke.
3. Routinely clean areas of the home that promote mold growth, such as shower stalls, basements, and window sills (mold sensitivity).
4. Have cooking systems in the home checked periodically for mold growth.
5. Avoid locations that promote the growth of molds, such as damp, poorly ventilated areas.
6. Avoid sleeping in a bedroom located in a basement or attic.
7. Use air conditioning to reduce humidity and decrease temperature. Keep windows closed to avoid contact with outdoor allergens (house dust mite and pollen sensitivity).
8. Encase pillows, mattresses, and even box springs in zippered protective encasings (house dust mite sensitivity).
9. Replace heavily mite-infested mattresses and pillows. Use foam pillows instead of down or feather pillows (house dust mite sensitivity).
10. Launder bedding regularly, including mattress pads and blankets, in hot water (140°F) (house dust mite sensitivity).
11. Vacuum carpets and clean floors regularly; if possible, remove carpeting from bedroom, or treat carpet with acaricide (house dust mite sensitivity).
12. Minimize dust-collecting surfaces, such as shelves, stuffed animals, books, stored blankets, and woolens.

chenille spreads, bed pads, and stuffed toys from the bedroom allows more complete control. Steam cleaning (129) or acaricides (130) help reduce mite numbers in carpets. Acaricidal treatment (131,132) with benzyl benzoate has shown symptomatic improvement in perennial allergic rhinitis. The effect is mild and should be accompanied by a comprehensive dust mite prevention program. Since high levels of humidity within the home are essential for dust mite population growth, reducing humidity may be an effective control method. However, there is variable efficacy with humidity reduction in homes with low and high dust mite infestation.

Cockroach infestation is an important cause of allergic sensitization particularly in inner-city substandard apartment complexes (133). Major allergens have been identified in the digestive secretions and on the body parts of the insects. Although there have been no studies to evaluate the effect of cockroach eradication on rhinitis, most experts recommend remediation for this allergen.

Approaches to the extermination of cockroaches are based on eliminating suitable environments. Because cockroaches depend on water and food sources to survive, the highest allergen levels are found in the kitchen or bathrooms, although high allergy levels may be detected in other areas of the home, including the bedroom. Effective methods of extermination include using safe, odorless insecticides and gel formulations that can be precisely placed in kitchens and other rooms. Cockroaches hide in cracks and crevices, and therefore the allergen collects in reservoirs. To remove allergens successfully from indoor environments, extensive cleaning after extermination is required (134,135). Effective treatment also requires behavioral changes to reduce the chance of reinfestation.

Overview of Pharmacologic Treatment

With mild intermittent allergic rhinitis, the suggested initial pharmacologic therapy consists of an oral antihistamine, an intranasal antihistamine, or an oral decongestant. When intermittent disease is moderate or severe, intranasal corticosteroids provide an alternative to the aforementioned agents. Persistent mild allergic rhinitis is usually treated in a similar fashion as moderate or severe intermittent allergic rhinitis. When symptoms are persistent and moderate or severe, intranasal corticosteroids should be the first class of medications employed. Investigation into the presence of allergic conjunctivitis should also take place so that appropriate intraocular H_1 blockers or intraocular chromones may be added to the therapeutic program. With all grades of severity, appropriate follow-up should occur in a reasonable period, and therapy intensified or stepped down, as indicated.

Pharmacologic Therapy

Intranasal Coriticosteroids

Intranasal corticosteroids represent the single most effective class of medications for allergic rhinitis and improve all nasal symptoms, including nasal congestion, rhinorrhea, itching, and sneezing. Guidelines recommend intranasal corticosteroids as first-line treatment for moderate-to-severe allergic rhinitis (136). Corticosteroids are generally considered the most effective medications for the management of the inflammatory component of allergic rhinitis. Their efficacy is most likely related to multiple pharmacologic actions. Corticosteroids have specific effects on the inflammatory cells and chemical mediators. Intranasal glucocorticoids inhibit the uptake and/or processing, but not the presentation of antigen by airway Langerhans cells (*137,138*). The significant reduction of Langerhans cells by intranasal corticosteroids reduces the secondary inflammatory response and symptoms of allergic rhinitis. Intranasal corticosteroids reduce eosinophils and their products and there is evidence for decreased eosinophil survival. There is also a reduction in the influx of basophils and mast cells in the epithelial layers of the nasal mucosa by intranasal corticosteroids. They also reduce T cells and subclasses in the epithelium. Intranasal corticosteroids reduce the levels of mRNA and protein for IL-3, IL-4, IL-5, and IL-13, and their receptors (*139,140*). They may also reduce the release of preformed and newly generated mediators, such as histamine (*141*), tryptase, prostanoids (*142*), and leukotrienes (*143*). Intranasal corticosteroids can also act on IgE production and inhibit seasonal increases in ragweed-specific IgE antibodies (*144*).

Studies in patients with allergic rhinitis have demonstrated that these effects of intranasal steroids on rhinitis symptoms are dependent on local activity of the steroids (*145*). When administered topically, the steroid molecule diffuses across the target cell membrane and enters the cytoplasm, where it binds to the glucocorticoid receptor. After the association of corticosteroid and receptor, the activated glucocorticoid receptor enters the cell nucleus, where it attaches as a dimer to specific sites on DNA in the promoter region of steroid-responsive genes. The effect of this interaction is to either induce or suppress gene transcription. The mRNA transcripts induced during this process then undergo posttranscriptional processing and are transported to the cytoplasm for translation by ribosomes, with subsequent production of new proteins. After posttranslational processing occurs, the new proteins are either released for extracellular activity or retained by the cell for intracellular activity. In addition, the activated glucocorticoid receptors may interact directly with other transcription factors in the cytoplasm and alter the steroid responsiveness of the target cell.

At the present time, several nasal corticosteroids are available for treating allergic rhinitis. These include beclomethasone dipropionate, flunisolide, triamcinolone acetonide, budesonide, fluticasone propionate, fluticasone furoate, mometasone furoate, and soon ciclesonide will be released. With the exception of beclomethasone dipropionate, these drugs are quickly metabolized to less active metabolites, have minimal systemic absorption, and have been associated with few systemic side effects. The total bioavailability of intranasal budesonide is 20% (*146*). The total bioavailability of intranasal mometasone is 0.1%, and that of fluticasone propionate is 2% (*147*). The bioavailability of fluticasone furoate is 0.5% (*148*). The intranasal bioavailability of intranasal triamcinolone acetonide is unknown. There are no reliable data regarding the bioavailability of beclomethasone dipropionate by any route. Unlike other intranasal steroids, beclomethasone dipropionate is metabolized to an active metabolite, beclomethasone-17-monopropionate, and a relatively inactive metabolite, beclomethasone-21-monopropionate and beclomethasone (149,150). Ciclesonide is a prodrug that is enzymatically converted to the active molecule desciclesonide (Des-CIC). The active molecule has an affinity for the glucocorticoid receptor that is 120 times higher than the parent compound. Des-CIC is 99% protein bound. There is a high first-pass effect that contributes to the overall low bioavailability of Des-CIC (undetectable) (151).

In terms of systemic side effects, laboratory evaluations of the hypothalamic-pituitary-adrenal axis by multiple means have shown minimal or no suppression (152). When compared with placebo, osteocalcin, a marker of bone turnover, and eosinophilia were unaffected by a variety of intranasal corticosteroids. This suggests that the systemic glucocorticoid burden was insignificant (153). In octogenarians using intranasal corticosteroids, there was no increase in bone fracture regardless of the dose (154). There are not enough data to draw a definite conclusion on the effects of intranasal corticosteroids in the eyes. However, a recent retrospective chart review study of 12 patients showed that intranasal corticosteroid use resulted in an increase in intraocular pressure. There were significant reductions in intraocular pressures observed after discontinuation of intranasal corticosteroids (155). In another study, similar effects on intraocular pressure were observed with intranasal or inhaled beclomethasone dipropionate (157). A 2006 position statement review by the Joint Task Force for the American Academy of Allergy, Asthma and Immunology and the American College of Allergy, Asthma and Immunology on the safety of intranasal corticosteroids stated that the effects of intranasal corticosteroids on eyes and bone are inconclusive because of the lack of sufficient data (157). However, it was strongly recommended that a physician should monitor the use of intranasal corticosteroids because adverse effects from their use can be insidious and may not be evident for many years. Patients may be using other topical corticosteroids which may increase their total steroid burden.

Long-term use of intranasal steroids does not appear to cause significant risk for adverse morphologic effects in the nasal mucosa. In a study of patients with perennial rhinitis treated with mometasone for 12 months, nasal biopsy specimens showed a decrease in focal metaplasia, no change in epithelial thickness, and no sign of atrophy (*158*). In a study of intranasal steroid treatment in 90 patients with perennial rhinitis, nasal biopsy specimens revealed normalization of the nasal mucosa at the end of the 12-month study period (*159*).

Although intranasal corticosteroids may vary in their sensory attributes (e.g., taste or smell) and thus in degree of patient acceptance and adherence, there do not appear to be any clear clinically relevant differences in efficacy among them (160). Intranasal steroids have been helpful in relieving the common allergic symptoms of the upper airway, such as sneezing, congestion, and rhinorrhea. In addition, they may be of value in relieving throat pruritus, cough associated with allergic rhinitis, watery itchy eyes associated with allergic conjunctivitis, and improvement of asthma (161).

The major side effects of intranasal steroids include local dryness or irritation in the form of sting, burning, or sneezing (Table 26.4). Prolonged administration of intranasal corticosteroids, warrants periodic examination of the nasal cavity, especially in patients who experience nasal crusting or bleeding. Hemorrhagic crusting and perforation of the nasal septum are more common in patients who improperly point the spray toward the septal wall. This complication can be reduced by (a) tilting the head downward, (b) using a mirror when spraying into the nose, (c) using the new actuators for nasal sprays, and (d) having the right hand spray the device into the left nostril and the left hand spray the device into the right nostril. The risk of perforation is usually greatest during the first 12 months of treatment. The majority of cases involve young women (162). The development of aqueous formulations has reduced the incidence of local irritation with intranasal steroids; the subsequent reduction in local irritation with those preparations has increased their use in children.

Initially, some patients may require topical decongestants before administering intranasal steroids. In some patients, the congestion is so severe that a 3- to 5-day course of oral corticosteroids is required to allow delivery of the intranasal steroids. In contrast to decongestant nasal sprays, it is suggested that patients be informed that intranasal steroids should be used prophylactically as the maximum benefit is not immediate and may take weeks. Although a delayed onset of action with intranasal steroids may occur in some patients, many patients have a clinically evident onset of action during the first day of administration (163, 164, 165). Some studies suggest using intranasal steroids on an as-needed basis by many patients, but for some patients, optimal effectiveness is achieved only with regular use 166, 167). Fluticasone dipropionate nasal spray delivered on an as-needed basis has been shown to be more effective than as needed H_1-receptor antagonists in the treatment of seasonal allergic rhinitis (168).

Intranasal Corticosteroid Injection

Intranasal corticosteroid injections are used in the management of patients with common allergic and nonallergic nasal conditions such as nasal polyposis. A recent study reported that intrapolyp steroid injection is associated with a significantly lower rate of complications than surgical excision of sinonasal polyps. Steroid injections also may decrease the need for further surgical intervention for polyps (169). However, with the advent of newer and safer intranasal steroids, the use of this technique has decreased in recent years. Turbinate injections have two major adverse effects that are not seen with intranasal corticosteroid sprays: (a) adrenal suppression secondary to absorption of the steroid, and (b) absorption of steroid emboli, which may lead to transient or permanent loss of vision.

Systemic Corticosteroids

Many allergists regard systemic corticosteroids as inappropriate therapy for patients with mild-to-moderate allergic rhinitis. Although rhinitis is not a threat to life, it can seriously impair the quality of it, and some patients respond only to corticosteroids. In addition, when the topical steroid cannot be adequately distributed in the nose because of marked obstruction, it will not be effective. In such cases, the blocked nose can be opened by giving systemic corticosteroid for 3 to 7 days, and the improvement can then be maintained by topical corticosteroid spray. It is essential always to relate the risk for side effects to the dosage given, and especially to the length of the treatment period. When short-term systemic steroid treatment is given for 1 to 2 weeks, it can be a valuable and safe supplement to topical treatments in the management of severe allergic rhinitis or nasal polyposis. As in the use of topical corticosteroids, however, systemic steroids should be reserved for severe cases that cannot be controlled by routine measures. They should be used for a limited period and never on a chronic basis.

TABLE 26.4   COMPLICATIONS OF NASAL CORTICOSTEROID SPRAYS

Systemic Reactions
  Common (>5% incidence)
    Headaches
  Uncommon (<5% incidence)
    Nausea and vomiting
    Loss of sense of taste and smell
    Dizziness and light-headedness
    Nasal bleeding
  Rare
    Increased intraocular pressure (with very high doses)

Local Reactions
  Nasal burning and stinging
  Sneezing, sinus congestion, watery eyes, throat irritation, bad taste in the mouth
  Drying of the mucous membranes with epistaxis or bloody discharge
  Perforation of nasal septum (more likely from sinusitis or after septal repair)

Antihistamines

Antihistamines are the foundation of symptomatic therapy and are most useful in controlling the symptoms of sneezing, rhinorrhea, and pruritus that occur in allergic rhinitis. Antihistamines are compounds of varied chemical structure that have the property of antagonizing some of the actions of histamine. Histamine acts through four receptors referred to as H_1, H_2, H_3, and H_4. Stimulation of the H_1 receptor produces many of the symptoms of rhinitis and asthma, including smooth muscle contraction, increased vascular permeability, increased mucous production, and activation of sensory nerves that cause itching and sneezing. Stimulation of the H_2 receptor causes gastric acid secretion and some vascular dilation. The H_3 receptor appears to be localized exclusively to nerve endings in the brain where it has an autoregulatory role in histamine secretion (170). The H_4 receptor is a recently described histamine receptor, expressed on hematopoietic cells, and may be linked to the pathologic pathways of allergy (171).

H_1 and H_2 receptors belong to the larger family of G-protein coupled receptors involved in cell signal transduction. Antihistamines are competitive antagonists of the histamine H_1 receptor. By occupying the H_1 receptor sites on effector cells without activating the cells, antihistamines block H_1 receptor binding and activation by histamine. Newer studies have shown that antihistamines function by way of constitutive signaling of G-protein coupled receptors, whereby continued activation of the H_1 receptor is downregulated, rather than blocked by antihistamines. The H_1 receptor antagonists have been reclassified as inverse agonists, because of their ability to stabilize the inactive conformation of the H_1 receptor (172).

The first-generation antihistamines (e.g., chlorpheniramine, diphenhydramine tripelennamine, and clemastine fumarate) are effective H_1-receptor antagonists. Problems associated with their use relate to side effects, which are numerous and can be severe in some patients. The most common and most important effects are anticholinergic, including dry mouth and eyes, urinary retention, and CNS effects (primarily sedation, and impairment of motor and cognitive functions). The patient may not be aware of having reduced cognitive ability, since it can occur independently of sedation (173). Large doses of first-generation antihistamines, such as diphenhydramine, are reported to cause torsades de pointes. Populations that require caution are those taking more than one antihistamine, patients with hypertension who require a diuretic, patients with hypokalemia or hypomagnesemia, and patients taking antiarrhythmic agents (174).

The central nervous system side effects can be problematic in any patient, particularly those who need to drive motor vehicles or operate complex machinery, or pay attention and learn in school. Often under recognized are the potentiating effects of alcohol and other CNS depressing drugs such as sedatives, hypnotics, and antidepressants.

Because the newer second-generation antihistamines do not appreciably penetrate the blood-brain barrier, most studies show a lack of sedation. These medications are free of anticholinergic side effects, such as dry mouth, constipation, difficulty voiding, and blurry vision. Older patients, who may have benign prostatic hypertrophy or xerostomia, usually tolerate these drugs. Because fatal cardiac arrhythmias occurred when terfenadine and astemizole were given concomitantly with erythromycin (a macrolide antibiotic), imidazole antifungal agents (ketoconazole and itraconazole), or medications that inhibit the cytochrome P450 system (175,176), these drugs have been removed from the U.S. market. The other second-generation antihistamines, loratadine, desloratadine, fexofenadine, cetrizine, and levocetrizine, have not been associated with cardiac toxicity. Second-generation antihistamines have a rapid onset of action that allows them to be taken as needed.

Azelastine is a selective H_1 receptor antagonist with structural and chemical differences that distinguish it from currently available antihistamines. Azelastine is 10 times more potent than chlorpheniramine at the H_1-receptor site (*177*). In addition to this H_1-blocking action, azelastine has demonstrated an inhibitory response on cells and chemical mediators of the inflammatory response. Azelastine prevents leukotriene generation from mast cells and basophils, and modulates the activity of eosinophils and neutrophils, macrophages, and cytokines. Azelastine has a low incidence of somnolence and does not seem to result in psychomotor impairment.

Azelastine is free of drug interactions and is a possible alternative to oral antihistamines. In certain patients, this drug may be used as a replacement for the antihistamine–intranasal corticosteroid combination (*178*). It may also demonstrate synergism when combined with an intranasal steroid (179).

Olopatadine nasal spray is another useful intranasal antihistamine. Like azelastine, it has a fast onset of action (180), and has shown efficacy in seasonal allergic rhinitis. An unpleasant taste is its most common side effect, but overall, olopatadine has been well tolerated (181).

Sympathomimetic Agents

Sympathomimetic drugs are used as vasoconstrictors for the nasal mucous membranes. The current concept regarding the mechanism of action of these agents includes two types of adrenergic receptors called á and β receptors. Activation of the á receptors results in constriction of smooth muscle in the vessels of the skin, viscera, and mucus membranes. Activation of the β receptors induces dilation of vascular smooth muscle, relaxation of bronchial smooth muscle, and cardiac stimulation. By taking advantage of drugs that stimulate á receptors, the edema of the nasal mucus membranes in allergic rhinitis can be reduced by topical or systemic administration. In large doses, these drugs induce elevated blood pressure, nervousness, and insomnia. These agents should be used with caution in patients who have hypertension, organic heart disease, angina pectoris, and hyperthyroidism. The sympathomimetic agents are also combined with antihistamines in many oral preparations to decrease the drowsiness that often accompanies antihistamine therapy.

Nose drops or nasal sprays containing sympathomimetic agents may be over used. The topical application of these drugs is often followed by a "rebound" phenomenon in which the nasal mucous membranes become even more congested and edematous. This leads the patient to use the drops or spray more frequently and in higher doses to obtain relief from nasal obstruction. The condition is called *rhinitis medicamentosa*. The patient must abruptly discontinue their use to alleviate the condition. Other measures, including a course of topical corticosteroids for a few weeks is often helpful to decrease the nasal congestion or until this distressing side effect disappears. Because of the duration of seasonal or perennial allergic rhinitis, it is best not to use topical vasoconstrictors in the allergic patient, except temporarily during periods of infectious rhinitis. The systemic use of sympathomimetic drugs has not been associated with rhinitis medicamentosa.

Leukotriene-Receptor Antagonists

The leukotriene-receptor antagonist montelukast is superior to placebo in relieving nasal symptoms in patients with allergic rhinitis (182). However, the drug is relatively weak as monotherapy. A meta-analysis demonstrated that, as compared with placebo, montelukast induced a moderate but significant reduction in scores for daily symptoms of rhinitis. In comparison, nasal corticosteroids induced a significant and substantial reduction in symptom scores (182). Thus, montelukast's role is generally as an adjunct in the treatment of a patient who does not have an adequate response to an antihistamine, a nasal corticosteroid, or both. However, there are no clear data demonstrating that leukotriene-receptor antagonists combined with either antihistamines or nasal corticosteroids reduce symptom scores more than the antihistamines or corticosteroids alone. Leukotriene-receptor antagonists, however, have shown efficacy in aspirin-sensitive rhinitis (183), and in patients who have the combination of seasonal allergic rhinitis and mild asthma 184).

Anticholinergics

Parasympathetic fibers originate in the superior salivatory nucleus of the brainstem, and relay in the sphenopalatine ganglion before distributing to the nasal glands and blood vessels. Parasympathetic stimulation causes a watery secretion, mediated by the classical autonomic transmitter acetylcholine, and a vasodilatation of blood vessels serving the glands. The muscarinic receptors of the sero-mucinous glands can be blocked by the anticholinergic drug ipratropium bromide. Ipratropium bromide, a quaternary derivative of isopropyl noratropine, is poorly absorbed by the nasal mucosa because of a low lipid solubility and does not cross the blood-brain barrier. Ipratropium bromide is effective in controlling watery nasal discharge, but it does not affect sneezing or nasal congestion in perennial allergic and nonallergic rhinitis. The drug is effective treatment for the common cold (185), gustatory rhinitis, and rhinorrhea in elderly patients. Topical side effects, due to anticholinergic action, are uncommon and usually dose-dependent in their severity. Nasal dryness, irritation and burning are the most prominent effects, followed by a stuffy nose, dry mouth, and headache. Since patients with perennial rhinitis usually suffer also from nasal congestion, itching, and sneezing, other drugs are preferable as first-line agents to ipratropium in the vast majority of cases of allergic rhinitis. Ipratropium combination with an intranasal glucocorticosteroid or an H_1-antihistamine may be considered in patients where rhinorrhea is the predominant symptom, or in patients with rhinorrhea who are not fully responsive to other therapies.

Intranasal Cromolyn

Cromolyn sodium is a derivative of the natural product khellin. The proposed mechanism of action of cromolyn in allergic rhinitis is to stabilize mast cell membranes, apparently by inhibiting calcium transmembrane flux and thereby preventing antigen-induced degranulation. It is effective in the management of seasonal and perennial allergic rhinitis. Cromolyn can be effective in reducing sneezing, rhinorrhea, nasal pruritus, and in a limited number of patients with nasal polyps. It has little effect on mucociliary transport. Cromolyn often prevents the symptoms of both seasonal and perennial allergic rhinitis, and diligent prophylaxis can significantly reduce both immediate and late symptoms after allergen exposures.

Adverse effects are rare and mostly include sneezing, nasal stinging, nasal burning, transient headache, and an unpleasant aftertaste. For management of seasonal rhinitis, treatment should begin 2 to 4 weeks before contact with the offending allergens, and should be continued throughout the period of exposure. Because cromolyn has a delayed onset, concurrent antihistamine therapy is usually necessary to control symptoms. It is essential for the patient to understand the rate and extent of response to be expected from intranasal cromolyn and that, because the product is prophylactic, it must be used on a regular basis for maximum benefit. In the United States, cromolyn nasal spray is available without prescription.

Several studies have compared the therapeutic efficacy of cromolyn nasal solution with that of the intranasal corticosteroids in allergic rhinitis. In both perennial and seasonal allergic rhinitis, intranasal steroids are reported to be more effective than cromolyn. Cromolyn is usually less effective than oral or intranasal antihistamines (*186*).

Immunotherapy

Allergen immunotherapy is defined as the repeated administration of specific allergens to patients with IgE-mediated conditions to provide protection against the allergic symptoms and inflammatory reactions associated with natural exposure to these allergens (187). Other terms that have been used for allergen immunotherapy include h*yposensitization, allergen-specific desensitization*, and the lay terms, *allergy shots* or *allergy injections*.

The immunologic changes associated with immunotherapy are complex. Allergen immunotherapy generates T-reg cells, IL-10 and TGF-B (188,189). Data indicate that increased production of IL-12, a strong inducer of T_H1 responses, contributes to this shift. Successful immunotherapy results in generation of a population of T-reg cells, which are $CD4^+CD25^+$ T-lymphocytes producing IL-10, TGF-β, or both (190–192). IL-10 reduces proinflammatory cytokine release from mast cells, eosinophils, and T cells, and illicits tolerance to T cells by means of selective inhibition of the CD28 costimulatory pathway (191,192).

In patients receiving immunotherapy, initially there is an increase in specific IgE antibody levels, followed by a gradual decrease to a level that is still higher than that present before treatment. Clinical improvement in many patients develops before decreases in their IgE antibody levels occur, or in other patients whose IgE antibody levels never decrease. This demonstrates that efficacy is not dependent on reductions in specific IgE levels (*193,194*). Immunotherapy does diminish the seasonal increase in specific IgE levels (*195*). Suppression of late-phase inflammatory responses in the skin and respiratory tract generally also occur with allergen immunotherapy (196). Allergen-specific IgG induced from immunotherapy can block IgE-dependent histamine release and allergen IgE complexes that present to B cells (197).

The severity of allergic rhinitis and its complications is a spectrum varying from minimal to marked symptoms, and from short to prolonged durations. Indications for immunotherapy, a fairly long-term treatment modality, are relative rather than absolute. Allergen immunotherapy should be considered for patients who (a) continue to have moderate-to-severe symptoms despite therapy, (b) require systemic corticosteroids, (c) have an inadequate response to the recommended doses of nasal corticosteroids, or (d) have coexisting conditions such as asthma or chronic sinusitis.

A frequent cause of treatment failure is that a patient expects too much, too soon, and thus prematurely discontinues the injection program because of dissatisfaction. The magnitude of symptom reduction during immunotherapy is variable, although in some trials, patients had a reduction of more than two-thirds in symptoms and medication scores (198). In one study of adults with allergic rhinitis who were treated with immunotherapy, a reduction of two-thirds in symptoms and medication scores persisted for at least 3 years after the termination of treatment (198). In a study of children with allergic rhinitis between the ages of 6 and 14 years, those who were treated with immunotherapy had a significantly lower rate of the development of asthma up to 7 years after completing immunotherapy (199). In the subgroup of children who were sensitized to only a single allergen (house dust mite), as distinguished from those sensitized to multiple allergens, the likelihood that IgE antibodies would develop to new allergens was markedly lower among patients who had undergone immunotherapy than among those who had not (200,201). Allergy immunotherapy is a cost-effective therapy which results in long-term benefits (202). It is the only intervention for allergic rhinitis that alters the natural history of the disease. However, a major drawback to use of this treatment is the risk of systemic reactions. Approximately 5% to 10% of patients who receive allergen immunotherapy have systemic reactions, which are moderately severe in 1% to 3% of patients. Rarely, patients have died from anaphylaxis secondary to allergy immunotherapy (203).

Allergen immunotherapy can also be administered sublingually. Although mild oral and sublingual itching and swelling occurs, systemic reactions are rare. A recent review of subcutaneous vs. sublingual therapy determined that, although sublingual is safer than subcutaneous therapy, sublingual therapy (SLIT) is only about one-half as effective (204). Given the safety profile of SLIT, it would be potentially beneficial in high-risk and pediatric patients. Currently within the United States, there is no approved form of SLIT and there is no consensus on a therapeutic dose or overall feasibility of employing multiple allergens as opposed to treatment with grass pollen extracts as immunotherapy.

Another potential approach to immunotherapy involves the use of agents that stimulate the innate immune system through specialized toll-like receptors (TLRs): either TLR-9 (stimulated by immunostimulatory sequences of DNA) (205) or TLR-4 (206), or immunization with peptides of allergens.

Omalizumab (anti-IgE antibody) has also been studied in the treatment of allergic rhinitis. Omalizumab is effective in both allergen challenge studies and clinical trials. Multiple randomized, double-blind, placebo-controlled studies have shown efficacy of omalizumab in seasonal (207,208) and perennial allergic rhinitis (209,210). In an open-label study of dust mite allergic rhinitis, even a low dose of omalizumab led to a significant reduction of nasal mean total symptom scores after nasal challenge with dust mites (211). Unfortunately, at present, the cost of omalizumab is prohibitive for the routine treatment of allergic rhinitis. It is primarily indicated in the treatment of severe persistent allergic asthma.

■ REFERENCES

1. Dykewicz MS, Fineman S. Executive summary of joint task force practice parameters on diagnosis and management of rhinitis. *Ann Allergy Asthma Immunol.* 1998;81:463–468.

2. Bousquet J, Van Cauwenberge P, Khaltaev N. ARIA Workshop Group, World Health Organization. Allergic rhinitis and its impact on asthma. *J Allergy Clin Immunol.* 2001;108:S147–S334.

11. Arshad SH, Bateman B, Sadeghnejad A, et al. Prevention of allergic disease during childhood by allergen avoidance: the Isle of Wight prevention study. *J Allergy Clin Immunol.* 2007;119:307–313.

12. Skoner DP. Allergic rhinitis: definition, epidemiology, pathophysiology, detection, and diagnosis. *J Allergy Clin Immunol.* 2001;108 (Suppl):S2–S8.

20. Graf N, Johansen P, Schindler C, et al. Analysis of the relationship between pollinosis and date of birth in Switzerland. *Int Arch Allergy Immunol.* 2007;143:269–275.

21. Morais-Almeida M, Gaspar A, Pires G, et al. Risk factors for asthma symptoms at school age: an 8-year prospective study. *Allergy Asthma Proc.* 2007;28:183–189.

23. Piippo-Savolainen E, Remes S, Korppi M. Does early exposure or sensitization to inhalant allergens predict asthma in wheezing infants? A 20-year follow-up. *Allergy Asthma Proc.* 2007; 28:454–461.

26. Stempel DA, Woolf R. The cost of treating allergic rhinitis. *Curr Allergy Asthma Resp.* 2002;2:223–230.

27. Leynaert B, Neukirch C, Liard R, et al. Quality of life in allergic rhinitis and asthma. A population-based study of young adults. *Am J Respir Crit Care Med.* 2000;162:1391–1396.

28. Nathan RA. The burden of allergic rhinitis. *Allergy Asthma Proc.* 2007;28:3–9.

29. Casale TB, Dykewicz MS. Clinical implications of the allergic rhinitis-asthma link. *Am J Med Sci.* 2004;327:127–138.

30. Nayak AS. The asthma and allergic rhinitis link. *Allergy Asthma Proc.* 2003;24:395–402.

36. Spector SL, Nicklas RA, Chapman JA, et al. Symptom severity assessment of allergic rhinitis: part 1. *Ann Allergy Asthma Immunol.* 2003;91:105–114.

37. Blaiss MS. Important aspects in management or allergic rhinitis. Compliance, costs, and quality of life. *Allergy Asthma Proc.* 2003; 24:231–238.

38. Lamb CE, Ratner PH, Johnson CE, et al. Economic impact of workplace productivity losses due to allergic rhinitis compared with select medical conditions in the United States from an employer perspective. *Curr Med Res Opin.* 2006;22:1203–1210.

39. Schoenwetter WF, Dupclay L Jr, Appajosula S, et al. Economic impact and quality-of-life burden of allergic rhinitis. *Curr Med Res Opin.* 2004;20:305–317.

41. van Beijsterveldt CE, Boomsma DI. Genetics of parentally reported asthma, eczema and rhinitis in 5-yr-old twins. *Eur Respir J.* 2007;29:516–521.

42. Ober C. Susceptibility genes in asthma and allergy. *Curr Allergy Asthma Rep.* 2001;1:174–179.

44. Slavin RG. The allergist and the workplace: occupational asthma and rhinitis. *All Asthma Proc.* 2005;26:255–261.

45. Niggemann B, Beyer K. Pitfalls in double-blind, placebo-controlled oral food challenges. *Allergy.* 2007;62:729–732.

46. Bush RK. Approach to patients with symptoms of food allergy. *Am J Med.* 2008;121:376–378.

47. Sicherer SH. Clinical implicaton of cross reaction food allergens. *J Allergy Clin Immunol.* 2001; 108:881–890.

48. Rolland JM, O'Hehir RE. Latex allergy: a model for therapy. *Clin Exp Allergy.* 2008;38:898–912.

49. Peden DB. Effect of pollutants in rhinitis. *Curr Allergy Asthma Rep.* 2001;1:242–246.

52. Greenberger PA. Interactions between rhinitis and asthma. *Allergy Asthma Proc.* 204;25:89–93.

53. Takizawa R, Pawankar R, Yamagishi S, et al. Increased expression of HLA-DR and CD86 in nasal epithelial cells in allergic rhinitis: antigen presentation to T cells and up-regulation by diesel exhaust particles. *Clin Exp Allergy.* 2007;37:420–433.

54. Godthelp T, Fokkens WJ, Kleinjan A, et al. Antigen presenting cells in the nasal mucosa of patients with allergic rhinitis during allergen provocation. *Clin Exp Allergy.* 1996;26:677–688.

55. Chomarat P, Banchereau J. Interleukin-4 and interleukin-13: their similarities and discrepancies. *Int Rev Immunol.* 1998;17:1–52.

56. Jabara HH, Chaudhuri J, Dutt S, et al. B-cell receptor cross-linking delays activation-induced cytidine deaminase induction and inhibits class-switch recombination to IgE. *J Allergy Clin Immunology.* 2008; 121:191–196.

57. Rosenwasser L. New insights into the pathophysiology of allergic rhinitis. *Allergy Asthma Proc.* 2007;28:10–15.

59. Iwasaki M, Saito K, Takemura M, et al. TNF-alpha contributes to the development of allergic rhinitis in mice. *J Allergy Clin Immunol.* 2003;112:134–140.

60. Cates EC, Gajewska BU, Goncharova S, et al. Effect of GM-CSF on immune, inflammatory, and clinical responses to ragweed in a novel mouse model of mucosal sensitization. *J Allergy Clin Immunol.* 2003;111:1076–1086.

61. Salib RJ, Kumar S, Wilson SJ, et al. Nasal mucosal immunoexpression of the mast cell chemoattractants TGF-beta, eotaxin, and stem cell factor and their receptors in allergic rhinitis. *J Allergy Clin Immunol.* 2004;114:799–806.

62. Togias A. Unique mechanistic features of allergic rhinitis. *J Allergy Clin Immunol.* 2000;105:S599–S604.

63. Hansen I, Klimek L, Mosges R, et al. Mediators of inflammation in the early and late phase of allergic rhinitis. *Curr Opin Allergy Clin Immunol.* 2004;4:159–163.

66. Ponikau JU, Sherris DA, Kephart GM, et al. Striking deposition of toxic eosinophil major basic protein in mucus: implications for chronic rhinosinusitis. *J Allergy Clin Immunol.* 2005;116:362–369.

71. Greiff L, Andersson M, Erjefalt JS, et al. Airway microvascular extravasation and luminal entry of plasma. *Clin Physiol Funct Imaging.* 2003;23:301–306.

72. Tos M. Distribution of mucus producing elements in the respiratory tract. Differences between upper and lower airway. *Eur J Respir Dis Suppl.* 1983;128:269–279.

75. Schwindt CD, Hutcheson PS, Leu SY, et al. Role of intradermal skin tests in the evaluation of clinically relevant respiratory allergy assessed using patient history and nasal challenges. *Ann Allergy Asthma Immunol.* 205;94:627–633.

83. Malm L, Gerth van Wijk R, Bachert C. Guidelines for nasal provocations with aspects on nasal patency, airflow, and airflow resistance. International Committee on Objective Assessment of the Nasal Airways, International Rhinologic Society. *Rhinology.* 2000;38:1–6.

84. Stubner UP, Gruber D, Berger UE. The influence of female sex hormones on nasal reactivity in seasonal allergic rhinitis. *Allergy.* 1999;54:865–871.

87. Szczeklik A, Stevenson DD. Aspirin-induced asthma: advances in pathogensis, diagnosis, and management. *J Allergy Clin Immunol.* 2003;111:913–921.

88. Varga EM, Jacobson MR, Masuyama K, et al. Inflammatory cell populations and cytokine mRNA expression in the nasal mucosa in aspirin-sensitive rhinitis. *Eur Respir J.* 1999;14:610–615.

89. Corrigan C, Mallett K, Ying S, et al. Expression of the cysteinyl leukotriene receptors LT (1) and cys LT(2) in aspirin sensitive and aspirin–tolerant chronic rhinosinusitis. *J Allergy Clin Immunol.* 2005; 115:316–322.

92. Gluck JC. The change of asthma course during pregnancy. *Clin Rev Allergy Immunol.* 2004;26:171–180.

94. Ricketti AJ, Cleri DJ, Porwancher RB, et al. Cerebrospinal fluid leak mimicking allergic rhinitis. *Allergy Asthma Proc.* 2005; 26:125–128.

95. Abuabara A. Cerebrospinal fluid rhinorrhea: diagnosis and management. *Med Oral Patol Oral Cir Bucal.* 2007;12:E397–E400.

96. Daudia A, Biswas D, Jones NS. Risk of meningitis with cerebrospinal fluid rhinorrhea. *Ann Otol Rhinol Laryngol.* 2007;116:902–905.

98. Meco C, Oberascher G. Comprehensive algorithm for skull base dural lesion and cerebrospinal fluid fistula diagnosis. *Laryngoscope.* 2004; 114:991–999.

99. Roche PH, Paris J, Regis J, et al. Management of invasive juvenile nasopharyngeal angiofibromas: the role of a multimodality approach. *Neurosurgery.* 2007;61:768–777.

101. Noone PG, Leigh MW, Sannuti A, et al. Primary ciliary dyskinesia: diagnostic and phenotypic features. *Am J Resp Crit Care Med.* 2004; 169:459–467.

105. Keh SM, Facer P, Simpson KD, et al. Increased nerve fiber expressions of sensory sodium channels Nav 1.7, Nav 1.8, Nav 1.9 in rhinitis. *Laryngoscope.* 2008;118:573–579.

106. Garcia GJ, Bailie N, Martins DA, et al. Atopic rhinitis: a CFD study of air conditioning in the nasal cavity. *J Appl Physiol.* 2007;103:1082–1092.

107. Berger WE, Schonfeld JE. Nonallergic rhinitis in children. *Curr Allergy Asthma Resp.* 2007;7:112–116.

108. Euler AR. Upper respiratory tract complications of gastroesophageal reflux in adult and pediatric-age patients. *Dig Dis.* 1998;16:111–117.

109. Halstead LA. Role of gastroesophageal reflux in pediatric upper airway disorders. *Otolaryngol Head Neck Surg.* 1999;120:208–214.

110. Marple BF. Allergic fungal rhinosinusitis: current theories and management strategies. *Laryngoscope.* 2001;111:1006–1019.

111. Schubert MS, Goetz DW. Evaluation and treatment of allergic fungal sinusitis. I. Demographics and diagnosis. *J Allergy Clin Immunol.* 1998;102:387–394.

112. Manning SC, Holman M. Further evidence for allergic pathophysiology in allergic fungal sinusitis. *Laryngoscope.* 1988;108:1485–1496.

113. Huchton DM. Allergic fungal sinusitis: an otorhinolaryngologic perspective. *Allergy Asthma Proc.* 2003;24:307–311.

116. Burgess JA, Walters EH, Byrnes GB, et al. Childhood allergic rhinitis predicts asthma incidence and persistence to middle age: a longitudinal study. *J Allergy Clin Immunol.* 2007;120:863–869.

117. von Mutius E, Weiland SK, Fritzsch C, et al. Increasing prevalence of hay fever and atopy among children in Leipzig, East Germany. *Lancet.* 1998;351:862–866.

124. Canova CR, Downs SH, Knoblauch A, et al. Increased prevalence of perennial allergic rhinitis in patients with obstructive sleep apnea. *Respiration.* 2004;71:138–143.

125. Ohashi Y, Nakai Y, Tanaka A, et al. Soluble intercellular adhesion molecule-1 level in sera is elevated in perennial allergic rhinitis. *Laryngoscope.* 1997;107:932–935.

126. Custovic A, Green R, Taggart SC, et al. Domestic allergens in public places. II. Dog (Can f 1) and cockroach (Bla g 2) allergens in dust and mite, cat, dog and cockroach allergens in the air in public buildings. *Clin Exp Allergy.* 1996:26:1246–1252.

127. Perzanowski MS, Ronmark E, Nold B, et al. Relevance of allergens from cats and dogs to asthma in the northern-most province of Sweden: schools as a major site of exposure. *J Allergy Clin Immunol.* 1999;103:1018–1024.

128. Almqvist C, Larsson PH, Egmar AC, et al. School as a risk environment for children allergic to cats and a site for transfer of cat allergen to homes. *J Allergy Clin Immunol.* 1999;103:1012–1017.

133. Chew GL, Carlton EJ, Kass D, et al. Determinants of cockroach and mouse exposure and associations with asthma in families and elderly individuals living in New York City public housing. *Ann Allergy Asthma Immunol.* 2006;97:502–513.

134. Eggleston PA, Wood RA, Rand C, et al. Removal of cockroach allergen from inner-city homes. *J Allergy Clin Immunol.* 1999;104:842–846.

135. Gergen PJ, Mortimer KM, Eggleston PA, et al. Results of the National Cooperative Inner-City Asthma Study (NCICAS) environmental intervention to reduce cockroach allergen exposure in inner-city homes. *J Allergy Clin Immunol.* 1999;103:501–506.

136. van Cauwenberge P, Bachert C, Passalaqua G, et al. Consensus statement on the treatment of allergic rhinitis. European Academy of Allergology and Clinical Immunology. *Allergy.* 2000;55:116–134.

147. Daley-Yates PT, Kunka RL, Yin Y, et al. Bioavailability of fluticasone propionate and mometasone furoate aqueous nasal sprays. *Eur J Clin Pharmacol.* 2004;60:265–268.

148. Allen A, Down G, Newland A, et al. Absolute bioavailability of intranasal fluticasone furoate in healthy subjects. *Clin Ther.* 2007;29:1415–1420.

149. Falcoz C, Kirby SM, Smith J, et al. Pharmacokinetics and systemic exposure of inhaled beclomethasone dipropionate. *Eur Resp J.* 1996; 9(Suppl 23):162S.

150. Daley-Yates PT, Price AC, Sisson JR, et al. Beclomethasone dipropionate: absolute bioavailability, pharmacokinetics, and metabolism following intravenous, oral, intranasal, and inhaled administration in man. *Br J Clin Pharmacol.* 2001;51:400–409.

151. Nave R, Wingertzahn MA, Brookman S, et al. Safety, tolerability and exposure of ciclesonide nasal spray in healthy and asymptomatic subjects with seasonal allergic rhinitis. *J Clin Pharmacol.* 2006;46: 461–467.

152. Wilson AM, McFarlane LC, Lipworth BJ. Effect of repeated once daily dosing of three intranasal corticosteroids on basal and dynamic measurements of hypothalamic-pituitary-adrenal axis activity. *J Allergy Clin Immunol.* 1998;101:470–474.

153. Wilson AM, Sims EJ, McFarlane LC, et al. Effects of intranasal corticosteroids on adrenal, bone, and blood markers of systemic activity in allergic rhinitis. *J Allergy Clin Immunol.* 1998;102:598–604.

154. Suissa S, Baltzan M, Kremer R, et al. Inhaled and nasal corticosteroid use and the risk of fracture. *Am J Respir Crit Care Med.* 2004;169:83–88.

155. Bui CM, Chen H, Shyr Y, et al. Discontinuing nasal steroids might lower intraocular pressure in glaucoma. *J Allergy Clin Immunol.* 2005;116:1042–1047.

157. Bielory L, Blaiss M, Fineman SM, et al. Concerns about intranasal corticosteroids for over-the-counter use: position statement of the Joint Task Force for the American Academy of Allergy, Asthma and Immunology. *Ann Allergy Asthma Immunol.* 2006;96:514–525.

160. Meltzer EO. Intranasal steroids: managing allergic rhinitis and tailoring treatment to patient preference. *Allergy Asthma Proc.* 2005;26:445–451.

161. Adams RJ, Fuhlbrigge AL, Finkelstein JA, et al. Intranasal steroids and the risk of emergency department visits for asthma. *J Allergy Clin Immunol.* 2002;109:636–642.

164. Selner JC, Weber RW, Richmond GW, et al. Onset of action of aqueous beclomethasone dipropionate nasal spray in seasonal allergic rhinitis. *Clin Ther.* 1995;17:1099–1109.

168. Kaszuba SM, Baroody FM, deTineo M, et al. Superiority of an intranasal corticosteroid compared with an oral antihistamine in the as-needed treatment of seasonal allergic rhinitis. *Arch Intern Med.* 2001;161:2581–2587.

169. Becker SS, Rasamny JK, Han JK, et al. Steroid injection for sinonasal polyps: the University of Virginia experience. *Am J Rhinol.* 2007;21:64–69.

170. Morisset S, Rouleau A, Ligneau X, et al. High constitutive activity of native H_3 receptors regulates histamine neurons in brain. *Nature.* 2000;408:860–864.

171. Thurmond RL, Gelfand EW, Dunford PJ. The role of histamine H1 and H4 receptors in allergic inflammation: the search for new antihistamines. *Nat Rev Drug Discov.* 2008;7:41–53.

172. Bakker RA, Wieland K, Timmerman H, et al. Constitutive activity of the histamine H1 receptor reveals inverse agonism of histamine H1 receptor antagonists. *Eur J Pharmacol.* 2000;387:R5–R7.

173. Bower EA, Moore JL, Moss M, et al. The effects of single-dose fexofenadine, diphenhydramine, and placebo on cognitive performance in flight personnel. *Aviat Space Environ Med.* 2003;74:145–152.

174. Weiler JM, Bloomfield JR, Woodworth GG, et al. Effects of fexofenadine, diphenhydramine, and alcohol on driving performance. *Ann Intern Med.* 2000;132:354–363.

175. Taglialatela M, Castaldo P, Pannaccione A, et al. Cardiac ion channels and antihistamines: possible mechanisms of cardiotoxicity. *Clin Exp Allergy.* 1999;29:182–189.

176. Simons FE. Advances in H1-antihistamines. *N Engl J Med.* 2004:351:2203–2217.

179. Bernstein JA. Azelastine hydrochloride: a review of pharmacology, pharmacokinetics, clinical efficacy and tolerability. *Curr Med Res Opin.* 2007;23:2441–2452.

180. Patel D, Garadi R, Brubaker M, et al. Onset and duration of action of nasal sprays in seasonal allergic rhinitis patients: olopatadine hydrochloride versus mometasone furoate monohydrate. *Allergy Asthma Proc.* 2007;28:592–599.

181. Fairchild CJ, Meltzer EO, Roland PS, et al. Comprehensive report of the efficacy, safety, quality of life, and work impact of olopatadine 0.6% and olopatadine 0.4% treatment in patients with seasonal allergic rhinitis. *Allergy Asthma Proc.* 2007;28:716–723.

182. Wilson AM, O'Byrne PM, Parameswaran K. Leukotriene receptor antagonist for allergic rhinitis: a systematic review and meta-analysis. *Am J Med.* 2004;116:338–344.

183. Parnes SM. The role of leukotriene inhibitors in patients with paranasal sinus disease. *Curr Opin Otolaryngol Head Neck Surg.* 2003;11:184–191.

184. Baena-Cagnani CE, Berger WE, DuBuske LM, et al. Comparative effects of desloratadine versus montelukast on asthma symptoms and use of beta 2-agonists in patients with seasonal allergic rhinitis and asthma. *Int Arch Allergy Immunol.* 2003;130:307–313.

187. Lox L, Ji JT, Nelson H, et al. Allergen immunotherapy: a practice parameters second update. *J Allergy Clin Immunol.* 2007;120:S25–S85.

188. Akdis M, Adkis CA. Mechanisms of allergen-specific immunotherapy. *J Allergy Clin Immunol.* 2007;119:780–791.

189. Till SJ, Francis JN, Nouri-Aria K, et al. Mechanisms of immunotherapy. *J Allergy Clin Immunol.* 2004;113:1025–1034.

190. Blaser K, Akdis CA. Interleukin-10, T regulatory cells and specific allergy treatment. *Clin Exp Allergy.* 2004;34:328–331.

191. Francis JN, Till SJ, Durham SR. Induction of IL-10$^+$CD4$^+$CD25$^+$ T cells by grass pollen immunotherapy. *J Allergy Clin Immunol.* 2003;111:1255–1261.

192. Jutel M, Akdis M, Budak F, et al. IL-10 and TGF-beta cooperate in the regulatory T cell response to mucosal allergens in normal immunity and specific immunotherapy. *Eur J Immunol.* 2003;33:1205–1214.

196. Rak S, Lowhagen O, Venge P. The effect of immunotherapy on bronchial hyperresponsiveness and eosinophil cationic protein in pollen allergic patients. *J Allergy Clin Immunol.* 1988;82:470–480.

197. Wachholz PA, Soni NK, Till SJ, et al. Inhibition of allergen-IgE binding to B cells by IgG antibodies after grass pollen immunotherapy. *J Allergy Clin Immunol.* 2003;112:915–922.

198. Durham SR, Walker SM, Varga EM, et al. Long-term clinical efficacy of grass-pollen immunotherapy. *N Engl J Med.* 1999;341:468–475.

199. Jacobsen L, Niggemann B, Dreborg S, et al. Specific immunotherapy has long-term preventive effect of seasonal and perennial asthma: 10-year follow-up on the PAT study. *Allergy.* 2007;62:943–948.

200. Des Roches A, Paradis L, Menardo JL, et al. Immunotherapy with a standardized Dermatophagoides pteronyssinus extract. VI. Specific immunotherapy prevents the onset of new sensitizations in children. *J Allergy Clin Immunol.* 1997;99:450–453.

201. Pajno GB, Barberio G, DeLuca F, et al. Prevention of new sensitizations in asthmatic children monosensitized to house dust mite by specific immunotherapy. A six-year follow-up study. *Clin Exp Allergy.* 2001;31:1392–1397.

202. Dykewicz MS, Fineman S, Skoner DP, et al. Diagnosis and management of rhinitis: complete guidelines of the Joint Task Force on Practice Parameters in Allergy, Asthma and Immunology. *Ann Allergy Asthma Immunol.* 1998;81:478–518.

203. Joint Task Force on Practice Parameters; American Academy of Allergy, Asthma and Immunology; American College of Allergy, Asthma and Immunology; Joint Council of Allergy, Asthma and Immunolgy. The diagnosis and management of anaphylaxis: an updated practice parameter. *J Allergy Clin Immunol.* 2005;115(3 Suppl 2):S483–S523.

204. Nelson H. Allergen immunotherapy: where is it now? *J Allergy Clin Immunol.* 2007;119:769–779.

205. Simons FE, Shikishima Y, Van Nest G, et al. Selective immune redirection in humans with ragweed allergy by injecting Amb a 1 linked to immunostimulatory DNA. *J Allergy Clin Immunol.* 2004;113:1144–1151.

206. Wheeler AW, Woroniecki SR. Allergy vaccines—new approaches to an old concept. *Expert Opin Biol Ther.* 2004;4:1473–1481.

207. Casale TB. Anti-IgE (omalizumab) therapy in seasonal allergic rhinitis. *Am J Respir Crit Care Med.* 2001;164:Sl8–S21.

208. Casale TB, Busse WW, Kline JN, et al. Omalizumab pretreatment decreases acute reactions after rush immunotherapy for ragweed-induced seasonal allergic rhinitis. *J Allergy Clin Immunol.* 2006; 117:134–140.

209. Chervinsky P, Casale T, Townley R, et al. Omalizumab, an anti-IgE antibody, in the treatment of adults and adolescents with perennial allergic rhinitis. *Ann Allergy Asthma Immunol.* 2003;91:160–167.

210. Vignola AM, Humbert M, Bousquet J, et al. Efficacy and tolerability of anti-immunoglobulin E therapy with omalizumab in patients with concomitant allergic asthma and persistent allergic rhinitis: SOLAR. *Allergy.* 2004;59:709–717.

211. Corren J, Diaz-Sanchez D, Saxon A, et al. Effects of omalizumab, a humanized anti-IgE antibody, on nasal reactivity to allergen and local IgE synthesis. *Ann Allergy Asthma Immunol.* 2004;93:243–248.

CHAPTER 27

Nasal Polyposis, Sinusitis, and Nonallergic Rhinitis

TOLLY G. EPSTEIN AND DAVID I. BERNSTEIN

■ NASAL POLYPS

Nasal polyps (NPs) have been recognized and treated since ancient times. The occurrence of nasal polyps in association with asthma and aspirin sensitivity, otherwise known as the *aspirin triad*, was first identified in 1911 (1). NPs are associated with chronic mucosal inflammation; a condition often referred to as chronic hyperplastic rhinosinusitis. In most cases, NPs arise from the mucosa of the middle meatus and clefts of the ethmoid region (2,3). Polyp tissue is generally characterized by chronic eosinophilic infiltration, but plasma cells, lymphocytes, and mast cells are also typically present (4,5). Polypoid tissue is rich in ground substance containing acid mucopolysaccharide (6).

The prevalence of nasal polyposis in the general population is estimated at 2% to 4% (7,8). A recent large population based study did not reveal any gender differences (9). NPs are diagnosed more often during the third and fourth decades of life. Most clinical data indicate that there is no greater prevalence of nasal polyps among atopic compared with normal populations, however, the coexistence of allergic rhinitis may render symptom control more challenging (10,11). In a study of an adult allergy clinic population, 4.2% of patients had NPs; 71% of polyp patients had asthma; and 14% had aspirin intolerance (12). NPs are less common in children. The discovery of NPs in a child should prompt an evaluation for cystic fibrosis (CF), in which the prevalence of NPs is 6.7% to 46%. NPs are also reported to affect 37% of adults with CF (13).

Clinical Presentation

Patients with nasal polyposis present with perennial nasal congestion, rhinorrhea, and anosmia (or hyposmia). Nasal and osteomeatal obstruction may result in purulent nasal discharge and chronic sinusitis. Enlargement of NPs may lead to broadening of the nasal bridge, and rarely, encroachment into the orbit, resulting in compression of ocular structures and unilateral proptosis, falsely suggesting an orbital malignancy (14).

A thorough examination with a nasal speculum is necessary for identification of NPs. More complete visualization can be accomplished by flexible rhinoscopy. NPs appear as bulbous translucent to opaque growths, often extending from the middle and inferior nasal turbinates, causing partial or complete obstruction of the nasal canals. Frontal, ethmoidal, and maxillary tenderness with purulent nasal discharge from the middle meatus indicate concurrent acute or chronic paranasal sinusitis. Sinus radiographic studies are rarely needed to identify NPs. Common radiographic changes include widening of the ethmoid labyrinths; mucoceles or pyoceles within the paranasal sinuses; and generalized loss of translucence in the maxillary, ethmoid, and frontal sinuses (15).

Etiology

While multiple theories regarding the etiology of nasal polyposis have been proposed, the pathogenesis remains poorly defined. Allergic mechanisms have been investigated, but no consistent association has been established between atopy and nasal polyposis. Patients with NPs are less likely to be sensitized to perennial allergens than those diagnosed with allergic rhinitis (16). Mast cells and mast cell mediators are abundant in polyp tissue and eosinophils are present in 70% to 90% of cases (4). $CD8^+$ T cells are increased in polyp tissue when compared with healthy controls (17). Immunoglobulin G (IgG), IgM, IgA, and IgE levels are also elevated in polyp fluid (18).

Growth factors and cytokines that can stimulate *in vitro* proliferation of basophils, mast cells, and eosinophils are present in NP tissue (19). The potential roles of T_H1 (T-helper cell type 1) and T_H2 (T-helper cell type 2) cytokines are under investigation (20). Total IgE and IL-5 levels are higher in nasal tissue of patients having chronic rhinosinusitis (CRS) with nasal polyps (CRSwNP), compared with CRS patients without NP (CRSsNP) (21). The pathophysiology of CF-related polyp disease may be different from that of non-CF-related polyps. For example, myeloperoxidase and IL-8 are increased in polyp tissue from CF patients, whereas ECP, eotaxin, and IgE are elevated in NPs of patients without CF (22).

Microbial pathogens have been postulated to play a role in the pathogenesis of NPs by promoting inflammation. In particular, *Staphylococcus aureus*-derived toxins may act as conventional allergens, leading to production of specific IgE, or as superantigens that can nonspecifically activate T cells (23). Patou et al. showed that Staph-derived protein A induces mast cell degranulation, while enterotoxin B can induce release of T_H2 cytokines, including IL-4, IL-5, and IL-13, and the regulatory cytokine, IL-10 in nasal polyp tissue (24).

The role of oxidative stress has also been investigated. Free oxygen radicals have been identified in NP tissue. Increased severity of nasal polyposis and bronchial hyperresponsiveness correlate with levels of free oxygen radicals in polyp tissue (25).

Aspirin intolerance is generally associated with severe nasal polyposis and chronic sinusitis that is less responsive to treatment (26). The link between aspirin sensitivity, asthma, and NPs has been attributed to enhanced production of leukotrienes from arachidonic acid. Patients with nasal polyposis generally have elevated levels of urinary LTE4 at baseline (27). Aspirin-sensitive patients demonstrate increased levels of urinary leukotriene E4 (LTE4) after oral aspirin challenge (28). In addition, LTC_4 synthase is overexpressed in NPs of patients with aspirin exacerbated respiratory disease (AERD)(29).

Treatment

Intranasal glucocorticoids are the treatment of choice for nasal polyposis and are often more effective than surgical polypectomy; intranasal steroids significantly reduce polyp size, nasal congestion, rhinorrhea, and increase nasal airflow (30, 31). Aggressive treatment of NPs with intranasal corticosteroids has also been reported to reduce the need for surgery (32). The effectiveness of intranasal steroids on improving olfactory dysfunction is variable; the best results may be obtained using a short course of oral corticosteroids (30 mg to 35 mg of prednisone daily for 5 to 7 days) followed by maintenance therapy with intranasal steroids (33,34). Optimal delivery of intranasal steroids is achieved by positioning the head in the downward and forward position. Higher doses of intranasal corticosteroids may be more effective. Coexistent sinus infections, which may reduce responsiveness to intranasal steroids, should be treated appropriately.

Limited data exist regarding the use of leukotriene antagonists to treat nasal polyposis. In a double-blind study of 40 post-operative patients with nasal polyps, there was no difference in the recurrence rate of polyps between patients treated with montelukast versus nasal beclomethasone for 1 year (35). However, intranasal steroids exhibited superiority in treating olfactory deficits and nasal congestion. Another small, double-blind study found significant improvement in health-related-quality-of-life in polyps patients on montelukast versus placebo for 4 weeks (36). Larger, controlled trials are needed to assess the usefulness and comparative efficacy (i.e., montelukast versus zileuton) of these drugs in treating NPs.

Surgical treatment for nasal polyposis should be considered when optimal medical therapy has failed. Simple polypectomy may be indicated for complete nasal obstruction, which causes extreme discomfort. If NPs are associated with persistent ethmoid sinusitis with obstruction of the osteomeatal complex, a more extensive surgical procedure may be considered. Several randomized controlled trials have shown equivalent outcomes at 1 year of follow-up after surgical versus medical management of NPs (37,38). Nasal polyps frequently recur after simple surgical polypectomy, and long-term recurrence rates may be as high as 60% following functional endoscopic sinus surgery (FESS) for severe disease (39). While further studies evaluating the role of long-term nasal steroids after surgery are needed, their administration in this setting should be considered to prevent recurrence (40).

Outcomes of FESS are generally less favorable among AERD patients compared with patients with chronic sinusitis who are aspirin-insensitive (41). In a retrospective study, patients with AERD had more extensive sinus disease based on radiologic findings, and 39% required surgical revisions versus 9% of sinusitis patients without aspirin sensitivity (41). The addition of aspirin following surgery may improve long-term outcomes in selected patients with nasal polyposis and AERD (42). Long-term aspirin desensitization has been reported to reduce the number of episodes of acute sinusitis, corticosteroid use, and requirement for polypectomies and sinus surgery (43). Because of the risk of provoking severe asthmatic attacks, this procedure should be performed exclusively by an experienced practitioner in an appropriate setting, and considered only in aspirin-sensitive patients refractory to conventional therapies (44).

■ SINUSITIS

Sinusitis affects approximately 16% of the population (45). The estimated annual health care costs for sinusitis exceed $3.5 billion annually, not including the costs incurred by missed work days (45). Sinusitis is an inflammatory disorder of the mucosal lining of the paranasal sinuses that may be initiated by infectious or noninfectious factors. Viral upper respiratory infections often precede acute bacterial sinus infections. Given that most viral infections resolve within 7 to 10 days, acute bacterial sinusitis is typically diagnosed when symptoms persist beyond 7 days (46). Rhinosinusitis is referred to as *chronic* when it persists for more than 8 to 12 weeks (47). Noninfectious triggers for sinusitis include environmental exposures to fumes or chemical vapors. Bacterial sinusitis has long been considered a complication of seasonal or perennial allergic rhinitis (48,49). Individuals with exposure to tobacco smoke and those with nonallergic rhinitis are also more susceptible to recurrent or chronic sinusitis (50,51).

Regardless of initiating events, the four physiologic derangements that contribute to the evolution of infectious sinusitis are: (a) reduced patency of the sinus ostia; (b) a decrease in the partial pressure of oxygen within the sinus cavities; (c) diminished mucociliary transport; and (d) compromise of microcirculation blood flow in the mucosa (52). Edematous obstruction of the sinus ostia is a consistent finding in both acute and chronic sinusitis; this condition causes a low-oxygen environment within the sinus cavity, which results in decreased mucociliary transport and favors the growth of common bacterial pathogens, including *Streptococcus pneumoniae, Haemophilus influenzae,* and anaerobic bacteria (53).

Biopsies of sinus mucosa from patients with purulent, nonpurulent, and recurrent sinusitis reveal basement membrane thickening, atypical gland formation, goblet cell hyperplasia, inflammatory cell infiltration, and subepithelial edema (52). Increasing chronicity of disease is associated with greater basement membrane thickening and an increase in the number and size of secretory glands (54). Neutrophils are elevated in the sinus fluid of patients with CRS, and IL-8, a strong chemoattractant for neutrophils is elevated in the mucosa of patients with acute sinusitis (19). Other inflammatory cells including eosinophils can also be found; however, these are more prominently associated with accompanying nasal polyposis (55).

Causative Microorganisms

Microbial pathogens implicated in acute maxillary sinusitis have been studied extensively. Identification of bacterial pathogens by endoscopically directed middle meatal cultures closely approximates results obtained via needle puncture of the maxillary sinus (56). However, cultures obtained by nasopharyngeal swab do not reflect bacterial isolates in the sinuses. A meta-analysis of cultures obtained by middle meatal sampling or maxillary sinus puncture for acute bacterial sinusitis in adults from 1990 to 2006 revealed that the most common pathogens were: *Streptococcus pneumoniae* (32.7%), *Haemophilus influenzae* (31.6%), *Staphylococcus aureus* (10.1%), and *Moraxella catarrhalis* (8.8%) (57). Another study, conducted in 1992, of 339 adult

patients with acute sinusitis found that viruses were cultured from 8% of aspirates, whereas 15% to 40% of antral aspirates were sterile. Common isolates included rhinovirus, influenza type A, and parainfluenza viruses (58). With the advent of molecular techniques, detectable viruses during sinusitis exceed 50% and include rhinovirus (18%), RSV (15%), adenovirus (3%), and enterovirus (3%) (59).

In children with acute maxillary sinusitis, *S. pneumoniae, H. influenzae, and M. catarrhalis* have been identified as the predominant pathogens; since the advent of Prevnar, the 7-valent pneumococcal vaccine, the proportion of sinusitis caused by *S. pneumoniae* has declined, while that caused by *H. influenzae* has increased (60).

Microbial pathogens involved in CRS may be quite different from those involved in acute disease. Anaerobic bacteria play a large role in CRS in adults, but are rarely identified in children. One series found that 88% of antral aspirates of adult patients with CRS were positive for anaerobes. Predominant aerobic pathogens include *S. pneumoniae* and *S. aureus.* There is also increasing concern for drug resistant gram-negative organisms in CRS, particularly *Pseudomonas aeruginosa* (56,57).

Immunocompromised individuals may develop sinusitis involving unusual or opportunistic organisms. A full discussion is beyond the scope of this text (61). Molecular techniques have revolutionized the rapidity with which diagnoses can be made (62). Mucormycotic sinusitis is caused by fungi of the family *Mucoraceae* (*Mucor*), which are zygomycetes. These organisms are saprophytic, abundant in the natural environment, and may be isolated from the throat and stools of normal individuals. Mucormycotic sinusitis is potentially fatal in diabetic, leukemic, or otherwise immunosuppressed patients. Similarly, invasive aspergillosis may involve the paranasal sinuses, primarily in the immunocompromised host, with rare cases occurring in immunocompetent individuals. Invasive aspergillosis involving the sphenoid sinus is particularly difficult to treat, even in immunocompetent patients, and can result in severe neurologic complications (63). Rarely, tuberculosis can cause infectious sinusitis, particularly in immunocompromised patients. Atypical mycobacteria have been reported to cause sinusitis in patients with acquired immunodeficiency syndrome (64).

Allergic fungal sinusitis is an increasingly recognized syndrome occurring in immunocompetent atopic patients with hypertrophic rhinitis and NPs, which may result from local hypersensitivity responses to a variety of mold spores colonizing the sinus cavities. Abundant mucin found within the sinuses demonstrates numerous eosinophils and Charcot-Leyden crystals; fungal stains reveal the presence of noninvasive hyphae (65). The disease occurs primarily in adults, but should be considered in atopic children with refractory sinus disease (66). While *Aspergillus* species are frequently involved, dematiaceous fungi have also been implicated. Patients generally exhibit high total serum IgE levels and have positive skin tests to fungal allergens (65).

Clinical Presentation

Episodes of acute sinusitis are most commonly preceded by symptoms suggestive of viral upper respiratory tract infections or other environmental stimuli, which can cause mucosal inflammation, hypertrophy, and obstruction of the sinus ostia. Common presenting symptoms include frontal or maxillary head pain, fever, and mucopurulent or bloody nasal discharge. Other clinical features include general malaise, cough, hyposmia, mastication pain, and changes in the resonance of speech. Pain cited as coming from the upper molars may represent an early symptom of acute maxillary sinusitis. Children with acute maxillary sinusitis present most often with cough, nasal discharge, and fetid breath, while fever is less common (50).

Symptoms associated with CRS are less fulminant; facial pain and/or pressure, headache, and postnasal discharge are common. The clinician should be aware that chronic maxillary sinusitis may result from primary dental infections (i.e., apical granuloma of the molar teeth, periodontitis) (55). Pain associated with temporomandibular dysfunction may be incorrectly diagnosed as CRS. Individuals with sinusitis may experience severe facial pain associated with rapid changes in position (e.g., lying supine or bending forward) or with rapid changes in atmospheric pressure that occur during air travel.

Episodes of acute or chronic sinusitis may be manifestations of other underlying problems. Local obstruction by a deviated nasal septum, NPs, or occult benign or malignant neoplasm may explain recurrent sinus infections. Patients presenting with frequent sinus infections that respond poorly to antibiotics should be examined for primary or acquired immunodeficiency states. Humoral immune deficiencies that should be considered include Common Variable Immune Deficiency (CVID), complement deficiencies, and selective IgA deficiency in combination with IgG subclass deficiency, or, more likely, specific antibody deficiency with limited or absent response to polysaccharide encapsulated bacteria. (See Chapter 4 for more detailed information) (67). Disorders of ciliary dysmotility usually occur in male patients. Kartagener syndrome is characterized by recurrent sinusitis, nasal polyps, situs inversus, infertility, and bronchiectasis (68). Incomplete forms of ciliary dysmotility may occur without associated pulmonary or cardiac involvement. Nasal mucosal biopsy and electron microscopic examination to identify abnormalities in ciliary structure should be done in suspected cases. Wegener granulomatosis is a necrotizing vasculitis that presents with epistaxis, refractory sinusitis, serous otitis, nodular pulmonary infiltrates, and focal necrotizing glomerulonephritis (69). CRS or otitis media can precede pulmonary and renal manifestations for years before full expression of the disease. Early diagnosis and treatment of Wegener before development of renal disease can be life saving.

Diagnosis

Palpable tenderness, erythema, and warmth may be appreciated over inflamed frontal, ethmoid, or maxillary sinuses. Clinical history and physical examination can reliably identify purulent sinusitis in more than 80% of cases (46,47). Sinus imaging should be reserved for difficult diagnostic problems or for patients with sinusitis unresponsive to an initial course of antibiotics (70). Rhinoscopy can be useful in identifying purulent discharge in the middle meatus compatible with acute maxillary sinusitis. When cultures are needed to guide therapy, endoscopically guided middle meatal cultures are a viable alternative to traditional antral puncture techniques (53). Computed tomography (CT) of the sinuses has become the standard radiologic method for defining pathologic changes in the paranasal sinuses (53). CT is particularly useful for defining abnormalities in the anterior ethmoid and middle meatal areas (ostiomeatal unit), which cannot be visualized well on sinus roentgenograms. Sinus mucosal thickening of 8 mm or greater on CT scan is a sensitive, but not specific diagnostic marker of bacterial sinusitis. Minimal radiologic changes are common in sterile sinusitis and in asymptomatic individuals. The CT coronal views (Fig. 27.1) are much less costly than a complete sinus CT and are adequate for determining the patency of the ostiomeatal complex, which includes the ethmoid and maxillary ostia and infundibulum. Such information is essential for assessing the need for surgical intervention in the treatment of CRS (52–54).

Complications

In the age of antibiotics, severe life-threatening complications of acute sinusitis are relatively uncommon. However, the clinician must be able to recognize clinical manifestations of potentially fatal complications of sinusitis so that medical and surgical treatments can be initiated in a timely fashion.

Symptoms commonly associated with acute frontal sinusitis include frontal head pain, local erythema and swelling, fever, and purulent nasal discharge. Serious complications of frontal sinusitis may be attributed to the proximity of the frontal sinus to the roof of the orbit and anterior cranial fossa. Osteomyelitis can result from acute frontal sinusitis and may present as a localized subperiosteal abscess (Pott puffy tumor) (71). Sinus radiographs exhibit sclerotic changes in the bone contiguous to the frontal sinus. Intracranial complications of frontal sinusitis include extradural, subdural, and brain

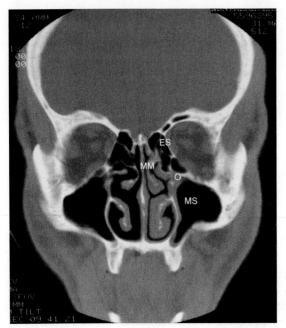

■ **FIGURE 27.1** Computed tomographic image of the paranasal sinuses. A coronal section exhibits significant sinus disease on the left with a relatively normal appearance on the right. The left middle meatus (*MM*) and maxillary ostium (*O*) are obstructed by inflamed tissue, causing significant obstruction of the left ethmoid (*ES*) and maxillary (*MS*) sinuses.

abscesses as well as meningitis and cavernous sinus thrombosis (53,72). (CT scans may be adequate to diagnose some complications of sinusitis, but magnetic resonance imaging [MRI] is superior to evaluate intracranial findings.) Acute ethmoiditis is encountered most commonly in children. Extension of inflammation into the orbit can result in unilateral orbital and periorbital swelling with cellulitis. This presentation can be distinguished from cavernous sinus thrombosis by the lack of focal cranial neurologic deficits, retroorbital pain, or meningeal signs. Affected patients usually respond to antibiotics, and surgical drainage is rarely necessary.

Cavernous sinus thrombosis is a complication of acute or chronic sinusitis, which demands immediate diagnosis and treatment. The cavernous sinuses communicate with the venous channels draining the middle one-third of the face. Cavernous sinus thrombosis often arises from a subcutaneous infection in the face or paranasal sinuses. Vital structures that course through the cavernous sinus include the internal carotid artery and the third, fourth, fifth, and sixth cranial nerves. Symptoms of venous outflow obstruction caused by cavernous sinus thrombosis include retinal engorgement, retrobulbar pain, and visual loss. Impingement of cranial nerves in the cavernous sinus can result in extraocular muscle paralysis and trigeminal sensory loss. If not treated promptly with high doses of parenteral

antibiotics, septicemia and central nervous system involvement can lead to a fatal outcome (73).

Acute sphenoid sinusitis is difficult to diagnose. A high index of suspicion and radiologic imaging with CT scan or MRI is essential (74). Affected patients report occipital and retroorbital pain, or the pain distribution may be nonspecific. Because of the posterior location of the sphenoid sinus, diagnosis of sphenoiditis may be delayed until serious complications are recognized. Extension of infections to contiguous structures may result in ocular palsies, orbital cellulitis, subdural abscess, meningitis, or hypopituitarism.

It has long been recognized that chronic or recurrent sinusitis may exacerbate asthma. A recent study demonstrated a strong correlation between sinus mucosal thickening and biomarkers of bronchial inflammation (e.g., sputum eosinophils, exhaled nitric oxide) in patients with severe asthma. Surgical treatment of chronic sinusitis may improve control in patients with difficult or refractory asthma (75). However, asthmatic and AERD patients tend to benefit less from sinus surgery in general (31,41).

Treatment of Acute Sinusitis

The primary goal of treatment should be facilitation of drainage of affected sinuses and elimination of causative organisms. Gwaltney studied 31 patients who presented with upper respiratory infection with significant CT abnormalities consistent with sinusitis (76). CT abnormalities spontaneously resolved in most patients 2 weeks later without antibiotics, suggesting that antibiotics are used unnecessarily in many patients. A recent Cochrane Review of 57 trials found that cure rates with antibiotics for acute, uncomplicated sinusitis were only slightly better than placebo. Judicious use of antibiotics is essential, especially in light of increasing problems with antibiotic resistance. Topical nasal vasoconstrictors (e.g., oxymetazoline) used prudently over the initial 2 to 3 days of treatment of acute sinusitis can facilitate drainage. Recent evidence suggests that topical vasoconstrictors may be safe when used for up to 4 weeks without causing rhinitis medicamentosa, although further studies are needed to support their widespread use in this fashion (77). Oxymetazoline and saline lavage used in combination for acute sinusitis have been shown to improve mucociliary clearance (78).

The use of nasal steroids either as monotherapy or in combination with antibiotics for acute sinusitis has been advocated. A meta-analysis involving patients with radiographic or endoscopically diagnosed acute sinusitis who were not receiving antibiotics reported that nasal steroids were more effective than placebo at relieving symptoms, with greater benefit seen at higher doses (130). A smaller trial looking at patients with acute sinusitis based on plain films or endoscopy concluded that nasal steroids used in combination with antibiotics (cefuroxime) were more effective than anti-biotics alone (80).

Antibiotics should be considered in those who fail the aforementioned drainage measures, or who have persistent symptoms for more than 7 to 10 days. The emergence of penicillin-resistant strains should be recognized. For treating acute sinusitis, amoxicillin (250 mg to 500 mg three times daily for 7 to 10 days) is still the antibiotic of choice in patients who are not at risk for resistant organisms. Appropriate first-line alterna-tives include trimethoprim-sulfamethoxazole (160 mg to 800 mg twice daily for 10 days) or doxycycline (100 mg twice daily for 1 day followed by 50 mg twice daily for 9 more days) (46). A study of 80 patients with acute sinusitis confirmed on radiographic imaging found that 3 days of trimethoprim-sulfamethoxazole may be just as effective as 10 days of treatment (81).

Antibiotic resistance can account for initial treat-ment failure and prompt a change in antibiotics. Infec-tion with a penicillin-resistant organism should be suspected in those patients who fail 14-day to 21-day courses of amoxicillin (53,57). In this situation, amoxi-cillin/clavulanic acid or an appropriate cephalosporin (e.g., cefuroxime), should be substituted (135). Modified macrolide antibiotics (e.g., clarithromycin, azithromycin) can also be used in treating patients unresponsive to amoxicillin. The clinical relevance of increasing resistance to macrolides has yet to be deter-mined. In general, use of fluoroquinolones is discour-aged based on lack of data showing superiority to less expensive agents in the treatment of acute sinusitis, and concerns for increasing bacterial resistance to these drugs (53,57) (82).

Treatment failures for acute sinusitis are not uncom-mon. Parenteral antibiotics should be instituted if local extension of infection (i.e., cellulitis or osteomyelitis) occurs, or if the infection is suspected to have spread to vital ocular or central nervous system structures. Surgi-cal drainage of infected sinuses may be indicated when fever, facial pain, and sinus imaging changes persist, and for complicated cases of acute sinusitis. FESS may be superior to open techniques, depending on the spe-cifics of a particular case (75). For patients with maxil-lary sinusitis who do not respond to conservative (medical) drainage measures and aggressive antibiotic therapy, resection of diseased tissue within the sinuses is recommended (53). Similar principles apply to the treatment of frontal, ethmoid, or sphenoid sinusitis; ethmoidectomy and sphenoidotomy can often be done endoscopically, which results in a quicker recovery and a shorter hospital stay (75).

Treatment of Chronic Rhinosinusitis

Sinusitis that persists beyond 8 weeks is termed *chronic rhinosinusitis* (CRS). The treatment approach to CRS and recurrent sinusitis should begin with identifying

contributing factors such as chronic allergic rhinitis, deviated nasal septum, immunodeficiency, NPs, concha bullosa, exposure to tobacco smoke, toxic irritants at work, and other environmental factors. Aggressive medical management has been shown to increase time to relapse in CRS (83). Daily maintenance therapy with oral decongestants alone or in combination with nasal steroids may be considered to improve ostial patency. One study showed improvements in nasal symptoms and nasal inspiratory flow in chronic sinusitis patients treated with intranasal budesonide for 20 weeks (84). Intranasal glucocorticoids are particularly effective in those with co-existing allergic rhinitis (47). Intermit-tent use of topical decongestants (oxymetazoline) in combination with nasal steroids may be a useful ad-junctive treatment for exacerbations of CRS (77,85).

Treatment of predisposing conditions is more likely to be effective than multiple rounds of increasingly more broad-spectrum antibiotics. If indicated, prolonged treatment (3 to 6 weeks) with antibiotics is thought to be more effective than shorter courses (86). When incom-plete resolution of exacerbations occurs, endoscopic or surgically obtained cultures can be helpful to guide anti-biotic choices, particularly when broad-spectrum antibi-otics such as fluoroquinolones are being considered (53).

When all attempts at pharmacologic management have failed, surgery may be required for chronic or recurrent sinusitis. FESS has supplanted older surgical procedures such as maxillary Caldwell-Luc antrostomy. The basic principle of endoscopic techniques is to resect the inflamed tissues that obstruct the ostiomeatal complex and the anterior ethmoids, and thus directly interfere with normal physiologic drainage (75). Because FESS is less invasive, postoperative morbidity has been reduced markedly in comparison with for-merly used surgical techniques. Multiple studies have demonstrated short-term improvements in symptoms after surgery for chronic or recurrent sinusitis (31). A recent prospective study of 82 patients who underwent FESS after failing medical management reported signifi-cant initial improvements in self-reported symptoms (87). However, there was a trend toward recurrence of presenting complaints by 3 years. Those patients with nasal polyps, aspirin sensitivity, and asthma were less likely to experience long-term benefits.

■ NONALLERGIC RHINITIS

Symptoms of nonallergic rhinitis often are indistin-guishable from those associated with perennial allergic rhinitis. Nonallergic rhinitis is defined as inflammation of the nasal mucosa that is not due to IgE-mediated sen-sitization. Lack of allergic causation should be proven by the absence of skin test reactivity to a panel of com-mon aeroallergens. A recent community-based Danish study of over 1,000 adults found that approximately 25% of chronic rhinitis sufferers had nonallergic rhinitis (88). Women were twice as likely to have nonallergic rhinitis as men, and symptom severity was indistinguishable between allergic and nonallergic rhinitics. Onset after age 40 is more likely associated with nonallergic versus allergic rhinitis.

Table 27.1 presents a classification for the nonallergic nasal disorders, which includes the differential diagnosis for conditions that may mimic rhinitis (88). Evaluation begins with a careful history and examination with a nasal speculum. Nasal septal deviation is usually obvious. Pale, boggy nasal turbinates characteristic of allergic rhinitis may also be seen in a patient with NARES (nonallergic rhinitis with eosinophilia syndrome) or NPs. The nasal mucosa appear beefy red or hemorrhagic in patients with rhinitis medicamentosa. Cytologic examination of a nasal mucus smear may reveal an abundance of neutrophils, which is suggestive of infectious rhinitis. Nasal eosinophils are consistent with allergic rhinitis, NARES, or nasal polyposis (89).

Vasomotor rhinitis or idiopathic, nonallergic noninfectious rhinitis is the most common of these disorders, excluding viral upper respiratory infections. Symptoms include perennial nasal congestion, rhinorrhea, and postnasal discharge. Pruritus is rare in the absence of allergic rhinitis. Ocular symptoms can be present in nonallergic rhinitis, although they tend to be more prominent in allergic rhinitis (90). Typically, nasal symptoms are triggered by irritants in tobacco smoke, chemical fumes, perfumes, or various scents and noxious odors. Symptoms are classically triggered by rapid changes in temperature. Although the pathophysiology of this condition is not well understood, it has been postulated that environmental factors may trigger neurogenic reflex responses, or that symptoms are a consequence of an imbalance in parasympathetic and sympathetic tone. Increased numbers of nerve fibers containing sensory neuropeptides characterize both allergic and nonallergic rhinitis (91). Gustatory rhinitis is a form of vasomotor rhinitis in which clear rhinorrhea is provoked by eating, particularly when eating hot or spicy foods (92). Other subtypes of vasomotor rhinitis are listed in Table 27.1.

NARES is an inflammatory nasal disorder in which eosinophils are detectable on a nasal smear (>5% to >20% nasal eosinophils), but skin tests to relevant aeroallergens are negative (93). The cause of this condition is unknown. Primary atrophic rhinitis is a disorder of unknown origin, which is characterized by formation of thick, malodorous, dry crusts that obstruct the nasal cavity (94). Secondary atrophic rhinitis is more common in the Western world, and is associated with granulomatous disease, nasal irradiation, trauma, and prior sinonasal surgery. Removal of the middle and/or inferior turbinates in particular may predispose to development of secondary atrophic rhinitis (95).

Rhinitis medicamentosa can result from the chronic use or abuse of topical decongestants, or from cocaine use. Excessive use of topical vasoconstrictor agents

TABLE 27.1 NONALLERGIC NASAL DISORDERS

SUBTYPES OF NONALLERGIC RHINITIS	CONDITIONS THAT MAY MIMIC SYMPTOMS OF RHINITIS
Vasomotor rhinitis	Nasal polyps
Gustatory rhinitis	Structural/mechanical factors
Irritant triggered (e.g., chlorine)	Deviated septum/septal wall anomalies
Cold air	Adenoidal hypertrophy
Exercise (e.g., running)	Trauma
Undetermined or poorly defined triggers	Foreign bodies
NARES	Nasal tumors
(nonallergic rhinitis with eosinophilia syndrome)	Benign
Atrophic rhinitis	Malignant
Rhinitis medicamentosa (topical vasocontrictors)	Choanal atresia
Drug-induced rhinitis (oral medications)	Cleft palate
Hormonally-induced rhinitis	Pharyngonasal reflux
Pregnancy rhinitis	Acromegaly (excess growth hormone)
Menstrual-cycle related	Rhinitis associated with inflammatory-immunologic
Infectious rhinitis	disorders
Acute	Granulomatous infections
Chronic	Wegener granulomatosis
	Sarcoidosis
	Midline granuloma
	Churg-Strauss
	Relapsing polychondritis
	Amyloidosis
	Cerebrospinal fluid rhinorrhea
	Ciliary dyskinesia syndrome

such as neosynephrine or oxymetazoline can result in epistaxis, "rebound" nasal congestion, and rarely cause nasal septal perforation (96). Intranasal cocaine use can result in the same signs and symptoms. Benzalkonium chloride, a preservative commonly used in over-the-counter and prescription aqueous products, might play a causative role in rhinitis medicamentosa, but this is highly speculative (97).

Drug-induced rhinitis occurs as an adverse effect of certain oral medications (Table 27.2) (98). In addition to older antihypertensive agents (not listed), some newer antihypertensives are also associated with drug-induced rhinitis. In particular, angiotensin-converting enzyme inhibitors (ACE inhibitors) have been reported to cause rhinorrhea and vasomotor symptoms in association with chronic cough, which resolve after withdrawal of the drug (99). Other oral medications associated with drug-induced rhinitis include phosphodiesterase type 5 inhibitors (e.g., sildenafil), NSAIDs such as aspirin, certain psychotropic medications, gabapentin, and alpha-antagonists used for benign prostatic hypertrophy (98,100).

Nasal congestion and rhinorrhea are common during pregnancy. This may be related to underlying allergic rhinitis, sinusitis, rhinitis medicamentosa, or may be due to vasomotor rhinitis of pregnancy ("pregnancy rhinitis"). "Pregnancy rhinitis" occurs in approximately one-fifth of pregnant women and manifests primarily as nasal congestion that occurs in the last 6 weeks of pregnancy and resolves within 2 weeks of delivery (101). It may be due to estrogen-induced nasal vasodilation and enhancement of mucus secretion, or possibly to placental growth hormone (101,102).

Conditions that mimic rhinitis must be considered in the differential diagnosis. A grossly deviated nasal septum, nasal tumors, or a foreign body can be the source of unilateral nasal obstruction refractory to medical treatment. Cerebral spinal fluid (CSF) rhinorrhea is characterized by clear nasal discharge. It occurs in 5% of all basilar skull fractures but can be present in patients with no history of trauma. The use of glucose oxidase paper tests may result in an erroneous diagnosis. Detection of β_2 transferrin in the CSF is useful in confirming the diagnosis (103).

Treatment

Selection of therapy for vasomotor rhinitis is empiric, and there are variable responses to different regimens. Azelastine hydrochloride (Astelin) is a topical antihistamine that has been shown to decrease nasal congestion and post-nasal drip associated with vasomotor rhinitis in multiple randomized controlled trials (104). Intranasal steroids are beneficial for some cases of vasomotor rhinitis (105). The combination of a topical nasal antihistamine with an intranasal steroid such as fluticasone proprionate provides greater symptomatic relief than either agent alone (104,106). When not contraindicated

TABLE 27. 2 CAUSTIVE AGENTS FOR DRUG-INDUCED RHINITIS

Antihypertensives
  Amiloride
  ACE inhibitors[a]
  ARBs[b]
  Beta blockers
  Chlorothiazide
  Clonidine
  Hydralazine
  Hydrochlorothiazide
  Methyldopa
Alpha-adrenergic antagonists[c]
  Prazosin
  Doxazosin
  Phentolamine
  Terazosin
  Tamsulosin
Phosphodiesterase type 5 inhibitors
  Sildenafil
  Tadalafil
  Verdenafil

Psychotropic agents
  Chlordiazepoxide-amitryptyline
  Chlorpromazine
  Risperidone
  Thioridazine
Ovarian hormonal agents
  Oral contraceptives[d]
  Exogenous estrogens
Pain relievers
  Aspirin
  Non-steroidal anti-inflammatory drugs
Miscellaneous
  Cocaine[e]
  Gabapentin

[a]Angiotensin converting enzyme inhibitors; [b]Angiotensin receptor blockers (114); [c]Used for hypertension or benign prostatic hypertrophy depending on specific drug; [d]May not apply to modern oral contraceptives (115); [e]Mechanism may be similar to other topical vasoconstrictors

(Adapted from Ramey JT, Bailen E, Lockey RF. Rhinitis medicamentosa. *J Investig Allergol Clin Immunol* 2006. 16(3): p. 148–155 [167]))

by co-existing medical conditions, oral decongestants are often effective for congestion caused by vasomotor rhinitis when given as 12-hour slow-release preparations (e.g., pseudoephedrine). Phenylephrine may not be as effective as an oral decongestant in commonly used doses (107). Nasal ipratropium, an anticholinergic agent, is proven to be effective in treating rhinorrhea associated with nonallergic rhinitis, and is the treatment of choice for gustatory and cold air induced rhinitis (92,108). Environmental triggers such as tobacco smoke and irritants encountered at home or work should be avoided.

NARES responds best to intranasal glucocorticoids (105). Atrophic rhinitis is treated chronically with saline irrigation, with topical and systemic antibiotics prescribed for acute infections. Patients with rhinitis medicamentosa should discontinue offending medications. Intranasal glucocorticoids may be of considerable benefit in these patients in decreasing mucosal edema (109).

For vasomotor rhinitis of pregnancy, medication use should be minimized. Saline rinses, mechanical nasal alar dilators, and limited use of decongestants may be appropriate. If necessary, intranasal budesonide may be safe and effective for controlling chronic allergic rhinitis symptoms encountered during pregnancy, but do not have proven efficacy for treating pure pregnancy rhinitis (101,110). Nasal ipratropium could also be considered to treat associated rhinorrhea (108,111).

Nasal obstruction caused by a severely deviated septum requires septoplasty. Some patients with CSF rhinorrhea recover spontaneously, or with medical treatment alone (112). When persistent, intravenous antibiotics should be started to prevent meningitis, and endoscopic or open surgery often is required to repair a dural tear (113).

■ REFERENCES

1. Moloney JR, Collins J. Nasal polyps and bronchial asthma. *Br J Dis Chest.* 1977;71(1):1–6.
2. Stammberger H. Surgical treatment of nasal polyps: past, present, and future. *Allergy.* 1999;54 (Suppl 53):7–11.
3. Andrews AE, Bryson JM, Rowe-Jones JM. Site of origin of nasal polyps: relevance to pathogenesis and management. *Rhinology.,* 2005;43(3):180–184.
4. Di Lorenzo G, Drago A, Esposito Pellitteri M, et al. Measurement of inflammatory mediators of mast cells and eosinophils in native nasal lavage fluid in nasal polyposis. *Int Arch Allergy Immunol.* 2001;125(2):164–175.
5. Kim JW, Hong SL, Kim YK, et al. Histological and immunological features of non-eosinophilic nasal polyps. *Otolaryngol Head Neck Surg.* 2007;137(6):925–930.
6. Weisskopf A, Burn HF. Histochemical studies of the pathogenesis of nasal polyps. *Ann Otol Rhinol Laryngol.* 1959;68(2):509–523.
7. Johansson L, Akerlund A, Holmberg K, et al. Prevalence of nasal polyps in adults: the Skovde population-based study. *Ann Otol Rhinol Laryngol.* 2003;112(7): 625–629.
8. Hedman J, Kaprio J, Poussa T, et al. Prevalence of asthma, aspirin intolerance, nasal polyposis and chronic obstructive pulmonary disease in a population-based study. *Int J Epidemiol.* 1999;28(4):717–722.
9. Klossek JM, Neukirch F, Pribil C, et al. Prevalence of nasal polyposis in France: a cross-sectional, case-control study. *Allergy.* 2005;60(2):233–237.
10. Settipane GA. Nasal polyps and immunoglobulin E (IgE). *Allergy Asthma Proc.* 1996;17(5):269–273.
11. Alobid I, Benitez P, Valero A, et al. The impact of atopy, sinus opacification, and nasal patency on quality of life in patients with severe nasal polyposis. *Otolaryngol Head Neck Surg.* 2006;134(4):609–612.
12. Settipane GA, Chafee FH. Nasal polyps in asthma and rhinitis. A review of 6,037 patients. *J Allergy Clin Immunol.* 1977;59(1):17–21.
13. Watelet JB, van Cauwenberge P, Bachert C. The nose in cystic fibrosis. *Eur Resp Mon.* 2001. 18:47–56.
14. Rupa V, Jacob M, Mathews MS. Atopy, proptosis and nasal polyposis. *Postgrad Med J.* 2001;77:343–344.
15. Lund VJ, Lloyd GA. Radiological changes associated with benign nasal polyps. *J Laryngol Otol.*1983; 97(6):503–510.
16. Van Lancker JA, Yarnold PA, Ditto AM, et al. Aeroallergen hypersensitivity: comparing patients with nasal polyps to those with allergic rhinitis. *Allergy Asthma Proc.* 2005; 26(2):109–112.
17. Conley DB, Tripathi A, Seiberling KA, et al. Superantigens and chronic rhinosinusitis: skewing of T-cell receptor V beta distribution in polyp derived CD4+ and CD8+ T cells. *Am J Rhinol.*2006; 20:534–539.
18. Biewenga J, Stoop AE, van der Heijden HA, et al. Albumin and immunoglobulin levels in nasal secretions of patients with polyps treated with endoscopic sinus surgery and topical corticosteroids. *J Allergy Clin Immunol.* 1995;96:334–340.
19. Rudack C, Stoll W, Bachert C. Cytokines in nasal polyposis, acute and chronic sinusitis. *Am J Rhinol.* 1998;12(6):383–388.
20. Danielsen A, Tynning T, Brokstad KA, et al. Interleukin 5, IL6, IL12, IFN-gamma, RANTES and Fractalkine in human nasal polyps, turbinate mucosa and serum. *Eur Arch Otorhinolaryngol.* 2006;263(3):282–289.
21. Riechelmann H, Deutschle T, Rozsasi A, et al. Nasal biomarker profiles in acute and chronic rhinosinusitis. *Clin Exp Allergy.* 2005;35(9):1186–1191.
22. Claeys S, Van Hoecke H, Holtappels G, et al. Nasal polyps in patients with and without cystic fibrosis: a differentiation by innate markers and inflammatory mediators. *Clin Exp Allergy.* 2005;35(4):467–472.
23. Tripathi A, Kern R, Conley DB, et al. Staphylococcal exotoxins and nasal polyposis: analysis of systemic and local responses. *Am J Rhinol.* 2005;19(4):327–333.
24. Patou J, Gevaert P, Van Zele T, et al. Staphylococcus aureus enterotoxin B, protein A, and lipoteichoic acid stimulations in nasal polyps. *J Allergy Clin Immunol.* 2008;121(1):110–115.
25. Kang BH, Huang NC, Wang HW. Possible involvement of nitric oxide and peroxynitrite in nasal polyposis. *Am J Rhinol.* 2004;18(4):191–196.
26. Ceylan E, Gencer M, San I. Nasal polyps and the severity of asthma. *Respirology.* 2007;12(2):272–276.
27. Higashi N, Taniguchi M, Mita H, et al. Clinical features of asthmatic patients with increased urinary leukotriene E4 excretion (hyperleukotrienuria): involvement of chronic hyperplastic rhinosinusitis with nasal polyposis. *J Allergy Clin Immunol.* 2004;113(2):277–283.
28. Swierczynska M, Nizankowska-Mogilnicka E, Zarychta J, et al. Nasal versus bronchial and nasal response to oral aspirin challenge: clinical and biochemical differences between patients with aspirin-induced asthma/rhinitis. *J Allergy Clin Immunol.* 2003;112(5):995–1001.
29. Adamjee J, Suh YJ, Park HS, et al. Expression of 5-lipoxygenase and cyclooxygenase pathway enzymes in nasal polyps of patients with aspirin-intolerant asthma. *J Pathol.* 2006;209(3):392–399.
30. Small CB, Hernandez J, Reyes R, et al. Efficacy and safety of mometasone furoate nasal spray in nasal polyposis. *J AllergyClin Immunol.* 2005;116:1275–1281.
31. Wright ED, Agrawal S. Impact of perioperative systemic steroids on surgical outcomes in patients with chronic rhinosinusitis with polyposis: evaluation with the Novel Perioperative Sinus Endoscopy (POSE) scoring system. *Laryngoscope.* 2007;117:1–28.
32. Aukema AA, Mulder PG, Fokkens WJ. Treatment of nasal polyposis and chronic rhinosinusitis with fluticasone propionate nasal drops reduces need for sinus surgery. *J Allergy Clin Immunol.* 2005; 115(5):1017–1023.
33. Benitez P, Alobid I, de Haro J, et al. A short course of oral prednisone followed by intranasal budesonide is an effective treatment of severe nasal polyps. *Laryngoscope.* 2006;116(5):770–775.
34. Alobid I, Benitez P, Pujols L, et al. Severe nasal polyposis and its impact on quality of life. The effect of a short course of oral steroids followed by long-term intranasal steroid treatment. *Rhinology.* 2006;44(1):8–13.

35. Mostafa BE, Abdel Hay H, Mohammed HE, et al. Role of leukotriene inhibitors in the postoperative management of nasal polyps. *ORL J Otorhinolaryngol Relat Spec.* 2005;67(3):148–153.

36. Pauli C, Fintelmann R, Klemens C, et al. (Polyposis nasi–improvement in quality of life by the influence of leukotrien receptor antagonists). *Laryngorhinootologie.* 2007;86(4):282–286.

37. Alobid I, Benitez P, Bernal-Sprekelsen M, et al. Nasal polyposis and its impact on quality of life: comparison between the effects of medical and surgical treatments. *Allergy.* 2005;60(4):452–458.

38. Ragab SM, Lund VJ, Scadding G. Evaluation of the medical and surgical treatment of chronic rhinosinusitis: a prospective, randomised, controlled trial. *Laryngoscope.* 2004;114(5):923–930.

39. Wynn R, Har-El G. Recurrence rates after endoscopic sinus surgery for massive sinus polyposis. *Laryngoscope.* 2004;114(5):811–813.

40. Rowe-Jones JM, Medcalf M, Durham SR, et al. Functional endoscopic sinus surgery: 5 year follow up and results of a prospective, randomised, stratified, double-blind, placebo controlled study of postoperative fluticasone propionate aqueous nasal spray. *Rhinology.* 2005;43(1):2–10.

41. Amar YG, Frenkiel S, Sobol SE. Outcome analysis of endoscopic sinus surgery for chronic sinusitis in patients having Samter's triad. *J Otolaryngol.* 2000;29(1):7–12.

42. Stevenson DD, Simon RA. Selection of patients for aspirin desensitization treatment. *J Allergy Clin Immunol.* 2006;118(4):801–804.

43. McMains KC, Kountakis SE. Medical and surgical considerations in patients with Samter's triad. *Am J Rhinol.* 2006;20:573–576.

44. Macy E, Bernstein JA, Castells MC, et al. Aspirin challenge and desensitization for aspirin-exacerbated respiratory disease: a practice paper. *Ann Allergy Asthma Immunol.* 2007;98(2):172–174.

45. Anand VK. Epidemiology and economic impact of rhinosinusitis. *Ann Oto Rhino & Laryngology.* 2004;193:S3–S5.

46. Piccirillo JF. Clinical practice. Acute bacterial sinusitis. *N Engl J Med.* 2004;351(9):902–910.

47. Cherry WB, Li JT. Chronic rhinosinusitis in adults. *Am J Med.* 2008.121(3):185–189.

48. Steele RW. Rhinosinusitis in children. *Curr Allergy Asthma Rep.* 2006;6(6):508–512.

49. Cirillo I, Marseglia G, Klersy C, et al. Allergic patients have more numerous and prolonged respiratory infections than nonallergic subjects. *Allergy.* 2007;62(9):1087–1090.

50. Duse M, Caminiti S, Zicari AM. Rhinosinusitis: prevention strategies. *Pediatr Allergy Immunol.* 2007;18(Suppl 18):71–74.

51. Ebbert JO, Croghan IT, Schroeder DR, et al. Association between respiratory tract diseases and secondhand smoke exposure among never smoking flight attendants: a cross-sectional survey. *Environ Health.* 2007;6:28–36.

52. Kaliner M. Medical management of sinusitis. *Am J Med Sci.* 1998;316:21–28.

53. Slavin RG, Spector SL, Bernstein IL, et al. The diagnosis and management of sinusitis: a practice parameter update. *J Allergy Clin Immunol.* 2005; 116:S13-S47.

54. Rehl RM, Balla AA, Cabay RJ, et al. Mucosal remodeling in chronic rhinosinusitis. *Am J Rhinol.* 2007;21(6):651–657.

55. Bachert C, van Cauwenberge P. Nasal polyps and sinusitis. In: Adkinson NF, Bochner BS, Yunginer JW, et al., eds. *Middleton's Allergy Principles & Practice.* 6th ed. Philadelphia: Mosby; 2003: 1432–1433.

56. Benninger MS, Payne SC, Ferguson BJ, et al. Endoscopically directed middle meatal cultures versus maxillary sinus taps in acute bacterial maxillary rhinosinusitis: a meta-analysis. *Otolaryngol Head Neck Surg.* 2006;134(1):3–9.

57. Payne SC, Benninger MS. Staphylococcus aureus is a major pathogen in acute bacterial rhinosinusitis: a meta-analysis. *Clin Infect Dis.* 2007;45(10):e121–127.

58. Gwaltney JM Jr, Scheld WM, Sande MA, et al. The microbial etiology and antimicrobial therapy of adults with acute community-acquired sinusitis: a fifteen-year experience at the University of Virginia and review of other selected studies. *J Allergy Clin Immunol.* 1992; 90(3 Pt 2):457–461; discussion 462.

59. Loens K, Goosens H, de Laat C, et al. Detection of rhinoviruses by tissue culture and two independent amplification techniques, nucleic acid sequence-based amplification and reverse transcription-pcr, in children with acute respiratory infections during a winter season. *J Clin Microbiol.* 2006;44:166–171.

60. Brook I, Gober AE. Frequency of recovery of pathogens from the nasopharynx of children with acute maxillary sinusitis before and after the introduction of vaccination with the 7-valent pneumococcal vaccine. *Int J Pediatr Otorhinolaryngol.* 2007;71(4):575–579.

61. Parikh SL, Venkatraman G, DelGaudio JM. Invasive fungal sinusitis: a 15-year review from a single institution. *Am J Rhinol.* 2004;18(2):75–81.

62. Willinger B, Obradovic A, Selitsch B, et al. Detection and identification of fungi from fungus balls of the maxillary sinus by molecular techniques. *J Clin Microbiol.* 2003;41:581–585.

63. Akhaddar A, Gazzaz M, Albouzidi A, et al. Invasive Aspergillus terreus sinusitis with orbitocranial extension: case report. *Surg Neurol.* 2008;69(5):490–495; discussion 495.

64. Naguib MT, Byers JM, Slater LN. Paranasal sinus infection due to atypical mycobacteria in two patients with AIDS. *Clin Infect Dis.* 1994;19(4):789–791.

65. Katzenstein AL, Sale SR, Greenberger PA. Allergic Aspergillus sinusitis: a newly recognized form of sinusitis. *J Allergy Clin Immunol.* 1983;72(1):89–93.

66. Campbell JM, Graham M, Gray HC, et al. Allergic fungal sinusitis in children. *Ann Allergy Asthma Immunol.* 2006;96(2):286–290.

67. Vanlerberghe L, Joniau S, Jorissen M. The prevalence of humoral immunodeficiency in refractory rhinosinusitis: a retrospective analysis. *B-ENT.* 2006;2(4):161–66.

68. Eliasson R, Mossberg B, Camner P, et al. The immotile-cilia syndrome. A congenital ciliary abnormality as an etiologic factor in chronic airway infections and male sterility. *N Engl J Med.* 1977;297(1):1–6.

69. Abraham-Inpijn L. Wegener's granulomatosis, serous otitis media and sinusitis. *J Laryngol Otol.* 1980;94(7):785–788.

70. Mudgil SP, Wise SW, Hopper KD, et al. Correlation between presumed sinusitis-induced pain and paranasal sinus computed tomographic findings. *Ann Allergy Asthma Immunol.* 2002. 88(2):223–226.

71. Raja V, Low C, Sastry A, et al. Pott's puffy tumor following an insect bite. *J Postgrad Med.* 2008; 53:114–116.

72. Betz CS, Issing W, Matschke J, et al. Complications of acute frontal sinusitis: a retrospective study. *Eur Arch Otorhinolaryngol.* 2008. 265(1):63–72.

73. Cannon ML, Antonio BL, McCloskey JJ, et al. Cavernous sinus thrombosis complicating sinusitis. *Pediatr Crit Care Med.* 2004;5(1):86–88.

74. Grillone GA, Kasznica P. Isolated sphenoid sinus disease. *Otolaryngol Clin North Am.* 2004. 37(2):435–451.

75. Scadding GK, Durham SR, Mirakian R, et al. BASCI guidelines for the management of rhinosinusitis and nasal polyposis. *Clin Exp Allergy.* 2007;38:260–275.

76. Gwaltney JM Jr, Phillips CD, Miller RD, et al. Computed tomographic study of the common cold. *N Engl J Med.* 1994;330(1):25-30.

77. Watanabe H, Foo TH, Djazaeri B, et al. Oxymetazoline nasal spray three times daily for four weeks in normal subjects is not associated with rebound congestion or tachyphylaxis. *Rhinology.* 2003;41(3):167–174.

78. Inanli S, Oztürk O, Korkmaz M, et al. The effects of topical agents of fluticasone propionate, oxymetazoline, and 3% and 0.9% sodium chloride solutions on mucociliary clearance in the therapy of acute bacterial rhinosinusitis in vivo. *Laryngoscope.* 2002;112(2):320–325.

79. Zalmanovici A, Yaphe J. Steroids for acute sinusitis. *Cochrane Database Syst Rev.* 2007;(2):CD005149.

80. Dolor RJ, Witsell DL, Hellkamp AS, et al. Comparison of cefuroxime with or without intranasal fluticasone for the treatment of rhinosinusitis. The CAFFS Trial: a randomized controlled trial. *JAMA.* 2001;286(24):3097–3105.

81. Williams JW Jr, Simel DL, Roberts L, et al. Randomized controlled trial of 3 vs 10 days of trimethoprim/sulfamethoxazole for acute maxillary sinusitis. *JAMA.* 1995;273(13):1015–1021.

82. Ahovuo-Saloranta A, Borisenko OV, Kovanen N, et al. Antibiotics for acute maxillary sinusitis. *Cochrane Database Syst Rev.* 2007;(2):CD000243. DOI: 10.1002/14651858.CD000243.pub2

83. Subramanian HN, Schechtman KB, Hamilos DL. A retrospective analysis of treatment outcomes and time to relapse after intensive medical treatment for chronic sinusitis. *Am J Rhinol.* 2002;16(6):303–312.

84. Lund VJ, Black JH, Szabó LZ, et al. Efficacy and tolerability of budesonide aqueous nasal spray in chronic rhinosinusitis patients. *Rhinology.* 2004; 42(2):57–62.

85. Tas A, Yaqiz R, Yalcin O, et al. Use of mometasone furoate aqueous nasal spray in the treatment of rhinitis medicamentosa: an experimental study. *Otolaryngol Head Neck Surg.* 2005;132(4):608–612.

86. Dubin MG, Kuhn FA, Melroy CT. Radiographic resolution of chronic rhinosinusitis without polyposis after 6 weeks vs 3 weeks of oral antibiotics. *Ann Allergy Asthma Immunol.* 2007;98(1):32–35.

87. Young J, Frenkiel S, Tewfik MA, et al. Long-term outcome analysis of endoscopic sinus surgery for chronic sinusitis. *Am J Rhinol.* 2007;21(6):743–747.

88. Wallace DV, Dykewicz MS, Bernstein DI, et al. The diagnosis and management of rhinitis: an updated practice parameter. *J Allergy Clin Immunol.* 2008;122(2 Suppl):S1–84.

89. Ciprandi G, Vizzaccaro A, Cirillo I, et al. Nasal eosinophils display the best correlation with symptoms, pulmonary function and inflammation in allergic rhinitis. *Int Arch Allergy Immunol.* 2005;136(3):266–272.

90. Bielory L. Vasomotor (perennial chronic) conjunctivitis. *Curr Opin Allergy Clin Immunol.* 2006;6(5):355–360.

91. Garay, R. Mechanisms of vasomotor rhinitis. *Allergy.* 2004;59 (Suppl 76):4–9; discussion 9–10.

92. Raphael G, Raphael MH, Kaliner M. Gustatory rhinitis: a syndrome of food-induced rhinorrhea. *J Allergy Clin Immunol.* 1989; 83(1):110–115.

93. Ellis AK, Keith PK. Nonallergic rhinitis with eosinophilia syndrome and related disorders. *Clin Allergy Immunol.* 2007;19:87–100.

94. Dutt SN, Kameswaran M. The aetiology and management of atrophic rhinitis. *J Laryngol Otol.* 2005;119(11):843–852.

95. Moore EJ, Kern EB. Atrophic rhinitis: a review of 242 cases. *Am J Rhinol.* 2001;15(6):355–361.

96. Keyserling HF, Grimme JD, Camacho DL, et al. Nasal septal perforation secondary to rhinitis medicamentosa. *Ear Nose Throat J.* 2006;85(6):376,378–379.

97. Marple B, Roland P, Benninger M. Safety review of benzalkonium chloride used as a preservative in intranasal solutions: an overview of conflicting data and opinions. *Otolaryngol Head Neck Surg.* 2004;130(1):131–141.

98. Ramey JT, Bailen E, Lockey RF. Rhinitis medicamentosa. *J Investig Allergol Clin Immunol.* 2006;16(3):148–155.

99. Berkin KE. Respiratory effects of angiotensin converting enzyme inhibition. *Eur Respir J.* 1989;2(3):198–201.

100. Wilt TJ, MacDonald R, Rutks I. Tamsulosin for benign prostatic hyperplasia. *Cochrane Database Syst Rev.* 2003;(1):CD002081.

101. Ellegard EK. The etiology and management of pregnancy rhinitis. *Am J Respir Med.* 2003;2(6):469–475.

102. Ellegard EK. Clinical and pathogenetic characteristics of pregnancy rhinitis. *Clin Rev Allergy Immunol.* 2004;26(3):149–159.

103. Ryall RG, Peacock MK, Simpson DA. Usefulness of beta 2-transferrin assay in the detection of cerebrospinal fluid leaks following head injury. *J Neurosurg.* 1992;77(5):737–739.

104. Bernstein JA. Azelastine hydrochloride: a review of pharmacology, pharmacokinetics, clinical efficacy and tolerability. *Curr Med Res Opin.* 2007;23(10):2441–2452.

105. Webb DR, Meltzer EO, Finn AF Jr, et al. Intranasal fluticasone propionate is effective for perennial nonallergic rhinitis with or without eosinophilia. *Ann Allergy Asthma Immunol.* 2002;88(4):385–390.

106. Kaliner MA. A novel and effective approach to treating rhinitis with nasal antihistamines. *Ann Allergy Asthma Immunol.* 2007;99(5): 383–390; quiz 391–392,418.

107. Corey JP, Houser SM, Ng BA. Nasal congestion: a review of its etiology, evaluation, and treatment. *Ear Nose Throat J.* 2000;79(9):690–693,696,698 passim.

108. Bonadonna P, Senna G, Zanon P, et al. Cold-induced rhinitis in skiers–clinical aspects and treatment with ipratropium bromide nasal spray: a randomized controlled trial. *Am J Rhinol.* 2001;15(5):297–301.

109. Ferguson BJ, Paramaesvaran S, Rubinstein E. A study of the effect of nasal steroid sprays in perennial allergic rhinitis patients with rhinitis medicamentosa. *Otolaryngol Head Neck Surg.* 2001;125(3): 253–260.

110. Ellegard EK, Hellgren M, Karlsson NG. Fluticasone propionate aqueous nasal spray in pregnancy rhinitis. *Clin Otolaryngol Allied Sci.* 2001;26(5):394–400.

111. The use of newer asthma and allergy medications during pregnancy. The American College of Obstetricians and Gynecologists (ACOG) and The American College of Allergy, Asthma and Immunology (ACAAI). *Ann Allergy Asthma Immunol.* 2000;84(5):475–480.

112. Lindstrom DR, Toohill RJ, Loehrl TA, et al. Management of cerebrospinal fluid rhinorrhea: the Medical College of Wisconsin experience. *Laryngoscope.* 2004;114(6):969–974.

113. Daudia A, Biswas D, Jones NS. Risk of meningitis with cerebrospinal fluid rhinorrhea. *Ann Otol Rhinol Laryngol.* 2007;116(12):902–905.

114. Samizo K, Kawabe E, Hinotsu S, et al. Comparison of losartan with ACE inhibitors and dihydropyridine calcium channel antagonists: a pilot study of prescription-event monitoring in Japan. *Drug Saf,* 2002;25(11):811–821.

115. Wolstenholme CR, Philpott CM, Oloto EJ, et al. Does the use of the combined oral contraceptive pill cause changes in the nasal physiology in young women? *Am J Rhinol.* 2006;20(2):238–240.

CHAPTER 28

Allergic Diseases of the Eye and Ear

SEONG CHO, MICHAEL S. BLAISS, AND PHIL LIEBERMAN

■ THE EYE

The allergic eye diseases are contact dermatoconjunctivitis, acute allergic conjunctivitis, vernal conjunctivitis, and atopic keratoconjunctivitis (allergic eye diseases associated with atopic dermatitis). Several other conditions mimic allergic disease and should be considered in any patient presenting with conjunctivitis. These include the blepharoconjunctivitis associated with staphylococcal infection, seborrhea and rosacea, acute viral conjunctivitis, chlamydial conjunctivitis, keratoconjunctivitis sicca, herpes simplex keratitis, giant papillary conjunctivitis, vasomotor (perennial chronic) conjunctivitis, and the "floppy eye syndrome." Each of these entities is discussed in relationship to the differential diagnosis of allergic conjunctivitis. The allergic conditions themselves are emphasized.

In addition to the systematic discussion of these diseases, because the chapter is written for the nonophthalmologist, an anatomic sketch of the eye (Fig. 28.1) is included.

Diseases Involving the Eyelids

Contact Dermatitis and Dermatoconjunctivitis

There are two allergic conditions to be considered when the eyelids are involved. They are contact dermatitis and atopic keratoconjunctivitis. Because the skin of the eyelid is thin (0.55 mm), it is particularly prone to develop both immune and irritant contact dermatitis. When the causative agent has contact with the conjunctiva and the lid, a dermatoconjunctivitis occurs.

Clinical Presentation

Contact dermatitis and dermatoconjunctivitis affect women more commonly than men because women use cosmetics more frequently. Vesiculation may occur early, but by the time the patient seeks care, the lids usually appear thickened, red, and chronically inflamed. Peeling and scaling of the eyelids also occur with chronic exposure. If the conjunctiva is involved, there is erythema and tearing. A papillary response with vasodilation and chemosis occurs. Pruritus is the cardinal symptom of contact dermatitis, a burning sensation may also be present. Rubbing the eyes intensifies the itching; tearing can occur. An erythematous blepharitis is common, and in severe cases, keratitis can result.

Causative Agents

Contact dermatitis and dermatoconjunctivitis can be caused by agents directly applied to the lid or conjunctiva, aerosolized or airborne agents contacted by chance, and cosmetics applied to other areas of the body. In fact, eyelid dermatitis occurs frequently because of cosmetics (e.g., nail polish, hair spray) applied to other areas of the body (1). However agents applied directly to the eye are the most common causes. Contact dermatitis can be caused by eye makeup, including eyebrow pencil and eyebrow brush-on products, eye shadow, eye liner, mascara, artificial lashes, and lash extender. These products often contain coloring agents, lanolin, paraben, sorbitol, paraffin, petrolatum, and other allergenic substances such as vehicles and perfumes (1). Brushes and pads used to apply these cosmetics also can produce dermatitis. In addition to agents applied directly only to the eye, soaps and face creams can also produce a selective dermatitis of the lid because of the thin skin in this area. Cosmetic formulations are frequently altered (1). Therefore, a cosmetic previously used without ill effect can become a sensitizing agent.

Any medication applied to the eye can produce a contact dermatitis or dermatoconjunctivitis. Ophthalmic preparations contain several sensitizing agents, including benzalkonium chloride, chlorobutanol, chlorhexidine, ethylenediaminetetraacetate (EDTA), and phenylmercuric salts. EDTA cross-reacts with ethylenediamine, so that patients sensitive to this agent are subject to develop dermatitis as a result of several other

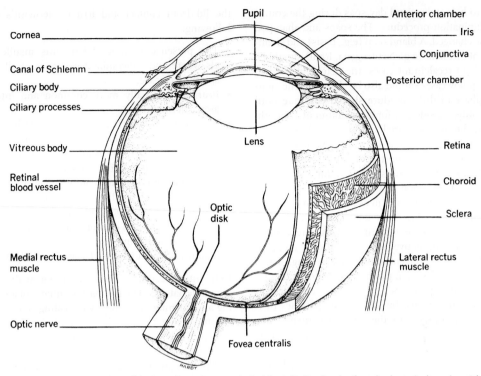

■ FIGURE 28.1 Transverse section of the eye. (From Brunner L, Suddarth D. *Textbook of medical-surgical nursing.* 4th ed. Philadelphia: JB Lippincott, 1980, with permission.)

medications. Today, antibiotics, antivirals, and anti-glaucoma drugs are probably the major causes of iatro-genic contact dermatoconjunctivitis. Several other topically applied medications, however, have been reported to cause dermatoconjunctivitis. These include antihistamines and sympathomimetics such as antazo-line, as well as atropine, pilocarpine, phenylephrine, epinephrine, and topical anesthetics.

Of increasing importance is the conjunctivitis asso-ciated with the wearing of contact lenses, especially soft lenses. Reactions can occur to the lenses themselves or to the chemicals used to treat them. Both toxic and immune reactions can occur to contact lens solutions. Thimerosal, a preservative used in contact lens solu-tions, has been shown to produce classic, cell-medi-cated contact dermatitis (2). Other substances found in lens solutions that might cause either toxic or immune reactions are the bacteriostatic agents (methylparaben, chlorobutanol, and chlorhexidine) and EDTA, which are used to chelate lens deposits. With the increasing use of disposable contact lenses, the incidence of con-tact allergy to lenses and their cleansing agents appears to be declining.

Dermatitis of the lid and conjunctiva can also result from exposure to airborne agents. Hair spray, volatile substances contacted at work, and the oleoresin moi-eties of airborne pollens have all been reported to pro-duce contact dermatitis and dermatoconjunctivitis.

Hair preparations and nail enamel frequently cause problems around the eye while sparing the scalp and the hands. Finally, *Rhus* dermatitis can affect the eye, producing unilateral periorbital edema, which can be confused with angioedema.

Diagnosis and Identification of Causative Agents

The differential diagnosis includes seborrheic dermati-tis and blepharitis, infectious eczematous dermatitis (especially chronic staphylococcal blepharitis), and rosacea. Seborrheic dermatitis usually can be differenti-ated from contact dermatitis on the basis of seborrheic lesions elsewhere and the lack of pruritus. Also, pruri-tus does not occur in staphylococcal blepharitis or rosa-cea. If the diagnosis is in doubt, an ophthalmology consultation should be obtained.

In some instances, the etiologic agent may be readily apparent. This is usually the case in dermatitis caused by the application of topical medications. However, many cases present as chronic dermatitis, and the cause is not readily apparent. In such instances, an elimina-tion-provocation procedure and patch tests can identify the offending substance. The elimination-provocation procedure requires that the patient stop using all sub-stances under suspicion. This is often difficult because it requires the complete removal of all cosmetics, hair sprays, spray deodorants, and any other topically applied substances. It should also include the cessation of visits to hair stylists and day spas during the course of the elimination procedure. The soaps and shampoo should be changed. A bland soap (e.g., Basis) and shampoo free of formalin (e.g., Neutrogena, Ionil) should be employed. In recalcitrant cases, the detergent used to wash the pillowcases should also be changed. The elimination phase of the procedure should continue until the dermatitis subsides, or for a maximum of 1 month. When the illness has cleared, cosmetics and other substances can be returned at a rate of one every week. On occasion, the offending substances can be identified by the recurrence of symptoms on the reintroduction of the substance in question.

Patch tests can be helpful in establishing a diagnosis (3,4). However, the skin of the lid is markedly different from that of the back and forearm, and drugs repeatedly applied to the conjunctival sac concentrate there, producing high local concentrations of the drug. Thus, false-negative results from patch tests are common (1). Testing should be performed, not only to substances in standard patch test kits, but also to the patient's own cosmetics. In addition to the cosmetics themselves, tests can be performed to applying agents, such as sponges and brushes. Both open- and closed-patch tests are indicated when testing with cosmetics (1). Fisher (4) describes a simple test consisting of rubbing the substances into the forearm three times daily for 4 to 5 days, and then examining the sites. Because of the difficulty involved in establishing the etiologic agent with standard patch test kits, an ophthalmic patch test tray (Table 28.1) has been suggested (3).

Therapy

The treatment of choice is removal of the offending agent. On occasion, this can be easily accomplished. An example of this is the switch from chemically preserved to heat-sterilized systems in patients with contact lens–associated contact conjunctivitis. The offending agent, however, frequently cannot be identified, regardless of the diagnostic procedures applied. In these instances, chronic symptomatic therapy, possibly in conjunction with an ophthalmologist, is all that can be offered to the patient.

Symptomatic relief can be obtained with topical corticosteroid creams, ointments, and drops. Corticosteroid drops should be employed only under the direction of the ophthalmologist. Cool tap-water soaks and boric acid eye baths may help.

Atopic Dermatitis Ocular Involvement

Manifestations of atopic involvement of the eyelids are similar to immune and irritant contact dermatitis of the lids. Chronic scaling, pruritus, and lichenification of the lids are most commonly due to these two disorders, and both should be considered in the differential diagnosis. The features that distinguish atopic dermatitis of the lid from contact and irritant dermatitis are the following:

- The presence of atopic dermatitis manifestations elsewhere and concomitant existence of allergic respiratory disease.
- Pruritus is usually more common and intense in atopic dermatitis.
- Madarosis (lash loss) and trichiasis (lash misdirection) are more common in atopic dermatitis.
- Involvement of the eye itself is also present in most cases of atopic dermatitis of the lid.
- The ocular findings are conjunctival erythema and swelling, limbal papillae, keratoconus (see below), anterior and posterior subcapsular cataracts, and occasionally corneal erosion with ulcers, neovascularization, and scarring.
- A family history of atopic disease is usually noted.

Dermatitis affecting the lids can present with a myriad of manifestations. The hallmark is intense bilateral itching and burning of the lids with scaling. There is often accompanying tearing and photophobia. Like vernal conjunctivitis, patients with ocular manifestations as well can exhibit a thick, ropy discharge.

The lids are often edematous, scaly, and thickened. There is a wrinkled appearance of the skin. Lichenification occurs with chronic involvement.; eyelid malpositions are common. Because of the chronic itching, the patient's rubbing and scratching of their lids leads to further changes such as fissures, which occur commonly near the lateral canthus (5).

Periorbital features of allergic disease have been described. The classic "Dennie-Morgan" fold is a crease extending from the inner canthus laterally to the mid-pupillary line of the lower lid. There is often periorbital darkening referred to as the *allergic shiner*. The lateral eyebrows are often absent (Hertoghe sign). Eyelid margin (blepharitis) involvement is characteristic. The findings resemble those of chronic bacterial blepharitis (see below), and indeed these findings may be due to bacterial overgrowth occurring with atopy. There is hyperemia and an exudate with crusting in the morning.

Due to misdirection of the lashes there is often contact of the lash with the conjunctivae, and this can be particularly bothersome to patients. As noted, bacterial colonization can be anticipated. *Staphylococcal aureus* is often the most common organism involved. Presumably, *Staphylococcus* colonizes the eye through contact with the hands. The phenotype of the *Staphylococcus* growing in the eye is the same as on the skin in the majority of instances (6).

Therapy

Therapy of the lids in atopic dermatitis is similar to that of allergic disease in general. Known environmental exacerbants should, of course, be avoided. Cool compresses and bland moisturizers are helpful. Vaseline

TABLE 28.1   SUGGESTED OPHTHALMIC TRAY FOR PATCH TESTING

COMPOUND	PATCH TEST CONCENTRATION (%)	VEHICLE
Preservatives		
Benzalkonium chloride	0.1	aq
Benzethonium chloride	1	aq
Chlorhexidine gluconate	1	aq
Cetalkonium chloride	0.1	aq
Sodium EDTA	1	aq
Sorbic acid	2.5	pet
Thimerosal	0.1;1	pet
β-Adrenergic blocking agents		
Befunolol	1	aq
Levobunolol HCl	1	aq
Metipranolol	2	aq
Metoprolol	3	aq
Timolol	0.5	aq
Mydriatics		
Atropine sulfate	1	aq
Epinephrine HCl	1	aq
Phenylephrine HCl	10	aq
Scopolamine hydrobromide	0.25	aq
Antibiotics		
Bacitracin	5	pet
Chloramphenicol	5	pet
Gentamicin sulfate	20	pet
Kanamycin	10	pet
Neomycin sulfate	20	pet
Polymyxin B sulfate	20	pet
Antiviral drugs		
Idoxuridine	1	pet
Trifluridine	5	pet
Antihistamines or antiallergic drug		
Chlorpheniramine maleate	5	pet
Sodium cromoglycate	2	aq
Anesthetics		
Benzocaine	5	pet
Procaine	5	aq
Oxybuprocaine	0.5	aq
Proxymetacaine	0.5	aq
Enzymatic cleaners		
Papain	1	pet
Tegobetaine	1	aq
Miotics		
Pilocarpine	1	aq
Tolazoline	10	aq
Echothiophate iodide	1	aq
Other		
Epsilon aminocaproic acid	1	aq

aq, aqueous; pet, petrolatum.

From Mondino B, Salamon S, Zaidman G. Allergic and toxic reactions in soft contact lens wearers. *Surv Ophthalmol* 1982;26:337–344, with permission.

and Aquaphor (Beiersdorf, Norwalk, Connecticut) are examples in this regard. Periodic exacerbations of lid inflammation can be treated with low-dose topical corticosteroid ointments. An example is fluorometholone 0.1% ophthalmic ointment. Care must be taken, however, because long-term administration can thin the skin of the eyelid and produce permanent cosmetic changes as vessels begin to show through the thin skin. The lowest dose for the shortest period of time should be employed. Tacrolimus and pimecrolimus topical preparation can also be helpful as in atopic dermatitis in general.

Pathophysiology

The pathogenesis of eye involvement in atopic dermatitis, like the pathophysiology underlying abnormalities in the skin, is complex. It certainly involves immunoglobulin E (IgE)- mediated mechanisms, but clearly other inflammatory pathways are active. Patients with atopic keratoconjunctivitis have elevated tear levels of interferon-γ, TNF-α, IL-2, IL-4, IL-5, and IL-10, thus indicating a combined T_H1 and T_H2 response (7). However, at least in animal models, there is a clear predominance of the T_H2 phenotype in terms of T cells. The characteristic ocular eosinophilia appears to be dependent on the presence of this T cell population (8). The active role of T cells in allergic disorders of the eye clearly explains the beneficial effect of cyclosporin in these diseases (9).

Acute Allergic Conjunctivitis

Pathophysiology

Acute allergic conjunctivitis is the most common form of allergic eye disease (10). It is produced by IgE-induced mast cell and basophil degranulation. As a result of this reaction, histamine, kinins, leukotrienes, prostaglandins, interleukins, chemokines, and other mediators are liberated (10). Patients with allergic conjunctivitis have elevated amounts of total IgE in their tears, and tear fluid also contains IgE specific for seasonal allergens (11). Eosinophils found in ocular scrapings are activated, releasing contents such as eosinophil cationic protein from their granules. These contents appear in tear fluid (12). Ocular challenge with pollen produces both an early- and a late-phase ocular response; in humans, the early phase begins about 20 minutes after challenge. The late phase is dose dependent, and large doses of allergen cause the initial inflammation to persist and progress (12). The late phase differs from that which occurs in the nose and lungs in that it is often continuous and progressive rather than biphasic (13). It is characterized by the infiltration of inflammatory cells, including neutrophils, eosinophils, and lymphocytes, with eosinophils predominating (13). In addition, during the late-phase reaction, mediators, including histamine, leukotrienes, and eosinophil contents are released continually (14).

Subjects with allergic conjunctivitis demonstrate a typical T_H2 (allergic) profile of cytokines in their tear fluid showing excess production of (IL-4) and IL-5. If the illness becomes chronic, however, there may be a shift in cytokine profile to a T_H1 pattern with excess production of interferon-γ, as seen in atopic keratoconjunctivitis (15) and atopic dermatitis.

Subjects with allergic conjunctivitis have an increased number of mast cells in their conjunctivae, and they are hyperresponsive to intraocular histamine challenge. Of interest is the fact that there is evidence of complement activation, with elevated levels of C3a des-Arg reported in tear fluid (16). The consequences of this immune reaction are conjunctival vasodilation and edema. The clinical reproducibility of the reaction is dependable. Instillation of allergen into the conjunctival sac was once used as a diagnostic test (17).

Clinical Presentation

Acute allergic conjunctivitis is usually recognized easily. Itching is always a prominent feature. Rubbing the eyes intensifies the symptoms. The findings are almost always bilateral. However, unilateral acute allergic conjunctivitis can occur because of manual contamination of the conjunctiva with allergens such as foods and animal dander. Ocular signs in some cases are minimal despite significant pruritus. The conjunctiva may be injected and edematous. In severe cases, the eye may be swollen shut. These symptoms of allergic conjunctivitis may be so severe as to interfere with the patient's sleep and work.

Allergic conjunctivitis rarely occurs without accompanying allergic rhinitis; the eye symptoms may be more prominent than nasal symptoms and can be the patient's major complaint. However, if symptoms or signs of allergic rhinitis are totally absent, the diagnosis of allergic conjunctivitis is doubtful. Allergic conjunctivitis also exists in a chronic form. Symptoms are usually less intense. As in acute allergic conjunctivitis, ocular findings on physical examination may not be impressive.

Diagnosis and Treatment

The diagnosis of allergic conjunctivitis can be made on the basis of history. Usually there is an atopic personal or family history; the disease is usually seasonal. At times, the patient may be able to define the offending allergen or season accurately. Skin tests are confirmatory. Stain of the conjunctival secretions may show numerous eosinophils, but the absence of eosinophils does not exclude the condition. Normal individuals do not have eosinophils in conjunctival scrapings; therefore, the presence of one eosinophil is consistent with the diagnosis (16). The differential diagnosis should include other forms of acute conjunctivitis, including viral and bacterial conjunctivitis, contact dermatoconjunctivitis, conjunctivitis sicca, and vernal conjunctivitis.

Treating allergic conjunctivitis is the same as for other atopic illness: avoidance, symptomatic relief, and immunotherapy, in that order. When allergic conjunctivitis is associated with respiratory allergic disease, the course of treatment is usually dictated by the more debilitating respiratory disorder. Avoiding ubiquitous aeroallergens is impractical, but avoidance measures outlined elsewhere in this text can be employed in the treatment of allergic conjunctivitis.

Effective symptomatic therapy for allergic conjunctivitis can usually be achieved with topical medications (18). The most significant change in the management of allergic eye disorders since the last edition of this text is the release of new topical agents to treat these disorders. Six classes of topical agents are now available. These are vasoconstrictors, "classic" antihistamines, "classic" mast cell stabilizers, new agents with multiple "antiallergic" activities, nonsteroidal anti-inflammatory agents, and corticosteroids. Selected examples of these agents are noted in Table 28.2. Corticosteroids are not discussed here because, as a result of their well-known side effects, patients should use them only when prescribed by the ophthalmologist.

TABLE 28.2 REPRESENTATIVE TOPICAL AGENTS USED TO TREAT ALLERGIC EYE DISORDERS

DRUG CLASS	REPRESENTATIVE TRADE NAME EXAMPLES	DOSAGE	COMMENTS
Vasoconstrictors			
Tetrahydrozoline, phenylephrine, oxymetazoline, naphazoline	Naphcon, Vasocon, Visine	1 to 2 drops every 4 hours as necessary (not more than q.i.d.)	Only helpful for eye redness. Does not relieve itch. Available without prescription. Some concern about "rebound." Contraindicated in narrow-angle glaucoma.
Antihistamines			
Levocabastine	Livostin	1 drop q.i.d.	Effective for itching. Available by prescription only. May be more potent than antihistamines available without prescription.
Emedastine	Emadine	1 drop q.i.d.	
Combination vasoconstrictor plus antistamine			
Antazoline, naphazoline	Vasocon-A	1 drop q.i.d.	Effective for eye redness and itch. Available without prescription.
Mast cell stabilizers			
Lodoxadine	Alomide	1 drop q.i.d.	Best when initiated before onset of symptoms
Cromolyn	Crolom	1 drop q.i.d.	
Nedocromil	Opticrom	1 drop q.i.d.	
Pemirolast	Allocril Alamast	1 drop q.i.d.	
Nonsteroidal anti-inflammatory			
Ketorolac	Acular	1 drop q.i.d.	Indicated for itching
Drugs with multiple "antiallergic" activities such as antihistamine, mast cell stabilizing, and antieosinophil effects			
Olopatadine	Patanol Pataday	1 to 2 drops b.i.d. 1 to 2 drops every day.	Prescription required
Ketotifen	Zaditor	1 drop every 8 to 12 hours	Available without prescription
Epinastine	Elestat	1 drop every 8 to 12 hours	Prescription required
Azelastine	Optivar	1 drop every 8 to 12 hours	Prescription required

b.i.d., twice daily; q.i.d., four times daily

Several preparations contain a mixture of a vasoconstrictor combined with an antihistamine (Table 28.2). These drugs can be purchased without prescription. The antihistamine is most useful for itching but also reduces vasodilation. Vasoconstrictors only diminish vasodilation and have little effect on pruritus. The two most frequently employed decongestants are naphazoline and phenylephrine. The two most common antihistamines available in combination products are antazoline and pheniramine maleate.

Levocabastine (Livostin) is an antihistamine available only by prescription. Levocabastine was specifically designed for topical application. In animal studies, it is 1,500 times more potent than chlorpheniramine on a molar basis (19). It has a rapid onset of action, is effective in blocking intraocular allergen challenge, and appears to be as effective as other agents, including sodium cromoglycate and terfenadine. Emedastine (Emadine) is also a selective H_1 antagonist with a receptor-binding affinity even higher than levocabastine. It appears to have a rapid onset of action (within 10 minutes) and a duration of activity of 4 hours (18).

As a rule, vasoconstrictors and antihistamines are well tolerated. However, antihistamines may be sensitizing. In addition, each preparation contains several different vehicles that may produce transient irritation or sensitization. Just as vasoconstrictors in the nose can cause rhinitis medicamentosa, frequent use of vasoconstrictors in the eye results in conjunctivitis medicamentosa. As a rule, however, these drugs are effective and well tolerated (10).

Four mast cell stabilizers are available for therapy. They are cromolyn sodium, nedocromil sodium, lodoxamide, and pemirolast. All are efficacious and usually well tolerated (18). They are more effective when started before the onset of symptoms and used regularly four times a day, but they can relieve symptoms if given shortly before ocular allergen challenge. Thus they are also useful in preventing symptoms caused by isolated allergen challenge such as occurs when visiting a home with a pet or mowing the lawn. In these instances, they should be administered immediately before exposure.

Ketorolac tromethamine (Acular) is a nonsteroidal anti-inflammatory agent that is most effective in controlling itching but also ameliorates other symptoms. Its effect results from its ability to inhibit the formation of prostaglandins, which cause itching when applied to the conjunctiva (20).

Four agents for the treatment of allergic eye disorders have broad-based antiallergic or anti-inflammatory effects in addition to their antihistamine activity. These are azelastine (Optivar), olopatadine (Patanol and Pataday), ketotifen (Zaditor), and epinastine (Elestat). They prevent mast cell degranulation, reduce eosinophil activity, and downregulate the expression of adhesion molecules as well as inhibit the binding of histamine to the H_1 receptor (10,18). Because of the efficacy and low incidence of side effects, these agents have become the most frequently prescribed class of drugs to treat allergic conjunctivitis.

Allergen immunotherapy can be helpful in treating allergic conjunctivitis. A study designed to assess the effect of immunotherapy in allergic rhinitis demonstrated improvement in ocular allergy symptoms as well (21). Immunotherapy can exert an added beneficial effect to pharmacotherapy (22). Finally, immunotherapy has been demonstrated to reduce the sensitivity to ocular challenge with grass pollen (21).

Vernal Conjunctivitis

Clinical Presentation

Vernal conjunctivitis is a chronic, bilateral, catarrhal inflammation of the conjunctiva most commonly arising in children during the spring and summer. It can be perennial in severely affected patients. It is characterized by very intense itching, burning, and photophobia.

The illness is often seen during the preadolescent years and resolves at puberty. Male patients are affected about three times more often than female patients when the onset precedes adolescence, but when there is a later onset, female patients predominate. In the later-onset variety, the symptoms are usually less severe. The incidence is increased in warmer climates. It is most commonly seen in the Middle East and along the Mediterranean Sea.

Vernal conjunctivitis presents in palpebral and limbal forms. In the palpebral variety, which is more common, the tarsal conjunctiva of the upper lid is deformed by thickened, gelatinous vegetations produced by marked papillary hypertrophy. This hypertrophy imparts a cobblestone appearance to the conjunctiva, which results from intense proliferation of collagen and ground substance along with a cellular infiltrate (22). The papillae are easily seen when the upper lid is everted. In severe cases, the lower palpebral conjunctiva may be similarly involved. In the limbal form, a similar gelatinous cobblestone appearance occurs at the corneal–scleral junction. Trantas' dots—small, white dots composed mainly of eosinophils—are often present. Usually, there is a thick, stringy exudate full of eosinophils. This thick, ropey, white or yellow mucous discharge has highly elastic properties and produces a foreign-body sensation. It is usually easily distinguished from the globular mucus seen in seasonal allergic conjunctivitis or the crusting of infectious conjunctivitis. The patient may be particularly troubled by this discharge, which can string out for more than 2.5 cm (1 inch) when it is removed from the eye. Widespread punctate keratitis may be present. Severe cases can result in epithelial ulceration with scar formation.

Pathophysiology and Cause

The cause of and pathophysiologic mechanisms underlying vernal conjunctivitis remain obscure (23). Several features of the disease, however, suggest that the atopic state is related to its pathogenesis. The seasonal occurrence, the presence of eosinophils, and the fact that most of the patients have other atopic disease (24) are circumstantial evidence supporting this hypothesis. In addition, several different immunologic and histologic findings are consistent with an allergic etiology. Patients with vernal conjunctivitis have elevated levels of total IgE, allergen-specific IgE, histamine, and tryptase in the tear film. In addition, histologic studies support an immune origin. Patients with vernal conjunctivitis have markedly increased numbers of eosinophils, basophils, mast cells, and plasma cells in biopsy specimens taken from the conjunctiva. The mast cells are often totally degranulated. Elevated levels of major basic protein are found in biopsy specimens of the conjunctiva. Also, in keeping with the postulated role of IgE-mediated hypersensitivity is the pattern of cytokine secretion and T cells found in tears and on biopsy specimens. A T_H2 cytokine profile with increased levels of IL-4 and IL-5 has been found (23). Finally, ocular shields, designed to prevent pollen exposure, have been reported to be therapeutically effective (25). A role for cell-mediated immunity has been proposed and is supported by the findings of increased $CD4^+/CD29^+$ helper T cells in tears during acute phases of the illness. Also in keeping with this hypothesis is the improvement demonstrated during therapy with topical cyclosporine (26).

Fibroblasts appear to participate in the pathogenesis as well. They may be activated by T-cell or mast cell products. When stimulated with histamine, fibroblasts from patients with vernal conjunctivitis produce excessive amounts of procollagen I and II (23). In addition, they appear to manufacture constitutively increased amounts of transforming growth factor-β (TGF-β), IL-1, IL-6, and tumor necrosis factor-α (TNF-α) *in vitro*. The increased levels of cytokines noted *in vitro* are accompanied by increased serum levels of IL-1 and TNF-α as well (23). This over-expression of mediators both locally and systemically probably accounts for the upregulation of adhesion molecules on corneal epithelium noted in this disorder.

The eosinophilic cellular infiltrate in vernal conjunctivitis may contribute to corneal complications. Eosinophils secrete gelatinase B and polycationic toxic proteins such as major basic protein and eosinophilic cationic protein. *In vitro* these can cause epithelial damage with desquamation and cellular separation (23). Enzymatic activity may contribute to the pathophysiology of vernal conjunctivitis since elevated levels of urokinase and metalloproteinases have been reported (27).

Vasomotor complications can occur in this disorder and perhaps produce a hyperreactivity of the conjunctivae. Increased expression of muscarinic and adrenergic receptors and neural transmitters have been shown to occur in vernal conjunctivitis. These abnormalities could possibly result in hypersecretion and corneal hyperreactivity (28).

Diagnosis and Treatment

Vernal conjunctivitis must be distinguished from other conjunctival diseases that present with pruritus or follicular hypertrophy. These include acute allergic conjunctivitis, conjunctivitis, and keratoconjunctivitis associated with atopic dermatitis, the giant papillary conjunctivitis associated with soft contact lenses and other foreign bodies, the follicular conjunctivitis of viral infections, and trachoma (rarely found in the United States).

In most instances, the distinction between acute allergic conjunctivitis and vernal conjunctivitis is not difficult. However, in the early phases of vernal conjunctivitis or in mild vernal conjunctivitis, giant papillae may be absent. In such instances, the distinction may be more difficult because both conditions occur in atopic individuals, and pruritus is a hallmark of each. However, in vernal conjunctivitis, the pruritus is more intense, and the tear film contains a significantly greater concentration of histamine and greater numbers of eosinophils. The conjunctival epithelium has more abundant mast cells. Also, the cornea is not involved in acute allergic conjunctivitis.

The conjunctivitis and keratoconjunctivitis associated with atopic dermatitis can be similar to vernal conjunctivitis. In atopic dermatitis, the conjunctivitis can produce hypertrophy and opacity of the tarsal conjunctiva; a form of keratoconjunctivitis with papillary hypertrophy and punctate keratitis can occur (29). Many of these patients have signs and symptoms typical of vernal conjunctivitis, including giant follicles and pruritus. In addition, vernal conjunctivitis and atopic dermatitis can occur together in the same patient. However, because the treatment of both conditions is similar, the distinction, except for its prognostic value, may not be essential.

The giant papillary conjunctivitis caused by the wearing of soft contact lenses is similar to that of vernal conjunctivitis. Patients complain of itching, mucous discharge, and a decreasing tolerance to the lens. Symptoms usually begin 3 to 36 months after lenses are prescribed (30). The syndrome can occur with hard and soft lenses and can be seen with exposed sutures and plastic prostheses (30). Thus, chronic trauma to the lid appears to be the common inciting agent. Several features distinguish this entity from vernal conjunctivitis. Lens-associated papillary conjunctivitis causes less intense itching and shows no seasonal variation. It resolves with discontinuation of lens use.

Viral infections can be distinguished from vernal conjunctivitis by their frequent association with systemic symptoms and the absence of pruritus. A slit-lamp examination can produce a definitive distinction between these two entities.

Patients with mild vernal conjunctivitis can be treated with cold compresses and topical vasoconstrictor-antihistamine preparations. Levocabastine has been shown to be effective in a double-blind, placebo-controlled trial of 46 patients over a period of 4 weeks (31). Oral antihistamines may be of modest help. Cromolyn sodium and lodoxamide have been used effectively not only for milder but also for more recalcitrant, chronic forms of the condition (23). Cromolyn has been found to decrease conjunctival injection, punctate keratitis, itching, limbal edema, and tearing when administered regularly. It may be more effective in patients who are atopic. In a multicenter, double-blind 28-day study, another mast cell stabilizer, lodoxamide, was found to be more effective than cromolyn sodium (32).

Aspirin (33) has been found to be helpful in a dose of 0.5 g to 1.5 g daily. Ketorolac tromethamine has not been approved for use in vernal conjunctivitis, but based on the studies of aspirin, it might be an effective agent in this regard. Acetylcysteine 10% (Mucomyst) has been suggested as a means of counteracting viscous secretions. In severe cases, cyclosporine has been used (34). None of the above medications is universally effective, however, and topical corticosteroids often are necessary. If topical corticosteroids are needed, the patient should be under the care of an ophthalmologist. Fortunately, spontaneous remission usually occurs at puberty.

Other Eye Manifestations Associated with Atopic Dermatitis

Atopic dermatitis is associated with several manifestations of eye disease (35). These include lid dermatitis, blepharitis, conjunctivitis, keratoconjunctivitis, keratoconus, cataracts, and a predisposition to develop ocular infections, especially with herpes simplex and vaccinia viruses. Lid involvement has been discussed in detail previously.

Atopic dermatitis patients with ocular complications can be distinguished from those without ocular disease in that they have higher levels of serum IgE and more frequently demonstrate IgE specific to rice and wheat. Those with associated cataract formation have the highest levels of IgE. Patients with ocular complications also have increased tear histamine and LTB$_4$ levels compared with atopic dermatitis subjects without ocular complications.

As with other allergic eye conditions, subjects with atopic keratoconjunctivitis have cells in ocular tissue that exhibit a T$_H$2 cytokine profile with increased expression of messenger RNA for IL-4 and IL-5. Subjects with allergic keratoconjunctivitis, however, are different from those with vernal conjunctivitis in that they also express increased levels of interferon-γ and IL-2, indicating that in later stages of this disease, an element of T$_H$1 involvement is occurring. Lid involvement

can resemble contact dermatitis as they become thickened, edematous, and coarse; the pruritus may be intense.

Conjunctivitis may vary in intensity with the degree of skin involvement of the face. It resembles acute allergic conjunctivitis and to some extent resembles vernal conjunctivitis. It actually may be allergic conjunctivitis occurring with atopic dermatitis. Atopic keratoconjunctivitis usually does not appear until the late teenage years. The peak incidence is between 30 and 50 years of age. Male patients are affected in greater numbers than female patients.

Atopic keratoconjunctivitis is bilateral. The major symptoms are itching, tearing, and burning. The eyelids may be red, thickened, and macerated. There is usually erythema of the lid margin and crusting around the eyelashes. The palpebral conjunctiva may show papillary hypertrophy. The lower lid is usually more severely afflicted and more often involved. Punctate keratitis can occur, and the bulbar conjunctiva is chemotic.

Atopic keratoconjunctivitis must be differentiated from chronic blepharitis of nonallergic origin and vernal conjunctivitis. This may be difficult in the case of blepharitis. Indeed, staphylococcal blepharitis often complicates this disorder. Vernal conjunctivitis is usually distinguished from atopic keratoconjunctivitis by the fact that it most often involves the upper rather than lower lids and is more seasonal. It also occurs in a younger age group. The papillae in vernal conjunctivitis are larger. Cromolyn sodium is helpful in treating atopic keratoconjunctivitis. Topical corticosteroids often are needed; their use should be under the direction of the ophthalmologist.

Keratoconus occurs less frequently than conjunctival involvement. The cause of the association between atopic dermatitis and keratoconus is unknown, but there appears to be no human leukocyte antigen (HLA) haplotype that distinguishes atopic dermatitis patients with keratoconjunctivitis from patients without it or from controls (29).

The incidence rate of cataract formation in atopic dermatitis has been reported to range from 0.4% to 25%. These cataracts may be anterior or posterior in location, as opposed to those caused by administering corticosteroids, which are usually posterior. They have been observed in both children and adults. They may be unilateral or bilateral. Their presence cannot be correlated with the age of onset of the disease, its severity, or its duration. The pathophysiology involved in the formation of cataracts is unknown, but may involve genetic polymorphisms (36). Patients with atopic cataracts have higher serum IgE levels and have elevated levels of major basic protein in aqueous fluid and the anterior capsule, which is not found in senile cataracts.

Eyelid disorders may be the most common ocular complaint in patients with atopic dermatitis (37). Dermatitis of the lid produces itching with lid inversion.

The skin becomes scaly, and the skin of the eyes around the lid may become more wrinkled. The skin is extremely dry. The lesion is pruritic, and the disorder can be confused with contact dermatitis of the lid. Herpes keratitis is more common in patients with atopic dermatitis. This condition may be recurrent, and recalcitrant epithelial defects can occur.

Blepharoconjunctivitis (Marginal Blepharitis)

Blepharoconjunctivitis (marginal blepharitis) refers to any condition in which inflammation of the lid margin is a prominent feature of the disease. Conjunctivitis usually occurs in conjunction with the blepharitis. Three illnesses are commonly considered under the generic heading of blepharoconjunctivitis: bacterial (usually *Staphylococcal*) blepharoconjunctivitis, seborrheic blepharoconjunctivitis, and rosacea. They often occur together. Blepharoconjunctivitis accounts for 4.5% of all ophthalmologic problems presenting to the primary care physician (38).

Staphylococcal Blepharoconjunctivitis

The *Staphylococcal* organism is probably the most common cause of conjunctivitis and blepharoconjunctivitis. The acute bacterial conjunctivitis is characterized by irritation, redness, and mucopurulent discharge with matting of the eyelids. Frequently, the conjunctivitis is present in a person with low-grade inflammation of the eyelid margins.

In the chronic form, symptoms of *Staphylococcal* blepharoconjunctivitis include erythema of the lid margins, matting of the eyelids on awakening, and discomfort, which is usually worse in the morning. Examination frequently shows yellow crusting of the margin of the eyelids, with collarette formation at the base of the cilia, and disorganized or missing cilia. If the exudates are removed, ulceration of the lid margin may be visible. Fluorescein staining of the cornea may show small areas of dye uptake in the inferior portion. It is believed that exotoxin elaborated by *Staphylococcus* organisms is responsible for the symptoms and signs. Because of the chronicity of the disease and the subtle findings, the entity of chronic blepharoconjunctivitis of *Staphylococcal* origin can be confused with contact dermatitis of the eyelids and contact dermatoconjunctivitis. The absence of pruritus is the most important feature distinguishing *Staphylococcal* from contact dermatoconjunctivitis.

Seborrheic Dermatitis of the Lids

Staphylococcal blepharitis can also be confused with seborrheic blepharitis. Seborrheic blepharitis occurs as part of seborrheic dermatitis. It is associated with oily skin, seborrhea of the brows, and usually scalp involvement. The scales, which occur at the base of the cilia, tend to be greasy, and if these are removed, no ulceration is seen. There is no pruritus.

Rosacea

Rosacea involving the eyes can be severe even if the skin involvement is minor (35). Patients present with an "angry," erythematous chronic conjunctivitis. The eyelid margin is involved with erythema and meibonium gland dysfunction. The glands are dilated and their orifices plugged. Pressure on the eyelids below the gland openings will often produce a toothpaste-like secretion. Chronic inflammation can result in loss of secretion and conjunctivitis sicca. Complications include hordeola, chalazia, and telangiectasia. Of course, there are cutaneous manifestations of telangiectasia with flushing as well.

The blepharitis is manifested by collarettes, loss of lashes, discoloration, and whitening and misdirection of the lashes. There is usually marked erythema of the lid margin. Vessels that are telangiectatic may be seen crossing the eyelid margin. Patients often present with these manifestations thinking they are allergy related, and therefore this condition must always be kept in mind when making a differential diagnosis. It is important to be aware of the disorder since it can result in corneal erosions with neovascularization, and there can be an associated episcleritis and iritis.

Diagnosis and Treatment of Blepharoconjunctivitis

In all three forms of blepharoconjunctivitis, the cardinal symptoms are burning, redness, and irritation. True pruritus is usually absent or minimal. The inflammation of the lid margin is prominent. The discharge is usually mucopurulent, and matting in the early morning may be an annoying feature. In the seborrheic and rosacea forms, cutaneous involvement elsewhere is present.

All three forms are usually chronic and are often difficult to manage. In staphylococcal blepharoconjunctivitis, lid scrubs using a cotton-tipped applicator soaked with baby shampoo and followed by the application of a steroid ointment may be helpful. Commercially available lid scrubs specifically designed to treat this condition are also available. Control of other areas of seborrhea is necessary. Tetracycline or doxycycline can be beneficial in the therapy of rosacea. Ophthalmologic and dermatologic consultation may be needed.

Infectious Conjunctivitis/Keratitis

Viral Conjunctivitis

Viral conjunctivitis is the most common cause of red eye. It has several characteristics that distinguish it from allergic and bacterial disease. They include:

- Profuse watery discharge without purulence
- Usually occurs during an upper respiratory tract infection (latter stages)

- Possible palpable preauricular node
- Absence of itching

Viral conjunctivitis is usually of abrupt onset, frequently beginning unilaterally and involving the second eye within a few days. Conjunctival injection, slight chemosis, watery discharge, and enlargement of a preauricular lymph node help to distinguish viral infection from other entities. Clinically, lymphoid follicles appear on the conjunctiva as elevated avascular areas, which are usually grayish. These correspond to the histologic picture of lymphoid germinal centers. Viral conjunctivitis is usually of adenoviral origin and is frequently associated with a pharyngitis and low-grade fever in pharyngoconjunctival fever.

Epidemic keratoconjunctivitis presents as an acute follicular conjunctivitis, with a watery discharge and preauricular adenopathy. This conjunctivitis usually runs a 7- to 14-day course and is frequently accompanied by small corneal opacities. Epidemic keratoconjunctivitis can be differentiated from allergic conjunctivitis by the absence of pruritus, the presence of a mononuclear cellular response, and a follicular conjunctival response. The treatment of viral conjunctivitis is usually supportive, although prophylactic antibiotics are frequently used. If significant corneal opacities are present, the application of topical steroid preparations has been suggested.

Acute Bacterial Conjunctivitis

The most prominent distinguishing feature of acute bacterial conjunctivitis is purulent discharge. Patients may also have a sensation mimicking a foreign body in the eye, and lid edema is not uncommon. The most common culprits are *Streptocossas* pneumonia, *Haemophilus influenzae*, *Staphylococcal aureus*, and *Moraxella catarrhalis*. Gonococcal conjunctivitis bears special mention because of the fact that it can be invasive and cause permanent damage. In gonococcal conjunctivitis, the typical symptoms are usually far more pronounced. There is often a very copious purulent discharge. Treatment consists of warm compresses and ocular antibiotics. A follow-up visit within two days should be scheduled to re-evaluate.

Chlamydial (Inclusion) Conjunctivitis

In adults, inclusion conjunctivitis presents as an acute conjunctivitis with prominent conjunctival follicles and a mucopurulent discharge. There is usually no preceding upper respiratory infection or fever. This process occurs in adults who may harbor the chlamydial agent in the genital tract, but with no symptoms referable to this system. A nonspecific urethritis in men and a chronic vaginal discharge in women are common. The presence of a mucopurulent discharge and follicular conjunctivitis, which lasts more than 2 weeks, certainly suggests inclusion conjunctivitis. A Giemsa stain of a conjunctival scraping specimen may reveal intracytoplasmic inclusion bodies and helps to confirm the diagnosis. The treatment of choice is systemic tetracycline for 10 days.

Herpes Simplex Keratitis

Up to 500,000 cases of ocular herpes simplex are seen in the United States each year (38). A primary herpetic infection occurs subclinically in many patients. However, acute primary keratoconjunctivitis may occur with or without skin involvement. The recurrent form of the disease is seen most commonly. Patients usually complain of tearing, ocular irritation, blurred vision, and occasionally photophobia. Fluorescein staining of the typical linear branching ulcer (dendrite) of the cornea confirms the diagnosis. Herpetic keratitis is treated with antiviral compounds or by debridement. After the infectious keratitis has healed, the patient may return with a geographic erosion of the cornea, which is known as *metaherpetic (trophic) keratitis*. In this stage, the virus is not replicating, and antiviral therapy is usually not indicated. If the inflammation involves the deep corneal stroma, a disciform keratitis may result and may run a rather protracted course, leaving a corneal scar. It is important to distinguish herpetic keratitis from allergic conjunctivitis. The absence of pruritus and the presence of photophobia, blurred vision, and a corneal staining area should alert the clinician to the presence of herpetic infection. Using corticosteroids in herpetic disease only spreads the ulceration and prolongs the infectious phase of the disease process (39).

Herpes Zoster

Herpes zoster can occur typically with the appearance of ocular symptoms as the first manifestation, prior to the onset of skin involvement. Therefore the diagnosis should always be kept in mind. The ocular symptoms occur when the ophthalmic division of the trigeminal nerve is involved. The presence of a vessicle at the tip of the nose (Hutchinson's sign) may appear as a sentinel lesion. Like herpes infection, zoster also produces a dendritic keratitis. The distinction between the two therefore may be dependent on the typical skin lesions.

Keratoconjunctivitis Sicca

Keratoconjunctivitis sicca is a chronic disorder characterized by a diminished tear production. This is predominately a problem in menopausal or postmenopausal women and may present in patients with connective tissue disease, particularly rheumatoid arthritis. Although keratoconjunctivitis sicca may present as an isolated condition affecting the eyes only, it may also be associated with xerostomia (Sjögren syndrome).

Symptoms may begin insidiously and are frequently confused with a mild infectious or allergic process. Mild conjunctival injection, irritation, photophobia, and mucoid discharge may be present. Corneal epithelial damage can be demonstrated by fluorescein or rose Bengal staining, and hypolacrimation can be confirmed by inadequate wetting of the Schirmer test strip. Frequent application of artificial tears can be helpful. Cyclosporin eye drops (Restasis) are indicated in patients not adequately responding to artificial tears.

Giant Papillary Conjunctivitis

Giant papillary conjunctivitis, which is characterized by the formation of large papillae (larger than 0.33 mm in diameter) on the upper tarsal conjunctiva, has been associated with the wearing of contact lenses, prostheses, and sutures (30). Although it is most commonly caused by soft contact lenses, it can also occur with gas-permeable and rigid lenses. Patients experience pruritus, excess mucus production, and discomfort when wearing their lenses. There is decreased lens tolerance, blurred vision, and excessive lens movement (frequently with lens displacement). Burning and tearing are also noted. The patient develops papillae on the upper tarsal conjunctiva. These range from 0.3 mm to greater than 1 mm in diameter. The area involved correlates with the type of contact lens worn by the patient (40).

The mechanism of production of giant papillary conjunctivitis is unknown. One hypothesis is that the reaction is caused by an immunologic response to deposits on the lens surface. Deposits consist not only of exogenous airborne antigens but also of products in the tear film such as lysozyme, IgA, lactoferrin, and IgG. However, the amount of deposits does not clearly correlate with the presence of giant papillary conjunctivitis, and all lenses develop deposits within 8 hours of wear (30). More than two-thirds of soft lens wearers develop deposits within 1 year of wear. Evidence suggesting an immune mechanism in the production of giant papillary conjunctivitis is based on several observations. The condition is more common in atopic subjects. Patients with giant papillary conjunctivitis have elevated, locally produced tear IgE (41). Eosinophils, basophils, and mast cells are found in giant papillary conjunctivitis in greater amounts than in acute allergic conjunctivitis. There are elevated levels of major basic protein in conjunctival tissues of patients with giant papillary conjunctivitis and elevated levels of LTC_4, histamine, and tryptase in their tears. Further evidence for an IgE-mediated mechanism is the observation that ocular tissues from patients with giant papillary conjunctivitis exhibit increased messenger RNA for IL-4 and IL-5 (42) and have increased levels of major basic protein and eosinophilic cationic protein in tears (30).

Non-IgE-mediated immune mechanisms have also been incriminated in the production of this disorder. In fact, since the condition clearly occurs in nonallergic patients, other mechanisms must be a cause. For example,

the tear cytokine profile in giant papillary conjunctivitis differs considerably from that found in vernal keratoconjunctivitis. It is clear therefore that microtrauma of the conjunctivitis is the major causative factor in this condition. Although eosinophils appear to play a strong role in vernal conjunctivitis and atopic keratoconjunctivitis, they seem to be less important in giant papillary conjunctivitis (42).

Treatment of giant papillary conjunctivitis is usually carried out by the ophthalmologist. Early recognition is important because discontinuation of lens wear early in the stage of the disease and prescription of appropriate lens type and edge design can prevent recurrence. It is also important to adhere to a strict regimen for lens cleaning and to use preservative-free saline. Enzymatic cleaning with papain preparations is useful to reduce the coating of the lenses by antigens. Disposable lenses may also be beneficial. Both cromolyn sodium and nedocromil sodium have been found to be helpful (43).

Floppy Eye Syndrome

Floppy eye syndrome is a condition characterized by lax upper lids and a papillary conjunctivitis resembling giant papillary conjunctivitis. Men older than 30 years of age constitute the majority of patients. The condition is thought to result from chronic traction on the lax lid produced by the pillow at sleep. It may be unilateral or bilateral (44).

Vasomotor (Perennial Chronic) Conjunctivitis

Vasomotor (perennial chronic) conjunctivitis is a poorly defined condition not mediated by IgE. It refers to a conjunctivitis characterized by "vasomotor" instability. The term has been used to apply to patients who have chronic conjunctival findings exacerbated by irritant, and perhaps weather, stimulants in whom other disorders of the eye have been ruled out. It has been estimated that vasomotor stimuli may be involved in 25% of chronic conjunctivitis cases (45). It can be considered the ocular analogue of "vasomotor" rhinitis.

Approach to the Patient with an Inflamed Eye

The physician examining a patient with acute or chronic conjunctivitis should first exclude diseases (not discussed in this chapter) that may be acutely threatening to the patient's vision. These include conditions such as acute keratitis, uveitis, acute angle-closure glaucoma, and endophthalmitis. The two most important symptoms pointing to a threatening condition are a loss in visual acuity and pain. These are signs that the patient could have an elevated intraocular pressure, keratitis, endophthalmitis, or uveitis. On physical examination, the presence of unreactive pupils and/or circumcorneal hyperemia (dilatation of the vessels adjacent to the corneal edge or limbus) are warning signals that indicate a potentially threatening problem, and require immediate ophthalmologic consultation. These findings, especially circumcorneal hyperemia, are present in four threatening conditions: keratitis, uveitis, acute angle-closure glaucoma, and endophthalmitis. This contrasts with the pattern of vasodilation seen in acute allergic conjunctivitis, which produces erythema that is more pronounced in the periphery and decreases as it approaches the cornea.

If the physician believes that the patient does not have a threatening eye disease, the next step is to differentiate between allergic and nonallergic diseases of the eye (Table 28.3). The differential diagnosis between allergic and nonallergic diseases of the eye can usually be made by focusing on a few key features. Five cardinal questions should be asked in this regard:

1. Does the eye itch? This is the most important distinguishing feature between allergic and nonallergic eye disorders. All allergic conditions are pruritic. Nonallergic conditions usually do not itch. The physician must be certain that the patient understands what is meant by itching because burning, irritated, "sandy feeling" eyes are often described as "itchy" by the patient.
2. What type of discharge, if any, is present? A purulent discharge with early morning matting is not a feature of allergic disease and points toward infection.
3. Is the lid involved? Lid involvement indicates the presence of atopic dermatitis, contact dermatitis, or occasionally seborrhea or rosacea. Often, the patient complains of "eye irritation," which may mean the lid, conjunctiva, or both. The physician should be careful to ascertain which area of the eye is involved.
4. Are other allergic manifestations present? Examples include atopic dermatitis, asthma, and rhinitis.
5. Are there other associated nonallergic conditions? Nonallergic conditions include dandruff and rosacea.

■ THE EAR: OTIC MANIFESTATIONS OF ALLERGY

The most common otologic problem related to allergy is otitis media with effusion (OME). The potential role of allergic disease in the pathogenesis of OME is explored in the following discussion.

Otitis media is a general term defined as any inflammation of the middle ear with or without symptoms and usually associated with an effusion. It is one of the most common medical conditions seen in children by primary care physicians (46). In 1996 it was estimated that total costs for otitis media in the United States

approximated $5 billion (47). The classification of otitis media can be confusing. The First International Symposium on Recent Advances in Middle Ear Effusions includes the following types of otitis media: (a) acute purulent otitis media, (b) serous otitis media, and (c) mucoid or secretory otitis media. Chronic otitis media is a condition displaying a pronounced, retracted tympanic membrane with pathologic changes in the middle ear, such as cholesteatoma or granulation tissue. The acute phase of otitis media occurs during the first 3 weeks of the illness, the subacute phase between 4 and 8 weeks, and the chronic phase begins after 8 weeks. For this review, *acute otitis media* (AOM) applies to the classic ear infection, which is rapid in onset and associated with a red, bulging, and painful tympanic membrane. Fever and irritability usually accompany AOM. The presence of middle ear fluid without signs or symptoms of infection is OME. In many of these patients, hearing loss accompanies the condition. Other commonly used names for OME are serous otitis media and secretory otitis media.

In the United States, there are 24.5 million office visits for OME annually (47), and this condition results in the one of the most commonly performed surgeries in the United States: tympanostomy tube placement (47). OME is of major importance in children because the effusion can lead to a mild-to-moderate conductive hearing loss of 20 dB or more (48). It has been theorized that chronic conductive hearing loss in the child may lead to poor language development and learning disorders. There are many epidemiologic factors in the development of recurrent and chronic OME in children, with age at first episode being a major risk factor (49). Other risk factors include male sex, bottle feeding, day care atendance, allergy, race (Native American and Inuit), lower socioeconomic status, pacifier use, prone sleep position, winter season, and passive smoke exposure (47,50). In addition, diseases of the antibody-mediated immune system, primary ciliary dyskinesia, Down syndrome, and craniofacial abnormalities, especially cleft palate, can all contribute to chronic OME. In evaluation of the patient with recurrent or chronic OME, each of these conditions needs to be considered.

Pathogenesis of Otitis Media with Effusion

It appears that multiple factors influence the pathogenesis of OME. Most studies link OME with eustachian tube dysfunction, viral and bacterial infections, abnormalities of mucociliary clearance, immature immune system, and allergy (Table 28.4).

Eustachian Tube Anatomy and Physiology

The nasopharynx and middle ear are connected by the eustachian tube. The production of middle ear effusions appears to be related to functional or anatomic

TABLE 28.3   DIFFERENTIAL FEATURES TO BE CONSIDERED IN DIAGNOSING ALLERGIC EYE DISEASE

CLINICAL FEATURE	SEASONAL	ITCHING	SCRATCHY (SANDY) IRRITATION	SKIN OF LIDS AND/OR MARGIN INVOLVED	BILATERAL	TEARING	DISCHARGE	REMARKS
Acute allergic conjunctivitis	Yes	Prominent	Not usual	No	Yes	Increased	Mucoid	Itching is cardinal feature; rhinitis is present.
Vernal conjunctivitis	Yes	Prominent	Not usual	No	Yes	Slightly increased	Stringy and tenacious	Seasonal—spring and summer, more common in children.
Conjunctivitis sicca	No	No	Prominent	No	Yes	Markedly decreased	Slight mucoid	Dry mouth, associated with autoimmune disease, especially Sjögren syndrome.
Acute viral conjunctivitis	Variable, usually is not	No	Variable	No	Variable	Normal to slightly increased	Watery	Follicular conjunctivitis, prominent injection, may have preauricular node enlargement, concomitant upper respiratory tract infection.
Acute bacterial conjunctivitis	No	No	Variable	Matting, lid edema	Variable	Normal to increased	Mucopurulent	Exudate most prominent feature. Patient may have sensation of foreign body.
Contact Dermato-conjunctivitis	No	Yes	No	Variable	Usually	Normal to increased	Variable	Itching usually is a helpful diagnostic feature.
Blepharoconjunctivitis (bacterial/seborrheic/rosacea)	No	No	No	Yes	Usually	Normal	Early morning matting	Crusting of lids, loss of cilia, signs of seborrhea, rosacea seen elsewere (face, scalp), scaling, telangiectasia, etc.

Note: These conditions are to be considered in the absence of significant pain, photophobia, vision loss or blurring, poorly reactive pupils, and/or a limbal flush (circum corneal hyperemia). Any of these manifestations can indicate an elevated intraocular pressure or the presence of uveitis or other threatening ocular conditions (see text).

TABLE 28.4 RISK FACTORS FOR CHRONIC AND RECURRENT OTITIS MEDIA WITH EFFUSION

1. Age—children with OME in the first year of life have increased incidence of recurrence
2. Males > females
3. Bottle-fed infants
4. Passive smoking exposure
5. Allergy
6. Lower socioeconomic status
7. Race—Native Americans and Eskimos > whites > African Americans
8. Day care centers
9. Season—winter > Summer
10. Genetic predisposition—if siblings have OME, higher risk
11. Down syndrome
12. Primary immunodeficiency disorders
13. Primary and secondary ciliary dysfunction
14. Craniofacial abnormalities

OME, otitis media with effusion

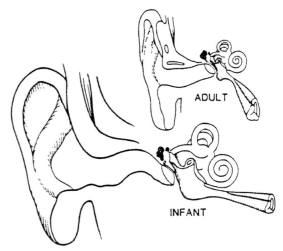

■ **FIGURE 28.2** Illustration showing difference in angles of eustachian tubes in infants and adults.

abnormalities of this tube. Under normal conditions, the eustachian tube has three physiologic functions: (a) ventilation of the middle ear to equilibrate pressure and replenish oxygen; (b) protection of the middle ear from nasopharyngeal sound pressure and secretions; and (c) clearance of secretions produced in the middle ear into the nasopharynx.

The eustachian tube of the infant and the young child differs markedly from that of the adult. These anatomic differences predispose infants and young children to middle ear disease. In infancy, the tube is wide, short, and more horizontal in orientation. As growth occurs, the tube narrows, elongates, and develops a more oblique course (Fig. 28.2). Usually after the age of 7 years, these physical changes lessen the frequency of middle ear effusion (47). In the normal state, the middle ear is free of any significant amount of fluid and is filled with air. Air is maintained in the middle ear by the action of the eustachian tube. This tube is closed at the pharyngeal end except during swallowing, when the tensor veli palatini muscle contracts and opens the tube by lifting its posterior lip (Fig. 28.3A). When the eustachian tube is opened, air passes from the nasopharynx into the middle ear, and this ventilation system equalizes air pressure on both sides of the tympanic membrane (Fig. 28.3B).

When the eustachian tube is blocked by either functional or anatomic defects, air cannot enter the middle ear, and the remaining air is absorbed. This results in the formation of negative pressure within the middle ear and subsequent retraction of the tympanic membrane (Fig. 28.3C). High negative pressure associated with ventilation may result in aspiration of nasopharyngeal secretions into the middle ear, producing acute otitis media with effusion (Fig. 28.3D). Prolonged negative pressure causes fluid transudation from the middle ear mucosal blood vessels (Fig. 28.3E). With chronic OME, there is infiltration of lymphocytes and macrophages, along with production of different inflammatory mediators. Also, there is an increased density of goblet cells in the epithelium of the eustachian tube. It is thought that many children with middle ear effusions, without a demonstrable cause of eustachian tube obstruction, have a growth-related inadequate action of the tensor veli palatini muscle. Another possibility is functional obstruction from persistent collapse of the tube owing to increased tubal compliance.

Nasal obstruction, either from adenoid hypertrophy or from infectious or allergic inflammation, may be involved in the pathogenesis of middle ear effusion by the Toynbee phenomenon (51). Studies have reported that, when the nose is obstructed, there is an increased positive nasopharyngeal pressure followed by a negative nasopharyngeal pressure on swallowing. The increased positive nasopharyngeal pressure may predispose to insufflation of secretions into the middle ear, and the secondary negative pressure in the nasopharynx may further be a factor in the inadequate opening of the eustachian tube, thereby causing obstruction.

Infection

Respiratory bacterial and viral infections are significant contributors to the pathogenesis of otitis media. Bacteria have been cultured in about 70% of middle ear effusions during tympanocentesis for otitis media in children (52). The three most common bacterial isolates in AOM and OME are *Streptococcus pneumoniae*, nontypeable *Haemophilus influenzae* (NTHI), and *Moraxella catarrhalis* (47). *Streptococcus pyogenes* and anaerobic cocci are isolated in less than 5% of the

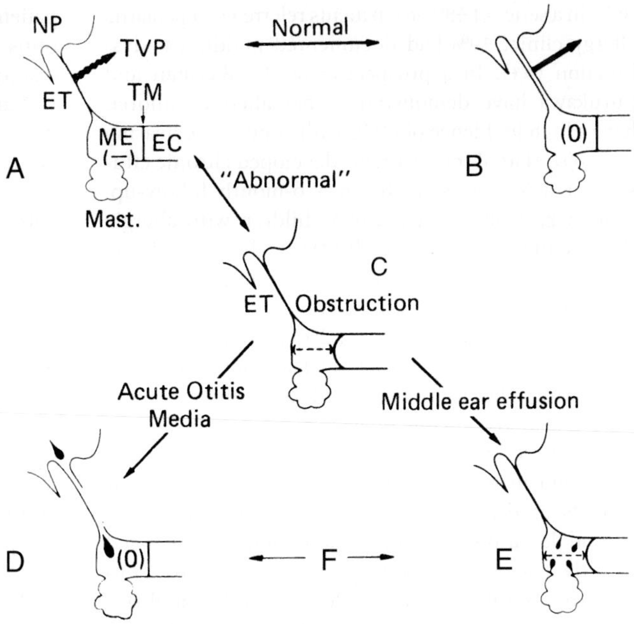

FIGURE 28.3 Proposed pathogenic mechanisms of middle ear effusion. *NP,* nasopharynx; *ET,* eustachian tube; *TVP,* tensor veli palatini muscle; *ME,* middle ear; *Mast.,* mastoid; *TM,* tympanic membrane; *EC,* external canal. (From Bluestone CD. Eustachian tube function and allergy in otitis media. *Pediatrics* 1978;61:753, with permission.)

patients with AOM. In 1999, *Alloiococcus otitis* was noted to be a significant bacterial pathogen in relationship with otitis media with effusion (53). The predominant anaerobes are gram-positive cocci, pigmented *Prevotella* and *Porphyromonas* species, *Bacterioides* species, and *Fusobacterium* species. The predominant organisms isolated from chronic otitis media are *Staphylococcus aureus, Pseudomonas aeruginosa,* and anaerobic bacteria. In neonates, group B streptococci and gram-negative organisms are common bacterial pathogens causing otitis media. Most patients with chronic OME have sterile middle ear effusions.

Post and associates used a polymerase chain reaction (PCR) to detect bacterial DNA in middle ear effusions in children who had failed multiple courses of antibiotics and therefore were undergoing myringotomy and tube placement (54). Of the 97 specimens, 75 (77.3%) were PCR positive for one or more of the following bacteria: *Streptococcus pneumoniae,* NTHI, and *Moraxella catarrhalis.* This suggests that active bacterial infection may be occurring in many children with chronic OME.

Viral agents are not commonly cultured from middle ear effusions. Most studies report positive viral cultures in less than 5% of the aspirates from the middle ear, with respiratory syncytial virus (RSV) being the most common isolate (55). However, using molecular techniques such as PCR, viral RNA can be detected in about 75% of children with AOM; common isolates include rhinovirus, coronavirus, and RSV (56,57).

Mucociliary Dysfunction

Mucociliary dysfunction from either a genetic defect or an acquired infectious or environmental condition can lead to OME. Investigations suggest that the mucociliary transfer system is an important defense mechanism in clearing foreign particles from the middle ear and the eustachian tube (58). Goblet and secretory cells provide a mucous blanket to aid ciliated cells in transporting foreign particles toward the nasopharynx for phagocytosis by macrophages, or to the lymphatics and capillaries for clearance. Respiratory viral infections are associated with transient abnormalities in the structure and function of cilia (59). Primary ciliary dyskinesia, an autosomal recessive syndrome, has been linked to more than 20 different structural defects in cilia, which lead to ciliary dysfunction (60). Both of these conditions can lead to inefficient ciliary transport, which results in mucostatics and can contribute to eustachian tube obstruction and the development of middle ear effusion.

Allergy and Immunology

There is considerable debate about whether allergic disorders are a factor in the pathogenesis of OME. Many investigators believe that allergic disorders play a prominent role, either as a cause or contributory factor; whereas others state that there is no convincing evidence that allergy leads to otitis media. Allergy has been implicated as a causative factor in otitis media with effusion by (a) double-blind placebo-control nasal challenge studies with histamine and allergens; (b) studies on allergic children; and (c) studies on randomly selected children with OME referred to specialty clinics (61,62). Kraemer compared risk factors of OME among children with tympanostomy tubes compared with controls matched for age and reported atopy as a risk factor

(63). In a series of 488 new patients referred to a pediatric allergy clinic, 49% had documented middle ear dysfunction (64). In a prospective study, Bierman and Furukawa have demonstrated that allergic children have a high incidence of OME with conductive hearing loss (65). Half of their patients developed chronic effusion or acute otitis media in a 6-month follow-up. Tomonaga et al. evaluated 605 children with allergic rhinitis and found 21% with OME. They also determined that 50% of 259 children with diagnosed OME had allergic rhinitis (66). Bernstein and Reisman reviewed the clinical course of 200 randomly selected children with OME who had at least one tympanostomy with tube insertion (67). Twenty-three percent were considered allergic by history, physical examination, and allergy skin testing.

In human studies, Friedman et al. evaluated eight patients, aged 18 to 29 years, with seasonal rhinitis but no middle ear disease. Patients were blindly challenged with the pollen to which the patient was sensitive or to a control. Nasal function was determined by nasal rhinomanometry and eustachian tube function by the nine-step-deflation tympanometric test. The results from this and other studies (68) showed that eustachian tube dysfunction can be induced by antigen and histamine challenge (68), although no middle ear effusions occurred. Osur evaluated 15 children with ragweed allergy and measured eustachian tube dysfunction before, during, and after a ragweed season (69). There was a significant increase in eustachian tube dysfunction during the pollen season, but it did not lead to OME. It appears that other variables need to be present for effusion to develop.

Work by Hurst et al. has provided the most conclusive evidence of the role of allergy in OME. These researchers evaluated 89 patients for allergy who required the placement of tympanostomy tubes because of persistent effusion. Radioallergosorbent test (RAST), serum IgE levels, and skin tests were performed. Atopy was present in 97% of the patients with OME by skin testing. Significant levels of eosinophil cationic protein and eosinophils were found in the effusions, suggesting allergic inflammation in the middle ear (70). These investigators also determined that IgE in middle ear effusion is not a transudate but more likely reflects an active localized process in atopic patients (71) and that tryptase, a reflection of mast cell activity, is found in most ears of patients with chronic effusion who were atopic (72). These findings and others (73) support the hypothesis that middle ear mucosa is capable of an allergic response and that the inflammation within the middle ear of most OME patients is allergic in nature.

Acute and chronic suppurative otitis media are commonly part of a primary or secondary immunodeficiency syndrome. The middle ear is usually one of many locations for infection in immunodeficient patients. Of the primary immunodeficiency conditions, otitis media is more common in the humoral or B-cell disorders, such as X-linked hypogammaglobulinemia, common variable immunodeficiency, and selective IgA deficiency. A patient's incapacity to produce antibodies against pneumococcal polysaccharide antigens and a related IgG2 subclass deficiency has been associated with the development of recurrent otitis media in children (74).

Diagnosis

Acute otitis media usually presents with fever, otalgia, vomiting, diarrhea, and irritability. In young children, pulling at the ear may be the only manifestation of otalgia. Otorrhea, discharge from the middle ear, may occur if spontaneous perforation of the tympanic membrane occurs. It is not uncommon for AOM to be preceded by an upper respiratory infection. The pneumatic otoscope is an important tool for making accurate diagnosis of AOM. Classically, the tympanic membrane is erythemic and bulging without a light reflex or the ossicular landmarks visualized. Pneumatic testing fails to elicit any movement of the tympanic membrane on applying positive and negative pressure.

Most children with OME do not have symptoms. Others may complain of stopped-up or popping ears or a feeling of fullness in the ear. Older children may even note a hearing loss. Their teachers and parents detect the condition in many younger children because they are noted to be inattentive, loud talkers, and slow learners. Other children may be discovered with OME in screening tests done for hearing at school. When middle ear effusions become chronic, there may be significant diminution of language development and auditory learning, with resultant poor academic achievement. On pneumatic otoscopic examination of patients with OME, the tympanic membrane may appear entirely normal. At other times, air-fluid levels and bubbles may be apparent. There is often retraction of the tympanic membrane, and the malleus may have a chalky appearance. As the disease progresses, the tympanic membrane takes on an opaque amber or bluish gray color. Alteration of the light reflex is commonly present. Mild retraction of the tympanic membrane may indicate only negative ear pressure without effusion. In more severe retraction, there is a prominent lateral process of the malleus with acute angulation of the malleus head. Tympanic membrane motility is generally poor when positive and negative pressures are applied by the pneumatic otoscopy.

Tympanometry is commonly used as a confirmatory test for OME. It is a tool for indirect measuring of the compliance or mobility of the tympanic membrane by applying varying ear canal pressure from 200 mm H_2O to 400 mm H_2O. Patients with OME have a flat (type B) curve because of failure of the tympanic membrane to move with the changing pressure. Audiometric examination in OME often discloses a mild to moderate degree of conduction hearing impairment of 20 dB to 40 dB. The guidelines for the treatment of OME in young children from the Agency for Health Care Policy and Research recommends that an otherwise healthy child with bilateral OME for 3 months should have a hearing evaluation (75). Acoustic reflectometry, a test that involves a tone sweep in the patient's ear and measuring reflected sound pressure to assess effusion, and tuning fork tests can also be used in the diagnosis and evaluation of OME.

The physical examination of the patient with OME should not stop at the tympanic membrane. Craniofacial anomalies, such as Down syndrome, submucous cleft palate, and bifid uvula, may be present that predispose to OME. Stigmata of an allergic diathesis should be sought in each patient. Eye examination may illustrate injected conjunctiva seen in patients with allergic conjunctivitis. Pale, boggy turbinates with profuse serous rhinorrhea are commonly found with allergic rhinitis. When chronic middle ear effusions are associated with the signs and symptoms of allergic disease, a standard allergic evaluation is indicated. A nasal smear for eosinophils, peripheral eosinophil count, and cutaneous tests for specific allergens may be of diagnostic importance.

In patients with recurrent or chronic otitis media in whom middle ear disease is just one of many sites of infection, screening of the immune system should be considered. Laboratory studies, such as IgG, IgA, and IgM, naturally occurring antibodies such as isohemagglutinins, and specific antibody titers to antigens previously given in vaccines, such as tetanus, are useful in evaluation of humoral immune status. Measuring specific antibody levels before and after administration of a pneumococcal polyvalent vaccine is an effective means of evaluating humoral immune function. Another possible condition to consider in children with multiple sites of recurrent infection is primary ciliary dyskinesia. Examination of the cilia by electron microscopy can illustrate abnormalities of the cilia ultrastructure, which can lead to ciliary dysfunction and its related chronic otitis.

Management

Management of the patient with OME requires appropriate pharmacologic and surgical intervention. It is important to understand the natural history of AOM and OME. Usually, the symptoms of AOM resolve in 48 to 72 hours if the organism is sensitive to the prescribed antibiotic. Two weeks into treatment, 70% of patients have a middle ear effusion. One month after treatment, 40% continue to have effusion, but after 3 months, only 10% of patients continue to have a persistent effusion (47). In patients with OME in which allergy may be a contributing factor, appropriate allergy treatment of avoidance of particular allergens, medication, and immunotherapy may be indicated.

Pharmacotherapy

Antimicrobial agents are the first-line therapy in AOM and may be beneficial in OME because bacteria are found in many cases. Amoxicillin is recommended as the first-line agent to treat uncomplicated AOM. For clinical treatment failures after 3 days of amoxicillin, recommended antimicrobial agents include oral amoxicillin/clavulanate, cefuroxime axetil, cefprozil, cefpodoxime proxetil, and intramuscular ceftriaxone (47). Intramuscular ceftriaxone should be reserved for severe cases or patients in whom noncompliance is expected. Tympanocentesis for identification of pathogens, and susceptibility to antimicrobial agents is recommended for selection of third-line agents (76). Resistant bacteria are an increasing problem in the management of children with otitis media. Sutton reported penicillin resistance in the middle ear fluid of 38.2% of *S. pneumoniae* cultures at the time of tympanostomy tube surgery (77). β-Lactamase production was found in 65.1% and 100% of *H. influenzae* and *M. catarrhalis* specimens, respectively, in that study. The Agency of Health Care Policy and Research, in its guidelines on OME in young children, revealed by meta-analysis of the literature that there was a 14% increase in the probability that OME would resolve when antibiotic therapy was given as compared with no treatment (76). Another management option advocated for OME is observation of the patient for up to 4 months because of the natural history of resolution of OME in most patients. In patients with recurrent episodes of otitis media, several studies have reported that prophylactic regimens may be effective. The suggested duration for prophylactic antibiotics is 3 to 6 months with amoxicillin 20 mg/kg given once a day or sulfisoxazole 75 mg/kg given once a day (78).

Another therapeutic modality prescribed in patients with OME is oral corticosteroids. Many studies have evaluated corticosteroids alone and in combination with antibiotics in clearing of middle ear effusions. The panel from the Agency of Health Care Policy and Research Guidelines on OME in young children reviewed 10 studies on the use of oral corticosteroids with and without antibiotics in OME and came to the conclusion that corticosteroid therapy is not effective in treating these children (76). At present, the data do not support the use of intranasal corticosteroids, antihistamines, or decongestants in the management of OME (47).

Environmental Control

When allergic rhinitis is associated with OME, environmental control of allergens and irritants should be advised. The most significant irritant is cigarette smoke. The parents must be urged to avoid exposure of their children to cigarette smoke in the home, car, restaurant, and day care facilities. Environmental inhalant allergens are more important to younger children because of the greater time spent in the home. Specific instructions for the avoidance of house dust mites, cockroaches, animal dander, and house mold spores should be given when indicated.

Vaccination

The heptavalent pneumococcal conjugate vaccine has been effective in significantly decreasing the number of episodes of otitis media in children. Black et al. demonstrated that children who received the pneumococcal conjugate vaccine were 20.1% less likely to require insertion of tympanostomy tubes than were controls (79). It is estimated to prevent up to 1,000,000 episodes of AOM per year, leading to cost savings of $160 per otitis media episode prevented (80). Similar results have been reported by Canadian investigators (81).

Surgical Treatment

Refractory cases that continue to have middle ear fluid after a 4-month trial of observation or medical management often need surgical intervention. Chronic middle ear effusion has been associated with the development of cholesteatomas, atrophy of the tympanic membrane, facial paralysis, and retention pockets. The Agency of Health Care Policy and Research Guidelines recommend myringotomy with the insertion of tympanostomy tubes for children with OME between the ages of 1 and 3 years who have bilateral hearing loss of at least 20 dB for 4 to 6 months. This procedure is effective in removing the effusion and restoring normal hearing in the child. A number of studies (47,82) have demonstrated the beneficial effect of tympanostomy tubes in OME. It is usually recommended that tympanostomy tubes remain in place for 6 to 18 months. The longer the tube remains in the tympanic membrane, the greater the chance of complications. These include tympanosclerosis, persistent perforation, otorrhea, and occasionally cholesteatoma. Adenoidectomy has been suggested in the treatment of OME to remove blockage of the eustachian tube and improve ventilation. The Agency of Health Care Policy and Research Guidelines do not recommend adenoidectomy for children between 1 and 3 years of age with OME, although older children may benefit from the surgery. Gates et al. demonstrated that adenoidectomy improved and reduced recurrence of OME in children older than 4 years of age (83). They reported that the size of the adenoids did not relate to improvement of OME with adenoidec-

tomy. Recently, the use of CO_2 laser myringotomy has been shown to be more efficacious than incisional myringotomy with adenoidectomy in OME (84). Tonsillectomy is not recommended in the management of children with OME (47,85).

Immunotherapy

Immunotherapy has been proved to be effective in the therapy for allergic rhinitis, when avoidance of the allergen is not possible or the symptoms are uncontrolled by medication. Many have the clinical impression that immunotherapy may be of help in OME in children with allergic rhinitis. However, there have been no controlled studies to verify this clinical impression.

In conclusion, the prognosis in OME is usually good. As the child gets older, the incidence of OME tends to decrease. The medical and surgical intervention outlined for OME helps to control the condition until the child "outgrows" this disease.

■ REFERENCES

1. Bashir SJ, Maibach HI. Compound allergy: an overview. *Contact Dermatitis.* 1997;36:179–183.
2. Marsh R, Towns S, Evans K. Patch testing in ocular drug allergies. *Trans Ophthalmol Soc UK.* 1978;98:278–280.
3. Mondino B, Salamon S, Zaidman G. Allergic and toxic reactions in soft contact lens wearers. *Surv Ophthalmol.* 1982;26:337–344.
4. Rietschel RL, Fowler JF. The role of patch testing. In: Rietschel RL, Fowler JF, eds. *Fisher's Contact Dermatitis.* 4th ed. Baltimore: Williams & Wilkins;1995:11–32.
5. Eiseman AS. The ocular manifestations of atopic dermatitis and rosacea. *Curr Allergy Asthma Rep.* 2006;6:292–298.
6. Inoue Y. Ocular infections in patients with atopic disease. *Intl Ophthalmol Clin.* 2002;42:55–69.
7. Leonardi A, De Dominicis C, Motterle L. Immunopathogenesis of ocular allergy: a schematic approach to different clinical entities. *Curr Opin in Allergy Clin Immunol.* 2007;7:429–435.
8. Fukushima A. Roles of T-cells in the development of allergic conjunctival diseases. *Cornea.* 2007;26:536–540.
9. Fukushima A, Yamaguchi T, Ishida W. Cyclosporin A inhibits eosinophilic infiltration into the conjunctivae mediated by type IV allergic reactions. *Clin Experiment Ophthalmol.* 2006;34:347–353.
10. Schultz BL. Pharmacology of ocular allergy. *Curr Opin Allergy Clin Immunol.* 2006;6(5):383–389.
11. Stahl, JL, Cook. EB, Barney, NP, et al. Pathophysiology of ocular allergy: the roles of conjunctival mast cells and epithelial cells. *Curr Allergy Asthma Rep.* 2002;2:332–339.
12. Bonini S. Allergic conjunctivitis: the forgotten disease. *Chem Immunol Allergy.* 2006;91:110–120.
13. Bonini S, Tomassini M, Adriani E, et al. The eosinophil has a pivotal role in allergic inflammation of the eye. *Int Arch Allergy Immunol.* 1992;99:354–358.
14. Bonini S, Bonini S. IgE and non-IgE mechanisms in ocular allergy. *Ann Allergy.* 1993;71:296–299.
15. Bielory L, Bonini S, Sonini S. Allergic eye disorders. *Clin Allergy Immunol.* 2002;16:311–323.
16. Bielory L, Friedlaender MH. Allergic conjunctivitis. *Immunol Allergy Clin North Am.* 2008;28:43–48.
17. Woods A. Ocular allergy. *Am J Ophthalmol.* 1949;32:1457–1461.
18. Bielory L, Katelaris CH, Lightman S, et al. Treating the ocular component of allergic rhinoconjunctioitis and relted eye disorders. *Med Gen Med.* 2007 9:35–50.
19. Dechant K, Goa K. Levocabastine: a review of its pharmacological properties and therapeutic potential as a topical antihistamine in allergic rhinitis and conjunctivitis. *Drugs.* 1991;41:202–224.

20. Woodward D, Bogardus AM, Donello JE, et al. Acular: studies on its mechanism of action in reducing allergic conjunctival itching. *J Allergy Clin Immunol.* 1995;95:360–366.

21. Powell RJ, Frew AJ, Corrigan CJ, et al. Effect of grass pollen immunotherapy on quality of life in seasonal allergic rhinoconjunctivitis. *Allergy.* 2007;62:1335–1338.

22. Moages R, Hassan H, Wenzel M. Optimal use of topical agents for allergic conjunctivitis. *BioDrugs.* 1997;8(4):250–262.

23. Leonardi A. Vernal keratoconjunctivitis, pathogenesis and treatment. *Prog Retin Eye Res.* 2002;21:319–339.

24. Abelson M, George M, Garofalo C. Differential diagnosis of ocular allergic disorders. *Ann Allergy.* 1993;70:95–113.

25. Little EC. Keeping pollen at bay. *Lancet.* 1968;2:512–513.

26. Scheinfeld N. A review of deferasirox, bortezomib, dasatinib, and cyclosporine eye drops: possible uses and known side effects in cutaneous medicine. *J Drugs Dermatol.* 2007;6:352–355.

27. Leonardi A, Brun P, Sartori MT, et al. Urokinase plasminogen activator, uPA receptor and its inhibitor in vernal keratoconjunctivitis. *Invest Ophthalmol Dis Sci.* 2005;46:1364–1370.

28. Motterle L, Diebold Y, Enriquez de Salamanca A, et al. Altered expression of neurotransmitter receptors and neuromediators in vernal keratoconjunctivitis. *Arch Ophthalmol.* 2006; 124:462-468.

29. Oshinskie L, Haine C. Atopic dermatitis and its ophthalmic complications. *J Am Ophthalmic Assoc.* 1982; 53:889–894.

30. Bozhurt G, Akyurek N, Irkec M, et al. Immunohistochemical findings in prosthesis associated giant papillary conjunctivitis. *Clin Experiment Ophthalmol.* 2007;35:535–540.

31. Goes F, Blockhuys S, Janssens M. Levocabastine eye drops in the treatment of vernal conjunctivitis. *Doc Ophthalmol.* 1994;87: 271–281.

32. Caldwell D, Verin P, Hartwich-Young R, et al. Efficacy and safety of iodoxamide 0.1% vs. cromolyn sodium 4% in patients with vernal keratoconjunctivitis. *Am J Ophthalmol.* 1992;113:632–637.

33. Meyer E, Kraus E, Zonis S. Efficacy of antiprostaglandin therapy in vernal conjunctivitis. *Br J Ophthalmol.* 1987;71:497–499.

34. Trocme S, Raizman M, Bartley G. Medical therapy for ocular allergy. *Mayo Clin Proc.* 1992;67:557–565.

35. Eiseman AS. The ocular manifestations of atopic dermatitis and rosacea. *Curr Allergy Asthma Rep.* 2006;6(4):292–298.

36. Matsuda A, Ebihara N, Kumagai N, et al. Genetic polymorphisms in the promoter of the interferon gamma receptor 1 gene are associated with atopic cataracts. *Invest Ophthal; Vis Sci.* 2007;48:583–389.

37. Garrity J, Liesegang T. Ocular complications of atopic dermatitis. *Can J Ophthalmol.* 1984;19:21–24.

38. Kerns B, Mason J. Red eye: a guide through the differential diagnosis. *Emerg Med.* 2004; 36(9):31-40.

39. Pavan-Langston D. Diagnosis and management of herpes simplex ocular infection. *Int Ophthalmol Clin.* 1975;15:19–35.

40. Katelaris C. Giant papillary conjunctivitis: a review. *Acta Ophthalmol Scand.* 1999;77:17–20.

41. Irkec M, Orhan M, Erdener U. Role of tear inflammatory mediators in contact lens associated giant papillary conjunctivitis in soft contact lens wearer. *Ocul Immunol Inflamm.* 1999;7(1):35–38.

42. Shoji J, Inada N, Sawa M. Antibody array generated cytokine profiles of tears of patients with vernal keratoconjunctivitis or giant papillary conjunctivitis. *Jpn J Ophthalmol.* 2006;50:195–204.

43. Bailey C, Buckley R. Nedocromil sodium in contact-lens-associated papillary conjunctivitis. *Eye.* 1993;7(Suppl):29–33.

44. Culbertson W, Ostler B. The floppy eyelid syndrome. *Am J Ophthalmol.* 1981;92:568–574.

45. Bielory L. Vasomotor (perennial chronic) conjunctivitis. *Curr Opin Allergy Clin Immunol.* 2006; 6:355–360.

46. Schappert S. *Office visits for otitis media: United States, 1975–90, advance data from vital and health statistics.* Hyattsville, MD: National Center for Health Statistics: 1992.

47. Werkhaven JA. Otitis media. In: Rakel RE, Bope ET, eds. *Conn's Current Therapy.* Philadelphia: Elsevier/Saunders;2004:196–198.

48. Dempster J, MacKenzie K. Tympanometry in the detection of hearing impairments associated with otitis media with effusion. *Clin Otolaryngol.* 1991;16:157–159.

49. Engel J, Anteunist L, Volovics A, et al. Risk factors of otitis media with effusion during infancy. *Int J Pediatr Otorhinolaryngol.* 1999;48(3):239–249.

50. Rovers M, Straatman H, Ingels K, et al. Prognostic factors for persistent otitis media with effusion in infants. *Arch Otolaryngol Head Neck Surg.* 1999;125(11):1203–1207.

51. Bellioni P, Cantani A, Salvinelli F. Allergy: a leading role in otitis media with effusion. *Allergol Immunopathol.* (Madr) 1987;15(4):205–208.

52. Riding K, Bluestone C, Michaels R, et al. Microbiology of recurrent and chronic otitis media with effusion. *J Pediatr.* 1978;93(5):739–743.

53. Hendolin P, Karkkainen U, Himi T, et al. High incidence of alloiococcus otitis in otitis media with effusion. *Pediatr Infect Dis J.* 1999;18(10):860–865.

54. Post J, Preston R, Aul J. Molecular analysis of bacterial pathogens in otitis media with effusion. *JAMA.* 1995;273:1598–1604.

55. Brook I, Van de Heyning P. Microbiology and management of otitis media. *Scand J Infect Dis.* 1994;(Suppl 93)(1):20–32.

56. Pitkäranta A, Jero J, Arruda E, et al. Polymerase chain reaction-based detection of rhinovirus, respiratory syncytial virus, and coronavirus in otitis media with effusion. *J Pediatr.* 1998;133:390–394.

57. Heikkinen T, Thint M, Chonmaitree T. Prevalence of various respiratory viruses in the middle ear during acute otitis media. *N Engl J Med.* 1999;340:260–264.

58. Ohashi Y, Nakai Y. Current concepts of mucociliary dysfunction in otitis media with effusion. *Acta Otolaryngol.* 1991;(Suppl 486):149–161.

59. Carson J, Collier A, Hu S. Acquired ciliary defects in nasal epithelium of children with acute viral upper respiratory infections. *N Engl J Med.* 1985;312:463–468.

60. Schidlow D. Primary ciliary dyskinesia (the immotile cilia syndrome). *Ann Allergy.* 1994;73(6):457–468;quiz, 468–470.

61. Bernstein J. The role of IgE-mediated hypersensitivity in the development of otitis media with effusion: a review. *Otolaryngol Head Neck Surg.* 1993;109(3 Pt 2):611–620.

62. Caffareli C, Savini E, Giordano S, et al. Atopy in children with otitis media with effusion. *Clin Exp Allergy.* 1998;28(5):591–596.

63. Kraemer M, Richardson M, Weiss N, et al. Risk factors for persistent middle-ear effusions: otitis media, catarrh, cigarette smoke exposure, and atopy. *JAMA.* 1983;249(8):1022–1025.

64. Marshall S, Bierman C, Shapiro G. Otitis media with effusion in childhood. *Ann Allergy.* 1984;53(5):370–378.

65. Bierman C, Furukawa C. Medical management of serous otitis in children. *Pediatrics.* 1978;61:768–774.

66. Tomonaga K, Kurono Y, Mogi G. The role of nasal allergy in otitis media with effusion: a clinical study. *Acta Otolaryngol.* 1988;(Suppl 458):41–47.

67. Bernstein J, Reisman R. The role of acute hypersensitivity in secretory otitis media. *Trans Am Acad Ophthalmol Otolaryngol.* 1974;78:120–127.

68. Friedman R, Doyle WJ, Casselbrant ML, et al. Immunologic-mediated eustachian tube obstruction: a double-blind crossover study. *J Allergy Clin Immunol.* 1983;71:442–447.

69. Osur S, Volovitz B, Bernstein J. Eustachian tube dysfunction in children with ragweed hayfever during natural pollen exposure. *Allergy Proc.* 1989;10:133–139.

70. Hurst D. Association of otitis media with effusion and allergy as demonstrated by intradermal skin testing and eosinophil cationic protein levels in both middle ear effusions and mucosal biopsies. *Laryngoscope.* 1996;106(9 Pt 1):1128–1137.

71. Hurst D, Weekley M, Ramanarayanan M. Evidence of possible localized specific immunoglobulin E production in middle ear fluid as demonstrated by ELISA testing. *Otolaryngol Head Neck Surg.* 1999;121(3):224–230.

72. Hurst D, Amin K, Seveus L, et al. Evidence of mast cell activity in the middle ears of children with otitis media with effusion. *Laryngoscope.* 1999; 109(3):471–477.

73. Luong A, Roland PS. The link between allergic rhinitis and chronic otitis media with effusion in atopic patients. *Otolaryngol Clin North Am.* 2008;41:311–323.

74. Umetsu D, Ambrosino D, Quinti I, et al. Recurrent sinopulmonary infection and impaired antibody response to bacterial capsular polysaccharide antigen in children with selective IgG-subclass deficiency. *N Engl J Med.* 1985;313:1247–1251.

75. Stool S, Berg A, Berman S. Otitis media with effusion in young children. In: *Clinical Practice Guidelines.* 1994(12), DHHS publication no (AHCRP) 94-0622.

76. Aronovitz G. Antimicrobial therapy of acute otitis media: review of treatment recommendations. *Clin Ther.* 2000;22(1):29–39.

77. Sutton D, et al. Resistant bacteria in middle ear fluid at the time of tympanostomy tube surgery. *Ann Otol Rhinol Laryngol.* 2000;109(1):24–29.

78. Williams R, Chambers T, Stange K. Use of antibiotics in preventing recurrent acute otitis media and in treating otitis media with effusion: a meta-analytic attempt to resolve the brouhaha. *JAMA.* 1993;270:1344–1351.

79. Black S, Shinefield H, Fireman B, et al. Efficacy, safety and immunogenicity of heptavalent pneumococcal conjugate vaccine in children. *Pediatr Infect Dis J.* 2000;19:187–195.

80. Lieu T, Ray A, Black S, et al. Projected cost-effectiveness of pneumococcal conjugate vaccination of healthy infants and young children. *JAMA.* 2000;283(11):1460–1468.

81. McClure CA, Ford MW, Wilson JB, et al. Pneummococcal conjugate vaccination in Canadian infants and children younger than five years of age; recommendations and expected benefits. *Can J Infec Dis Med Microbiol.* 206;17:19–26.

82. Rosenfeld R, Bhyer M, Bower C, et al. Impact of tympanostomy tubes on child quality of life. *Arch Otolaryngol Head Neck Surg.* 2000;126(5):585–592.

83. Gates G, Avery C, Prihoda T, et al. Effectiveness of adenoidectomy and tympanostomy tubes in the treatment of chronic otitis media with effusion. *N Engl J Med.* 1987;317(23):1444–1451.

84. Szeremeta W, Parameswaran M, Isaacson G. Adenoidectomy with laser or incisional myringotomy for otitis media with effusion [In process citation]. *Laryngoscope.* 2000;110(3 Pt 1):342–345.

85. Stewart I. Evaluation of factors affecting outcome of surgery for otitis media with effusion in clinical practice. *Int J Pediatr Otorhinolaryngol.* 1999;49(Suppl 1):S243–S245.

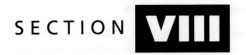

SECTION VIII

Cutaneous Allergic Disease

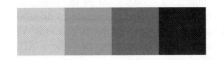

CHAPTER **29**

Atopic Dermatitis
PECK Y. ONG AND DONALD Y.M. LEUNG

■ INTRODUCTION

Atopic dermatitis (AD) is the most common chronic inflammatory skin disease in childhood. The disease is characterized by itch and frequent skin infections. Affected individuals, particularly those with moderate-to-severe disease, often have disruption in sleep, daily activities, school, or work (1). The stress in taking care of children with moderate-to-severe AD is equivalent to that associated with the care of children who require home enteral feeding (2). AD also results in a significant number of physician visits, and cost to the patients and health care system ($3.8 billion/year) (3,4,5). There is currently no curative therapy for AD. The current chapter will discuss an integrative approach in the management of this condition involving preventive measures, trigger avoidance, symptomatic treatments and patient education.

■ EPIDEMIOLOGY AND NATURAL HISTORY

The worldwide prevalences of AD range from 2% to 20% (6). In the United States, AD constitutes about 17% of school children (7). The severity of AD may be categorized into mild (80%), moderate (18%), and severe (2%) (8). Eighty percent of AD patients have

onset of their disease before 5 years, but most (60%), particularly those with mild AD, outgrow it by adolescence (9). Patients with moderate-to-severe AD (77% to 91%) have persistent disease into their adulthood (10). A significant proportion of AD children (more than 60%) are at risk for developing allergic rhinitis and/or asthma (11).

■ PATHOGENESIS

Genetics clearly play an important role in the pathogenesis of AD, as the concordance rate of AD in identical twins and fraternal twins are seven-fold and three-fold, respectively, as compared to the general population (12). Various genetic polymorphisms involving skin barrier defects and immune functions have been associated with AD. Genetic variations in the epidermal differentiation complex (EDC) on chromosome 1q21 have been found in AD (13). EDC contains a cluster of genes, including filaggrin, involucrin, loricrin, and S100 proteins, that are crucial in epidermal functions. Most notably, two loss-of-function mutations in the filaggrin gene have been associated with AD (14). Polymorphisms in 5q31, which contains a cluster of T helper (T_H) 2 cytokine genes including IL-4, IL-5, and IL-13, have also been linked to AD (13). Clinically, increased expression of IL-4 and IL-13 is pathognomonic of acute

519

AD lesions (15). More recently, IL-31, another T_H2 cytokine, has also been found to be increased in acute AD lesions (16). Thymic stromal lymphopoietin, a IL-7-like cytokine, is produced by keratinocytes and may lead to the production of T_H2 chemokines and cytokines (17). *Staphylococcus aureus* (*S. aureus*) is capable of inducing atopic skin inflammation via the effects of superantigens and superantigen-specific immunoglobulin E (IgE) (18).

■ DIAGNOSIS

Although elevated total serum IgE and multiple allergic sensitizations to food and inhalant allergens are often associated with AD children, it is important to note that about 25% of these patients have normal total serum IgE and have no allergic sensitization to food or inhalant allergens. The diagnosis of AD is based on a constellation of clinical signs and symptoms. The U. K. diagnostic criteria have been shown to be the most validated diagnostic criteria for AD (Table 29.1) (19). Older children or adults with new-onset AD should raise suspicion for other differential diagnoses, which are summarized in Table 29.2.

■ CLINICAL EVALUATION AND MANAGMENT

Evaluation of Severity

Validated scoring systems such as SCOring of Atopic Dermatitis (SCORAD) and Eczema Area and Severity Index (EASI) are often used in the research setting for grading the severity of AD (20). In the clinical setting, patients with recurrent flares of AD, needing escalation of treatment (e.g., from low- to mid-potency topical corticosteroids) or seeking additional medical advice (21), should prompt further evaluation or referral. In addition, patients with total or near-total body involvement of AD, recent history of hospitalization, or use of systemic corticosteroids for AD, eczema herpeticum, or ocular involvement should also be evaluated further by AD specialists.

Routine Daily Skin Care

Daily bath or shower for 10 to 20 minutes followed by application of topical moisturizer and/or medications is recommended to improve skin hydration (22). Such preventive care is crucial in restoring skin barrier function in AD patients. More recently, a number of barrier repair creams have been developed. These include Atopiclair, Mimyx, and Epiceram. These medications have been marketed as medical devices and therefore require prescriptions.

Topical Corticosteroids

Topical corticosteroids remain the first-line of treatment for AD. Table 29.3 shows some of the common topical corticosteroids in different potencies. For mild AD, low-potency topical corticosteroids (Groups VI or VII) may suffice. But for moderate-to-severe AD, mid-potency topical corticosteroids (e.g., Groups IV and V) should be prescribed in adequate quantity. Undertreatment of moderate-to-severe AD with low-potency topical corticosteroids due to concern with side effects may lead to persistent AD, and may further enhance parents' or patients' fear regarding the safety of topical corticosteroids, which in turn increases noncompliance (23). In spite of numerous studies showing the efficacy and safety of topical corticosteroids in AD (23–26), adherence with topical corticosteroids remains poor (27,28), and reluctancy in prescribing these medications is prevalent (3). These problems often arise from unfounded fear of side effects of topical corticosteroids which include skin atrophy, telangiectasias, and adrenal suppression (23). There continues to be a need for patient education regarding the safety of topical corticosteroids and the consequences of undertreatment, i.e., sleep loss, adverse psychosocial and academic development, decreased work productivity, chronic dermatitis, and skin wounds (29–31). For the minority of patients with severe AD who are chronically dependent on mid- to high-potency topical corticosteroids, other treatment options may be considered including topical calcineurin inhibitors.

TABLE 29.1 DIAGNOSTIC CRITERIA FOR ATOPIC DERMATITIS

The presence of itchy skin in the past 12 months, plus three or more of the following:

1. Onset of the skin condition under 2 years (not used in children under 4 years)
2. History of itchy skin involving flexural areas (elbows, behind the knees, front of ankles, or around the neck)
3. History of generalized dry skin
4. Personal history of asthma or allergic rhinitis (for children under 4 years, history of atopic disease in a first-degree relative may be included)
5. Visible flexural dermatitis

Reference: Williams HC, Burney PG, Pembroke AC, et al. The U.K. Working Party's diagnostic criteria for atopic dermatitis. III. Independent hospital validation. *Br J Dermatol* 1994; 131:406–416.

TABLE 29.2   DIFFERENTIAL DIAGNOSES OF ATOPIC DERMATITIS

Dermatologic diseases
Seborrheic dermatitis, irritant or allergic contact dermatitis, psoriasis, nummular dermatitis, keratosis pilaris, lichen simplex chronicus, pityriasis rosea, ichthyosis

Neoplastic diseases
Cutaneous T-cell lymphoma (mycosis fungoides, Sézary syndrome), Letterer-Siwe disease (Langerhans cell histocytosis), necrolytic migratory erythema associated with pancreatic tumor

Immunodeficiencies
Hyper-IgE syndrome, Wiskott-Aldrich syndrome, severe combined immunodeficiency, Omenn syndrome, IPEX (Immune dysregulation, polyendocrinopathy, enteropathy X-linked) syndrome

Infectious diseases
Human immunodeficiency virus–associated eczema, scabies, candidiasis, tinea versicolor

Congenital and metabolic disorders
Netherton syndrome, phenylketonuria, acrodermatitis enteropathica, essential fatty acid deficiency, biotin deficiency, infantile-onset multiple carboxylase deficiency

Reference: Krol A, Krafchik B. The differential diagnosis of atopic dermatitis in childhood. *Dermatol Ther* 2006; 19: 73–82.

Management of Itch and Sleep

Itch is one of the most distressing symptoms of AD. It can adversely affect sleep and activity. The mechanism for itch in AD is not fully understood and does not appear to be histamine-mediated. The use of first-generation antihistamines in AD relies mainly on their sedative effects. Therefore, these medications are best used at bedtime. The nonsedative second-generation antihistamines have not been proven to be effective in controlling itch in AD. Other sedative medications that have been used, but not approved for AD, include doxepin, benzodiazepines, nonbenzodiazepine hypnotics, chloral hydrate, and clonidine (32). There is increasing evidence that neuropeptides and opioid receptors may be involved in the pathogenesis of itch in AD (33). A recent placebo-controlled trial showed that topical naltrexone, an opioid receptor antagonist, may be effective in relieving pruritus in AD patients (34). However, the role of neuropeptides and opioid receptors in the pathogenesis of itch, and the use of antagonists for these receptors in AD, require further studies.

Evaluation and Management of Food Allergies

Food allergy affects up to 40% of children with moderate-to-severe AD (35). Clinical history is an important factor in evaluating food allergies. Patients or parents should be asked on the timing of reaction (immediate versus delayed) and types of symptoms (hives, increased itching, difficulty breathing, vomiting, or diarrhea). Allergy to cow's milk, egg, soybean, wheat, peanut, tree nuts, or shellfish accounts for more than 90% of all food allergies. Therefore, asking specific questions regarding the ingestion of these foods and consistency of symptom recurrence can be helpful in ruling out most food allergies. In young children, negative allergy skin tests to foods are highly predictive of a negative IgE-mediated reaction (>95%) (36). On the other hand, positive skin tests to foods are less helpful, with a positive predictive value of only 50% (36). Serum specific IgE levels, as measured by ImmunoCAP, have more than 95% positive predictive value for some of the common food allergens (36,37). These values are useful in deciding whether an oral food challenge is necessary, especially when restriction of specific food(s) can adversely affect the child's nutritional status and growth. Oral food challenges should be performed in a setting that is well-prepared for managing anaphylaxis. Double-blind, placebo-controlled oral food challenges are considered to be the gold standard for diagnosing food allergy (36). AD patients with proven food allergy, as demonstrated by history and specific IgE, and/or oral food challenge, should avoid the specific food allergen(s), regardless of whether the food allergen(s) trigger AD symptoms. For AD children with multiple food allergies, a dietary consultation is useful in guiding food avoidance and nutritional supplements.

The Role of Aeroallergens

The role of aeroallergens as a trigger for AD has been controversial. Randomized, double-blind placebo studies have shown conflicting results on the role of house dust mites (HDM) as a trigger for AD (38,39). However, more recent studies showing an improvement of AD with HDM immunotherapy support the role of HDM in AD (40). Since respiratory allergies are common in AD patients and HDM preventive measures using mite-impermeable bed covers have been shown to improve respiratory allergies (41), these measures may be

TABLE 29.3   TOPICAL CORTICOSTEROID POTENCIES

Group I (most potent)
Betamethasone dipropionate 0.05% (Diprolene)
  (cream, ointment)
Diflorasone diacetate 0.05% (Psorcon)(ointment)
Clobetasol propionate 0.05% (Temovate)
  (cream, ointment)
Halobetasol dipropionate 0.05% (Ultravate)
  (cream, ointment).

Group II
Amcinonide 0.1% (Cyclocort)(ointment)
Betamethasone dipropionate 0.05% (Diprosone)
  (cream, ointment)
Mometasone furoate 0.1% (Elocon)(ointment)
Halcinonide 0.1% (Halog)(cream)
Fluocinonide 0.05% (Lidex)(gel, cream, ointment)
Desoximetasone (Topicort)(0.05% gel, 0.25% cream,
  ointment).

Group III
Fluticasone propionate 0.005% (Cutivate)(ointment)
Amcinonide 0.1% (Cyclocort)(lotion, cream)
Diflorasone diacetate 0.05% (Florone)(cream)
Betamethasone valerate 0.1% (Valisone)(ointment).

Group IV
Mometasone furoate 0.1% (Elocon)(cream)
Triamcinolone acetonide 0.1% (Kenalog)(cream)
Fluocinolone acetonide 0.025% (Synalar)(ointment).

Group V
Fluticasone propionate 0.05% (Cutivate)(cream)
Fluocinolone acetonide 0.025% (Synalar)(cream)
Desonide 0.05% (Tridesilon)(ointment)
Betamethasone valerate 0.1% (Valisone)(cream)
Hydrocortisone valerate 0.2% (Westcort)(cream).

Group VI
Alclometasone dipropionate 0.05% (Aclovate)
  (cream, ointment)
Flucinolone acetonide 0.01% (Synalar)
  (solution, cream)
Desonide 0.05% (Tridesilon)(cream and aqueous
  gel).

Group VII (least potent)
Hydrocortisone 1%/2.5% (Hytone)(lotion, cream,
  ointment).

Reference: Stoughton RB. Vasoconstrictor assay—specific applications. In Maibach HI, Surber C, eds. *Topical Corticosteroids*. Basel, Switzerland: Karger; 1992; p. 42–53.

considered in AD patients with HDM allergies and concurrent respiratory symptoms. Other dust mite control measures include frequent vacuuming (e.g., once a week) and washing linens in hot water. There have been fewer studies on the role of pet dander and pollens as a trigger for AD. Evidence supporting the role of these aeroallergens in AD have come from case reports

and atopy patch testing (42,43). More recently, ingestion of birch pollen-related foods (e.g., apple, celery, carrot) were shown to exacerbate AD (44). Although more controlled studies are needed to confirm the role of aeroallergens in AD, the potential role of these allergens should be considered on an individual basis.

Evaluation and Management of Infections

S. aureus frequently colonizes AD lesions and causes infection in AD patients. Although there is clear evidence that *S. aureus* plays an important role in triggering AD symptoms, routine use of antibiotics in the absence of clinical signs of infection is not recommended due to concern of causing bacterial resistance. For AD patients with isolated areas of skin infections, topical mupirocin may be used. But for more wide-spread skin infection, oral antibiotics are usually needed. Due to the increasing prevalence of methicillin-resistant *S. aureus*, skin wound cultures should be considered to assess antibiotic sensitivity before starting systemic antibiotics. For infants with extensive secondary skin infection or patients with persistent fever, further work-up for more invasive infections (e.g., bacteremia, endocarditis, arthritis, osteomyelitis, bursitis) (45) and hospital admission for intravenous antibiotics should be considered.

Herpes simplex virus (HSV) can cause life-threatening eczema herpeticum in AD patients. Patients with eczema herpeticum may present with fever, malaise, and widespread vesicles (46). However, some HSV-superinfected AD lesions may not appear vesicular, but rather as punched-out lesions with an erythematous base. HSV DNA polymerase chain reaction (PCR), Tzanck smear, or viral culture should be obtained from the lesion while the patient is started on systemic acyclovir. Patients with periocular or ocular involvement should be evaluated by an ophthalmologist emergently.

Eczema vaccinatum refers to a life-threatening reaction from vaccinia virus in AD patients, who have been in contact with a recently vaccinated person. The site of the smallpox vaccination can drain and shed virus for up to 3 weeks. Thus, subjects who are vaccinated with vaccinia, must not be allowed to be in contact with AD patients. In addition, AD patients (even if just a history of childhood eczema) should be deferred from vaccinia immunization.

Other Treatment Options

Topical Calcineurin Inhibitors

Tacrolimus ointment (Protopic, Astellas) 0.03% and pimecrolimus cream (Elidel, Novartis) 1% are approved for children 2 years and above with AD, and tacrolimus ointment 0.1% for adults with AD. However, FDA has issued a "black box" warning for continuous use of both tacrolimus ointment and pimecrolimus cream due to concerns for possible development of malignancies from long-term use. The Topical Calcineurin Inhibitor Task Force of the American College of Allergy, Asthma and Immunology and the American Academy of Allergy, Asthma and Immunology have reviewed all available data and concluded that the risk/benefit ratio of topical pimecrolimus and tacrolimus were similar to those of most conventional therapies for the treatment of chronic relapsing AD (47). FDA currently recommends the use of these medications up to twice daily in minimal amount on affected areas only. As topical calcineurin inhibitors do not cause skin atrophy, they remain useful as alternative agents for treatment of AD involving atrophy-prone areas including the face, groin, and axillae.

Wet-wrap Treatment

Wet-wrap with topical corticosteroids is effective for symptomatic treatment of severe AD patients (48). Detailed procedures of different wet-wrap regimens have recently been described in a review article (49). However, wet-wrap treatment is labor-intensive, and may be associated with potential secondary skin infection, therefore it should be carried out under the supervision of experienced physicians. Large prospective studies and objective efficacy parameters are needed in comparing its efficacy to conventional AD treatments.

Systemic Treatments

Systemic corticosteroids are an alternative treatment for symptomatic relief of flare in severe AD. However, a short 1-week course of systemic corticosteroids should be followed by a taper over a few days and more intensive daily skin care (i.e., increase bathing frequency and the amount of topical corticosteroids), due to the potential of rebound AD symptoms off systemic corticosteroids (50). The side effects of repeat or prolonged courses of systemic corticosteroids include adrenal suppression, growth retardation in children, osteoporosis, hypertension, peptic ulcer, glaucoma, cataracts, and infections due to immunosuppression. Other systemic immunosuppressants including cyclosporin A, azathioprine, methotrexate, and mycophenolate mofetil have also been shown to be effective in the symptomatic control of severe AD patients (51,52). Among these immunosuppressants, cyclosporine A has been the best studied in treating severe AD (52). Potential long-term side effects of these systemic immunosuppressants include malignancy, renal damage, and hepatotoxicity (51). These agents are generally not recommended for children with AD due to insufficient long-term safety data.

Phototherapy

Ultraviolet phototherapies have also been shown to be effective in treating both adults and children with severe AD (53,54). However, there is insufficient data on the long-term risk of skin cancer in AD patients who undergo phototherapy. Further studies are needed regarding the risk-and-benefit ratio of phototherapy for AD, particularly in children.

Experimental Treatments

Probiotics have not been proven to be effective for AD (55,56). The efficacy of Chinese medicinal herbs for the treatment of AD has also not been confirmed (52). There is currently no convincing data to support the use of intravenous immunoglobulin (IVIG) (51,52) or Omalizumab (Xolair) (57) in AD. Controlled trials are needed to study the use of these agents in AD. Double-blind, placebo-controlled trials have failed to show the efficacy of montelukast in AD (58,59). Allergen immunotherapy (subcutaneous or sublingual), on the other hand, has shown some promising results in the treatment of AD (40,60,61). The most convincing benefits in these studies were found in HDM-sensitized AD patients. The potential side effects of allergen immunotherapy include anaphylaxis and worsening of AD. Further studies are needed to compare this therapy with conventional AD treatment.

■ SUMMARY AND CONCLUSIONS

AD remains a challenging condition to treat. In spite of the safety and efficacy of topical corticosteroids, adherence with these medications continues to be a problem. Patient education regarding the risks and benefits of topical corticosteroids, and preventive care with skin hydration is a crucial component in the care of AD patients. For patients who are chronically dependent on mid- to high-potency topical corticosteroids, further evaluation for food allergies, inhalant allergies, and infections are indicated. Other treatment options for these patients include topical calcineurin inhibitors, wet-wrap treatment, systemic immunosuppressants, and phototherapy. Promising experimental treatments include allergen immunotherapy and anti-IgE for AD.

■ ACKNOWLEDGMENTS

Dr. Ong is supported in part by Grant # MO1 RR00046, Children's Hospital Los Angeles General Clinical Research Center (GCRC), and the Saban Research Institute Clinical Research Award (5-MOI RR00004346). Dr. Leung is supported by NIH grants 3M01 RR00051 and 5 R01 AR41256.

■ REFERENCES

1. Meltzer LJ, Moore M. Sleep disruptions in parents of children and adolescents with chronic illnesses: prevalence, causes, and consequences. *J Pediatr Psychol.* 2008;33:279–291.
2. Faught J, Bierl C, Barton B, et al. Stress in mothers of young children with eczema. *Arch Dis Child.* 2007; 92:683-686.

3. Horii KA, Simon SD, Liu DY, et al. Atopic dermatitis in children in the United States, 1997–2004: visit trends, patient and provider characteristics, and prescribing patterns. *Pediatrics.* 2007;120:e527–534.

4. Emerson RM, Williams HC, Allen BR. What is the cost of atopic dermatitis in preschool children? *Br J Dermatol.* 2001;144:514–522.

5. Ellis CN, Drake LA, Prendergast MM, et al. Cost of atopic dermatitis and eczema in the United States. *J Am Acad Dermatol.* 2002; 46: 361–370.

6. Schultz Larsen F, Hanifin JM. Epidemiology of atopic dermatitis. *Immunol Allergy Clin North Am.* 2002;22:1–24.

7. Laughter D, Istvan JA, Tofte SJ, et al. The prevalence of atopic dermatitis in Oregon schoolchildren. *J Am Acad Dermatol.* 2000;43:649–655.

8. Ben-Gashir MA, Seed PT, Hay RJ. Predictors of atopic dermatitis severity over time. *J Am Acad Dermatol.* 2004;50:349–356.

9. Williams HC, Wuthrich B. The natural history of atopic dermatitis. In: Williams HC, eds. *Atopic Dermatitis. The Epidemiology, Causes and Prevention of Atopic Eczema.* Cambridge, UK: Cambridge University Press;2000:41–59.

10. Lammintausta K, Kalimo K, Raitala R, et al. Prognosis of atopic dermatitis. A prospective study in early adulthood. *Int J Dermatol.* 1991;30:563–568.

11. Kapoor R, Menon C, Hoffstad O, et al. The prevalence of atopic triad in children with physician-confirmed atopic dermatitis. *J Am Acad Dermatol.* 2008;58:68–73.

12. Thomsen SF, Ulrik CS, Kyvik KO, et al. Importance of genetic factors in the etiology of atopic dermatitis: a twin study. *Allergy Asthma Proc.* 2007;28:535–539.

13. Morar N, Willis-Owen SA, Moffatt MF, et al. The genetics of atopic dermatitis. *J Allergy Clin Immunol.* 2006;118:24–34.

14. Palmer CN, Irvine AD, Terron-Kwiatkowski A, et al. Common loss-of-function variants of the epidermal barrier protein filaggrin are a major predisposing factor for atopic dermatitis. *Nat Genet.* 2006; 38:441–446.

15. Hamid Q, Boguniewicz M, Leung DY. Differential *in situ* cytokine gene expression in acute versus chronic atopic dermatitis. *J Clin Invest.* 1994;94:870–876.

16. Bilsborough J, Leung DY, Maurer M, et al. IL-31 is associated with cutaneous lymphocyte antigen-positive skin homing T cells in patients with atopic dermatitis. *J Allergy Clin Immunol.* 2006;117:418–425.

17. Liu YJ. Thymic stromal lymphopoietin and OX40 ligand pathway in the initiation of dendritic cell-mediated allergic inflammation. *J Allergy Clin Immunol.* 2007; 120:238–244.

18. Leung DY, Boguniewicz M, Howell MD, et al. New insights into atopic dermatitis. *J Clin Invest.* 2004;113:651–657.

19. Brenninkmeijer EE, Schram ME, Leeflang MM, et al. Diagnostic criteria for atopic dermatitis: a systematic review. *Br J Dermatol.* 2008;158:754–765.

20. Schmitt J, Langan S, Williams HC, et al. What are the best outcome measurements for atopic eczema? A systematic review. *J Allergy Clin Immunol.* 2007;120:1389–1398.

21. Langan SM, Thomas KS, Williams HC. What is meant by a "flare" in atopic dermatitis? A systematic review and proposal. *Arch Dermatol.* 2006;142:1190–1196.

22. Gutman AB, Kligman AM, Sciacca J, et al. Soak and smear: a standard technique revisited. *Arch Dermatol.* 2005;141:1556–1559.

23. Charman CR, Morris AD, Williams HC. Topical corticosteroid phobia in patients with atopic eczema. *Br J Dermatol.* 2000;142:931–936.

24. Friedlander SF, Hebert AA, Allen DB; Fluticasone Pediatrics Safety Study Group. Safety of fluticasone propionate cream 0.05% for the treatment of severe and extensive atopic dermatitis in children as young as 3 months. *J Am Acad Dermatol.* 2002;46:387–393.

25. Lucky AW, Grote GD, Williams JL, et al. Effect of desonide ointment, 0.05%, on the hypothalamic-pituitary-adrenal axis of children with atopic dermatitis. *Cutis.* 1997;59:151–153.

26. Eichenfield LF, Basu S, Calvarese B, et al. Effect of desonide hydrogel 0.05% on the hypothalamic-pituitary-adrenal axis in pediatric subjects with moderate to severe atopic dermatitis. *Pediatr Dermatol.* 2007;24:289–295.

27. Zuberbier T, Orlow SJ, Paller AS, et al. Patient perspectives on the management of atopic dermatitis. *J Allergy Clin Immunol.* 2006;118:226–232.

28. Krejci-Manwaring J, Tusa MG, Carroll C, et al. Stealth monitoring of adherence to topical medication: adherence is very poor in children with atopic dermatitis. *J Am Acad Dermatol.* 2007; 56:211–216.

29. Daud LR, Garralda ME, David TJ. Psychosocial adjustment in preschool children with atopic eczema. *Arch Dis Child.* 1993;69:670–676.

30. Absolon CM, Cottrell D, Eldridge SM, et al. Psychological disturbance in atopic eczema: the extent of the problem in school-aged children. *Br J Dermatol.* 1997;137:241–245.

31. Holm EA, Esmann S, Jemec GB. The handicap caused by atopic dermatitis–sick leave and job avoidance. *J Eur Acad Dermatol Venereol.* 2006;20:255–259.

32. Kelsay K. Management of sleep disturbance associated with atopic dermatitis. *J Allergy Clin Immunol.* 2006;118:198–201.

33. Bigliardi-Qi M, Lipp B, Sumanovski LT, et al. Changes of epidermal mu-opiate receptor expression and nerve endings in chronic atopic dermatitis. *Dermatology.* 2005;210:91–99.

34. Bigliardi PL, Stammer H, Jost G, et al. Treatment of pruritus with topically applied opiate receptor antagonist. *J Am Acad Dermatol.* 2007;56:979–988.

35. Eigenmann PA, Sicherer SH, Borkowski TA, et al. Prevalence of IgE-mediated food allergy among children with atopic dermatitis. *Pediatrics.* 1998;101:E8.

36. Bock SA. Diagnostic evaluation. *Pediatrics.* 2003;111:1638–1644.

37. Sampson HA. The evaluation and management of food allergy in atopic dermatitis. *Clin Dermatol.* 2003;21:183–192.

38. Tan BB, Weald D, Strickland I, et al. Double-blind controlled trial of effect of housedust-mite allergen avoidance on atopic dermatitis. *Lancet.* 1996;347:15–18.

39. Oosting AJ, de Bruin-Weller MS, Terreehorst I, et al. Effect of mattress encasings on atopic dermatitis outcome measures in a double-blind, placebo-controlled study: the Dutch mite avoidance study. *J Allergy Clin Immunol.* 2002;110:500–506.

40. Bussmann C, Maintz L, Hart J, et al. Clinical improvement and immunological changes in atopic dermatitis patients undergoing subcutaneous immunotherapy with a house dust mite allergoid: a pilot study. *Clin Exp Allergy.* 2007;37:1277–1285.

41. van den Bemt L, van Knapen L, de Vries MP, et al. Clinical effectiveness of a mite allergen-impermeable bed-covering system in asthmatic mite-sensitive patients. *J Allergy Clin Immunol.* 2004;114:858–862.

42. Endo K, Hizawa T, Fukuzumi T, et al. Keeping dogs indoor aggravates infantile atopic dermatitis. *Arerugi.* 1999;48:1309–1315.

43. Darsow U, Vieluf D, Ring J. Evaluating the relevance of aeroallergen sensitization in atopic eczema with the atopy patch test: a randomized, double-blind multicenter study. Atopy Patch Test Study Group. *J Am Acad Dermatol.* 1999;40:187–193.

44. Bohle B, Zwolfer B, Heratizadeh A, et al. Cooking birch pollen-related food: divergent consequences for IgE- and T cell-mediated reactivity in vitro and in vivo. *J Allergy Clin Immunol.* 2006;118:242–249.

45. Benenson S, Zimhony O, Dahan D, et al. Atopic dermatitis–a risk factor for invasive Staphylococcus aureus infections: two cases and review. *Am J Med.* 2005;118:1048–1051.

46. Wollenberg A, Wetzel S, Burgdorf WH, et al. Viral infections in atopic dermatitis: pathogenic aspects and clinical management. *J Allergy Clin Immunol.* 2003;112:667–674.

47. Fonacier L, Spergel J, Charlesworth EN, et al. Report of the Topical Calcineurin Task Force of the American College of Allergy, Asthma and Immunology and the American Academy of Allergy, Asthma and Immunology. *J Allergy Clin Immunol.* 2005;115:1249–1253.

48. Devillers AC, Oranje AP. Efficacy and safety of 'wet-wrap' dressings as an intervention treatment in children with severe and/or refractory atopic dermatitis: a critical review of the literature. *Br J Dermatol.* 2006;154:579–585.

49. Oranje AP, Devillers A, Kunz B, et al. Treatment of patients with atopic dermatitis using wet-wrap dressings with diluted steroids and/or emollients. An expert panel's opinion and review of the literature. *J Eur Acad Dermatol Venereol.* 2006;20:1277–1286.

50. Forte WC, Sumita JM, Rodrigues AG, et al. Rebound phenomenon to systemic corticosteroid in atopic dermatitis. *Allergol Immunopathol* (Madr). 2005;33:307–311.

51. Akhavan A, Rudikoff D. The treatment of atopic dermatitis with systemic immunosuppressive agents. *Clin Dermatol.* 2003;21:225–240.

52. Schmitt J, Schakel K, Schmitt N, et al. Systemic treatment of severe atopic eczema: a systematic review. *Acta Derm Venereol.* 2007;87:100–111.

53. Meduri NB, Vandergriff T, Rasmussen H, et al. Phototherapy in the management of atopic dermatitis: a systematic review. *Photodermatol Photoimmunol Photomed.* 2007;23:106–112.

54. Clayton TH, Clark SM, Turner D, et al. The treatment of severe atopic dermatitis in childhood with narrowband ultraviolet B phototherapy. *Clin Exp Dermatol.* 2007;32:28–33.

55. Williams HC. Two "positive" studies of probiotics for atopic dermatitis: or are they? *Arch Dermatol.* 2006;142:1201–1203.

56. Lee J, Seto D, Bielory L. Meta-analysis of clinical trials of probiotics for prevention and treatment of pediatric atopic dermatitis. *J Allergy Clin Immunol.* 2008;121:116–121.

57. Beck LA, Saini S. Wanted: a study with omalizumab to determine the role of IgE-mediated pathways in atopic dermatitis. *J Am Acad Dermatol.* 2006;55:540–541.

58. Friedmann PS, Palmer R, Tan E, et al. A double-blind, placebo-controlled trial of montelukast in adult atopic eczema. *Clin Exp Allergy.* 2007;37:1536–1540.

59. Veien NK, Busch-Sorensen M, Stausbol-Gron B. Montelukast treatment of moderate to severe atopic dermatitis in adults: a randomized, double-blind, placebo-controlled trial. *J Am Acad Dermatol.* 2005;53:147–149.

60. Bussmann C, Bockenhoff A, Henke H, et al. Does allergen-specific immunotherapy represent a therapeutic option for patients with atopic dermatitis? *J Allergy Clin Immunol.* 2006;118:1292–1298.

61. Pajno GB, Caminiti L, Vita D, et al. Sublingual immunotherapy in mite-sensitized children with atopic dermatitis: a randomized, double-blind, placebo-controlled study. *J Allergy Clin Immunol.* 2007;120: 164–170.

CHAPTER 30

Contact Dermatitis

ANDREW J. SCHEMAN

A skin condition commonly encountered by physicians is allergic contact dermatitis. With new chemical sensitizers being introduced into our environment constantly, physicians will be evaluating more instances of this disease. Contact dermatitis is the most common occupational disease and, as such, is of importance to both the individual and to society. The patient with allergic contact dermatitis may be very uncomfortable and have poor quality of life. Inability to pursue employment or recreation is common, especially if there is a delay in diagnosis and removal from exposure.

■ IMMUNOLOGIC BASIS

The classification of immunologic hypersensitivity reactions is reviewed in Chapter 17 on drug allergies. Allergic contact dermatitis is a type IVa_1, T-cell–mediated hypersensitivity. Type IVa_1 allergy is also referred to as delayed-type hypersensitivity, reflecting the fact that typical reactions occur 5 to 25 days after initial exposure (1) and 12 to 96 hours after subsequent exposures. In contrast, immediate hypersensitivity is a type I immunoglobulin E(IgE) humoral antibody-mediated reaction, generally occurring withing 1 hour or less.

Whereas the typical skin lesion in immediate hypersensitivity is urticarial, typical allergic contact dermatitis is eczematous (1). Thus, skin lesions can include vesicles, bullae, and poorly-demarcated erythematous scaly plaques acutely and, when chronic, lichenification. It is important to realize that contact allergy is often morphologically and histologically identical to other forms of eczema, including atopic dermatitis and irritant contact dermatitis, which is defined as nonimmunologic damage to the skin caused by a direct toxic effect. Therefore, patch testing is usually needed to distinguish contact allergy from other types of eczema.

Typically, immediate hypersensitivity is caused by parenteral exposure through ingestion or respiratory exposure through inhalation. An exception is immunologic contact urticaria, in which a type I reaction is induced by topical exposure. The typical type IV_{a1} contact allergy is induced by topical exposure. An exception occurs with systemic ingestion of a contact allergen that reproduces skin lesions caused by a previous external exposure to the same or a similar substance; this is termed *systemic contact dermatitis*. The list of substances capable of causing type I allergy is different from the list of substances capable of causing type IVa_1 allergy. There are a few substances, such as penicillin, quinine, sulfonamides, mercury, and arsenic that have can cause both IVa_1 contact hypersensitivity and type I immediate hypersensitivity reactions.

Although atopic individuals are prone to type I allergies, they been generally considered not to be more likely to develop type IVa_1 allergy than nonatopic individuals. On the other hand, it has been clearly demonstrated that atopic persons are much more likely to have a lowered threshold for developing irritant contact dermatitis.

Sensitization

The inductive or afferent limb of contact sensitivity begins with the topical application to the skin of a chemically reactive substance called a hapten. The hapten may be organic or inorganic and is generally of low molecular weight (<500 daltons)(1). Its ability to sensitize depends on penetrating the skin and forming covalent bonds with proteins. The degree of sensitization is directly proportional to the stability of the hapten–protein coupling. In the case of the commonly used skin sensitizer dinitrochlorobenzene, the union of the chemical hapten and the tissue protein occurs in the Malpighian layer of the epidermis, with the amino acid sites of lysine and cysteine being most reactive (2). It has been suggested that skin lipids might exert an adjuvant effect comparable with the myoside of mycobacterium tuberculosis.

There is strong evidence that Langerhans cells are of crucial importance in the induction of contact sensitivity (3). These dendritic cells in the epidermis cannot be identified on routine histologic sections of the skin by light microscopy, but they can be easily visualized using special stains. They possess MHC class II and B7 homology receptors B7(CD80/86).

Elicitation

Langerhans cells are dendritic epidermal cells that possess MHC Class II antigen on their surface. The Langerhans cell ingests the hapten–protein complex, processes it, and then produces a resulting peptide that binds to the HLA-DR antigen on the surface of the cell. The peptide is then presented to a CD4$^+$ helper T-cell type 1 (T_H1) with specific complementary surface receptors.

The binding of the T_H1 cell induces the Langerhans cell to release cytokines including interleukin-1(IL-1). IL-1 in turn activates the bound T_H1 cell to release interleukin-2 which leads to T-cell proliferation. The proliferating T cells magnify the response by releasing interferon-γ, which leads to increased HLA-DR display on Langerhans cells and increased cytotoxicity of T cells, macrophages, and natural killer cells. The sensitized T_H1 cells also result in an anamnestic response to subsequent exposure to the same antigen. Type IVa$_1$ hypersensitivity can be transferred with sensitized T_H1 cells (4).

Contact allergy involves both T effector cells leading to hypersensitivity and T suppressor cells leading to tolerance. The net effect is the balance of these two opposing inputs. Cutaneous exposure tends to induce sensitization, whereas oral or intravenous exposure is more likely to induce tolerance. Once sensitivity is acquired, it usually persists for many years; however, it occasionally may be lost after only a few years. Hardening refers to either a specific or generalized loss of hypersensitivity due to constant low-grade exposure to an antigen. This type of deliberate desensitization has been successful only in rare instances and is therefore not recommended as a therapeutic strategy.

Histopathology

The histologic picture in allergic contact dermatitis reveals that the dermis is infiltrated by mononuclear inflammatory cells, especially about blood vessels and sweat glands (2). The epidermis is hyperplastic with mononuclear cell invasion. Frequently, intraepidermal vesicles form, which may coalesce into large blisters. The vesicles are filled with serous fluid containing granulocytes and mononuclear cells. In Jones-Mote contact sensitivity, in addition to mononuclear phagocyte and lymphocyte accumulation, basophils are found. This is an important distinction from hypersensitivity reactions of the T_H1 type, in which basophils are completely absent.

■ CLINICAL FEATURES

History

Allergic contact dermatitis occurs most frequently in middle-aged and elderly persons, although it may appear at any age. In contrast to the classical atopic diseases, contact dermatitis is as common in the population at large as in the atopic population, and a history of personal or family atopy is not a risk factor.

The interval between exposure to the responsible agent and the occurrence of clinical manifestations in a sensitized subject is usually 12 to 96 hours, although it may be as early as 4 hours and sometimes longer than 1 week. The incubation or sensitization period between initial exposure and the development of skin sensitivity may be as short as 2 to 3 days in the case of a strong sensitizer such as poison ivy, or several years for a weak sensitizer such as chromate. The patient usually will note the development of erythema, followed by papules, and then vesicles. Pruritus follows the appearance of the dermatitis and is uniformly present in allergic contact dermatitis.

Physical Examination

The appearance of allergic contact dermatitis depends on the stage at which the patient presents. In the acute stage, erythema, papules, and vesicles predominate, with edema and occasionally bullae (Fig. 30.1). The boundaries of the dermatitis are generally poorly marginated. Edema may be profound in areas of loose tissue such as the eyelids and genitalia. Acute allergic contact dermatitis of the face may result in a marked degree of periorbital swelling that resembles angioedema. The presence of the associated dermatitis should allow the physician to make the distinction easily. In the subacute phase, vesicles are less pronounced, and crusting, scaling, and early signs of lichenification may be present. In the chronic stage, few papulovesicular lesions are evident, and thickening, lichenification, and scaliness predominate.

Different areas of the skin vary in their ease of sensitization. Pressure, friction, and perspiration are factors that seem to enhance sensitization. The eyelids, neck, and genitalia are among the most readily sensitized areas, whereas the palms, soles, and scalp are more

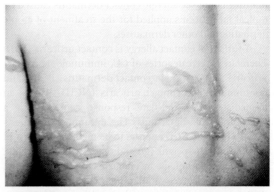

■ **FIGURE 30.1**   The acute phase of contact dermatitis due to poison ivy. Note the linear distribution of vesicles. (Courtesy of Dr. Gary Vicik.)

resistant. Tissue that is irritated, inflamed, or infected is more susceptible to allergic contact dermatitis. A clinical example is the common occurrence of contact dermatitis in an area of stasis dermatitis that has been treated with topical medications or sensitizing chemicals.

Differential Diagnosis

The skin conditions most frequently confused with allergic contact dermatitis are seborrheic dermatitis, atopic dermatitis, psoriasis, and primary irritant dermatitis. In seborrheic dermatitis, there is a general tendency toward oiliness of the skin, and a predilection of the lesions for the scalp, the T-zone of the face, mid-chest, and inguinal folds.

Atopic dermatitis (Chapter 29) often has its onset in infancy or early childhood. The skin is dry, although pruritus is a prominent feature, it appears before the lesions and not after them, as in the case of allergic contact dermatitis. The areas most frequently involved are the flexural surfaces. The margins of the dermatitis are indefinite, and the progression from erythema to papules to vesicles is not seen.

Psoriasis is characterized by well demarcated erythematous plaques with white to silvery scales; pruritus is often mild or absent. Lesions are often distributed symmetrically over extensor surfaces such as the knee or elbow.

The dermatitis caused by a primary irritant is a simple chemical or physical insult to the skin. For example, what is commonly called *dishpan hands* is a dermatitis caused by household detergents. A prior sensitizing exposure to the primary irritant is not necessary, and the dermatitis develops in a large number of normal persons. The dermatitis begins shortly after exposure to the irritant, in contrast to the 12 to 96 hours after exposure in allergic contact dermatitis. Primary irritant dermatitis may be virtually indistinguishable in its physical appearance from allergic contact dermatitis. It should be emphasized that skin conditions may coexist. It is not unusual to see allergic contact dermatitis caused by topical medications applied for the treatment of atopic dermatitis and other dermatoses.

A variant of contact allergy is contact urticaria (CU). There are three categories of CU: immunologic contact urticaria (ICU), protein contact dermatitis (PCD), and nonimmunologic contact urticaria (NCU). ICU is an immediate wheal-and-flare response generated by a wide variety of contactants. The immunopathogenesis of both ICU and PCD appears to be mediated at least in part by antigen-specific IgE and type I hypersensitivity. The immunopathologic mechanisms in PCD other than type I are unclear. Several authors have reported Type IV cutaneous reactions corroborated by positive patch tests (5). NCU is caused by some allergens such as fragrances and benzyl alcohol known to cause immunologic reaction; however, in the case of NCU, the etiology is unclear.

■ IDENTIFYING THE OFFENDING AGENT

History and Physical Examination

Once the diagnosis of allergic contact dermatitis is made, vigorous efforts should be directed toward determining the cause. A careful, thorough history is absolutely mandatory. The temporal relationship between exposure and clinical manifestations must be kept in mind as an exhaustive search is made for exposure to a sensitizing allergen in the patient's occupational, home, or recreational environment. The location of the dermatitis most often relates closely to direct contact with a particular allergen. At times this is rather straightforward, such as dermatitis of the feet, caused by contact sensitivity to shoe materials or dermatitis from jewelry appearing on the wrist, the ear lobes, or the neck. The relationship of the dermatitis to the direct contact allergen may not be as obvious at other times, and being able to associate certain areas of involvement with particular types of exposure is extremely helpful. Contact dermatitis of the face, for example, is often due to cosmetics directly applied to the area. One must keep in mind other possibilities, however, such as hair dye, shampoo, and hair-styling preparations. Contact dermatitis of the eyelid, although often caused by eye shadow, mascara, and eye liner, also may be caused by nail polish. Involvement of the thighs may be caused by keys or coins in pants pockets. Therefore, it is vital that the physician be familiar with various distribution patterns of contact dermatitis that may occur in association with particular allergens.

Frequently, the distribution of the skin lesions may suggest a number of possible sensitizing agents, and patch testing is of special value. Certain allergens may be airborne, and exposure may occur by this route. Dermatitis among farmers caused by ragweed oil sensitivity occurs occasionally. Smoke from burning the poison ivy plant may contain the oleoresin as particulate matter, and thus expose the sensitive individual. Forest fire fighters develop generalize allergic contact dermatitis from smoke from the burning branches and leaves containing urushiol. Another route of acquiring poison ivy contact dermatitis without touching the plant is by indirect contact with clothing or animal fur containing the oleoresin. It should be remembered also that systemic administration of a drug or a related drug that has been previously used topically and to which the patient has been sensitized can elicit a localized or generalized eruption. An example is sensitivity to ethylenediamine. A patient may have developed localized contact dermatitis to topically applied ethylenediamine hydrochloride previously used as a stabilizer in such compounds as Mycolog cream. After being sensitized, a localized or generalized eruption may then occur when aminophylline is administered orally (6).

The oral mucosa also may be the site of a localized allergic contact reaction resulting in contact stomatitis or stomatitis venenata (7). The relatively low incidence of contact stomatitis compared with contact dermatitis is attributed to the brief duration of surface contact, the diluting and buffering action of saliva, and the rapid dispersal and absorption because of extensive vascularity. Agents capable of producing contact stomatitis include dentifrices, mouthwashes, dental materials such as acrylic and epoxy resins, and foods. The clinical response is most commonly inflammation of the lips, but cases of "burning mouth" syndrome have also been attributed to contact allergy.

Patch Testing

Principle

Patch testing or epicutaneous testing is the diagnostic technique of applying a specific substance to the skin with the intention of producing a small area of allergic contact dermatitis. It can be thought of as reproducing the disease in miniature. The patch test is generally kept in place for 48 hours (although reactions may appear after 24 hours in markedly sensitive patients), and then observed for the gross appearance of a localized dermatitis (most commonly after 48 and 96 hours). The same principles of proper interpretation of a positive patch test apply as in the case of the immediate wheal and erythema skin test reaction (Chapter 4). A positive patch test is not absolute proof that the test substance is the actual cause of dermatitis. It may reflect a previous episode of dermatitis, or it may be without any clinical relevance at all. The positive patch test must always correlate with the patient's history and physical examination.

Allergic Contact Dermatitis and Indications for Patch Testing

All unexplained cases of eczema that either do not respond to treatment or recur after treatment may be due to contact allergy and should be considered for patch testing (9). Currently, patch testing is the only accepted scientific proof of contact allergy. If patch testing is successful at identifying a causative allergen, avoidance often will be curative. Alternatively, if the causative agent is not identified, it is likely that the patient will need ongoing treatment and that treatment will be less than optimal.

A thorough history and physical examination should be performed with emphasis on the distribution and timing of the clinical lesions. Once this information is obtained, an exhaustive history should be taken to identify all potential allergens that had opportunity to come in contact with the skin of the patient. A tray of patch test materials is then assembled.

Most physicians doing patch testing use the TRUE Test, a ready-made series of 23 common allergens that can be easily applied in a busy office setting (Table 30.1). Since a recent study reported that less than 26% of contact allergy problems will be fully solved using the TRUE Test, patients often need referral to a physician specializing in patch testing. These specialists will generally have a wide array of allergens relevant to most occupations and exposures and are familiar with where these allergens are found and alternatives to avoid exposure. Testing is usually performed with an expanded standard tray and additional allergens individualized to the patient exposure.

The physician should become familiar with the potent sensitizers and with the various modes of exposure. It is important to keep in mind the possibility of cross-reactivity to other allergens because of chemical similarities. Sensitivity to paraphenylenediamine, for example, also may indicate sensitivity to para-aminobenzoic acid and other chemicals containing a benzene ring with an amino group in the "para" position.

The most common cause of Type IVa_1-delayed hypersensitivity allergic contact dermatitis in the United States is *Toxicodendron* (poison ivy, poison oak, poison sumac). In contrast, latex-induced contact dermatitis is a Type I contact uriticaria which affects health

TABLE 30.1   ALLERGENS ON THE TRUE TEST STANDARD TRAY LISTED BY FUNCTION

Metals	Nickel sulfate, potassium dichromate Cobalt chloride
Medications	Benzocaine, neomycin sulfate, thimerosol, ethylenediamine
Cosmetic fragrances	Fragrance mix, balsam of Peru
Cosmetic preservatives	Paraben mix, quaternium 15, Kathon CG, formaldehyde
Other cosmetic ingredients	Colophony (rosin), paraphenylenediamine, lanolin (wool wax) alcohol
Rubber ingredients	Mercaptobenozothiazole, mercapto mix, carba mix (carbamates), thiuram mix, black rubber paraphenylenediamine mix
Adhesives	Epoxy resin, paratertiarybutylphenol formaldehyde resin

care workers, patients with spina bifida, and manufacturing employees who prepare latex-based products. Table 30.2 is a list of some of the most potent sensitizers and agents that contain them. It is by no means complete, and is not intended as a general survey. More detailed information on other sensitizers, environmental exposures, and preparation of testing material is contained in several standard references (10–12).

Techniques

The two most common types of patch test chambers, the aluminum Finn chamber and the plastic IQ chamber, come in strips that hold 10 allergens (9). Allergens are placed into the chambers as a drop of liquid on filter paper or as a 1-cm cylinder of allergen in petrolatum from a syringe. With the patient standing erect, the patch test strips are applied starting at the bottom and pressing each allergen chamber firmly against the skin as it is applied. The skin surrounding the patch test strips is then outlined with either fluorescent ink or gentian violet marker. Reinforcing tape, and sometimes a medical adhesive such as Mastisol, is then used to further affix the patches in place. The patch test series is documented in the medical records clearly showing the position of each allergen. The patient should be instructed to keep the patch test sites dry and avoid vigorous physical activity until after patch test reading is completed. The allergens are removed and read 48 hours after application and the patient returns for a second reading of the patch tests commonly at 72 or 96 hours, with the 96-hour test being preferred by this author. Some physicians also do readings at 1 week after application to identify more delayed reactions.

It is essential that the skin of the back be free of eczema at the time of testing to avoid false-positive reactions due to what has been called the *angry back syndrome*. It is also important that the testing site has not been exposed to topical steroids or ultraviolet light during the preceding week. Oral steroids should be avoided when possible; however, some strong patch test reactions can be obtained even when a patient is taking up to 20 mg prednisone daily.

Photoallergy and Photopatch Testing

When an eruption is observed in a sun-exposed distribution, photoallergic contact dermatitis should be considered. Photoallergy is identical to allergic contact dermatitis with the exception that the allergen in contact with the skin must be exposed to ultraviolet A (UVA) light for the reaction to occur. Photopatch testing is performed similar to routine patch testing, but a second identical set of allergens is also applied to the back. Approximately 24 hours after application, one set of allergens is uncovered and exposed to 15 joules of

TABLE 30.2   EXAMPLES OF ANTIGENS AND EXPOSURE COMMONLY CAUSING CONTACT DERMATITIS

CONTACTANT	EXPOSURE
Carba mix	Rubber, nitrile rubber, lawn and garden fungicides
Copper	Coins, alloys, insecticides, fungicides
Epoxy resin	Adhesives
Formalin (formaldehyde)	Cosmetics, insecticides, fabrics containing cotton and/or rayon
Ethylenediamine hydrochloride	Aminophylline, hydroxyzine, antihistamines
Imidazolidinyl urea	Preservative in skin/hair/cosmetic products and topical medications
Mercaptobenzothiazole	Rubber, nitrile rubber, anticorrosion agent
Mercury	Topical ointments, disinfectants, insecticides
Nickel	Jewelry, buckles, clasps, door handles
Paraben	Preservative in skin/hair/cosmetic products and topical medications
Paraphenylenediamine	Hair dye
Phenylbetanaphthylamine	Rubber compounds (antioxidant)
Potassium dichromate	Leather (chrome tanning), cement
P-tert-butylphenol formaldehyde resin	Leather adhesive
Thiuram mix	Rubber, nitrile rubber, lawn and garden fungicides

UVA light. The patches are then carefully reapplied. All patches are then removed at 72 hours and read at 96 hours. A photoallergy is confirmed if only the site exposed to UVA light shows a reaction. If both the exposed and unexposed sites show equal reactions, a standard contact allergy is confirmed. A stronger reaction at the site exposed to UVA indicates contact allergy augmented by coexisting photoallergy.

Patch Testing Reading and Interpretation

The patch tests are read using a template that is aligned inside the marker lines on the back to show the exact position of each allergen. The sites are then graded as 1+ (erythema), 2+ (edema or vesiculation of <50% of the patch test site), 3+ (edema or vesiculation of >50% of the patch test site), ± or ? (questionable), or Ir (irritant). Strong irritant reactions sometimes result in a sharply demarcated, shiny, eroded patch test site. Weak irritant and allergic reactions are often morphologically indistinguishable.

One of the most important aspects of patch testing is to determine if patch test reactions are relevant to the patient's clinical condition. Some patch test reactions merely indicate sensitization from an exposure that occurred many years prior. In addition, false-positive reactions are not uncommon. Pustular patch test reactions can occur with metal salts and do not indicate contact allergy. Some allergens, such as nickel, formaldehyde, and potassium dichromate, are tested at levels that can also cause an irritant reaction. In addition, when a test site is strongly positive or if the patient experiences severe irritation from tape, nearby sites may show false-positive reactions due to the angry back syndrome. When in doubt, a "use test" can be performed by applying a suspected substance twice daily for 1 week to the antecubital fossa to confirm or exclude an allergic reaction.

Reactions to Cosmetics and Skin Care Products

Although most skin care products available are quite safe, allergic reactions can occur occasionally to almost any cosmetic product. The most common causative agents are fragrance and preservative ingredients. A discussion of some common cosmetic allergens follows.

Fragrance

Fragrance is found in a wide variety of cosmetic products. It is responsible for a relatively large number of allergic reactions to cosmetics (13–15). This is partially because fragrance is not a single ingredient, but is, instead, a general name that includes a variety of individual fragrance ingredients. Individual ingredients in fragrance are usually not listed on ingredient labels. It is important to read the actual ingredient list on products and avoid products that contain fragrance, perfume, or essential oils. Essential oils (i.e., cinnamon oil, clove oil, rosewood oil) often are used as fragrance ingredients. Labels that claim that the product is "unscented" or "fragrance-free" can be misleading. Unscented products may contain a masking fragrance designed to eliminate odors, and fragrance-free products can sometimes include essential oils that the manufacturer may not consider as fragrance. Also, consumers should beware of other less obvious fragrance ingredients that may be listed on the label, such as benzyl alcohol, benzaldehyde, and ethylene brassylate.

There are two materials in the TRUE test patch test tray that screen for allergy to fragrance. Fragrance mix I is a mixture of eight common fragrance ingredients and 20 years ago was reported to be able to identify about 80% of individuals allergic to fragrance (16). Balsam of Peru is an extract from a South American tree in the Myroxylon genus; it contains many constituents used commonly in fragrances and was originally thought to identify 50% of fragrance-allergic patients (16). In the mid-1990s, it was believed that these two screening substances Fragrance mix I and Balsam of Peru, together would identify over 90% of all fragrance allergy (17). Balsam of Peru is used in the artificial flavoring industry and individuals allergic to the substance may have reactions to sweet junk foods, condiments, mouthwashes, toothpaste, cough medicines, liqueurs, and spiced teas. It also can cross-react with citrus peels and tomatoes. It is rarely used directly in the fragrance industry (18). As newer fragrance ingredients have been introduced into the fragrance industry, these screening ingredients are estimated to identify only 60% to 70% of individuals allergic to fragrance (19).

Formaldehyde-releasing Preservatives

Formaldehyde is still the most effective cosmetic preservative against gram-negative bacteria. Substances that release formaldehyde are therefore still commonly used in skin care and cosmetic products (20). Currently used formaldehyde-releasing preservatives include quaternium 15, imidazolidinyl urea, diazolidinyl urea, DMDM hydantoin, and 2-bromo-2-nitropropane-1,3-diol (Bronopol). Individuals allergic to one of these ingredients may cross-react to any of the other formaldehyde-releasing preservatives. Therefore, it is often good advice to avoid all of these substances if patch testing results to one of them are clearly positive.

Parabens

Parabens are the most commonly used preservatives in facial cosmetics and are relatively infrequent sensitizers. A person who has an allergic reaction to parabens may still be able to use paraben-containing products if they are only applied to undamaged skin. That is, almost all paraben allergic reactions occur on inflamed or cracked skin; this has been termed the *paraben paradox* (21).

Parabens are also found in syrups, milk products, soft drinks, candies, jellies, and some systemic medications. However, no sensitization has been reported by ingestion of parabens. Foods containing various preservatives that are known to be topical contact allergens have been occasional causes of hand dermatitis in cooks and bakers.

Kathon CG

Kathon CG (methylisothiazolinone and methylchloroisothiazoline) is a preservative system that has become a common sensitizer (22). In addition to being used in skin, hair, and cosmetic products, it is also found in oils and cutting fluids used by machinists.

Euxyl K400

Euxyl K400 (phenoxyethanol and methyldibromoglutaronitrile) is a preservative system that frequently causes contact allergy (23). It has not achieved a strong market presence in the United States and is being used less frequently now that it has been identified as a frequent sensitizer. Methyldibromoglutaronitrile is the usual sensitizer.

Iodopropynylbutylcarbamate

Iodopropynylbutylcarbamate is a preservative used in skin care and cosmetic products which has been an occasional cause of contact allergy (24). It is also used as an antifungal agent in paints.

Sorbic Acid

Sorbic acid is another cosmetic preservative that only occasionally causes allergic reactions (25). Persons allergic to sorbic acid also may react to potassium sorbate. Sorbic acid has often been used to replace thimerosol in sensitive eye products. Sorbic acid can also cause non-immunologic contact urticaria.

Thimerosol

Thimerosol is primarily found in liquid products for use in the eyes, nose, and ears (26). In cosmetics, it is mostly used in mascaras. It is an ingredient in some vaccines, eye drops, contact lens products, nose sprays, nose drops, and ear drops. Aside from its use in vaccines, it is now used only in occasional products.

Benzocaine

Benzocaine cross-reacts with other benzoate ester anesthetics, such as procaine, tetracaine, and cocaine (26).

It also may cross-react with other para compounds such as para-aminosalicylic acid, para-aminobenzoic acid (PABA), paraphenylenediamine, procainamide, and sulfonamides. Cross-reaction with amide anesthetics, such as lidocaine, dibucaine, mepivacaine, and cyclomethycaine, is uncommon.

Paraphenylenediamine

Another well recognized contact sensitizer, paraphenylenediamine (PPD), is an ingredient in permanent, demipermanent, and semipermanent hair dyes (27). This ingredient can be avoided by use of certain temporary hair dyes, metallic hair dyes, henna, or occasional other dye products without PPD. Persons allergic to this ingredient also may react to similar "para compounds" such as PABA and its derivatives (found in sunscreens), benzocaine (found in skin anesthetics such as sunburn medications), procaine, sulfonamides, para-aminosalicylic acid, and azo dyes (in synthetic clothing fabrics). Allergy to hair dye can be problematic for hair colorists because PPD penetrates readily through latex gloves.

Glyceryl Thioglycolate

Glyceryl thioglycolate is found in the acid permanent wave products used in salons (27). This is a common cause of contact allergy in hairdressers because it can permeate latex gloves. The alkaline permanent waves predominate in retail stores and are also commonly used in salons. These products and many depilatories contain ammonium thioglycolate, which rarely crossreacts with glyceryl thioglycolate.

Lanolin

Lanolin is a moisturizing substance obtained from the sebaceous secretions of sheep (28). The alcohol fraction of lanolin is the primary sensitizing portion. Individuals allergic to lanolin need to also avoid products displaying the European names wool wax and wool wax alcohol (synonymous with lanolin and lanolin alchohol, respectively).

Propylene Glycol

Propylene glycol is a versatile ingredient that is both a solvent and a humectant (29). It can be an irritant that stings when applied to inflamed or cracked skin. Less commonly, it can cause true allergic reactions.

Toluene Sulfonamide/Formaldehyde Resin

Toluene sulfonamide/formaldehyde resin is found in nail polish and is the most common cause of eyelid contact allergy (30). Nail polishes containing other resins in place of this ingredient can be used by persons who are allergic to toluene sulfonamide/formaldehyde resin.

Cocamidopropyl Betaine

There have been a number of reports of contact allergy to cocamidopropyl betaine (31). This ingredient is used in baby shampoos due to its gentleness and the fact that it does not sting when it gets onto the eyes. It has been used more widely in many types of shampoos and cleansers. The sensitizer appears to be impurities formed in the manufacture of the ingredient (31).

Sunscreen Ingredients

Sunscreen ingredients that can cause allergic reactions include PABA and its derivatives, benzophenone, cinnamates, and Parsol 1789 (also called avobenzone or butylmethoxydibenzoylmethane) (32). These sunscreen ingredients are also found in many other cosmetic products, including foundations, pressed powders, antiaging products, lip and nail products, and toners.

One common cause of sunscreen allergy is PABA and its derivatives. The derivatives of PABA include glyceryl PABA and octyl dimethyl PABA, also called Padimate O. Unfortunately, there are products on the market that claim to be PABA-free but which include PABA derivatives. PABA and its derivatives are being used less commonly in products available currently.

The benzophenones, especially oxybenzone, are now the most common cause of contact allergy to sunscreens. There are numerous cases of persons allergic to benzophenones who have assumed they were allergic to PABA and have switched to another PABA-free sunscreen only to discover they react poorly to the substitute because it also contains benzophenones. Benzophenones are also found in nail products, hair products, textiles, and plastics. Parsol 1789 is a newer UVA sunscreen that can cause both contact allergy and photoallergy. Cinnamates are occasional photosensitizers. Salicylates rarely have also caused contact allergy.

Colophony (Rosin)

Colophony or rosin is distilled oil of turpentine (33). It is used in some cosmetics, adhesives (commonly in shoe adhesives), tape, flypaper, epilating wax, rosin bags, furniture polish, price labels, varnish, glue, ink, recycled paper, and waxes for cars or floors. Colophony cross-reacts with abietic acid, abitol, and hydrobietic acid, which are also used in cosmetic products.

Medications That Are Sensitizers

A number of medications have been reported to cause allergic contact dermatitis. In the case of topical products, it is important to consider vehicle ingredients as possible contact allergens in addition to the active drug.

Topical Steroids

It is now appreciated that topical steroids are a fairly frequent cause of contact allergy (34,35). The two best screening ingredients for topical steroid allergy are believed to be tixocortol pivalate and budesonide. The European literature divides topical steroids into four structural groups: group A (tixocortol pivalate, hydrocortisone, prednisone); group B (budesonide, triamcinolone acetonide); group C (dexamethasone, desoximetasone); group D (clobetasol-17-propionate, hydrocortisone-17-butyrate). Cross reactions between structural groups can occur; for example, Groups B and D often cross-react (35).

Ethylenediamine-related Drugs

Ethylenediamine was most commonly found in Mycolog cream, but is not in the current Mycolog II. It is still found in a small number of topical products. Ethylenediamine cross-reacts with aminophylline (which contains 33% ethylenediamine by weight as a stabilizer), ethylenediamine and piperazine antihistamines such as hydroxyzine and cetirizine, ethylenediamine-related motion sickness medications, menstrual analgesics, and some antiparasitics (36). Ethylenediamine is also used as a stabilizer in the manufacture of dyes, rubber accelerators, fungicides, waxes, and resins. However, these sources of exposure are uncommon causes of contact dermatitis.

Neomycin and Bacitracin

Bacitracin and neomycin often cause contact allergy because they are used on injured skin with damaged barrier function (37). Neomycin may cross-react with gentamcin and other aminoglycosides. Bacitracin is recognized to be a frequent cause of contact allergy. Many patients are allergic to both neomycin and bacitracin. This probably does not represent a true cross-reaction but rather reflects the fact that these two ingredients are often in the same products.

Mercurials

Mercurials are divided into organics or inorganics (38). Organics include Merthiolate (thimerosol) and Mercurochrome (merbromin). Inorganics include mercury (thermometers), yellow oxide of mercury, ammoniated mercury (found in Unguentum Bossi and Mazon cream for psoriasis), and phenylmercuric acetate (a spermicidal agent and an occasional preservative in eye solutions). Cross-reactions can occur between organic and inorganic mercury substances. Also, systemic administration of mercurials can induce a severe systemic allergic reaction in a person topically sensitized to mercury.

Metals

Metals can cause both allergic and irritant contact dermatitis. Reactions to metal are most common when moisture such as sweat is present. Also, moisture under jewelry from repeated hand washing is a common cause of irritant dermatitis to metals. The most common cause of skin discoloration to metals is due to the abrasive action of powders in cosmetic products on metal jewelry. The resulting black powder creates what has been called *black dermatographism*.

Nickel

Nickel is the most common cause to allergic contact dermatitis in patients undergoing patch testing (39). Sweat will act on nickel to create a green/black tarnish that can induce an allergic contact dermatitis. Sensitization often occurs via ear or body piercing. Metal jewelry that contains a significant amount of nickel can be identified using a dimethylglyoxime nickel test kit. Many alloys of steel can cause nickel contact allergy. The nickel in stainless steel is so often firmly bound that reactions may only occur with prolonged contact and sweat.

A significant amount of nickel is found not only in jewelry but also in keys, blue jean buttons, bobby pins, safety pins, some non-U.S. coins, eyeglass frames, zippers, bra and garter snaps, doorknobs, scissors, pens, and shoelace eyelets. Nickel is also used in many alloys of chrome and white gold.

Chromium

Chromium causes both allergic and irritant reactions; however, allergic reactions are more common (39). Allergy to chrome or chrome-plated objects is uncommon. When reactions to chrome products occur, the reaction is usually due to nickel in the product.

Most allergic reactions to chromium are to chromates in tanned leather or cement, and these reactions tend to be chronic dermatitis. Chromates are the most common cause of contact allergy to leather and are used in soft tanned leather of the type commonly found on shoe uppers. Potassium dichromate and other chromates are also found in cement, matches, bleach, phosphate-containing detergents, antirust compounds, varnish, orange or yellow paint, spackle, and green tattoos. Chromate reactions in cement workers are often severe, chronic, and may persist many years after exposure to cement has ended.

Cobalt

Objects containing nickel often also contain cobalt (39). It is found in the adhesive of flypaper, light brown hair colors, hard metals, polyester resins, paints, cements, pottery, ceramics, pigments, lubricating oils, and blue tattoos. Occupational exposure includes masons, construction workers, tile workers, dentists, printers, mechanics, and machinists.

Gold

Positive reactions to gold on patch testing are not uncommon (40). However, many individuals who test positive to gold will tolerate gold jewelry. Contact allergy to gold can sometimes occur on the face rather than at the site where gold jewelry is worn.

Tattoos

Several metals used in tattoos can cause allergic contact dermatitis: red tattoos contain mercury sulfide (red cinnabar); green tattoos contain chromium; blue tattoos contain cobalt aluminate; yellow tattoos contain cadmium yellow (a possible cause of phototoxic reactions) (41).

Rubber-related Compounds

Latex products can cause type I allergy as well as type IVa_1 allergy (42). Type I latex allergy to gloves may present as a localized contact urticaria that can mimic an allergic contact dermatitis. Alternatively, latex protein can be inhaled on particles of powder from gloves and cause widespread urticaria and anaphylaxis. *In vitro* testing can be used to screen for type I allergy to latex but does not have 100% sensitivity. Therefore, the skin-prick test is still the gold standard for type I latex allergy testing. Unfortunately, no U.S. Food and Drug Administration-approved latex extract is available yet in the United States for skin-prick testing.

Alternatively, chemicals used to process rubber frequently cause type IVa_1 allergy to latex products and artificial rubber (nitrile rubber). Mercaptobenzothiazole and other mercapto compounds are rubber accelerators that frequently are allergic sensitizers.

Tetramethylthiuram and disulfiram are also rubber accelerators that can cause allergic contact dermatitis. Thiurams are also used in insecticides and fungicides and are often found on lawns and garden plants. Disulfiram is also the active ingredient in Antabuse. Carbamates are rubber accelerators that are common sensitizers and are closely related to thiurams. They are also found in similar products such as rubber and pesticides. Currently, carbamates are the most common accelerators used in latex and nitrile medical gloves.

Black rubber paraphenylenediamine is an antioxidant used in the manufacture of black rubber. This is fortunately a relatively uncommon sensitizer because avoidance of this ubiquitous substance is difficult. Thioureas and naphthyl compounds are rubber accelerators that are less common causes of allergy.

Clothing-related Dermatitis

Most clothing fibers are nonsensitizers or rare sensitizers (43). Dyes used in clothing and shoes can cause allergic reactions. The disperse dyes, such as azo and anthraquinone dyes, which are used on synthetic fabrics, are most problematic. Some persons reacting to azo dyes cross-react with PPD and PABA.

Fabrics containing cotton or rayon usually contain formaldehyde resins and a small amount of free formaldehyde. Allergy to free formaldehyde has become less common because manufacturers have reduced levels of free formaldehyde in fabrics. However, it is possible to have contact allergy to the formaldehyde resins used in these fabrics. These individuals may or may not react to formaldehyde.

Because allergy to clothing is not usually identified using a standard patch test, testing requires specialized nonstandard allergens. Other causes of clothing dermatitis include reactions to rubber used in elastic. Spandex (except some from Europe which contains mercaptobenzothiazole) and Lycra are good substitutes.

Plastic-related Dermatitis

Plastics that can sensitize include epoxies (before full hardening occurs), paratertiary butyphenol formaldehyde resin (commonly used in leather adhesives), and acrylate and methacrylate monomers (44,45). Household adhesives may contain both formaldehyde resins and epoxy.

Acrylic monomers, used in about 95% of dentures in the United States, are a common cause of contact allergy in dentists and their patients. The allergen can penetrate rubber gloves. If the material fully polymerizes and hardens, it is no longer allergenic. Acrylic sculptured nails, nail products, and acrylic prostheses also can cause sensitization. Cyanoacrylate adhesives can occasionally cause contact allergy.

Plants

Allergic contact dermatitis to plants is most commonly due to the oleoresin fraction, especially the essential oil fraction. In contrast, type I reactions to plants are most commonly due to pollen and other plant proteins.

Toxicodendron (Rhus)

Rhus dermatitis (poison ivy, oak, and sumac) is the most common form of allergic contact dermatitis seen in both children and adults in the United States (46,47). Rhus plants have now been reclassified as toxicodendron. Cross-reactions can occur with other anacardiaceae such as Japanese lacquer tree, marking-nut tree of India, cashew nutshells, mango, Ginkgo tree fruit pulp, and the Rengas (black varnish) tree.

Ragweed

Ragweed dermatitis generally affects older individuals and rarely occurs in children (48). Men are affected twenty times more often than women. Affected persons are not usually atopic. The allergic contact reaction is a type IVa$_1$ hypersensitivity to the oil-soluble fraction. Type I reactions to the protein fraction lead to allergic rhinitis. Contact allergy occurs in Chicago from mid-August to late September. A rash involving exposed areas may develop from airborne ragweed exposure.

Compositae

Compositae are ubiquitous in many parts of the world (48). This large family of plants includes chrysanthemums, daisies, asters, arnica, artichokes, burdock, chamomile, chicory, cocklebur, feverfew, lettuce, marigold, marsh elder, pyrethrum, ragweed, sagebrush, sunflower, tansy, and yarrow. The sensitizers in these plants are sesquiterpene lactones. Although a sesquiterpene lactone mix is available for patch testing and will be positive in many cases of compositae allergy, it will miss some cases because sesquiterpene lactones may not be cross-reactive.

Alstromeria

Alstromeria (Peruvian lilly) is the most common cause of contact allergy in florists and is due to tuliposide-A (α butyrolactone) (49). Cross-reactions may occur from handling tulip bulbs.

Photoreactions

Phototoxic reactions are due to nonimmunologic mechanisms, usually occur on first exposure, and tend to resemble sunburn (50). The action spectrum of two common causes, tar and psoralens, is primarily UVA. Other topical phototoxic agents include phenothiazines, sulfanilamide, anthraquinone dyes, eosin, and methylene blue.

Phytophotodermatitis

Phytophotodermatitis is a phototoxic reaction to UVA light due to furocoumarins in several families of plants, especially Umbelliferae (51). The Umbelliferae family includes carrots, celery, parsnips, fennel, dill, parsley, caraway, anise, coriander, and angelica. Also, Rutaceae plants (orange, lemon, grapefruit, lime, and bergamot lime) and some members of Compositae (yarrow) and Moraceae (figs) are also possible causes. Photocontact dermatitis on the neck is caused by perfumes containing oil of bergamot (bergapten or 5-methoxy-psoralens). Bartenders handling Persian limes also can develop phytophotodermatitis.

Photoallergic Contact Reactions

Type IVa$_1$ hypersensitivity mediates photoallergic contact reactions (52). The most common cause in the past was halogenated salcylanides in soaps and cleansers; however, these are no longer used in the United States or Europe. Hexachlorophene, a halogenated phenol, also can cause photoallergy and can cross-react with these compounds.

Today sunscreen ingredients such as PABA, benzophenones, cinnamates, and avobenzone are common causes of photoallergy. Fragrances are another common cause.

Phenothiazines are used in insecticides and can cause topical photoallergy and phototoxic reactions. This does not occur by the oral route, with the exception of chlorpromazine, which can cause phototoxic reactions.

Most topical sulfonamides are not photosensitizers, but sulfanilamide can cause both photoallergic and phototoxic reactions. Oral sulfonamides, tetracyclines, fluoroquinolones, hypoglycemics, and thiazides can cause both photoallergic and phototoxic reactions.

Precautions

Several precautions must be observed in patch testing. The application of the test material itself may in very rare cases sensitize the patient. Potent materials that may sensitize on the first application include plant oleoresins, PPD, and methylsalicylate. Patch testing and, especially, repeated patch testing should not be performed unnecessarily. In testing, one has to avoid provoking nonspecific inflammation. The testing material must be dilute enough to avoid a primary irritant effect. This is especially important when testing with a contactant not included in the standard patch test materials. To be significant, a substance must elicit a reaction at a concentration that will not cause reactivity in a suitable number of normal controls. Patch testing should ideally not be performed in the presence of an acute or widespread contact dermatitis since false-positive reactions may be obtained because of increased reactivity of the skin. In addition, a positive patch test reaction with the offending agent may cause a flare-up of the dermatitis. As mentioned earlier, an anaphylactoid reaction can occur when testing for immunologic contact urticaria.

■ COMPLICATIONS

The most common complication of allergic contact dermatitis is secondary infection caused by the intense pruritus and subsequent scratching. An interesting but poorly understood complication is the occasional occurrence of the nephrotic syndrome and glomerulonephritis in severe generalized contact dermatitis caused by poison ivy or poison oak (53).

■ MANAGEMENT

General management strategies are outlined in Table 30.3 (54).

■ SYMPTOMATIC TREATMENT

The inflammation and pruritus of allergic contact dermatitis necessitate symptomatic therapy. For limited, localized allergic contact dermatitis, cool tap water compresses and a topical corticosteroid are the preferred modalities. It is safest to use hydrocortisone on the face, however, its use should be limited to a maximum of a few days on the eyelids.

When the dermatitis is particularly acute or widespread, systemic corticosteroids should be used. In instances when further exposure can be avoided, such as poison ivy dermatitis, there should be no hesitation in administering systemic corticosteroids. This is a classic example of a self-limited disease that will respond to a course of oral corticosteroid therapy. The popular use of a 4- to 5-day decreasing steroid regimen often results in a flare-up of the dermatitis several days after discontinuing the steroids. It is often necessary to continue the treatment for 10 to 14 days or longer. The response to systemic corticosteroids is generally dramatic, with improvement apparent in only a few hours. Three rules that might be applied to systemic corticosteroid therapy in acute contact dermatitis are (a) use an inexpensive preparation such as prednisone; (b) use enough (1 mg/kg); and (c) avoid prolonged administration (i.e., more than 2 weeks of therapy if possible).

For secondary infection resulting from scratching because of the pruritus of allergic contact dermatitis, antibiotics may be needed. In addition to oral antibiotics, topical mupirocin can be helpful since this medication rarely causes contact allergy.

TABLE 30.3   MANAGEMENT OF THE ALLERGIC CONTACT DERMATITIS

Limited, localized reaction	Cool tap water compress Topical corticosteroid cream
Extensive, acute reaction	Oral prednisone: 40 mg to 60 mg per day initially (adult); allow taper over 2 weeks
Prophylaxis	Antigen avoidance Protective clothing Barrier cream

■ PROPHYLAXIS

The physician has a responsibility to his or her patients not only to treat disease but also to prevent it. For that reason, avoid topical applications of medications that have a high index of sensitization. Included in this group are benzocaine, most topical antihistamines, neomycin, and bacitracin.

When the offending agent causing allergic contact dermatitis is discovered, careful instruction must be given to the patient so as to avoid it in the future. The physician should discuss all of the possible sources of exposure, and when dealing with occupational dermatitis, should have knowledge about suitable jobs for patients. In the case of chemical sensitivity, this list of exposure sources may be quite extensive. When dealing with a plant sensitizer, the patient should be instructed in the proper identification of the offending plant.

Patient education is of paramount importance when treating contact allergy. It has been reported that if the patient is aware of the allergen and informed about the variety of substances that contain it, they are more likely to improve (55).

There may be instances in which exposure cannot be avoided, either because of the patient's occupation or because of the ubiquitous nature of the allergen. The use of protective clothing is sometimes beneficial, however, barrier creams often will not be useful. Early diagnosis and avoidance of further allergen exposure are critical if chronic, debilitating dermatitis is to be prevented (56).

■ REFERENCES

1. Rietschel RL, Fowler JF. The pathogenesis of allergic contact hypersensitivity. In: Rietschel RL, Fowler JF, eds. *Fisher's Contact Dermatitis.* 4th ed. Baltimore: Williams & Wilkins;1995:1–10.

2. Ray MC, Tharp MD, Sullivan TJ, et al. Contact hyper-sensitivity reactions to dinitrofluorobenzene mediated by monoclonal IgE anti-DNP antibodies. *J Immunol.* 1983;131:1096–1102.

3. Silberberg-Sinakin I, Gigli I, Baer RL, et al. Langerhans cells: role in contact hypersensitivity and relationship to lymphoid dendritic cells and to macrophages. *Immunol Rev.* 1980;53:203–232.

4. Belsito DV. The pathophysiology of allergic contact dermatitis. *Clin Rev Allergy.* 1989;7:347.

5. Amaro C, Goossens A. Immunologic occupational contact urticaria and contact dermatitis from proteins: a review. *Contact Dermatitis.* 2008;58(2): 67–75.

6. Fisher AA. New advances in contact dermatitis. *Int J Dermatol.* 1977:16:552–568.

7. LeSuer BW, Yiannias JA. Contact stomatitis. *Dermatol Clin.* 2003; 21(1);105–114.

8. Rietschel RL. Is patch testing cost effective? *J Am Acad Dermatol.* 1989;21:885–887.

9. Rietschel RL, Fowler JF. The role of patch testing. In: Rietschel RL, Fowler JF, eds. *Fisher's Contact Dermatitis.* 4th ed. Baltimore: Williams & Wilkins;1995:11–32.

10. Belsito DV. The diagnostic evaluation treatment, and prevention of allergic contact dermatitis in the new millennium. *J Allergy Clin Immunol.* 2000;3:409–420.

11. Krasteva M, Kehren J, Sayag M, et al. Contact dermatitis: clinical aspects and diagnosis. *Eur J Dermatol.* 1999;9:144–159.

12. Belsito DV. Allergic contact dermatitis. In: Freedberg IM, Eisen AZ, Wolff K, et al., eds. *Fitzpatrick's Dermatology in General Medicine.* 6th ed. New York: McGraw Hill;2003.

13. Paulsen E, Andersen KE. Colophonium and compositae mix as markers of fragrance allergy: cross-reactivity between fragrance terpenes, colophonium and Compositae plant extracts. *Contact Dermatitis.* 2005; 53:285–291.

14. Larsen WG. How to instruct patients sensitive to fragrances. *J Am Acad Dermatol.* 1989;21:880–884.

15. Katsarma G, Gawkrodger DJ. Suspected fragrance allergy requires extended patch testing to individual fragrance allergens. *Contact Dermatitis.* 1999;41:193–197.

16. Larsen WG. Perfume dermatitis. *J Am Acad Dermatol.* 1985;12:1–9.

17. Larsen W, Nakayama H, Lindberg M, et al. Fragrance contact dermatitis: a worldwide multicenter investigation (part I). *Am J Contact Dermatitis.* 1996;7:77–83.

18. Api AM. Only Peru Balsam extracts or distillates are used in perfumery. *Contact Dermatitis.* 2006;54:179.

19. Larsen W, Nakayama H, Fischer T, et al. Fragrance contact dermatitis—a worldwide multicenter investigation (part III). *Contact Dermatitis.* 2002;46:141–144.

20. Fransway AF. The problem of preservation in the 1990s. I. Statement of the problem, solution(s) of the industry, and the current use of formaldehyde and formaldehyde-releasing biocides. *Am J Contact Dermatitis.* 1991;2:6–22.

21. Jackson EM. Paraben paradoxes. *Am J Contact Dermatitis.* 1993;4: 69–70.

22. Mowad CM. Methylchloro-isothiazolinone revisited. *Am J Contact Dermatitis.* 2000;11:115–118.

23. Zachariae C, Johansen JD, Rastogi SC, et al. Allergic contact dermatitis from methyldibromo glutaronitrile—clinical cases from 2003. *Contact Dermatitis.* 2005;52:6–8.

24. Schnuch A, Geier J, Brasch J, et al. The preservative iodopropynyl butylcarbamate: frequency of allergic reactions and diagnostic considerations. *Contact Dermatitis.* 2002;46:153–156.

25. Fisher AA. Sorbic acid: a cause of immediate nonallergenic facial erythema: an update. *Cutis.* 1998;61:17.

26. Scheman AJ. Contact allergy alternatives. *Cutis.* 1996;57: 235–240.

27. Scheman AJ. New trends in hair products: an update for dermatologists. *Cosmetic Derm.* 1998;11:17–21.

28. Matthieu L, Dockx P. Discrepancy in patch test results with wool wax alcohols and Amerchol L-101. *Contact Dermatitis.* 1997;36:150–151.

29. Jackson EM. Propylene glycol: irritant, sensitizer or neither? *Cosmetic Derm.* 1995;8:43–45.

30. Rosenzweig R, Scher RK. Nail cosmetics: adverse reactions. *Am J Contact Dermatitis.* 1993;4:71–77.

31. Fowler JF, Zug KM, Taylor JS, et al. Allergy to cocamidopropyl betaine and amidoamine in North America. *Dermatitis.* 2004;15:5–6.

32. Schauder S, Ippen H. Contact and photocontact sensitivity to sunscreens: review of a 15-year experience and of the literature. *Contact Dermatitis.* 1997;37:221–232.

33. Downs AMR, Sansom J. Colophony allergy: a review. *Contact Dermatitis.* 1999;41:305–310.

34. Isaksson M, Bruze M. Corticosteroids. *Dermatitis.* 2005;16:3–5.

35. Jacob SE, Steele T. Corticosteroid classes: a quick reference guide including patch test substances and cross-reactivity. *J Am Acad Dermatol.* 2006;54:723–727.

36. Ash S, Scheman A. Systemic contact dermatitis to hydroxzine. *Am J Contact Dermat.* 1997;8:2–5.

37. Gette MT, Marks JG, Maloney ME. Frequency of postoperative allergic contact dermatitis to topical antibiotics. *Arch Dermatol.* 1992;128:365–367.

38. Wekkeli M, Hippman G, Rosenkranz AR, et al. Mercury as a contact allergen. *Contact Dermatitis.* 1990;22:295–296.

39. Kiec-Swierczynska M. Allergy to chromate, cobalt and nickel in Lodz 1977–1988. *Contact Dermatitis.* 1990;8:95–104.

40. Bruze M, Edman B, Björkner B, et al. Clinical relevance of contact allergy to gold sodium thiosulfate. *J Am Acad Dermatol.* 1994;31:579–583.

41. Levy J, Sewell M, Goldstein N. II. A short history of tattooing. *J Derm Surg Oncol.* 1979;5:851–856.

42. Cohen DE, Scheman AJ, Stewart L, et al. American Academy of Dermatology's position paper on latex allergy. *J Am Acad Dermatol.* 1998;39:98–106.

43. Scheman AJ, Carroll PA, Brown KH, et al. Formaldehyde-related textile allergy: an update. *Contact Dermatitis.* 1998;38:332–336.

44. Holness DL, Nethercott JR. Results of patch testing with a specialized collection of plastic and glue allergens. *Am J Contact Dermatitis.* 1997;8:121–124.

45. Kanerva L, Jolanki R, Estlander T. Ten years of patch testing with the (meth)acrylate series. *Contact Dermatitis.* 1997;37:255–258.

46. Fisher AA. Poison ivy/oak dermatitis. Part I: prevention—soap and water, topical barriers, hyposensitization. *Cutis.* 1996;57:384–386.

47. Fisher AA. Poison ivy/oak/sumac. Part II: specific features. *Cutis.* 1996;58:22–24.

48. Warshaw EM, Zug KA. Sesquiterpene lactone allergy. *Am J Contact Dermatitis.* 1996;7:1–23.

49. Marks JG. Allergic contact dermatitis to *Alstromeria. Arch Dermatol.* 1988;124:914–916.

50. MacFarlane DF, DaLeo VA. Phototoxic and photoallergic dermatitis. In: Guin JD, ed. *Practical Contact Dermatitis.* New York: McGraw-Hill:1995:83–92.

51. Pathak MA. Phytophotodermatitis. *Clin Dermatol.* 1986;4:102–121.

52. DaLeo VA, Suarez SM, Maso MJ. Photoallergic contact dermatitis: results of photopatch testing in New York, 1985 to 1990. *Arch Dermatol.* 1992;128:1513–1518.

53. Rytand DA. Fatal anuria, the nephrotic syndrome and glomerular nephritis as sequels of the dermatitis of poison oak. *Am J Med.* 1968;5:548–560.

54. Slavin RG. Allergic contact dermatitis. In: Fireman P, Slavin RG, eds. *Atlas of Allergies.* 2nd ed. Philadelphia: JB Lippincott;1996.

55. Breit R, Turk RBM. The medical and social fate of the dichromate allergic patient. *Br J Dermatol.* 1976;94:349–350.

56. Rietschel RL. Occupational contact dermatitis. *Lancet.* 1997;349:1093–1095.

CHAPTER 31

Urticaria, Angioedema, and Hereditary Angioedema

CAROL A. SALTOUN

The earliest texts called urticaria and angioedema "a vexing problem" (1). Little has changed since that assessment. Today's clinician is still faced with a common syndrome that affects 20% of the population at some time in their lives (2), but there is no cohesive understanding of the many clinical mechanisms, presentations, or clinical management of the urticarias. For the clinician, this requires a broad knowledge of the many clinical forms of urticaria and an even more extensive familiarity with the creative ways that medications and treatment can be applied. Modern concepts of allergen-induced cellular inflammation, late-phase cutaneous responses, adhesion molecules, cytokines, inflammatory autocoids, and autoantibodies are leading to a better understanding of pathogenesis and treatment. Meanwhile, clinicians should formulate a rational approach to the care of patients with these conditions.

Urticarial lesions can have diverse appearances. Generally they consist of raised, erythematous skin lesions that are markedly pruritic, tend to be evanescent in any one location, are usually worsened by scratching, and always blanch with pressure. Individual lesions typically resolve within 24 hours and leave no residual skin changes. This description does not cover all forms of urticaria, but it includes the features necessary for diagnosis in most clinical situations. Angioedema is associated with urticaria in 40% of patients, but the two may occur independently (3). Angioedema is similar to urticaria, except that it occurs in deeper tissues and is often asymmetric. Because there are fewer mast cells and sensory nerve endings in these deeper tissues, pruritus is less common with angioedema, which more typically involves a tingling or burning sensation. Although urticaria may occur on any area of the body, angioedema most often affects the perioral region, periorbital regions, tongue, genitalia, and extremities. In this review, angioedema and urticaria are discussed jointly except where specified.

The incidence of acute urticaria is not known. Although it is said to afflict 10% to 20% of the population at some time during life, it is most common in young adults (1). Chronic urticaria occurs more frequently in middle-aged persons, especially women. In a family practice office, its prevalence has been reported to be 30% (4). If patients have chronic urticaria for more than 6 months, 40% will continue to have recurrent wheals 10 years later (5). The presence of angioedema, severity of symptoms, and evidence of autoimmune mechanism have been shown to prognosticate longer duration of disease; however, race, education, smoking, comorbidity and atopy did not influence duration (3,6,7). It is possible that the true prevalence of urticaria is higher than reported owing to many acute, self-limited episodes that do not come to medical attention.

Acute urticaria is arbitrarily defined as persisting for less than 6 weeks, whereas chronic urticaria refers to episodes lasting more than 6 weeks. When considering chronic urticaria, an etiologic agent or precipitating cause such as a physical urticaria is established in up to 30% of patients who are thoroughly evaluated (8). However, most chronic urticaria is idiopathic. Success rates of determining an inciting agent are higher in acute forms. Because of the sometimes extreme discomfort and cosmetic problems associated with chronic urticaria, a thorough evaluation to search for etiologic factors is recommended. This evaluation should rely primarily on the history and physical examination as well as response to therapy; limited laboratory evaluation may be indicated based on history and physical exam findings (Fig. 31.2). In a study of 238 consecutive new patients with chronic urticaria and/or angioedema, subjects were initially worked up with a questionnaire and limited laboratory tests. Subsequently they were evaluated with a rigorous screening program including biopsy, extensive blood tests, radiography, provocation tests, and elimination diets. After the rigorous workup, only one patient was found to have a cause for their urticaria that would not have been found with the initial workup alone (9).

PATHOGENESIS

There is no unifying concept to account for all forms of urticaria; however, because erythema, edema, and localized pruritus are mimicked by intracutaneous injection of histamine, its release is thought to be the underlying mediator. The hypothesis that histamine is the central mediator of urticaria is bolstered by (a) the cutaneous response to injected histamine; (b) the frequent clinical response of various forms of urticaria to therapeutic antihistamines; (c) the documented elevation of plasma histamine or local histamine release from "urticating" tissue in some forms of the condition; and (d) the apparent degranulation of skin mast cells. Tissue resident mast cells or circulating and/or tissue-recruited basophils continue to be the presumed source of the released histamine. Understanding the mechanisms responsible for the release of histamine in the various forms of urticaria continues to be the focus of current research.

Several potential mechanisms for mast cell activation in the skin are summarized in Table 31.1 and include (a) immunoglobulin E (IgE) immediate hypersensitivity such as occurs with penicillin or foods, (b) activation of the classical or alternative complement cascades such as occurs in immune complex disease like serum sickness or collagen vascular disease, (c) direct mast cell membrane activation such as occurs with injection of morphine or radio contrast media, and (d) generation of thrombin from the extrinsic coagulation pathway with mast cell activation and increase in vascular permeability (10). The presence of major basic protein in biopsy samples of chronic urticaria (11) makes the eosinophil suspect as an effector cell. Prolonged response to histamine, but not leukotrienes, in the skin of patients with chronic urticaria may suggest abnormal clearance of mediators locally (12).

Recent efforts in studying the pathogenesis of chronic urticaria has resulted in the belief that serological mediators such as autoantibodies or histamine-releasing factors (HRFs) which are not autoantibodies in addition to/or an alteration in mast cell or basophil responsiveness to histamine-releasing agents can lead to chronic urticaria. Evidence for an autoimmune cause of chronic urticaria came to light when it was reported that 14% of patients with chronic idiopathic urticaria (CIU) had antithyroid antibodies (13). Treatment of

TABLE 31.1 POTENTIAL MECHANISMS OF MAST CELL ACTIVATION IN URTICARIA OR ANGIOEDEMA

TYPE	CAUSE	MEDIATORS
IgE immediate hypersensitivity	Allergens Modified IgE IgG Autoimmune anti-IgE or FcεRIα FcεRII (CD23) on platelets, lymphocytes, or eosinophils	Histamine, leukotrienes PGD2, PAF, ECF-A, HRF
Activation of classical pathway of complement	Antigen-antibody complexes (IgM IgG1, IgG2, or IgG3)	C3a, C4a, C5a (anaphylatoxins) cause release of mast cell mediators
Activation of alternative pathway of complement	IgA-antigen complexes, complex polysaccharides, lipopolysaccharides	C3a, C4a, C5a (anaphylatoxins) cause release of mast cell mediators
Direct activation of mast cell membrane	Morphine, codeine, polymyxin antibiotics, thiamine, radiocontrast media, certain foods causing histamine release (strawberries)	Opiates act through specific receptors to release histamine Others nonspecifically activate cell membrane to release or generate mast cell mediators
Plasma-kinin generating system	Activation of plasma and/or tissue Kallikrein or coagulation pathway Negatively charges surfaces, collagen vascular basement membrane, or endotoxin	Bradykinin; thrombin activation; especially for HAE and some cases of CIU

these patients with thyroid hormone has not changed the natural course of the disease, but it may have variable benefit to severity and duration of urticarial lesions (14). Because of the association between autoimmune thyroid disease and urticaria, other autoantibodies in patients with chronic urticaria were sought. Greaves reported a 5% to 10% incidence of anti-(IgE) antibodies in these patients (15). Next, the high affinity IgE receptor (FcεRI) was identified and isolated. Shortly thereafter, it was reported that 45% to 50% patients with CIU have anti–IgE-receptor antibodies that bind to the α subunit of the IgE receptor, causing activation of mast cells or basophils (16). A more recent study of 78 patients with CIU found that one-third of patients had functional (histamine releasing) autoantibodies directed against either (17). Patients with CIU and presence of these autoantibodies are now classified as chronic autoimmune urticaria (CAU) by some investigators.

The presence and clinical relevance of autoantibodies to FcεRI or IgE can be identified by both *in vivo* and *in vitro* tests. The autologous serum skin test (ASST) consists of a cutaneous injection of autologous serum resulting in a wheal-and-flare at 30 minutes; however, healthy patients without urticaria have been found to have positive ASST(18). Due to the occurrence of immunoreactive but nonhistamine releasing autoantibodies in some CIU patients and their presence in patients with autoimmune connective tissue diseases without CIU, immunoassays for these antibodies have not been useful. Instead, methods for measuring the release of histamine have been developed where the sera of patients with CIU is incubated with donor basophils, then measured directly for histamine or indirectly through basophil activation marker CD203c (19). These assays are limited by the variability of releasibility between donor basophils from different sources and it has yet to be proven that the presence of functional autoantibodies in CIU patients are pathogenic.

The suggestion of the presence of a nonantibody HRF such as complement, chemokines, or cytokines, comes from the finding that over 50% of CIU patients do not have autoantibodies. In support of this notion, it has been shown that IgG-depleted serum can cause a positive ASST (20). Evidence for alterations in basophil function comes from the finding of 2 basophil phenotypes in patients with CIU with differing IgE receptor responsiveness (21). In addition to differences in histamine releasability, patients with CIU have been found to have decreased numbers of serum basophils which suggests that basophils are recruited to the skin in CIU (22). This was confirmed by observations that both lesional and nonlesional skin of patients with CAU contained increased basophils after ASST compared to healthy controls (23).

Products from the kinin-generating system are now known to be important in hereditary angioedema (HAE) (24) and angioedema resulting from angiotensin-

converting enzyme (ACE) inhibitors (25). In addition, bradykinin has been reported to be capable of causing a wheal-and-flare reaction when injected into human skin. Aspirin and nonsteroidal anti-inflammatory drugs (NSAIDs) are capable of altering arachidonic acid metabolism and can result in urticaria without specific interaction between IgE and the pharmacologic agent.

Nonspecific factors that may aggravate urticaria include fever, heat, alcohol ingestion, exercise, emotional stress, peri-menopausal status, and hyperthyroidism. Anaphylaxis and urticaria due to progesterone have been described (26) but seem to be exceedingly rare, and progesterone has been used to treat chronic cyclic urticaria and eosinophilia (27). Certain food additives such as tartrazine or monosodium glutamate have been reported to aggravate chronic urticaria (25,28). Many experts experienced in urticaria believe that progesterone is not a cause or a treatment and that food preservatives do not aggravate chronic urticaria. There have been studies showing no relationship between urticaria and monosodium glutamate as well as aspartame (29,30).

■ BIOPSY

Biopsy of urticarial lesions has accomplished less than expected to improve our understanding of the pathogenesis of urticaria, but may help guide therapy in refractory cases. Three major patterns are currently recognized (Table 31.2). Acute and physical urticarias

TABLE 31.2 BIOPSY PATTERNS OF URTICARIAL AND ANGIOEDEMA LESIONS

TYPE	DESCRIPTION
Acute urticaria/ angioedema	Dilation of small venules and capillaries in superficial dermis (urticaria) or subcutaneous tissue (angioedema); flattening of rete pegs; swollen collagen fibrils
Chronic idiopathic urticaria	Mild cellular inflammation including activated T-lymphocytes, monocytes, and mast cells; delayed-onset urticaria may be mediated by cytokines; e.g., IL-1, 3, 5, or HRF
Urticarial vasculitis	Neutrophil infiltration with vessel wall necrosis; occasional deposition of immunoglobulin and complement

CONTINUUM OF ACUTE URTICARIA TO URTICARIAL VASCULITIS

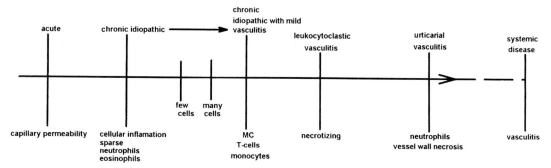

■ **FIGURE 31.1**   A hypothetical model for describing the range of histology of chronic idiopathic urticaria.

show only dermal edema without cellular infiltrate, whereas chronic urticaria typically shows a perivascular mononuclear or lymphocytic infiltrate with an increased number of mast cells. Urticarial vasculitis—in which lesions last more than 24 hours, may be purpuric, and may heal with residual hyperpigmentation—show neutrophil infiltration and vessel wall necrosis with or without immunoprotein deposition. A subset of patients (up to 19% in one study) with acute or chronic urticaria will have a neutrophil predominant dermal infiltrate without evidence of vasculitis (31). Further studies may determine if these several pathologic forms of urticaria represent a continuum of disease (Fig. 31.1) or separate pathophysiologic entities.

Studies of the cellular infiltrate of CIU patients both with and without functional antibodies to FcεRIα found no difference in either the type or number of inflammatory cells or the cytokine pattern between the two groups. In addition, the histological findings were similar to that of the late-phase reaction in atopic individuals. CIU skin biopsies demonstrated increased levels of IL-4, IL-5, and INF-γ while late-phase reactions biopsies revealed increased IL-4, IL-5, but not IFN-γ, suggesting the involvement of a mixture of T_H1 and T_H2 cells or alternatively T_H0 cells in CIU (32).

■ CLASSIFICATION

Classification in terms of known causes is helpful in evaluating patients with urticaria. Table 31.3 presents one classification that may be clinically useful. Additional knowledge of precipitating events or mechanisms may simplify this classification (33).

Nonimmunologic

Physical Urticaria

The physical urticarias are a unique group that constitute up to 17% of chronic urticarias and several reviews have been published (34–36). They are frequently missed as a cause of chronic urticaria, and more than one type may occur together in the same patient. Most forms, with the exception of delayed pressure urticaria (DPU), occur as simple hives without inflammation, and individual lesions resolve within 24 hours. As a group, they can be reproduced by various physical stimuli that have been standardized in some cases (Table 31.4).

Dermographism literally means "write on skin." This phenomenon, also called factitious urticaria, may be detected unexpectedly on routine examination, or patients may complain of pruritus and rash, frequently characterized by linear wheals. When questioned carefully, they may state that itching precedes the rash, causing them to scratch and worsen the condition. The cause of this lesion is unknown. Because it appears in approximately 5% of people, it may be a normal variant. Its onset has been described following severe drug reactions and may be confused with vaginitis in evaluating genital pruritus (37). A delayed form has been recognized with onset of lesions 3 to 8 hours after stimulus to the skin, which may be related to DPU. It may accompany other forms of urticaria. The lesion is readily demonstrated by lightly stroking the skin of an affected patient with a pointed instrument or tongue depressor. This produces erythema, pruritus, and linear streaks of edema or wheal formation. No antigen, however, has been shown to initiate the response, but dermographism has been passively transferred with plasma. Antihistamines usually ameliorate symptoms if they are present. Cutaneous mastocytosis may be considered under the heading of dermographism, because stroking the skin results in significant wheal formation (Darier sign). This disease is characterized by a diffuse increase in cutaneous mast cells. The skin may appear normal, but is usually marked by thickening and accentuated skin folds.

Delayed pressure urticaria, with or without angioedema, is clinically characterized by the gradual onset of wheals or edema in areas where pressure has been applied to the skin. Onset is usually 4 to 6 hours after exposure, but wide variations may be noted. An immediate form of pressure urticaria has been observed. The

TABLE 31.3   CLASSIFICATION OF URTICARIA

Nonimmunologic		
Physical Uriticarias	Hereditary urticaria	Miscellaneous
Dematographism	Hereditary angioedema	Infections
Adrenergic	Hereditary vibratory angioedema	Vasculitis
Pressure	Urticaria, deafness, amyloidosis syndrome	Neoplasm
Vibratory	Familial localized heat urticaria	Anaphylaxis
Solar	C3b inactivator deficiency	Recurrent idiopathic
Cholinergic	Porphyria	Exercise-induced
Local heat	Papular urticaria	
Cold	Urticaria pigmentosa	
Immunologic		
Food	Transfusion reactions	
Drugs	Schnitzler syndrome (119)	
Autoimmune anti-IgE and/or anti-FcεRI	Atopy	
Insect stings	Acquired C1 INH deficiency	
Identifiable agents (uncertain mechanisms)		
Aspirin	Radiocontrast media	
Opiates		

lesion of DPU can be reproduced by applying pressure with motion for 20 minutes (38). DPU lesions can be pruritic and/or painful and may be associated with malaise, fever, chills, arthralgias, and leukocytosis. The mechanism of these reactions is unknown, but biopsy samples of lesions show a predmoninantly eosinophilic cell infiltrate located in the deep dermis (39). In addition, increased levels of TNF-α have been found in many cell types of patients with DPU (40). A recent case report demonstrated successful treatment of DPU with anti-TNF-α, suggesting that TNF-α may play an important role in DPU (41). The incidence of DPU has been reported as 2% of all urticarias; however, one recent study has found that 37% of patients with CIU have associated DPU (9,42). Treatment is based on avoidance of situations that precipitate the lesions. Antihistamines are generally ineffective, and a low-dose, alternate-day corticosteroid may be necessary for the more severe cases. NSAIDs (43), dapsone, montelukast, and colchicine have occasionally been helpful in case reports (42).

Solar urticaria is clinically characterized by development of pruritus, erythema, and edema within minutes of exposure to light. The lesions are typically present only in exposed areas. Diagnosis can be established by using broad-spectrum light with various filters or a spectrodermograph to document the eliciting wavelength (44). Treatment includes avoidance of sunlight and use of protective clothing and various sunscreens or blockers, depending on the wavelength eliciting the lesion (45). An antihistamine taken 1 hour before exposure may be helpful in some forms, and induction of tolerance is possible.

Cholinergic urticaria (generalized heat), a common form of urticaria (5% to 7%), especially in teenagers and young adults (11.2%), is clinically characterized by small, punctate hives surrounded by an erythematous flare, the so-called "fried egg" appearance. These lesions may be clustered initially, but can coalesce and usually become generalized in distribution, primarily over the upper trunk and arms. Pruritus is generally severe. The onset of the rash is frequently associated with hot showers, sudden temperature change, exercise, sweating, or anxiety. A separate entity with similar characteristic lesions induced by cold has been described (46). Rarely, systemic symptoms may occur. The mechanism of this reaction is not certain, but cholinergically mediated thermodysregulation resulting in a neurogenic reflex has been postulated, because it can be reproduced by increasing core body temperature by 0.7°C to 1°C (47). Histamine and other mast cell mediators have been documented in some patients (48) and increased muscarinic receptors have been reported in lesional sites of a patient with cholinergic urticaria (49). The appearance and description of the rash are highly characteristic and are reproduced by an intradermal methacholine skin test, but only in one-third of the patients. Exercise in an occlusive suit or submersion in a warm bath is a more sensitive method of reproducing the urticaria. Passive heat can be used to differentiate this syndrome from exercise-induced urticaria or anaphylaxis. Nonsedating antihistamines are the treatment of choice; however, some patients require combination treatment including a first-generation antihistamine such as hydroxyzine.

A form of "autonomic" urticaria called *adrenergic urticaria* has been described and can be reproduced by intracutaneous injection of noradrenaline (3–10 ng in 0.02 ml saline) (50). This unique form of urticaria is characterized by a "halo" of white skin surrounding a small papule. It may have been previously misdiagnosed as cholinergic urticaria because of its small lesions and its association with stress. In this case, however, relief can be provided with β blockers.

Local heat urticaria, a rare form of heat urticaria (51), may be demonstrated by applying localized heat to the skin. A familial localized heat urticaria also has been reported (52) and is manifested by a delay in onset of urticarial lesions of 4 to 6 hours following local heat exposure.

Cold urticaria is clinically characterized by the rapid onset of urticaria or angioedema after cold exposure. Lesions are generally localized to exposed areas, but sudden total body exposure, as in swimming, may cause hypotension and result in death (53). Although usually idiopathic (primary acquired cold urticaria), cold urticaria has been associated with cryoglobulinemia, cryofibrinogenemia, cold agglutinin disease, and paroxysmal cold hemoglobinuria (secondary acquired

cold urticaria) (54). The mechanism of cold urticaria is not known. Release of histamine and several other mediators has been demonstrated in selected patients following cold exposure (13). A recent case report describes the successful treatment of cold-induced urticaria with anti-IgE, suggesting a possible role for IgE and FcεRI in its pathogenesis (55). In patients with abnormal proteins, passive transfer of the cold sensitivity has been accomplished using plasma (56,57). Some cryoprecipitates can fix complement, and thus may induce anaphylatoxin production. Diagnosis of cold urticaria frequently can be confirmed by placing an ice cube on the forearm for 4 minutes (Table 31.4). Several coexisting cold-induced urticarias do not respond to an ice cube test (58). If cryoglobulins are present, a search should be performed for an underlying cause, e.g., hepatitis B or C infection or lymphoreticular malignancy. Treatment should consist of limited cold exposure (e.g., the patient should enter swimming pools cautiously), proper clothing, and oral cyproheptadine (59), although other antihistamines are useful (60). In cases in which an abnormal protein is present, treatment of the underlying disease may be indicated and curative. Delayed-onset hypersensitivity to cold also has been reported (61).

Inherited Angioedema

Hereditary angioedema (HAE) is clinically characterized by recurrent spontaneous or trauma-induced episodes of angioedema involving any part of the body. Urticaria is not a feature of this disease. Laryngeal edema is common and is the major cause of death. Angioedema of the gastrointestinal tract may cause abdominal discomfort and can mimic an acute abdomen. HAE type I is inherited as an autosomal dominant trait,

TABLE 31.4   TEST PROCEDURES FOR PHYSICAL AND CHRONIC IDIOPATHIC URTICARIA

URTICARIA TYPE	PROCEDURE
Dermographism	Firmly stroke interscapular skin with tongue blade or dermatographometer.
Delayed pressure urticaria	Hang 15-pound weight across shoulder while walking for 20 min.
Solar urticaria	Expose skin to defined wavelengths of light.
Cholinergic urticaria	1. Methacholine skin test 2. Immersion in hot bath (42°C) to raise body temperature 0.7°C
Local heat urticaria	Apply warm compress to forearm.
Cold urticaria	1. Apply ice cube to forearm for 4 min; observe rewarming for 10 min. 2. Exercise in cold and observe for cholinergic-like urticaria (cold-induced cholinergic urticaria).
Aquagenic	Apply water compress (35°C) for 30 min.
Vibratory	Laboratory vortex applied gently to mid-forearm for 4 min
Autoimmune	Intradermal injection of autologous serum

manifested by a decrease in expression of C1-inhibitor (C1-INH) in the plasma. HAE type II is characterized by expression of a dysfunctional C1-INH with normal plasma levels. A recently described HAE type III demonstrates normal C1-INH plasma levels and activity and occurs uniquely in women (62). Because C1-INH regulates the classical complement cascade, the mechanism of edema formation in HAE was initially thought to be due to unhindered complement activation. Subsequently, it was demonstrated that C1-INH also plays a role in controlling the production of bradykinin via the contact system by inactivation of plasma kallikrein and factor XIIa. This knowledge paired with the finding of increased bradykinin levels in the plasma of patients with HAE during attacks suggest that the primary mediator of HAE is bradykinin produced through the contact system (63). The specific trigger that initiates the angioedema remains unknown.

The diagnosis of HAE usually is established by a history of angioedema, a family history of similar disease or early death because of laryngeal obstruction, and appropriate complement studies (Table 31.5). The usual forms of treatment for angioedema, including epinephrine, corticosteroids, and antihistamines, are generally ineffective for HAE. Tracheostomy may be necessary in urgent situations where laryngeal edema has occurred. Supportive therapy, such as intravenous fluids or analgesics, may be required for other manifestations of the disease.

Attenuated androgens such as Danazol (64) and stanozolol (65) have been used successfully on a chronic basis to treat HAE. Each of these attenuated androgens appears to upregulate the synthetic capability of hepatic cells that make C1-INH with a corresponding increase in C4 level and reduction of the number and severity of acute exacerbations. Often, sufficient clinical improvement may be obtained with minimal doses such that the C4 level is normalized, but the C1 inhibitor level is not significantly increased. Initial treatment with 200 mg/day of Danazol or 2 mg/day to 4 mg/day of stanozolol should be used to control symptoms, then decreased as tolerated. Long-term low (minimal) dose stanozolol at 0.5 mg/day to 2 mg/day or 4 mg every other day or Danazol at 200 mg/day is remarkably safe (66), however stanolozol is currently unavailable in the United States. Side effects of attenuated androgens include abnormal liver function, lipid abnormalities, weight gain, amenorrhea, acne, hirsutism, and rarely peliosis hepatitis. One woman given attenuated androgens during the last 8 weeks of pregnancy experienced no ill effects, and virilization of the infant was transient (67).

Severe, acute attacks of HAE have been treated with esterase-inhibiting drugs such as epsilon amino caproic acid (5 g every 6 hours) and tranexamic acid (not available in the United States, but given orally) in efforts to slow complement activation; however, these agents require up to 48 hours to have an affect (68,69). Fresh frozen plasma, which contains C1-INH can also be used

TABLE 31.5   DIAGNOSIS OF THE DIFFERENT FORMS OF HEREDITARY AND ACQUIRED ANGIOEDEMA

	MECHANISM	DIAGNOSIS
HAE type I (85% of HAE)	Autosomal codominant Deficiency of C1-INH Bradykinin mediated angioedema	Low C4 when asymptomatic Low or absent C2 during an attack Low or absent C1-INH level and function
HAE type II (15% of HAE)	Functionally inactive C1-INH	Normal level of C1-INH, but low functional activity (functional assay required) Low C4 Low or absent C2 during attacks
HAE type III	Unknown, affects women only, suggesting X-linked dominant	Normal C4 Normal C1-INH level and function
Acquired angioedema	Reduced C1q levels by excessive activation of C1 (e.g., lymphoma) through autoimmune immunoglobulin	Low C1q levels Low C1-INH level Low C4 Absent family history
Autoimmune acquired angioedema	Autoantibody (IgG) against C1-INH	Low C1q Low C1-INH Low C4 Absent family history

in acute attacks, but rarely can cause worsening of symptoms because it also contains high-molecular-weight kininogen, which can increase bradykinin production. Although not yet available in the United States, purified pooled plasma C1-INH has been used safely and succesfully for the treatment of acute attacks of HAE, prophylaxis in surgery, and in children and pregnant women in Europe (66,70). Its use is limited by infectious disease issues that are of concern with all blood products, such that a recombinant C1-INH is currently being developed (71). Promising new therapies for acute attacks of HAE currently under development include the kallikrein inhibitor, ecallatide (72), which prevents bradykinin generation, and icatibant (73), the bradykinin receptor-2 antagonist which blocks the bradykinin receptor (74). Both products seemingly prevent the bradykinin-induced formation of angioedema. In the absence of C1-INH therapy, at the very first sign of angioedema, patients should initiate Danazol 600 mg to 800 mg (or stanozolol 6 mg to 8 mg if available) and seek medical care in the emergency department.

Acquired forms of C1 inhibitor deficiency result from increased destruction or metabolism of C1 inhibitor. Destruction occurs when autoantibodies directed against the C1 inhibitor are produced, bind to its active site, and cause inactivation (75). Alternatively, anti-idiotypic antibodies are produced against specific B-cell surface immunoglobulins, leading to immune complex formation and continuous C1 activation (76). Large quantities of C1 inhibitor are subsequently consumed, causing a deficit and thus the symptoms of C1 inhibitor deficiency. This acquired type of deficiency is usually associated with rheumatologic disorders or B-cell lymphoproliferative disorders such as multiple myeloma, leukemia, and essential cryoglobulinemia. These patients may require larger doses of androgens to control symptoms, but therapy should be directed at the underlying lymphoproliferative or autoimmune disorder. As in the hereditary forms of the disease, C1 inhibitor, C2, and C4 are low, but only in the acquired forms is C1q also depressed.

Hereditary vibratory angioedema is clinically characterized by localized pruritus and swelling in areas exposed to vibratory stimuli (77). It appears to be inherited as an autosomal-dominant trait, and generally is first noted in childhood. The mechanism is not certain, but histamine release has been documented during experimental induction of a lesion (78). Treatment consists of avoidance of vibratory stimuli and use of antihistamines in an attempt to reduce symptoms.

Other Forms of Urticaria Angioedema

Papular urticaria is clinically characterized by slightly erythematous, highly pruritic linear papular lesions of various sizes. Each lesion tends to be persistent, in contrast to most urticarial conditions. The lower extremities are involved most often, although the trunk also may be affected, especially in young children. The mechanism is unknown, but the rash is thought to be caused by hypersensitivity to the saliva, mouth parts, or excreta of biting insects such as mosquitoes, bedbugs, fleas, lice, and mites. Treatment is supportive: antihistamines are given, often prophylactically, in an attempt to reduce pruritus. Good skin care is essential to prevent infection caused by scratching. Examination of a person's sleeping quarters and children's play areas for insects may provide a clue to the etiology. Pruritic urticaria papules and plaques of pregnancy are an extremely pruritic condition of primigravida women that occurs in the third trimester. Lesions begin in the striae distensae and spread up and around the umbilicus, thighs, and buttocks. In some atypical cases, biopsy should be performed to distinguish the diagnosis from herpes gestationis (25).

Urticaria Pigmentosa

Urticaria pigmentosa is characterized by persistent, red-brown, maculopapular lesions that urticate when stroked (Darier sign). These lesions generally have their onset in childhood. Rare familial forms have been described. Biopsy shows mast cell infiltration. The diagnosis may be established by their typical appearance, Darier sign, and skin biopsy. Occasionally, it has been noted to complicate other forms of anaphylaxis such as *Hymenoptera* venom sensitivity, causing very severe reactions with sudden vascular collapse. These cutaneous lesions may occur in patients with systemic mastocytosis, a generalized form of mast cell infiltration into bone, liver, lymph nodes, and spleen.

The remaining forms of urticaria are associated with many diverse etiologies (Table 31.3). Diagnosis is established by history and physical examination based on knowledge of the possible causes. Laboratory evaluation is occasionally helpful in establishing a diagnosis and identifying the underlying disease. Treatment is based on the underlying problem, and may include avoidance, antihistamines, and corticosteroid therapy or other forms of anti-inflammatory drugs.

Clinical Approach

History

The clinical history is the single most important aspect of evaluating patients with urticaria. The history generally provides important clues to the etiology; therefore, an organized approach is essential.

If the patient has no rash at the time of evaluation, urticaria or angioedema usually can be established historically with a history of hives, welts, or wheps resembling mosquito-bite–like lesions; raised, erythematous, pruritic lesions; evanescent symptoms; potentiation of lesions by scratching; and lesions that may coalesce. By contrast, angioedema is asymmetric, often involves nondependent areas, recurs in different sites, is transient, and is associated with little pruritus. Urticaria and angioedema may occur together. Cholinergic or adrenergic urticaria, papular urticaria, dermographism, urticaria pigmentosa, and familial cold urticaria, however, do not fit the typical pattern.

Both papular urticaria and urticaria pigmentosa most often arise in childhood. HAE and hereditary vibratory angioedema also may occur during childhood, but are readily recognized by the absence of urticaria in both diseases. Other etiologic factors in childhood urticaria have been reviewed (36,79,80).

Once the diagnosis of urticaria is established on the basis of history, etiologic mechanisms should be considered. The patient with dermographism usually reports a history of rash after scratching. Frequently, the patient notices itching first, scratches the offending site, and then develops linear wheals. Stroking the skin with a pointed instrument without disrupting the integument confirms the diagnosis. With most patients, the physical urticarias may be eliminated quickly as a possible diagnosis merely by asking about the temporal association with light, heat, cold, pressure, or vibration, or by using established clinical tests (Table 31.4). Cholinergic urticaria is usually recognized by its characteristic lesions and relationship to rising body temperature or stress. Hereditary forms of urticaria are rare. Familial localized heat urticaria is recognized by its relationship to the local application of heat, and familial cold urticaria by the unusual papular skin lesions and the predominance of a burning sensation instead of pruritus. Thus, after a few moments of discussion with a patient, a physical urticaria or hereditary form usually can be suspected or established.

The success of determining an etiology for urticaria is most likely a function of whether it is acute or chronic, because a cause is discovered much more frequently when it is acute. Each of the items in Table 31.3 may be involved. Food may be identified in acute urticaria. Great patience and effort are necessary, along with repeated queries to detect drug use. Over-the-counter preparations are not regarded as drugs by many patients, and must be specified when questioning the patient. While penicillins are a common cause of urticaria, aspirin and other nonselective NSAIDs can trigger acute urticaria within minutes to 3 hours after ingestion or can cause exacerbations of chronic idiopathic urticaria in some patients. Drug-induced episodes of urticaria are usually of the acute variety. Another recognized offender causing angioedema is the group of ACE inhibitor drugs used primarily for hypertension or heart failure. Reactions to ACE inhibitors usually occur within 1 week of initiating therapy, but can occur at any time. Angiotensin II receptor blockers are believed to have no effect on bradykinin production. Although

theoretically they should not cause angioedema and are considered a safe alternative, several case reports have been published (81,82). Infections documented as causes of urticaria include infectious mononucleosis, viral hepatitis (both B and C), and fungal and parasitic invasions. Chronic infection as a cause of chronic urticaria is a rare event, although chronic hepatitis has been postulated to cause chronic urticaria (83). If the history does not reveal significant clues, the patient's urticaria generally is labeled CIU. Most patients with chronic urticaria fall into this category.

Physical Examination

A complete physical examination should be performed on all patients with urticaria. The purpose of the examination is to identify typical urticarial lesions, if present; to establish the presence or absence of dermographism; to identify the characteristic lesions of cholinergic and papular urticaria; to characterize atypical lesions; to determine the presence of jaundice, urticaria pigmentosa (Darier sign), or familial cold urticaria; to exclude other cutaneous diseases; to exclude evidence of systemic disease; and to establish the presence of coexisting diseases.

Diagnostic Studies

It is difficult to outline an acceptable diagnostic program for all patients with urticaria. Each diagnostic workup must be individualized, depending on the results of the history and physical examination. An algorithm may become a useful adjunct in this often unrewarding diagnostic endeavor (Fig. 31.2).

Foods

Five diagnostic procedures may be considered when food is thought to be a cause of urticaria (Table 31.6). These include (a) avoidance, (b) restricted diet, (c) diet diary, (d) skin testing with food extracts or fresh foods, and (e) food challenge.

Skin Tests

Routine food skin tests used in evaluating urticaria are of unproven value at best. Because the etiology of chronic urticaria is established in only an additional 5% of patients (47), and only some of these cases will be related to food, the diagnostic yield from skin testing is very low. In unselected patients, the positive predictive value of skin tests is low. Important studies of food-induced atopic dermatitis (84) have revealed a few selected foods that are most commonly associated with symptoms. These include eggs, peanuts, fish, soy, pork, milk, wheat, beef, and chicken. If no food skin test results are positive, then foods are probably not a cause. If all food skin test results are positive, dermagraphism

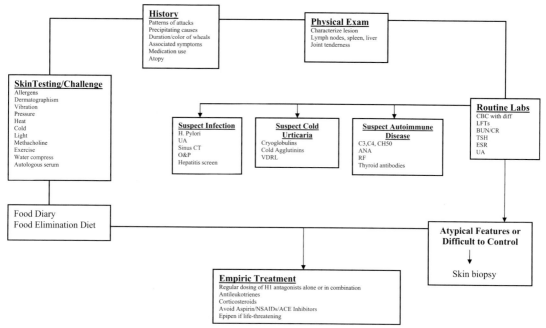

■ FIGURE 31.2 This algorithm suggests a potential method for evaluating and treating chronic urticaria. The method includes challenge procedures and laboratory data that may be considered but are not always indicated. Empiric treatment should generally follow the cumulative, sequential use of the medications shown. Avoidance of aspirin, nonsteroidal anti-inflammatory drugs, and angiotensin-converting enzyme inhibitors is essential. Corticosteroids may be useful for a brief time during the initial treatment until the severity of the urticaria is controlled.

is probably present. Second, for patients in whom a mixed food (combination of ingredients) is thought to be the problem, food tests may isolate the particular item (e.g., soybeans). At present, an extensive battery of food tests cannot be recommended on a routine basis, and must be used with clinical discretion. Commercially prepared extracts frequently lack labile proteins responsible for IgE-mediated sensitivity to many fruits and vegetables. If the clinical history is convincing for a food allergy, but skin testing with a commercially prepared extract is negative, testing should be repeated with the fresh food before concluding that food allergen-specific IgE is absent (85). Additionally, certain foods have been shown to cross-react with pollen allergens (86) or latex allergens (87) to which a patient may be exquisitely sensitive. Radioallergosorbent testing (RAST) may be used in place of skin testing. Although it is considered less sensitive, it may be necessary when a patient has an exquisite sensitivity to a certain food or significant dermographism or when antihistmines cannot be discontinued.

Drugs

With the exception of penicillins, foreign sera, and recombinant proteins such as insulin, there are no

reliable diagnostic tests for predicting or establishing clinical sensitivity to a drug. In patients with urticaria, drugs must always be considered as etiologic agents. The only evaluation of value is avoidance of the drug. This can be accomplished safely and effectively in most patients, even when multiple drugs are involved and coexisting diseases are present. Substitute drugs with different chemical structures are frequently available and may be used. Not all drugs need to be stopped simultaneously unless the allergic reaction is severe.

Infections

As noted previously, viral infections such as Hepatitis B and C, bacterial infections, fungal infections, and parasites have all been reported to cause urticaria (88). Patients with infectious mononucleosis or hepatitis or *H. pylori* colonization generally have other symptoms, and appropriate laboratory studies confirm the diagnosis. The demonstration of anti-H. pylori IgG or IgM antibodies has been found in as many as 70% of patients with chronic idiopathic urticaria, but treatment has not resolved the urticarial lesions. Thus, this finding questions a shared pathogenic mechanism such as molecular mimicry. Routine physical examination should include a search for tinea pedis, capitas, or thrush to

TABLE 31.6   DIAGNOSTIC STUDIES OF FOOD-INDUCED URTICARIA

Avoidance (acute)	Use patient history	Eliminate 1 or 2 foods; urticaria should clear
Restricted diet (chronic relapsing)	Use standardized rice/lamb or other restrictive diets; elemental diet may be useful	Reinstitute one food every 3 to 5 days; repeat if successful
Diet diary intermittent episodes for extended period	List all foods and events for 24 hours prior to episode on several occasions	Eliminate suspected food
Skin tests (chronic unknown etiology)	Use a brief battery of food skin tests based on patient's history; certain inhalant or latex allergens may suggest cross-reacting foods	Eliminate suspected test positive foods; a battery of negative skin tests suggests no food hypersensitivity
Double-blind, placebo-controlled food challenge	Gold standard; especially useful when the patients' perceptions may bias accurate symptom assessment	

rule out fungal infection as the possible cause. Many of the parasitic infections will be associated with peripheral blood eosinophilia, high serum IgE concentrations, or positive stool specimens. An extensive search for occult infection is of no value. If history or examination suggests undiagnosed infection, appropriate laboratory studies should be undertaken (Fig. 31.2).

Penetrants

The medical literature is filled with numerous case reports of urticaria following contact. The only tests to be performed involve actual contact with the agent and demonstration of a localized skin eruption in the area of contact. Usually, these cases of urticaria result from penetration of the skin by antigen or a mediator-releasing substance from animal hairs or stingers. Examples of agents causing such urticaria include latex, drugs, and occupationally used chemicals (89).

Insect Stings

Urticaria may present as a result of insect stings, and this history generally is obtained easily. Appropriate skin tests with *Hymenoptera* venoms may be indicated in cases of generalized urticaria and anaphylaxis to demonstrate immediate hypersensitivity. One should consider fire ant stings due to their continued migration into more northern latitudes. Whole body extract skin testing or a RAST for venom may be helpful diagnostically.

Neoplasm

If neoplasm is suspected by history or examination, standard evaluation should be undertaken and perhaps repeated on several occasions.

Vasculitis

In a patient who has urticarial lesions that last for more than 24 hours, cause burning rather than pruritus, leave residual scarring, or appear petechial in nature, vasculitis should be suspected. A complete blood count (CBC), sedimentation rate, urinalysis, and tissue biopsy are indicated. Tests for antinuclear antibody and rheumatoid factor, complement studies, and screening for hepatitis and mononucleosis are generally indicated. Urticarial vasculitis must be differentiated from CIU (90).

Serum Sickness

Acute urticaria in association with arthralgias, fever, and lymphadenopathy developing 1 to 3 weeks following drug exposure, insect sting, or heterologous serum administration is suspicious for serum sickness. CBC, urinalysis, and a sedimentation rate are indicated. Serum concentrations of C3, C4, and total hemolytic complement are depressed, indicating that immune complexes are involved in the pathogenesis of this disease.

Idiopathic Chronic Urticaria

The more difficult and more common problem regarding diagnostic tests relates to those patients who appear to have idiopathic disease. Laboratory studies are probably unnecessary in the absence of abnormal features in the history or physical examination (91). Most of these episodes are self-limited and resolve spontaneously.

In some patients with CIU, the discomfort, inconvenience, and disfigurement of the disease generally warrant further evaluation. The following tests should be considered but not necessarily performed in all patients: CBC with differential; urinalysis; sedimentation rate; complement studies; examination of stool for ova and parasites; antinuclear antibody; Venereal Disease Research Laboratory (VDRL) testing; hepatitis screen; and skin biopsy. Because thyroid disease (particularly Hashimoto thyroiditis) is more common in chronic urticaria, thyroid function testing (T3, T4, ultrasensitive thyroid stimulating hormone [TSH]; antibodies for thyroglobulin and microsomes) may be considered in anyone with a palpable goiter, family history of thyroid disease, or evidence of thyroid dysfunction (14). In some cases of CIU that are not responsive to usual treatment, an ASST or an *in vitro* test for histamine release may be considered to determine the presence of functional autoantibodies before initiating immunomodulatory therapy.

Urinalysis (cells or protein), CBC (anemia, leukocytosis, or eosinophilia), TSH, and transaminases are the most likely tests to demonstrate significant abnormalities. The sedimentation rate may be elevated in active vasculitis. Circulating hepatitis-related antibodies may indicate acute or chronic disease. Although complement abnormalities are common in reports of CIU, the underlying mechanisms are unclear and their relevance is uncertain. Thus, the need for complement assays should be reserved for difficult to treat cases.

Skin biopsy is currently suggested for CIU that is difficult to manage, and it is probably indicated in patients with connective tissue disease or a complement abnormality. Acute urticaria probably does not warrant biopsy when laboratory studies are normal.

Therapy

Pharmacologic therapy is the main form of treatment for urticaria and angioedema (Table 31.7). However, as in other forms of allergic disease, if an allergen or specific trigger has been identified, avoidance is the most effective treatment. Avoidance techniques for specific forms of urticaria have been reviewed previously (25). For most urticaria patients, three types of drugs are adequate to obtain symptomatic control: sympathomimetic agents, antihistamines, and corticosteroids.

The sympathomimetic agents, notably epinephrine, has α agonist properties that causes vasoconstriction in superficial cutaneous and mucosal surfaces, which directly opposes the effect of histamine on these end organs. Normally, it is used for severe acute urticaria and episodes of life-threatening angioedema.

Antihistamines (H_1 blockers) are the mainstay of symptomatic improvement or control of urticaria and angioedema. Antihistamines are useful in most cases of urticaria. They have been thought of as competitive inhibitors of histamine, reducing the end-organ effect of histamine even if histamine release continues. Recent experiments have demonstrated that the H_1 antagonists actually are "inverse agonists" of the H_1 receptor and decrease the H_1 response in the absence of the agonist histamine (92). The newer antihistamines offer some

TABLE 31.7 TREATMENT OF CHRONIC IDIOPATHIC URTICARIA

Avoidance of triggers
Keep diary of flares
Regular use of low-sedating antihistamine with or without sedating antihistamine at night
Add leukotriene modifiers
Add doxepin/increase antihistamine doses
Add ketotifen if available
β blockers (adrenergic urticaria only)
Cautious use of corticosteroids
Consider adding immunomodulating agent

valuable options because they are long-acting and cause little sedation. Fexofenadine (93,94), cetirizine (95–97), levocetirizine (98), and desloratidine (99) are well tolerated and effective in most cases of chronic urticaria. Ketotifen (100,101) is another effective alternative for the treatment of chronic urticaria and physical urticarias because in addition to being a histamine antagonist, it can inhibit mast cell degranulation. While the oral formulation is currently not on the market in the United States, ketotifen is available in 2-mg tablets in many countries. Low-dose antidepressants, especially doxepin (102), are unique in having very potent H_1- and H_2-antagonist effects and inhibit other mediators such as platelet-activating factor. The main side effect is sedation, but when administered in small doses (10 mg to 30 mg) at bedtime, this may be avoided. A trial of therapy with representative agents from the different classes of antihistamines may be required to select the proper drug.

Hydroxyzine has clinical antihistaminic effects as well as experimental anticholinergic and antiserotoninergic effects. This agent is considered the drug of choice for cholinergic urticaria, and is also very effective in many other forms of chronic urticaria. Often, the initially effective dose can be reduced or used only at night for chronic therapy. A combination of a nonsedating second-generation antihistamine given in the morning with a first-generation agent given at night or low-sedating antihistamines given over licensed dosages might be necessary in patients with more persistent urticaria. Additionally, an effort should be made to determine what period of the day each patient is most symptomatic (usually evening or early morning) to maximize therapy at that time.

Cyproheptadine is thought to be a serotonin and histamine antagonist, and to have anticholinergic effects. Its mechanism of action in urticaria is uncertain, but it appears to be effective in some cases. It is most commonly used to treat cold urticaria (59), but it can stimulate the appetite and result in significant weight gain. Leukotriene modifiers such as montelukast and zileuton have been reported to help control chronic urticaria as well as reduce corticosteroid requirements in an undefined small subset of patients (103–105). These agents work best when given in combination with antihistamines. Limited benefit has been reported from using a combination of H_1 and H_2 antihistamines for both acute and chronic urticaria (106).

Corticosteroids, such as oral prednisone, used in combination with antihistamines may be necessary in the management of urticaria. Because of their potential for significant long-term side effects, these drugs should be used to control urticaria only after a demonstrated failure of both high-dose and combination antihistamine therapy. Based on clinical experience, moderate-dose steroid therapy (30 mg to 40 mg prednisone) may be required initially to control the urticaria. Thereafter, alternate-day therapy generally provides control on a long-term basis, often with decreasing doses. As in all forms of therapy, the risk:benefit ratio must be assessed when using steroid therapy for long-term treatment. Short-term prednisone has limited side effects, and is often useful for control of acute urticaria not responding to antihistamines. DPU frequently may require the use of low-dose or alternate-day corticosteroids to maintain the patient's activity, and a cautious trial of a nonsteroidal anti-inflammatory drug may be helpful.

The choice of agents and the route of administration of drugs is dependent on the clinical situation. The adult patient who presents in an emergency room or physician's office within hours of the onset of significant urticaria can be treated with epinephrine 0.3 mL (1:1,000) intramuscularly, as well as hydroxyzine 25 mg to 50 mg or cetirizine 10 mg orally. Such an approach gives prompt relief from symptoms in many patients. After evaluation for a precipitating agent (e.g., drug or food), the patient may be released with instructions to take hydroxyzine or cetirizine for 24 to 48 hours. A brief "burst" of corticosteroids and prolonged observation may be judicious, and is essential if there have been associated signs of anaphylaxis. Ambulatory medical follow-up should be required.

The patient who presents with urticaria of several days' duration may be treated with regular doses of antihistamines. The combination of cetirizine 10 mg every morning and hydroxyzine 25 mg at bedtime is quite useful. Leukotriene modifiers, oral albuterol, or H_2 antagonist may be prescribed with the initial antihistamine. Failure to respond in a few days to this therapy may indicate the need for a short course of prednisone. Many patients respond to this therapy, but the antihistamines should be continued for a period after the prednisone is stopped.

The patient with a history of chronic urticaria presents a more complicated therapeutic problem. Following evaluation for an etiology, therapy is usually initiated with regular dosing of a potent antihistamine (often hydroxyzine, fexofenadine, cetirizine, or doxepin) and possibly a leukotriene modifier. Failure to respond suggests that moderate-dose prednisone should be initiated if the symptoms are sufficiently severe. Every effort to use alternate-day therapy should be made, but this is often initially inadequate. When control is achieved, the steroids are slowly withdrawn to determine whether chronic steroid therapy is required. For those patients who are unable to discontinue corticosteroid therapy, use of a steroid sparing agent should be considered. In patients thought to have CAU with the presence of functional antibodies, low-dose cyclosporine (2.5 mg/kg/day) given for 3 to 4 months has been shown to be effective and safe (107,108); however, blood pressure, renal function, as well as serum lipids need to be monitored throughout treatment.

Other anti-inflammatory medications have been reported in small studies or case reports to be useful in refractory patients. Stanozolol (109), hydroxychloroquine (110), dapsone (111), colchicine and other immunomodulatory drugs, including methotrexate (112), tacrolimus (113), and mycophenolate mofetil (114) have been used experimentally for chronic urticaria. Omalizumab has also been reported to be beneficial in refractory chronic idiopathic urticaria patients with both normal and high total IgE levels (115,116). Sulfasalazine has been effective in case studies for DPU (117,118).

Patients with urticaria can be very uncomfortable, have difficulty sleeping, and sometimes avoid social/work situations due to cosmetic appearance. Aggressive and consistent therapy for at least several months provides relief in many cases. Every effort should be made to find the best regimen with the least amount of side effects to control their symptoms.

In summary, CIU may be unpleasant, frustrating, and frightening to a patient. Often these patients seek help from various physicians for an allergen that does not exist. At times, they undergo expensive, inappropriate tests and treatments that are of no value and perhaps dangerous. These patients need reassurance. While the duration of CIU is highly variable, treatment with prednisone in doses that will induce a remission followed by 3 to 6 months of a nightly dose of a potent antihistamine often yields a good outcome.

■ REFERENCES

1. Sheldon JM, Mathews KP, Lovell RG. The vexing urticaria problem: present concepts of etiology and management. *J Allergy.* 1954;25:525–560.

2. Mathews KP. Urticaria and angioedema. *J Allergy Clin Immunol.* 1983;72:1–14.

3. Toubi E, Kessel A, Avshovich E, et al. Clinical and laboratory parameters in predicting chronic urticaria duration: a prospective study of 139 patients. *Allergy.* 2004;59:869–873.

4. Cooper KD. Urticaria and angioedema: diagnosis and evaluation. *J Am Acad Dermatol.* 1991;25:166–176.

5. Champion RH, Roberts SOB, Carpenter RG, et al. Urticaria and angioedema: a review of 554 patients. *Br J Dermatol*. 1969;81:588–597.

6. Van der Valk PGM, Moret G, Kiemeney LALM. The natural history of chronic urticaria and angioedema in patients visiting a tertiary referral centre. *Br J Dermatol*. 2002;146:110–113.

7. Kozel M, Mekkes J, Bossuyt P, et al. Natural course of physical and chronic urticaria and angioedema in 220 patients. *J Am Acad Dermatol*. 2001;45:387–391.

8. Green GR, Koelsche GA, Kierland RR. Etiology and pathogenesis of chronic urticaria. *Ann Allergy*. 1965;23:30–36.

9. Kozel M, Mekkes J, Bossuyt P, et al. The effectiveness of a history-based diagnostic approach in chronic urticaria and angioedema. *Arch Dermatol*. 1998;134:1575–1580.

10. Asero R, Tedeschi A, Coppola R, et al. Activation of the tissue factor pathway of blood coagulation in patients with chronic urticaria. *J Allergy Clin Immunol*. 2007;119:705–710.

11. Peters MS, Schroeter AL, Kaphart GM, et al. Localization of eosinophilic granule major basic protein in chronic urticaria. *J Invest Dermatol*. 1983;81:39–43.

12. Maxwell DL, Atkinson BA, Spur BW, et al. Skin responses to intradermal histamine and leukotrienes C4, D4 and E4 in patients with chronic idiopathic urticaria and in normal subjects. *J Allergy Clin Immunol*. 1990;86:759–765.

13. Lexnoff A, Sussman GL. Syndrome of idiopathic chronic urticaria and angioedema with thyroid autoimmunity: a study of 90 patients. *J Allergy Clin Immunol*. 1989; 84:66–71.

14. O'Donnell BF, Francis DM, Swana GT, et al. Thyroid autoimmunity in chronic urticaria. *Br J Dermatol*. 2005;153:331–335.

15. Greaves MW. Chronic urticaria. Current concepts. *N Engl J Med*. 1995;332:1767–1772.

16. Tong LJ, Balakrishman G, Kochan JP, et al. Assessment of autoimmunity in patients with urticaria. *J Allergy Clin Immunol*. 1997;99: 461–465.

17. Sabroe RA, Greaves MW. Chronic idiopathic urticaria with functional autoantibodies: 12 years on. *Br J Dermatol*. 2006;154:813–819.

18. Sabroe RA, Grattan CEH, Francis DM, et al. The autologous serum skin test: a screening for autoantibodies in chronic idiopathic urticaria. *Br J Dermatol*. 1999;140:446–452.

19. Yasnowsky KM, Dreskin SC, Efaw B, et al. Chronic urticaria sera increase basophil CD203c expression. *J Allergy Clin Immunol*. 2006;117:1430–1434.

20. Fagiolo U, Kricek R, Ruf C, et al. Effects of complement inactivation and IgG depletion on skin reactivity to autologous serum in chronic idiopathic urticaria. *J Allergy Clin Immunol*. 2000;106:567–572.

21. Vonakis M, Vasagar K, Gibbons SP, et al. Basophil FcεR1 histamine release parallels expression of Src-homology 2-containing inositol phosphatases in chronic idiopathic urticaria. *J Allergy Clin Immunol*. 2007;119:441–448.

22. Grattan CEH, Dawn G, Gibbs S, et al. Blood basophil numbers in chronic ordinary urticaria and healthy controls: diurnal variation, influence of loratadine and prednisolone and relationship to disease activity. *Clin Exp Allergy*. 2003;33:337–341.

23. Caproni M, Giomi B, Volpi W, et al. Chronic idiopathic urticaria infiltrating cells and related cytokines in autologous serum induced wheals. *Clin Immunol*. 2005;114:284–292.

24. Fields T, Ghebrehiwet B, Kaplan AP. Kinin formation in hereditary angioedema plasma: evidence against kinin derivation from C2 and in support of "spontaneous" formation of bradykinin. *J Allergy Clin Immunol*. 1983;72:54–60.

25. Charlesworth EN. Urticaria and angioedema: A clinical spectrum. *Ann Allergy Asthma Immunol*. 1996;76:484–95.

26. Meggs WJ, Pescovitz OR, Metcalfe DD, et al. Progesterone sensitivity as a cause of recurrent anaphylaxis. *N Engl J Med*. 1984; 311:1236–1238.

27. Mittman RJ, Berstein DI, Steinberg DR, et al. Pro-gesterone-responsive urticaria and eosinophilia. *J Allergy Clin Immunol*. 1989; 84:304–310.

28. Park H, Park C, Park S, et al. Dermatologic adverse reactions to 7 common food additives in patients with allergic diseases: a double-blind, placebo-controlled study. *J Allergy Clin Immunol*. 2008; 121:1059–1061.

29. Geha RS, Beiser A, Ren C, et al. Multicenter, double-blind, placebo-controlled, multiple-challenge evaluation of reported reactions to monosodium glutamate. *J Allergy Clin Immunol*. 2000;106:973–980.

30. Geha R, Buckley CE, Greenberger P, et al. Aspartame is no more likely than placebo to cause urticaria/angioedema: results of a multicenter, randomized, double-blind, placebo controlled, crossover study. *J Allergy Clin Immunol*. 1993;92:513–520.

31. Toppe E, Haas N, Henz BM. Neutrophilic urticaria: clinical features, histological changes and possible mechanisms. *Br J Dermatol*. 1998;248–253.

32. Ying S, Kikuchi Y, Meng Q, et al. T_H1/T_H2 cytokines and inflammatory cells in skin biopsy specimens from patients with chronic idiopathic urticaria: comparison with the allergen-induced late-phase cutaneous reaction. *J Allergy Clin Immunol*. 2002;109:694–700.

33. Vaughn MP, DeWalt AC, Diaz JD. Urticaria associated with systemic disease and psychological factors. *Immunol Allergy Clin North Am*. 1995;15:725–743.

34. Greaves MW. The physical urticarias. *Clin Exp Allergy*. 1991;21(suppl 1):284–289.

35. Schafer CM. Physical urticaria. *Immunol Allergy Clin North Am*. 1995;15:679–699.

36. Khakoo G, Sofianou-Katsoulis A, Perkin MR, et al. Clinical features and natural history of physical urticaria in children. *Pediatr Allergy Immunol*. 2008;19:363-366.

37. Sherertz EF. Clinical pearl: symptomatic dermatographism as a cause of genital pruritus. *J Am Acad Dermatol*. 1994;31:1040–1041.

38. Ryan TJ, Shim-Young N, Turk JL. Delayed pressure urticaria. *Br J Dermatol*. 1968;80:485–490.

39. Hass N, Toppe E, Henz BM. Microscopic morphology in different types of urticaria. *Arch Dermatol*. 1998;134:41–46.

40. Margerl M, Philipp S, Manasterski M, et al. Successful treatment of delayed pressure urticaria with anti-TNF-α. *J Allergy Clin Immunol*. 2007;119:752–754.

41. Hermes B, Prochazka A, Haas N, et al. Upregulation of TNF-α and IL-3 expression in lesional and uninvolved skin in different types of urticaria. *J Allergy Clin Immunol*. 1999;103:307–314.

42. Kobza-Black A. Delayed pressure urticaria. *J Invest Dermatol Symposium*. 2001;6:148–149.

43. Sussman GL, Harvey RP, Schocket AL. Delayed pressure urticaria. *J Allergy Clin Immunol*. 1982;70:337–342.

44. Roelandts R. Diagnosis and treatment of solar urticaria. *Dermatol Ther*. 2003;16:52–56.

45. Grundmann SA, Stander S, Luger TA, et al. Antihistamine combination treatment for solar urticaria. *Br J Dermatol*. 2008;158:1384–1386.

46. Kaplan AP, Garofalo J. Identification of a new physically induced urticaria. Cold-induced cholinergic urticaria. *J Allergy Clin Immunol*. 1981;68:438–441.

47. Kaplan AP. Urticaria and angioedema. In: Adkinson NA, Yunginger JW, Busse WM, et al., eds. *Allergy: Principles and Practice*. 6th ed. Philadelphia: Mosby; 2003:1537–1558.

48. Kaplan AP, Gray L, Shaff RE. *In vivo* studies of mediator release in cold urticaria and cholinergic urticaria. *J Allergy Clin Immunol*. 1975;55:394–402.

49. Shelley WB, Shelley ED, Ho AK. Cholinergic urticaria: acetylcholine-receptor–dependent immediate-type hypersensitivity reaction to copper. *Lancet*. 1983;843–846.

50. Shelley WB, Shelley EO. Adrenergic urticaria: a new form of stress induced hives. *Lancet*. 1985;2:1031–1033.

51. Kaplan AP. Urticaria and angioedema. In: Frank MM, Austen KF, Claman HN, et al., eds. *Samter's Immunologic Diseases*. 5th ed. Boston: Little, Brown; 1995:1329–1343.

52. Michaelson G, Ros A. Familial localized heat urticaria of delayed type. *Acta Derm Venereal (Stockh.)* 1971;51: 279–283.

53. Horton BT, Brown GE, Roth GM. Hypersensitivities to cold with local and systemic manifestations of a histamine-like character: its amenability to treatment. *JAMA*. 1936;107:1263–1269.

54. Lee CW, Sheffer AL. Primary acquired cold urticaria. *Allergy and Asthma Proc*. 2003;24:9–12.

55. Boyce JA. Successful treatment of cold-induced urticaria/anaphylaxis with anti-IgE. *J Allergy Clin Immunol*. 2006;117:1415–1418.

56. Costanzi JJ, Coltman JR Jr, Donaldson VH. Activation of complement by a monoclonal cryoglobulin associated with cold urticaria. *J Lab Clin Med*. 1969;74:902–910.

57. Costanzi JJ, Coltman JR Jr. Kappa chain precipitable immunoglobulin G (IgG) associated with cold urticaria. I. Clinical observations. *Clin Exp Immunol*. 1967;2:167–168.

58. Kaplan AP. Urticaria and angioedema. In: Kaplan AP, ed. *Allergy*. 2nd ed. Philadelphia: WB Saunders; 1997:573–592.

59. Sigler RW, Evans R, Hoarkova Z, et al. The role of cyproheptadine in the treatment of cold urticaria. *J Allergy Clin Immunol*. 1980;65: 309–312.

60. Bentley B II. Cold-induced urticaria and angioedema: diagnosis and management. *Am J Emerg Med*. 1993;11:43–46.

61. Sarkany I, Turk JL. Delayed type hypersensitivity to cold. *Proc R Soc Med*. 1965;58:622–623.

62. Bork K, Barnstedt S, Koch P, et al. Hereditary angioedema with normal C1-inhibitor activity in women. *Lancet*. 2000;356:213–217.

63. Davis AE. Hereditary angioedema: a current state-of-the-art review, III: mechanisms of hereditary angioedema. *Ann Allergy Asthma Immunol*. 2008;100(suppl 2):S7–S12.

64. Gelfand JA, Sherins RJ, Alling DW, et al. Treatment of hereditary angioedema with danazol: reversal of clinical and biochemical abnormalities. *N Engl J Med*. 1976;295:1444–1448.

65. Sloane DE, Lee CW, Sheffer AL. Hereditary angioedema: safety of long-term stanozolol therapy. *J Allergy Clin Immunol*. 2007;120:654–658.

66. Farkas H, Jakab L, Tmesszentandrasi G, et al. Hereditary angioedema: a decade of human C1-inhibitor concentrate therapy. *J Allergy Clin Immunol*. 2007;120:941–947.

67. Cicardi M, Bergamaschini L, Cugno M, et al. Long-term treatment of hereditary angioedema with attenuated androgens: a survey of a 13-year experience. *J Allergy Clin Immunol*. 1991;87:768–773.

68. Frank M, Gelfand JA, Alling DW, et al. Episolon aminocaproic acid for HAE. *N Eng J Med*. 1977;21:1235–1236.

69. Sheffer AL, Austen KF, Rosen FS. Transexamic acid therapy in hereditary angioneurotic edema. *N Eng J Med*. 1972;9:452–454.

70. Bork K, Witzke G. Long-term prophylaxis with C1-inhibitor (C1 INH) concentrate in patients with recurrent angioedema caused by hereditary and acquired C1-inhibitor deficiency. *J Allergy Clin Immunol*. 1989;83:677–682.

71. van Doorn MB, Buffraat J, van Dam T, et al. A phase I study of recombinant human C1-inhibitor in asymptomatic patients with hereditary angioedema. *J Allergy Clin Immunol*. 2005;4:876–883.

72. Schneider L, Lumry W, Vegh A, et al. Critical role of kallikrein in hereditary angioedema pathogenesis: a clinical trial of ecallantide, a novel kallikrein inhibitor. *J Allergy Clin Immunol*. 2007;120:416–422.

73. Bork K, Frank J, Grundt B, et al. Treatment of acute edema attacks with a bradykinin receptor-2 antagonist (Icatibant). *J Allergy Clin Immunol*. 2007;119:1497–1503.

74. Frank MM, Jiang H. New therapies for hereditary angioedema: disease outlook changes dramatically. *J Allergy Clin Immunol*. 2008;121:272–280.

75. Gelfand JA, Boss GR, Conley CL, et al. Acquired C1 esterase inhibitor deficiency and angioedema: a review. *Medicine*. 1979;58:321–328.

76. Frigas E. Angioedema with acquired deficiency of the C1 inhibitor: a constellation of syndromes. *Mayo Clin Proc*. 1989;64:1269–1275.

77. Patterson R, Mellies CJ, Blankenship ML, et al. Vibratory angioedema: a hereditary type of physical hypersensitivity. *J Allergy Clin Immunol*. 1972;50:174–182.

78. Metzger WJ, Kaplan AP, Beaven MA, et al. Hereditary vibratory angioedema: confirmation of histamine release in a type of physical hypersensitivity. *J Allergy Clin Immunol*. 1976;57:605–608.

79. Ghosh S, Kanwar AJ, Kaur S. Urticaria in children. *Pediatr Dermatol*. 1993;10:107–110.

80. Volonakis M, Katsarou-Katsari A, Stratigos J. Etiologic factors in childhood chronic urticaria. *Ann Allergy*. 1992;69:61–65.

81. Malde B, Regalado J, Greenberger PA. Investigation of angioedema associated with the use of angiotensin-converting enzyme inhibitors and angiotensin receptor blockers. *Ann Allergy Asthma Immunol*. 2007;98:57–63.

82. Irons BK, Kumar A. Valsartan-induced angioedema. *Ann Pharmacother*. 2003;37:1024–1027.

83. Vaida GA, Goldman MA, Bloch KJ. Testing for hepatitis B in patients with chronic urticaria and angioedema. *J Allergy Clin Immunol*. 1983;72:193–198.

84. Sampson HA. The role of food allergy and mediation release in atopic dermatitis. *J Allergy Clin Immunol*. 1988;81:635–645.

85. Sampson H. Food allergy. Part 2: diagnosis and management. *J Allergy Clin Immunol*. 1999;103:987–989.

86. Bush RK, Helfe SL. Lessons and myths regarding cross-reacting foods. *Allergy Proc*. 1995;16:245–246.

87. Dompmartin A, Szczurko C, Michel M, et al. Two cases of urticaria following fruit ingestion, with cross-sensitivity to latex. *Contact Dermatitis*. 1994;30:250–252.

88. Wedi B, Raap U, Kapp A. Chronic urticaria and infection. *Curr Op Allergy Clin Immunol*. 2004:4:387-396.

89. Vonkrog HG, Maiback HI. Contact urticaria. In: Adams RM, ed. *Occupational Skin Disease*. New York: Grune & Stratton; 1983:58–69.

90. Brown NA, Carter JD. Urticarial vasculitis. *Curr Rheumatol*. 2007;9:312–319.

91. Kozel MM, Bossuyt PM, Mekkes JR, et al. Laboratory tests and identified diagnoses in patients with physical and chronic urticaria and angioedema: a systematic review. *J Am Acad Dermatol*. 2003;48:409–416.

92. Bakker RA, Nicholas MW, Smith TT, et al. In vitro pharmacology of clinically used central nervous system-active drugs as inverse H$_1$ receptor agonists. *J Pharmacol Exp Ther*. 2007;332:172–179.

93. Nelson HS, Reynolds R, Mason J. Fexofenadine HC1 is safe and effective for the treatment of chronic idiopathic urticaria. *Ann Allergy Asthma Immunol*. 2000;84:517–522.

94. Finn AF, Kaplan AP, Fretwell R, et al. A double-blind, placebo controlled trial of fexofenadine HCl in treatment of chronic urticaria. *J Allergy Clin Immunol*. 1999;103:1071–1078.

95. Campoli-Richards DM, Buckley MM, Fitton A. Cetirizine: a review of its pharmacological properties and clinical potential in allergic rhinitis, pollen-induced asthma, and chronic urticaria. *Drugs*. 1990;40:762–781.

96. Breneman D, Bronsky EA, Bruce S, et al. Cetirizine and astemizole therapy for chronic idiopathic urticaria: a double-blind, placebo-controlled, comparative trial. *J Am Acad Dermatol*. 1995;33:192–198.

97. Townley RG. Cetirizine: a new H$_1$ antagonist with antieosinophilic activity in chronic urticaria. *J Am Acad Dermatol*. 1991;25:668–674.

98. Dubuske LM. Levocetirizine: the latest treatment option for allergic rhinitis and chronic idiopathic urticaria. *Allergy Asthma Proc*. 2007;28:724–734.

99. Dubuske LM. Desloratidine for chronic idiopathic urticaria: a review of clinical efficacy. *Am J Clin Dermatol*. 2007;8:271–283.

100. Hutson DP, Bressler RB, Kaliner M, et al. Prevention of mast-cell degranulation by ketotifen in patients with physical urticarias. *Ann Intern Med*. 1986;104:507–510.

101. Egan CA, Rallis TM. Treatment of chronic idiopathic urticaria with ketotifen. *Arch Dermatol*. 1997;133:147–149.

102. Greene SL. Reed CE, Schroeter AL. Double-blind crossover study comparing doxepin with diphenhydramine for the treatment of chronic idiopathic urticaria. *J Am Acad Dermatol*. 1985;12:669–675.

103. Ellis MH. Successful treatment of chronic urticaria with leukotriene antagonist. *J Allergy Clin Immunol*. 1998;102:876–877.

104. Erbagci Z. The leukotriene receptor antagonist montelukast in the treatment of chronic idiopathic urticaria: A single-blind, placebo-controlled, crossover clinical study. *J Allergy Clin Immunol*. 2002;110:484-488.

105. Di Lorenzo G, Pacor ML, Mansueto P, et al. Is there a role for anti-leukotrienes in urticaria? *Clin Exp Dermatol*. 2006;31:327–334.

106. Lin RV, Curry A, Pesola GR, et al. Improved outcomes in patients with acute allergic syndromes who are treated with combined H$_1$ and H$_2$ antagonists. *Ann Emerg Med*. 2000;36:5:462–468.

107. Grattan CEH, O'Donnell BF, Francis DM, et al. Randomized double blind study of cyclosporin in chronic idiopathic urticaria. *Br J Dermatol*. 2000;143:365–372.

108. Serhat Inaloz H, Ozturk S, Akcali C, et al. Low-dose and short-term cyclosporine treatment in patients with chronic idiopathic urticaria: a clinical and immunological evaluation. *J Dermatol*. 2008;35:276–282.

109. Brestel EP, Thrush LB. The treatment of glucocorticosteroid-dependent chronic urticaria with stanozolol. *J Allergy Clin Immunol*. 1988;82:265–269.

110. Reeves GE, Boyle MJ, Bonfield J, et al. Impact of hydroxychloriquine therapy on chronic idiopathic: chronic autoimmune urticaria study and evaluation. *Intern Med J*. 2004;34:182–186.

111. Criado RF, Criado PR, Martins JE, et al. Urticaria unresponsive to antihistaminic treatment: an open study of therapeutic options based on histopathologic features. *J Dermatol Treat*. 2008;19:92–96.

112. Weiner MJ. Methotrexate in corticosteroid-resistant urticaria. *Ann Intern Med*. 1989;110:848.

113. Kessel A, Bamberger E, Toubi E. Tacrolimus in the treatment of severe chronic idiopathic urticaria: an open-label prospective study. *J Am Acad Dermatol*. 2005;52:145–148.

114. Shahar E, Bergman R, Guttman-Yassky E, et al. Treatment of severe chronic idiopathic urticaria with oral mycophenolate mofetil in patients not responding to antihistamines and/or corticosteroids. *Internat J Dermatol*. 2006;45:1224–1227.

115. Spector SL, Tan RA. Effect of omalizumab on patients with chronic idiopathic urticaria. *Ann Allergy Asthma Immunol*. 2007;99:190–193.

116. Sands MF, Blume JW, Schwartz SA. Successful treatment of 3 patients with recurrent idiopathic angioedema with omalizumab. *J Allergy Clin Immunol*. 2007;120:979–978.

117. Engler RJ, Squire E, Benson P. Chronic sulfasalazine therapy in the treatment of delayed pressure urticaria and angioedema. *Ann Allergy Asthma Immunol*. 1995; 74:155–159.

118. Jaffer AM. Sulfasalazine in the treatment of corticosteroid-dependent chronic idiopathic urticaria. *J Allergy Clin Immunol*. 1991; 88:964–965.

119. Berdy SS, Bloch KJ. Schnitzler's syndrome: a broader clinical spectrum. *J Allergy Clin Immunol*. 1991;87:849–854.

CHAPTER 32

Approach to the Patient with Pruritus

DAVID C. REID AND ANNE E. LAUMANN

■ INTRODUCTION

Pruritus, or itching, is a common, complex, and often debilitating sensation that, if sufficiently strong, will provoke either conscious or reflex scratching, or the desire to scratch. The word, *pruritus*, originates from the Latin prurire (to itch). The suffix "itus" is not to be confused with the Greek-derived "itis," meaning "inflammation of." While the temporary discomfort of itch, such as that which develops after an insect bite, is common, pruritus that is generalized, severe, or persistent can be an incapacitating symptom and a sign of internal disease.

Itching is the most common dermatologic symptom. When it is symptomatic of a visible skin problem, the etiology may be discerned from physical examination and/or biopsy. Pruritus in the absence of cutaneous findings, however, is a diagnostic challenge, and effective therapy may be elusive. This chapter begins with an overview of pruritus, and then discusses the investigation and management of the individual with itching in the absence of visible skin disease.

■ CLASSIFICATION

There is no universally accepted classification of pruritus, and nomenclature is variable. Generally, itching is described as "cutaneous" (due to skin disease) or essential (lacking skin findings). It may also be distinguished based on source: dermatologic or pruritoceptive (originating in the skin due to localized irritation), systemic (arising from pathology in internal organs), neurogenic/neuropathic (due to diseases of the central or peripheral nervous system), and psychogenic (due to psychiatric disease).

In 2007, the International Forum for the Study of Itch formed a clinically based classification of pruritic diseases (1):

 I. Pruritus on diseased (inflamed) skin
 II. Pruritus on nondiseased (noninflamed) skin
III. Pruritus with severe secondarily scratched lesions

This chapter focuses on group II. It is important to note, however, that the presence of skin findings does not exclude an underlying systemic cause, and the absence of rash does not equate with systemic disease.

■ PATHOPHYSIOLOGY

It was long thought that nociceptors in the skin mediate both pruritus (through weak activation) and pain (through stronger activation), but more recent evidence suggests that specific receptors and nerves selectively signal itch. The triggering sensation is transmitted by a functionally distinct subset of afferent, unmyelinated C-fibers (2). These neurons respond to histamine, interleukin-2, μ- and κ-opioid system changes, and substance P (3). They are insensitive to mechanical stimuli. Different receptors may be responsible for itching resulting from electrical stimuli or friction. After reaching dorsal horn neurons in the spinal cord, the stimulus travels to the thalamus and cerebral cortex, producing the itch sensation and, through activation of the motor cortex, the desire to scratch.

■ ETIOLOGY

Itching without skin lesions can be due to underlying systemic disease, stem from neurologic or psychologic disorders, or result from pharmacologic therapy. Ten to fifty percent of patients with pruritus have an underlying systemic disease, chronic renal disease, cholestasis, hematologic malignancies, thyroid dysfunction, HIV infection, and carcinoid syndrome being the most common (4).

■ HISTORY

A detailed history is essential. In the absence of visible skin disease, temporal associations, environmental factors, and systemic symptoms are important pointers. No particular clinical characteristic helps define the probability of an underlying disease, but some predication can be made from the summation of features. Sometimes multiple office visits and review of patient self-kept journals are necessary.

Leading questions are suggested in Table 32.1. Abrupt onset of severe itching is uncommon for systemic disease, which usually presents insidiously. Systemic diseases often produce generalized, symmetric itching, whereas a localized distribution suggests a neuropathic etiology, such as brachioradial pruritus (5), or notalgia paresthetica. Prior to direct questioning, the patient may not realize that the itching occurs at specific times of day or related to particular activities, such as bathing or exercise. Most itching is more problematic at night so this diurnal variation is of limited diagnostic value.

The feeling of insects crawling or biting under the skin is called formication, and may be a symptom of depression, but the presence of a psychologically localized, fixed, and immutable belief that the discomfort stems from parasitic infestation, despite a lack of objective evidence, portends the condition, delusions of parasitosis. A tell-tale sign is the appearance in the doctor's office of small bags or boxes of lint, skin flakes, and textile fibers for microscopic examination. Delusions of parasitosis is related to the recently identified Morgellons disease (6).

Medications known to cause or worsen pruritus are listed in Table 32.2. Interestingly, some drugs known to exacerbate itching in one situation may help the symptom in another. These include aspirin, used together with paroxetine for pruritus associated with polycythemia vera (7,8), and indomethacin, sometimes helpful for HIV infection-induced pruritus (9).

TABLE 32.1 HISTORICAL QUESTIONS FOR THE PRURITIC PATIENT

- **Distribution:** generalized, localized, acral (cholestasis)
- **Nature/quality:** burning, pain, numbness, formication
- **Periodicity:** paroxysmal, constant, diurnal, nocturnal
- **Duration:** days, weeks, months, years
- **Intensity:** mild, moderate, severe, interference with daily activities and sleep
- **Instigating/exacerbating factors:** environment, exercise, occupational factors, bathing
- **Past medical history:** atopic diathesis, known allergies, systemic illnesses, renal, liver, endocrine, hematologic disorders
- **Review of systems:** fever, chills, weight loss, fatigue, jaundice, temperature intolerance
- **Medications:** systemics, over-the-counter products, herbal supplements, topicals, illicit drugs
- **Social history:** occupation, living situation, travel history, sexual history

TABLE 32.2 COMMON SYSTEMIC CAUSES OF GENERALIZED PRURITUS

Chronic Renal Failure
Hepatic Cholestasis (obstructive hepatic disease of all types):
- Primary biliary cirrhosis
- Primary sclerosing cholangitis
- Choledocolithiasis
- Bile duct carcinoma
- Viral hepatitis
- Drug-induced hepatitis
- Pregnancy-associated cholestasis

Endocrine
- Functional thyroid or parathyroid disorder

Malignancy
- Hodgkin disease
- Non-Hodgkin lymphoma
- Myeloid and lymphatic leukemia
- Myelodysplasia
- Solid tumors, carcinoid tumors

Hematological
- Polycythemia vera
- Paraproteinemia
- Mastocytosis

Pharmacological
- Chloroquine, clonidine, gold, lithium, β-blockers, tamoxifen, captopril, sulfonamides, retinoids, tramadol, aspirin, nonsteroidal anti-inflammatory agents, codeine, cocaine, morphine, hydroxyethyl starch[*]

Psychogenic
- Depression
- Generalized anxiety disorder
- Obsessive compulsive disorder
- Delusions of parasitosis

Neurologic
- Notalgia paresthetica
- Brachioradial pruritus
- Postherpetic neuralgia

[*] Hydroxyethyl starch is a component of colloid plasma volume expanders (56)

The review of systems may help uncover systemic illness. Fever, weight loss, and fatigue may point to a malignancy, such as lymphoma. Common symptoms of thyroid disease include heat or cold intolerance, diarrhea or constipation, and hair loss or change. Neurologic symptoms in the presence of paroxysmal pruritus suggest multiple sclerosis (10). Information about sexual behavior, the use of illicit chemicals, blood transfusions, personal living situations, and travel may lead to the identification of infections and infestations, not visibly apparent in the early stages.

■ PHYSICAL EXAM

In most cases of itching, an obvious primary skin disorder, such as atopic dermatitis, urticaria, or arthropod reaction will be manifest. The absence of readily visible findings does not exclude the possibility of a primary cutaneous cause. Xerosis and scabies, for example, can be easily overlooked; careful inspection is required to identify fine scaling and papules, and burrows, respectively. Given the intermittency of urticaria, wheals are often absent during an office visit, although the presence of dermatographism may be helpful. Active cutaneous fibrosis in systemic sclerosis is often itchy. The skin may appear smooth and tight. It is important not to mistake excoriations, prurigo nodules, or lichenification (thickened skin with increased skin markings) for primary cutaneous findings. These secondary lesions result from rubbing, picking, or scratching. Given the transient or episodic nature of some cutaneous diseases, re-examination over time may lead to diagnostic findings.

To identify systemic disease, a standard physical examination is helpful including assessments for cachexia, pallor, jaundice, palpable lymph nodes, liver, and spleen. Examination of the nails may reveal findings, such as half and half nails (renal disease), Terry's white nails (hepatic disease or endocrinopathy), koilonychia (iron deficiency anemia), or distal onycholysis (hyperthyroidism). System-specific signs are detailed in the section, Pruritus in Systemic Disease.

■ LABORATORY AND IMAGING STUDIES

Screening laboratory tests may not be necessary at initial presentation. If the history and physical examination do not suggest a systemic disease, a trial of antipruritic therapy is reasonable (see treatment section). Ongoing itching that is nonresponsive to such therapy should lead to investigation for systemic disease (see Table 32.3).

A skin biopsy may occasionally help to evaluate for underlying skin diseases such as cutaneous mastocytosis that can have subtle physical findings. However, in the absence of clinically apparent disease, a skin biopsy should be avoided to prevent over diagnosis, such as the finding of dermal mast cells without other evidence for mastocytosis.

■ DIFFERENTIAL DIAGNOSIS

The differential diagnosis for systemic causes of generalized pruritus is broad, including conditions affecting the renal, hepatic, hematologic, and endocrine systems. Several malignancies and drugs are known to produce pruritus. Neurologic and psychogenic disorders must also be considered. The most common underlying disorders are listed in Table 32.2.

■ TREATMENT

Despite recent advances, therapy is often frustrating. Clinical studies assessing efficacy are difficult to interpret, as the placebo effect ranges from 50% to 66% (11). Of course, at times, therapy specific for the particular systemic disease is highly effective. Reduction of stress and anxiety, as well as physical exercise and relaxation techniques may be beneficial.

Topical Therapy

The use of appropriate topical therapy is crucial, together with the avoidance of scratching and rubbing. The latter may be so pleasurable, almost erotic, that strict behavior modification in the form of encouraging frequent daily application of emollients is essential. Bathing, showering, and the use of soap often aggravate itching, even when there is a systemic cause. Occlusive agents, such as petrolatum, mineral oil, and lanolin, act as barriers to decrease water loss from the skin. Glycerin, urea, and alpha-hydroxy acids are examples of humectants, which help deliver water to the stratum corneum. Some newer moisturizers contain ceramide, a natural component of the skin's lipid bilayer, which enhances hydration. Thick, greasy products are generally the most effective, but the unpleasing texture and

---

TABLE 32.3 SUGGESTED LABORATORY EVALUATION FOR GENERALIZED PRURITUS OF UNKNOWN ORIGIN

Recommended
- Complete blood count, including differential
- Chemistry profile, with blood urea nitrogen, creatinine, and fasting glucose
- Liver function: transaminases, alkaline phosphatase, total and direct bilirubin, gamma-glutamyl transpeptidase
- Thyroid function: thyroid stimulating hormone; if abnormal, thyroxine (T4) and triiodothyronine (T3)
- Erythrocyte sedimentation rate, C-reactive protein

Optional as indicated by results of above or from examination
- Chest X-ray
- Stool examination for ova, parasites, occult blood
- Human immunodeficiency virus testing
- Viral hepatitis testing
- Parathyroid function: parathyroid hormone, calcium, phosphate
- Serum tryptase, 24-hour urine histamine
- Serum protein electrophoresis with immunofixation
- Urine protein electrophoresis with immunofixation
- Abdominal ultrasound/CT scan
- Iron studies: serum iron, serum ferritin, transferrin (total iron binding capacity)
- Skin biopsy is rarely helpful and may cause diagnostic confusion

appearance may affect patient compliance, so combination regimens may help, such as the use of a nonoily cream during the day and a thicker messier ointment at night. Use after bathing helps prevent xerosis of the stratum corneum caused by water evaporation.

Other mainstays of topical treatment include cooling counterirritants (menthol, phenol, or camphor), topical anesthetics (lidocaine or pramoxine), and capsaicin, a naturally occurring alkaloid, which initially induces release of substance P from peripheral sensory neurons producing a burning pain, but after repeated application, depletes the neuron of substance P, and prevents its reaccumulation, thus reducing sensation. A topical formulation of naltrexone, an opioid receptor antagonist that modifies epidermal μ-opiate receptor expression, has also shown great promise (12). Topical diphenhydramine should be avoided related to a high risk of sensitization, and topical doxepin can be problematic related to systemic side effects.

Topical steroids can help break the itch-scratch cycle that produces eczema or lichenification, but should not be used indiscriminately. Moderate potency steroids, such as triamcinolone acetonide 0.1% ointment, are reserved for the trunk and extremities, while more mild agents, like 1% hydrocortisone cream, are appropriate for the face, groin, or axilla, where skin is thin and more prone to atrophy. Recently, topical calcineurin inhibitors (tacrolimus, pimecrolimus) have emerged as immunomodulating agents that exhibit comparable efficacy to mild corticosteroids. They often cause temporary burning skin discomfort themselves, but lack the long-term adverse effects of steroids.

Systemic Therapy

H_1 antihistamines are often used to control the pruritus associated with urticaria, a histamine-mediated problem. However, when used to control itch without any other skin manifestations, the main effect is probably soporific rather than truly antipruritic (13). Consequently, first-generation, sedating, H_1 antihistamines may be used, but H_2 and H_3 antagonists are not indicated.

Opioid receptor antagonists, such as the orally administered naltrexone, have been used for generalized itching due to both dermatologic and systemic causes (14), but are most useful for cholestatic pruritus (15,16). Naloxone infusions can be used for acute exacerbations (17).

Gabapentin and its successor, pregabalin, structural analogs of γ-aminobutyric acid, modulate central nervous system pathways of itch and pain. Titrated slowly upward, they may be helpful for chronic pruritus (18).

Of the selective serotonin reuptake inhibitors, only paroxetine has been shown to improve pruritus related to systemic disease (19,20), suggesting its benefit may be elicited through a nonserotoninergic mechanism. Nausea is common, and abrupt cessation can cause severe pruritus and acute anxiety. Mirtazapine, a tetra-

cyclic antidepressant that works centrally by increasing release of norepinephrine and serotonin, is also an antagonist of serotonin, H_1 histamine, peripheral α_1-adrenergic, and muscarinic antagonist receptors. It may be especially helpful for difficult cases of nocturnal pruritus (21)

More rarely, thalidomide, a tumor necrosis factor-α inhibitor and immune modulator, may be used, but its use is limited by the almost universal development of peripheral neuropathy. Cholestyramine, an anion-exchange resin that binds bile acids in the GI tract, thus interrupting their enterohepatic circulation, has been used for many years to relieve cholestatic pruritus (22,23), but nowadays, rifampin, an hepatic enzyme inducer, is considered first-line therapy (24–26). The atypical antipsychotic pimozide, and more recently olanzepine, have been used for delusions of parasitosis (27,28), but mirtazapine or pregabalin may be safer and easier options.

Broad-band or narrow-band ultraviolet light (UVB) therapy, typically given for a few minutes three times weekly, is considered the treatment of choice for renal pruritus (29), and has shown efficacy in cholestatic pruritus, aquagenic pruritus, pruritus of HIV infection, and polycythemia vera (30). UV-B therapy decreases dermal mast cells (31), presumably through inducing apoptosis (32), and can induce remission in as few as six to eight treatments (33).

Given the association of pruritus and stress-related mediators, it is not surprising that psychologic approaches reduce itch intensity. Behavioral therapy, biofeedback, and so-called alternative therapies, including acupuncture, may improve symptoms and quality of life (34).

■ PRURITUS IN SYSTEMIC DISEASE

Although there are few definitive associations between particular symptoms and/or signs and specific systemic causes of pruritus, some associations can be made.

Pruritus and Renal Disease (Uremic Pruritus)

At least 30% and possibly, at times, 90% of those in chronic renal failure suffer from ongoing itch (35). In contrast, acute renal failure rarely causes pruritus, suggesting that, as with other uremic symptoms, elevated serum urea or creatinine is not causative. Instead, elevated levels of histamine, serotonin, and divalent ions, such as calcium, phosphate, magnesium, and aluminum, as well as imbalance of the μ- and κ-opioid receptors on lymphocytes have been implicated. In addition, uremic patients with pruritus have more dermal degranulated mast cells than those without itch (36,37). The initiation of dialysis does not necessarily alleviate pruritus, presumably because there is some persistent solute retention (38). For unknown reasons, those on hemodialysis are more often affected than those on continuous ambulatory peritoneal dialysis (4). The involvement of immunologic dysfunction is imputed from the absence of itch in those with a poorly functioning transplanted kidney until such time as immunosuppression is discontinued. Nephrogenic systemic fibrosis, a recently recognized and rare condition that affects only those with end-stage renal disease (GFR < 30 mL/min/1.73m²) and a history of gadolinium- containing contrast agent exposure, can be very itchy during the early stages of active fibrosis (39).

Renal pruritus is an independent marker for mortality (40,41), possibly related to the negative impact on sleep quality. It is typically prolonged (lasting 6 months or more), and frequent, with nearly 50% of patients experiencing daily symptoms (35). The distribution is usually symmetric and generalized, but symptoms may be localized to the back, abdomen, scalp, and shunt arms (35,42). The itch intensity may increase during nighttime, summer months, or immediately following hemodialysis sessions. On physical exam, xerosis, decreased mental acuity (uremia), and peripheral neuropathy may be evident. See Table 32.4 for a list of therapies for generalized pruritus.

Pruritus and Liver Disease (Cholestatic Pruritus)

Cholestatic itching is related to impaired bile secretion and occurs with all types of obstructive liver disease (43) (see Table 32.2). Although intracutaneous injections of bile acids produce pruritus (44), the deposition of bile salts in the skin is not, as once believed, the causative factor. Instead, elevated histamine levels, accumulation of pruritogenic intermediates in bile salt synthesis, the release of pruritogenic substances, such as opioid receptors, from the injured liver cells as well as from epidermal cells and macrophages are implicated (45). Seventy percent of patients with primary biliary cirrhosis suffer from itching (46), and pruritus is often the presenting symptom. The spontaneous disappearance of pruritus in patients with hepatitis may signify a severe deterioration in hepatic function with a parallel worsening of prognosis (47). Itching associated with liver disease is insidious in onset, mild in severity, and begins acrally, later progressing to more generalized involvement. Hot spots on the hands and feet, or on areas restricted by tight-fitting clothing, may persist. Only rarely are the head, neck, or genitalia involved. Scratching does not relieve the sensation, and patients may scratch until they bleed (48).

The stigmata of liver failure seen on physical exam are well established and include icterus, ascites, dilated abdominal wall vessels, purpura, palmar erythema, spider angiomas, gynecomastia, small muscle wasting, Dupuytren contractures and hepatosplenomegaly.

Malignancy-associated Pruritus

Solid malignancies are infrequently associated with pruritus. Gastric carcinoids, through serotonin release, produce episodic, itchy episodes of intense flushing. In other cases of solid malignancy, the dorsal arms and anterior legs are preferentially affected. Specific tumors may be associated with localized itching, e.g., brain tumors and itching in the nostrils (49). However, a full investigation for solid tumors in patients with generalized pruritus is not warranted, as the incidence of solid malignancies is the same as in the general population (50).

More common than solid tumors is the association with hematologic malignancies, in particular Hodgkin

---

TABLE 32.4 THERAPIES FOR GENERALIZED PRURITUS

Pharmacologic
- *Topical:* Emollients, menthol, phenol, eucalyptus, calamine, capsaicin, pramoxine, doxepin, naltrexone
- *Oral:*
  Sedating antihistamines: H1 only
  Opiate antagonists: naltrexone, naloxone
  Neurologic: gabapentin, pregabalin
  Psychiatric: mirtazapine, paroxetine
  Immunomodulatory: thalidomide

Nonpharmacologic
- Phototherapy (narrow-band UVB, broad-band UVB, psoralen, and UVA)
- Cognitive behavioral therapy, stress reduction, biofeedback
- Acupuncture
- Cutaneous field stimulation (localized pruritus only)

Cause-specific
- *Renal Pruritus:*
  UVB phototherapy (three times weekly)
  Naltrexone (50 mg to 100 mg by mouth daily)
  Gabapentin (200 mg to 300 mg after hemodialysis sessions)
  Thalidomide (100 mg by mouth daily)
- *Cholestatic Pruritus:*
  Rifampin (300 mg to 600 mg by mouth daily)
  Cholestyramine (4 g to 16 g by mouth daily)
  Naltrexone (25 mg to 250 mg by mouth daily)
  Naloxone (infusion slowly titrated to .2μg/kg/min)
  Thalidomide (100 mg by mouth daily)
- *Polycythemia Vera:*
  Aspirin (325 mg by mouth daily to three times daily)
- *HIV Pruritus:*
  Indomethacin (25 mg three times daily), UVB phototherapy (three times weekly)
- *Malignancy-associated Pruritus:*
  Paroxetine (5 mg to 30 mg by mouth daily)
  Mirtazapine (7.5 mg to 30 mg by mouth daily)

lymphoma, leukemias, other lymphomas, and polycythemia vera. Severe, relentless itching, coupled with systemic symptoms (fever, chills, night sweats) suggest lymphoma. Up to 30% of patients with Hodgkin lymphoma itch, an important clue as itching may precede diagnosis by as much as 5 years (45). The distribution is usually generalized, although it can localize to areas draining the involved lymphatic channels. Sometimes there is also a strong burning sensation.

Other itch-associated hematologic malignancies include non-Hodgkin lymphoma (10% of patients), rare cases of cutaneous T-cell lymphoma, mastocytosis, multiple myeloma, and the leukemias (most often chronic lymphocytic leukemia). The pruritus of leukemia is milder than that of lymphoma.

Endocrine Pruritus

The excess thyroid hormone in thyrotoxicosis leads to sympathetic overactivity, vasodilation, elevation of skin temperature, activation of kinin pathways, and lowering of the itch threshold resulting in generalized pruritus in 4% to 11% of patients (51). On the other hand, the itch of hypothyroidism, which affects up to 90% of patients, is not metabolic in origin but related to xerosis. The hypothyroid individual may have coarse, thick, flaky skin; diffuse alopecia with thick brittle hair; ptosis; and loss of the lateral one-third of the eyebrows. The thyrotoxic patient may have smooth skin with hyperhidrosis, a fine tremor, diffuse telogen hair loss with thin hairs, proptosis, onycholysis, and, at times, urticaria.

Despite popular conception, generalized itching is not found more commonly in those with diabetes than in the general population (52). In fact, advanced peripheral neuropathy may prevent any feeling at all. Localized areas of itch may result from cutaneous candidiasis, lichen simplex chronicus, or nummular eczema.

Pruritus without Skin Signs Related to Infectious Disease

Pruritus may be the presenting sign of HIV infection. Severe itching occurs with progressive infection (CD4 count <50), possibly through the effect of viral proteins on nociceptive neurons. Other signs of HIV are equally nonspecific, but include weight loss, seborrheic dermatitis, and coexisting infections (53).

Hematological Pruritus

Itching occurs in up to 50% of those with polycythemia vera. It often predates the diagnosis by several years and is characteristically aquagenic, i.e., an intense pricking itch occurs on contact with water of any temperature (54). A sudden drop in ambient temperature may produce similar symptoms. Plasma histamine, the numbers of circulating basophils and degranulated skin mast cells are increased (51). Physical exam may reveal splenomegaly, hepatomegaly, and plethora—a ruddy complexion in the face, mucosa, and conjunctiva. Despite old reports, iron deficiency alone does not produce itch (55).

■ REFERENCES

1. Stander S, Weisshaar E, Mettang T, et al. Clinical classification of itch: a position paper of the International Forum for the Study of Itch. *Acta Derm Venereol*. 2007;87(4):291–294.
2. Schmelz M, Schmidt R, Bickel A, et al. Specific C-receptors for itch in human skin. *J Neurosci*. 1997;17(20):8003–8008.
3. Twycross R, Greaves MW, Handwerker H, et al. Itch: scratching more than the surface. *QJM*. 2003;96(1):7–26.
4. Bernhard JD. *Itch: Mechanisms and Management of Pruritus*. New York: McGraw-Hill; 1994.
5. Lane JE, McKenzie JT, Spiegel J. Brachioradial pruritus: a case report and review of the literature. *Cutis*. 2008;81(1):37–40.
6. Harvey WT. Morgellons disease. *J Am Acad Dermatol*. 2007;56(4):705–706.
7. Jackson N, Burt D, Crocker J, et al. Skin mast cells in polycythaemia vera: relationship to the pathogenesis and treatment of pruritus. *Br J Dermatol*. 1987;116(1):21–29.
8. Tefferi A, Fonseca R. Selective serotonin reuptake inhibitors are effective in the treatment of polycythemia vera-associated pruritus. *Blood*. 2002;99(7):2627.
9. Smith KJ, Skelton HG, Yeager J, et al. Pruritus in HIV-1 disease: therapy with drugs which may modulate the pattern of immune dysregulation. *Dermatology*. 1997;195(4):353–358.
10. Koeppel MC, Bramont C, Ceccaldi M, et al. Paroxysmal pruritus and multiple sclerosis. *Br J Dermatol*. 1993;129(5):597–598.
11. Yosipovitch G, David M. The diagnostic and therapeutic approach to idiopathic generalized pruritus. *Int J Dermatol*. 1999;38(12): 881–887.
12. Bigliardi PL, Stammer H, Jost G, et al. Treatment of pruritus with topically applied opiate receptor antagonist. *J Am Acad Dermatol*. 2007;56(6):979–988.
13. Krause L, Shuster S. Mechanism of action of antipruritic drugs. *Br Med J (Clin Res Ed)*. 1983;287(6400):1199–1200.
14. Metze D, Reimann S, Beissert S, et al. Efficacy and safety of naltrexone, an oral opiate receptor antagonist, in the treatment of pruritus in internal and dermatological diseases. *J Am Acad Dermatol*. 1999; 41(4):533–539.
15. Wolfhagen FH, Sternieri E, Hop WC, et al. Oral naltrexone treatment for cholestatic pruritus: a double-blind, placebo-controlled study. *Gastroenterology*. 1997;113(4):1264–1269.
16. Terg R, Coronel E, Sorda J, et al. Efficacy and safety of oral naltrexone treatment for pruritus of cholestasis, a crossover, double blind, placebo-controlled study. *J Hepatol*. 2002;37(6):717–722.
17. Bergasa NV, Alling DW, Talbot TL, et al. Effects of naloxone infusions in patients with the pruritus of cholestasis. A double-blind, randomized, controlled trial. *Ann Intern Med*. 1995;123(3):161–167.
18. Ehrchen J, Stander S. Pregabalin in the treatment of chronic pruritus. *J Am Acad Dermatol*. 2008;58(2 Suppl):S36–S37.
19. Zylicz Z, Krajnik M, Sorge AA, et al. Paroxetine in the treatment of severe non-dermatological pruritus: a randomized, controlled trial. *J Pain Symptom Manage*. 2003;26(6):1105–1112.
20. Zylicz Z, Smits C, Krajnik M. Paroxetine for pruritus in advanced cancer. *J Pain Symptom Manage*. 1998;16(2):121–124.
21. Hundley JL, Yosipovitch G. Mirtazapine for reducing nocturnal itch in patients with chronic pruritus: a pilot study. *J Am Acad Dermatol*. 2004;50(6):889–891.
22. Datta DV, Sherlock S. Cholestyramine for long term relief of the pruritus complicating intrahepatic cholestasis. *Gastroenterology*. 1966;50(3):323–332.
23. Datta DV, Sherlock S. Treatment of pruritus of obstructive jaundice with cholestyramine. *Br Med J*. 1963;1(5325):216–219.
24. Ghent CN, Carruthers SG. Treatment of pruritus in primary biliary cirrhosis with rifampin. Results of a double-blind, crossover, randomized trial. *Gastroenterology*. 1988;94(2):488–493.
25. Podesta A, Lopez P, Terg R, et al. Treatment of pruritus of primary biliary cirrhosis with rifampin. *Dig Dis Sci*. 1991;36(2):216–220.

26. Khurana S, Singh P. Rifampin is safe for treatment of pruritus due to chronic cholestasis: a meta-analysis of prospective randomized-controlled trials. *Liver Int.* 2006;26(8):943–948.

27. Damiani JT, Flowers FP, Pierce DK. Pimozide in delusions of parasitosis. *J Am Acad Dermatol.* 1990;22(2 Pt 1):312–313.

28. Meehan WJ, Badreshia S, Mackley CL. Successful treatment of delusions of parasitosis with olanzapine. *Arch Dermatol.* 2006; 142(3):352–355.

29. Szepietowski JC, Schwartz RA. Uremic pruritus. *Int J Dermatol.* 1998;37(4):247–253.

30. Seckin D, Demircay Z, Akin O. Generalized pruritus treated with narrowband UVB. *Int J Dermatol.* 2007;46(4):367–370.

31. Cohen EP, Russell TJ, Garancis JC. Mast cells and calcium in severe uremic itching. *Am J Med Sci.* 1992;303(6):360–365.

32. Szepietowski JC, Morita A, Tsuji T. Ultraviolet B induces mast cell apoptosis: a hypothetical mechanism of ultraviolet B treatment for uraemic pruritus. *Med Hypotheses.* 2002;58(2):167–170.

33. Gilchrest BA, Rowe JW, Brown RS, et al. Ultraviolet phototherapy of uremic pruritus. Long-term results and possible mechanism of action. *Ann Intern Med.* 1979;91(1):17–21.

34. Fried RG. Nonpharmacologic treatments in psychodermatology. *Dermatol Clin.* 2002;20(1):177–185.

35. Zucker I, Yosipovitch G, David M, Gafter U, Boner G. Prevalence and characterization of uremic pruritus in patients undergoing hemodialysis: uremic pruritus is still a major problem for patients with end-stage renal disease. *J Am Acad Dermatol.* 2003;49(5):842–846.

36. Matsumoto M, Ichimaru K, Horie A. Pruritus and mast cell proliferation of the skin in end stage renal failure. *Clin Nephrol.* 1985; 23(6):285–288.

37. Szepietowski J, Thepen T, van Vloten WA, et al. Pruritus and mast cell proliferation in the skin of haemodialysis patients. *Inflamm Res.* 1995;44(Suppl 1):S84–S85.

38. Gilchrest BA, Stern RS, Steinman TI, et al. Clinical features of pruritus among patients undergoing maintenance hemodialysis. *Arch Dermatol.* 1982;118(3):154–156.

39. Knopp EA, Cowper SE. Nephrogenic systemic fibrosis: early recognition and treatment. *Semin Dial.* 2008;21(2):123–128.

40. Wikstrom B. Itchy skin—a clinical problem for haemodialysis patients. *Nephrol Dial Transplant.* 2007;22(Suppl 5):v3–7.

41. Pisoni RL, Wikstrom B, Elder SJ, et al. Pruritus in haemodialysis patients: international results from the Dialysis Outcomes and Practice Patterns Study (DOPPS). *Nephrol Dial Transplant.* 2006;21(12): 3495–3505.

42. Stahle-Backdahl M. Uremic pruritus. Clinical and experimental studies. *Acta Derm Venereol Suppl (Stockh).* 1989;145:1–38.

43. Bergasa NV. The pruritus of cholestasis. *Semin Dermatol.* 1995;14(4):302–312.

44. Varadi DP. Pruritus induced by crude bile and purified bile acids. Experimental production of pruritus in human skin. *Arch Dermatol.* 1974;109(5):678–681.

45. Etter L, Myers SA. Pruritus in systemic disease: mechanisms and management. *Dermatol Clin.* 2002;20(3):459–472,vi–vii.

46. Heathcote J. The clinical expression of primary biliary cirrhosis. *Semin Liver Dis.* 1997;17(1):23–33.

47. Bergasa NV. Update on the treatment of the pruritus of cholestasis. *Clin Liver Dis.* 2008;12(1):219–234,x.

48. Rishe E, Azarm A, Bergasa NV. Itch in primary biliary cirrhosis: a patients' perspective. *Acta Derm Venereol.* 2008;88(1):34–37.

49. Adreev VC, Petkov I. Skin manifestations associated with tumours of the brain. *Br J Dermatol.* 1975;92(6):675–678.

50. Paul R, Jansen CT. Itch and malignancy prognosis in generalized pruritus: a 6-year follow-up of 125 patients. *J Am Acad Dermatol.* 1987;16(5):1179–1182.

51. Charlesworth EN, Beltrani VS. Pruritic dermatoses: overview of etiology and therapy. *Am J Med.* 2002;113(Suppl 9A):25S–33S.

52. Neilly JB, Martin A, Simpson N, et al. Pruritus in diabetes mellitus: investigation of prevalence and correlation with diabetes control. *Diabetes Care.* 1986;9(3):273–275.

53. Shapiro RS, Samorodin C, Hood AF. Pruritus as a presenting sign of acquired immunodeficiency syndrome. *J Am Acad Dermatol.* 1987;16(5 Pt 2):1115–1117.

54. Steinman HK, Greaves MW. Aquagenic pruritus. *J Am Acad Dermatol.* 1985;13(1):91–96.

55. Lewiecki EM, Rahman F. Pruritus. A manifestation of iron deficiency. *JAMA.* 1976;236(20):2319–2320.

56. Haught JM, Jukic DM, English JC 3rd. Hydroxyethyl starch-induced pruritus relieved by a combination of menthol and camphor. *J Am Acad Dermatol.* 2008;59(1):151–153.

Pharmacology

Antihistamines
JONATHAN A. BERNSTEIN

■ INTRODUCTION

Histamine, a low-molecular amine, is produced by the reaction of histidine decarboxylase on L-histidine (1,2). This enzyme is located in cells found throughout the body including the central nervous system, gastric parietal cells, mast cells, and basophils (1,2). As a result of its ubiquitous presence in the body, it is not surprising that histamine has a wide range of biologic effects. Currently it is known that histamine exerts these effects through four histamine receptors (HRs). Histamine is involved in sleeping and waking, energy and endocrine homeostasis, cognition and memory through histamine receptor 1 (H_1R), regulation of gastric acid secretion through H_2R, modulation of neurotransmitter release through H_3R, and facilitation of pro-inflammatory activities through H_4R (Table 33.1) (1). HR antagonists (antihistamines) can be categorized in terms of their structure, pharmacokinetics, pharmacodynamics, and clinical utility (Table 33.1) (1). Histamine binding to H_1Rs causes itching, pain, vasodilatation, vascular permeability, hypotension, flushing, headache, tachycardia, bronchoconstriction, stimulation of airway vagal afferent nerves and cough receptors, and decreased atrioventricular-node conduction time (1,2). Histamine binding to H_2Rs causes increased gastric acid secretion, vascular permeability, hypotension, flushing, headache, tachycardia, chronotropic and inotropic activity, bronchodilation, and airway mucus production (1,2). Histamine binding to H_3Rs prevents excessive bronchoconstriction and mediates pruritus through nonmast cell pathways (1,2). Finally, histamine binding to H_4Rs is important for differentiation of myeloblasts and promyelocytes. Histamine has been shown to have a number of immunomodulatory effects through these various receptors. Clinically, selective antagonists are available for blocking H_1 and H_2 receptors (Table 33.1) (1). Nonselective H_3- and H_4-receptor antagonists are available as research tools but not for clinical use at the present time (Table 33.1) (1). Second-generation antihistamines, many of which have been derived from first-generation agents, are more selective for H_1Rs and have added a new dimension to the treatment of allergic disorders. Over the last several years, additional second-generation antihistamines have been introduced to the market and others, still under investigation may become available in the near future. This chapter will provide an overview of the immunologic and clinical effects of histamine so that the reader can appreciate the evolving role of histamine-antagonists in a broad spectrum of clinical disorders.

■ THE DISCOVERY OF HISTAMINE AND HISTAMINE RECEPTORS: A HISTORICAL PERSPECTIVE

Histamine or β-imidazolylethylamine was first synthesized by Windaus and Vogt in 1907 (3). The term *histamine* was adopted because of its prevalence in animal and human tissues (*hist:* relating to tissue) and its amine structure (Figure 33.1) (4,5). Dale and Laidlaw (6) in 1910 were the first to report histamine's role in anaphylaxis when they observed a dramatic bronchospastic and

TABLE 33.1 CHARACTERISTICS OF HISTAMINE RECEPTORS

CHARACTERISTIC	H_1	H_2	H_3	H_4
Receptor described/ human gene cloned	1966/1993	1972/1991	1983/1999	1994/2000
Best characterized function	Acute allergic reactions	Gastric acid secretion	Neurotransmitter modulation	Immunomodulator
Receptor proteins in humans	487 amino acids, 56kD	359 amino acids, 40kD	445 amino acids, 70kD	390 amino acids
Chromosomal location in humans	3p25, 3p14-21	5q35.3	20q13.33	18q11.2
Receptor expression	Widespread (neurons, endothelial, smooth muscle)	Widespread (gastric parietal cells, smooth muscle, heart)	Histaminergic neurons	Bone marrow, peripheral hematopoietic cells (dendritic cells, mast cells, eosinophils, monocytes, basophils and T cells
G-protein coupling	$G\alpha_q$	$G\alpha_s$	$G\alpha_{i/o}$	$G\alpha_{i/o}$
Major signally pathway	Increases in Ca^{2+}	Increases in cAMP	Inhibition of cAMP	Increases in Ca^{2+}
Histamine pK_i	4.2	4.3	7.8	8.1
Diphenhydramine pK_i	7.9	>10,000	<5	<5
Loratadine pK_i	6.8	ND	ND	<5
Cetirizine pK_i	8.0	ND	ND	<5
Fexofenadine pK_i	8.3	ND	ND	<5
Ranitidine pK_i	<4	7.1	<5	<5
Cimetidine pK_i	<5	6.2	<5	<5
Thioperamide pK_i	<5	<4	7.3	7.2
JNJ 7777120 pK_i	<5	>4.5	5.3	8.4

From Thurmond RL, Glefand EW, Dunford PJ. The role of histamine H_1 and H_4 receptors in allergic inflammation: the search for new antihistamines. *Nat Rev Drug Discov* 2008;7:41–53. Simons FE. Advances in H_1-antihistamines. *N Engl J Med* 2004;351:2203–2217.

cAMP, cyclic adenosine monophosphate; pK_i, negative log of the dissociation constant; ND,not determined

vasodilatory effect in animals injected intravenously with this compound. Subsequently, histamine was found to be synthesized from L-histidine by L-histidine decarboxylase and metabolized by histamine N-methyltransferase to form N-methylhistidine or by diamine oxidase to form imidazole acetic acid (7). However, only the N-methyltransferase pathway is active in the central nervous system. Originally, histamine's classic physiologic actions of bronchoconstriction and vasodilation were believed responsible for the symptoms of allergic diseases through its action at one type of HR. In 1966, Ash and Schild were the first to recognize that histamine-mediated reactions occurred through more than one receptor based on observations that histamine had an array of actions such as contraction of guinea pig ileal smooth muscle, inhibition of rat uterine contractions, and suppression of gastric acid secretion (8). This speculation was confirmed in 1972 by Black et al., who used the experimental histamine antagonists, mepyramine

and burimamide, to block histamine-induced reactions in animals (9). They observed that each of these antagonists inhibited different physiologic responses, suggesting that there were at least two histamine receptors, now referred to as H_1 and H_2 (9). Arrang et al., discovered a third histamine receptor (H_3) with unique physiologic properties, raising the possibility that additional, yet unrecognized, histamine receptors exist (10). Table 33.1 summarizes the pharmacodynamic effects after activation of the known histamine receptors and their common agonists and antagonists (5,10,11). Characterizing histamine receptors has been essential in discovering histamine's physiologic actions on target cells which include increased mucus secretion, increased nitrous oxide formation, endothelial cell contraction leading to increased vascular permeability, gastric acid secretion, bronchial relaxation, and suppressor T-cell stimulation. Finally, the H_4R was discovered based on a genomic approach using the H_3R sequence.

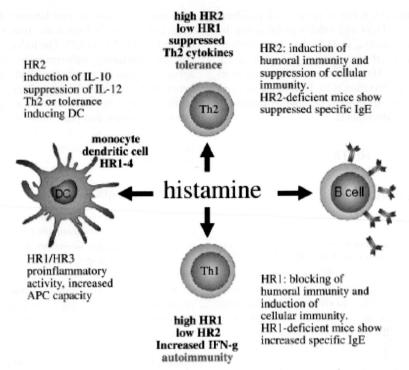

high HR2
low HR1
suppressed
Th2 cytokines
tolerance

HR2: induction of
humoral immunity and
suppression of cellular
immunity.
HR2-deficient mice show
suppressed specific IgE

HR2
induction of IL-10
suppression of IL-12
Th2 or tolerance
inducing DC

monocyte
dendritic cell
HR1-4

histamine

Th2

B cell

DC

Th1

HR1/HR3
proinflammatory
activity, increased
APC capacity

HR1: blocking of
humoral immunity and
induction of
cellular immunity.
HR1-deficient mice show
increased specific IgE

high HR1
low HR2
Increased IFN-g
autoimmunity

■ **FIGURE 33.1** Function of histamine on histamine receptors. (Reproduced with permission from Simons FER, Simons KJ. The pharmacology and use of H1-receptor-antagonist drugs. *NEJM* 1994; 330:1663.)

As mentioned, this receptor is expressed more selectively on dendritic cells, mast cells, eosinophils, monocytes, basophils, and T cells; therefore, it is believed to have an important immunoregulatory role (12). Figure 33.1 illustrates the actions of histamine on histamine receptors in allergic inflammation (13).

■ THE ROLE OF HISTAMINE IN ALLERGIC INFLAMMATION

Histamine is stored in the cytoplasm of mast cells and basophils, attached to anionic carboxylate and sulfate groups on secretory granules (13,14). Histamine is released from mast cell and basophil secretory granules after aggregation of high-affinity immunoglobulin E (IgE) receptors. IgE receptors are coupled to G-proteins which when activated lead to a sequence of chemical reactions with the end result being histamine release. However, histamine can be released spontaneously by activation of mast cells and basophils by histamine releasing factors, which include chemokines (RANTES, MCP-1, and MIP-1 α) and several cytokines (IL-1, IL-3, IL-5, IL-6, IL-7) (7).

Histamine's inflammatory action depends on which histamine receptors are activated, the level of histamine receptor expression, and the effector cells involved (1,2). For example, H_1R expression is increased during the differentiation of monocytes to macrophages and H_1R expression can be increased by a number of inflam-

matory stimuli (1,2,12,13). Furthermore, histamine has varying effects on different inflammatory cells. For example, mast cells express H_1, H_2, and H_4 receptors (1,2,12,13). Although histamine does not appear to have a direct effect on mast cell degranulation, by binding to H_4Rs it can act synergistically with chemoattractants such as CXCL12 (1). In contrast, histamine binding to H_2 receptors on mast cells can act to inhibit histamine release and modulate cytokine production (1,2,13).

Low concentrations of histamine via H_4 receptors can induce eosinophil chemotaxis but at higher concentrations via H_2 receptors can attenuate this effect (1,2,14). Histamine binding to H_4 receptors can stimulate upregulation of adhesion molecules and reorganization of actin polymers, whereas binding to H_1 receptors can induce superoxide production and complement receptor upregulation in eosinophils (1,2,12,13).

Dendritic cells express H_1, H_2, and H_4 receptors (1,13). Histamine can cause chemotaxis of dendritic cells by binding primarily to H_4Rs and to a lesser extent to H_1Rs (1). Furthermore, T-cell polarization may be regulated by histamine binding via H_1 and H_4 receptors on dendritic cells in conjunction with other chemokines: CCL17, thymus and activation regulated chemokine (TARC); CCL22; CCL3 macrophage inflammatory protein 1 α (MIP1α).

Histamine can have direct effects on T cells via H_1, H_2, and H_4 receptors which are expressed on $CD4^+$ and $CD8^+$ T cells (1). The effect of histamine on T-cell proliferation varies (1). It can increase T-cell proliferation by binding to H_1Rs and inhibit proliferation by binding to H_2Rs. Binding to H_2Rs has been demonstrated to inhibit T-cell production of IL-2, IL-4, IL-13, and interferon γ (1). However, the role of histamine in regulating T-cell proliferation is likely much more complicated than can be explained by the counter-regulatory roles of cytokine production (1).

■ H_1-RECEPTOR HISTAMINE ANTAGONISTS

First-Generation Agents

Structure

The first histamine antagonist was accidentally discovered in 1937 by Bovet and Staub who found that a drug originally being studied for its adrenergic antagonistic properties in guinea pigs also had potent antihistaminic activity (5). By 1942, safe and effective antihistamines developed for human use became available. Many of these agents, such as pyrilamine maleate, tripelennamine, and diphenhydramine, are still widely prescribed today (2,5).

The chemical structure of H_1-antagonists differs substantially from histamine (Figure 33.2) (1). Histamine is composed of a single imidazole heterocyclic ring linked to an ethylamine group, whereas H_1 antagonists consist of one or two heterocyclic or aromatic rings joined to a "linkage atom" (nitrogen, oxygen, or carbon) (Table 33.2) (1,5). The linkage atom is important in structurally differentiating these groups of agents, whereas the number of alkyl substitutions and heterocyclic or aromatic rings determines their lipophilic nature (1,5). The ethylenediamines, phenothiazines, piperazines, and piperidines all contain nitrogen as their linkage atom, whereas the ethanolamines contain oxygen and the alkylamines contain carbon as their linkage atoms (2,5).

Pharmacokinetics

Accurate pharmacokinetic data on first-generation antihistamines are now available in children and adults because of sensitive detection techniques, such as gas-liquid chromatography, mass spectrometry, and high-performance liquid chromatography (2,5,11). Generally, these compounds are rapidly absorbed orally or intravenously, resulting in peak serum concentrations within 2 to 3 hours and symptomatic relief within 30 minutes. They have large volumes of distribution, slow clearance rates, and are metabolized primarily by hydroxylation in the hepatic cytochrome P450 system. The vast majority of the parent drug is excreted as inactive metabolites in the urine within 24 hours of dosing. As a rule, serum half-lives ($t_{1/2}$) are longer in adults than they are for children. Their lipophilic nature

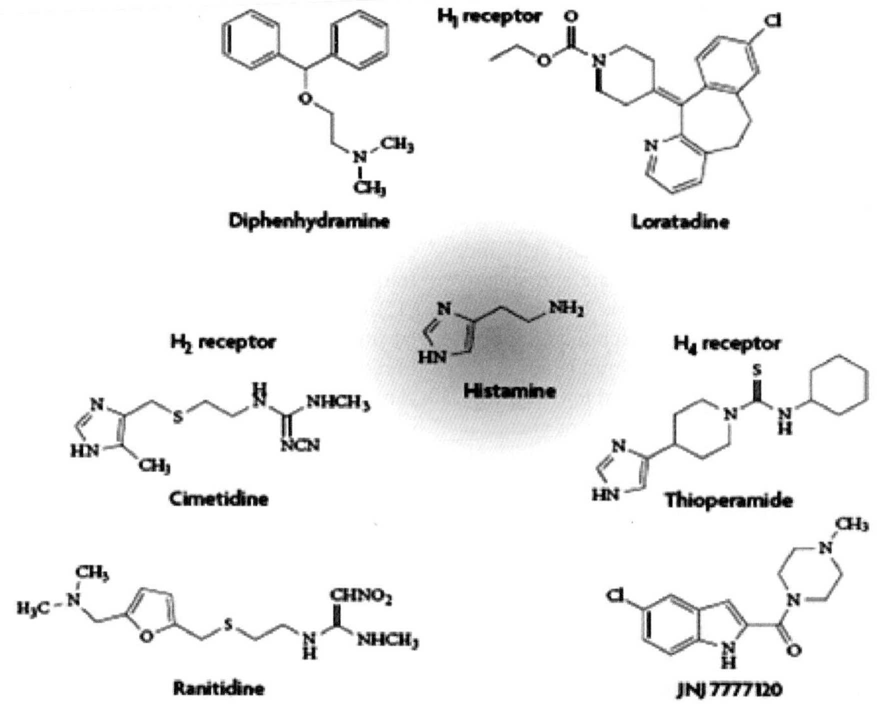

■ **FIGURE 33.2** Structure of histamine and representative histamine receptor ligands. (Reproduced with permission from Thurmond RL, Glefand EW, Dunford PJ. The role of histamine H_1 and H_4 receptors in allergic inflammation: the search for new antihistamines. *Nature Reviews/Drug Discovery* 2008;7:41–53.)

TABLE 33.2   CLASSIFICATION OF COMMON H₁-(FIRST-GENERATION) ANTAGONISTS[11]

STRUCTURAL CLASS/ LINKAGE ATOM	GENERIC NAME	TRADE NAME
Ethanolamines/"O" (oxygen)	Diphenhydramine hydrochloride	Benadryl
	Dimenhydrinate	Dramamine
	Clemastine fumorate	Tavist
Alkylamines/"C" (carbon)	Chlorpheniramine maleate	Chlortrimeton, Teldrin
	Brompheniramine maleate	Dimetane
	Dexchlorpheniramine maleate	Polaramine
	Dexbrompheniramine maleate	Drixoral*
	Triprolidine HCl	Actifed*
	Chlorpheniramine tannate/ pyrilamine tannate	Rynatan+
	Pheniramine maleate/ pyrilamine maleate	Triaminic TR+
Ethylenediamines/ "N"(nitrogen)	Tripelennamine HCl	Pyribenzamine HCl
	Tripelennamine citrate	PBZ
	Pyrilamine maleate	Allertoc
	Antazoline phosphate	Vasocon-A
Piperazines/"N"(nitrogen)	Hydroxyzine HCl	Atarax/Vistaril
	Meclizine HCl	Antivert/Bonine
Phenothiazines/ "N"(nitrogen)	Promethazine HCl	Phenergan
	Trimiprazine tartrate	Temaril
Piperidines/"N"(nitrogen)	Cyproheptadine HCl	Periactin
	Azatadine maleate	Optamine/Trinalin*

*With decongestant

+Combination ethylenediamine/alkylamine compound.

From Simons FER. H₁ receptor antagonists: chemical pharmacology and therapeutics. *J Allergy Clin Immunol* 1989;84:845, with permission.

allows them to cross the placenta and the blood–brain barrier. This access into the central nervous system is responsible for many of the side effects experienced by patients. These agents are also excreted in breast milk (2,5,11). Table 33.3 summarizes pharmacokinetic and pharmacodynamic data for the most commonly used first- and second-generation agents (2,5,14).

Pharmacodynamics

The first-generation H_1 antagonists are thought to compete with histamine for binding to histamine receptors. This competitive inhibition is believed to be reversible and, therefore, highly dependent on free drug plasma concentrations. As these agents are metabolized and excreted into the urine as inactive metabolites, the histamine receptors become desaturated, allowing surrounding histamine to bind. This mechanism emphasizes the need to instruct patients on using these agents on a regular basis to achieve a maximal therapeutic benefit (2,5,14). Experimental findings suggest another

mechanism for the effects of H_1R antagonists. It has been speculated that H_1R antagonists are "inverse agonists," implying that they could decrease constitutive receptor responses (15). The H_1R antagonist is described as having "negative intrinsic activity," despite the release of histamine from mast cells or basophils.

Pharmacy

Table 33.4 summarizes the pediatric and adult dosing schedules of commonly prescribed antihistamines (11,14,16). Prior to the availability of pharmacokinetic data, these agents were believed to have short half-lives which necessitated frequent dosing intervals to be effective (15). Since chlorpheniramine, brompheniramine, and hydroxyzine have serum half-lives greater than 20 hours in adults, it may be feasible to administer these agents only once or twice a day to achieve similar efficacy. The availability of sustained-release preparations of shorter half-life agents has also allowed less frequent

TABLE 33.3   PHARMACOKINETICS AND PHARMACODYNAMICS OF ORAL H₁-ANTAGONISTS IN HEALTHY YOUNG ADULTS

H1-ANTIHISTAMINE (METABOLITE)	T_{max}* AFTER A SINGLE DOSE (HR)	TERMINAL ELIMINATION HALF-LIFE	% ELIMINATION UNCHANGED IN URINE/FECES	DRUG-DRUG INTERACTION	ONSET, DURATION OF ACTION (HOURS)**	USUAL ADULT DOSE	DOSE ADJUSTMENT
First generation drug (±SD)							
Chlorpheniramine	2.8±0.8	27.9±8.7	–	Possible	3,24	4 mg tid to qid or 12 mg sustained release qd to bid	–
Dipenhydramine	1.7±1.0	9.2±2.5	–	Possible	2,12	25 mg to 50 mg up to qid	Hepatic impairment
Doxepin	2	13	–	Possible	–	25 mg to 50 mg up to tid	Hepatic impairment
Hydroxyzine	2.1±0.4	20.0±4.1	–	Possible	2,24	25 mg to 50 mg up to qid	Hepatic impairment
Second generation drug (±SD)							
Acrivastine	1.4±0.4	1.4–3.1	59/0	Unlikely	1,8	8 mg tid	–
Cetirizine	1.0±0.5	6.5–10	60/10	Unlikely	1,24	5 mg to 10 mg qd	Renal and hepatic impairment
Loratadine (descarboethoxy-loratadine)	1.2±0.3 (1.5±0.7)	7.8±4.2 (24±9.8)	Trace	Unlikely	2,24	10 mg qd	Hepatic impairment
Fexofenadine	2.6	14.4	12/80	Unlikely	2,24	60 mg bid, 120 qd or 180 qd	Renal impairment
Desloratadine	1–3	27	0	Unlikely	2,24	5 mg qd	Renal and hepatic impairment
Levocetirizine	0.8±0.5	7±1.5	86/13	Unlikely	1,24	5 mg qd	Renal and hepatic impairment
Second-generation drugs not approved in the US for oral use							
Ebastine (carebastine)	(2.6–5.7)	(10.3–19.3)	(75–90/0)	–	2,24	10 mg to 20 mg qd	Renal and hepatic impairment
Mizolastine	1.5	12.9	0.5/0	–	1,24	10 mg qd	–

From Thurmond RL, Glefand EW, Dunford PJ. The role of histamine H₁ and H₄ receptors in allergic inflammation: the search for new antihistamines. *Nat Rev Drug Discov* 2008;7:41–53. Simons FE. Advances in H₁-antihistamines. *N Engl J Med* 2004;351:2203–2217.

Simons FE. Antihistamines. In: Middleton E, Reed CE, Ellis EF, et al., eds. 5th ed. *Allergy Principles and Practice*. St Louis: CV Mosby; 1998:612–637.

Bid, twice daily; qd, daily; qid, four times daily; tid, three times daily

*T_{max} – time from oral intake to peak plasma concentration; **Onset and duration of action are based on wheal-and-flare studies

dosing, thereby improving patient compliance and minimizing side effects. It remains unclear whether treatment with sustained-released formulations of conventional agents with shorter half-lives offers any advantages over conventional agents with longer half-lives when dosed similarly (17).

Second-Generation Agents

Structure

The new H_1R selective, nonsedating class of antihistamines is categorized as second-generation. Their structural and pharmacokinetic profiles are responsible for their milder side effects and better tolerance among patients (2,5,18). Fexofenadine and loratadine are piperidines; cetirizine and levocetirizine are piperazines. Table 33.4 lists the chemical derivations of these agents in addition to other similar compounds undergoing investigation and Figure 33.2 illustrates their structures in comparison to first-generation agents (2,5,11,18). The five currently available second-generation agents in the United States are fexofenadine, loratadine, desloratidine, cetirizine, and levocetirizine.

Terfenadine and astemizole are no longer available in the United States because of safety concerns. Both of these agents were associated with serious interactions with drugs that were also metabolized by the liver cytochrome P450 enzyme 3A4, such as erythromycin and ketoconazole. This led to accumulation of the parent compound, which caused cardiac side effects such as torsade de pointes (2,5). Although this was a rare occurrence and dose-dependent, the advent of newer antihistamine drug metabolites that were not dependent on cytochrome oxidase metabolism made them expendable. Loratadine has not been demonstrated to induce these cardiovascular side effects most likely because it is metabolized by two isoenzymes (CYP2D6 and CYP3A4) (38,39). Therefore, loratidine can be safely taken with macrolide antibiotics (i.e., erythromycin) and oral antifungal agents (i.e., ketoconazole) (38). It should be emphasized that terfenadine and astemizole were very safe and effective drugs which were able to be used in the vast majority of clinical circumstances. Cetirizine, fexofenadine, levocetirizine, or desloratadine do not affect the Ik or cause QTc prolongation (2).

Post-surveillance monitoring was essential for identifying these severe adverse cardiac effects of terfenadine and astemizole. As a result, we have gained a better appreciation for the roles of pharmacodynamics/kinetics and metabolism in drug development and pharmacoepidemiology (18). In fact, investigations into the adverse drug reactions associated with the second-generation agent, terfenadine, have served as prototypes for the design of current long-term surveillance studies monitoring the safety of drugs in a variety of clinical situations.

Pharmacokinetics

The pharmacokinetic data available for second-generation agents are summarized in comparison to first-generation agents in Table 33.3 (2,5,14,19). Fexofenadine, loratadine, and cetirizine are well absorbed from the gastrointestinal tract, with peak serum concentrations occurring within 1 to 2 hours after oral administration (2,5,14,19). Data on humans on volumes of distribution for these agents are not available (2,5,14).

Loratadine is metabolized by the cytochrome P450 CYP3A4 enzyme to form descarbethoxyloratadine. However, if the CYP3A4 enzyme is inhibited, loratadine can be alternatively metabolized by the CYP2D6 enzyme, thereby preventing increased levels of the unmetabolized parent compound. Astemizole undergoes oxidative dealkylation, aromatic hydroxylation, and glucoronidation through the P450-CYP3A4 pathway to form several metabolites (18). The major active metabolite of astemizole is N-desmethylastemizole which has a half-life of 9.5 days. This metabolite, which does not have the same potential cytochrome oxidase enzyme interactions as its parent compound, underwent trials in the United States but has yet to be approved by the FDA. Terfenadine is exclusively metabolized by oxidation and oxidative N-dealkylation through the P450-CYP3A4 pathway to form an active acid metabolite, fexofenadine and an inactive metabolite (MDL 4829), respectively (5).

Cetirizine and fexofenadine are not extensively metabolized in the cytochrome P450 system and are therefore less likely to compete for elimination with other medications metabolized by the same cytochrome P450 enzyme systems. Over 50% of cetirizine is eliminated unchanged in the urine. Its elimination can be impaired in patients with hepatic and renal insufficiency. Most of fexofenadine is eliminated in the urine and feces unchanged. Its elimination can be also impaired in patients with renal insufficiency (2,5).

Desloratidine (Clarinex), a metabolite of loratidine, is completely metabolized whereas for Levocetirizine (Xyzal), the active enantiomer of cetirizine, 86% is excreted unchanged in the urine and 13% in the feces (2). Both drugs have low likelihood of drug–drug interactions but have to be dose-adjusted in patients with renal and hepatic impairment (Table 33.3) (2).

Pharmacodynamics

In contrast to first-generation agents, second-generation agents do not operate by simple competitive inhibition. Instead, these agents bind to and dissociate from H_1 receptors slowly in a noncompetitive fashion. They are not displaced from H_1Rs in the presence of high histamine concentrations (2). Although the second-generation antagonists are potent suppressors of the wheal-and-flare responses, this feature has not been established as a useful method for comparing the clinical

TABLE 33.4   FORMULATIONS AND DOSAGES OF REPRESENTATIVE H$_1$-RECEPTOR ANTAGONISTS.

H$_1$-RECEPTOR ANTAGONIST	FORMULATION	RECOMMENDED DOSE
First Generation		
Chlorpheniramine maleate (Chlor-Trimeton)	Tablets: 4 mg, 8 mg, 12 mg Syrup: 2.5 mg/5 mL Parenteral solution: 10 mg/mL	Adult: 8 mg to 12 mg 2x/day Child: 0.35 mg/kg/24 hours
Hydroxyzine hydrochloride (Atarax)	Capsules: 10 mg, 25 mg, 50 mg Syrup: 10 mg/5 mL	Adult: 25 mg to 50 mg 2x/day (or once a day at bedtime) Child: 2 mg/kg/24 hours
Diphenhydramine hydrochloride (Benadryl)	Capsules: 25 mg, 50 mg Elixir: 12.5 mg/5 mL Syrup: 6.25 mg/5 mL Parenteral solution: 50 mg/mL	Adult: 25 mg to 50 mg 3x/day Child: 5 mg/kg/24 hr
Second Generation		
Fexofenadine (Allegra)*	Tablets: 30 mg, 60 mg, 180 mg Liquid: 30 mg/5mL	Adult: 60 mg 2x/day or 180 mg/day Child: 7 to 12 years, 30 mg 2x/day
Loratadine (Claritin, Alavert)*	Tablets and reditabs: 10 mg PO or sublingual Syrup: 1 mg/mL	Adult: 10 mg/day Child: >3 years <30 kg = 5 mg PO/day; >3 years >30 kg = 10 mg PO/day)
Cetirizine hydrochloride (Zyrtec)	Tablets: 5 mg, 10 mg, 5 mg/mL syrup	Adult and children 6 to 12 years: 5 mg to 10 mg/day Children 2 to 5 years: 2.5 mg/day
Acrivastine (Semprex)*	Tablets: 8 mg	Adult: 8 mg 3x/day
Ketotifen fumarate (Zatidor)	Eye drops: 0.025%	Allergic conjunctivitis 1 drop in each eye 2x/day
Levocetirizine (Xyzal)	Tablets: 5 mg Liquid: 2.5 mg/5 mL	Adult: 5 mg/day Children 6-11: 2.5 mg/day
Desloratadine (Clarinex)	Tablets: 5 mg Syrup: 2.5 mg/5 mL	Adult: 5 mg/day Child: 2.5 mg/day
Azelastine hydrochloride (Astelin)	Nasal solution: 0.1% 0.137 mg/spray	Topical: 1 to 2 sprays/nostril/ 1 to 2x/day
Levocabastine hydrochloride (Livostin)	Eye drops: 0.05%	Topical: 1 drop in each eye 2 to 4x/day
Olopatadine hydrochloride (Patanol)	Eye drops: 0.1%	Topical: 1 to 2 drops each eye 2x/day
(Patanase)	Nasal solution: 0.6%	Topical: adults & children >11 yrs 2 sprays each nostril 2x/day

From *Physicians' Desk Reference.* 62nd ed. Montrale, NJ:Thomson Healthcare; http://www.PDR.net.

PO, by mouth

*Formulation available also with decongestant

potencies of the different agents currently available (20). Their lipophobic properties prevents them from crossing the blood–brain barrier, and thus their activity on H$_1$-receptors is restricted to the peripheral nervous system (2,21). They have very little affinity for non-H$_1$Rs (2,5).

Pharmacy

Second-generation antihistamines are only available as oral formulations (tablets and liquid). They all have convenient dosing once or twice daily (Table 33.5) (11,14). Studies have shown that a single dose of fexofenadine (180 mg) is equally effective as 60 mg twice a day at improving allergic rhinitis symptom scores and suppressing histamine-induced wheal-flare responses. All of the available second-generation antihistamines have comparable antihistaminic potency; however, a head-to-head comparison study between levocetirizine and desloratadine using an environmental exposure unit reported that levocetirizine had a more rapid onset

TABLE 33.5   CHEMICAL DERIVATIONS OF SECOND-GENERATION H_1-ANTAGONISTS AND DUAL-ACTION ANTIHISTAMINES

ANTIHISTAMINES	CHEMICAL FAMILY DERIVATION
Terfenadine* (Seldane)	Butyrophenone related to haloperidol
Astemizole* (Hismanal)	Aminopiperidinyl-benzimidazole
Loratadine (Claritin, Alavert)	Piperidine derivative of azatadine
Fexofenadine (Allegra)	Acid metabolite of terfenadine
Cetirizine (Zyrtec)	Cyclizine derivative of hydroxyzine
Acrivastine	Acrylic acid derivative of tripolidine
Mequitazine	Derivative of phenothiazine
Temelastine (SKF 93944)	Derivative of pyrilamine
Levocabastine (R 50547)	Stereoisomer of a cyclohexylpiperdine
Azelastine**	Phthalazinone derivative
Ketotifen**	Benzocycloheptathiophene
Oxatamide**	Related to cinnarizine
Norastemizole	Metabolite of astemizole
Levocetirizine	Isomer of cetirizine
Desloratadine	Metabolite of loratadine

*No longer available for clinical use in the United States

**Dual-action antihistamines

of action (1 hour versus 3 hours) and resulted in greater symptomatic relief after 24 hours compared to desloratidine (22).

■ DUAL-ACTION ANTIHISTAMINES

A number of agents currently not available for oral administration in the United States have been found to have a number of clinical effects in addition to their antihistaminic properties; examples are ketotifen, olopatadine, and azelastine. The derivation of these compounds are summarized in Table 33.4 (5,18). Although many of their mechanisms of action are unknown, they have been hypothesized to act on mast cells and basophils by preventing calcium influx or intracellular calcium release which interferes with activation and release of potent bioactive mediators (23). Azelastine has been demonstrated to inhibit superoxide generation by eosinophils and neutrophils which may represent one of its important anti-inflammatory mechanisms (24). These drugs can bind to H_1-receptors in a competitive and noncompetitive fashion (5,50–52). In addition to their calcium-antagonistic activity, they have variable amounts of antiserotonin, anticholinergic, and antileukotriene activities (18,24,25).

Pharmacokinetic information for oral antihistamines is summarized in Table 33.3 (2,16). Cetirizine, azelastine, and ebastine may have modest antiasthma effects that are not mediated through H_1Rs. These effects include inhibition of eosinophil chemotaxis, their adherence to endothelial cells, and their recruitment into the airways after allergen challenge (5,26). Olopatadine (Patanol, Pataday, Patanase) is a compound that has been demonstrated to have strong mast cell stabilization and H_1R-antagonistic properties; it is available as an ophthalmologic solution or a nasal spray (27).

■ OTHER AGENTS WITH ANTIHISTAMINE PROPERTIES

Tricyclic antidepressants originally synthesized for their antihistaminic properties in the 1950s, were never fully developed as antihistamines once they were recognized to have impressive antidepressant effects (18). Because doxepin has a very high H_1-receptor affinity, it has become an acceptable alternative agent for the treatment of chronic idiopathic urticaria (28).

■ CLINICAL USE OF ANTIHISTAMINES

The ideal H_1-receptor antagonist should provide complete and rapid relief of allergic symptoms, have a moderate duration of action, and be devoid of adverse effects. Unfortunately this type of agent does not exist (2). In general, first- and second-generation agents have fairly comparable antihistaminic effects in relieving common allergic symptoms, but all have poor decongestant capabilities (2,15). H_1 antagonists have proven useful in the treatment of allergic rhinitis, allergic conjunctivitis, atopic dermatitis, urticaria, asthma, and anaphylaxis (2,5,11,14). The treatment of these disorders is discussed in other chapters of this book.

Numerous studies have compared the antihistaminic efficacy of second-generation antagonists with that of first-generation antagonists in the treatment of allergic rhinitis. Results have uniformly shown these agents to be more effective than placebo, but just as effective as first-generation agents, such as chlorpheniramine, using comparable dosing schedules (29,30). Studies comparing second-generation agents to one another have found no dramatic differences in their clinical effects (29,31,32).

Studies have reported that topical eye preparations of H_1-antagonists are very effective for the treatment of allergic conjunctivitis (2,5,33). While many clinicians have their favorite regimens for chronic idiopathic urticaria, all of the first- and second-generation agents have been reported to be effective for patient treatment (34,35). Some types of urticaria respond better to a given antihistamine; cyproheptadine as the preferred treatment for cold-induced urticaria is an example (36).

A position paper from the American Academy of Allergy, Asthma and Immunology addressing the use of antihistamines in asthmatics has served to clarify controversy surrounding their use in patients with this disease (37). Previously it had been believed that the anticholinergic properties (i.e., dryness of the airways) of these antagonists could contribute to asthma exacerbations; it is now known that antihistamines, including some of the dual-action compounds, may actually serve a beneficial role in the treatment of asthma because of their bronchodilator and anti-inflammatory activities (24,38). Although, these agents are not considered first-line therapy for asthma, they are certainly not contraindicated in asthma patients who require them for concomitant allergic problems (38). The *Physicians' Desk Reference* has subsequently modified warnings stating they should be used cautiously in patients with concomitant asthma (16).

Histamine is increased during the early and late airway response after specific allergen provocation and during spontaneous asthma exacerbations. Histamine can exert many of the physiologic sequelae leading to asthma including cough by direct stimulation of the sensory nerves, smooth muscle constriction, mucous hypersecretion, increased permeability of the pulmonary epithelium, vasodilation, and extravasation of fluid at the postcapillary venule level (2,5). Many studies have shown that antihistamines are bronchoprotective

depending on the stimulus. For example, antihistamines attenuate bronchospasm induced by adenosine by 80%, but have little or no effect against methacholine, leukotriene, agonists, or neurokinin A (2,5,26,39).

Antihistamines serve as important adjuncts in the management of anaphylaxis, but should never replace the first-line therapy, which by general consensus is epinephrine (11). Antihistamines are commonly used to treat atopic dermatitis, but are no more effective than placebo (40). The sedating first-generation antihistamines such as diphenhydramine and hydroxyzine are often more effective than nonsedating agents for controlling pruritus because they allow the patient to sleep (40,41).

As with any other medication, antihistamines should be used cautiously during pregnancy (11). Long-term clinical experience using antihistamines during pregnancy has shown that tripelennamine, chlorpheniramine, and diphenhydramine cause no greater risk for birth defects than experienced by the normal population (42,43). Chlorpheniramine, diphenhydramine, loratadine, and cetirizine are all classified as Pregnancy Category B, indicating that no birth defects have been observed in animal models (16). Antihistamines are excreted in breast milk and therefore infants of nursing mothers who were taking first-generation antihistamines have been reported to experience drowsiness and irritability; the antihistamines loratadine, cetirizine, and fexofenadine have not been reported to cause symptoms in babies being breastfed by mothers on these medications (44).

Antihistamines are also useful in treating nonallergic disorders such as nausea, motion sickness, vertigo, extrapyramidal symptoms, anxiety, and insomnia (2,5). Studies evaluating these agents in the treatment of children with otitis media and upper respiratory infections have found they offer no significant benefit when used as solo agents (45,46). However, children with recurrent otitis media and a strong family history for allergies should be evaluated by an allergist to identify potential environmental triggers and implementation of treatment with avoidance measures and a combination of antihistamines, decongestants, cromolyn, and/or topical intranasal corticosteroids, to reduce inflammation and secretions which could be contributing to recurrent infections.

The use of second-generation over first-generation antagonists as first-line agents has previously been considered premature by many experts. If a first-generation agent is taken on a regular basis at bedtime, its sedative side effects are often well tolerated by many patients. Of equal importance is their substantially lower cost. However, since some patients do not tolerate these agents, they require treatment with second-generation nonsedating agents. These agents have been well documented to consistently cause less impairment of cognitive and psychomotor skills such as learning, reaction times, driving, memory, tracking, perception, recognition and processing (2,5). Impairment of these functions increases indirect costs associated with the treatment of allergic rhinitis including missed days from work or school and decreased concentration and performance while at work resulting in overall decreased productivity (2,5). The Joint Task Force on Practice Parameters for the diagnosis and management of rhinitis has recommended that second-generation, nonsedating antihistamines be first-line treatment of perennial and seasonal allergic rhinitis to avoid potential central nervous system side effects (47). However, if individuals have nonallergic rhinitis with or without an allergic component manifested as severe postnasal drainage, it may be necessary to use first-generation antihistamines with or without decongestants to take advantage of their anticholinergic drying effects. In these situations, it is best to dose the sedating antihistamine at bedtime as the sedative carry-over effect the following morning of these agents does not usually cause impaired cognitive performance. In general, it is important to educate the patient about the advantages and disadvantages of sedating and nonsedating antihistamines in the management of specific allergic diseases. Use of either or both agents should be appropriately tailored to the patient's individual needs and tolerance.

■ ADVERSE EFFECTS OF H₁-ANTAGONISTS

The numerous side effects of first-generation antihistamines have been attributed to their affinity for P glycoprotein and their lipophilicity resulting in the ability to cross the blood–brain barrier (48). In addition, they are relatively nonselective resulting in anticholinergic activity (49). The side effects of first-generation antihistamines vary in character and severity among the structural subclasses. For instance, the ethylenediamines (PBZ) have more pronounced gastrointestinal side effects, whereas the ethanolamines such as diphenhydramine have increased antimuscarinic activity and cause a greater degree of sedation in patients. The alkylamines such as chlorpheniramine have milder central nervous system (CNS) side effects and are generally the best tolerated among the first-generation agents (50).

Specific side effects of first-generation agents include impaired cognition, slowed reaction times, decreased alertness, confusion, dizziness, tinnitus, anorexia, nausea, vomiting, epigastric distress, diarrhea, and constipation. Associated anticholinergic side effects include dry mouth, blurred vision, and urinary retention; first-generation agents also potentiate the effects of benzodiazepines and alcohol (11,50). Cyproheptadine, a piperidine derivative, has the effect of causing weight gain in some patients (14).

Intentional and accidental overdose, although uncommon, has been reported with these drugs (11).

Adults usually manifest symptoms of CNS depression, whereas children may exhibit an excitatory response manifested as hyperactivity, irritability, insomnia, visual hallucinations, and seizures. Even with normal doses, it is not unusual for children to experience a paradoxic excitatory reaction. Malignant cardiac arrhythmias have been known to occur with overdoses, emphasizing the need to act expeditiously to counteract the toxic effect of these agents (11,50). Caution should be exercised using antihistamines in elderly patients or in those with liver dysfunction because of their slower clearance rates and increased susceptibility to overdose (11). Because these agents are secreted in breast milk, caution should be exercised using these agents in lactating women (44, 50).

The second-generation agents have substantially fewer associated side effects. Sedation and other side effects associated with first-generation agents, have been noted to occur, but generally at a rate similar to placebo (11). No longer available in the United States, terfenadine and astemizole were very occasionally associated with torsades de points. Newer second-generation antihistamines, such as fexofenadine and loratadine, have not been reported to cause cardiotoxicity (5). Cetirizine is considered a low-sedating antihistamine but is generally well tolerated by most patients, especially if dosed at bedtime. The newer second-generation antihistamines desloratadine and levocetirizine have thus far been demonstrated to be very safe and well tolerated.

■ TOLERANCE

Tolerance to antihistamines is a common concern of patients taking these agents chronically. This phenomenon has been speculated to occur due to autoinduction of hepatic metabolism, resulting in an accelerated clearance rate of the antihistamine. However, studies have failed to confirm this hypothesis and most reports of tolerance to antihistamines are now believed to be secondary to patient noncompliance because of intolerable drug side effects or breakthrough symptoms due to severity of disease (18). Short-term studies evaluating tolerance to second-generation agents have found no change in their therapeutic efficacy after 6 to 8 weeks of regular use (11,18). Studies up to 12 weeks found no evidence that second-generation agents cause autoinduction of hepatic metabolism leading to rapid excretion rates and drug tolerance. The clinical efficacy of these agents in the skin and treatment of allergic rhinitis does not decrease with chronic use (50).

■ SYMPATHOMIMETICS

Many of the first-generation antihistamines, and now second-generations have been formulated in combination with decongestants. The decongestants currently used in most preparations include phenylephrine hydrochloride or pseudoephedrine hydrochloride. These agents have saturated benzene rings without 3- or 4-hydroxyl groups, which is the reason for their weak α-adrenergic effect, improved oral absorption, and duration of action. Compared with other decongestants, these agents have less effect on blood pressure and are less apt to cause CNS excitation manifested as insomnia or agitation. Phenylpropanolamine was removed from the U.S. market because of concerns regarding hemorrhagic stroke in women taking this medication. Pseudoephedrine, the most effective of the α-adrenergic agonists, has been designated as a Schedule V over-the-counter drug product because of issues with individuals using this compound to manufacture methamphetamines; several studies have reported fewer visits to the emergency department for methamphetamine-related burn incidents due to illicit lab fires since this law went into effect [51]. Phenylephrine is a weaker α-adrenergic agonist available in many over-the-counter cough and cold formulations. Recently, questions have been raised regarding safety of these agents in children; in addition, their efficacy in clinical trials at the dose available in these preparations is unclear [52].

■ H$_2$-ANTAGONISTS

H$_2$-histamine antagonists were first synthesized in 1969 for the purpose of developing a drug capable of inhibiting gastric acid secretion [53]. These agents have a close structural resemblance to histamine, because most are simple modifications of the histamine molecule itself [54]. Histamine's affinity for H$_1$-receptors is ten-fold greater than for H$_2$-receptors [54]. H$_2$-antagonists are weak bases with water-soluble hydrochloride salts and tend to be less lipophilic than H$_1$-antagonists [5]. Cimetidine (Tagamet, SmithKline, Philadelphia, PA) was introduced to the United States in 1982 and has been proven safe and effective in the treatment of peptic ulcer disease [54]. Cimetidine and oxmetidine resemble the earliest agents structurally, as they have an imidazole ring similar to histamine's structure. The newer agents vary structurally by having different internal ring components. For example, ranitidine (Zantac, Glaxo, Research Triangle Park, NC) has a furan ring, whereas famotidine (Pepcid, Merck Sharp & Dohme, West Point, PA), and nizatidine (Axid, Eli Lilly and Company, Indianapolis, IN) are composed of thiozole rings [54]. H$_2$-antagonists act primarily by competitive inhibition of the H$_2$-receptors, with the exception of famotidine, which works noncompetitively [54]. The four available agents all have potent H$_2$-antagonistic properties; they vary in their pharmacokinetics and adverse effects such as drug interactions. Several H$_2$–antagonists are now available over the counter [5,54].

Numerous studies have been undertaken to examine the clinical utility of H$_2$-antagonists in allergic and immunologic diseases. Although several studies report these agents have promising immunologic changes *in vitro*, these findings have not been substantiated clinically [5,55]. Generally, H$_2$-antagonists have limited or no utility in treating allergen-induced and histamine-mediated diseases in man [55]. One notable exception to this rule may be their use in combination with H$_1$-antagonists in the treatment of chronic idiopathic urticaria [56]. The studies evaluating the H$_2$-antagonists' clinical efficacy in allergic and immunologic disorders are extensively reviewed elsewhere [5,54].

■ H$_3$-RECEPTOR ANTAGONISTS

H$_3$-receptors act as presynaptic autoreceptors that inhibit synthesis and release of histamine from neurons in the CNS. H$_3$-receptors also exist as receptors on nonhistaminergic neurons, regulating the release of neurotransmitters such as dopamine and noradrenaline. Subsequent studies have been directed toward finding a selective H$_3$-antagonist. Two such agents have been synthesized: JNJ7777120 and thioperamide, a derivative of imidazolylpiperidine. They both have demonstrated H$_3$-receptor selectivity, but are available only for experimental use [10].

■ H$_4$-RECEPTOR ANTAGONISTS

The H$_4$ receptor is primarily expressed on immunologic cells such as eosinophils, mast cells, T cells, and dendritic cells. The H$_4$ receptor is approximately 35% homologous with the H$_3$ receptor. Many of the known H$_3$ agonists and antagonists also bind the H$_4$ receptor; examples include thioperamide and JNJ7777120.

■ CONCLUSIONS

The discovery of H$_1$-receptor antagonists has proven to be a significant breakthrough in the treatment of allergic diseases. Chemical modifications of these early agents have yielded the second-generation antihistamines, which are of equal antagonistic efficacy but with fewer side effects. Newer nonsedating antihistamines, which are metabolites or isomers of existing agents, are now under development. H$_2$-receptor antagonists have been found extremely useful in the treatment of peptic ulcer disease. However, they have not proven to be very useful in the treatment of allergic and immunologic disorders in humans. Due to better side effect profiles, newer, selective nonsedating H$_1$-antagonists and dual-action antihistamines have provided therapeutic advantages over first-generation agents for long-term management of allergic diseases including rhinitis, conjunctivitis, and urticaria.

■ REFERENCES

1. Thurmond RL, Glefand EW, Dunford PJ. The role of histamine H_1 and H_4 receptors in allergic inflammation: the search for new antihistamines. *Nat Rev Drug Discov.* 2008;7:41–53.

2. Simons FE. Advances in H_1-antihistamines. *N Engl J Med.* 2004;351:2203–2217.

3. Windaus A, Vogt W. Syntheses des imidazolylathylamines. *Ber Dtsch Chem Ges.* 1907;3:3691.

4. Fried JP, ed. *Dorland's Illustrated Medical Dictionary.* Philadelphia: WB Saunders; 1974.

5. Simons FE. Antihistamines. In: Middleton E, Reed CE, Ellis EF, et al., eds. 5th ed. *Allergy Principles and Practice.* St Louis: CV Mosby; 1998:612–637.

6. Dale HH, Laidlaw PP. The physiological action of α-imidazolylethylamine. *J Physiol.* 1910;41:318–344.

7. Pearce FL. Biological effects of histamine: an overview. *Agents Actions.* 1991;33:4–7.

8. Ash ASF, Schild HO. Receptors mediating some actions of histamine. *BR J Pharmacol Chemother.* 1966;27:427–439.

9. Black JW, Duncan WAM, Durant CJ, et al. Definition and antagonism of histamine H_2 receptors. *Nature.* 1972;236:385–390.

10. Arrang JM, Garbarg M, Lancelot JC, et al. Highly potent and selective ligands for histamine H_3 receptors. *Nature.* 1987;327:117–123.

11. Simons FER. H_1 receptor antagonists: clinical pharmacology and therapeutics. *J Allergy Clin Immunol.* 1989;84:845–861.

12. Sugata Y, Okano M, Fujiwara T, et al. Histamine H4 receptor agonists have more activities than H4 agonism in antigen-specific human T-cell responses. *Immunology.* 2007;121:266–275.

13. Akdis CA, Simms FE. Histamine receptors are hot in immunopharmacology. *Eur J Pharmacol.* 2006;533:69–76.

14. Simons FER, Simons KJ. The pharmacology and use of H_1-receptor-antagonist drugs. *N Engl J Med.* 1994;330:1663–1670.

15. Bakker RA, Nicholas NW, Smith TT, et al. In vitro pharmacology of clinically used central nervous system-active drugs as inverse H_1 receptor agonists. *J Pharmacol Exp Ther.* 2007;322: 172–179.

16. *Physicians' Desk Reference.* 62nd ed. Montrale, NJ:Thomson Healthcare; http://www.PDR.net.

17. Kotzan JA, Vallner JJ, Stewart JT, et al. Bioavailability of regular and controlled release chlorpheniramine products. *J Pharm Sci.* 1982;71:919.

18. Simons FER. Advances in H_1 antihistamines. *N Engl J Med.* 2004;351:2203–2217.

19. Honig PK, Wortham DC, Lazarev A, et.al. Grapefruit juice alters the systemic bioavailability and cardiac repolarization of terfenadine in poor metabolizers of terfenadine. *J Clin Pharmacol.* 1996;36:345–351.

20. Simons FE, McMillan JL, Simons KJ. A double-blind, single-dose, crossover comparison of cetirizine, terfenadine, loratadine, astemizole and chlorpheniramine versus placebo: suppressive effects on histamine-induced wheals and flares during 24 hours in normal subjects. *J Allergy Clin Immunol.* 1990;86:540–547.

21. Roth T, Roehrs T, Koshorck G, et al. Sedative effects of antihistamines. *J Allergy Clin Immunol.* 1987;80:94–98.

22. Day JH, Briscoe MP, Rafeiro E, et al. Comparative clinical efficacy, onset and duration of action of levocetirizine and desloratadine for symptoms of seasonal allergic rhinitis in subjects evaluated in the Environmental Exposure Unit (EEU). *Int J Clin Pract.* 2004;58:109–118.

23. Tasaka K, Mio M, Okamoto M. Intracellular calcium release induced by histamine releasers and its inhibition by antiallergic drugs. *Ann Allergy.* 1986;56:464–469.

24. Bernstein JA. Azelastine hydrochloride: a review of pharmacology, pharmacokinetics, clinical efficacy and tolerability. *Curr Med Res Opin.* 2007; 23:2441–2452.

25. Ohmori K, Ishii H, Kubota T, et al. Inhibitory effects of oxatomide on several activities of SRS-A and synthetic leukotrienes in guinea pigs and rats. *Arch Int Pharmacodyn Ther.* 1985;275:139–150.

26. Roquet A, Dahlen B, Kumlin M, et.al. Combined antagonism of leukotrienes and histamine produces predominant inhibition of allergen induced early and late phase airway obstruction in asthmatics. *Am J Respir Crit Care Med.* 1997;155:1856–1863.

27. Rosenwasser LJ, O'Brien T, Weyne J. Mast cell stabilization and antihistamine effects of olopatadine ophthalmic solution: a review of

pre-clinical and clinical research. *Curr Med Res Opin.* 2005;21:1377–1387.

28. Goldsobel AB, Rohr AS, Siegel SC, et al. Efficacy of doxepin in the treatment of chronic idiopathic urticaria. *J Allergy Clin Immunol.* 1986;78:867–873.

29. Holgate ST, Canonica GW, Simons FE, et al. Consensus Group on New Generation Antihistamines (CONGA): present status and recommendations. *Clin Exp Allergy.* 2003;33:1305–1342.

30. Theunissen EL, Vermeeren A, Ramaekers JG. Repeated-dose effects of mequitazine, cetirizine and dexchlorpheniramine on driving and psychomotor performance. *Br J Clin Pharmacol.* 2005;61:79–86.

31. Frossard N. Pharmacodynamics of H_1 antihistamines: from concept to reality. *Clin Exp Allergy Rev.* 2003;3:87–89.

32. Simons FE. Comparative pharmacology of H_1 antihistamines: clinical relevance. *Am J Med.* 2002;16:38S–46S.

33. Bielory L. Ocular allergy treatment. *Immunol Allergy Clin North Am.* 2008;28:189–224.

34. Black AK, Greaves MW. Antihistamines in urticaria and angioedema. *Clin Allergy Immunol.* 2002 17:249–286.

35. Jauregui I, Ferrer M, Montoro J, et al. Antihistamines in the treatment of chronic urticaria. *J Investig Allergol Clin Immunol.* 2007; 17(Suppl 2): 41S–52S.

36. Bentley B. Cold-induced urticaria and angioedema: diagnosis and management. *Am J Emerg Med.* 1993;11:43–46.

37. Sly MR, Kemp JP, Anderson JA, et al. Position statement: the use of antihistamines in patients with asthma. *J Allergy Clin Immunol.* 1988;82:481.

38. Lordan JL, Holgate ST. H_1-antihistamines in asthma. *Clin Allergy Immunol.* 2002;17:221–248.

39. Phillips GD, Rafferty P, Beasley R, et al. Effect of oral terfenadine on the broncho constrictor response to inhaled histamine and adenosine 5'-monophospate in non-atopic asthma. *Thorax.* 1987;42:939–945.

40. Klein PA, Clark RA. An evidence-based review of the efficacy of antihistamines in relieving pruritus in atopic dermatitis. *Arch Dermatol.* 1999;135:1522–1525.

41. Hanifin JM, Cooper KD, Ho VC, et al. Guidelines for the care of atopic dermatitis. *J Am Acad Dermatol.* 2004;50:391–404.

42. Gilbert C, Mazzotta P, Loebstein R, et al. Fetal safety of drugs used in the treatment of allergic rhinitis: a critical review. *Drug Saf.* 2005;28:707–719.

43. Keles N. Treatment of allergic rhinitis during pregnancy. *Am J Rhinol.* 2004;18:23–28.

44. Incaudo GA, Takach P. The diagnosis and treatment of allergic rhinitis during pregnancy and lactation. *Immunol Allergy Clin North Am.* 2006;26:137–154.

45. Sutter AI, Lemiengre M, Campbell H, et al. Antihistamines for the common cold. *Cochrane Database Syst Rev.* 2003;3:CD001267.

46. Griffin GH, Flynn C, Bailey RE, et al. Antihistamines and/or decongestants for otitis media with effusion (OME) in children. *Cochrane Database Syst Rev.* 2006;4:CD003423.

47. Wallace DV, Dykewicz MS, Bernstein DI, et al. The diagnosis and management of rhinitis: an updated practice parameter. *J Allergy Clin Immunol.* 2008;122:S1–S84.

48. Montoro J, Sastre J, Bartra J, et al. Effect of H_1 antihistamines upon the central nervous system. *J Investig Allergol Clin Immunol.* 2006;16(Suppl 2):24S–28S.

49. Liu H, Farley JM. Effects of first and second generation antihistamines on muscarinic induced mucus gland cell ion transport. *BMC Pharmacology.* 2005;5:8.

50. Simons FE. H_1 receptor antagonists. Comparative tolerability and safety. *Drug Saf.* 1994;10:350–380.

51. Burke BA, Lewis RW, Latenser BA, et al. Pseudoephedrine legislation decreases methamphetamine laboratory-related burns. *J Burn Care Res.* 2008;29:138–140.

52. Traynor K. Nonprescription cold remedies unsafe for young children, FDA advisers say. *Am J Health Syst Pharm.* 2007;64:2408–2410.

53. Duncan WAM, Parsons ME. Reminiscences of the development of cimetidine. *Gastroenterology.* 1980;78:620–625.

54. Lipsy RJ, Fennerty B, Fagan TC. Clinical review of histamine₂ receptor antagonists. *Arch Intern Med.* 1990;150:745–751.

55. Parsons ME, Ganellin CK. Histamine and its receptors. *Br J Pharmacol.* 2006;147:S127–S135.

56. Harvey RP, Schocket AL. The effect of H_1 and H_2 blockade on cutaneous histamine response in man. *J Allergy Clin Immunol.* 1980;65:136–139.

β Agonists

JACQUELINE A. PONGRACIC

Since bronchoconstriction has long been regarded to be a hallmark of asthma, bronchodilation has become an important component of asthma therapy. Among the various agents available for this purpose, β-adrenergic agonists have played a prominent role. Short-acting β agonists are the mainstay of rescue therapy. The more recent availability of long-acting preparations has changed the way β agonists may be used.

■ HISTORICAL PERSPECTIVES

Sympathomimetic agents have been used for asthma for thousands of years. Ephedrine, which is found in Ma huang (*Ephedra sinica*), has been used by the Chinese since 3000 BC. Because its therapeutic benefits were noted to wane over time, while adverse reactions such as central nervous system stimulation increased, new and improved sympathomimetic agents were highly desired. Subcutaneous injections of adrenaline were used in the early 1900s but were also associated with unacceptable side effects. It was only 60 years ago that the first β-adrenergic agonist, isoproterenol, appeared on the scene (1). As a potent, nonselective β agonist, isoproterenol was associated with many side effects but fewer than occurred with adrenaline. These toxicity issues and the identification of α and β adrenoreceptors led to the development of the β_2-selective agonist, albuterol, in the 1960s. Since then, a variety of other β_2-selective agonists have been developed as well. Pirbuterol, terbutaline, and fenoterol are short, rapidly acting β agonists (SABA). Fenoterol is potent, but less β_2 selective than the others, and it is not available in the United States. In response to continued concerns about side effects, further examination and refinements in these molecules have led to the production of an enantiomeric form of albuterol, called *levalbuterol*. Long-acting β agonists (LABA) have also become available. Salmeterol and formoterol represent this newer class of β-adrenergic agonists.

■ MECHANISM OF ACTION AND PHARMACOLOGY

β-Adrenergic agonists exert their effects through interactions with membrane-bound receptors. Three types of β-adrenergic receptors have been characterized: β_1, β_2, and β_3. The β_1 receptors predominate in the heart, whereas β_3 receptors are found in adipose tissue. The β_2 receptors are ubiquitous; in the lung, residing in smooth muscle, submucosal glands, epithelium, and alveoli as well as in smooth muscle and endothelium of the pulmonary arterial system. Radioligand binding studies and computed tomographic imaging have shown that these receptors are present in greater concentrations in the central lung and alveoli. There are β_2 receptors also found on a variety of inflammatory cells commonly associated with asthma, including mast cells, macrophages, neutrophils, eosinophils, and lymphocytes. β_2 adrenoceptors are present in very high concentrations in airway smooth muscle, and less so in epithelial cells, endothelial cells, type II cells, and mast cells.

The β_2-adrenergic receptor, illustrated in Figure 34.1, is a member of a superfamily of 7-transmembrane G-protein–coupled receptors encoded by a gene on chromosome 5 (2). Until recently, a lock-and-key mechanism by which β agonists engaged the receptor was hypothesized. However, it appears that β_2-adrenergic receptors vacillate between inactive and active states (3) and β agonists may shift the equilibrium to favor the activated state. An agonist drug, such as albuterol binds to the extracellular domain of the receptor and induces a conformational change so that the intracellular regions of the receptor may bind to a G protein. As a result, adenylyl cyclase is activated and causes an increase in cyclic adenosine monophosphate (cAMP). cAMP acts as a second messenger by activating protein kinase A, which causes phosphorylation with resultant relaxation of airway smooth muscle. cAMP also augments intracellular calcium ion stores leading to relaxation of airway smooth muscle.

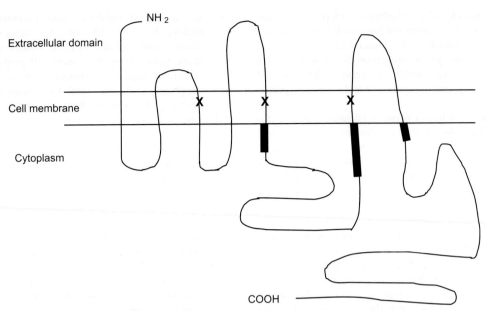

■ FIGURE 34.1 The structure of the human β$_2$-adrenergic receptor. Regions involved in G protein coupling are bolded. Sites involved in β$_2$-agonist binding are marked as X.

Review of the development of β adrenergic agents highlights the functional differences among these medications. The early β agonists were initially modeled after adrenaline and noradrenaline. Structural modifications of these catecholamines were noted to impart functional changes in these compounds. For example, substitutions in the hydroxyl groups on the benzene ring reduce inactivation by the gastrointestinal enzyme catechol *O*-methyltransferase, as is the case for albuterol, terbutaline, metaproterenol, and fenoterol. These specific alterations increase duration of action and allow for oral administration. Modifications of the side-chain increase selectivity for the β$_2$ receptor, reduce inactivation by monoamine oxidase, and extend duration of action, as is seen for albuterol, terbutaline, pirbuterol, and procaterol. Salmeterol and formoterol have much larger lipophilic side chains that account for their long-lasting β$_2$-selective effects. Despite their structural and functional similarities, salmeterol and formoterol have different mechanisms of action at the cellular level (4). Salmeterol, which is highly lipophilic, is rapidly taken up into the cell after which it gradually diffuses out to interact with the receptor. Its side chain engages with an exocite of the receptor acting as an anchor to prevent dissociation of the agonist from the receptor while the rest of the molecule engages and disengages the active site of the receptor like a hinge (2).

The response to agonists also varies by polymorphisms of the β$_2$-adrenoceptor. There are two genes for the receptor so that individuals may be homozygous or heterozygous for any given polymorphism. Studies have found nine distinct polymorphisms characterized by a single base alteration. Some, but not all, studies have shown that mutations at codons 16 and 27 are associated with altered bronchodilator responses (5,6) and pulmonary function (7,8).

■ SHORT-ACTING β AGONISTS

SABAs induce relaxation of airway smooth muscle quickly. For example, albuterol produces bronchodilation within 5 minutes of inhalation. Its pharmacologic effects peak after 60 to 90 minutes and last 4 to 6 hours. Because β$_2$ receptors are also found on a variety of inflammatory cells, investigators have postulated that β$_2$ agonists may also possess anti-inflammatory effects. Albuterol inhibits histamine release from activated mast cells *in vitro* (9). Inhibitory effects have also been demonstrated on eosinophils (10–13), lymphocytes (14–16), and neutrophils (17,18). *In vivo* studies of albuterol have failed to uphold an anti-inflammatory effect and, in fact, show a potentiated late-phase response, elevation in sputum eosinophils, and increased number of activated eosinophils in bronchial biopsy specimens (19,20).

Until recently, all SABAs in clinical use have been racemic mixtures of two mirror-image stereoisomers, called R and S, in equal parts. (R)-isomers induce bronchodilator responses, whereas (S)-isomers do not. Studies performed in humans have demonstrated that regular use of racemic albuterol is associated with increases in airway responsiveness to allergen (19,21). *In vitro*, (R)-albuterol induces bronchodilation in isolated human trachea (22), whereas (S)-albuterol augments contractile responses to histamine and leukotriene C4 in bronchial tissue (23). In isolated smooth muscle cells, (S)-albuterol increases calcium influx (24,25). (S)-albuterol has much less affinity for β_2 receptors than does (R)-albuterol (26). (S)-albuterol appears to have proinflammatory effects as well, with evidence of eosinophil activation demonstrated through elevations in superoxide and eosinophil peroxidase (27,28).

In vivo, differences between (R)-albuterol and (S)-albuterol are also evident. (S)-albuterol is metabolized 10 times more slowly than (R)-albuterol (29–31) and is detectable in the blood stream for up to 24 hours after administration of racemic albuterol (30). Formulations of (R)-albuterol, called levalbuterol, are available for nebulized and metered-dose inhaler (MDI) administration. The safety and efficacy of levalbuterol in adults and children has been well documented. A multicenter randomized study in 362 teenagers and adults with moderate-to-severe asthma reported that 0.63 mg of levalbuterol was as effective as 2.5 mg of racemic albuterol over 4 weeks of administration (32). Because of the flat dose–response curve, this study failed to show a significant difference with regard to efficacy between levalbuterol and racemic albuterol. Similarly, there was no difference in dose-dependent side effects between levalbuterol and racemic albuterol. In a smaller study of levalbuterol and racemic albuterol in children, lower doses of levalbuterol were as effective as 2.5 mg of racemic albuterol, and all treatments were equally well tolerated in terms of side effects (33). Other studies have addressed whether levalbuterol has a bronchoprotective effect. Using methacholine challenge, a small randomized, double-blind, placebo-controlled study showed a small, sustained bronchoprotective effect for levalbuterol as compared with (S)-albuterol and racemic albuterol (34). A small increase in airway hyperresponsiveness was seen for (S)-albuterol. Other investigations have not confirmed this finding (35,36), yet regular treatment with (R)-albuterol and racemic albuterol results in partial loss of bronchoprotection after methacholine challenge (36).

■ LONG-ACTING β AGONISTS

LABAs provide bronchodilation for 12 hours, much longer than that seen with SABAs. Interestingly, salmeterol and formoterol differ in time to onset of action. Salmeterol effects are seen in 10 to 20 minutes, whereas formoterol actions begin in as little as 1 to 3 minutes. In addition to their bronchodilatory properties, LABA have bronchoprotective effects. This has been shown for bronchoprovocation with methacholine (37–39), histamine (40), exercise (41), hyperventilation (42,43), sulfur dioxide (44), and distilled water (45).

Salmeterol and formoterol also inhibit allergen-induced early- and late-phase airway responses and accompanying bronchial hyperresponsiveness (46–48).

This has led to speculation about potential anti-inflammatory effects by LABA. *In vitro* studies support these effects. Salmeterol inhibits antigen-induced mediator release from human lung mast cell preparations (49) and thromboxane B_2 synthesis from human alveolar macrophages (50). Salmeterol and formoterol also inhibit neutrophil leukotriene B4 production (51). Several *in vivo* studies of salmeterol in humans have documented no anti-inflammatory effect as measured by bronchoalveolar lavage (52,53), bronchial biopsy (54), sputum or circulating eosinophils or eosinophilic cationic protein (ECP) (55–57), or urinary leukotriene E4 excretion (58), despite improvements in peak expiratory flow rates and decreased need for rescue therapy. Other studies have documented reductions in sputum eosinophils (59), ECP in bronchoalveolar lavage (60), serum ECP (61), and airway mucosal mast cells and eosinophils (62). Most evidence suggests that despite their anti-inflammatory effects *in vitro*, LABA do not exhibit significant anti-inflammatory effects *in vivo*. When used in combination with inhaled corticosteroids, LABAs do not appear to offer additional anti-inflammatory effects in most studies (63–65). It is important to note that these agents do not appear to enhance airway inflammation.

■ CLINICAL USE OF β AGONISTS IN ASTHMA

Current national guidelines promote the regular daily use of anti-inflammatory, or "controller," agents for persistent asthma (66). Despite the use of controller therapy, some individuals may develop breakthrough symptoms or acute exacerbations of their disease. SABAs are recommended for the relief of acute asthma symptoms and also for prevention of exercise-induced bronchospasm. SABAs are preferred over other bronchodilators, such as methylxanthines and anticholinergic agents, because SABAs exhibit faster onset of action without significant adverse effects when used appropriately. These guidelines also suggest that the frequency with which SABAs are needed for symptom relief serves as a useful marker of asthma control and of the need for adjusting anti-inflammatory therapy. In fact, SABA prescription refills have been shown to be a good marker for asthma morbidity, with refills typically occurring on or the day after asthma-related emergency department visits, and hospitalizations (67).

SABA may also be used to confirm the diagnosis of asthma by establishing whether reversible bronchospasm exists (66).

SABA are also effective for the prevention of symptoms, such as exercise-induced bronchospasm, when used 5 to 15 minutes before exercise (68,69). Given their short duration of action, SABA are not well suited for the prevention of nocturnal symptoms.

Similar to other SABAs, levalbuterol should be used for rescue and prevention of exercise-induced bronchoconstriction but not for maintenance therapy. Randomized controlled trials of levalbuterol versus albuterol conducted in the emergency department have shown conflicting results for superiority of levalbuterol on hospitalization rates (70), time to discharge (71), and clinical improvement (72). Levalbuterol may be a suitable alternative for patients who experience intolerable side effects from racemic β agonists although there does not appear to be a clear consistent advantage in the literature. Whether levalbuterol offers superior efficacy over racemic albuterol remains hotly debated.

The regular daily use of SABAs is generally not recommended, but this has been a source of controversy for many years. Although some reports maintain that routine use of SABAs is safe and effective, other studies have reported detrimental effects. Several studies have demonstrated a reduction in forced expiratory volume in 1 second (FEV_1) after regular SABA use (73–78). Increases in bronchial reactivity have also been noted (73–81). Although some prospective studies of regular inhaled SABA use failed to demonstrate deterioration in asthma (82–85), other studies have shown deleterious effects in as little as 3 weeks (78). Because there has been no evidence that regular use of SABAs improves long-term asthma control, their regular use is not advised. Consensus panel reports clearly state that antiinflammatory treatment should be considered when β agonists are needed on a frequent, regular basis (66).

The situation appears to be quite different for LABAs. In light of their slower onset of action, LABAs are not recommended for relief of acute symptoms (86). This class should be used daily to improve asthma control. LABAs block exercise-induced bronchoconstriction (87,88). Regular LABA provides protection of exercise-induced symptoms for up to 5 hours (66). Given their onset of action, they should be administered at least 30 to 60 minutes before exercise (89) but frequent use for prevention of exercise symptoms is not recommended (66). This class is also better suited for control of nocturnal asthma (86,89). Despite the ability to prevent such symptoms, LABAs should be used as adjunctive therapy to inhaled corticosteroids and should not be used as monotherapy (66). In randomized control trials of inhaled corticosteroid versus salmeterol, the salmeterol group experienced more asthma exacerbations and treatment failures (90–92). In fact, many studies have demonstrated that the combined use of inhaled corticosteroids with salmeterol or formoterol is associated with improvements in pulmonary function and symptom control (93–100). Moreover, a recent *Cochran Review* confirmed that adding LABA to inhaled corticosteroids reduces the risk of asthma exacerbations compared to using similar doses of inhaled corticosteroids (101). Another such review showed that the combination of LABA and inhaled corticosteroid allows for the use of lower doses of inhaled corticosteroid to maintain asthma control (102). Based on the benefits demonstrated in these studies, LABAs should be used in conjunction with inhaled corticosteroids for the management of asthma that is inadequately controlled with low-dose inhaled corticosteroids (66).

■ ADVERSE EFFECTS

A variety of side effects have been described with the use of β agonists. It is important to note that most of the adverse effects associated with β agonists are reduced when these drugs are administered through inhalation. Tolerance to systemic (nonbronchodilator) effects occurs as well (103,104). Given the widespread distribution of β_2 receptors, many organ systems may be affected. The most common complaint is tremor, which is due to stimulation of β_2 receptors in skeletal muscle. Restlessness is also commonly reported. Often associated with oral or intravenous administration, tachycardia and palpitations are much less frequent when usual doses are administered through inhalation. Mediated by β vascular relaxation in skeletal muscle, cardiac stimulation occurs as a result of decreased peripheral resistance with resultant sympathetic output. It is also important to note that prolongation of the QT interval as seen on an EKG may lead to arrhythmias or myocardial ischemia in susceptible patients. Transient decreases in PaO_2 may occur when vascular dilation and increased cardiac output enhance perfusion to underventilated areas of lung (105). Abdominal complaints are sometimes seen in children receiving aggressive therapy for management of severe, acute asthma. Metabolic effects include hyperglycemia (due to glycogenolysis) and reductions in serum potassium and magnesium. Intracellular potassium shifts occur as a result of direct stimulation of the Na^+-K^+ pump. Magnesium also moves in this fashion, but increased urinary excretion further contributes to the reduction in this cation. Recent randomized controlled trials comparing albuterol and levalbuterol have found the frequency and types of adverse events to be similar (70,72,106).

Paradoxical bronchospasm may occur after the use of β agonists. A review noted that despite the low frequency with which this occurs, these reactions may be quite severe, even life-threatening (107). This report found that warmth, flushing, pruritus, nasal obstruction, and laryngeal wheeze frequently accompanied acute bronchospasm. It has been suggested that a lack of efficacy to β agonists may also be attributed to this phenomenon. Paradoxical bronchospasm was associated with use of new MDIs and bottles of nebulized solutions. Propellants have been implicated because they account for 58% to 99% of the composition of MDIs (107). For nebulized solutions, other possible factors

TABLE 34.1   UNTOWARD EFFECTS ASSOCIATED WITH THE REGULAR USE OF β AGONISTS

PROBLEM	SABA	LABA
Tolerance (↓ bronchodilator response)	Y	Y
↓ FEV₁	Y	N
↑ Response to bronchial challenge	Y	Y
Loss of bronchoprotection	Y	Y
↓ Protection against EIB	Y	Y
Cardiac toxicity	Y	N
↓ Response to SABA	Y	Conflicting results

have been suggested, such as acidity, osmolality, and preservatives, specifically benzalkonium chloride, ethylenediamine tetraacetic acid, and sulfites (108). Contamination of nebulized solutions, particularly from multidose bottles may also contribute to this problem. Finally, investigations suggest that the detrimental effects of (S)-albuterol may account for paradoxical bronchospasm (109).

Short-term loss of effectiveness, or tachyphylaxis, occurs for β agonists as it commonly does with agonist–cell surface receptor interactions. This occurs in response to continuous or frequent, repetitive use. Whether clinically relevant tachyphylaxis to bronchodilatory effect exists remains controversial. Tolerance has also been demonstrated in some, but not all, studies of long-term, inhaled β-agonist use (110–113). Tolerance occurs after as little as 3 weeks of repeated use and appears to affect the duration rather than peak response (110–112). Table 34.1 summarizes problems associated with the regular use of β agonists.

■ β AGONISTS AND ASTHMA MORTALITY

Two major epidemics within the past 40 years prompted international concern and investigation into the relationships between β agonists and asthma deaths. As a result, the safety of β agonists has been hotly debated. The first epidemic occurred in the 1960s, when a 2- to 10-fold increase in asthma mortality rates was noted in six countries, including the United Kingdom and Norway. Initial evaluation did not find the rise to be related to changes in diagnosis, disease classification, or death certificate information (114). Because MDI β-agonist preparations had been introduced in the early 1960s, investigators pursued the possibility of a new treatment effect. A high-dose isoproterenol forte preparation was in use in the affected countries at the time, and the epidemics occurred only in those countries. Case series analysis revealed that many of those who died of asthma used

excessive amounts of this high-dose product (115). Removal of this product from the market was followed by a reduction in mortality. It was thought that the deaths had been due to cardiac toxicity of this nonspecific β agonist. Despite what had been learned, another epidemic occurred in New Zealand 10 years later. Epidemiologic studies found that the risk for asthma death was increased in those patients who had been treated with another potent but less β₂-selective agent, fenoterol (116–118). Case-control studies found that it had been prescribed more often to those who died, but some investigators believed that these findings may have been confounded by asthma severity. After removing the product from the market, mortality declined. Subsequent studies have attempted to address whether this is a specific effect of fenoterol or a class effect of rapid-acting β agonists. The Saskatchewan studies suggest a general class effect (119,120), although their methods have been contested (121–123). Other studies have demonstrated increased risk for death in asthmatic children receiving fenoterol (124). The mechanism by which various β agonists may cause increased asthma mortality remains unclear. Several possible mechanisms have been proposed suggesting proinflammatory effects, differential tolerance and a recent hypothesis of a dual effect of rebound bronchoconstriction and bronchial hyperresponsiveness along with development of tolerance to therapeutic effects (125).

Studies have tried to assess similar risks for long-acting β agonists. The Serevent National Surveillance Project enrolled more than 25,000 adults but had insufficient power to establish relative risk because of the low number of deaths from asthma (126). Another large-scale study, which tracked prescription events, lacked a control group, and no causal association could be established between salmeterol and asthma death (127). A much smaller, case-control study of salmeterol and near-fatal asthma suggested that salmeterol confers no increased risk (128). The Salmeterol Multicenter Asthma Research Trial showed a small increase in respiratory and asthma-related deaths in the salmeterol group (versus placebo). These fatalities occurred mostly in African Americans and in those who were not using inhaled corticosteroids at baseline (129). Overall, the evidence suggests that mortality outcomes may have been due to other factors, such as reliance on β agonists and failure to seek medical care early (130).

LABA/INHALED CORTICOSTEROID OR SABA/INHALED CORTICOSTEROID FOR RELIEVER AND CONTROLLER THERAPY

Although not approved by the U.S. Food and Drug Administration (FDA) in the United States, the combinations of an inhaled corticosteroid with either formoterol or albuterol have been reported in studies utilizing the combination inhaler for both maintenance and reliever therapy (131–135). The concept is based on early "symptom-driven" intervention and may not be applicable for all patients. The studies have used patients with either mild (135), mild-moderate asthma (131–133), or moderate-severe (134) and employed budesonide/formoterol (131–134) and beclomethasone dipropionate/albuterol (135). During exacerbations, the use of more than 8 inhalations/day of budesonide/formoterol was less than in patients receiving either scheduled budesonide/formoterol with terbutaline for relief or higher doses of budesonide with terbutaline for relief (131,132). The number of courses of prednisone also was reduced, and there was no evidence that the exacerbations that occurred were more severe in the patients receiving combination therapy as reliever. These data suggest that combination therapy may have a role in the initial management of exacerbations of asthma or when there is a change in respiratory status. It remains to be determined if this approach will be approved by the FDA or will have application to greater numbers of patients with asthma.

SUMMARY

β-Agonists occupy a pivotal role in asthma management. Refinements in their chemical structure have led to improvements in efficacy, safety, and tolerance. Short-acting agents are indicated for the treatment of mild, intermittent asthma and for initial management of acute asthma symptoms in patients with persistent asthma. This class is also effective for the prevention of exercise-induced bronchospasm. Regular use of SABAs is not recommended. Levalbuterol, the enantiomer of racemic albuterol, may offer some benefit for acute management of asthma. Long-acting β agonists have a delayed, but prolonged, onset of action. Consequently, these agents are best used for asthma control, e.g., prevention of symptoms. LABAs should not be used as monotherapy for asthma, and current guidelines emphasize their position as adjunctive therapy in combination with inhaled corticosteroids.

REFERENCES

1. Tattersfield AE. Current issues with β₂-adrenoceptor agonists: historical background. *Clin Rev Allergy Immunol.* 2006;31:107–118.
2. Johnson M. Molecular mechanisms of β₂-adrenergic receptor function, response, and regulation. *J Allergy Clin Immunol.* 2006;117:18-24.
3. Liggett SB. Update on current concepts of the molecular basis of β₂-adrenergic receptor signaling. *J Allergy Clin Immunol.* 2002;110:S223–S228.
4. Johnson M. Mechanisms of action of β₂-adrenergic agonists. In: Busse WW, Holgate ST, eds. *Asthma and Rhinitis.* Oxford, UK: 2nd ed. Oxford, UK: Blackwell; 2000:1541–1557.
5. Martinez FD, Graves PE, Baldini M, et al. Association between genetic polymorphisms of the β₂-adrenoceptor and response to albuterol in children with and without a history of wheezing. *J Clin Invest.* 1997;100:3184–3188.
6. Cho SH, Oh SY, Bahn JW, et al. Association between bronchodilating response to short-acting beta-agonist and non-synonymous single-nucleotide polymorphisms of β₂-adrenoceptor gene. *Clin Exp Allergy.* 2005;35:1162–1167.
7. Israel E, Drazen JM, Liggett SB, et al. The effect of polymorphisms of the beta(2)-adrenergic receptor on the response to regular use of albuterol in asthma. *Am J Respir Crit Care Med.* 2000;162:75–80.
8. Israel E, Chinchilli VM, Ford JG, et al. National Heart, Lung, and Blood Institute's Asthma Clinical Research Network. Use of regularly scheduled albuterol treatment in asthma: genotype-stratified, randomised, placebo-controlled cross-over trial.[see comment]. *Lancet.* 2004;364:1505–1512.
9. Church MK, Hiroi J. Inhibition of IgE-dependent histamine release from human dispersed lung mast cells by antiallergic drugs and salbutamol. *Br J Pharmacol.* 1987;90:421–429.
10. Yukawa T, Ukena D, Chanez P, et al. Beta-adrenergic receptors on eosinophils: binding and functional studies. *Am Rev Respir Dis.* 1990;141:1446–1452.
11. Rabe KF, Giembycz MA, Dent G, et al. β2-Adrenoceptor agonists and respiratory burst activity in guinea pig and human eosinophils. *Fundam Clin Pharmacol.* 1991;5:A402.
12. Munoz NM, Vita AF, Neely SP, et al. Beta adrenergic modulation of formyl-methionone-leucine-phenylalanine stimulate secretion of eosinophil peroxidase and leukotriene C4. *J Pharmacol Exp Ther.* 1994;268:1339–1343.
13. Hadjokas NE, Crowley JJ, Bayer CR, et al. Beta-adrenergic regulation of the eosinophil respiratory burst as detected by lucigenin-dependent luminescence. *J Allergy Clin Immunol.* 1995;95:735–741.
14. Didier M, Aussel C, Ferrua B, et al. Regulation of interleukin 2 synthesis by cAMP in human T cells. *J Immunol.* 1987;139:1179–1184
15. Feldman RD. β-Adrenergic receptor-mediated suppression of interleukin-2 receptors in human lymphocytes. *J Immunol.* 1987;139:3355–3359.
16. Borger P, Hoekstra Y, Esselink MT, et al. Beta-adrenoceptor-mediated inhibition of IFN-gamma, IL-3, and GM-CSF mRNA accumulation in activated human T lymphocytes is solely mediated by the β₂-adrenoceptor subtype. *Am J Respir Cell Mol Biol.* 1998;19:400–407.
17. Busse WW, Sosman JM. Isoproterenol inhibition of isolated neutrophil function. *J Allergy Clin Immunol.* 1984;73:404–410.
18. Bloemen PG, van den Tweel MC, Henricks PA, et al. Increased cAMP levels in stimulated neutrophils inhibit their adhesion to human bronchial epithelial cells. *Am J Physiol.* 1997;272:L580–587.
19. Gauvreau GM, Jordana M, Watson RM, et al. Effect of regular inhaled albuterol on allergen-induced late responses and sputum eosinophils in asthmatic subjects. *Am J Respir Crit Care Med.* 1997;156:1738–1745.
20. Manolitsas DN, Wang J, Devalia JL, et al. Regular albuterol, nedocromil sodium, and bronchial inflammation in asthma. *Am J Respir Crit Care Med.* 1995;151:1925–1930.
21. Cockcroft DW, McParland CP, Britto SA, et al. Regular inhaled salbutamol and airway responsiveness to allergen. *Lancet.* 1993;342:833–838.
22. Prior C, Leonard MB, McCullough JR. Effects of enantiomers of beta 2-agonists on Ach release and smooth muscle contraction in the trachea. *Am J Physiol.* 1998;274:L32–38.

23. Templeton AGB, Chapman ID, Chilverws E, et al. Effect of (S)-albuterol on isolated human bronchus. *Pulm Pharmacol.* 1998;11:1–6.

24. Yamaguchi H, McCullough J. S-albuterol exacerbates calcium responses to carbachol in airway smooth muscle cells. *Clin Rev Allergy Immunol.* 1996;14:47–55.

25. Mitra S, Ugur M, Ugur O, et al. (S)-albuterol increases intracellular free calcium by muscarinic receptor activation and a phospholipase C-dependent mechanism in airway smooth muscle. *Mol Pharmacol.* 1998;53:347–354.

26. Penn RB, Frielle T, McCullough JR, et al. Comparison of R-, S-, and RS-albuterol interaction with human beta 1- and beta 2-adrenergic receptors. *Clin Rev Allergy Immunol.* 1996;14:37–45.

27. Volcheck GW, Gleich GJ, Kita H. Pro- and anti-inflammatory effects of beta adrenergic agonists on eosinophil response to IL-5. *J Allergy Clin Immunol.* 1998;101:S35.

28. Leff AR, Herrnreiter A, Naclerio RM, et al. Effect of enantiomeric forms of albuterol on stimulated secretion of granular protein from human eosinophils. *Pulm Pharmacol Ther.* 1997;10:97–104.

29. Walle T, Eaton Ea, Walle UK, et al. Stereoselective metabolism of RS-albuterol in humans. *Clin Rev Allergy Immunol.* 1996;14:101–113.

30. Gumbhir-Shah K, Kellerman D, DeGraw S, et al. Pharmacokinetics and pharmacodynamics of cumulative single doses of inhaled salbutamol enantiomers in asthmatic subjects. *Pulm Pharmacol Ther.* 1999(12):353–362.

31. Koch P, McCullough JR, DeGraw SS, et al. Pharmacokinetics and safety of (R)-, (S)-, and (RS)-albuterol following nebulization in healthy volunteers. *Am J Respir Crit Care Med.* 1997;155:A279.

32. Nelson HS, Bensch G, Pleskow WW, et al. Improved bronchodilation with levalbuterol compared with racemic albuterol in patients with asthma. *J Allergy Clin Immunol.* 1998;102:943–952.

33. Gawchik SM, Saccar CL, Noonan M, et al. The safety and efficacy of nebulized levalbuterol compared with racemic albuterol and placebo in the treatment of asthma in pediatric patients. *J Allergy Clin Immunol.* 1999;103:615–621.

34. Perrin-Fayolle M, Blum PS, Morley J, et al. Differential responses of asthmatic airways to enantiomers of albuterol. *Clin Rev Allergy Immunol.* 1996;14:139–147.

35. Cockroft DW, Swystun VA. Effect of single doses of S-albuterol, R-albuterol, racemic albuterol, and placebo on the airway response to methacholine. *Thorax.* 1997;52:845–848.

36. Cockroft DW, Davis BE, Swystun VA, et al. Tolerance to the bronchoprotective effect of β2-agonists: comparison of the enantiomer of albuterol with racemic albuterol and placebo. *J Allergy Clin Immunol.* 1999;103:1049–1053.

37. Ramsdale EH, Otis J, Kline PA, et al. Prolonged protection against methacholine-induced bronchoconstriction by the inhaled β2-agonist formoterol. *Am Rev Respir Dis.* 1991;143:998–1001.

38. Derom EY, Pauwels RA, Van Der Straeten MEF. The effect of inhaled salmeterol on methacholine responsiveness in subjects with asthma up to 12 hours. *J Allergy Clin Immunol.* 1992;89:811–815.

39. Verberne AAPH, Hop WCJ, Bos AB, et al. Effect of a single dose of inhaled salmeterol on baseline airway caliber and methacholine-induced airway obstruction in asthmatic children. *J Allergy Clin Immunol.* 1993;91:127–134.

40. Gongora HC, Wisniewski AFZ, Tattersfield AE. A single-dose comparison of inhaled albuterol and two formulations of salmeterol on airway reactivity in asthmatic subjects. *Am Rev Respir Dis.* 1991;144:626–629.

41. Newnham DM, Ingram CG, Earnshaw J, et al. Salmeterol provides prolonged protection against exercise-induced bronchoconstriction in a majority of subjects with mild, stable asthma. *Respir Med.* 1993;87:439–444.

42. Malo J-L, Cartier A, Trudeau C, et al. Formoterol, a new inhaled β2-adrenergic agonist, has a longer blocking effect than albuterol on hyperventilation-induced bronchoconstriction. *Am Rev Respir Dis.* 1990;142:1147–1152.

43. Nowak D, Jorres R, Rabe KF, et al. Salmeterol protects against hyperventilation-induced bronchoconstriction over 12 hours. *Eur J Clin Pharmacol.* 1992;43:591–595.

44. Gong H, Linn WS, Shamoo DA, et al. Effect of inhaled salmeterol on sulfur dioxide induced bronchoconstriction in asthmatic subjects. *Chest.* 1996;110:1229–1235.

45. Bootsma GP, Dekhuijzen PNR, Festen J, et al. Sustained protection against distilled water provocation by a single dose of salmeterol in patients with asthma. *Eur Respir J.* 1997;10:2230–2236.

46. Twentyman OP, Finnerty JP, Harris A, et al. Protection against allergen-induced asthma by salmeterol. *Lancet.* 1990;336:1338–1342.

47. Pedersen B, Dahl R, Larsen BB, et al. The effect of salmeterol on the early and late phase reaction to bronchial allergen and postchallenge variation in bronchial reactivity, blood eosinophils, serum eosinophil cationic protein and serum eosinophil protein X. *Allergy.* 1993;48:377–382.

48. Palmqvist M, Balder B, Lowhagen O, et al. Late asthmatic reaction decreased after pretreatment with salbutamol and formoterol, a new long-acting β2-agonist. *J Allergy Clin Immunol.* 1992;89:844–849.

49. Butchers PR, Vardey CJ, Johnson M. Salmeterol: a potent and long-acting inhibitor of inflammatory mediator release from human lung. *Br J Pharmacol.* 1991;104:672–676.

50. Baker AJ, Palmer J, Johnson M, et al. Inhibitory actions of salmeterol on human airway macrophages and blood monocytes. *Eur J Pharmacol.* 1994;264:301–306.

51. Johnson M. The pharmacology of salmeterol. *Lung.* 1990;168(Suppl.):115–119.

52. Gardiner PV, Ward C, Booth H, et al. Effect of eight weeks treatment with salmeterol on bronchoalveolar lavage inflammatory indices in asthmatics. *Am J Respir Crit Care Med.* 1994;150:1006–1011.

53. Kraft M, Wenzel SE, Bettinger CM, et al. The effect of salmeterol on nocturnal symptoms, airway function, and inflammation in asthma. *Chest.* 1997;111:1249–1254.

54. Roberts JA, Bradding P, Britten KM, et al. The long-acting β2-agonist salmeterol xinafoate: effects on airway inflammation in asthma. *Eur Respir J.* 1999;14:275–282.

55. Weersink EJM, Aalbers R, Koeter GH, et al. Partial inhibition of the early and late asthmatic response by a single dose of salmeterol. *Am J Respir Crit Care Med.* 1994;150:1261–1267.

56. Pizzichini MMM, Kidney JC, Wong BJO, et al. Effect of salmeterol compared with beclomethasone on allergen-induced asthmatic and inflammatory responses. *Eur Respir J.* 1996;9:449–455.

57. Turner MO, Johnston PR, Pizzichini E, et al. Anti-inflammatory effects of salmeterol compared with beclomethasone in eosinophilic mild exacerbations of asthma: a randomized, placebo controlled trial. *Can Respir J.* 1998;5(4):261–268.

58. Taylor IK, O'Shaughnessy KM, Choudry NB, et al. A comparative study in atopic subjects with asthma of the effects of salmeterol and salbutamol on allergen-induced bronchoconstriction, increase in airway reactivity, and increase in urinary leukotriene E4 excretion. *J Allergy Clin Immunol.* 1992;89:575–583.

59. Dente FL, Bancalari L, Baaci E, et al. Effect of a single dose of salmeterol on the increase in airway eosinophils induced by allergen challenge in asthmatic subjects. *Thorax.* 1999;54:622–624.

60. Dahl R, Pederson B. The influence of inhaled salmeterol on bronchial inflammation: a bronchoalveolar lavage study in patients with bronchial asthma. *Eur Respir Rev.* 1991;1:277–285.

61. DiLorenzo G, Morici G, Norrito F, et al. Comparison of the effects of salmeterol and salbutamol on clinical activity and eosinophil cationic protein serum levels during the pollen season in atopic asthmatics. *Clin Exp Allergy.* 1995;25:951–956.

62. Wallin A, Sandström T, Söderber M, et al. The effects of regular inhaled formoterol, budesonide, and placebo on mucosal inflammation and clinical indices in mild asthma. *Am J Respir Crit Care Med.* 1998;158:79–86.

63. Lee DK, Jackson CM, Currie GP, et al. Comparison of combination inhalers vs inhaled corticosteroids alone in moderate persistent asthma. *Br J Clin Pharmacol.* 2003;56:494–500.

64. Aziz I, Wilson AM, Lipworth BJ. Effects of once-daily formoterol and budesonide given alone or in combination on surrogate inflammatory markers in asthmatic adults. *Chest.* 2000;118:1049–1058.

65. Overbeek SE, Mulder PG, Baelemans SM, et al. Formoterol added to low-dose budesonide has no additional antiinflammatory effect in asthmatic patients. *Chest.* 2005;128:1121–1127.

66. National Asthma Education and Prevention Program. Expert Panel Report 3 (EPR-3): Guidelines for the Diagnosis and Management of Asthma-Summary Report 2007. *J Allergy Clin Immunol.* 2007;120:S94–S138.

67. Naureckas ET, Dukic V, Bao X, et al. Short-acting β-agonist prescription fills as a marker for asthma morbidity. *Chest.* 2005;128:602–608.

68. Anderson S, Seale JP, Ferais L, et al. An evaluation of pharmacotherapy for exercise induced asthma. *J Allergy Clin Immunol.* 1979;64:612–624.

69. Godfrey S, Konig P. Inhibition of exercise-induced asthma by different pharmacological pathways. *Thorax.* 1976;31:137–143.

70. Carl JC, Myers TR, Kirchner HL, et al. Comparison of racemic albuterol and levalbuterol for treatment of acute asthma. *J Pediatr.* 2003;143:731–736.

71. Nowak R, Emerman C, Hanrahan JP, et al. XOPENEX Acute Severe Asthma Study Group. A comparison of levalbuterol with racemic albuterol in the treatment of acute severe asthma exacerbations in adults. *Am J Emerg Med.* 2006;24:259–267.

72. Qureshi F, Zaritsky A, Welch C, et al. Clinical efficacy of racemic albuterol versus levalbuterol for the treatment of acute pediatric asthma. *Ann Emerg Med.* 2005;46:29–36.

73. Vathenen AS, Knox AJ, Higgens JR, et al. Rebound increases in bronchial responsiveness after treatment with inhaled terbutaline. *Lancet.* 1988;1(8585):554–558.

74. Sears MR, Taylor CG, Print DC, et al. Regular inhaled beta-agonist treatment in bronchial asthma. *Lancet.* 1990;336:1391–1396.

75. Taylor DR, Sears MR, Herbison GP, et al. Regular inhaled beta agonists in asthma: effects on exacerbations and lung function. *Thorax.* 1993;48:134–138.

76. Van Schayck CP, Dompeling E, van Herwaarden CLA, et al. Bronchodilator treatment in moderate asthma or chronic bronchitis: continuous or on demand? A randomised controlled study. *Br Med J.* 1991;303:1426–1431.

77. Harvey JE, Tattersfield AE. Airway response to salbutamol: effect of regular salbutamol inhalation in normal, atopic and asthmatic subjects. *Thorax.* 1982;37:280–287.

78. Wahedna I, Wong CS, Wisniewski AF, et al. Asthma control during and after cessation of regular beta$_2$-agonist treatment. *Am Rev Respir Dis.* 1993;148:707–712.

79. Van Schayck CP, Graafsma SJ, Visch MB, et al. Increased bronchial responsiveness after inhaling salbutamol during 1 year is not caused by subsensitization to salbutamol. *J Allergy Clin Immunol.* 1990;86: 793–800.

80. Kerrebijn KF, von Essen-Zandvliet EEM, Neijens JJ. Effect of long-term treatment with inhaled corticosteroids and beta agonists on the bronchial responsiveness in children with asthma. *J Allergy Clin Immunol.* 1987;79:653–659.

81. Kraan JG, Koeter GH, Van der Mark TW, et al. Changes in bronchial hyperreactivity induced by 4 weeks of treatment with antiasthmatic drugs in patients with allergic asthma: a comparison between budesonide and terbutaline. *J Allergy Clin Immunol.* 1985;76: 628–636.

82. Drazen JM, Israel E, Boushey HA, et al. Comparison of regularly scheduled with as-needed use of albuterol in mild asthma. *N Engl J Med.* 1996;335:841–847.

83. Vandewalker ML, Kray KT, Weber RW, et al. Addition of terbutaline to optimal theophylline therapy: double blind crossover study in asthmatic patients. *Chest.* 1986;90:198–203.

84. Pearlman DS, Chervinsky P, LaForce C, et al. A comparison of salmeterol with albuterol in the treatment of mild-to-moderate asthma. *N Engl J Med.* 1992;327:1420–1425.

85. D'Alonzo GE, Nathan RA, Henochowicz S, et al. Salmeterol xinafoate as maintenance therapy compared with albuterol in patients with asthma. *JAMA.* 1994;271:1412–1416.

86. Nelson HS. B-adrenergic bronchodilators. *N Engl J Med.* 1995;333(8):499–506.

87. Kemp JP, Dockhorn RJ, Busse WW, et al. Prolonged effect of inhaled salmeterol against exercise-induced bronchospasm. *Am J Respir Crit Care Med.* 1994; 150:1612–1615.

88. Boner AL, Spezia E, Piovesan P, et al. Inhaled formoterol in the prevention of exercise-induced bronchoconstriction in asthmatic children. *Am J Respir Crit Care Med.* 1994;149:935–939.

89. Busse WW. Long- and short-acting β$_2$-adrenergic agonists effects on airway function in patients with asthma. *Arch Intern Med.* 1996;156:1514–1520.

90. Lazarus SC, Boushey HA, Fahy JV, et al. Asthma Clinical Research Network for the National Heart, Lung, and Blood Institute. Long-acting beta2-agonist monotherapy vs continued therapy with inhaled corticosteroids in patients with persistent asthma: a randomized controlled trial.[see comment]. *JAMA.* 2001;285:2583–2593.

91. Simons FE. A comparison of beclomethasone, salmeterol, and placebo in children with asthma. Canadian Beclomethasone Dipropionate-Salmeterol Xinafoate Study Group. *N Engl J Med.* 1997;337:1659–1665.

92. Verberne AA, Frost C, Roorda RJ, et al. One year treatment with salmeterol compared with beclomethasone in children with asthma. The Dutch Paediatric Asthma Study Group. *Am J Respir Crit Care Med.* 1997;156:688–695.

93. Greening AP, Ind PW, Northfield M, et al. Added salmeterol versus higher-dose corticosteroid in asthma patients with symptoms on existing inhaled corticosteroid. *Lancet.* 1994;344:219–224.

94. Woolcock A, Lundback B, Ringdal N, et al. Comparison of addition of salmeterol to inhaled steroids with doubling the dose of inhaled steroids. *Am J Respir Crit Care Med.* 1996;153:1481–1488.

95. Wilding P, Clark M, Coon JT, et al. Effect of long term treatment with salmeterol on asthma control: a double blind, randomised crossover study. *Br Med J.* 1997;314:1441–1446.

96. Russell G, Williams DAJ, Weller P, et al. Salmeterol xinafoate in children on high dose inhaled steroids. *Ann Allergy Asthma Immunol.* 1995;75:423.

97. Pauwels RA, Lofdahl CG, Postma DS, et al. Effect of inhaled formoterol and budesonide on exacerbations of asthma. *N Engl J Med.* 1997;337:1405–1411.

98. Condemi JJ, Goldstein S, Kalberg C, et al. The addition of salmeterol to fluticasone propionate versus increasing the dose of fluticasone propionate in patients with persistent asthma. *Ann Allergy Asthma Immunol.* 1999;82:383–389.

99. Pearlman DS, Stricker W, Weinstein S, et al. Inhaled salmeterol and fluticasone: a study comparing monotherapy and combination therapy in asthma. *Ann Allergy Asthma Immunol.* 1999;82:257–265.

100. Verberne AAPH, Frost C, Duiverman EJ, et al. Addition of salmeterol versus doubling the dose of beclomethasone in children with asthma. *Am J Respir Crit Care Med.* 1998;158:213–219.

101. Gibson PG, Powell H, Ducharme FM. Differential effects of maintenance long-acting beta-agonist and inhaled corticosteroid on asthma control and asthma exacerbations. *J Allergy Clin Immunol.* 2007;119: 344–350.

102. Gibson P, Powell H, Ducharme F, et al. Long-acting β$_2$-agonists as an inhaled corticosteroid-sparing agent for chronic asthma in adults and children. *Cochrane Database Syst. Rev.* CD005076 2005.

103. Maconochie JG, Minton NA, Chilton JE, et al. Does tachyphylaxis occur to the non-pulmonary effects of salmeterol? *Br J Clin Pharmacol.* 1994;37:199–204.

104. Newnham DM, Grove A, McDevitt DG, et al. Subsensitivity of bronchodilator and systemic β$_2$-adrenoceptor responses after regular twice daily treatment with eformoterol dry powder in asthmatic patients. *Thorax.* 1995;50:497–504.

105. Wagner PD, Dantzker DR, Iacovoni VE, et al. Ventilation-perfusion inequality in asymptomatic asthma. *Am Rev Respir Dis.* 1978;118:511–524.

106. Hamilos DL, D'Urzo A, Levy RJ, et al. Long-term safety study of levalbuterol administered via metered-dose inhaler in patients with asthma. *Ann Allergy Asthma Immunol.* 2007;99:540–548.

107. Nicklas RA. Paradoxical bronchospasm associated with the use of inhaled beta agonists. *J Allergy Clin Immunol.* 1990;85:959–964.

108. Asmus MJ, Sherman J, Hendeles L. Bronchoconstrictor additives in bronchodilator solutions. *J Allergy Clin Immunol.* 1999;104: S53–S60.

109. Handley D. The asthma-like pharmacology and toxicology of (S)-isomers of β-agonists. *J Allergy Clin Immunol.* 1999;104: S69–S76.

110. Newnham DM, McDevitt DG, Lipworth BJ. Bronchodilator subsensitivity after chronic dosing with formoterol in patients with asthma. *Am J Med.* 1984;97:29–37.

111. Weber RW, Smith JA, Nelson HS. Aerosolized terbutaline in asthmatics: development of subsensitivity with long-term administration. *J Allergy Clin Immunol.* 1982;70:417–422.

112. Repsher LH, Anderson JA, Bush RU, et al. Assessment of tachyphylaxis following prolonged therapy of asthma with inhaled albuterol aerosol. *Chest.* 1984;85:34–38.

113. Holgate ST, Baldwin CJ, Tattersfield AE. β-Adrenergic agonists resistance in normal human airways. *Lancet.* 1977;2:375–377.

114. Speizer FE, Doll R, Heaf P. Observations on recent increases in mortality from asthma. *Br Med J.* 1968;1(5588):335–339.

115. Fraser PM, Speizer FE, Waters DM, et al. The circumstances preceding death from asthma in young people in 1968 to 1969. *Br J Dis Chest.* 1971;65:71–84.

116. Crane J, Pearch N, Flatt A, et al. Prescribed fenoterol and death from asthma in New Zealand, 1981–83: case-control study. *Lancet.* 1989;1:917–922.

117. Pearce N, Grainger J, Atkinson M, et al. Case-control study of prescribed fenoterol and death from asthma in New Zealand, 1977–1981. *Thorax.* 1990;45:170–175.

118. Grainger J, Woodman K, Pearch N, et al. Prescribed fenoterol and death from asthma in New Zealand, 1981–1987: a further case-control study. *Thorax.* 1991;46:105–111.

119. Spitzer WD, Suissa S, Ernst P, et al. The use of beta agonists and the risk of death and near death from asthma. *N Engl J Med.* 1992; 326:501–506.

120. Suissa S, Ernst P, Boivin JF, et al. A cohort analysis of excess mortality in asthma and the use of inhaled β-agonists. *Am J Respir Crit Care Med.* 1994;149:604–610.

121. Beasley R, Pearce N, Crane J, et al. B-agonists: what is the evidence that their use increases the risk of asthma morbidity and mortality? *J Allergy Clin Immunol.* 1999;103:S18–S30.

122. Pearce N, Hensley MJ. Epidemiologic studies of beta agonists and asthma deaths. *Epidemiol Rev.* 1998;20:173–186.

123. Barrett TE, Strom BL. Inhaled beta-adrenergic receptor agonists in asthma: more harm than good? *Am J Respir Crit Care Med.* 1995; 151:574–577.

124. Matsui T. Asthma deaths and B2-agonists. In: Shimomiya K, ed. *Current Advances in Paediatric Allergy and Clinical Epidemiology: Selected Proceedings from the 32nd Annual Meeting of the Japanese Society of Paediatric Allergy and Clinical Immunology.* Tokyo: Churchill Livingstone, 1996:161–164.

125. Hancox RJ. Concluding remarks: can we explain the association of β-agonists with asthma mortality? A hypothesis. *Clin Rev Allerg Immunol.* 2006;31:279–288.

126. Castle W, Fuller R, Hall J, et al. Serevent nationwide surveillance study: comparison of salmeterol with salbutamol in asthmatic patients who require regular bronchodilator treatment. *Br Med J.* 1993;306: 1034–1037.

127. Mann RD, Kubota K, Pearch G, et al. Salmeterol: a study by prescription event monitoring in a UK cohort of 15,407 patients. *J Clin Epidemiol.* 1996;49:247–250.

128. Williams C, Crossland L, Finnerty J, et al. Case-control study of salmeterol and near-fatal attacks of asthma. *Thorax.* 1998;53:7–13.

129. Nelson HS, Weiss ST, Bleecker ER, et al. SMART Study Group. The Salmeterol Multicenter Asthma Research Trial: a comparison of usual pharmacotherapy for asthma or usual pharmacotherapy plus salmeterol. *Chest.* 2006;129:15–26.

130. Nelson HS. Is there a problem with inhaled long-acting β-adrenergic agonists. *J Allergy Clin Immunol.* 2006;117:3–16.

131. O'Byrne PM, Bisgaard H, Godard PP, et al. Budesonide/formoterol combination therapy as both maintenance and reliever medication in asthma. *Am J Respir Crit Care Med.* 2005;171:129–136.

132. Bisgaard H, Le Roux P, Bjamer D, et al. Budesonide/formoterol maintenance plus reliever therapy: a new strategy in pediatric asthma. *Chest.* 2006;130:1733–1743.

133. Rabe KF, Pizzichini E, Stallberg B, et al. Budesonide/formoterol in a single inhaler for maintenance and relief in mild-to-moderate asthma: a randomized, double-blind trial. *Chest.* 2006;129:246–256.

134. Rabe KF, Atienza T, Magyar P, et al. Effect of budesonide in combination with formoterol for reliever therapy in asthma exacerbations: a randomized controlled, double-blind study. *Lancet.* 2006;368:744–753.

135. Papi A, Canonica GW, Maestrelli P, et al. Rescue use of beclomethasone and albuterol in a single inhaler for mild asthma. *N Engl J Med.* 2007;356:2040–2052.

Corticosteroids in Treatment of Allergic Diseases

SAI R. NIMMAGADDA

■ HISTORY OF CORTICOSTEROIDS

Corticosteroids—the synthetic analogs of the glucocorticoid hormones of the adrenal cortex—have emerged as the single most effective class of drugs for treatment of inflammatory diseases. Although it was as early as 1885 that Addison described a "wasting disease" after destruction of the adrenal gland (1), it wasn't until the 20th century that researchers defined the activity of the adrenal steroids (2). In 1949, Hench et al. introduced corticosteroid treatment for arthritis and other diseases (3,4), which soon expanded to the use of corticosteroids as treatments for nearly all inflammatory diseases. Enthusiasm for systemic corticosteroid therapy waned with the discovery that chronic use caused numerous debilitating adverse effects, but the 1957 introduction of topically active corticosteroids with greatly diminished side effects (5) renewed interest in their widespread use.

Inhaled corticosteroid (ICS) therapy was introduced in the 1970s, initially targeted to patients with severe asthma who required treatment with oral corticosteroids (6,7). Later, ICS therapy was extended to patients for whom sympathomimetics and methylxanthines were ineffective (8), but the major focus was still on patients with severe disease.

The recognition of asthma as an inflammatory disease changed treatment strategy. Reports showing similarities in infiltrations of lymphocytes, mast cells, and eosinophils in the bronchial mucosa, regardless of the severity of asthma (9,10), extended ICS use to populations with only mild persistent disease (11). Clinical reports showing greater reductions in bronchial hyperresponsiveness with the regular use of an ICS in comparison with the regular use of an inhaled β_2 agonist (12,13) added to the impetus. In 1991, the *Guidelines for the Diagnosis and Management of Asthma of the National Asthma Education and Prevention Program* (NAEPP) recommended ICS therapy for patients with both severe and moderate asthma (14). By 1997, the recommendations also included patients with mild persistent disease (15), and the 2007 Guidelines state that ICSs are the most consistently effective long-term control medications at all steps of care for persistent asthma in both children and adults, regardless of severity (16).

■ PHARMACOLOGY OF CORTICOSTEROIDS

There are two general classes of corticosteroids: mineralocorticoids (MCs) and glucocorticoids (GCs). MCs principally affect the regulation of fluid and electrolyte balance and have no clinical use in the treatment of allergic disease. However, MC activity in corticosteroid medications may produce fluid and electrolyte side effects, so they are not entirely without relevance.

The basic chemical structure of GCs consists of 21 carbon atoms with a total of four rings, three six-carbon rings and a five-carbon ring (17). Hydrocortisone (cortisol) is the parent molecule from which other natural and synthetic GCs derive. Essential features of the anti-inflammatory GC consist of the following: (a) a two-carbon chain at the 17th position, (b) methyl groups at carbons 10 and 13, (c) a ketone oxygen at C3, (d) an unsaturated bond between C-4 and C-5, (e) a ketone oxygen at C-20, and (f) a hydroxyl group at C-11. Modifications of either the nucleus or the side chains produce different GC agents with varying anti-inflammatory and MC activity as compared to cortisol. Further alterations at the C-17 and C-21 positions result in corticosteroids with high topical activity and minimal systemic adverse effects.

Cortisol secretion results from a cascade of stimulatory events in the hypothalamic-pituitary-adrenal (HPA) axis (18). The process begins in the hypothalamus with the secretion of corticotropin-releasing factor (CRF), which stimulates the release of adrenocorticotropic hormone (ACTH), a product of the basophil cells of the anterior pituitary gland. In turn, ACTH stimulates the production of GCs, which are primarily produced in the zona fasciculata of the adrenal cortex. Cortisol and ACTH secretion normally reaches peak levels in the early morning, then declines throughout the day to a low point in the early-to-late evening (2). Daily secretion of cortisol is about 10 mg to 20 mg (28 μmol to 55 μ (mol), but environmental stress or increased circulating levels of cytokines, such as interleukin (IL)-1, IL-2, IL-6, or tumor necrosis factor-α (TNFα), can raise levels to as high as 400 mg to 500 mg (19).

At least 90% of circulating cortisol is protein-bound, principally to cortisol-binding globulin or transcortin (17). The unbound fraction is biologically active and may bind to transcortin (high affinity/low capacity) or to serum albumin (low affinity/high capacity). Transcortin has a binding capacity of only 0.7 μmol (250 μg) cortisol per liter serum. Thus at low concentrations, approximately 90% of cortisol is plasma-protein-bound, and at higher concentrations of cortisol, transcortin binding becomes saturated. Some synthetic GCs, such as dexamethasone, exhibit little or no binding to transcortin. Because pharmacologic actions, metabolism, and excretion of corticosteroids all relate to unbound steroid concentrations, the binding of circulating steroids to transcortin and albumin play important roles in modifying GC potency, half-life, and duration of effects (2).

The intrinsic pharmacokinetic properties of GCs are described by their volume of distribution (absorption) and clearance (metabolism, half-life, or excretion). Other factors may also include pro-drug conversion by pulmonary esterases to an active GC metabolite. For a specific corticosteroid, bioavailability is also part of the equation (Tables 35.1 and 35.2).

Natural and synthetic steroids are lipophilic compounds readily absorbed after intravenous, oral, subcutaneous, or topical administration. However, lipophilicity varies among preparations. In general, the systemic availability of both oral and intravenous GC preparations is high and is limited by first-pass liver metabolism rather than by incomplete absorption. However, with inhaled GCs, the pharmacokinetic profile and the method of delivery determine the extent and time to systemic absorption of a given GC. A portion of a dose of ICS is swallowed—unless rinsed out—and absorbed from the gastrointestinal (GI) tract. The rest reaches the lower airways and exerts the desired effect. The ratio of desirable/undesirable effects depends on:

- Topical activity of drug in the airways (GC receptor-binding affinity)
- Percentage of oropharyngeal *versus* lower airway deposition
- Systemic activity of drug after absorption by the GI tract or lungs and first-pass metabolism (20)
- Activation or conversion of a GC to an active metabolite or compound

Catabolism of corticosteroids is mainly in the liver, although other organs such as the kidney, placenta, lung, muscle, and skin may contribute to the metabolism of endogenous and synthetic GCs. Enzymatic coupling with a sulfate or glucuronic acid forms water-soluble compounds, which leads to renal excretion. There is minimal excretion via the biliary and fecal routes.

■ MOLECULAR AND ANTI-INFLAMMATORY MECHANISMS OF GLUCOCORTICOID ACTION

As anti-inflammatory agents, GCs exert both direct and indirect inhibitory effects on multiple inflammatory genes (encoding cytokines, chemokines, adhesion molecules, inflammatory enzymes, receptors, and proteins) that have been activated during the inflammatory process (21).

Glucocorticoids diffuse readily across cell membranes and bind to glucocorticoid receptors (GRs) in the cytoplasm (22). The GR is a 94-kD protein which exists in the cytoplasm as a multiprotein complex

TABLE 35.1 PHARMACOKINETIC VARIABLES AND EQUIVALENT DOSES OF COMMON ORAL GLUCOCORTICOSTEROIDS

ORAL GCS	PLASMA HALF-LIFE (h)	CLEARANCE (L/min)	BINDING AFFINITY	VOLUME OF DISTRIBUTION (L/kg)	SYSTEMIC BIOAVAILABILITY COMPARATIVE %	DOSE (mg)
Cortisol	0.5	ND	0.04	1.4	40 to 70	20
Prednisone	1	0.2	1.6	2.5	25	5
Prednisolone	3.5	0.2	1.6	0.4 to 0.8	21	5
Methylprednisolone	3	0.4	4.2	0.8 to 1.1	39	4
Dexamethasone	3.5	0.4	1.0	0.7 to 1.4	20	0.75

TABLE 35.2 PHARMACOKINETIC VARIABLES OF COMMON INHALED AND INTRANASAL GLUCOCORTICOIDS

INHALED GCS	ON-SITE ACTIVATION	PLASMA HALF-LIFE (h)	CLEARANCE (L/min)	BINDING AFFINITY	VOLUME OF DISTRIBUTION (L/kg)	SYSTEMIC BIOAVAILABILITY (%)	
						INHALED	ORAL
BDP	Somewhat	0.1 to 0.5	3.8	0.4	NA	20	<20
BUD	No	2.8	1.4	9.4	2.7 to 4.3	25	6 to 13
FLN	No	1.6	1.0	1.8	1.8	39	21
FP	No	3.1 to 7.8	0.9 to 1.1	18	3.7 to 8.9	20	<1
FF	No	7.7 to 14	0.8 to 1.1	29	NA	NA	<0.05
MF	No		0.80 to 1.0	22			<0.1
TA	No	1.5	0.7 to 1.2	3.6	2.1	21	10 to 22
CIC	Yes	0.36 to 3.4	2.5 to 3.8	12		NA	<1

BDP, beclomethasone dipropionate; BUD, budesonide; FLN, flunisolide; FP, fluticasone propionate; FF, fluticasone furoate; MF, mometasone furoate, TA, triamcinolone acetonide; CIC, ciclesonide. NA, not available

containing several heat shock proteins (Hsp90, Hsp70, Hsp56, and Hsp40) (23). These heat shock proteins protect the receptor and prevent its nuclear localization by covering the sites on the receptor that are needed for transport across the nuclear membrane into the nucleus (23). Once corticosteroids have bound to GRs, changes in the receptor structure result in rapid transport of the GR-corticosteroid complex into the nucleus where it binds as a homodimer to specific DNA-binding sites, i.e., glucocorticoid responsive elements (GREs) (24). The relative potency of GCs is dependent on plasma protein-binding, intracellular receptor affinity, and receptor dissociation from activated receptors.

After binding to GREs in the DNA, GCs can promote (transactivate) or inhibit (transrepress) gene expression (25). The number of genes directly regulated by GRs in any given cell is unknown, but studies place the number of steroid-responsive genes per cell at 10 to 100 (26,27). In addition, many genes are indirectly regulated through an interaction with other transcription factors and co-activators. The mechanisms of action of GCs are mediated by genomic effects, secondary nongenomic effects, and interactions with cellular-membrane-bound GRs (28). The classic genomic mechanism of GC action results in the following:

- Transactivation: production of Annexin-1 (lipocortin-1) SLPI (secretory leukoprotease inhibitor), MKP-1 (mitogen-activated kinase phosphatase-1), IκB-α, glucocorticoid-induced leucine zipper protein (GILZ), and the ß2 adrenoceptor (21).
- Transrepression: upregulation or downregulation of transcription factors that alter specific messenger ribonucleic acid (mRNA) production, which results in increased production of anti-inflammatory mediators and proteins and decreased production of proinflammatory mediators, including cytokines, chemokines, and adhesion molecules (21). Theoretically, high levels of transcription factors could suppress GC action by neutralizing receptors. This occurrence could be a potential mechanism of GC resistance (21).
- Cisrepression: GR homodimer interaction with GREs to suppress genes associated with side effects of GC. These include: proopiomelanocortin (POMC), corticotrophin-releasing factor-1 (CRF-1), osteocalcin, and keratin (21).

These mechanisms are now thought to be among the most important in explaining GC anti-inflammatory action, but other factors come into play as well. Glucocorticoids hinder the recruitment and activation of T-lymphocytes, eosinophils, dendritic cells, macrophages, and other inflammatory cells, and they inhibit the survival of mast cells at the airway surface, though they do not prevent their activation (29). Airway epithelial cells are likely major targets for inhaled GCs because these cells release numerous inflammatory mediators (29).

■ CORTICOSTEROID THERAPY

Regardless of the route of administration, a general rule of thumb with GC therapy is that clinicians should use the lowest possible effective dose for the shortest time, and patients should undergo frequent reevaluation with the goal of eliminating GCs or reducing dosages. Complications of GC therapy relate to the pharmacology of the agent, dose, dosing interval, and duration of use. Local administration—topical cutaneous or inhaled nasal/bronchial—is recommended where possible to avoid or reduce systemic side effects. These eight broad principles apply:

1. If possible, treatment agents should have little or no MC activity.
2. Patients with nonlife-threatening disorders, e.g., atopic dermatitis or nasal polyps, should undergo long-term systemic GC therapy only when alternative and more conservative therapy has failed.
3. To facilitate rapid, safe reductions in dose and use of prolonged courses of systemic GC therapy, patients should receive concurrent maximal doses of topical preparations.
4. Single-dose oral GCs should be given in the morning to minimize disruption of the HPA axis.
5. Acute allergic disease exacerbations can usually be safely treated with 5- to 10-day courses of moderate-dose daily systemic GC therapy without significant adverse effects.
6. For alternate-day systemic GC therapy, the best choices are oral agents with tissue half-lives in the 12- to 36-hour (intermediate) range, such as prednisone, prednisolone, and methylprednisone.
7. Children receiving GC therapy should be regularly evaluated for growth, especially those using both intranasal and inhaled GC therapy.
8. All patients on GC treatment should undergo frequent reevaluation to attempt to reduce the dosage or eliminate steroids altogether.

Inhaled Corticosteroids and Asthma

The National Heart, Lung and Blood Institute Expert Panel Report 3 (EPR-3) guidelines recommend a stepwise approach for the treatment of persistent asthma (16,30). The guidelines stress (a) assessing severity before initiating treatment and (b) periodically assessing asthma control to adjust therapy, stepping up if necessary, and stepping down if possible (30,31). In almost all patients, with the possible exception of those with mild, intermittent symptoms, ICS therapy remains the first-line treatment in patients of all ages. Treatment with ICSs reduces local inflammation and bronchial hyperresponsiveness, improves pulmonary function, reduces or eliminates the need for oral steroids, decreases hospitalizations, and asthma mortality (30,32). It has been reported that low-dose ICSs reduced the risk of death in asthma by 50% when patients used at least six canisters per year of ICS (33).

While GCs have been known to reduce inflammation and control symptoms of asthma, there is mounting evidence that they are not disease-modifying agents. Studies have suggested that early use of GCs in children as young as 2 years of age can reduce symptoms and exacerbations (34). However, 2 years of GC therapy did not change the development of asthma symptoms or lung function after treatment was discontinued. Early use of inhaled fluticasone propionate for wheezing in preschool children had no effect on the natural history of asthma or wheeze later in childhood (35). Furthermore, it appears that ICSs do not prevent lung function decline or reduce airway reactivity in preschool children (34,36).

Current knowledge of the mechanisms of asthma suggests that the prudent treatment strategy is early introduction and relatively high initial doses of ICSs to gain maximum control quickly, followed by dose reduction to the minimum needed to maintain control. Contrary to the earlier belief that appropriate treatment would reverse airway obstruction, current evidence suggests that "airway remodeling," i.e., structural changes and irreversible airway obstruction, occurs with chronic inflammation (37–42).

Some recent research postulates that inflammation and airway remodeling may not be as closely connected as many have believed. Bush suggests that eosinophilic inflammation and airway remodeling are parallel processes and that the primary abnormality is not airway inflammation but some form of disordered airway repair (43). In a review, Warner and Knight also found evidence that features of remodeling such as angiogenesis, goblet cell hyperplasia, and thickened lamina reticularis occur early in the disease and independently of inflammation (44). Another study presented evidence that the airway epithelium in asthma is fundamentally abnormal and has increased susceptibility to environmental injury and impaired repair (45).

Clearly, the study of the cause and effects of airway remodeling is still in its infancy. However, current research favors the early introduction of ICS therapy in all patients, given that irreversible damage can occur and that permanent changes may be preventable. Even in patients with mild persistent disease, studies show that the lowest effective dose of ICS therapy is safe, well-tolerated, and cost-effective (46–49).

Inhaled Corticosteroid Preparations

Seven ICS preparations are currently available for the treatment of asthma in the United States. They are: beclomethasone dipropionate (BDP), flunisolide (FL), fluticasone propionate (FP), triamcinolone acetonide (TA), budesonide (BUD), mometasone furoate (MF), and ciclesonide (CIC).

Not all ICSs have the same efficacy and safety profiles, however. Their efficacy and safety are shaped by their pharmacokinetic and pharmacodynamic effects. Characteristics that enhance the efficacy of ICSs include high glucocorticoid-receptor-binding affinity, small particle size, prolonged pulmonary residence time, and lipid conjugation (50). Characteristics that enhance the safety of an ICS include minimal oral bioavailability, onsite activation in the lung, low oropharyngeal exposure, high protein binding, and rapid systemic clearance (30,50). Clinicians should consider these characteristics when choosing an appropriate ICS. Pharmacokinetic variables are summarized in Table 35.2.

Reviews of the literature are helpful, but clinicians should interpret comparative studies with caution because study parameters may differ in their methods of measuring adverse effects and their choices of delivery device. Either of these can result in false comparisons. A better method of comparing various ICSs or a single drug in different formulations is the therapeutic index, which is the ratio of desirable-to-undesirable effects. Desirable topical effects would include potency, the amount of GCs delivered to the lung, and pro-drug conversion. Undesirable effects would be due to mineralocorticoid activity, rate of clearance from the body, and the bioavailability of the GC after lung and gastrointestinal absorption. First-pass metabolism of the swallowed fraction of the GC is also of great importance in determining drug choice in asthma therapy.

Most newer ICS products have low oral bioavailability (Table 35.2). Budesonide, MF, and FP have a lower oral bioavailability than BDP because of their extensive hepatic first-pass metabolism, but studies suggest that the oral deposition of CIC is significantly less than with either FP (51) or BUD (52). The lower the oral bioavailability, the fewer the systemic side effects at equivalent doses. The relative anti-inflammatory potency of the ICS from most-potent to least-potent can be summarized as follows: CIC = FP = MF > BUD = BDP >TA = FL.

Delivery Devices

The type of delivery device plays an important role in determining the amount of drug delivered to the lungs; Chapter 38 reviews delivery devices in more detail. Lung deposition is influenced by the inhalation device, propellant, particle size, i.e., mass mean aerodynamic diameter (MMAD), and by whether the solution is an aerosol or suspension. Delivery devices are the metered-dose inhaler (MDI), dry powder inhaler (DPI), and the nebulizer (for infants, young children, and the elderly). Ease of use and less-frequent dosing are other factors to consider, as they lead to better compliance (Tables 35.3 and 35.4). Some devices have multidose capabilities. In MDIs, which may be either breath-activated or pressurized, hydrofluoroalkane (HFA) propellants have largely replaced chlorofluorocarbon (CFC) propellants due to a worldwide mandate. A spacer may be used with CFC/HFA-propelled MDIs to reduce oropharyngeal deposition.

One study that compared delivery of FL via an HFA MDI (with a built-in spacer) to delivery via a CFC MDI found that HFA FL was similarly efficacious at one-third the dosage (53). The authors noted that aerosol particle size in the new FL HFA solution is smaller than the FL CFC suspension (1.2 versus 3.8 MMAD). Because aerosol particle size is a key determinant of lung deposition and regional distribution of inhaled drugs, the HFA MDI improved distal lung deposition.

The dose of drug delivered to the lungs differs between MDIs and DPIs and among devices delivering different ICSs (Table 35.3), so clinicians should consider these differences when choosing a device. For maintenance asthma therapy in young children over 5 years of age, the pressurized MDI (pMDI) in combination with a spacer is the first choice for delivering aerosols (54), and it is the most cost-effective (55). A face mask can be attached if necessary, but a good seal is crucial to avoid a dramatic reduction in delivered dose. Using a pMDI with extra-fine particles can improve lung deposition. A cooperative patient is also essential. During crying, the dose to the lungs is minimal (54).

Nebulizers deliver relatively low doses of drug to the lungs. An *in-vitro* study comparing two nebulizers found that both delivered 9% to 15% of the nominal dose of FL to the breathing simulator (56). The characteristics of the facemask, the seal, and the breathing pattern all affect the amount of drug delivered.

Dose-Response Considerations

Drug deposition in the lungs should predict clinical response, but the flat nature of dose-response curves often masks this relationship (57). With regard to improved lung function, several recent meta-analyses of the literature report that low-to-medium doses of ICS produced nearly maximal benefit—up to 90% in one study—compared with high doses (58,59). However, though there appears to be little relationship between ICS dose and forced expiratory volume in 1 second (FEV_1), there may be a dose-related favorable response with regard to other outcomes, such as bronchial hyperresponsiveness (60), cortical suppression (61), and reduction in oral steroid dose (62).

There is a much steeper dose-response curve for systemic effects, however, so the smaller proportional additional benefits of higher doses must be weighed against the risks in individual patients. The principal adverse effects are adrenal suppression, reduced bone mineral density, and steroid purpura. The loss of bone mineral density is of particular concern in patients who may require lifelong asthma treatment. One must also consider the severity of the patient's asthma. Patients with very mild asthma have relatively minimal airflow obstruction and little room for improvement, so low doses potentially provide maximal improvement. Patients with unstable or more severe asthma have significantly greater airflow obstruction and therefore may show a greater response to increasing doses.

Clinical Use of Inhaled Corticosteroid Therapy

Inhaled corticosteroid therapy is recommended as first-line treatment for all patients with persistent symptoms. The clinician should begin ICS in any patient

TABLE 35.3 COMPARISON OF DRUG DEPOSITION WITH METERED-DOSE INHALERS/ HYDROFLUOROALKANE AND DRY-POWDER INHALERS (%)

DRUG	FORMULATION	MMAD (μ–M)	MDI	DPI	NEBULIZER
BDP	MDI-HFA solution	1.1	18.6	NA	NA
BUD	DPI/nebulized suspension	NA	NA	34	10% to 20%
FLN	MDI-HFA solution	1.2	68	NA	NA
FP	DPI/MDI-HFA solution	DPI-NA/MDI-2.4 to 3.2	13-18	16	NA
MF	Dry powder		NA	14	NA
TA	Suspension	NA	20	NA	NA
CIC	Solution		52	NA	NA

BDP used a Volumatic spacer; BUD used a Nebuhaler spacer; TA used a built-in spacer.

BDP used Clickhaler; BUD used Turbuhaler; FP used Diskus.

DPI, dry powder inhaler; MDI, metered-dose inhaler; HFA, hydrofluoroalkane; MMAD, mass mean aerodynamic diameter

who requires a β_2-agonist inhaler more than two times per week or uses more than two β_2-agonist canisters per year. The current approach is to start with a dose of ICS corresponding to the asthma severity classification based on the EPR-3 (30) (Table 35.5 for comparative doses for adults and children). Step-up therapy with additional controller agents and/or a change of device, ICS, or preparation may control symptoms when single ICS therapy is ineffective. A short course of oral systemic GC may also be used to gain faster control. Once control is achieved, the dose should be stepped down to the lowest possible dose necessary for optimal control, which is defined as best/normal lung function and only occasional need for a short-acting β_2-agonist inhaler. Long-acting β_2 agonists (LABAs) may be used in combination with ICSs for long-term control and prevention of symptoms in moderate or severe persistent asthma. Adding a LABA more consistently reduces impairment compared with increasing the dose of ICS (30).

Dose changes should be gradual, at 3-month intervals or longer. An MDI with a large-volume spacer or mouth rinsing after use of a DPI helps to reduce the risk of local and systemic effects. Twice-a-day dosing is standard for older preparations, but in unstable asthma, four-times-a-day will achieve better control (63), and once-a-day will not reduce efficacy for doses of 400 µg or less (64). The newer ICSs—FP, CIC, and MF—may be given as once-daily doses.

Systemic Glucocorticoid Therapy and Acute Severe Asthma

The EPR-3 recommends systemic GC therapy for exacerbations that are not responsive to therapy with inhaled β_2 agonists (30). In moderate-to-severe exacerbations, systemic GC treatment should be initiated immediately after recognition of an acute attack. Systemic GC therapy reduces hospitalizations and prevents relapses, especially in patients at high risk for fatal asthma (65,66). Administration can be by oral, intravenous (IV), or intramuscular routes. Commonly used IV-administered GCs include hydrocortisone, betamethasone, methylprednisolone, and dexamethasone (67). There are no clinical studies to date that suggest

TABLE 35.4 COMPARISON FACTORS FOR RISK/BENEFIT RATIOS OF GLUCOCORTICOIDS AND DELIVERY SYSTEMS*

PHARMACOKINETICS	PHARMACODYNAMICS	DELIVERY DEVICE CHARACTERISTICS
Receptor affinity	Dose-response characteristics	Output
Plasma half-life	Duration of action	Particle-size distribution
Volume of distribution		Efficiency of lung delivery
Plasma clearance		Ease of use
Rate of first-pass metabolism		

*Cost could also be relevant.

TABLE 35.5   COMPARATIVE ICS DOSAGES FOR ADULTS (>12 YEARS) AND CHILDREN (0 TO 4 YEARS AND 5 TO 11 YEARS)

DRUG (μg PER PUFF)	LOW DOSE (μg)	MEDIUM DOSE (μg)	HIGH DOSE (μg)
Beclomethasone HFA 40 or 80	Adults 80 to 240 Children 80 to 160	Adults >240 to 480 Children >160 to 320	Adults >480 Children >320
Budesonide DPI 90 or 180 Respules 0.25 mg, 0.5 mg, 1.0 mg (0 to 4 yr)	Adults 180 to 600 Children 180 to 400 Children (0 to 4) 0.25 mg to 0.5 mg	Adults 600 to 1,200 Children 400 to 800 Children (0 to 4) 0.5mg to 1.0 mg	Adults >1,200 Children >800 Children: (0 to 4) >1.0 mg
Flunisolide HFA 80	Adults 320 Children 160	Adults 320 to 640 Children 320	Adults >640 Children >640
Triamcinolone HFA 100	Adults 300 to 750 Children 300 to 600	Adults >750-1,500 Children >600 to 900	Adults >1,500 Children >900
Fluticasone HFA 44, 110, 220 DPI 50, 100, 250	Adults 88 to 264 Children 88 to 176 Children (0 to 4) 176	Adults 264 to 440 Children 176 to 352 Children (0 to 4) 176 to 352	Adults >440 Children >352 Children (0 to 4) >352
Mometasone DPI 110 or 220	Adults 220 Children 110	Adults 440 Children 220 to 330	Adults >440 Children >330
Ciclesonide	Adults 320	Adults 320 to 640	Adults >640

pharmacological advantages translate to clinical differences among the commonly used IV preparations (68). However, methylprednisolone, because of its greater anti-inflammatory potency, lower mineralocorticoid activity, and lower price by comparison with hydrocortisone, may be the drug of choice for IV therapy (68).

For acutely ill asthmatic adults, 10 mg/kg to 15 mg/kg/24 hours intravenously of hydrocortisone (or its equivalent) may be appropriate. This would equate to a comparable dose of 600 mg to 900 mg of hydrocortisone (4 mg/kg to 6 mg/kg in children), 150 mg to 225 mg of prednisone (1 mg/kg to 1.5 mg/kg in children) or 120 mg to 180 mg per day of methylprednisolone (1 mg/kg every 6 hours in children for 48 hours then 1 mg/kg/day to 2 mg/kg/day) for an average adult asthmatic (66–69). For maximum therapeutic benefit, treatment should be maintained for 48 hours depending on the clinical response. Dosing intervals depend on the clinical condition of the acutely ill asthmatic. However, intervals may begin at every 4 to 6 hours. When signs and symptoms improve, doses can be tapered to twice daily, then to a single morning daily dose. Patients who require IV GCs can be switched to oral GCs once stable. The total duration of IV therapy is dependent on both subjective and objective improvement in respiratory status and responsiveness to adrenergic bronchodilator therapy (67).

Oral glucocorticoids in moderately high doses may be required in severe chronic asthma or in acute exacerbations. In most hospitalized patients without risk of impending ventilatory failure, oral prednisone,

prednisolone, or methylprednisolone are as effective as IV treatments (69). Prednisone 60 mg/day to 80 mg/day (1 mg/kg/day to 2 mg/kg/day in children) or methylprednisolone 7.5 mg/day to 60 mg/day (0.25 mg/kg/day to 2.0 mg/kg/day in children) may be given in single or divided doses. In patients with mild asthma who are typically well controlled, an asthma exacerbation may require a 3- to 10-day course of oral GCs (66–71). Patients who need to continue oral GC treatment for longer periods should convert to alternate-day administration to reduce the risk of side effects. The clinician should attempt to reduce the dose by 5 mg to 10 mg every two weeks until the lowest clinically effective dose is reached. The goal is to discontinue systemic GC therapy if possible.

Allergic reactions to systemic corticosteroids have been reported and are more common in aspirin-sensitive asthmatics (72). Worsening asthma despite systemic corticosteroid therapy may be mediated by immunoglobulin E (IgE) mechanisms (73,74). Skin-prick testing and *in vitro* IgE levels are used for confirming this very rare diagnosis (72). Commonly implicated GCs include hydrocortisone, prednisone, and methylprednisolone. Patients who have confirmed allergy to GCs should undergo challenge testing with an alternative preparation such as dexamethasone or prednisone (75).

Intranasal Glucocorticoids and Allergic Rhinitis

Guidelines for the treatment of both perennial and seasonal allergic rhinitis recommend intranasal GCs as safe and effective therapy. These anti-inflammatory medications have prolonged local action, few local side effects, and few, if any, systemic effects (76). Currently, there are eight intranasal ICS preparations available for treatment of allergic rhinitis in the United States: BDP, FL, FP, fluticasone furoate (FF), TA, BUD, MF, and ciclesonide (CIC). All have similar safety profiles, and all are similarly efficacious in controlling symptoms (Table 35.2).

All intranasal GCs act directly on inflammation to reduce the symptoms of allergic rhinitis—nasal congestion, itching, sneezing, and rhinorrhea. They reduce fluid exudation and the number of circulating inflammatory cells, including basophils, lymphocytes, mast cells, eosinophils, neutrophils, and macrophages. These preparations have rapid onsets, short half-lives, and rapid first-pass hepatic metabolism (77). CIC, the newest of these drugs, compares favorably with other newer intranasal GCs in its ability to effectively reduce symptoms without producing local or systemic side effects (78–80).

A review of randomized controlled trials suggests that combining antihistamines and intranasal GCs in the treatment of allergic rhinitis provides no additional benefit (81). However, intranasal FF appears to reduce daily reflective total ocular-symptom scores in patients with seasonal allergic rhinitis (82). Further research is needed to determine the role of combination therapy of antihistamines and intranasal GC in seasonal allergic rhinitis.

Treatment with intranasal GCs is best begun days before allergen exposure—usually about 2 weeks before the beginning of allergy season—and may be maintained for another 2 weeks after the end of the season to control residual mucosal hyperreactivity. Therapy should be used regularly, rather than as needed. Guidelines recommend tapering the dose to the lowest level required to maintain symptom relief after reaching initial control (83).

Most adverse effects are mild and do not warrant discontinuation of treatment. Epistaxis occurs in 5% to 8% of patients and is usually self-limiting. Atrophy or thinning of the nasal tissue with long-term use is not a problem with the newer intranasal GCs. The potential for systemic absorption and HPA-axis suppression is a concern in children since systemically absorbed GC may interrupt or retard growth. However, studies have generally found no difference between intranasal GCs and placebo in their effects on HPA-axis function in either children or adults (84,85). One study did find significantly slower growth rates after 1 year in children treated with intranasal BDP versus placebo, beginning as early as 1 month after treatment began (86). Other intranasal GCs do not appear to affect growth (84). Clinicians should be aware, however, that this finding applies to the use of intranasal GCs alone and in recommended doses, not to higher doses or treatments that combine intranasal GCs with ICSs or other topical corticosteroids. Such patients should always be monitored for growth. Even if children are treated only with intranasal GCs, however, it is prudent to observe the growth rate.

Corticosteroids for Other Allergic Diseases

Nasal Polyposis

Topical and systemic GCs are accepted medical adjuncts to surgery in patients who have nasal polyposis (87–89). Medical polypectomy may be achieved by oral prednisolone 0.5 mg/kg/day for 5 to 10 days plus betamethasone nasal drops three times daily in each nostril in the "head upside down" position for 5 days, then twice daily until the bottle runs out (87). Maintenance therapy with topical corticosteroids, such as BDP, BUD, MF, or FL helps in ameliorating rhinitis symptoms and reducing polyp size (90,91). In mild cases, topical GCs can be used alone as long-term therapy, which will have fewer systemic effects than betamethasone nasal drops (90,91).

Atopic Dermatitis and Allergic Contact Dermatitis

The use of high-potency topical GCs has led to improved treatment for dermatologic conditions that have an inflammatory etiology, such as urticaria and atopic dermatitis (AD) (Chapter 29 on atopic dermatitis) (92,93). The choice of topical corticosteroid potency depends on the severity and distribution of AD. Although using the least potent corticosteroid is typically a good rule to follow, this approach should be weighed against the possibility that treatment with a preparation that is too weak may result in persistence or worsening of AD, which can result in decreased adherence or the need for high-potency topical or systemic corticosteroids. A more effective strategy may be to use a stepped approach starting with a mid-potency preparation (except for eczema involving the face, axillae, or groin) and, with clinical improvement, switching to a lower-potency preparation. High-potency corticosteroids may be needed for severe hand and foot eczema. Only mild-to-moderate potency steroid preparations should be used in children. In severe cases of atopic dermatitis, oral GC may be used sparingly (94). Severe allergic contact dermatitis that fails to respond to topical treatment may improve with once-daily, then alternate-day oral prednisone at doses of 30 mg to 60 mg for 1 to 2 weeks (95).

Ocular Allergy

Nonsteroidal anti-inflammatory agents, antihistamines, and mast-cell stabilizers are the typical treatments for mild-to-moderate allergic conjunctivitis, but in severe cases, topical corticosteroids—preferably those with reduced side effects—may be necessary (96). Loteprednol etabonate (LE) has been found effective for treating ocular allergy and inflammation (97). LE eye drops are available as either 0.5% or 0.2% suspensions, but several randomized trials confirm that the lower dose is effective in reducing redness and itching without causing significant changes in intraocular pressure, even with long-term use (98).

Treatments for vernal keratoconjunctivitis, a severe but transient form of ocular allergy, include LE, fluorometholone 0.1%, nedocromil 2%, and sodium cromoglycate 2% (96,97). Because it potentiates the tendency for paclitaxel to induce full-thickness skin necrosis, fluorometholone should not be used in patients receiving treatment with Taxol (99).

Idiopathic Anaphylaxis and Urticaria

Idiopathic anaphylaxis in both adults and children has been successfully treated with systemic prednisone, hydroxyzine, and albuterol to control symptoms and induce remission (100). It should be noted, however, that systemic administration of steroids, notably methylprednisolone, can very rarely induce anaphylaxis (73).

Management of acute and chronic urticaria typically includes H_1- and H_2-type of antihistamines (101). In refractory cases of chronic urticaria additional measures are needed to control symptoms. Initial therapy with GC may start with 30 mg to 40 mg of prednisone to control symptoms, and then alternate day therapy with a taper as clinically indicated (101). Delayed pressure urticaria may respond more favorably to oral corticosteroids (101).

Adverse Effects of Glucocorticoid Therapy

Potentially, there are many adverse effects associated with GC therapy (Table 35.6), particularly with oral and parenteral routes of administration, so patients on

chronic steroid therapy should be monitored closely. Tests may include those for suppression of the HPA axis, cataracts, hyperglycemia, hypertension, and osteoporosis. Complications attributable to steroid use are directly related to dose, variability of individual response, dosing schedule, route of administration, and duration of therapy.

Patients who are subjected to long-term oral GC therapy develop an increased risk of osteoporosis, which is associated with a high risk of bone fractures (102). Several studies of ICS use in children suggest that, at currently recommended doses, there is no significant reduction in bone mineral density (103,104). However, in adult asthmatics evidence indicates that long-term ICS use affects bone mineral density and risk of fractures in a dose-dependent fashion that appears significant at high doses (1,000 µg to 2,000 µg BDP daily) (105). Steroid-induced osteoporosis appears to be irreversible (106), so it is important to limit systemic steroid use as much as possible in susceptible patients. Attention to good bone health in patients receiving CS is advisable as most patients are not usually ingesting sufficient quantities of vitamin D or calcium.

Administration of exogenous corticosteroids can result in HPA suppression. Since there is significant patient-to-patient variability, it is difficult to determine the smallest dose or duration that would suppress the HPA axis. High doses (15 mg/day to 50 mg/day) of prednisone in short duration (i.e., <30 days) or low dosage (0.09 mg/kg/day to 0.15 mg/kg/day of prednisone equivalent) prescribed for over 1 year may induce adrenal insufficiency. Initial studies with ICS suggested that adrenal suppression occurred only with inhaled doses over 1,500 µg/day to 2,000 µg/day BDP or equivalent for 1 year (107), but more recent data suggest that further studies are necessary to determine the cumulative effect (108).

Patients who develop acute adrenal insufficiency can present with dehydration, shock, electrolyte abnormalities, severe abdominal pain, and lethargy (109). This is a medical emergency that requires prompt diagnosis and rapid treatment with intravenous

TABLE 35.6   POTENTIAL ADVERSE EFFECTS OF GLUCOCORTICOIDS*

Hypertension	Cataracts	Myopathy
Osteoporosis; fractures	Growth retardation	Hypokalemia
Diabetes	Pancreatitis	Recurrent infections
Peptic ulcer disease	Hypoadrenalism	Hypoglycemia
Immunosuppression	Avascular necrosis	Poor wound healing
Glaucoma	Muscle wasting	HPA-axis suppression
Weight gain	Fluid retention	
Behavioral symptoms	Cushing syndrome	

*Using the minimal effective dose and duration of GCs will reduce potential adverse effects.

hydrocortisone (100 mg every 8 hours until the patient becomes stabilized and can tolerate oral therapy) (109). All adrenally suppressed individuals should receive hydrocortisone at the time of any surgical procedure or at times of acute stress. Complete recovery from adrenal suppression can take as long as 12 months after cessation of long-term GC therapy.

The effect of ICSs on linear growth remains the greatest concern in pediatric patients. A review conducted by the EPR-3 found that most studies did not demonstrate an effect on growth (30). Consensus panels have concluded the following:

- ICSs are associated with a decrease in short-term growth rates in children, but the overall effect is small and may not be sustained with long-term ICS therapy.
- The final adult height attained by asthmatic children treated with ICSs is not different from that of non-asthmatic children.
- There is insufficient information on the difference between steroid formulations to derive definitive comparative conclusions.
- Poorly controlled asthma might have a greater impact on growth than ICS.

Physicians should be cautious: step down therapy when possible and closely monitor children's growth rates. Risk of adverse effects is minimized by using the lowest effective dosage, by limiting systemic availability of the drug through careful selection of the inhalation device and proper technique, by the adjunct use of alternative anti-inflammatory agents, and, when higher doses are required, by choice of ICS medication. The lowest effective dose of ICS should be prescribed and additional add-on therapy for steroid-sparing agents (i.e., long-acting β-agonists or leukotriene-modifying agents) should be explored. Additional treatments such as concomitant oral GC may further impact growth rates if used on a frequent basis.

The principal local adverse effects of GC and ICS therapy include oral candidiasis, dysphonia, throat irritation, and cough. Oral candidiasis and hoarseness appear to be dose-dependent. These problems are not sufficient reasons to discontinue ICS treatment. A spacer and/or a change to an MDI preparation may alleviate both oral candidiasis and hoarseness. GC-induced candidiasis responds to oral antifungal preparations, such as nystatin or fluconazole. Gargling and mouth rinsing after inhalation can reduce future occurrences. There is no evidence for atrophy of the lining of the airway or of an increase in lung infections (including tuberculosis) after ICS use.

Steroid-resistant, Steroid-dependent Asthma

Most physicians recognize that certain patients do not respond to even high doses of GCs. Some may initially seem to do so but subsequently develop resistance. Resistance to the therapeutic effects of GC treatment is also recognized in other inflammatory and autoimmune diseases, including inflammatory bowel disease (110). Studies indicate a spectrum of GC responsiveness, with rare resistance at one end and relative resistance in patients who require high doses of inhaled and oral GC (50,111).

Glucocorticoid-resistant asthma is defined as failure to improve FEV_1 or peak expiratory flow by more than 15% after treatment with oral prednisolone 20 mg twice daily for 2 weeks (112). It is important to determine that the patient has asthma and not another disease, such as chronic obstructive pulmonary disease, which may not respond to GC treatment (113). The clinician should also investigate the possibility of instigating factors, such as allergens, other medications, or psychological problems that could increase the severity of asthma and its resistance to treatment (114,115). In clinical practice, any patient not responding to 40 mg to 60 mg daily of prednisone for 3 weeks should be suspected of having GC-resistance asthma.

A poor response to GC therapy could be related to reduced numbers of GCRs, altered affinity for the ligand for GCRs, reduced ability of the GCRs to bind DNA, or increased expression of inflammatory transcription factors, such as AP-1, that compete for DNA binding (116). Other factors contributing to GC resistance include poor absorption, reduced metabolism, corticosteroid allergy with aspirin sensitivity, and ongoing allergen exposure.

The glucocorticoid receptor has more than one phenotype: GCR-β will not bind to glucocorticoids but does interfere with the movement of GCR-α to the nucleus and with gene activation (117). Abnormal GCR binding may be due to cytokine-driven alternative splicing of exon 9 of the CR gene which gives rise to increased levels of GR-β (118). Increased expression of GR-β has been noted in fatal asthma and nocturnal asthma and in patients with emphysema, chronic sinusitis, and ulcerative colitis (118). It is unknown whether there is any downregulation of GRs in the airways with treatment with topical GC (116).

Some alternative treatments are so-called "corticosteroid-sparing" drugs because they may reduce GC requirements. These include methotrexate, oral gold, cyclosporine-A, intravenous immunoglobulin (IVIG), etanercept, furosemide, lidocaine, macrolide antibiotics, and omalizumab. Methotrexate, an antimetabolite, has been extensively studied (119–121). Methotrexate has both immunosuppressive and anti-inflammatory mechanisms, but there is little evidence of immunosuppressive effects at low doses. Etanercept, furosemide, lidocaine, macrolide antibiotics, IVIG, and cyclosporine-A have been shown to have marginal benefits in oral GC reduction in steroid-dependent asthmatics (111). These treatments all have adverse effects that can cause problems of their own, so they are recommended for treatment in asthma patients only when there is no alternative.

Omalizumab, a recombinant humanized monoclonal antibody against IgE represents a novel therapeutic approach to allergic asthma. By binding the high-affinity receptor for the IgE molecule, omalizumab prevents IgE production by B-lymphocytes and sensitization of the mast cell. Treatment has been shown to improve quality of life in difficult-to-control asthma, when compared with guideline-directed therapy. Patients who experience two exacerbations requiring a hospitalization in a 12-month period or who fail to respond to oral corticosteroids should be considered for a 6-month trial of omalizumab (122).

■ REFERENCES

1. Addison T. *On the Constitutional and Local Effects of Disease of the Suprarenal Capsules.* London: Samuel Higley; 1855.

2. Schleimer RP, Busse WW, O'Byrne PM. *Inhaled Glucocorticoids in Asthma, Mechanisms and Clinical Actions.* New York: Marcel Dekker; 1997.

3. Hench PS, Kendall EC, Slocumb CH, et al. The effect of a hormone of the adrenal cortex (17-hydroxy-11-dehydrocortiscosterone; compound E) and of pituitary adrenocorticotropic hormone on rheumatoid arthritis. *Proc Staff Meet Mayo Clinic.* 1949;24:181–197.

4. Hench PS, Kendall EC, Slocumb CH, et al. Effects of cortisone acetate and pituitary ACTH on rheumatoid arthritis, rheumatic fever and certain other conditions. *Arch Intern Med.* 1950;85:545–666.

5. Khoo BP, Leow YH, Ng SK, et al. Corticosteroid contact hypersensitivity screening in Singapore. *Am J Contact Dermat.* 1998;9(2):87–91.

6. Gaddie J, Reid IW, Skinner C, et al. Aerosol beclomethasone dipropionate: a dose response study in chronic bronchial asthma.*Lancet.* 1973;2:280–281.

7. Davies G, Thomas P, Broder I, et al. Steroid-dependent asthma treated with inhaled beclomethasone dipropionate—a long-term study. *Ann Intern Med.* 1977;86:549–553.

8. Johnson CE. Aerosol corticosteroids for the treatment of asthma. *Drug Intell Clin Pharm.* 1987;21(10):784–790.

9. Djukanovic R, Roche WR, Wilson JW, et al. State of the art: mucosal inflammation in asthma. *Am Rev Respir Dis.* 1990;142:434–437.

10. Laitinen LA, Heino M, Laitinen A, et al. Damage of the airway epithelium and bronchial reactivity in patients with asthma. *Am Rev Respir Dis.* 1985;131:599–606.

11. Boushey HA. Effects of inhaled corticosteroids on the consequences of asthma. *J Allergy Clin Immunol.* 1998;102:S5–S16.

12. Kraan J, Koeter GH, van der Mark TW, et al. Changes in bronchial hyperreactivity induced by 4 weeks of treatment with antiasthmatic drugs in patients with allergic asthma: a comparison between budesonide and terbutaline. *J Allergy Clin Immunol.* 1985;76:628–636.

13. Kerrebijn KF, van Essen-Zandvliet EEM, Neijens HJ. Effect of long-term treatment with inhaled corticosteroids and beta-agonists on the bronchial responsiveness in children with asthma. *J Allergy Clin Immunol.* 1987;79:653–659.

14. National Asthma Education Program. *Expert Panel Report: Guidelines for the Diagnosis and Management of Asthma.* Bethesda, MD: NIH/National Heart, Lung, and Blood Institute; 1991. Publication 91–3042.

15. National Asthma Education and Prevention Program. *Expert Panel Report 2: Guidelines for the Diagnosis and Management of Asthma.* Bethesda, MD: NIH/National Heart, Lung, and Blood Institute; April 1997. Publication 97–4051.

16. National Asthma Education and Prevention Program. *Expert Panel Report 3: Guidelines for the Diagnosis and Management of Asthma.* Bethesda, MD: NIH/National Heart, Lung, and Blood Institute; November 2007. Publication 08–4051.

17. Orth DN, Kovacs WJ, DeBold CR. The adrenal cortex. In: Wilson JD, Forster DW, eds. *Williams Textbook of Endocrinology.* 8th ed. Philadelphia: WB Saunders; 1991:489–619.

18. Jackson RV, Bowman RV. Corticosteroids. *Med J Aust.* 1995;162:663–665.

19. Esteban NV, Laughlin T, Yergey AI, et al. Daily cortisol production rate in man determined by stable isotope dilution/mass spectrometry. *J Clin Endocrinol Metab.* 1991;72:39–45.

20. Pedersen S, O'Byrne P. A comparison of the efficacy and safety of inhaled corticosteroids in asthma. *Allergy.* 1997;52(suppl 39):1–34.

21. Barnes PJ. How corticosteroids control inflammation: Quinteles Prize lecture 2005. *Br J Pharmacol.* 2006;148(3):245–254.

22. Stahn C, Lowenberg M, Hommes DW, et al. Molecular mechanisms of glucocorticoid action and selective glucocorticoid receptor agonists. *Mol Cell Endocrinol.* 2007;275(1–2):71–78.

23. Wikstrom AC. Glucocorticoid action and novel mechanisms of steroid resistance: role of glucocorticoid receptor-interacting proteins for glucocorticoid responsiveness. *J Endocrinol.* 2003;178:331–337.

24. Kassel O, Herrlich P. Crosstalk between the glucocorticoid receptor and other transcription factors: molecular aspects. *Mol Cell Endocrinol.* 2007;275(1–2):13–29.

25. Dostert A, Heinzel T. Negative glucocorticoid receptor response elements and their role in glucocorticoid action. *Curr Pharm Des.* 2004;10(23):2807–2816.

26. Jee YK, Gilmour J, Kelly A, et al. Repression of interleukin-5 transcription by the glucocorticoid receptor targets GATA3 signaling and involves histone deacetylase recruitment. *J Biol Chem.* 2005;280(24):23243–23250.

27. Wilson SJ, Wallin A, Della-Cioppa G, et al. Effects of budesonide and formoterol on NF-kappaβ, adhesion molecules, and cytokines in asthma. *Am J Resp Crit Care Med.* 2001;164(6):1047–1052.

28. Tasker JG, Di S, Malcher-Lopes R. Minireview: rapid glucocorticoid signaling via membrane-associated receptors. *Endocrinology.* 2006;147(12):5549–5556.

29. Barnes PJ. Molecular mechanisms and cellular effects of glucocorticosteroids. *Immunol Allergy Clin North Am.* 2005;25(3):451–468.

30. National Asthma Education and Prevention Program. Expert Panel Report 3 (EPR-3): guidelines for the diagnosis and management of asthma—summary report 2007. *J Allergy Clin Immunology.* 2007;120(5 Suppl):S94–S138.

31. Kroegel C. Global initiative for asthma management and prevention–GINA 2006. *Pneumologie.* 2007;61(5):295–304.

32. Cerasoli Switch F Jr. Developing the ideal corticosteroid. *Chest.* 2006;130:548–648.

33. Suissa S, Ernst P, Benayoun S, et al. Low-dose inhaled corticosteroids and the prevention of death from asthma. *N Engl J Med.* 2000;343(5):332–336.

34. Murray CS, Woodcock A, Langley SJ, et al. Secondary prevention of asthma by the use of inhaled fluticasone propionate in wheezy infants (IFWIN): double-blind, randomized, controlled study. *Lancet.* 2006;368:754–762.

35. Guilbert TW, Morgan WJ, Zeiger RS, et al. Long-term inhaled corticosteroids in preschool children at high risk for asthma. *New Engl J Med.* 2006;354:1985–1997.

36. Murray CS. Can inhaled corticosteroids influence the natural history of asthma? *Curr Opin Allergy Clin Immunol.* 2008;8(1):77–81.

37. Munakata, M. Airway remodeling and airway smooth muscle in asthma. *Allergol Int.* 2006;55(3):235–243.

38. Sears MR. Consequences of long-term inflammation. The natural history of asthma. *Clin Chest Med.* 2000;21(2):315–329.

39. Djukanovic R. Asthma: a disease of inflammation and repair. *J Allergy Clin Immunol.* 2000;105(2Pt2):S522–S526.

40. Vignola AM, Chanez P, Bonsignore G, et al. Structural consequences of airway inflammation in asthma. *J Allergy Clin Immunol.* 2000;105(2Pt2):S514–S517.

41. Fahy JV, Corry DB, Boushey HA. Airway inflammation and remodeling in asthma. *Curr Opin Pulm Med.* 2000;6(1):15–20.

42. Homer RJ, Elias JA. Consequences of long-term inflammation. Airway remodeling. *Clin Chest Med.* 2000;21(2):331–343.

43. Bush A. How early do airway inflammation and remodeling occur? *Allergol Int.* 2008;57(1):11–19.

44. Warner SM, Knight DA, Airway modeling and remodeling in the pathogenesis of asthma. *Curr Opin Allergy Clin Immunol.* 2008;8(1):44–48.

45. Holgate ST. The airway epithelium is central to the pathogenesis of asthma. *Allergol Int.* 2008;57(1):1–10.

46. Sheffer AL, Silverman M, Woolcock AJ, et al. Long-term safety of once-daily budesonide in patients with early-onset mild persistent asthma: results of the Inhaled Steroid Treatment as Regular Therapy in Early Asthma (START) study. *Ann Allergy Asthma Immunol.* 2005;94(1):48–54.

47. Silverman M, Sheffer AL, Diaz PV, et al. Safety and tolerability of inhaled budesonide in children in the Steroid Treatment as Regular Therapy in early asthma (START) trial. *Pediatr Allergy Immunol.* 2006;17(17Suppl):14–20.

48. Navarro RP, Parasuraman B. Cost effectiveness of asthma controller therapies: influence of disease severity and other variables. *Manag Care Interface.* 2005;18(6):31–40.

49. Fuhlbrigge AL, Bae SJ, Weiss ST, et al. Cost-effectiveness of inhaled steroids in asthma: impact of effect on bone mineral density. *J Allergy Clin Immunol.* 2006;117(2):359–366.

50. Derendorf H, Nave R, Drollmann A, et al. Relevance of pharmacokinetics and pharmacodynamics of inhaled corticosteroids to asthma. *Eur Respir J.* 2006;28(5):1042–1050.

51. Richter K, Kanniess F, Biberger C, et al. Comparison of the oropharyngeal deposition of inhaled ciclesonide and fluticasone propionate in patients with asthma. *J Clin Pharmacol.* 2005;45: 146–152.

52. Nave R, Zech K, Bethke TD. Lower oropharyngeal deposition of inhaled ciclesonide via hydrofluoralkane metered-dose inhaler compared with budesonide via chlorofluorocarbon metered-dose inhaler in healthy subjects. *Eur J Clin Pharmacol.* 2005;61(3):203–208.

53. Waugh J, Goa KL. Flunisolide HFA. *Am J Respir Med.* 2002; 1(5):369–372.

54. Janssens HM, Tiddens HA. Aerosol therapy: the special needs of young children. *Pediatr Respir Rev,* 2006; 7 Suppl 1:S83–S85.

55. Brocklebank D, Wright J, Cates C. Systematic review of clinical effectiveness of pressurized metered dose inhalers versus other hand held inhaler devices for delivering corticosteroids in asthma. *BMJ.* 2001;323(7318):896–900.

56. O'Callaghan C, White J, Jackson J, et al. The output of flunisolide from different nebulisers. *J Pharm Pharmacol.* 2002;54(4): 565–569.

57. Newman SP. Deposition and effects of inhaled corticosteroids. *Clin Pharmacokinet.* 2003;42(6):529–544.

58. Donohue JF, Ohar JA. Effects of cortocosteroids on lung function in asthma and chronic obstructive pulmonary disease. *Proc Am Thorac Soc.* 2004;1:152–160.

59. Masoli M, Holt S, Weatherall M. Dose-response relationship of inhaled budesonide in adult asthma: a meta-analysis. *Eur Respir J.* 2004;23:552–558.

60. Currie GP, Fowler SJ, Lipworth BJ. Dose response of inhaled corticosteroids on bronchial hyperresponsiveness: a meta-analysis. *Ann Allergy Asthma Immunol.* 2003;90(2):194–198.

61. Martin RJ, Szefler SJ, Chinchilli VM, et al. Systemic effect comparison of six inhaled corticosteroid preparations. *Am J Respir Crit Care Med.* 2002;165(10):1377–1383.

62. Miyamoto T, Takahashi T, Nakajima S, et al. A double blind, placebo-controlled steroid-sparing study with budesonide turbuhaler in Japanese oral steroid-dependent asthma patients. *Respirology.* 2000; 5:231–240.

63. Malo J, Cartier A, Merland N, et al. Four-times-a-day dosing frequency is better than twice-a-day regimen in subjects requiring a high-dose inhaled steroid, budesonide, to control moderate to severe asthma. *Am Rev Respir Dis.* 1989;140:624–628.

64. Jones AH, Langdon CG, Lee PS, et al. Pulmicort Turbohaler once daily as initial prophylactic therapy for asthma. *Respir Med.* 1994; 88:293–299.

65. Rowe BH, Edmonds ML, Spooner CH, et al. Corticosteroid therapy for acute asthma. *Respir Med.* 2004;98:275–284.

66. Rowe BH, Spooner CH, Ducharme FM, et al. Corticosteroids for preventing relapse following acute exacerbations of asthma. *Cochrane Database Syst Rev.* 2007;8(3):CD000195.

67. McFadden ER. Dosages of corticosteroids in asthma. *Am Rev Respir Dis.* 1993;147:1306–1310.

68. Fiel SB, Vincken W. Systemic corticosteroid therapy for acute asthma exacerbations. *J Asthma.* 2006;43:321–331.

69. Cunnington D, Smith N, Steed K, et al. Oral versus intravenous corticosteroids in adults hospitalized with acute asthma. *Pul Pharmacol Ther.* 2005;18(3):207–212.

70. Spahn JD, Szefler SJ. Steroid therapy for asthma in children. *Curr Opin Pediatr.* 2007;19:300–305.

71. Heldeles, L. Selecting a systemic corticosteroid for acute asthma in young children. *J Pediatr,* 2003;142(2 Suppl):S40–S44.

72. Sheth A, Reddymasu S, Jackson R. Worsening of asthma with systemic corticosteroids. A case report and review of the literature. *J Gen Intern Med.* 2006;21(2):C11–C13.

73. Mendelson LM, Meltzer EO, Hamburger RN. Anaphylaxsis-like reactions to corticosteroid therapy. *J Allergy Clin Immunol.* 1974; 54:125–131.

74. Burgdoff T, Venemalm L, Vogt T, et al. IgE mediated anaphylactic reaction induced by succinate ester of methylprednisolone. *Ann Allergy Asthma Immunol.* 2002;89:425–428.

75. Ventura MT, Calogiuri GR, Matino MG, et al. Alternative glucocorticoids for use in cases of adverse reaction to systemic glucocorticoids: a study on 10 patients. *Br J Dermatol.* 2003;148:139–141.

76. Dupclay L Jr, Doyle J. Assessment of intranasal corticosteroid use in allergic rhinitis: benefits, costs, and patient preferences. *Am J Manag Care.* 2002;8:S335–S340.

77. Baena-Cagnani CE. Safety and tolerability of treatments for allergic rhinitis in children. *Drug Saf.* 2004;27(12):883–898.

78. Ratner, PH, Wingertzahn MA, van Bavel JH, et al. Efficacy and safety of ciclesonide nasal spray for the treatment of seasonal allergic rhinitis. *J Allergy Clin Immunol.* 2006;118(5):1142–1148.

79. Meltzer EO, Kunjibettu S, Hall N, et al. Efficacy and safety of ciclesonide, 200 microg once daily, for the treatment of perennial allergic rhinitis. *Ann Allergy Asthma Immunol.* 2007;98(2):175–181.

80. Chervinsky P, Kunjibettu S, Miller DL, et al. Long-term safety and efficacy of intranasal ciclesonide in adult and adolescent patients with perennial allergic rhinitis. *Ann Allergy Asthma Immunol.* 2007; 99(1):69–76.

81. Nielsen LP, Dahl R. Comparison of intranasal corticosteroids and antihistamines in allergic rhinitis: review of randomized, controlled trials. *Am J Respir Med.* 2003;2(1):55–65.

82. Kaiser HB, Naclerio RM, Given J, et al. Fluticasone furoate nasal spray: a single treatment option for the symptoms of seasonal allergic rhinitis. *J Allergy Clin Immunol.* 2007;119(6):1430–1437.

83. Scadding GK, Durham SR, Mirakian R, et al. BSACI guidelines for the management of allergic and non-allergic rhinitis. *Clin Exp Allergy.* 2008;38:19–42.

84. Boner AL. Effects of intranasal corticosteroids on the hypothalamic-pituitary-adrenal axis in children. *J Allergy Clin Immunol.* 2001;108(1 Suppl):S32–S39.

85. Galant SP, Melamed IR, Nayak AS, et al. Lack of effect of fluticasone propionate aqueous nasal spray on the hypothalamic-pituitary-adrenal axis in 2- and 3-year-old patients. *Pediatrics.* 2003;112(1 Pt 1): 96–100.

86. Skoner DP, Rachelefsky GS, Meltzer EO, et al. Detection of growth suppression in children during treatment with intranasal beclomethasone dipropionate. *Pediatrics.* 2000;105(2):E23.

87. Scadding GK, Durham SR, Mirakian R, et al. BSACI guidelines for the management of rhinosinusitis and nasal polyposis. *Clin Exp Allergy.* 2007;38:260–275.

88. Hissaria P, Smith W, Wormald PJ, et al. Short course of systemic corticosteroids in sinonasal polyposis: a double-blind, randomized, placebo-controlled trial with evaluation of outcome measures. *J Allergy Clin Immunol.* 2006;118(1):128–133.

89. Patiar S, Reece, P. Oral steroids for nasal polyps. *Cochrane Database Syst Rev.* 2007;24(1):CD005232.

90. Valera FC, Anselmo-Lima WT. Evaluation of efficacy of topical corticosteroids for the clinical treatment of nasal polyposis: searching for clinical events that may predict response to treatment. *Rhinology.* 2007;45:59–62.

91. Small CB, Hernandez J, Reyes A, et al. Efficacy and safety of mometasone furoate nasal spray in nasal polyposis. *J Allergy Clin Immunol.* 2005;116:1275–1281.

92. Leung DY, Nicklas RA, Li JT, et al. Disease management of atopic dermatitis: an update practice parameter. Joint Task Force on Practice Parameters. *Ann Allergy Asthma Immunol.* 2004;93(3 Suppl 2):S1–S21.

93. Szczepanowska J, Reich A, Szepietowski JC. Emollients improve treatment results with topical corticosteroids in childhood atopic dermatitis: a randomized comparative study. *Pediatr Allergy Immunol.* 2008 Jan 18 [Epub ahead of print].

94. Ong PY, Boguniewicz M. Atopic dermatitis. *Prim Care.* 2008; 35(1):105–117.

95. Jacob SE, Castanedo-Tardan MP. Pharmacotherapy for allergic contact dermatitis. *Expert Opin Pharmacother.* 2007;8(16):2757–2774.

96. Bielory L, Katelaris CH, Lightman S, et al. Treating the ocular component of allergic rhinoconjunctivitis and related eye disorders. *MedGenMed.* 2007;9(3):35.

97. Pavesio CE, Decory HH. Treatment of ocular inflammatory conditions with loteprednol etabonate. *Br J Ophthalmol.* 2008 Feb 1 [Epub ahead of print].

98. Novack GD, Howes J, Crockett RS, et al. Changes in intraocular pressure during long-term use of loteprednol etabonate. *J Glaucoma.* 1998;7(4):266–269.

99. Aboolian A, Tornambe R, Ricci M. Skin necrosis in the presence of paclitaxel and fluorometheolone. *Support Care Cancer.* 1999;7(3): 158–159.

100. Greenberger PA. Idiopathic anaphylaxis. *Immunol Allergy Clin North Am.* 2007;27(2):273–293.

101. Amar SM, Dreskin SC. Urticaria. *Prim Care*. 2008;35(1):141–157.

102. Van Staa TP, Laan RF, Barton IP, et al. Bone density threshold and other predictors of vertebral fracture in patients receiving oral glucocorticoid therapy. *Arthritis Rheum*. 2003;48(11):3224–3229.

103. Allen, DB. Effects of inhaled steroids on growth, bone metabolism, and adrenal function. *Adv Pediatr*. 2006;53:101–110.

104. Allen DB, Bielory L, Derendorf H, et al. Inhaled corticosteroids: past lessons and future issues. *J Allergy Clin Immunol*. 2003;112(3 Suppl):S1–S40.

105. Che M, Ettinger B, Nguyen MT, et al. High-dose corticosteroid exposure and osteoporosis intervention in adults. *Ann Allergy Asthma Immunol*. 2006;97(4):497–501.

106. Devogelaer JP, Goemaere S, Boonen S. et al. Evidence-based guidelines for the prevention and treatment of glucocorticoid-induced osteoporosis: a consensus document of the Belgian Bone Club. *Osteoporos Int*. 2006;17(1):8–19.

107. Brown PH, Blundell G, Greening AP, et al. Hypothalamo-pituitary-adrenal axis suppression in asthmatics inhaling high dose corticosteroids. *Respir Med*. 1991;85(6):501–510.

108. Zollner EW. Hypothalamic-pituitary-adrenal axis suppression in asthmatic children on inhaled corticosteroids (Part 2)—the risk as determined by gold standard adrenal function tests: a systematic review. *Pediatr Allergy Immunol*. 2007;18(6):469–474.

109. Bouillon R. Acute adrenal insufficiency. *Endocrinol Metab Clin N Am*. 2006;35:767–775.

110. Chikanza IC, Kozaci D, Chernajovsky Y. The molecular basis of corticosteroid resistance. *J Endocrinol*. 2003;179:301–310.

111. Randhawa I, Klaustermeyer WB. Oral corticosteroid-dependent asthma: a 30 year review. *Ann Allergy Asthma Immunol*. 2007;99(4):291–302.

112. Leung DYM, Bloom JW. Update on glucocorticoid action and resistance. *J Allergy Clin Immunol*. 2003;111:3–22.

113. Adcock IM, Ito K. Steroid resistence in asthma: a major problem requiring novel solutions or a non-issue? *Current Opin Pharm*. 2004;4(3):257–262.

114. Ito K, Fan Chung K, Adcock I. Update on glucocorticoid action and resistance. *J Allergy Clin Immunol*. 2006;117:522–543.

115. Sheth A, Reddymasu S, Jackson R. Worsening of asthma with systemic corticosteroids. *J Gen Intern Med*. 2006;21:C11–C13.

116. Kelly A, Bowen H, Lavender P, et al. The glucocorticoid receptor β isoform can mediate transcriptional repression by recruiting histone deacetylases. *J Allergy Clin Immunol*. 2008;121:203–208.

117. Lewis Tuffni LJ, Cidlowski JA. The physiology of human glucocorticoid receptor β (hGRβ) and glucocorticoid resistance. *Ann NY Acad Sci*. 2006;1069:1–9.

118. Loke T-K, Sousa AR, Corrigan CJ, et al. Glucocorticoid-resistant asthma. *Curr Allergy Asthma Rep*. 2002;2:144–150.

119. Mullarkey MF, Lammert JK, Blumenstein BA. Long-term methotrexate treatment in corticosteroid-dependent asthma. *Ann Intern Med*. 1990;112:577–581.

120. Comet R, Domingo C, Larrisa M, et al. Benefits of low weekly doses of methotrexate in steroid dependent asthmatic patients: a double blind, randomized, placebo controlled study. *Respir Med*. 2006;100:411–419.

121. Dyer PD, Vaughan TR, Weber RW. Methotrexate in the treatment of steroid-dependent asthma. *J Allergy Clin Immunol*. 1991;88:208–212.

122. Thompson PJ, Misso NL, Woods J. Omalizumab (Xolair) in patients with steroid-resistant asthma: lessons to be learnt. *Respirology*. 2007;12(Suppl 3):S29–S34.

CHAPTER 36

Other Antiallergic Drugs: Cromolyn, Nedocromil, Antileukotrienes, Anticholinergics, and Theophylline

CAROL A. WIGGINS

There are many medications used in the treatment of allergic patients. Antihistamines, corticosteroids, and β agonists are discussed in Chapters 33, 35, and 34, respectively. A summary of drugs listed in 2007 National Heart, Lung, and Blood Institute/National Asthma Education and Prevention Program Expert Panel (NHLBI/NAEPP) report can be found in Table 36.1. Characteristics of other antiallergic drugs are cataloged in Table 36.2.

■ CROMOLYN AND NEDOCROMIL

Cromolyn and nedocromil are chemically dissimilar drugs with similar pharmacologic and therapeutic properties. These drugs, collectively referred to as cromones, are nonsteroidal anti-inflammatory medications with no significant adverse effects. Roger Altounyan et al. developed the cromones as synthetic analogues of the herbal remedy khellin. Although often classified as mast cell stabilizing drugs, the cromones possess a number of anti-inflammatory properties. These drugs have generally been replaced by other anti-inflammatory drugs as first-line therapy, but may play a useful adjunctive role in the treatment of asthma, allergic rhinitis, and conjunctivitis.

Pharmacology

Cromolyn and nedocromil have low oral bioavailability, and all of their pharmacologic effects in asthma result from topical deposition in the lung. Cromolyn has a very short plasma half-life of 11 to 20 minutes (1). Nedocromil has a longer plasma half-life of 1.5 to

2 hours (2). There are no significant drug interactions with the cromones (1,2). Neither drug relieves bronchospasm; both should be used preventively, as maintenance medications or prior to exercise or allergen exposure.

Mechanism of Action

The cromones block chloride transport channels in airway epithelial cells, neurons, and mucosal mast cells that appear to result in their anti-inflammatory effects (3). Mast cell degranulation is dependent on calcium channel activation that is blocked by cromolyn and nedocromil. Chloride transport channels, which are blocked by the cromones, provide the negative membrane potential necessary to maintain calcium influx and the sustained intracellular calcium elevation necessary for mast cell degranulation, and allow for changes in cell tonicity and volume. The ability of the cromones to block chloride transport also may be the underlying mechanism for their other anti-inflammatory effects (4).

The cromones have been reported to inhibit release of mediators such as histamine, prostaglandin D_2, and cytokines such as tumor necrosis factor-α from human mast cells (5,6). The cromones inhibit antigen- and anti–immunoglobulin E (IgE)-induced mast cell degranulation as well as mediator release triggered by calcium ionophore, phospholipase A, substance P, and compound 48/80 (1,5). Cromolyn inhibits mast cell degranulation in some tissue types better than others. Mediator release from human mast cells obtained from bronchoalveolar lavage is inhibited by much lower concentrations of cromolyn than is required to inhibit release from mast cells from human lung tissue

TABLE 36.1   ASTHMA MAINTENANCE DRUGS LISTED IN NHLBI/NAEPP 2007 REPORT

AGE	MEDICATIONS: ALTERNATIVES TO INHALED CORTICOSTEROIDS	ALTERNATIVE TO LABAS AS ADD-ON THERAPY
0 to 4 years	cromolyn, montelukast	Montelukast
5 to 11 years	cromolyn, LTRA, nedocromil, theophylline	LTRA, theophylline
>11 years	cromolyn, LTRA, nedocromil, theophylline	LTRA, theophylline or zileuton

LABA, long acting β agonist; LTRA, leukotriene receptor antagonist

fragments. The cromones suppress eosinophil chemotaxis and decrease eosinophil survival (7). Cromolyn and nedocromil inhibit neutrophil activation and migration (8). The cromones also inhibit expression of adhesion molecules (9), as well as antigen-induced production of interleukin-5 (IL-5) from mast cells and mononuclear cells (9), granulocyte-macrophage colony-stimulating factor secretion (7), and IgE synthesis. (10,11).

Challenge Studies

Inhalation challenge studies have determined that the cromones inhibit both the early and late asthmatic reactions when administered prior to allergen challenge. Nedocromil also inhibits the late phase of inflammation when administered after the onset of the early phase reaction (12). Cromolyn and nedocromil also inhibit bronchial hyperresponsiveness to other stimuli, including fog, exercise, cold air, and sulfur dioxide (13). The cromones do not inhibit bronchospasm induced by histamine or methacholine in the acute setting but may inhibit bronchial hyperresponsiveness to methacholine after several weeks of therapy (14).

Efficacy

Cromolyn and nedocromil have been reported to improve clinical outcomes and lung function when started early in the course of the asthma (15–17). They are effective in both nonallergic and allergic asthma. Although at least one study suggested that nedocromil is superior to cromolyn, most studies have reported no significant difference in efficacy. However, nedocromil may be effective when used on a twice a day schedule; this would tend to improve patient compliance compared with cromolyn, which must be used four times daily for optimal benefit (18).

The cromones are less efficacious than inhaled corticosteroids in the treatment of asthma (16). Some studies have suggested that the cromones have modest corticosteroid-sparing properties (19); others have failed to demonstrate significant steroid-sparing effects (20). Studies have demonstrated that cromolyn and nedocromil are similar in efficacy to theophylline, with significantly fewer side effects (21,22). Cromolyn is less effective than inhaled β agonists for prevention of exercise-induced asthma (23).

There is a common perception that nedocromil may be particularly useful when cough is a major asthma symptom, presumably by virtue of inhibitory effects on neuropeptides. However, cromolyn also inhibits the effects of inflammatory neuropeptides. Inhaled corticosteroids are effective in reducing asthmatic cough, and there is no evidence that nedocromil is superior to inhaled corticosteroids in suppressing cough as an asthma symptom. The cromones may be helpful in reducing cough associated with angiotensin-converting enzyme inhibitors when there is not an alternative to this class of drugs (24).

Current NAEPP guidelines suggest that the cromones may be used as alternative medications for patients with mild persistent asthma, or as prophylaxis prior to exercise or allergen exposure (25).

Safety and Drug Interactions

Cromolyn and nedocromil have no known drug interactions, toxicity, or clinically significant adverse effects. Cough or paradoxical bronchospasm may occur with inhalers. Some patients experience a bad taste with nedocromil. Both are pregnancy category B.

Dosing and Preparations

Cromolyn is available as a metered-dose inhaler that delivers 1 mg per actuation, and in 20-mg/2-mL ampoules for nebulization. The recommended dose of cromolyn is two inhalations, or one ampoule every 4 hours, or 10 to 60 minutes prior to exercise or allergen exposure.

Cromolyn is also available as a nasal spray for treatment of allergic rhinitis. It is less effective than topical nasal steroids and must be used 4 to 6 times daily for optimal benefit. Cromolyn and nedocromil are available as ophthalmic preparations for treatment of allergic and vernal conjunctivitis. Cromolyn is also available as a 100 mg ampoule to be taken orally for systemic mastocytosis and eosinophilic gastroenteritis.

Nedocromil is available as a metered-dose inhaler that delivers 2 mg per actuation. The recommended dose for children 6 years of age and older and adults is

TABLE 36.2 CHARACTERISTICS OF OTHER ANTIALLERGIC DRUGS

DRUG	MOA	SAFETY	EFFICACY	DOSING: ADULTS (A) CHILDREN(C)	DRUG INTERACTIONS	PREGNANCY CATEGORY
Cromolyn	Blocks chloride transport channels in mast cells	Virtually no known clinically relevant side effects, except for cough due to irritant effect of inhaled particles	Nonallergic asthma Inhibits both early and late phase of allergic asthma Exercise-induced asthma.	A and C: MDI (1 mg/puff): 2 puffs qid Ampule (20 mg/amp) 1 amp nebulized qid	None reported	B
Nedocromil	Blocks chloride transport channels in mast cells	Virtually no known clinically relevant side effects, except for cough due to irritant effect of inhaled particles	Asthma, including cough variant asthma ACE inhibitor cough Exercise-induced asthma	A and C: MDI (2 mg/puff): 2 puffs qid	None reported	B
Zafirlukast	Blocks cysteinyl leukotriene receptor	Very rarely associated with onset of Churg-Strauss vasculitis; hepatic dysfunction has been reported	Mild-to-moderate asthma	Ages 12 and Over: 20 mg bid C 5 to 11 years: 10 mg bid	Increases warfarin half-life and prothrombin time by about 35%	B
Montelukast	Blocks cysteinyl leukotriene receptor	Very rarely associated with onset of Churg-Strauss vasculitis	Asthma Exercise-induced asthma Allergic rhinitis	C (2 to 6 years): 4 mg qd C (6 to 15 years): 5 mg qd Ages ≥15: 10 mg qd	None reported	B
Zileuton	Inhibits 5-lipoxygenase activity	Increases liver enzymes in 3%; monitoring of liver function required	Asthma	Ages ≥12yr: 600 mg bid	Increases blood levels of warfarin, theophylline, and propranolol	C
Ipratropium	Anticholinergic; blocks M1, M2, and M3 receptors	Dry mouth common; rarely causes glaucoma, dilated pupil, blurred vision, especially with direct eye contact	COPD	Adults: MDI 2 puffs qid (17 mcg/puff)	None reported	B
Tiotropium	Anticholinergic; blocks M1, M2, and M3 receptors	Dry mouth common; rarely causes glaucoma, blurred vision, urinary retention	COPD	Adults: 18 mcg/capsule which should be inhaled once a day with Handi-Haler device	None reported	C
Theophylline	Not known; probably related to phosphodiesterase inhibition resulting in smooth muscle relaxation	Narrow therapeutic index; <u>serious adverse effects including seizures and arrhythmias causing death have been reported</u>	Asthma COPD	All Ages: dosing must be individualized based on monitoring peak serum concentrations of theophylline	MANY: including (**NOT** limited to) allopurinol, cimetadine, ciprofloxacin, erythromycin, estrogen, interferon, lithium, phenobarbital, phenytoin, propranolol, rifampin, ticlopidine, verapamil	C

COPD, chronic obstructive pulmonary disease; bid, two times per day; qd, every day; qid, four times per day; MDI, metered-dose inhaler two inhalations up to four times daily. Nedocromil is available for treatment of allergic conjunctivitis in a 2% solution.

■ ANTILEUKOTRIENES

The leukotrienes, C_4, D_4, and E_4, previously identified as "the slow reacting substance of anaphylaxis," are known to be potent mediators of inflammation in asthma. Three antileukotriene drugs are available in the United States: zileuton, zafirlukast, and montelukast.

Leukotriene Formation and Biologic Activity of the Leukotrienes

The leukotrienes are formed from arachidonic acid. The initial steps in this process are catalyzed by an enzyme complex containing 5-lipoxygenase (5-LO). Separate pathways lead to production of leukotriene B_4 (LTB_4) or the cysteinyl leukotrienes: leukotriene C_4 (LTC_4), leukotriene D_4 (LTD_4), and leukotriene E_4 (LTE_4) (25).

The cysteinyl leukotrienes have a common receptor that is distinct from the LTB_4 receptor. The cysteinyl leukotrienes are potent mediators of bronchoconstriction, airway responsiveness, micro vascular permeability, and mucus secretion. LTB_4 is a well-recognized chemoattractant for neutrophils in the lung (25).

The leukotrienes are important mediators of aspirin-sensitive asthma. Aspirin-sensitive asthmatics have increased baseline levels of leukotrienes compared with nonaspirin-sensitive asthmatics, and develop markedly enhanced levels of leukotrienes in their lungs, nasal secretions, and urine following aspirin challenge (26). There are increased numbers of cysteine leukotriene receptor 1 in nasal biopsy samples from aspirin-intolerant patients with sinusitis.

Mechanism of Action of Antileukotrienes

The first antileukotriene to be approved was the 5-LO inhibitor zileuton. Zileuton directly inhibits the catalytic activity of 5-LO and inhibits production of LTB_4 as well as the cysteinyl leukotrienes. Zafirlukast and montelukast are competitive antagonists of the cysteinyl leukotriene receptor and therefore inhibit the activity of LTC_4, LTD_4, and LTE_4 (26). The antileukotrienes have been reported to inhibit influx of eosinophils into the airways and to reduce blood eosinophil levels (26). Montelukast and zafirlukast have demonstrated bronchodilator activity (27).

Challenge Studies

In one study, zafirlukast inhibited lymphocyte and basophil influx into bronchoalveolar lavage fluid following allergen challenge. Montelukast and zafirlukast inhibit both the early- and late-phase responses to allergen challenge (28,29). Zileuton does not significantly inhibit the airway response to allergen (30). The antileukotrienes have demonstrated protective effects against exercise-induced bronchoconstriction (31). Zafirlukast has been reported to inhibit sulfur dioxide-induced bronchospasm (32). Zafirlukast and zileuton inhibit bronchoconstriction induced by cold, dry air (33). Zileuton and montelukast have been reported to inhibit aspirin-induced bronchospasm in aspirin-sensitive asthma (34).

Efficacy

The antileukotrienes are generally well tolerated and result in fewer asthma symptoms and exacerbations, decreased use of rescue inhalers and improved lung function (35). They are typically less efficacious than inhaled corticosteroids (26), but may be suitable as monotherapy for selected asthma patients (25).

Antileukotrienes may result in improved asthma control as additional therapy in patients not adequately controlled by inhaled corticosteroids (26). Most of the data from randomized trials show that long acting β agonists are superior to antileukotrienes as add-on therapy to inhaled corticosteroids for asthma (36)

Antileukotrienes have been demonstrated to be similar in efficacy and tolerability to antihistamines for the treatment of allergic rhinitis (37,38). Fluticasone propionate has been shown to be superior to montelukast for the treatment of seasonal allergic rhinitis (39). There have been several small trials with conflicting results regarding the use of montelukast for the treatment of chronic urticaria (40).

Safety and Drug Interactions

The antileukotrienes are generally safe and well tolerated. Zileuton can cause liver toxicity, and significant elevations of hepatic transaminases have occurred in 3.2% of patients according to manufacturer's long-term surveillance data, although symptomatic hepatitis appears to be rare. Patients receiving zileuton should have serum alanine transaminases measured monthly for the first three months, quarterly for the next year, and at the discretion of the prescribing physician thereafter according to the manufacturer's recommendations (41). Zafirlukast and montelukast do not appear to cause hepatotoxicity at recommended doses.

There have been several reports of Churg-Strauss syndrome (CSS) developing after initiation of therapy with cysteinyl leukotriene receptor antagonists. All of the patients reported were patients with severe asthma, and most had previously received corticosteroids (42). It is not possible to rule out the possibility that these drugs cause this very rare condition, but it is far more likely that the drugs are to be used as treatment in severe asthma, which is, by definition, a part of CSS (43).

Zileuton and zafirlukast may prolong the prothrombin time in patients receiving warfarin (44). Zileuton may double serum theophylline concentrations. Theophylline dosages should be reduced and serum concentration monitored in patients taking both drugs (45). Montelukast has not demonstrated any clinically significant drug interactions. Zileuton is a category C drug in pregnancy. Zafirlukast and montelukast are category B drugs in pregnancy.

Dosage and Preparations

Zileuton is available in 600-mg tablets to be taken four times daily, and as a sustained released tablet to be taken as two 600-mg tablets twice a day. Zafirlukast is available in 20-mg tablets to be taken twice a day. Both zileuton and zafirlukast are approved for ages 12 and above. Montelukast is available in 4-mg and 5-mg chewable tablets (for ages 2 to 6 and 6 to 15, respectively), 4-mg oral granules (for ages 6 months and above) and 10-mg tablets for ages 15 and older. Montelukast is administered once a day in the evening, or as a single dose 2 hours prior to exercise to prevent exercise-induced bronchospasm.

■ ANTICHOLINERGICS

The naturally occurring anticholinergics, most notably atropine, have been used for centuries to treat asthma and a variety of other medical conditions. The toxicity of these drugs has long been recognized, and is reflected in the common Latin name *Atropa belladonna*, "deadly nightshade," the plant from which atropine is derived. Scopolamine, another naturally occurring anticholinergic, is now used primarily in the treatment of motion sickness. Methscopolamine, a quaternary ammonium derivative of scopolamine, lacks the central nervous system side effects of scopolamine, and is used in a variety of proprietary medications, usually in combination with antihistamines or decongestants. Ipratropium bromide, a synthetic congener of atropine, is the only anticholinergic with an FDA indication for use in asthma, and is also available as a nasal spray for allergic and nonallergic rhinitis. Tiotropium is a synthetic anticholinergic approved for treatment of chronic obstructive pulmonary disease.

Cholinergic Mechanisms in Asthma

The autonomic innervation of the airways is supplied by branches of the vagus nerve, which are found primarily in large- and medium-sized airways. The postganglionic terminals of the vagal fibers supply smooth muscles of the airways and vasculature. Release of acetylcholine from the parasympathetic postganglionic fibers, acting on muscarinic receptors, results in smooth muscle contraction and release of secretions from submucosal glands (46). The activity of the cholinergic fibers results in a constant, low level of tonic activity of the airways. A variety of stimuli, including irritants, exercise, cold dry air, histamine, and allergens can trigger irritant receptors of vagal afferent nerves, resulting in almost immediate reflex bronchoconstriction and mucus hypersecretion (46).

Mechanism of Action of Anticholinergics

The anticholinergic agents compete with acetylcholine at muscarinic receptors. There are three known subtypes of muscarinic receptors in the lung. M1 and M3 receptors promote bronchoconstriction and mucus secretion, whereas M2 receptors promote bronchodilatation (47). All of the currently available anticholinergics nonselectively inhibit all muscarinic receptor subtypes (46). The blockade of M2 receptors may potentiate bronchoconstriction, which antagonizes the bronchodilatory effect of M1 and M3 receptor blockade. This has led to a search for selective drugs that do not antagonize the bronchodilatory effects of M2 receptors, but none is currently available. Because muscarinic receptors are found primarily in the central airways, anticholinergic bronchodilatation occurs mostly in the larger airways (48).

The anticholinergics provide virtually complete protection against bronchoconstriction induced by cholinergic agonists such as methacholine. Anticholinergics provide varied or partial protection against bronchoconstriction induced by inflammatory stimuli, including histamine, irritants, exercise, and allergens (48).

Pharmacology

Atropine is well absorbed from mucosal surfaces and reaches peak serum levels within 1 hour. The bronchodilatory effects last for 3 to 4 hours. Atropine relaxes smooth muscle in the airways, gastrointestinal tract, iris, and peripheral vasculature. It inhibits relaxation of the urinary sphincter. It causes bradycardia at low doses and tachycardia at high doses. It reduces salivary secretions and mucociliary clearance in the airways. Atropine crosses the blood–brain barrier and can cause central nervous system side effects.

Ipratropium bromide is a quaternary ammonium congener of atropine. The quaternary ammonium structure allows for poor absorption across respiratory and other mucous membranes (49). This results in a lack of significant anticholinergic side effects and allows ipratropium to remain in the airways longer than atropine. Ipratropium does not cross the blood–brain barrier or inhibit mucociliary clearance. Bronchodilation induced by ipratropium bromide lasts 5 to 6 hours

(49). Tiotropium bromide, indicated for chronic obstructive pulmonary disease (COPD), also is poorly absorbed after oral inhalation (<20%). In COPD patients, increases in forced expiratory volume in 1 second (FEV_1) can be demonstrated within 30 minutes and can last for 24 hours (50).

Efficacy

Anticholinergics are less effective bronchodilators than β-adrenergic agonists. Ipratropium bromide has a much slower onset of action than albuterol. Peak bronchodilatation occurs 30 to 90 minutes after inhalation of ipratropium, compared with 5 to 15 minutes after inhalation of albuterol. Ipratropium bromide has a longer duration of action than albuterol. Some patients may respond better to ipratropium than to albuterol, but there are no reliable predictors for which patients respond well to ipratropium (51). Anticholinergic agents are superior to β-adrenergic agonists in preventing bronchospasm induced by beta blockers or psychogenic bronchospasm (51). Ipratropium may be a useful bronchodilator for patients in patients who are intolerant to short acting β agonists (25). Ipratropium does not appear to be useful as maintenance monotherapy therapy for chronic asthma (52,53). A number of studies have addressed the addition of ipratropium to albuterol in the management of acute severe asthma, and the results have been conflicting (54,55). Ipratropium bromide nasal spray relieves rhinorrhea associated with allergic or nonallergic rhinitis as well as rhinorrhea caused by viral upper respiratory infections (56).

Safety and Drug Interactions

Atropine may cause significant side effects, even at therapeutic doses. Warmth and flushing of the skin, impairment of mucociliary clearance, gastroesophageal reflux, and urinary retention are common. Central nervous system effects ranging from irritability to hallucinations and coma may occur. Tachyarrhythmias may occur at low doses, and atrioventricular dissociation may occur at high doses. Atropine may trigger angle-closure glaucoma (49). Because of the frequency of side effects, potential for severe toxicity, and availability of drugs with superior safety and efficacy, there is no role for atropine in the management of asthma; it is mainly used to treat symptomatic bradycardia and reverse organophosphate poisoning.

Ipratropium bromide has no severe adverse effects or drug interactions and is very well tolerated. Rare cases of acute angle-closure glaucoma, blurred vision, and dilatation of the pupil have occurred with nebulized ipratropium, presumably due to direct contact with the eye (57). Dry mouth is a common side effect, and some patients complain of a bad taste or worsening bronchospasm with ipratropium (49). Ipratropium is a category B drug in pregnancy.

Preparations and Dosing

Ipratropium bromide is available in a metered-dose inhaler, alone or in combination with albuterol, and is administered as two inhalations four times a day. Each actuation delivers 18 µg of ipratropium bromide. It is also available in unit dose vials for use in nebulizers as a 0.02% solution. Ipratropium bromide is available in a nasal spray, 0.03% for rhinitis and 0.06% for upper respiratory infections. The recommended dose is two sprays in each nostril two to three times a day. Atropine and scopolamine are incorporated in low doses in some combination tablets with antihistamines and decongestants to treat rhinitis symptoms.

■ THEOPHYLLINE

Theophylline was one of the first drugs to be used as maintenance therapy for asthma. However, the emphasis on treatment of inflammation in asthma, as well as the introduction of newer drugs with similar or superior efficacy and improved safety and tolerability, has led to decreased use of theophylline.

Pharmacology

Theophylline is a member of the methylxanthine family of drugs, which includes the naturally occurring alkaloid compounds caffeine and theobromine. The solubility of the methylxanthines is low unless they form salts or complexes with other compounds such as ethylenediamine (as in aminophylline). Theophylline is rapidly absorbed after oral, rectal, or parenteral administration, and maximum serum levels occur 2 hours after ingestion on an empty stomach. Most theophylline preparations in current use are sustained release and administered once or twice a day. Food generally slows the rate but not the amount of absorption (57).

The elimination rate of theophylline varies widely in individuals, depending on age, genetic, and environmental factors, as well as underlying diseases. Serum levels of theophylline are altered by many other medications. High-protein, low-carbohydrate diets and diets high in charcoal-grilled foods, as well as smoking tobacco and marijuana, may increase theophylline clearance and therefore decrease serum levels. Pregnancy, fever, older age, liver disease, congestive heart failure, and COPD with chronic hypoxemia may increase serum theophylline levels (57).

Mechanism of Action

The mechanism of action of theophylline is unclear. Theophylline inhibits cyclic adenosine monophosphate (cAMP)-specific phosphodiesterases at high concentrations, but this effect is negligible at therapeutic doses. Antagonism of adenosine receptors is thought to be a possible mechanism of theophylline, as adenosine and theophylline are structurally similar, and adenosine is a bronchoconstrictor. However, enprophfylline, another xanthine that is a more potent bronchodilator than theophylline, does not block the effects of adenosine (58). The clinical effects of theophylline are primarily relaxation of smooth muscle in pulmonary arteries and airways, increased respiratory drive during hypoxia, decreased fatigue of diaphragmatic muscles, increased mucociliary clearance, and decreased microvascular leakage of plasma into airways (57). In recent years, modest anti-inflammatory effects of theophylline have been described (59). Inhibition of eosinophil infiltration into the airways of asthmatics has been reported. Reduced influx of $CD8^+$ T cells and resulting decreased IL-4 expression in airways have also been attributed to theophylline.

Challenge Studies

Theophylline inhibits bronchial hyperresponsiveness to methacholine; it inhibits the early-phase but not the late phase response to inhaled allergen (60).

Efficacy

Studies have demonstrated that theophylline is similar in efficacy but less well tolerated than β agonists (61). A study comparing the leukotriene antagonist zileuton with theophylline found it to be as effective as theophylline and to have fewer unpleasant side effects (62). In comparison studies of theophylline with the long-acting β agonists salmeterol and formoterol, theophylline resulted in similar improvement in FEV_1, but less improvement in morning and evening peak flow rates and use of rescue inhalers. There were also more adverse events associated with the use of theophylline than with salmeterol or formoterol. Current practice guidelines suggest that sustained release theophylline may be alternative adjunctive therapy for patients whose asthma is not optimally controlled with inhaled corticosteroids alone (25). It is listed along with cromolyn, nedocromil, and leukotriene receptor antagonists.

Intravenous theophylline had been considered to be a standard therapy for status asthmaticus. However, most recent studies in adults and children have reported that theophylline offers little additional benefit to corticosteroids and $β_2$ agonists in hospitalized asthmatics and thus would be used in special situations only with a target of 5 mg/mL to 15 mg/mL (57).

Safety and Drug Interactions

Theophylline is a drug with a very narrow therapeutic index. Serum concentration should be monitored and maintained between 5 μg/mL and 15 μg/mL. Many common drugs can double or triple serum theophylline levels. Severe and fatal toxicity may occur when serum levels exceed 25 μg/mL. In a 10-year prospective study of theophylline overdoses referred to the Massachusetts Poison Control Center, there were 356 cases in which the theophylline level was greater than 30 μg/mL. Seventy-four patients had arrhythmias, and 29 had seizures; 15 subjects died (63). Analysis of recent surveillance data reported to poison control centers throughout the United States between 1992 and 2003 indicates that accidental overdose and prescribing errors of theophylline in elderly patients shows that theophylline continues to be one of the most common drugs causing serious adverse drug reactions including deaths (64). Other toxic effects of theophylline include hypokalemia, hyperglycemia, encephalopathy, hyperthermia, and hypotension (57).

In addition to potentially life-threatening side effects, theophylline has unpleasant side effects that patients may find intolerable. Side effects such as headache, irritability, nausea, and insomnia may occur even when serum levels are within the therapeutic range.

Drugs that significantly elevate theophylline levels include clarithromycin, erythromycin, most of the quinolone antibiotics, cimetidine, disulfiram, estrogen, fluvoxamine, interferon-α, mexiletine, pentoxiphylline, propafenone, propranolol, tacrine, ticlopidine, thiabendazole, verapamil, and zileuton. Theophylline may decrease the effects of adenosine, diazepam, flurazepam, lithium, and pancuronium. Carbamazapine, phenobarbital, phenytoin, rifampin, and sulfinpyrazone may decrease theophylline levels (57). Theophylline is a category C drug in pregnancy.

Preparations and Dosing

Theophylline is usually prescribed in long-acting tablets or capsules, which come in a number of different dosages, to be administered once or twice a day. It is also available as uncoated tablets, encapsulated sprinkles, in suspension, and as a rectal suppository.

The dosage of theophylline is based on body weight. For children older than 6 months and adults, the starting dose should be 10 mg/kg up to a maximum initial dose of 300 mg/day. The dosage may be increased every 3 days, if tolerated, up to 16 mg/kg with a maximum dose of 600 mg/day. A serum level should be measured after at least 3 days at the maximum dose. The peak serum level occurs 8 to 13 hours after the sustained-release preparations and should be 5 μg/mL to 15 μg/mL. Dosage requirements generally maintain stable, but concomitant medications and acute or chronic illness may alter serum levels (57).

■ REFERENCES

1. Murphy S, Kelly HW. Cromolyn sodium: a review of mechanisms and clinical use in asthma. *Drug Intel Clin Pharm.* 1987;2(Part 1): 22–35.

2. Parish RC, Miller L. Nedocromil sodium. *Ann Pharmacol*. 1993; 27:599–606.

3. Alton EW, Kingsleigh-Smith DJ, Munkonge FM, et al. Asthma prophylaxis agents alter the function of an airway epithelial chloride channel. *Am J Respir Cell Mol Biol*. 1996;14:380–387.

4. Norris AA, Alton EW. Chloride transport and the action of sodium cromoglycate and nedocromil sodium in asthma. *Clin Exp Allergy*. 1996;26:250–253.

5. Okayama Y, Benyon RC, Rees PH, et al. Inhibition profiles of sodium cromoglycate and nedocromil sodium on mediator release from mast cells of human skin, lung, tonsil, adenoid and intestine. *Clin Exp Allergy*. 1992;22:401–409.

6. Bissonette EY, Enisco JA, Befus AD. Inhibition of tumor necrosis factor release from mast cells by the anti-inflammatory drugs sodium cromoglycate and nedocromil sodium. *Clin Exp Immunol*. 1995;102: 78–84.

7. Roca-Ferrer J, Mullol J, Lopez E, et al. Effect of topical anti-inflammatory drugs on epithelial cell-induced eosinophil survival and GM-CSF secretion. *Eur Respir J*. 1997;10:1489–1495.

8. Hoshino M, Nakamura Y. The effect of inhaled sodium cromoglycate on cellular infiltration into the bronchial mucosal and the expression of adhesion molecules in asthmatics. *Eur Respir J*. 1997;10: 858–865.

9. Matsuse H, Shimoda T, Matsuo N, et al. Sodium cromoglycate inhibits antigen-induced cytokine production by peripheral blood mononuclear cells from atopic asthmatics in vitro. *Ann Allergy Asthma Immunol*. 1999; 83(Part 1):522–525.

10. Loh RK, Jabara HH, Geha RS. Disodium cromoglycate inhibits S_μ → S_ε deletion and switch recombination and IgE synthesis in human B cells. *J Exp Med*. 1994;180:663–671.

11. Loh RK, Jabara HH, Geha RS. Mechanisms of inhibition of IgE synthesis by nedocromil sodium: nedocromil sodium inhibits deletional switch recombination in human B cells. *J Allergy Clin Immunol*. 1996;97:1141–1150.

12. Calhoun WJ, Jarjour NN, Gleich GJ, et al. Effect of nedocromil sodium pretreatment on the immediate and late responses of the airway to segmental antigen challenge. *J Allergy Clin Immunol*. 1996;98(Part 2; suppl):46–50.

13. del Bufalo C, Fasano L, Patalano F, et al. Inhibition of fog-induced bronchoconstriction by nedocromil sodium and sodium cromoglycate in intrinsic asthma: a double-blind, placebo controlled study. *Respiration*. 1989;55:181–185.

14. Griffin MP, Macdonald N, McFadden ER. Short- and long-term effect of cromolyn sodium on the airway of asthmatics. *J Allergy Clin Immunol*. 1983;71:331–338.

15. Konig P. The effects of cromolyn sodium and nedocromil sodium in early asthma prevention. *J Allergy Clin Immunol*. 2000; 105(Part 2): 575–581.

16. Guevara JP, Ducharme FM, Keren R, et al. Inhaled corticosteroids versus sodium cromoglycate in children and adults with asthma. *Cochrane Database Syst Rev*. 2006;2:CD003558. DOI: 10.1002/14651858.CD003558.pub2.

17. Sridhar AV, McKean M. Nedocromil sodium for asthma in children. *Cochrane Database Syst Rev*. 2006;3:CD004108. DOI:10.1002/14651858.CD004108.pub2

18. Creticos P, Burk J, Smith L, et al. The use of twice daily nedocromil sodium in the treatment of asthma. *J Allergy Clin Immunol*. 1995;95:829–836.

19. O'Hickey SP, Rees PJ. High-dose nedocromil sodium as an addition to inhaled corticosteroids in the treatment of asthma. *Respir Med*. 1994;88:499–502.

20. Bone R, Kubik MM, Keany NP, et al. Nedocromil sodium in adults with asthma dependent on inhaled corticosteroids: a double blind, placebo controlled study. *Thorax*. 1989;44:654–659.

21. Crimi E, Orefice U, De Beneditto F, et al. Nedocromil sodium versus theophylline in the treatment of reversible obstructive airway disease. *Ann Allergy Asthma Immunol*. 1995;74:501–508.

22. Hendeles L, Harman E, Huang D, et al. Theophylline attenuation of airway response to allergen: comparison with cromolyn metered-dose inhaler. *J Allergy Clin Immunol*. 1995;95:505–514.

23. Rohr AS, Siegel SC, Katz RM, et al. A comparison of inhaled albuterol and cromolyn in the prophylaxis of exercise-induced bronchospasm. *Ann Allergy*. 1987;59:107–109.

24. Hargreaves MR, Benson MK. Inhaled cromoglycate in angiotensin-converting enzyme inhibitor cough. *Lancet*. 1995;345:13–16.

25. National Asthma Education Program Expert Panel Report 3. Guidelines for the diagnosis and management of asthma. Summary Report. *J Allergy Clin Immunol*. 2007;120(5):S113.

25a. Peters-Golden M, Henderson,WR. Leukotrienes. *New Eng J Med*. 2007;3571841–1854.

26. Scow DT, Luttermoser GK, Dickerson KS. Leukotriene inhibitors in the treatment of allergy and asthma *Am Fam Physician*. 2007;75: 65–70.

27. Green RH, Pavord ID. Leukotriene antagonists and symptom control in chronic persistent asthma. *The Lancet*. 2001;357:1991–1992.

28. Ducharme FM, Di Salvio F. Anti-leukotriene agents compared to inhaled corticosteroids in the management of recurrent and/or chronic asthma in adults and children. *Cochrane Database Syst Rev*. 2004;1: CD002314. DOI: 10.1002/14651858.CD002314.pub2.

29. Diamant Z, Grootendorst DC, Veseli-Charvat M, et al. The effect of montelukast (MK-0476), a cysteinyl leukotriene antagonist, on allergen-induced airway responses and sputum cell counts in asthma. *Clin Exp Allergy* 1999; 2:42–51.

30. Hui KP, Taylor GW, Rubin P. Effect of a 5-lipoxygenase inhibitor on leukotriene generation and airway responses after allergen challenge in asthmatic patients. *Thorax*. 1991;46:184–189.

31. Finnerty JP, Wood-Baker R, Thompson H, et al. Role of leukotrienes in exercise-induced asthma. Inhibitory effect of ICI 204.219, a potent leukotriene D_4 receptor antagonist. *Am Rev Respir Dis*. 1992; 145(Part 1):746–749.

32. Lazarus SC, Wong HH, Watts MJ, et al. The leukotriene receptor antagonist zafirlukast inhibits sulfur dioxide–induced bronchoconstriction in patients with asthma. *Am J Respir Crit Care Med*. 1997; 156:1725–1730.

33. Richter K, Jorres RA, Magnussen H. Efficacy and duration of the antileukotriene zafirlukast on cold air-induced bronchoconstriction. *Eur Respir J*. 2000;15:693–699.

34. Israel E, Fischer AR, Rosenberg MA, et al. The pivotal role of 5-lipoxygenase products in the reaction of aspirin-sensitive asthmatics to aspirin. *Am Rev Respir Dis*. 1993;148(Part 1):1447–1451.

35. Altman LC, Munk Z, Seltzer J, et al. A placebo-controlled, dose-ranging study of montelukast, a cysteinyl leukotriene-receptor antagonist. Montelukast Asthma Study Group. *J Allergy Clin Immunol*. 1998; 102:50–56.

36. Ducharme FM, Lasersson TJ, Cates CJ. Long-acting beta 2-agonists versus antileukotrienes as add-on therapy to inhaled corticosteroids for chronic asthma. *Cochrane Database Syst Rev* 2006; 4:CD0031137.

37. Nayak A, Langdon R. Monteleukast in the treatment of allergic rhinitis: an evidence-based review. *Drugs*. 2007;67(6):887–901.

38. Rodrigo GJ, Yanez A. The role of antileukotriene therapy in seasonal allergic rhinitis: a systematic review of randomized trials. *Ann Allergy Asthma Immunol*. 2006;96(6):779–786.

39. Martin BG, Andrews CP, van Bavel JH, et al. Fluticasone propionate is superior to montelukast for allergic rhinitis while neither affects overall asthma control. *Chest*. 2005;128(4):1910–1920.

40. NcBane TO, Siddall OM. Montelukast treatment of urticaria. *Ann Pharmacother*. 2006;40(5):939–942.

41. Zyflo CR. *Physicians' Desk Reference*. 62nd ed. Montvale, NJ: Medical Economics Co., 2008:1997–1998.

42. Keogh KA. Leukotriene receptor antagonists and Churg-Strauss syndrome: cause, trigger or merely an association? *Drug Saf*. 2007; 30(10):837–843.

43. Du Mouchel W, Smith ET, Beasley R, et al. Association of asthma therapy and Churg-Strauss syndrome: an analysis of post marketing surveillance data. *Clin Ther*. 2004;26(7):1092–1104.

44. Adkins JC, Brogden RN. Zafirlukast: a review of its pharmacology and therapeutic potential in the management of asthma. *Drugs*. 1998; 55:121–144.

45. Granneman GR, Braeckman RA, Locke CS, et al. Effect of zileuton on theophylline kinetics. *Clin Pharmacokinet*. 1995;29(suppl 2):77–83.

46. Jartti T. Asthma, asthma medication and autonomic nervous system dysfunction. *Clin Physiol*. 2001;21:260–269.

47. Fryer AD, el-Fakahany EE. Identification of three muscarinic receptor subtypes in rat lung using binding studies with selective antagonists. *Life Sci*. 1990;47:611–618.

48. Morris HG. Review of ipratropium bromide in induced bronchospasm in patients with asthma. *Am J Med*. 1986;81:36–44.

49. Brown JH, Taylor P. Muscarinic receptor agonists and antagonists. In: Hardman JG, Gilman AG, Limbird LE, eds. *Goodman and Gilman's The Pharmacological Basis of Therapeutics*. 11th ed. Online edition 2007;Chapter 7.

50. Dusser D, Bravo ML, Iacano P, et al. The effect of tiotropium on exacerbations and airflow in patients with COPD. *Eur Resp J*. 2006; 27:547–555.

51. Tee AK, Koh MS, Gibson PG, et al. Long- acting beta-agonists versus theophylline for maintenance treatment of asthma. *Cochrane Database Syst Rev.* 2007;(3):CD00120139:272–276.

52. Westby M, Benson M, Gibson P. Anticholinergic agents for chronic asthma in adults. *Cochrane Database Syst Rev.* 2004;(3) CD003269.

53. Everard ML, Bara A, Kurian M, et al. Anticholinergic drugs for wheeze in children under the age of two years. *Cochrane Database Syst Rev.* 2005;(3):CD001279.

54. Stoodley RG, Aaron SD, Dales RE. The role of ipratropium bromide in the emergency management of acute asthma exacerbation: a meta-analysis of randomized clinical trials. *Ann Emerg Med.* 1999;34: 8–18.

55. Salo D, Tulo M, Lavery RF, et al. A randomized, clinical trial comparing the efficacy of continuous nebulized albuterol (15 mg) versus continuous nebulized albuterol (15 mg) plus ipratroprium bromide (2 mg) for the treatment of acute asthma. *J Emerg Med.* 2006;31(4): 371–376.

56. *Management of Allergic and Non Allergic Rhinitis.* Summary, Evidence Report/Technology Assessment: Number 54, May 2002. Agency for Healthcare Research and Quality, Rockville, MD.; http://www.ahrq.gov/clinic/epcsums/rhinsum.htm.

57. Jusko WJ, Gardner MJ, Mangione A, et al. Factors affecting theophylline clearances: age, tobacco, marijuana, cirrhosis, congestive heart failure, obesity, oral contraceptives, benzodiazapines, and ethanol. *J Pharm Sci.* 1979;68:1358–1366.

58. Rabe KF, Magnussen H, Dent G. Theophylline and selective PDE inhibitors as bronchodilators and smooth muscle relaxants. *Eur Respir J.* 1995;8:637–642.

60. Schwartz HJ, Petty T, Dube LM, et al. A randomized controlled trial comparing zileuton with theophylline in moderate asthma. *Arch Intern Med.* 1998;158:141–148.

61. Tee AK, Koh MS, Gibson PG, et al. Long-acting beta-agonists versus theophylline for maintenance treatment of asthma. *Cochrane Database Syst Rev.* 2007(3):CD001201.

62. Mitra A, Bassler D, Goodman K, et al. Intravenous aminophylline for acute severe asthma in children over two years receiving inhaled bronchodilators. *Cochrane Database Syst Rev.* 2005;(2) CD001276.

63. Shannon M. Life-threatening events after theophylline overdose: a 10-year prospective analysis. *Arch Intern Med.*1999;159:989–994.

64. Cobaugh DJ, Krenzelok EP. Adverse drug reactions and therapeutic errors in older adults: a hazard factor analysis of poison control center data. *Am J Health System Pharm.* 2006;63(22):2228–2234.

CHAPTER 37

Delivery Devices for Inhaled Medications

UMBREEN S. LODI AND THEODORE M. LEE

■ **HISTORY OF INHALATION THERAPY**

Inhalation therapy for bronchial disorders has been used since ancient times. Centuries ago, the stramonium (a botanically derived antimuscarinic agent) cigarette was described as a treatment for acute asthma (1,2). Antecedents of contemporary inhalation therapy are grounded in the early part of the 20th century with the invention of the hand-held glass bulb nebulizer (3), followed by introduction of compressor-driven nebulizers (4). Inhalation therapy subsequently was revolutionized by the introduction of pressurized metered-dose inhalers (MDIs) containing isoproterenol or epinephrine into clinical practice in the 1950s (5). In Europe, albuterol MDIs were first marketed in 1969 and beclomethasone dipropionate MDIs in 1972. The first dry powder inhaler (DPI), containing cromolyn sodium, was launched in 1967 (6,7).

Inhalation devices in use today include conventional pressurized MDIs (used with or without spacers or breath-actuation accessories), DPIs, and nebulizers.

■ **AEROSOL PARTICLE CHARACTERISTICS**

A synopsis of the significance of particle behavior in inhalation therapy is a necessary preface to a clinically oriented discussion of aerosol devices. Deposition of aerosolized particles occurs as a result of inertial impaction, sedimentation, and diffusion (Table 37.1). The aerodynamic size of a particle describes its impaction and sedimentation characteristics and is the primary determinant of its capture in the airways. (8,9). Generally, the desirable aerodynamic size for pharmaceutical aerosols is 2 μm to 5 μm. Particles larger than 5 μm penetrate into the bronchi poorly, but potentially are absorbed systemically if swallowed. Particles under 2 μm are not deposited into the airways and are exhaled or are deposited in the alveoli (10,11) (Table 37.2) with minimal if any clinical benefit in the usual applications,

but with occurrence of undesirable systemic absorption. The term *fine particle mass* is used for the percentage of the emitted dose that is in the respirable range, less than or equal to 5 μm (12). With most devices for aerosol therapy, fine particle mass is 10% to 25%. Deposition into peripheral airways relative to central airways is maximal at 2 μm to 3 μm (13).

■ **METERED-DOSE INHALERS**

Propellants

Until recently, the propellants used in pressurized MDIs were chlorofluorocarbons (CFCs) known as Freon compounds. Manufacture of Freon compounds has been discontinued because of their role in depletion of the stratospheric ozone layer (14).

Chlorine free aerosol hydrofluoroalkane (HFA) propellants (15,16) which do not contribute to stratospheric ozone depletion have been developed. Because the surfactants used to stabilize suspensions in CFC MDIs are not compatible with HFA propellants, ensuring suspension stability was a significant challenge in the development of non-CFC MDIs (17). HFAs generally appear to be safe and effective alternatives to CFC propellants (18,19), although they are not necessarily absolutely interchangeable. For example, beclomethasone dipropionate (BDP) is in solution in HFA propellant, whereas CFC formulations of BDP were suspensions (20). BDP is at least twice as potent with HFA propellants, and the BDP HFA aerosol properties are more favorable for airway deposition (21). However, no significant differences in bronchodilating effects have been reported comparing CFC and HFA albuterol inhalers (14,22,23).

Some HFA MDIs contain excipients such as ethanol. Breath alcohol levels up to 35 μg per 100 mL have been detected for up to 5 minutes after 2 puffs of albuterol HFA MDIs containing ethanol (24). Because the infrared spectrums of HFAs overlap with commonly used

TABLE 37.1   MECHANISMS OF AEROSOL PARTICLE DEPOSITION

MODE OF CAPTURE	DESCRIPTION OF MECHANISM
Impaction	Particles caught at apex of flow bifurcation due to inertia
Sedimentation	Particles "rain out" from suspension in gas due to gravity
Diffusion	Particles collide with surrounding tissue due to Brownian motion

anesthetic gasses, HFA propellants may cause erroneous readings in anesthetic gas-monitoring systems (25).

The Respimat Soft Mist inhaler (Boehringer Ingelheim Pharmaceuticals, Inc.—not available in the United States at this writing) is an MDI device which does not utilize pressurized propellants. It uses a spring-driven mechanism significantly differing from conventional pressurized MDIs in design (*Fig. 37.1*) and output (*Fig. 37.2*) (26).

Technique of Use of Metered-Dose Inhalers

The pressurized MDI is comprised of several components including active drug, propellants/excipients, metering valve, actuator, and container (*Fig. 37.3*). Figure 37.4 shows a schematic diagram of the operation of an MDI. Prior to actuation, the propellant-drug formulation for the subsequent single dose is contained within the small metering chamber inside the MDI canister. During the actuation, the metering chamber briefly communicates with the atmosphere but is sealed off from the remainder of the formulation within the canister; at this time, the dose within the metering chamber exits the inhaler through the valve stem. Immediately after the dose is released, however, the valve blocks the connection of the metering chamber to the atmosphere but permits the chamber to communicate with the interior of the canister, allowing refilling of the metering chamber.

In most cases the active drug is not soluble in the propellant; therefore, micronized drug particles within the canister are in suspension rather than in solution. Shaking the canister prior to each actuation is essential to ensure that drug particles are re-suspended; otherwise, the aliquot of propellant that enters the metering chamber may not be a homogenous suspension and therefore may not contain the expected amount of drug. Inattention to shaking a budesonide MDI prior to actuation has been documented to result in a significant reduction in drug delivery to the airways (27). If the pause between shaking and actuation is excessive, the drug-propellant suspension will become inhomogeneous before it is drawn into the metering chamber. Several other details are important for proper use of an MDI. The canister must be held still and in the vertical position until the valve has completely returned to its resting position. Failure to do so may cause inconsistent dosing. The likelihood of such problems increases toward the end of canister life (28); this issue is less significant with the re-engineered HFA inhalers which provide improved dosing consistency. When a period of time elapses between actuations of an MDI, the suspension that entered the metering chamber at the time of last actuation may lose homogeneity, with some drug sticking to the walls of the metering chamber. When this occurs, the amount of drug delivered with the next dose actuation will be reduced (29,30), a phenomenon termed *loss of prime*. The patient may compensate for this by discarding the first 2 puffs prior to each use of MDI, a procedure termed *priming the inhaler* (30). Loss

TABLE 37.2   DEPOSITION OF AEROSOLS

PARTICLE DIAMETER (μM)	PERCENTAGE DEPOSITION			
	OROPHARYNX	TRACHEOBRONCHIAL	ALVEOLAR	EXHALED
1	0	0	16	84
2	0	2	40	58
3	5	7	50	38
4	20	12	42	26
5	37	16	30	17
6	52	21	17	10
7	56	25	11	8
8	60	28	5	7

Adapted from references 10, 11, and 75.

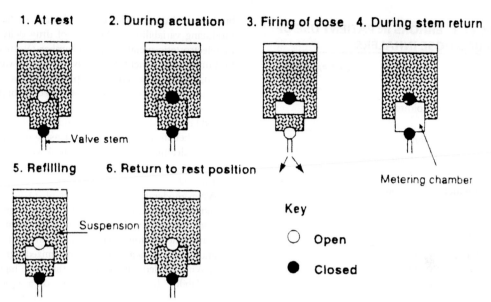

■ FIGURE 37.4   The operation of a propellant metered-dose inhaler valve. (Adapted from Purewal TS. Formulation of metered dose inhalers. In: Purewal TS, Grant DJW, eds. *Metered dose inhaler technology.* Buffalo Grove, IL: Interpharm; 1998:9–68.)

of prime was a significant issue with CFC MDIs; it is less significant with HFA MDIs (31). Breath holding increases drug deposition in the airways. Greater bronchodilation is found with a 10-second pause compared with a 4-second pause, but a 20-second pause appears to produce no further benefit (32).

When an MDI is used without a holding chamber, the issue of whether the lips should be closed around the inhaler mouthpiece or instead held several centimeters from the open mouth (33,34) is open to debate. Comparisons between the two techniques have not shown consistent superiority of either technique over the other (32,35–37). Another issue relevant to optimal inhaler technique regards the lung volume at which inhalation begins. Although it has been proposed that inhalation from functional residual capacity yields improved results as compared with inhalation from residual volume (37), the difference is probably minor (39).

Limitations of Metered-Dose Inhalers as a Delivery System for Inhaled Medications

Many studies have documented the prevalence of errors in patients' use of MDIs (40,41) (Table 37.3). Moreover, health care professionals often are not familiar with the details of appropriate use of the devices. Despite training, around 15% of individuals are not able to use inhalers properly without assistive devices. Of patients with initially inadequate technique who master proper technique with training, around 50% subsequently again develop significant deficiencies in technique over time (40). In patients with initially proper inhaler technique, 20% demonstrated incorrect usage at a later date.

In addition to suboptimal response to treatment due to incorrect inhaler technique, there is significant direct economic loss as a result of wasted aerosol medication (41,42).

■ SPACER DEVICES: ADJUNCTS TO METERED-DOSE INHALERS

Spacer devices are inhalation aids designed to overcome coordination difficulties, enhance aerosol deposition in the lower airways, and minimize oropharyngeal deposition (Fig. 37.5). There are three categories of spacers: (a) simple tubes which function as extensions of the actuator mouthpiece; (b) holding chambers with a one-way valve (43) to prevent the patient from blowing the dose away by exhaling into the chamber; and (c) reverse-flow reservoirs (44,45) in which the spray initially is actuated away from the patient into the spacer. Many spacer devices are available. They differ in a number of characteristics including volume (ranging from 20 mL to 750 mL), length, shape (cylinder, pear-shaped, etc.), construction material (plastic, metal), rigidity (rigid or collapsible), presence or absence of valves, and interface with airway opening (mouthpiece, face mask, adaptor to ventilator tubing). The Optihaler (Respironics, Inc.) holding chamber is designed to limit the patient's inhalation until the canister is depressed, coordinating actuation of the MDI with the beginning of inhalation (47). Figure 37.6 illustrates a variety of spacer devices available in the United States.

Slow inspiratory flow rates from spacer devices have been documented to result in improved efficacy of inhaled medications, probably as a result of reduced impact in the oral cavity, pharynx, and large central

TABLE 37.3   ERRORS IN PATIENT USE OF METERED-DOSE INHALERS

	% OF PATIENTS
Breath-hold too short	44
Excessively rapid inspiratory flow rate	34
Incomplete inhalation	23
Device not actuated at the beginning of inhalation	19
Multiple actuations with one inhalation	19
Actuation at the end of inhalation	18
Nasal inhalation after actuating MDI into mouth	12
Wrong position of inhaler	7
No inhalation	6
Failure to remove cap	0.4

Adapted from reference 40.

airways, with greater homogeneity of lung deposition (32,48). Laube et al., using radiolabeled cromolyn sodium, found that a mean of 11.8% of radiolabeled aerosol was deposited into the lungs with slow inspiration using a large-volume spacer, as compared with a mean of 8.6% with faster inspiration (48). Some spacer devices incorporate a whistle to alert patients when inspiratory flow is excessive; the patient is instructed to inhale slowly so that the whistle does not emit any sound (45).

A proportion of drug particles emitted by an MDI carry an electrostatic charge. Static electricity accumulates on plastic spacer devices, which may attract and bind these drug particles on the device's surface, thus producing variability in the dose of drug delivered. A nonelectrostatic metal holding chamber (Vortex, PARI Respiratory Equipment, Inc.) may obviate the variability in drug delivery observed with plastic devices (49). To minimize electrostatic effects, published recommendations suggest that before initial use, plastic spacers should be washed in warm water and diluted kitchen detergent, then air-dried rather than rinsing or wiping dry (50,51). Cleaning spacers every 1 to 4 weeks is recommended, as is replacement of plastic spacers every 12 months (52).

When moderate or high dosages of inhaled corticosteroids are administered via MDI, it is usual practice to routinely prescribe a spacer. As a result of reduced oropharyngeal deposition (*Figure 37.2*), local adverse effects of candidiasis and hoarseness are minimized significantly (53). With inhaled corticosteroids that have higher oral bioavailability (e.g., BDP), the use of a spacer also reduces potential systemic side effects due to reduction in swallowed medication (54). The decrease in systemic bioactivity due to reduced oral deposition exceeds the increase in systemic bioactivity resulting from pulmonary deposition because of use of the spacer. The net effect of the addition of the spacer device is reduced systemic bioactivity. However, when inhaled steroids with minimal oral bioavailability (e.g., fluticasone propionate) are used with a spacer, the net effect may instead be increased systemic bioactivity (55). It should be noted that the clinical trial data evaluating the effects of many inhaled corticosteroids at specific dosages have been generated without the use of spacer devices. The conclusions obtained from these studies with regard to efficacy and systemic effects of a particular inhaled-steroid MDI preparation at a specific dosage used without a spacer cannot necessarily be generalized to administration of the same drug formulation utilizing a spacer device.

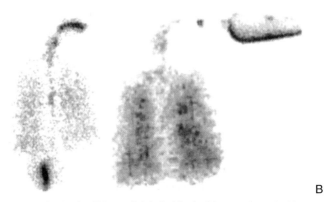

A   B

■ **FIGURE 37.5** Scintigraphic images obtained utilizing radiolabeled flunisolide; spacer used with pressurized MDI results in increased pulmonary delivery of aerosol with reduced oropharyngeal and gastric (swallowed drug) deposition; capture of aerosol particles on the walls of the spacer is noted. Images were obtained from the same subject on different days. **(A)** Pressurized MDI alone and **(B)**, MDI with 250 mL tube spacer. (Adapted from Newman SP, Steed KP, et al. Efficient delivery to the lungs of flunisolide aerosol from a new hand-held portable multidose nebulizer. *J Pharm Sci* 1996; 85:960–964.)

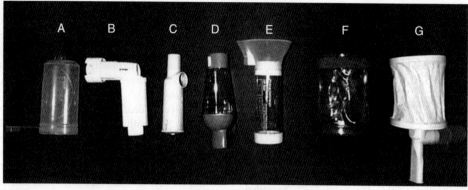

■ **FIGURE 37.6**   Various spacer devices. **(A)** Tube holding chamber (Ellipse, Glaxo Wellcome). **(B)** Tube holding chamber integrated with metered-dose inhaler actuator (Azmacort, KOS Pharmaceuticals). **(C)** Holding chamber with inspiratory control valve (Optihaler, Respironics). **(D)** Valved holding chamber with mouthpiece (Easivent, DEY). **(E)** Valved holding chamber with mask (Aerochamber with Mask, Monoghan Medical Corp.). **(F)** Large-volume collapsible bag holding chamber (E-Z Spacer, WE Pharmaceuticals). **(G)** Large-volume collapsible bag holding chamber with inspiratory flow auditory monitor (InspirEase, Schering-Plough).

A review of randomized controlled trials assessing the effects of holding chambers (spacers) compared to nebulizer for delivery of a β_2 agonist for acute asthma was compiled by Cates et al. (56). In adults, no differences were found between the two methods, while in children the length of stay in the emergency department was longer in the nebulizer group. MDI with spacer produced outcomes that were at least equivalent to nebulizer delivery. This review excluded patients with life-threatening asthma (56).

Whether bronchodilator MDIs always should be administered with a spacer is open to debate. Clearly, use of spacers with MDIs is absolutely necessary in young children and during acute bronchospastic episodes (57). In adults and older children with excellent inhaler technique, data have indicated only minimal additional clinical benefit compared to use of MDI alone. However, in patients with suboptimal inhaler technique, use of a spacer clearly results in additional clinical benefit (58).

Considerations for Metered-Dose Inhaler/Spacer Device Use in Infants and Young Children

Several important special considerations pertain to the use of MDIs with spacers in infants and toddlers: (a) a facemask rather than mouthpiece interface is required; (b) dosage of medication administered relative to body size differs greatly from that utilized in older patients; and (c) medication is delivered in multiple tidal breaths rather than in one deep inhalation. Because of these differences the only appropriate devices for utilization in these pediatric patients are small- or moderate-sized valved holding chambers equipped with properly designed facemasks. Valves in devices intended for

these patients should open at minimal inspiratory flows, and valve function should be visible.

It has been shown *in vitro* that even a small air leak in the face mask can dramatically reduce the efficiency of drug delivery. Spacer output did not depend on the position of the leak but lung dose was higher with leaks near the chin than for leaks near the nose (59,60). Aerosolized drug delivery with face mask may increase facial and eye deposition of aerosol with potential for local adverse effects. However, actual occurrence of such effects has been minimal in children (61). Delivery of drug by mouthpiece is more efficient than by facemask; patients should be transitioned to mouthpiece as early as possible (49).

The use of valved holding chambers with mask to deliver medications to infants and toddlers via tidal breathing differs considerably from the considerations that apply to the usual administration to older children and adults. Based on radionuclide studies conducted by Tal et al., in this situation only around 2% of the dose placed into the holding chamber is deposited into the patient's lungs, a roughly 10-fold reduction from what is typically observed in older patients (62). However, if the patient is crying during the administration of the aerosol, lung deposition of less than 0.35% was observed. Ideally inhalation should be administered when the patient is calm or asleep. The mask should remain sealed over the patient's face for 20 to 30 seconds of tidal breathing after actuation of the MDI. Tal et al. (using a plastic spacer without special precautions to reduce electrostatic charge) found longer periods of time to be useless because the aerosol adhered to the spacer after 30 seconds. Because of the expected 10-fold reduction in pulmonary deposition, the full adult dose of aerosol medication, typically at least two puffs, is administered (62). It may be appropriate to start with several puffs, a dose larger than would be typically used in older children and adults, then to reduce the dose once it is clear that the treatment is effective (63).

■ BREATH-ACTUATED METERED-DOSE INHALERS

The breath-actuated devices are alternatives to holding chambers developed to improve coordination of actuation of conventional pressured MDIs with inhalation. These devices are designed to actuate the MDI automatically with a spring mechanism as the patient inhales. In the United States, two breath-actuated MDI devices are available—the Autohaler (only provided bundled with pirbuterol MDI, Graceway Pharmaceuticals), and the MD Turbo (TEAMM Pharmaceuticals) which may be used with nearly all MDIs and includes a dose counter. Although these devices are of little additional benefit to patients with good inhaler coordination, use of a breath-actuated inhaler in those with poor coordination increased the deposition of radiolabeled aerosol into the lungs from a mean of 7.2% with a conventional MDI to a mean of 20.8% with breath-actuated inhaler; there was a corresponding dramatic improvement in change in forced expiratory volume in 1 second (FEV_1) after breath-actuated inhaler use as compared with measured after conventional MDI in these patients (64).

Dependence on inspiratory flow is a theoretical drawback of the breath-actuated inhaler. At least one case has been described in which a patient experiencing acute severe airway obstruction was not able to generate sufficient inspiratory flow to activate the device (65), suggesting that, in rare instances, this issue may be clinically significant.

■ DRY POWDER INHALERS

Currently the major alternative to the pressurized MDI (used alone or in conjunction with spacer or breath-actuated devices) is the DPI. In 2008, around 20 different DPIs had reached the worldwide market, and many more have been described in publications (66). In general, DPIs are easier to use effectively than MDIs because they are inherently breath-actuated. The current routinely available DPIs require an inspiratory flow rate of at least 60 L/min for optimal dispersion of the powdered medication into respirable particles (67); below 30 L/min, the fine particle output may be reduced by as much as 50% (68). Consequently, concerns have been raised regarding possible inadequacy of drug delivery to the airways from DPIs during severe exacerbations; in the United States, short-acting bronchodilators are not available in DPI form. Because of inspiratory flow dependency, small children as well as adults with cognitive impairment may not be able to use DPIs effectively. In one study, only 40% of preschool children with acute wheezing could

generate an inspiratory flow rate exceeding 28 L/min, although around 75% could exceed this inspiratory flow rate during periods of stable asthma (69). Error rates exceeding 80% in use of routinely available DPIs have been documented in elderly patients with severe airway obstruction who have not received any training in use of these devices (70).

Overall pulmonary deposition from DPIs is similar to that of an MDI with spacer; fine particle mass is around 20% with the available DPIs at the usual inspiratory flow rates (67,68). Because of differences in particle size, aerosols generated by DPIs show greater deposition in the central airways as compared with MDI and nebulizers (clinical relevance of this observation is uncertain) (71). Hoarseness and other undesirable oropharyngeal effects are common with high-dose inhaled corticosteroid preparations delivered via DPI but typically are not problematic with low-dose inhaled corticosteroids.

Currently available DPIs may be categorized into three groups.

1. *Single-dose DPI*: In a single dose device, each dose is loaded into the device before use. The drug is supplied in an individual single-dose capsule which is placed into the inhaler and is pierced by spears or severed by a twisting action; the powder is then inhaled by the patient. After use, the remains of the capsule are removed. The Aerolizer device supplied with formoterol (Schering Corporation) and the HandiHaler device supplied with tiotropium (Boehringer Ingelheim Pharmaceuticals, Inc.) are single-dose DPIs.
2. *Multiple-dose Reservoir DPI*: The first such inhaler to be developed was the Turbuhaler (Fig. 37.7), now replaced in the United States by a similar device, the Flexhaler (AstraZeneca). It contains a bulk supply of powdered drug from which individual doses are released with each actuation. The Novolizer (*Fig. 37.8*) (Meda AB) is a more recently designed multiple-dose reservoir device not available in the United States at the time of this writing.
3. *Multiple Unit-dose DPI*: These devices utilize individually prepared and sealed doses of drug. In the Diskhaler, the drug is provided in a series of packets on a disk. The Diskus device shown in Fig. 37.9 contains a coiled strip of 60 double foil-wrapped individual doses. The patient operates the inhaler by sliding a lever which moves the next dose-containing blister into place with simultaneous peeling apart of two layers of foil, exposing the dose ready for inhalation (72).

■ MONITORING DEVICES FOR INHALERS

Nearly all multiple-dose DPIs have integrated dose counters. Several MDI products incorporating integrated dose counters recently have been introduced. The MD Turbo breath-actuated device includes a dose counter

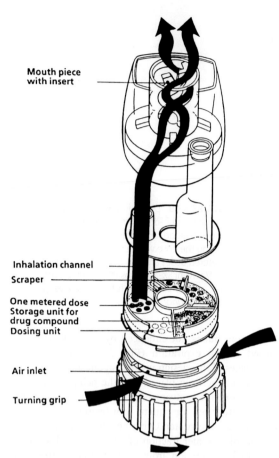

Mouth piece
with insert

Inhalation channel

Scraper

One metered dose
Storage unit for
drug compound
Dosing unit

Air inlet

Turning grip

■ **FIGURE 37.7** Turbuhaler is a cylindrical, multiple-dose reservoir dry powder inhaler device. Dosing is achieved by twisting the turning grip back and forth followed by deep inhalation. (From Vaswani SK, Creticos PS. Metered dose inhaler: past, present, and future. *Ann Allergy Asthma Immunol* 1998;80:11–21; with permission.)

(66,73). Several electronic monitoring devices which document the actual times and dates of actuation have been developed; these are attached externally to the MDI canisters or actuators (74). Currently they are used, primarily, to document medication adherence in pharmaceutical clinical trials.

■ NEBULIZERS

A device that simply sprays gas through a liquid resulting in aerosolization is termed an *atomizer*. In contrast, nebulizers are more complex devices which, by the incorporation of baffles, selectively remove particles that are too large to enter the lower airways. Most nebulizers used in aerosol drug therapy are *jet* nebulizers driven by air compressors. In the jet nebulizer, the compressed air moves through a narrow hole known as a venturi. Negative pressure pulls liquid up to the venturi by the Bernoulli Effect; at the venturi the liquid is

subsequently atomized. Many of the droplets initially atomized are much larger than the 5 μm maximum necessary for them to enter the smaller lower airways. These large particles impact on the nebulizer's baffles or the internal wall of the nebulizer and return to the reservoir for renebulization. Details of the baffle design have a major effect on the sizes of the particles produced. *Ultrasonic* nebulizers use a rapidly vibrating piezoelectric crystal to generate aerosol. Vibrations from the crystal are transmitted to the surface of the liquid in the nebulizer, where standing waves are formed. Droplets released from the crests of these waves produce the aerosol. The ultrasonic nebulizers are quieter and usually smaller than jet nebulizers but have the drawback of not nebulizing drug suspensions efficiently (75).

Many clinicians are surprised to learn that most of the drug placed into a nebulizer chamber never reaches the lungs. Of the approximately 30% to 50% that is emitted, some particles are too large to enter the lungs, and some are so small that they are not deposited into the airway, but are exhaled. With many nebulizer designs, much of the nebulized medication is released during expiration and is therefore dispersed into the room air. Typically, only 7% to 25% of medication placed into the nebulizer is delivered to the patient's airway (75,76).

For drugs that are relatively inexpensive and have a high therapeutic index such as bronchodilators, it is simple and effective to compensate for these issues by placing a large dose of medication into the nebulizer; provided that the dosage delivered to the patient is within the flat range of the dose-response curve, the precision and efficiency of delivery may not be a critical issue. However, these factors may become meaningful when medications that are expensive and have a greater potential for significant dose-dependent adverse effects, such as corticosteroids, are used. Such issues have served as an impetus for modifications in nebulizer design.

The traditional nebulizer design provides continuous flow of gas from the compressor into the nebulizer; the rate of aerosol outflow from the nebulizer is equal to the inflow rate from the compressor and does not change with the phases of respiration (Fig. 37.10). Modifications to the conventional design include the *open vent* design, the *dosimetric* design with a manually operated valve to interrupt gas flow into the nebulizer during expiration, combinations of the open vent and dosimetric features, and the most recent breath-assisted open vent nebulizers designed to combine the open vent design with the convenience of continuous operation and the efficiency of intermittent nebulization excluding the expiratory phase (77).

Open vent nebulizers provide a vent from the open atmosphere into the nebulizer. Negative pressure is generated as compressed air expands at the venturi and draws air in through the open vent, resulting in more

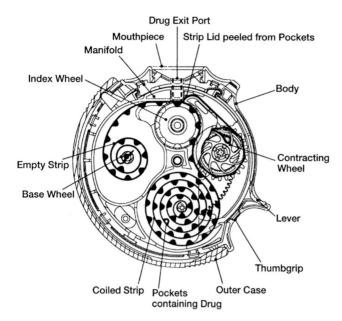

Drug Exit Port
Mouthpiece   Strip Lid peeled from Pockets
Manifold
Index Wheel
Body
Empty Strip
Contracting
Wheel
Base Wheel
Lever
Thumbgrip
Coiled Strip   Pockets   Outer Case
containing Drug

■ **FIGURE 37.9** Diskus is a disk-shaped, pocket-size, multiple unit-dose dry powder inhaler device. During inhalation, air is drawn through the device delivering the dose via the mouthpiece. It contains 60 metered doses and has a built-in dosage counter. (From Vaswani SK, Creticos PS. Metered dose inhaler: past, present, and future. *Ann Allergy Asthma Immunol* 1998;80:11–21; with permission.)

airflow through the chamber than provided by the compressor; therefore, more aerosol is generated in a given period of time. This nebulizer design has been combined with a manual interrupter that the patient operates to allow aerosol generation only during inspiration. For a given medication dose placed into the nebulizer, the use of a manual interrupter results in greater delivery to the airways but prolongs nebulization time (75).

With the breath-assisted open vent nebulizers, the vent is designed to be open only during inspiration, enhancing aerosol generation only during the inspiratory phase. Aerosol generation continues as a result of the continuous gas flow from the compressor during

expiration, but is not enhanced by the vent, which is closed during expiration (Fig. 37.11). The primary advantages of this design include significantly improved delivery of the drug placed into the nebulizer into the airway, and the convenience of continuous operation without the need for patient coordination of actuation of a manual interrupter. Other benefits include the generation of a greater fraction of smaller particles due to increased evaporation from droplets due to the additional airflow, and the need for less powerful compressors with this category of nebulizer (75).

For a single drug preparation, various nebulizers may give widely differing drug delivery that further varies depending on the patient's tidal volume during

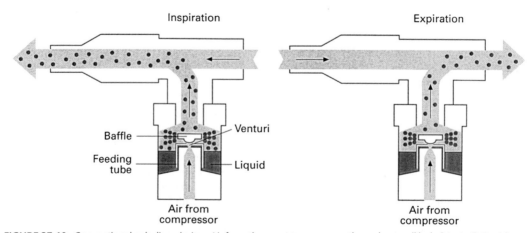

Inspiration   Expiration

Baffle   Venturi
Feeding   Liquid
tube

Air from   Air from
compressor   compressor

■ **FIGURE 37.10** Conventional nebulizer design. Air from the compressor passes through a small hole (Venturi). Rapid expansion of air causes a negative pressure, which sucks fluid up the feeding tube system, where it is atomized. Larger particles impact on baffles and the walls of the chamber and are returned for renebulization. Small aerosol particles are released continuously from the nebulizer chamber. On expiration, the nebulizer continues to generate aerosol, which is wasted. (From O'Callaghan C, Barry PW. The science of nebulized drug delivery. *Thorax* 1997;52(suppl 2):31–44; with permission.)

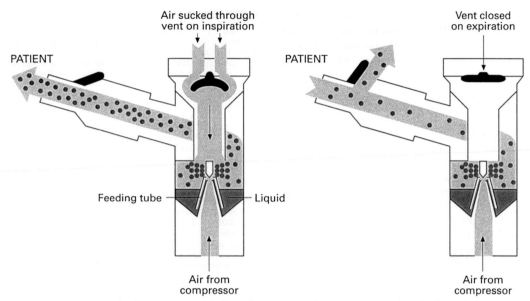

■ **FIGURE 37.11** An example of an open vent nebulizer, the Pari LC Jet Plus. On inspiration the valve located at the top of the chamber opens, allowing extra air to be sucked through the vent. The main effect of this is to pull more aerosol from the nebulizer on inspiration, increasing the dose to the patient. On expiration the vent closes and aerosol exits via a one-way valve near the mouthpiece. Aerosol lost from the nebulizer on expiration is thus proportionally less than that from a conventional nebulizer. Nebulization times will be faster and the drug dose received by the patient will be significantly greater than with conventional nebulizers. (From O'Callaghan C, Barry PW. The science of nebulized drug delivery. *Thorax* 1997;52[suppl 2]: 31–44; with permission.)

nebulization. In models of nebulization of budesonide suspension, using various nebulizer devices and tidal volumes ranging from 75 ml to 600 ml, the estimated percentage of the dosage placed into the nebulizer that is inhaled varied over a wide range depending on these factors; nonbreath-assisted open-vent nebulizers performed poorly in these models (76,77).

Effective drug delivery to the airways of infants and toddlers depends on proper nebulization techniques and minimization of crying. A point of controversy is

TABLE 37.4   RECOMMENDATIONS FOR AEROSOL DELIVERY DEVICES (UNITED STATES, 2008)

AGE (YEARS)	FIRST CHOICE(S)	SECOND CHOICE
0 to 3	MDI with spacer and facemask	Nebulizer
3 to 6	MDI with spacer	Nebulizer
6 to 12 (bronchodilators)	MDI with spacer or BAI	
> 12 (bronchodilators)	MDI with spacer or BAI	MDI alone*
> 6 (low-dose ICS with or without LABA)	DPI or MDI with spacer	
> 6 (high-dose ICS with or without LABA)	MDI with spacer	DPI
Acute bronchial obstruction (all ages)	MDI with spacer	Nebulizer
Continuous bronchodilator therapy prescribed in emergency department, intensive care unit (all ages)	Nebulizer	

*Only for those patients who demonstrate excellent technique with MDI alone

BAI = breath-actuated inhaler; ICS = inhaled corticosteroids the effectiveness of aerosolized medications delivered by hood or "blow-by" from a mask or extension tubing held in front of the patient's face (instead of delivery using a tightly fitting facemask, to which young patients often object). An *in vitro* study compared the inhaled fine particle dose from a T-piece nebulizer using close-fitting facemask, blow-by with mask, and blow-by with corrugated extension tube. In this model, blow-by via mask resulted in decreased lung dose at all tidal volumes, but blow-by via extension tube resulted in inhaled dosage similar to that from a close-fitting mask. These data suggest that blow-by with extension tube may be an acceptable alternative to a close-fitting mask, especially if it prevents crying or fussiness of the child (78). Aerosol therapy delivered to wheezing infants with a hood interface has been reported to be as efficient as that using a mask (79).

Most drugs used for nebulization are supplied in single-use ampoules, largely eliminating the need for preservative additives, some of which have been documented to have significant bronchoconstrictor effects. When multiple use vials are used, the clinician should be aware of the additives present and any bronchoconstrictor potential that they may have with repetitive dosing (80).

■ SUMMARY

The pressurized MDI has been available for more than 50 years and remains the most widely used inhaler device. The main limitation of the MDI is variability in airway deposition due to inadequate patient inhalation technique. These difficulties in coordination of actuation and inhalation with use of MDIs may be ameliorated by adjunctive devices—spacers and breath-actuating attachments. Multiple-use DPIs, which are simple to use, compact, and inherently breath-actuated are valuable alternatives to MDIs, but are dependent on adequate inspiratory flow rate and are available with fewer drug formulations than are MDIs. Although preferred by some patients and caregivers, nebulizers require longer treatment times and involve greater expense for device and medication.

A recent comprehensive review of the comparative efficacy of aerosol devices reported no significant consistent differences between devices in any outcome variable or patient group (81). When selecting a device for an individual patient (82), patient preferences as well as economic considerations must be taken into account. Age and medication-specific recommendations for choice of aerosol delivery devices are shown in Table 37.4.

Simplicity as the paramount clinical element cannot be overemphasized—minimizing the number and variety of daily doses of inhaled medications and categories of devices used is often dramatically effective in enhancing adherence and attaining control of asthma.

■ REFERENCES

1. Cooper S. A dissertation on the properties and effects of the *Datura stramonium*, or common thornapple [Dissertation]. Philadelphia: Smith, 1797:39.
2. Gandevia B. Historical review of the use of parasympatholytic agents in the treatment of respiratory disorders. *Postgrad Med J.* 1975;51(suppl 7):13–20.
3. Graeser JB, Rowe AH. Inhalation of epinephrine for relief of asthmatic symptoms. *J Allergy Clin Immunol.* 1935;6:415–420.
4. Wright BM. A new nebuliser. *Lancet.* 1958;2:24–25.
5. Freedman T. Medihaler therapy for asthma: a new type of aerosol therapy. *Postgrad Med.* 1956; 20:667–673.
6. Crompton G. A brief history of inhaled asthma therapy over the last fifty years. *Prim Care Respir J.* 2006;15,326–331.
7. Sanders M. Inhalation therapy: an historical review. *Prim Care Respir J.* 2007;16(2):71–81.
8. Coates AL. Guiding aerosol deposition in the lung. *N Engl J Med.* 2008;358:3,304–305.
9. Lewis D. Metered-dose inhalers: actuators old and new. *Expert Opin.* 2007;4(3):235–245.
10. Stalhofen W, Gebbert J, Heyder J. Experimental determination of the regional deposition of aerosol particles in the human respiratory tract. *Am Ind Hyg Assoc J.* 1980;41:385–399.
11. Task Group on Lung Dynamics. Deposition and retention models for internal dosimetry of the human respiratory tract. *Health Physics.* 1966;12:173–208.
12. Sheth KA, Kelly HW, Mitchell BH. *Innovations in Dry Powder Inhalers.* Meniscus Ltd., 2000.
13. Rudolph G, Kobrich R., Stalhofen W. Modeling and algebraic formulation of regional aerosol deposition in man. *J Aerosol Sci.* 1990; 21(suppl 1):306–406.
14. Hendeles L, Colice GL, Meyer, RJ. Withdrawal of albuterol inhalers containing chlorofluorocarbon propellants. *N Engl J Med.* 2007;356:1344–1351.
15. Leach CL. Preclinical safety of propellant HFA-134a and Airomir. *Br J Clin Pract.* 1995;79(suppl):10–12.
16. Taggart SCO, Custovic A, Richards DH, et al. GR106642X: a new nonozone depleting propellant for inhalers. *BMJ.* 1995;310:1639–1640.
17. Brindley A. The chlorofluorocarbon to hydrofluoroalkane transition: the effect on pressurized metered dose inhaler suspension stability. *J Allergy Clin Immunol.* 1999;104(suppl):221–226.
18. Dockhorn R, Vanden Burgt J, Ekholm B, et al. Clinical equivalence of a novel non-chlorofluorocarbon-containing salbutamol sulfate metered-dose inhaler and a conventional chlorofluorocarbon inhaler in patients with asthma. *J Allergy Clin Immunol.* 1995;96:50–56.
19. Parameswaran K. Concepts of establishing clinical bioequivalence of chlorofluorocarbon and hydrofluoroalkane B-agonists. *J Allergy Clin Immunol.* 1999;104(suppl):243–245.
20. Borgstrom L. The pharmacokinetics of inhaled hydrofluoroalkane formulations. *J Allergy Clin Immunol.* 1999;104(suppl):246–249.
21. Leach CL. Effect of formulation parameters on hydrofluoroalkane-beclomethasone diproprionate drug deposition in humans. *J Allergy Clin Immunol.* 1999;104(suppl):250–252.
22. Ramsdell JW, Colice GL, Ekholm BP, et al. Cumulative dose response study comparing HFA-134a albuterol sulfate and conventional CFC albuterol in patients with asthma. *Ann Allergy Asthma Immunol.* 1998;81:593–599.
23. Kleerup EC, Tashkin DP, Cline AP, et al. Cumulative dose-response study of non-CFC propellant HFA 134a salbutamol sulfate metered-dose inhaler in patients with asthma. *Chest.* 1996;109:702–707.
24. Barry PW, O'Callaghan C. New formulation metered dose inhaler increases breath alcohol levels. *Respir Med.* 1999;93:167–168.
25. Levin PD, Levin D, Avidan A. Medical aerosol propellant interference with infrared anaesthetic gas monitors. *Br J Anaesth.* 2004;92:865–869.
26. Hochrainer D, Holz H, Kreher C, et al. Comparison of the aerosol velocity and spray duration of Respimat Soft Mist Inhaler and pressurized metered dose inhalers. *J Aerosol Med.* 2005;18(3):273–282.
27. Thorsson L, Edsbacker S. Lung deposition of budesonide from a pressurized metered dose inhaler attached to a spacer. *Eur Respir J.* 1998;12:1340–1345.
28. Cummings RH. Pressurized metered dose inhalers: chlorofluorocarbon to hydrofluoroalkane transition-valve performance. *J Allergy Clin Immunol.* 1999;104(suppl):230–235.
29. Cyr TD, Graham SJ, Li R, et al. Low first-spray drug content in albuterol metered-dose inhalers. *Pharmacol Rev.* 1991;8:658–560.

30. Blake KV, Harman E, Hendeles L. Evaluation of a generic albuterol metered-dose inhaler: importance of priming the MDI. *Ann Allergy.* 1992;68:169–174.

31. Ross DL, Gabrio BJ. Advances in metered-dose inhaler technology with the development of a chlorofluorocarbon-free drug delivery system. *J Aerosol Med.* 1999;12:151–160.

32. Newman SP, Pavia D, Clarke SW. How should a pressurized beta-adrenergic bronchodilator be inhaled? *Eur J Respir Dis.* 1981;62:3–21.

33. Connolly CK. Methods of using pressurized aerosols. *BMJ.* 1975;2:21.

34. Dolovich M, Ruffin RE, Roberts RE, et al. Optimal delivery of aerosols from metered dose inhalers. *Chest.* 1981;80(suppl):911–915.

35. Lawford P, McKenzie D. Pressurized bronchodilator aerosol technique: influence of breath holding time and relationship of inhaler to mouth. *Br J Dis Chest.* 1982;76:229–233.

36. Thompson A, Traver GA. Comparison of three methods of administering a self-propelled bronchodilator [Abstract]. *Am Rev Respir Dis.* 1982;125(suppl 4):140.

37. NHLBI, NAEPP, *Expert Panel Report 3; How to Use MDI*, Section 3, Component 2, Fig 3-14, Page 128 at http://www.nhlbi.nih.gov/guidelines/asthma/05_sec3_comp2.pdf.

38. Riley DJ, Liu RT, Edelman NH. Enhanced responses to aerosolized bronchodilator therapy in asthma using respiratory maneuvers. *Chest.* 1979;76:501–507.

39. Newman SP, Clarke SW. The proper use of metered dose inhalers. *Chest.* 1984;86:342–344.

40. Giraud V, Roche N. Misuse of corticosteroid metered-dose inhaler is associated with decreased asthma stability. *Eur Respir J.* 2002; 19:246–251.

41. King D, Earnshaw, Delaney JC. Pressurized aerosol inhalers; the cost of misuse. *Br J Clin Pract.* 1991;45:10–11.

42. Newman SP, Principles of metered-dose inhaler design. *Respiratory Care.* 2005;50(9):1177–1190.

43. Dalby RN, Somaraju S, Chavan VS, et al. Evaluation of aerosol drug output from the Optichamber and Aerochamber spacers in a model system. *J Asthma.* 1998;35:173–177.

44. Tobin MJ. Use of bronchodilator aerosols. *Arch Intern Med.* 1985;145:1659–1663.

45. Tobin MJ, Jenouri G, Danta I, et al. Response to bronchodilator drug administration by a new reservoir aerosol delivery system and a review of other auxiliary delivery systems. *Am Rev Respir Dis.* 1982; 126:670–675.

46. Lavorini F, Fontana G, Pistolesi M. Drug delivery to the lungs—effects of spacer devices. *European Special Populations* 2006, http://www.touchbriefings.com/cdps/cditem.cfm?NID=2386.

47. Nelson H, Loffert DT. Comparison of the bronchodilator response to albuterol administered by OptiHaler, the AeroChamber, or by metered dose inhaler alone. *Ann Allergy.* 1994;72(4):337–340.

48. Laube BL, Edwards AM, Dalby RD, et al. The efficacy of slow versus faster inhalation of cromolyn sodium in protecting against allergen challenge in patients with asthma. *J Allergy Clin Immuno.* 1998; 101:465–483.

49. O'Callaghan C, Barry PW. How to choose delivery devices for asthma. *Arch. Dis. Child.* 2000; 82:185–187.

50. Janssen R, Weda M, Ekkelenkamp MB, et al. Metal versus plastic spacers: an in vitro and in vivo comparison. *Int J Pharm.* 2002;245 (1-2): 93–98.

51. Pierart F, Wildhaber JH, Vrancken I, et al. Washing spacers in household detergent reduces electrostatic charge and greatly improves delivery. *Eur. Respir. J.* 1999;13:673–678.

52. British Thoracic Society; Scottish Intercollegiate Guidelines Network. British guideline on the management of asthma. *Thorax.* 2003; 58:(suppl 1):1–94.

53. Toogood JH, Baskerville J, Jenning B, et al. Use of spacers to facilitate inhaled corticosteroid treatment of asthma. *Am Rev Respir Dis.* 1984; 129:723–729.

54. Brown, PH, Blundell G, Greening AP, et al. Do large volume spacer devices reduce the systemic effects of high dose inhaled corticosteroids? *Thorax.* 1990;45:736–739.

55. Dempsey OJ, Wilson AM, Coutie WJ, et al. Evaluation of the effect of a large volume spacer on the systemic bioactivity of fluticasone propionate metered-dose inhaler. *Chest.* 1999;116:935–940.

56. Cates CJ, Crilly JA, Rowe BH. Holding chambers (spacers) versus nebulizers for beta-agonist treatment of acute asthma. *Cochrane Database Syst Rev.* 2006; 2: CD000052.D01:10. 1002/14651858.CD000052.Pub 2.

57. McFadden ER. Therapy of acute asthma. *J Allergy Clin Immunol.* 1989;84:151–158.

58. Giannini D, DiFranco A, Bacci E, et al. The protective effect of salbutamol inhaled using different devices on methacholine bronchoconstriction. *Chest.* 2000;117:1319–1323.

59. Esposito-Festen JE, Ates b, van Vliet FJ, et al. Effect of a facemask leak on aerosol delivery from pMDI-spacer system. *J Aerosol Med.* 2004;17(1):1–6.

60. Erfinger S, Schueepp KG, Brooks-Wildhaber J, et al. Facemasks and aerosol delivery in vivo. *J Aerosol Med.* 2007;20(1):S78–S84.

61. Geller DE. Clinical side effects during aerosol therapy: cutaneous and ocular effects. *J Aerosol Med.* 2007;20(1):S100–109.

62. Tal A, Golan H, Grauer N, et al. Deposition pattern of radiolabeled salbutamol inhaled from a metered-dose inhaler by means of a spacer with mask in young children with airway obstruction. *J Pediatr.* 1996;128:479–484.

63. Gillies J. Overview of delivery system issues in pediatric asthma. *Pediatr Pulmonol.* 1997;(suppl 15):55–58.

64. Newman SP, Weisz AWB, Talace N, et al. Improvement of drug delivery with a breath actuated pressurised aerosol for patients with poor inhaler technique. *Thorax.* 1991;46:712–716.

65. Hannaway PJ. Failure of a breath-actuated bronchodilator inhaler to deliver aerosol during a bout of near fatal asthma [Letter]. *J Allergy Clin Immunol.* 1996;98:853.

66. Bell J, Neman S. The rejuvenated pressurized metered dose inhaler. *Expert Opin.* 2007;4(3):215–234.

67. Ollson B. Aerosol particle generation from dry powder inhalers: can they equal pressurized metered dose inhalers. *J Aerosol Med.* 1995;8(suppl 3):13–18.

68. Prime D, Grant AC, Slater AL, et al. A critical comparison of the dose delivery characteristics of four alternative inhalation devices delivering salbutamol: pressurized metered dose inhaler, Diskus inhaler, Diskhaler inhaler, and Turbuhaler inhaler. *Aerosol Med.* 1999;12:75–84.

69. Pedersen S, Hansen OR, Fuglsang G. Influence of inspiratory flow rate upon the effect of a Turbuhaler. *Arch Dis Child.* 1990;65: 308–310.

70. Wieshammer S, Dreyhaupt, J. Dry powder inhalers: which factors determine the frequency of handling errors? *Respiration.* 2008;75: 18–25.

71. Zainudin BMZ, Biddiscombe M, Tolfree SEJ, et al. Comparison of bronchodilator responses and deposition patterns of salbutamol inhaled from a pressurized metered dose inhaler, as a dry powder, and as a nebulized solution. *Thorax.* 1990;45:469–473.

72. Chrystyn H. The Diskus: a review of its position among dry powder inhaler devices. *Int J Clin Pract.* 2007;61(6):1022–1036.

73. Wasserman RL, Sheth K, Lincourt WR, et al. Real-world assessment of a metered-dose inhaler with integrated dose counter. *Allergy Asthma Proc.* 2006;27(6):486–492.

74. Burgess SW, Wilson SS, Cooper DM, et al. In vitro evaluation of an asthma dosing device: the Smart-inhaler. *Respir Med.* 2006;100:841–845.

75. O'Callaghan C, Barry W. The science of nebulised drug delivery. *Thorax.* 1997;52(suppl 2):31–44.

76. Smaldone GC, Cruz-Rivera M, Nikander K, et al.: In vitro determination of inhaled mass and particle distribution for budesonide nebulizing suspension. *J Aerosol Med.* 1998;11:113–125.

77. Barry PW, OCallaghan C. Drug output from nebulizers is dependent on the method of measurement. *Eur Respir J.* 1998;12:463–466.

78. Geller DE, Kesser B. Blow vs. face mask for nebulized drugs in young children. *J Allergy Clin Immunol.* 2004;113(2):532.

79. Shakked T, Broday DM, Katoshevski D, et al. Administration of aerosolized drugs to infants by a hood: a three-dimensional numerical study. *J Aerosol Med.* 2006;19(4):533–542.

80. Asmus MJ, Sherman J, Hendeles L. Bronchoconstrictor additives in bronchodilator solutions. *J Allergy Clin Immunol.* 1999;104(suppl): 53–60.

81. Dolovich MB, Ahrens RC, Hess DR, et al. Device selection and outcome of aerosol therapy: evidence-based guidelines. *Chest.* 2005;127: 335–371.

82. Blaiss MS. Part 11: Inhaler technique and adherence to therapy. *Curr Med Res Opin.* 2007;23(3):513–520.

CHAPTER 38

Novel Immunologic Therapies

LESLIE C. GRAMMER

Allergic diseases are very prevalent, afflicting up to 20% of the American population; novel immunologic approaches to their abatement are avidly pursued. These approaches generally can be divided into three strategies. One approach is to administer monoclonal antibodies against molecules, usually proteins, that have been reported to be key in mediating allergic inflammation. Another is to administer other monoclonal proteins that will interfere with the allergic inflammatory process. A final strategy is to modify allergen immunotherapy using innovative techniques to reduce allergenicity and maintain and/or enhance immunogenicity.

■ MONOCLONAL ANTIBODIES

Monoclonal Anti–immunoglobulin E

The elimination of immunoglobulin E (IgE) to provide an effective therapy for allergic diseases is based on the importance of IgE in both early- and late-phase reactions (1). Various strategies have been used to interfere with the binding of IgE to its receptors, thus abrogating allergic disease. Examples include inhibiting IgE production, use of IgE fragments to occupy the receptor, administration of soluble receptors to bind free IgE, and neutralizing antibodies against IgE. Polyclonal and monoclonal anti-IgE antibodies have been produced to study mechanisms of allergic disease (1). Omalizumab is a recombinant humanized monoclonal antibody that is reported to be effective for the treatment of patients with moderate-to-severe persistent asthma who have IgE-mediated disease not controlled by corticosteroids (2–4). In addition to reducing free IgE, other mechanisms of action, including changes in eosinophil and T cell function as well as reduction of FcεRI expression on dendritic cells, mast cells, and basophils, have been described (5).

In a ragweed rhinitis trial, some symptomatic improvement was described in patients who had markedly reduced free IgE levels and markedly increased bound IgE levels (6). Trials of omalizumab for atopic dermatitis have reported both positive and negative results (7,8). To date, there have been no reports of omalizumab inducing an antibody response in humans. While the most common side effect has been the development of urticarial eruptions, patients have developed other adverse effects, including the rare possibility of anaphylaxis (9,10).

Anti–interleukin-5

Interleukin-5 (IL-5) is a helper T-cell type 2 (T_H2) cytokine that is reported to be essential for the recruitment and proliferation of eosinophils in the allergic inflammatory response. In animal models, anti–IL-5 blocking antibody has been reported to inhibit eosinophil recruitment and ablate the late-phase response (11). A humanized anti–IL-5 blocking antibody (mepolizumab) is, at the time of this writing, in clinical trials for the treatment of hypereosinophilic syndrome (HES), eosinophilic esophagitis (EE), severe asthma, and nasal polyposis (12). Mepolizumab received orphan drug status for treatment of patients with HES in the United States and the European Union in 2004. It should be noted that there are subgroups of HES, individuals with FIP1L1-PDGFRA fusion gene (F/P+ variant) or increased IL-5 production by a clonally expanded T-cell population (lymphocytic variant), most frequently characterized by a CD3⁻CD4⁺ phenotype. For F/P+ patients, imatinib, a low-molecular-weight tyrosine kinase inhibitor, has become first-line therapy (13). Recent data suggest that mepolizumab is an effective corticosteroid-sparing agent for F/P-negative patients. Mepolizumab is in phase I/II clinical development for the treatment of EE. When administered intravenously to allergic asthmatic subjects, it reduced both blood and sputum eosinophilia, but did not reduce airway hyperresponsiveness or allergen-induced late-phase response. These results question the association between IL-5 and allergic disease, but do not preclude its importance in disorders that are known to be eosinophil-mediated (12).

Anti–tumor Necrosis Factor-α

It is well recognized that tumor necrosis factor-α (TNF-α) is involved in the inflammation of certain T_H1-associated diseases like Crohn, psoriasis, and rheumatoid arthritis. In those diseases, anti-TNF-α therapies have produced significant clinical improvement. In patients with severe, steroid dependent asthma, TNF-α may be upregulated as well, resulting in the recruitment of neutrophils and eosinophils into the airways (14). While there was initial enthusiasm for anti-TNF-α therapy, this has been dampened by concerns over safety. Moreover the efficacy of anti-TNF-α therapy is likely to be confined to a small subgroup of patients with severe asthma. There is an increasing recognition that there is considerable phenotypic heterogeneity in severe refractory asthma. Therefore, it seems that the utility of anti-TNF-α as a novel therapy will be limited to phenotypes that are highly selected (15). In severe, recalcitrant atopic dermatitis (AD), anti-TNF therapy may be a consideration (14).

Other Monoclonal Antibodies and Fusion Proteins

There are several monoclonal antibodies, developed and approved for other diseases, that have been reported to be efficacious in allergic diseases. In general, the intensity of the allergic disease is severe, thereby justifying the known adverse effects. In a small trial of anti-CD20 (rituximab) treatment, improvement in severe AD was reported (16). Although well tolerated, only two of nine patients with moderate-to-severe AD benefited from treatment with alefacept, a fusion protein which combines part of an antibody with a protein that blocks the growth of some types of T cells (17).

Integrins are validated drug targets that might be useful in a variety of inflammatory diseases (18). Monoclonal antibodies that antagonize integrin alphaIIbbeta3 (e.g., abciximab), integrin alphaIbeta2 (efalizumab), and integrin alpha4beta1 (natalizumab) are currently U.S. Food and Drug Administration (FDA)-approved for acute coronary syndromes, psoriasis, and multiple sclerosis, respectively. However, none has been approved for indications related to asthma and other allergic diseases. Since selectins and integrins play key roles in respiratory inflammation, it is possible that monoclonal antibodies against them may be of use in asthma and other allergic diseases (18).

Another important target for intervening in allergic disease emerged with the discovery that chemokines belonging to the CC family (which includes RANTES and MCP-1, -3, and -4) are potent eosinophil chemoattractants that use a common receptor, CCR3. A monoclonal antibody to CCR3 has been reported to cause inhibition of eosinophil migration (19). Using bacteriophage expression libraries and combinatorial chemistry, highly selective CCR3 antagonists have been discovered. Low-molecular-weight approaches have supplanted monoclonal antibodies; CCR3 antagonists have been associated with decreases in tissue eosinophilia and airway hyperreactivity in animal models (20,21).

■ OTHER MONOCLONAL PROTEINS

Soluble Interleukin-4 Receptor

Interleukin-4 (IL-4) plays an important proinflammatory role in asthma through several mechanisms, including stimulation of T_H2 lymphocytes, which results in production of IL-5, IL-13, and more IL-4. When IL-4 is absent, T_H2 lymphocyte differentiation is inhibited. Several studies have reported the results of using soluble IL-4 receptor (sIL-4R) as a treatment for allergic disease. In one such randomized, placebo-controlled trial of 25 moderate asthmatics, all requiring inhaled corticosteroids, there was improvement in forced expiratory volume in 1 second (FEV_1) on the fourth day of aerosolized sIL-4R treatment in the high-dose group (22). There were no serious side effects of sIL-4R. In another study, sIL-4R was evaluated in steroid dependent asthma patients following the withdrawal of inhaled corticosteroid (ICS) therapy (23). Anti-inflammatory activity was shown by a reduction in exhaled nitric oxide after a single sIL-4R dose; stabilization of asthma symptoms also occurred, despite ICS therapy withdrawal. When administered once weekly for 12 weeks, sIL-4R stabilized the FEV_1. However, the study discontinuation rate due to asthma exacerbation was similar between the sIL-4R and placebo groups. No recent clinical evaluation has been reported.

Interferons

Recombinant interferon-γ (IFN-γ) is available as a therapy approved by the FDA for chronic granulomatous disease. IFN-γ is known to suppress IgE production and to downregulate the function and proliferation of $CD4^+$ T_H2 cells (24). The role of interferons in IgE-mediated diseases probably will be restricted to very severely affected patients because the risk for side effects, including fever, chills, headache, rash, depression, and even suicide, generally outweigh any possible benefit (25). Clinical improvement has been reported in patients with severe atopic dermatitis (26).

■ MODIFIED ALLERGEN IMMUNOTHERAPY

Recombinant proteins that are allergen-specific are included in this section, not in the previous one describing recombinant proteins that are not allergen-specific. Allergic responses are strongly associated with T_H2-type immune responses, and modulation of the skewed T_H2

response toward a more balanced response is the major goal of allergen immunotherapy (IT) in allergic disorders. To achieve this goal, several approaches have been developed.

Immunoglobulin-allergen Fusion Protein

A human immunoglobulin (Ig) Fcγ-Fcε fusion protein has been reported; it directly cross-links FcεRI and FcγRIIb on human mast cells and basophils and is thereby able to inhibit degranulation (27). It has been hypothesized that human gamma-allergen fusion proteins would achieve a similar inhibitory effect in an allergen-specific fashion while preserving the immunogenicity of the allergen component. A human-cat chimeric fusion protein composed of the human Fcγ1 and the cat allergen *Fel d 1* (*Felis domesticus*) for cat allergen-specific IT has been produced. Another novel Fcγ-Fcε fusion protein has been created combining the human Fcγ chain and a major peanut allergen (27). The potential of these novel fusion proteins for allergen IT is being studied.

Engineered Recombinant Allergenic Proteins

The major advantage of recombinant DNA technology is the ability to produce single allergens of identical structure. The use of single allergens, instead of the currently available allergenic vaccines, would allow a potentially more precise diagnosis and patients could receive immunotherapy only with the proteins to which they are allergic. On the other hand, one advantage of natural vaccines is in their antigenic completeness. Isoforms are proteins with similar amino acid sequences that have very different allergenicity. Overcoming the problems of isoform variability presents difficulties using recombinant technology (28,29).

The real innovation that would be possible with recombinant technology is to use it to develop new forms of treatment. Recombinant allergens can be engineered by site-directed mutagenesis to produce "hypoallergens" that no longer bind IgE but do retain T-cell epitopes (30). Among the hypoallergens that have been reported are a grass allergen (*Ph1 p 5*), group 2 mite allergens, a tree allergen (*Bet v 1*) and a peanut allergen (*Ara h 2*) (31,32).

Attempts to treat peanut allergy using traditional methods of allergen desensitization are accompanied by a high risk of anaphylaxis. IgE-binding epitopes on the native *Ara h 2* allergen have been modified, creating *mAra h 2*. Native *Ara h 2* and *mAra h 2* proteins stimulated proliferation of T cells from peanut-allergic patients to similar levels. In contrast, the *mAra h 2* protein exhibited greatly reduced IgE-binding capacity compared to the native allergen (32). In addition, the

modified allergen released significantly lower amounts of beta-hexosaminidase, a marker for IgE-mediated degranulation, compared to the native allergen. The potential of *mAra h 2* for food allergy IT is being studied.

T Cell Peptides

T cells and B cells recognize different epitopes on the same protein. Whereas B cells recognize conformational epitopes via their immunoglobulin receptors, T cells recognize linear epitopes 8 to 22 amino acids in length via their T-cell receptors. These peptide fragments are associated with products of the major histocompatibility complex (MHC) expressed on the surface of antigen-presenting cells. CD4$^+$ T cells regulating IgE response by B cells are MHC class II restricted. At least 100 allergens have been sequenced, and identification of T-cell epitopes is a rapidly progressing endeavor (33).

The tolerizing property of T-cell peptides was tested in a murine model using *Fel d 1*. In animals with a pre-existing immune response to *Fel d 1*, subcutaneous injections of T-cell epitopes resulted in tolerance as measured by decreased IL-2 production when spleen cells were cultured with antigen. Several clinical trials have been initiated. Unfortunately some of the peptide vaccines cause late asthmatic reactions. delayed bronchoconstriction without evidence of enhanced inflammation (34). These reactions are IgE independent and MHC restricted. No recent trials have been published.

Immunotherapy Affecting Dendritic Cells

IT could be aimed at inducing a T$_H$1 response to allergens using dendritic cells. The ideal dendritic cell would be one that is producing high levels of IL-12 (35). There are various ways that IL-12 production by dendritic cells can be increased. One *in situ* possibility is to add a recall antigen, such as tetanus toxoid, to the allergen of interest. The presentation of recall antigen by dendritic cells results in stimulation of specific CD4$^+$ memory cells that rapidly upregulate CD40L, effectively conditioning the dendritic cell to increase its IL-12 production *in vivo*. T-cell activity after dendritic cell vaccination is dependent on the type of antigen and mode of delivery. Cancer, in particular, melanoma, appears to be potentially treatable with this approach (35,36). There are no recent data reporting the utility of this technique in the treatment of allergic disease.

Toll-like Receptor-directed Immunotherapy

Toll-like receptors (TLRs) are part of the innate immune system which provides rapid, nonspecific responses to pathogens. This is accomplished through highly conserved pattern-recognition receptors that bind pathogens. Engagement of the innate immune system receptors, such as the TLRs, results in a rapid host response that activates the innate, and subsequently, the adaptive immune response. TLRs, 10 of which have been described in humans, are located on the cell surface and within the cell. Although ligand binding to each TLR activates a different molecular cascade, many induce T_H1 cytokines such as IFN-γ and IL-12 (37).

TLR9 Agonist: DNA Sequence Oligodeoxynucleotides

A method of triggering maturation of dendritic cells and upregulation of their production of IL-12 is to administer a TLR9 ligand, such as CpG immunostimulatory DNA sequence oligodeoxynucleotides (ISS-ODNs) (38). Bacterial DNA contains a relatively high frequency of unmethylated CpG dinucleotides that exist at a much lower frequency and are methylated in the DNA of vertebrates. The innate human immunologic system has evolved pattern recognition receptors, such as TLR9, that distinguish procaryotic DNA from vertebrate DNA by detecting these unmethylated CpG dinuleotides, also called CpG motifs.

In studies of subhuman primates, there have been several reports that CpG motifs are potent adjuvants (39,40). Human trials using CpG as a vaccine adjuvant have reported efficacy (41,42). In the coming years, the potential role of CpG ISS-ODNs in IT for allergic disease should become much clearer.

TLR4 Agonists: Lipopolysaccharides and Monophosphoryl Lipids

The classic TLR4 agonist is lipopolysaccharide (LPS). In animal models, it has been shown that LPS exposure, in ovalbumin (OVA)-sensitized animals inhibits the OVA-induced airway hyperresponsiveness. It has also been reported that LPS abrogates the OVA-induced immediate and late phase allergic responses (43). Due to adverse reactions, LPS is not likely to be routinely used as an adjuvant for human allergen vaccines.

A potent vaccine adjuvant derived from *Salmonella minnesota*, monophosphoryl lipid A, was recently licensed in Europe as a component of an improved vaccine for hepatitis B. Monophosphoryl lipid, like LPS from which it is derived, signals via the TLR4/myeloid differentiation protein-2 (MD-2) complex. A series of synthetic TLR4 agonists have been produced (44). These TLR4 agonists are part of a class of compounds called aminoalkyl glucosamide phosphates. They can act as potent adjuvants for mucosal administration of vaccine antigens, enhancing both antigen-specific antibody and cell-mediated immune responses. Thus, by combining the adjuvant and innate resistance induction properties of aminoalkyl glucosamide phosphates it may be possible to generate mucosal vaccines that provide innate protection immediately following

administration together with long-term acquired immunity. Clinical trials are underway.

TLR7/8 Agonist: Imiquimod

Imiquimod (IQ) is an immune-response modifying agent, first approved by FDA for the topical treatment of external genital and perianal warts in 1997. IQ stimulates TLRs 7 and 8 which are localized on the surface of antigen-presenting cells; in response to stimulation, there is synthesis and release of several endogenous pro-inflammatory cytokines such as interferon-α (IFN-α), tumor necrosis factor-α (TNF-α), and interleukins (IL), namely IL-6 and IL-12 (45). In turn, those cytokines activate both the innate and acquired immune pathways, resulting in upregulation of natural antiviral and antitumor activity. IQ 5% cream has been used for the treatment of a wide variety of dermatologic conditions in which the immune system is thought to play a role in regression of the disease. In some disorders, such as genital and perianal warts, actinic keratoses, basal cell carcinomas, Bowen disease, and molluscum contagiosum, relative safety and efficacy are supported by randomized controlled trials of IQ. However, it is common for patients to experience local skin reactions, which can range from mild to severe in intensity, but usually resolve 1 to 2 weeks after interrupting treatment. Additional randomized trials are being conducted to assess safety and efficacy of IQ in the treatment of an even wider range of cutaneous disorders.

DNA Vaccines

There are many viral diseases for which efficient vaccines are not available. Using DNA that encodes for viral proteins results in a robust response in many situations. Swine immunized with naked DNA vaccines for the highly virulent foot-and-mouth disease were protected on subsequent exposure (46). In a phase I study of vaccination with a plasmid containing DNA encoding for hepatitis D surface antigen, a booster response—but not a primary response—was reported (47). A DNA vaccine for hepatitis E virus has been reported to be effective in mice (48). There are preclinical studies using DNA vaccines for house dust mite allergens in animal models of allergic disease such as asthma; positive results have been reported (49). Although these results are encouraging, the possibility of the DNA being incorporated into the genome at an inopportune position that might activate a promoter or oncogene is of concern.

Probiotics

According to the WHO Expert Consultation Report of 2001, probiotics are "live microorganisms which, when administered in adequate amounts, confer a health benefit on the host"(50). While there is a reasonable rationale for anticipating benefits from probiotics, there are currently insufficienct data to recommend probiotics as a treatment for any allergic condition. Furthermore, although there have been several studies reporting a benefit in prevention of atopic disease such as eczema, other studies have failed to support this (51). None of the studies has shown any clear preventive effect on sensitization, nor any benefit in any allergic disease other than atopic dermatitis.

The term *probiotic* is often used loosely to include bacterial strains with little documented immunomodulatory capacity or controlled studies to support the claims. It is not known whether effects in experimental systems have any clinical relevance. Finally, little is known about the large, complex gut ecosystem. Explanations for the varied results among studies include host factors such as genetic differences in microbial responses and allergic predisposition. The variable reported results may also be caused by environmental factors, including the pre-existing microbial gut flora, individual organisms chosen to include in the probiotic, diet, and treatment of the host with antibiotics.

Clinical studies continue to be performed and reported. Hopefully there will be a better understanding of which individuals will likely benefit from which probiotics, as studies, including careful characterization of subjects and probiotic composition, are conducted.

■ CONCLUSION

Novel immunologic therapies offer the hope of true revolutions in treatment of asthma and allergic-immunologic disorders. Knowledge gained from basic research has led to potential therapies, but the clinical effectiveness remains to be established. When an antagonist or biologic modifier becomes available, its administration helps to reinforce or minimize the contribution of the agonist or biologic reactant to disease processes. For example, platelet-activating factor (PAF) is known to be a bronchoconstrictor agent and is a potent chemotactic factor for eosinophils. To date, PAF antagonists have had modest effects on inhibiting allergen-induced as opposed to PAF-induced bronchial responses. Thus, the contribution of PAF to allergen-induced bronchial responses seems less than initially anticipated based on the potency of PAF as a bronchoconstrictor agonist.

Novel therapies need to be safe if widespread use is planned. Physicians will need to be aware of possible unexpected positive or negative effects when new therapies are used. For example, administration of novel immunologic therapy for patients with asthma and allergic rhinitis might concurrently exacerbate the patient's rheumatoid arthritis or vice versa. There will be opportunities to revolutionize therapy, and learning how best to use the novel agents will involve pharmacologic studies, clinical trials, effectiveness studies, and postlicensing surveillance.

■ REFERENCES

1. Gould HJ, Sutton BJ. IgE in allergy and asthma today. *Nat Rev Immunol.* 2008;8:205–217.
2. Busse W, Corren J, Lanier BQ, et al. Omalizumab, anti-IgE recombinant humanized monoclonal antibody, for the treatment of severe allergic asthma. *J Allergy Clin Immunol.* 2001;108:184–190.
3. Bousquet J, Cabrera P, Berkman N, et al. The effect of treatment with omalizumab, an anti-IgE antibody, on asthma exacerbations and emergency medical visits in patients with severe persistent asthma. *Allergy.* 2005; 60:302–308.
4. Niebauer K, Dewilde S, Fox-Rushby J, et al. Impact of omalizumab on quality-of-life outcomes in patients with moderate-to-severe allergic asthma. *Ann Allergy Asthma Immunol.* 2006; 96:316–326.
5. Noga O, Hanf G, Brachmann I, et al. Effect of omalizumab treatment on peripheral eosinophil and T-lymphocyte function in patients with allergic asthma. *J Allergy Clin Immunol.* 2006; 117:1493–1499.
6. Casale TB, Bernstein IL, Busse W, et al. Use of anti-IgE humanized monoclonal antibody in ragweed-induced allergic rhinitis. *J Allergy Clin Immunol.* 1997;100:100–110.
7. Lane JE, Cheyney JM, Lane TN, et al. Treatment of recalcitrant atopic dermatitis with omalizumab. *J Am Acad Dermatol.* 2006;54(1):68–72.
8. Krathen RA, Hsu S. Failure of omalizumab for treatment of severe adult atopic dermatitis. *J Am Acad Dermatol.* 2006;55(3):540–541.
9. Cox L, Platts-Mills TAE, Finegold I, et al. American Academy of Allergy, Asthma and Immunology/American College of Allergy, Asthma and Immunology Joint Task Force Report on omalizumab-associated anaphylaxis. *J Allergy Clin Immunol.* 2007 120:1373–1377.
10. Miller CW, Krishnaswamy N, Johnston C, et al. Severe asthma and the omalizumab option. *Clin Mol Allergy.* 2008;6:4.
11. Teran C. Chemokines and IL-5: major players of eosinophil recruitment in asthma. *Clin Exp Allergy.* 1999;29:287–290.
12. Anonymous. Mepolizumab: anti-IL-5 monoclonal antibody, SB 240563. *Drugs R D.* 2008;9:125–130.
13. Gleich GJ, Leiferman KM. The hypereosinophilic syndromes: still more heterogeneity. *Curr Opin Immunol.* 2005;17:679–684.
14. Brightling C, Berry M, Amrani Y. Targeting TNF-alpha: a novel therapeutic approach for asthma. *J Allergy Clin Immunol.* 2008; 121(1):5–10.
15. Jacobi A, Antoni C, Manger B, et al. Infliximab in the treatment of moderate to severe atopic dermatitis. *J Am Acad Dermatol.* 2005;52:522–526.
16. Simon D, Hosli S, Kostylina G, et al. Anti-CD20 (rituximab) treatment improves atopic eczema. *J Allergy Clin Immunol.* 2008;121(1):122–128.
17. Moul DK, Routhouska SB, Robinson MR, et al. Alefacept for moderate to severe atopic dermatitis: a pilot study in adults. *J Am Acad Dermatol.* 2008;58:984–989.
18. Woodside DG, Vanderslice P. Cell adhesion antagonists: therapeutic potential in asthma and chronic obstructive pulmonary disease. *Biodrugs.* 2008;22(2):85–100.
19. Heath H, Zin S, Rao P, et al. The importance of CCR-3 demonstrated using an antagonistic monoclonal antibody. *J Clin Invest.* 1997;99:178–184.
20. Morokata T, Suzuki K, Masunaga Y, et al. A novel, selective, and orally available antagonist for CC chemokine receptor 3. *J Pharmacol Exp Ther.* 2006; 317:244–250.
21. Wegmann M, Goggel R, Sel S, et al. Effects of a low-molecular-weight CCR-3 antagonist on chronic experimental asthma. *Am J Respir Cell Mol Biol.* 2007;36:61–67.
22. Borish LC, Nelson HS, Lanz MF, et al. Interleukin-4 receptor in moderate atopic asthma: a phase I/II randomized, placebo-controlled trial. *Am J Respir Crit Care Med.* 1999;160:1816–1823.
23. Borish LC, Nelson HS, Corren J, et al. Efficacy of soluble IL-4 receptor for the treatment of adults with asthma. *J Allergy Clin Immunol.* 2001;107:963–970.
24. Gajewski TF, Fitch FW. Anti-proliferative effect of IFN-gamma in immune regulation. I. IFN-gamma inhibits the proliferation of Th2 but not Th1 murine helper T lymphocyte clones. *J Immunol.* 1988; 140:4245–4252.
25. Pung YH, Vetro SW, Bellanti JA. Use of interferons in atopic (IgE-mediated) diseases. *Ann Allergy.* 1993;71:234–238.
26. Jang IG, Yang JK, Lee HJ, et al. Clinical improvement and immunohistochemical findings in severe atopic dermatitis treated with interferon gamma. *J Am Acad Dermatol.* 2000;42(6):1033–1040.
27. Zhang K, Zhu D, Kepley C, et al. Chimeric human fcgamma-allergen fusion proteins in the prevention of allergy. *Immunol Allergy Clin North Am.* 2007;27:93–103.

28. Breiteneder H, Ferreira F, Hoffmann-Sommergruber K, et al. Four recombinant isoforms of Cor a 1, the major allergen of hazel pollen, show different IgE-binding properties. *Eur J Biochem.* 1993;212:355–362.

29. Schenk S, Hoffmann-Sommergruber K, Breiteneder H, et al. Four recombinant isoforms of Cor A 1, the major allergen of hazel pollen, show different reactivity with allergen-specific T-lymphocyte clones. *Eur J Biochem.* 1994;224:717–722.

30. Linhart B, Valenta R. Molecular design of allergy vaccines. *Curr Opin Immunol.* 2005;17:646–655.

31. Pree I, Reisinger J, Focke M, et al. Analysis of epitope-specific immune responses induced by vaccination with structurally folded and unfolded recombinant Bet v 1 allergen derivatives in man. *J Immunol.* 2007;179:5309–5316.

32. King N, Helm R, Stanley JS, et al. Allergenic characteristics of a modified peanut allergen. *Mol Nutr Food Res.* 2005;49:963–971.

33. Larche M. Immunoregulation by targeting T cells in the treatment of allergy and asthma. *Curr Opin Immunol.* 2006;18:745–750.

34. Oldfield WL, Larche M, Kay AB. Effect of T-cell peptides derived from Fel d 1 on allergic reactions and cytokine production in patients sensitive to cats: a randomised controlled trial. *Lancet.* 2002; 360:47–53.

35. Lesterhuis WJ, Aarntzen EH, De Vries IJ, et al. Dendritic cell vaccines in melanoma: from promise to proof? *Crit Rev Oncol Hematol.* 2008; 66:118–134.

36. Benko S, Magyarics Z, Szabo A, et al. Dendritic cell subtypes as primary targets of vaccines: the emerging role and cross-talk of pattern recognition receptors. *Biol Chem.* 2008;389:469–485.

37. Tse K, Horner AA. Update on toll-like receptor-directed therapies for human disease. *Ann Rheum Dis.* 2007;66 (Suppl 3):iii77–80.

38. Hartmann G, Krieg AM. Mechanism and function of a newly identified CpG DNA motif in human primary B-cells. *J Immunol.* 2000;164:944–953.

39. Davis HL, Suparto I, Weeratna R, et al. Vaccination of orangutans at risk for hepatitis B infection: hyporesponsiveness to hepatitis B surface antigen overcome by CpG DNA. *Vaccine* (in press).

40. Hartmann G, Weeratna RD, Ballas ZK, et al. Delineation of a CpG phosphorothioate oligodeoxynucleotide for activation primate immune responses *in vitro* and *in vivo. J Immunol.* (in press).

41. Creticos PS, Cen YH, Schroeder JT. New approaches in immunotherapy: allergen vaccination with immunostimulatory DNA. *Immunol Allergy Clin North Am.* 2004;24:569–581.

42. Creticos PS, Schroeder JT, Hamilton RG, et al. Immunotherapy with a ragweed-toll-like receptor 9 agonist vaccine for allergic rhinitis. *N Engl J Med.* 2006;355:1445–1455.

43. Tulic MK, Holt PG, Sly PD. Modification of acute and late-phase allergic responses to ovalbumin with lipopolysaccharide. *Int Arch Allergy Immunol.* 2002;129:119–128.

44. Alderson MR, McGowan P, Baldride JR, et al. TLR4 agonists as immunomodulatory agents. *J Endotoxin Res.* 2006; 313–319.

45. Lacarrubba F, Nasca MR, Micali G. Advances in the use of topical imiquimod to treat dermatologic disorders. *Ther Clin Risk Manag.* 2008;4:87–97.

46. Beard C, Ward G, Reider E, et al. Development of DNA vaccines for foot-and-mouth disease, evaluation of vaccines encoding replication and non-replication nucleic acids in swine. *J Biotechnol.* 1999;73:243–249.

47. Tacket CO, Roy MJ, Widera G, et al. Phase I safety and immune response studies of a DNA vaccine encoding hepatitis B surface antigen delivered by a gene delivery device. *Vaccine.* 1999;17:2826–2869.

48. He J, Binn LN, Caudill JD, et al. Antiserum generated by DNA vaccine binds to hepatitis E virus (HEV) as determined by PCR and immune electron microscopy (IEM): application for HEV detection by affinity-capture RT-PCR. *Virus Res.* 1999;62:59–65.

49. Chua KY, Huangfu T, Liew LN. DNA vaccines and allergic diseases. *Clin Exp Pharmacol Physiol.* 2006;33:546–550.

50. FAO/WHO. *Health and Nutritional Properties of Probiotics in Food.* Report of a Joint FAO/WHO Expert Consultation on Evaluation of Health and Nutritional Properties of Probiotics in Food. 2001.

51. Prescott SL, Bjorksten B. Probiotics for the prevention or treatment of allergic diseases. *J Allergy Clin Immunol.* 2007;120:255–262.

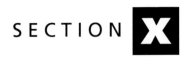
Special Situations

CHAPTER **39**

Allergic Disorders and Pregnancy
PAUL A. GREENBERGER

T he major conditions that the allergist-immunologist diagnoses and treats can occur in the context of gestation or in anticipation of pregnancy. Examples include asthma, allergic and nonallergic rhinitis, acute or chronic rhinosinusitis, nasal polyposis, urticaria, angioedema, anaphylaxis, and immunodeficiency. Goals of managing gravidas should include effective control of the underlying allergic-immunologic conditions, avoidance measures, guidance on medications, action plans or preparedness for emergencies such as acute severe asthma or anaphylaxis, and communication between the physician managing the allergic-immunologic conditions and the physician managing the pregnancy.

 **ASTHMA**

Asthma occurs in 3.7% to 8.4% of pregnancies in the United States (1–3) and in up to 12.4% of pregnancies in Australia (4). Asthma may have its onset during gestation and present as acute severe asthma, requiring hospitalization. Wheezing dyspnea may result in interrupted sleep, persistent coughing, hypoxemia, and even rib fractures during gestation. The sequelae of ineffectively controlled asthma on the gravida can be devastating in that maternal deaths may occur in the most extreme cases (5,6). Other untoward outcomes of asthma during gestation include fetal loss (abortions or stillbirths), increased rate of preterm deliveries (<37 weeks' gestation), intrauterine growth retardation (<2400 g), antepartum and postpartum

hemorrhage, gestational hypertension, pre-eclampsia, oligohydramnios, and hyperemesis gravidarum (1,2, 5,7,8–10,11–12,13–17). Not all studies report all the listed complications. There is a troubling report of acute exacerbations of asthma during the first trimester being associated with an increased risk of congenital malformations (18). Repeated episodes of acute severe asthma during gestation have resulted in hypoxemic effects on the fetus. There is a report of pregnancy termination because of life-threatening acute severe asthma (*19*). Conversely, with cooperation between the gravida and physician managing the asthma and effective asthma control, there can be successful outcomes for most women (8–10,*11*,13–17,20–22). Prevention of acute severe asthma has been associated with pregnancy outcomes approaching that of the general population (9). Use of inhaled cortiocosteroids (1,2,9,*11*,14,20,22,23) has been effective as has prednisone in managing even the most severe cases of asthma during gestation. Some studies have reported small (100 g to 200 g) reductions in birth weight in gravidas who had used prednisone. Other studies have found essentially normal outcomes despite administration of prednisone as long as there was avoidance of hospitalizations and emergency care (9,11).

Exacerbations of asthma during gestation may result in more hospitalizations than in nonpregnant patients with asthma. One mechanistic explanation is that there is reduced respiratory reserve in gravidas with asthma. It is also possible that they may receive less than recommended treatment because they are pregnant. When a comparison was made of emergency department treatment, 51 gravidas were compared with 500 nonpregnant women with asthma (24). Presentation peak expiratory flow rate (PEFR) was comparable (51% versus 53%) (24). However, corticosteroids were administered to 44% of gravidas compared with 66% of nonpregnant women (24). Hospitalization rates were similar (24% versus 21%). Unexpectedly, on discharge, oral corticosteroids were prescribed for 38% of gravidas and 64% of nonpregnant women (24). At the 2-week follow-up by telephone, asthma symptoms were reported by 35% of gravidas compared with 23% of nonpregnant women (24). Thus, pharmacotherapy was inadequate, in that oral corticosteroids were less likely to be prescribed with continued asthma symptoms at 2 weeks after emergency treatment. The 2008 American College of Obstetrics-Gynecology Practice Bulletin (2) and the National Asthma Education and Prevention Program Expert Panel Report (1,23) advise oral corticosteroids for treatment of acute episodes of asthma as part of a step-wise approach.

PHYSIOLOGIC CHANGES DURING GESTATION

Although the frequency of respiration is not changed, tidal volume increases in pregnancy (25,26). The minute ventilation rises 19% to 50% by late pregnancy (25–27). Vital capacity is unchanged, unless there is an exacerbation of asthma. Oxygen consumption increases by 20% to 32%. Large increases in progesterone and estrogen produce a respiratory alkalosis from greater minute ventilation attributable to increased carotid body sensitivity to hypoxia (28). These changes occur before there is significant enlargement of the uterus. Arterial blood gas concentrations reflect a compensated respiratory alkalosis with pH ranging from 7.40 to 7.47 and partial pressure of carbon dioxide (P_{CO2}) from 25 mm Hg to 32 mm Hg (29,30). The maternal partial pressure of oxygen (P_{O2}) ranges from 91 to as high as 106 mm Hg (30). The near-term alveolar-arterial oxygen gradient is 14 mm Hg in the sitting position compared with 20 mm Hg in the supine position. An explanation for the larger alveolar-arterial oxygen gradient when supine is decreased cardiac output because the enlarging uterus compresses the inferior vena cava which reduces venous return. In the third trimester, gravidas should try to avoid sleeping supine (29).

Total lung capacity is unchanged or reduced by 4% to 6%. The gravida breathes at reduced lung volumes because her residual volume and functional residual capacity are decreased. The diaphragm moves cephalad (27). As with the development of maternal hyperventilation, the residual volume and functional residual capacity decline before significant uterine enlargement occurs. The diaphragm flattens during gestation, and

there is less negative intrathoracic pressure reported in some studies. One could speculate that early airway closure would occur if there were less negative intrathoracic pressure. Because during episodes of acute asthma, the gravida with asthma generates large negative intrathoracic pressures to apply radial bronchodilating traction, any decline in ability to develop more negative inspiratory pressures would predispose gravidas with asthma to more sudden deterioration because of airway closure.

Bronchial responsiveness to methacholine does not change in a clinically important way; however, a statistically significant change has been reported with PC20 increasing from 0.35 to 0.72 mg/mL from pre-conception to postpartum (31). In this study of gravidas with mild asthma, the forced expiratory volume in 1 second (FEV_1) improved by 150 mL and the FEV_1 increased from 82% to 87% (31). The increase in serum progesterone concentration during gestation did not correlate with improvement in bronchial responsiveness (32). Although progesterone relaxes smooth muscles of the uterus and gastrointestinal tract, these findings suggest that factors other than progesterone contribute to changes in bronchial responsiveness.

Other Physiologic Changes

Cardiac output increases by 25% at 6 weeks and in later pregnancy can rise 30% to 60% because of the increase in heart rate and reduced vascular resistance (30,33,34). The latter results from estrogen supported generation of nitric oxide (35). The decrease in systemic vascular resistance is accompanied by an increase in the heart rate from 10 to 20 beats/minute. Stroke volume increases little; the uterine blood flow rises as much as 10-fold, from 50 mL/min to 500 mL/min at term (30). The blood volume increases an average of 1600 mL, and gravidas appear vasodilated as total body water expands by 1 L to 5 L (30,33,34,36). Gravidas are sensitive to overzealous fluid administration. Although correcting any dehydration is indicated, injudicious fluid replacement has resulted in acute pulmonary edema with normal cardiac function. During the latter half of gestation, these changes become manifest because the gravida has increased pre-load (mild volume overload with activation of the renin-angiotensin-aldosterone system), increased chronotropy, and reduced afterload (30,33,34).

Even though during gestation there is a 20% to 40% increase in erythrocyte mass, the maternal hemoglobin concentration decreases (28,30). The increase in erythrocyte mass is offset by the even larger increase of plasma volume resulting in relative anemia.

FETAL OXYGENATION

The vascular resistance of uterine vessels (progesterone effect) declines so that there can be the large increase in uterine blood flow (30,34). The fetus survives in a low-oxygen environment with little reserve oxygen store, should the supply of oxygen-rich uterine blood be compromised. Animal and human studies demonstrate reduced fetal oxygenation if there is reduced uterine blood flow that may occur with severe maternal hypotension, hypocarbia, or shock (30). Maternal hyperventilation can reduce venous return and shift the maternal oxyhemoglobin dissociation curve to the left. Modest declines in maternal oxygenation seem to be tolerated satisfactorily by the fetus, but substantial degrees of maternal hypoxemia may threaten survival of the fetus. Uterine vessels during gestation are dilated maximally based on experimental data, primarily from pregnant sheep and from some human studies. Uterine vessels do not vasodilate after β-adrenergic agonist stimulation, but do vasoconstrict from α-adrenergic agonists. Some obstetric anesthesiologists administer ephedrine 25 mg to 50 mg intravenously if hypotension occurs during epidural anesthesia. The β-adrenergic effects of ephedrine result in increased cardiac output, which increases systolic blood pressure and maintains uterine perfusion. Intramuscular epinephrine provides primarily β-adrenergic stimulation, whereas intravenous epinephrine results in mostly β and some α effects.

The fetal hemoglobin is 16.5 g/L and the oxygen pressure at which hemoglobin is 50% saturated is 22 mm Hg in the fetus, in contrast to 26 mm Hg to 28 mm Hg in the gravida (30,37). Fetal umbilical venous P_{O2} measurements at term average about 32 mm Hg, with P_{CO2} 49 mm Hg. There is a very large shunt effect of the uteroplacental circulation; this is demonstrated when the gravida inspires 100% oxygen in the absence of acute asthma, fetal umbilical venous P_{O2} increases to 40 mm Hg and P_{CO2} is 48 mm Hg (37). Such changes in P_{O2} can be quite important for the fetus in distress, although the uteroplacental shunt is large. For the same incremental increases in arterial P_{O2}, the leftward shift of the fetal hemoglobin oxygen dissociation curve results in larger increases in fetal oxygen saturation than in maternal blood.

In summary, fetal oxygen delivery depends on many factors, but most critical are blood flow (maternal cardiac output) to the uterus, integrity of the placenta, and maternal arterial oxygen content.

■ EFFECTS OF PREGNANCY ON ASTHMA

For the individual gravida, it is not always possible to predict the effects of pregnancy on asthma. Studies in the literature report varying degrees of improvement, deterioration, or no change in the clinical course (2,38). Over the past 3 decades, the published reports appear to be rather consistent, with approximately equal proportions of patients being unchanged, improving, or deteriorating. In a review from 1980 of nine studies involving 1,059 pregnancies, 49% of gravidas were unchanged in terms of severity of asthma, 29% improved, and 22% worsened (39). A prospective study of 198 pregnancies in 1988 recorded somewhat similar results in that 40% of gravidas had no change in medications, 18% of gravidas required fewer medications, but 42% required more medications (40). Similarly, using medication and symptom diary cards, during 366 gestations in 330 gravidas with mild or moderate asthma, asthma was unchanged in 33%, improved in 28%, and worsened in 35% (41). In a prospective study of 873 gravidas with asthma from 2003, 44% had no symptoms or treatment during the pregnancy, 32% had intermittent asthma, and 23% were considered to have persistent asthma (mild 13%, moderated 7%, and severe 4%) (13). How effective is the asthma control? In a series of 2,123 gravidas with asthma, about 33% had acute "unscheduled" care ranging from office visits to hospitalizations (42). It is not known if ineffectively controlled asthma contributed, but there is a report of an association between maternal asthma and intellectual disability in children (43). The association also was increased in the presence of maternal diabetes, renal or urinary tract conditions, and epilepsy (43).

Pregnancy in adolescents with asthma has been associated with many emergency department visits and hospitalizations for asthma (44). Some adolescents with severe asthma may not benefit from the prescription of anti-inflammatory medications because of poor adherence (45). The combination of poverty, inadequate or no prenatal care, limited education, and not being able to make control of asthma a priority can complicate pregnancies at any age of the gravida but especially during adolescent pregnancies.

Cigarette smoking during gestation can have long-term effects. Maternal smoking of 20 or more cigarettes/day *in utero* was associated with current asthma in 14-year-old girls but not in 14-year-old boys (46). These findings support the persistence of harmful effects of smoking *in utero* even if the gravida then quits after she delivers. Adverse effects on the child's lung function, FEV_1 and FEF_{25-75} and FEV_1/FVC, have been demonstrated in 7- to 18-year-olds whose mothers smoked during pregnancy or where another member (but not the gravida) smoked during the pregnancy (47). Clearly, gravidas must not smoke during gestation for their own well-being and that of their children.

■ CHOICE OF THERAPY

The approach to therapy includes making an assessment of the level of control, severity, and risks (1,2,23,48,49) (Table 39.1). Specifically, it should be determined (a) whether the gravida has near fatal (potentially fatal) asthma (48,49), (b) whether allergens in the home or workplace are contributing, and

TABLE 39.1 GOALS OF THERAPY FOR MANAGEMENT OF THE GRAVIDA WITH ASTHMA

- Prevent maternal fatalities and fetal demise
- Maximize asthma control
- Prevent hospitalizations, emergency department visits, and unscheduled care visits
- Prevent/reduce nocturnal asthma
- Prevent/reduce limitations of activities, school or work absenteeism/presenteeism
- Maximize respiratory status and pulmonary function
- Use appropriate medications
- Prepare an Action Plan for exacerbations

TABLE 39.2 APPROPRIATE MEDICATIONS DURING GESTATION

Anti-asthma Medications
Albuterol, levalbuterol
Salmeterol
Formoterol
Budesonide, beclomethasone dipropionate, fluticasone
Prednisone/methylprednisolone
Cromolyn
Montelukast/Zafirlukast
Nedocromil
Theophylline
Epinephrine (intramuscular)
Terbutaline
Ipratropium bromide

Allergen Immunotherapy

Tri-Valent Inactivated Influenza Vaccine

Anti-rhinitis Medications
Budesonide, beclomethasone dipropionate, fluticasone
Cromolyn
Loratadine
Cetirizine
Levocetirizine
Diphenhydramine
Chlorpheniramine
Pseudoephedrine (third trimester only, if at all)

Gastroesophageal Reflux Disease Medications
Lansoprazole
Esopmeprazole
Rabeprozole
cimetidine
Ranitidine
Famotidine

Antibiotics
Azithromycin
Penicillin derivatives
Cephalosporins
Clindamycin
Nitrofurantoin

(c) whether the gravida is likely to be adherent to the recommendations provided.

Avoidance Measures

General avoidance measures include cessation of smoking and preferably recommending that there be no second-hand smoking in the home environment. There should be no or very minimal consumption of alcoholic beverages, cessation of illicit drug use, and avoidance of drugs with teratogenic or harmful potential. Examples of these include tetracyclines (discoloration of infant's teeth from insufficient production of enamel), sulfonamides in the last trimester (glucose-6 phosphate dehydrogenase G6PD deficiency could cause hemolytic anemia), troleandomycin, clarithromcyin, methotrexate, mycophenolate mofetil, and antibiotics such as quinolones.

When there is allergic asthma, individual avoidance measures should be implemented for animals, dust mites, cockroaches, and fungi. Aspirin and nonsteroidal anti-inflammatory drugs should be withheld in the gravidas with aspirin exacerbated respiratory disease. However, nonselective anti-inflammatory drugs such as ibuprofen or naproxen (50) are considered appropriate for the first 32 weeks of gestation, if indicated for aspirin-tolerant gravidas. Acetaminophen is acceptable.

Medications

There are increasing data to justify the appropriate use of many medications for treatment of asthma and its comorbidities during gestation (Table 39.2) (1,2,13,14,16,21,23,50–53). Where feasible, it is preferable to use inhaled as opposed to oral medications; to some extent this point has become moot in that there are data to justify appropriate use of oral medications. In human gestation, organogenesis is proportionately relatively short (days 12 to 56) compared with animals. Drugs are infrequent causes of major congenital malfor-

mations, which have an overall rate of 3% to 7% depending on the studies and degree of ascertainment (54). About two-thirds of malformations are from unknown factors and an additional 25% are genetically determined. About 5% of malformations have been associated with environmental factors including medications, maternal infections, and radiation.

Examples of teratogenic agents include ethanol, isotretinoin, phenytoin, carbamazepine, valproic acid, angiotensin-converting enzyme inhibitors, diethylstil-bestrol (vaginal carcinoma), thalidomide, inorganic iodides, lithium carbonate, tetracycline, doxycycline, streptomycin, mycophenolate mofetil, and some anti-neoplastic drugs that have not caused fetal loss earlier. Erythromycin has been associated with an increase in cardiac malformations, and clarithromycin has a U.S. Food and Drug Administration (FDA) category C rating (50).

Most to almost all medications for use for asthma are considered appropriate for treatment in pregnancy. The strength of this statement varies depending on the first trimester data (1,2,13,14,18,20,21,23,50–53). There is only a single citation and limited experience with use of formoterol (51); there is more experience with salmeterol (23,53). Harm has not been described. The combination product of budesonide/formoterol has been used effectively as reliever and controller therapy in nonpregnant women (55). It is an FDA category C drug in the United States. It may well be an acceptable therapy during gestation as a reliever medication as data are accumulated.

Human data on the use of oral corticosteroids have not identified teratogenic effects for prednisone, methylprednisolone, or hydrocortisone, and they are recommended when indicated (1,2,9,11,22,23,53). The most published data for inhaled corticosteroids report on belcomethasone dipropionate and budesonide. Most gravidas with mild persistent and some with moderate persistent asthma will be managed effectively with budesonide or other inhaled corticosteroids such as beclomethasone dipropionate. The American College of Obstetricians and Gynecologists Practice Bulletin (2) concluded that "budesonide is the preferred inhaled corticocosteroid for use in pregnancy." The National Asthma Education and Prevention Program (NAEPP) Working Group took a view that "inhaled corticosteroids other than budesonide may be continued in patients who were well controlled by these agents prior to pregnancy especially if it was thought that changing formulations may jeopardize control"(1).

Oral steroids should be initiated early during exacerbations, as doubling of the inhaled corticosteroid from whatever was the controlling dosage often is ineffective unless the controlling dosage was "pediatric" such as budesonide 200 µg/day to 400 µg/day. In a study of nonpregnant patients who were managed with a mean dose of beclomethasone dipropionate of 710 µg/day, the approach tried was that of doubling the inhaled corticosteroid when there were 15% or greater reductions of peak expiratory flow rates or increased symptoms (56). This approach did not prevent the need for oral corticosteroids, which were initiated when the peak expiratory flow rate decreased by 40% (56). Therefore, the gravida should be aware that the inhaled corticosteroid, inhaled corticosteroid/albuterol, or inhaled corticosteroid/long-acting β_2 agonist combination may be inadequate for some exacerbations of asthma. Although this statement applies to gravidas with severe persistent asthma, it also applies to gravidas with mild or moderate persistent asthma who might experience a severe worsening of asthma when there is an upper respiratory infection.

Cromolyn (53,57) has a very long record of use for asthma (allergic rhinitis and allergic conjunctivitis) and can be recommended for intermittent or mild or moderate persistent asthma. It can be effective as prophylactic treatment before exercise, cold air and/or fume exposure, and for pet dander or mold exposures. Nedocromil (53) also inhibits early and late bronchial responses to allergens as does cromolyn and both are labeled FDA Category B.

Leukotriene antagonists, montelukast and zafirlukast, are designated as FDA Category B and are recommended (23) for moderate and persistent asthma as alternative treatments. It is informative that one series of 96 women did not identify an increased risk of teratogenicity (52).

Albuterol is recommended as the short acting β_2-adrenergic agonist of choice (2,23). The NAEPP Working Group advises that for acute exacerbations of asthma "up to 3 treatments of 2–4 puffs by MDI at 20 minute intervals or single nebulizer treatment" can be started at home (23). This author would suggest that albuterol be limited to 2 inhalations and prednisone 40 mg to 60 mg initiated instead of up to 12 inhalations in the first hour if there is no physician present. If the gravida remains quite dyspneic, she should seek emergency department or perhaps office assessment and care.

Some gravidas with severe asthma during pregnancy may require low to moderate dose prednisone administered on an alternate-day basis to maintain effective asthma control. Experience with alternate-day prednisone, along with intermittent courses of daily prednisone (40 mg to 60 mg each morning for 5 to 7 days) for exacerbations has resulted in avoidance of emergency department visits and hospitalizations and normal pregnancy outcomes such as newborn birth weight, head circumference, and length (9–10,11).

Theophylline is not contraindicated for treatment of asthma during gestation, but has a narrow therapeutic index and is considered an alternative therapy (2). Its metabolism is altered by many factors, and drug interactions must be considered. The peak serum concentration should be in the range of 5 µg/mL to 12 µg/mL.

Allergen Immunotherapy

Allergen immunotherapy can be continued or even initiated during pregnancy. The only recognized risk from allergen immunotherapy is anaphylaxis. There are no data to suggest that women are more likely to experience anaphylaxis from allergen immunotherapy when pregnancy occurs. Data from 121 pregnancies in 90 gravidas receiving allergen immunotherapy showed a low incidence of anaphylaxis (58). The Joint Task Force on Practice Parameters of the American Academy of Allergy, Asthma and Immunology (AAAAI); American College of Allergy, Asthma and Immunology (ACAAI); and Joint Council of Allergy, Asthma and Immunology advises that dosing of immunotherapy not be increased during pregnancy (59). This author believes that as long as the gravida is not having systemic reactions to immunotherapy, she can have the dosage increased in the normal manner. Indeed, the goal of immunotherapy is to reduce the symptoms and need for medications. Allergen immunotherapy does not protect the fetus from subsequent development of atopic disorders (58,60).

Acute Asthma

As in managing the nonpregnant patient with asthma, exacerbations of asthma should be reversed as quickly and effectively as possible. Acute severe asthma (status asthmaticus) has been associated with intrauterine growth restriction (retardation), stillbirths, maternal deaths, and untoward effects on the fetus such as cerebral palsy from inadequate oxygenation. The goal in treating the gravida with acute asthma is to minimize maternal hypoxemia, hypocarbia, or respiratory acidosis and to maintain adequate oxygenation for the fetus.

β_2-adrenergic agonists (such as albuterol) are the drugs of choice for home or emergency department/hospital use (1,2,23). If the gravida presents in the emergency department and the initial response to albuterol is incomplete, oral or intravenous corticosteroids should be administered promptly. Continued acute severe dyspnea may necessitate continued nebulized therapy or additional albuterol by metered-dose inhaler. There must be monitoring of oxygen and overall respiratory status. Ipratropium may be administered with albuterol but is not the primary treatment. Some gravidas with very severe dyspnea will not respond to albuterol administered by nebulizer or metered-dose inhaler; in that setting, epinephrine can be administered intramuscularly as 0.3 mL (1:1000). The justification for epinephrine is as follows: (a) it is synthesized endogenously, (b) it is not teratogenic, (c) it is metabolized rapidly, (d) its onset of action is rapid, and (e) variables associated with drug delivery by inhalation do not have to be considered. The use of epinephrine for acute asthma or anaphylaxis increases cardiac output, which can maintain uterine perfusion in contrast to the fear that epinephrine will cause fetal loss by decreasing uterine blood flow. The adverse effects of acute severe asthma (or anaphylaxis) can be a serious threat to the gravida or fetus.

The NAEPP Expert Panel Report suggested that home treatment of the acute exacerbation could include inhaled β_2-adrenergic agonist (albuterol) therapy from 2 to 4 inhalations every 20 minutes in the first hour or

as a single nebulizer treatment (23). With a good response defined as peak expiratory flow >80% of the personal best, no wheezing or shortness of breath, a response to the albuterol treatment lasting for 4 hours and no apparent drop in fetal kick counts, the gravida should continue the albuterol and double the inhaled corticosteroid for the next 7 to 10 days (23). If the gravida has an incomplete response, such as having continued wheezing and shortness of breath and the peak expiratory flow rate being 50% to 80%, an oral corticosteroid was recommended. A poor response to the initial treatment was defined as peak expiratory flow of <50%, marked wheezing and shortness of breath, and decreased fetal kick activity. The gravida, in that case, should begin the oral corticosteroid, repeat the albuterol, call for medical advice and proceed to the emergency department (23).

A personalized approach uses the level of asthma severity to guide therapy. How much medication and what types have been used in the past to control the asthma? How responsive has the asthma been? Have there been previous hospitalizations, intensive care unit admissions, or intubations? The latter two events imply a diagnosis of potentially (near) fatal asthma (48,49). If there was poor adherence in the past, it can be anticipated that guideline-type of control will not be achievable. Alternative treatment plans should be considered.

When the gravida presents with moderate or severe acute wheezing dyspnea, oral corticosteroids should be administered with the initial albuterol or albuterol/ipratropium treatment. For example, prednisone 40 mg to 60 mg is an appropriate dosage. The initial beneficial effects may be in 2 to 6 hours or longer. If the initial treatment is not effective over the first 2 hours, it is likely that acute severe asthma (status asthmaticus) has occurred. Hospitalization or treatment in an observation unit is indicated; theophylline has not been found to be superior to albuterol and intravenous methylprednisolone therapy. In some gravidas with acute severe asthma, it may be sufficient to monitor the pulse oxygenation measurements. In other gravidas, an arterial blood gas determination will be necessary to monitor the P_{CO2} and pH. Some gravidas require fetal heart monitoring during or before discharge.

Excessive fluid replacement is not indicated, but volume depletion should be corrected. The gravida can develop acute pulmonary edema (noncardiac) from excessive crystalloid administration as she is volume-expanded during gestation. The resultant acute dyspnea may be attributed to acute severe asthma when it is from fluid overload and noncardiac pulmonary edema.

When the gravida, who has experienced an exacerbation of asthma, is discharged from the emergency department, observation unit, or hospital, a short course of oral corticosteroid should be administered to prevent continued symptoms and signs of asthma

(1,2,23,61). In the rare setting of acute respiratory failure during acute severe asthma, an emergency cesarean delivery may be necessary (*19*,62).

■ PERSISTENT ASTHMA

Some types of persistent asthma during gestation are listed in Table 39.3. Should gravidas require daily medication, an allergy-immunology consultation is indicated to identify and address IgE-mediated triggers of asthma, to determine if allergic bronchopulmonary aspergillosis is present, and to provide expertise in the diagnosis and treatment of nasal polyps, cough, rhinitis, or rhinosinusitis. Avoidance measures are indicated to reduce bronchial hyperresponsiveness and the need for antiasthma medications.

The goals of management include maintaining a functional respiratory status, as well as minimizing wheezing dyspnea, nocturnal asthma, exercise intolerance, emergency department visits, acute severe asthma, and maternal fatalities or loss of the fetus (Table 39.1).

Dyspnea can be sensed during gestation in the absence of asthma during the first two trimesters (*63*). A respiratory rate of more than 18 breaths/min has been considered a warning sign for pulmonary pathology complicating "dyspnea during pregnancy" (*63*). A comorbidity to consider includes peripartum cardiomyopathy.

Many gravidas can be managed effectively with inhaled budesonide or beclomethasone dipropionate and inhaled albuterol for symptomatic relief. For gravidas who have intermittent asthma or mild persistent asthma, inhaled budesonide or beclomethasone diproprionate, cromolyn, leukotriene-receptor antagonists, or possibly theophylline are appropriate during gestation. A short-acting bronchodilator such as albuterol would be recommended if needed. If these drugs are ineffective because of worsening asthma, such as from an upper respiratory infection, a short course of prednisone such as 40 mg daily for 5 to 7 days may be administered. Antibiotics can be prescribed for secondary bacterial infections after viral upper respiratory infections, acute bronchitis, or exacerbations of chronic or subacute rhinosinusitis. Azithromycin, ampicillin, amoxicillin, amoxicillin-clavulanate, or cephalosporins are appropriate antibiotics (Table 39.2).

For severe persistent asthma, higher dosages of budesonide or other inhaled corticosteroids can be used as can fluticasone/salmeterol (23) or budesonide/formoterol. Higher doses of inhaled corticosteroids may produce systemic side effects. Proper inhalation technique is necessary and should be assessed periodically. Should asthma be managed ineffectively with avoidance measures and the inhaled corticosteroid/long-acting β_2-adrenergic agonist combination, then cromolyn, leukotriene-receptor antagonists, or theophylline can be considered (1,23).

If the gravida has significant wheezing on examination, nocturnal asthma, or major changes in spirometry or peak expiratory flow rates, a short course of prednisone may be indicated to relieve symptoms and improve respiratory status. If the gravida has improved after 1 week of prednisone, either the prednisone can be discontinued or it can be converted to alternate-day administration and tapered (9,*11*). The most effective antiasthma medications for chronic administration during gestation in order of efficacy are prednisone, inhaled corticosteroids, and then inhaled β-adrenergic agonists (albuterol, levalbuterol, or terbutaline), leukotriene-receptor antagonists, cromolyn, and theophylline. Theophylline has a low therapeutic index and for the most part, is not considered anti-inflammatory. In some gravidas with severe persistent asthma, bronchiectasis from allergic bronchopulmonary aspergillosis, or inhaled corticosteroid phobia, theophylline can be used. It is not teratogenic in humans. Comorbidities such as allergic rhinitis, rhinosinusitis, and gastroesophageal reflux disease should be addressed (Table 39.2).

Essentially all patients can be managed successfully during gestation. Some patients with potentially (near) fatal asthma are unmanageable because of noncompliance with physician advice, medications, or in keeping ambulatory clinical appointments. Such gravidas are considered to have malignant potentially fatal asthma. Long-acting methylprednisolone (80 mg to 120 mg intramuscularly) is of value to prevent repeated episodes of status asthmaticus or respiratory failure. This approach should be instituted to try to prevent fetal loss or maternal death in the nearly impossible-to-manage gravida. Adequate documentation in the medical record is needed. Psychologic, psychiatric, and social work evaluations may be obtained. Gravidas with malignant potentially fatal asthma, however, may refuse evaluation or necessary therapy. The serum glucose should be determined regularly because of hyperglycemia produced by long-acting methylprednisolone. Other antiasthma medications should be minimized to simplify the medication regimen.

TABLE 39.3 CLASSIFICATION OF ASTHMA DURING PREGNANCY

- Intermittent
- Persistent (allergic or nonallergic)
  - Mild
  - Moderate
  - Severe
- Potentially (near) fatal asthma
- Asthma with allergic bronchopulmonary aspergillosis
- Aspirin exacerbated respiratory disease (aspirin intolerant asthma)
- Adolescent asthma

■ LABOR AND DELIVERY

When asthma is controlled effectively, the gravida can participate in prepared childbirth methods without limitation. Minute ventilation increases to as great as 20 L/min during labor and delivery (37). Should cesarean delivery be necessary, complications from anesthesia should not create difficulty if asthma is well controlled. When the gravida has used inhaled corticosteroids or oral corticosteroids during gestation, predelivery corticosteroid coverage should include 100 mg hydrocortisone intravenously every 8 hours until postpartum, and other medications can be used. Parenteral corticosteroids suppress any asthma that might complicate anesthesia required for cesarean delivery. The prior use of recommended dosages of inhaled corticosteroids or alternate-day prednisone should not suppress the surge of adrenal corticosteroids associated with labor or during anesthesia.

When the gravida who requires regular moderate- to high-dose inhaled corticosteroids or daily or alternate-day prednisone plans to have a cesarean delivery, preoperative prednisone should be administered for 3 days before anesthesia. The gravida should be examined ideally 1 to 2 weeks before delivery to confirm stable respiratory status and satisfactory pulmonary function. In gravidas with persistent mild asthma, preanesthetic therapy can consist of 5 days of inhaled corticosteroid.

When the gravida presents in labor in respiratory distress, emergency measures such as inhaled albuterol and oral or intravenous corticosteroids should be administered promptly. Adequate oxygenation and fetal monitoring are essential.

■ RHINITIS DURING PREGNANCY

Intranasal obstruction and nasal secretions can be very troublesome during gestation and interfere with sleep. It has been reported that 18% to 61% of gravidas experience symptoms of rhinitis during some time during gestation (64). Nasal congestion during gestation may be influenced by (a) increased blood volume, (b) progesterone's effects causing smooth muscle relaxation of nasal vessels, (c) estrogen's effects causing mucosal edema, (d) production of nitric oxide, which is a vasodilator, from the maxillary sinuses, and (e) effects of vasodilating neuropeptides.

Nasal biopsy results from symptom-free gravidas showed glandular hyperactivity manifested by swollen mitochondria and increased number of secretory granules (65). Special stains demonstrated increased metabolic activity, increased phagocytosis, and increased acid mucopolysaccharides, thought to be attributed to high concentrations of estrogen. Similar findings were present in gravidas with nasal symptoms. Additional findings included increased (a) goblet cell numbers in the nasal epithelium, (b) cholinergic nerve fibers around glands and vessels, and (c) vascularity and transfer of metabolites through cell membranes (65). Women who used older (stronger) oral contraceptives but in whom no nasal symptoms had occurred had similar histopathologic and histochemical changes, as did symptom-free gravidas (66). Regarding post-nasal drainage, it has been estimated that in nonpregnant females, 700 mL to 900 mL of nasal secretions are generated per day for proper conditioning of inspired air. In some gravidas, this volume may be even greater and secretions are not reabsorbed, which results in symptoms of rhinitis, post-nasal drip, or cough.

Nasal congestion causing symptoms is likely to occur in the second and third trimesters. However, it may occur in the first trimester as well (64). The differential diagnosis for rhinitis of pregnancy includes allergic rhinitis, nonallergic rhinitis (including nonallergic rhinitis with eosinophilia), nasal polyposis, and rhinosinusitis or purulent rhinitis resulting from enlarged inferior turbinates that are occlusive with the nasal septum. There can be referred pain to the sinuses consistent with rhinologic or contact headache, a condition that mimics an exacerbation of rhinosinusitis. Rhinitis medicamentosa may be present when there has been excessive use of topical decongestants.

Treatment of nasal symptoms during gestation necessitates an accurate diagnosis, effective pharmacotherapy, and, in some cases, avoidance measures. For example, smoking and illicit drugs should be discontinued, as should topical decongestants. Intranasal budesonide or beclomethasone dipropionate are indicated to relieve nasal obstruction. There are published asthma data for budesonide and beclomethasone dipropionate; however, the very low bioavailability of other corticosteroids such as mometasone and fluticasone suggests that they also are appropriate during gestation. If large nasal polyps are present and topical corticosteroids are ineffective, a short course of prednisone should be prescribed. The blood glucose should be monitored because the gravida is prone to hyperglycemia.

Antihistamines help gravidas with milder degrees of allergic rhinitis and occasionally with some nonallergic types of rhinitis. As of 1977, there had been very long-term experience and safety for chlorpheniramine (1,070 exposures), diphenhydramine (595 exposures), and tripelennamine (121 exposures) (67). These first generation antihistamines remain appropriate (Table 39.2) but second generation antihistamines are acceptable and infrequently sedating. Loratadine was used in 2,147 pregnancies (68) and has the most published experience in pregnancy. By analogy, the metabolite of loratadine, desloratadine, should be appropriate as well. Cetirizine and its parent, hydroxyzine, were not associated with teratogenic effects in 39 and 53 pregnancies, respectively (69) or in 196 pregnancies, of which 153 women used cetirizine within 5 weeks of the last menstrual period (70). Data on cetirizine have shown that it is not teratogenic (69,70). A very conservative approach is to avoid its use during the first trimester or in women planning a pregnancy.

For perspective, the FDA classification system category B means that animal studies are negative but that human studies have not been conducted or that animal studies are positive but such findings of fetal risk have not been demonstrated in human pregnancies. FDA category C implies that animal studies have identified adverse fetal effects and that there are no controlled studies in human pregnancies or human data aren't available (50,71). The proviso is to use such medications only if the "potential benefit outweighs the potential risk to the fetus" (50,71). The FDA category B medications include chlorpheniramine, loratadine, and cetirizine whereas fexofenadine and azelastine are FDA category C (71). The leukotriene-receptor antagonists, montelukast and zafirlukast, are category B (71) and experience in 96 pregnancies did not identify harm (52). Intranasal (or ocular or orally inhaled) cromolyn is considered appropriate (57) and is FDA category B. Except for budesonide, nasal corticosteroids remain FDA category C, although their benefits outweigh any risks.

This author tries not to prescribe pseudoephedrine to avoid potential α-adrenergic stimulation of uterine vessels, even though it has not been found to be teratogenic (71,72). Phenylpropanolamine (not available in the United States) in 726 exposures was associated with significantly greater risk of malformations (ear and eye), whereas this risk was not detected with pseudoephedrine (39 exposures) or phenylephrine (1,249 exposures) (67).

Antibiotics for pregnant women with infectious rhinosinusitis or purulent rhinitis are listed in Table 39.2. Ampicillin, amoxicillin, amoxicillin-clavulanate, azithromycin, and cephalosporins are initial antibiotics, depending on the prior therapy of the gravida. Sulfonamides are contraindicated because of the possibility of G6PD deficiency in the fetus. Tetracyclines are contraindicated because of maternal fatty liver during gestation (third trimester) and staining of teeth in the infant. Human experience with clarithromycin is not available, so azithromycin should be used if it is indicated. FDA category B antibiotics include azithromycin, cephalosporins, clindamycin, erythromycin, and penicillins, which include ampicillin/sulbactam and amoxicillin/clavulanic acid. (71). FDA category C antibiotics consist of aminoglycosides, chloramphenicol, clarithromycin, quinolones, sulfonamides, tetracycline derivatives, and vancomycin (71).

Allergen immunotherapy helps reduce the need for medications in cases of allergic rhinitis or asthma. This therapy can be continued in pregnancy and, if symptoms are severe and the gravida agrees, immunotherapy may be initiated during gestation. During immunotherapy in 121 pregnancies in 90 gravidas, 6 gravidas experienced anaphylaxis (58). No abortions or other adverse effects occurred (58). The decision to begin immunotherapy after delivery often is made for the purpose of convenience and ability of the woman to present for injections in a timely fashion. Severe allergic rhinitis symptoms during gestation can be treated with intranasal corticosteroids and antihistamines.

As stated earlier, the dose of allergen immunotherapy can be increased in the absence of large local reactions or systemic reactions. There is no evidence that the incidence of anaphylaxis from allergen immunotherapy (or skin testing) is greater during the time of gestation.

Replacement immunoglobulin for gravidas with primary or secondary immunodeficiency should be continued or initiated during gestation. The dosage is at least 0.4 g/kg every 4 weeks.

■ URTICARIA, ANGIOEDEMA, AND ANAPHYLAXIS

Urticaria or angioedema should be evaluated and treated during gestation with little change from the nongravid state, detailed in Chapter 31. Some causes for urticaria and angioedema include foods, medications, infections (viral), and underlying autoimmune conditions such as collagen vascular disorders. Some episodes of urticaria are attributable to dermatographism or other physical urticarias, chronic (autoimmune) urticaria, or idiopathic acute urticaria. The differential diagnosis during gestation includes hereditary angioedema (HAE) (73–74,75–77), pruritic urticarial papules and plaques of pregnancy (PUPPP) (78), herpes gestationis (79), and prurigo of pregnancy.

In the series of Frank et al. (74), there was an increased frequency of attacks of HAE in only 2 of 25 gestations. No acute episodes of HAE occurred during delivery. In contrast, Chappatte and deSwiet reported on the unpredictability of HAE during gestation and a maternal fatality (73). From a series of 227 pregnancies in 107 women in the PREHAEAT project of the European Union, HAE worsened in 38% of women, was unchanged in 32%, and was less severe in 30% (77). It was reported that the course of HAE was usually similar to the prepregnancy course (77). The concentration of C1 inhibitor declines in normal pregnancy because of increased plasma volume. Some gravidas have worsening clinical symptoms and create major management problems. Contraception is advisable as a rule. Stanozolol or danazol result in a fourfold to fivefold increase in the concentration of C1 inhibitor and C4. Although stanozolol has been administered during gestation without masculinizing fetal effects or fetal loss (73), its use is discouraged in gravidas with HAE. Contraception should be used if a woman is receiving attenuated androgens for HAE. Genetic counseling is advisable for women with HAE because it is an autosomal-dominant condition, although there is incomplete penetrance.

For acute severe central episodes of HAE, rapid administration of intramuscular epinephrine has been used, but additional specific therapy will have to include danazol 600 mg to 800 mg immediately or stanozolol, 4 mg four times a day, and airway care measures (intubation or tracheostomy). Fresh frozen plasma also may be infused on an emergent basis in some situations. Although unavailable in the United States, a concentrate of C1 inhibitor for parenteral administration has proved effective, with onset of action in 10 to 60 minutes (76). Antifibrinolytic agents are considered unwise to use in pregnancy because of their potential thrombotic effects. Nevertheless, three pregnancies in one gravida occurred uneventfully despite use of ε-amino-caproic acid (80).

During gestation, no specific maintenance therapy is necessary in gravidas with peripheral HAE. Based on Frank's series of gravidas with peripheral or central (upper airway involvement) HAE, exacerbations during the time of tissue trauma, delivery, did not occur (74). In the PREHAEAT project, there were exacerbations of HAE postpartum or within 48 hours of delivery in just 6% of pregnancies (77). If an episode of upper airway obstruction occurs during a cesarean delivery, epinephrine, danazol, stanozolol, and intubation would be indicated. Use of C1 inhibitor concentrates, if available and of low risk, otherwise would be of value acutely.

The PUPPP syndrome occurs in the last trimester and begins on the abdomen with numerous extremely pruritic, erythematous, urticarial plaques and papules surrounded by pale halos (78). Topical corticosteroids are of value, and maternal or fetal complications are unlikely. The plaques and papules may last until 6 weeks postpartum. Herpes gestationis consists of intense pruritus followed by lesions that may be bullous, papulovesicular, or pustular (79). Some gravidas develop tense grouped vesicles on the abdomen or extremity.

Pharmacologic treatment of chronic urticaria or angioedema often is required. The antihistamines listed in Table 39.2 are recommended. Prednisone may be indicated for acute exacerbations of urticaria, angioedema, or anaphylaxis. Leukotriene-receptor antagonists are appropriate but often do not provide relief for urticaria in nonpregnant women.

Anaphylaxis during gestation has been described after penicillin (81), cefotetan (82), Hymenoptera stings (83), oxytocin (84), diclofenac (85), phytomenadione (86), fentanyl (87), ferric gluconate (88), antisnakebite venom (89), latex (90), and succinylcholine (91). Anaphylaxis during gestation has caused fetal distress, fetal encephalopathy, or fetal demise. Gravidas have experienced profound shock with reduced uterine blood flow during anaphylaxis as the fundamental insult to the fetus. As in other cases of anaphylaxis, prevention and emergency medications and therapy are needed. Epinephrine intramuscularly should be administered

promptly. If the gravida is hypotensive, then usual resuscitative measures should be instituted to maintain blood pressure and the airway. Obstetric assistance should be obtained immediately should cesarean delivery be indicated.

■ VENOM IMMUNOTHERAPY

Venom immunotherapy is a highly efficacious form of therapy to prevent future episodes of Hymenoptera anaphylaxis. Graft (92) reported a successful pregnancy in a gravida treated with maintenance dosages of wasp and mixed vespid venoms. Subsequently the Committee on Insects of the AAAAI reported 63 pregnancies in 26 gravidas with no definite systemic reactions (93). Five of 43 gestations resulted in spontaneous abortions, thought to be unrelated to stings or immunotherapy. One term infant (2.7%) had multiple congenital cardiovascular malformations; this incidence is within the range of expected congenital malformations. The Joint Task Force on Practice Parameters of the AAAAI, ACAAI, and the Joint Council of Allergy, Asthma and Immunology suggested that the dosages of venom not be increased during pregnancy (59). This author would take a more aggressive approach and continue to build up during the injections in the absence of systemic reactions or large local reactions (>8 cm). Other issues should be discussed with the gravida, such as avoidance measures and personal use of epinephrine.

■ REFERENCES

1. National Institutes of Health, National Heart, Lung and Blood Institute. *National Asthma Education and Prevention Program Working Group Report on Managing Asthma during Pregnancy: Recommendations for Pharmacologic Treatment*. U.S. Department of Health and Human Services, NIH publication 05–5236, March 2005.
2. ACOG Practice Bulletin: Clinical Management Guidelines for Obstetric-Gynecologists, number 90, February 2008. Asthma in pregnancy. *Obstet Gynecol*. 2008;111,457–464.
3. Kwon, HL, Belanger K, Bracken MB. Asthma prevalence among pregnancy and childbearing-aged women in the United States: estimates from national health surveys. *Ann Epidemiol*. 2003;13:317–324.
8. Liu S, Wen SW, Demissie K, et al. Maternal asthma and pregnancy outcomes: a retrospective cohort study. *Am J Obstet Gynecol*. 2001;184:90–96.
9. Greenberger PA, Patterson R. The outcomes of pregnancy complicated by severe asthma. *Allergy Proc*. 1988;9:539–543.
10. Triche EW, Saftlas AF, Belanger K, et al. Association of asthma diagnosis, severity, symptoms, and treatment risk of preeclampsia. *Obstet Gynecol*. 2004;104:585–93.
13. Bracken MB, Triche EW, Belanger K, et al. Asthma symptoms, severity, and drug therapy: a prospective study of effects on 2205 pregnancies. *Obstet Gynecol*. 2003;102:739–752.
14. Breton M-C, Martel M-J, Vilain A, et al. Inhaled corticosteroids during pregnancy: a review of methodologic issues. *Respir Med*. 2008;102:862–875.
15. Beckmann CA. The effect of asthma on pregnancy and perinatal outcomes. *J Asthma*. 2003;40:171–180.
16. Bakhireva LN, Schatz M, Jones KL, et al. Asthma control during pregnancy and the risk of preterm delivery or impaired fetal growth. *Ann Allergy Asthma Immunol*. 2008;101:137–143.
17. Schatz M, Dombrowski MP, Wise, R, et al. Asthma morbidity during pregnancy can be predicted by severity classification. *J Allergy Clin Immunol*. 2003;112:283–288.

18. Blais L, Forget A. Asthma exacerbations during the first trimester of pregnancy and the risk of congenital malformations among asthmatic women. *J Allergy Clin Immunol.* 2008;121:1379–1384.

20. Bakhireva LN, Jones KL, Schatz M, et al. Asthma medication use in pregnancy and fetal growth. *J Allergy Clin Immunol.* 2005;116:503–509.

21. Blais L, Beauchesne M-F, Rey E, et al. Use of inhaled corticosteroids during the first trimester of pregnancy and the risk of congenital malformations among women with asthma. *Thorax.* 2007;62:320–328.

22. Norjavaara E, de Verdier MG. Normal pregnancy outcomes in a population–based study including 2968 pregnancy women exposed to budesonide. *J Allergy Clin Immunol.* 2003;111:736–742.

23. NAEPP Expert Panel Report. Managing asthma during pregnancy: recommendations for pharmacologic treatment–2004 update. *J Allergy Clin Immunol.* 2005;115:34–46.

24. Cydulka RK, Emerman CL, Schreiber D, et al. Acute asthma among pregnant women presenting to the emergency department. *Am J Respir Crit Care Med.* 1999;160:887–892.

28. Vargus M, Vargas E, Julian CG, et al. Determinants of blood oxygenation during pregnancy in Andean and European residents of high altitude. *Am J Physiol Regul Integr Comp Physiol.* 2007; 293:R1303–R1312.

29. Cousins L. Fetal oxygenation, assessment of fetal well-being, and obstetric management of the pregnant patient with asthma. *J Allergy Clin Immunol.* 1999;103 (suppl):343–349.

33. Rang S, von Montfrans GA, Wolf H. Serial hemodynamic measurements in normal pregnancy, preeclampsia, and intrauterine growth restriction. *Am J Obstet Gynecol.* 2008;198:e1–19.

34. Bamfo JE, Kemetas NA, Chambers JB, et al. Maternal cardiac function in normotensive and pre-eclamptic intrauterine growth restriction. *Ultrasound Obstet Gynecol.* 2008;32(5):682–686.

35. Valensise H, Vasapollo B, Novelli GP, et al. Maternal and fetal hemodynamic effects induced by nitric oxide donors and plasma volume expansion in pregnancies with gestational hypertension complicated by intrauterine growth restriction with absent end-diastolic flow in the umbilical artery. *Ultrasound Obstet Gynecol.* 2008;31:55–64.

38. Kircher S, Schatz M, Long L. Variables affecting asthma course during pregnancy. *Ann Allergy Asthma Immunol.* 2002;89:437–438.

42. Schatz M. Dombrowski MP, Wise P, et al. Spirometry is related to perinatal outcomes in pregnant women with asthma. *Am J Obstet Gynecol.* 2006;194:120–126.

43. Leonard H, de Klerk N, Bourke J, et al. Maternal health in pregnancy and intellectual disability in the offspring: a population-based study. *Ann Epidemiol.* 2008;16:448–454.

46. Alati R, Al Mamun A, O'Callaghan M, et al. In utero and postnatal maternal smoking and asthma in adolescence. *Epidemiology.* 2006; 17:138–144.

47. Gilliland FD, Berhane K, Li YF, et al. Effects of early onset asthma and in utero exposure to maternal smoking on childhood lung function. *Am J Respir Crit Care Med.* 2003;167:917–924.

48. Story RE, Greenberger PA. Potentially fatal asthma. *Allergy Asthma Proc.* 2004;25:S29–S30.

49. National Heart, Lung, and Blood Institute: National Asthma Education and Prevention Program. *Expert Panel Report 3: Guidelines for the Diagnosis and Management of Asthma.* NIH Publication No. 07–4051. Bethesda (MD): NHLBI 2007.

50. Vlastarakos PV, Manolopoulos L, Ferekidis E, et al. Treating common problems of the nose and throat in pregnancy: what is safe? *Eur Arch Otorhinolaryngol.* 2008;265:499–508.

51. Tamasi L, Bohacs A, Pallinger E, et al. The management of bronchial asthma during pregnancy-Hungarian experiences. *Orv Hetil.* 2005;146:2305–2309.

52. Bakhireva LN, Jones KL, Schatz M, et al. Safety of leukotriene receptor antagonists in pregnancy. *J Allergy Clin Immunol.* 2007;119: 618–25.

53. Gluck JC, Gluck PA. Asthma controller therapy during pregnancy. *Am J Obstet Gynecol.* 2005;192:369–380.

54. Finnell RH. Teratology: general considerations and principles. *J Allergy Clin Immunol.* 1999;103 (suppl):337–342.

55. Kuna P, Peters MJ, Manjra AI, et al. Effect of budesonide/formoterol maintenance and reliever therapy on asthma exacerbations. *Int J Clin Pract.* 2007;61:725–736.

56. Harrison TW, Oborne J, Newton S, et al. Doubling the dose of inhaled corticosteroid to prevent asthma exacerbations: randomized controlled trial. *Lancet.* 2004;363:271–275.

59. Joint Task Force on Practice Parameters: American Academy of Allergy, Asthma and Immunology; American College of Allergy, Asthma and Immunology; Joint Council of Allergy, Asthma and Immunology. Allergen immunotherapy: a practice parameter second update. *J Allergy Clin Immunol.* 2007;120:S25–S85.

61. Rowe BH, Spooner CH, Ducharme FM, et al. Corticosteroids for preventing relapse following acute exacerbations of asthma. *Cochrane Database Syst Rev.* 2007; 3:CD000195. DOI: 10,1002/14651858. CD000195.pub2.

62. Siddiqui AK, Gouda H, Multz AS, et al. Ventilator strategy for status asthmaticus in pregnancy: a case-based review. *J Asthma.* 2005;42:159–162.

64. Ellegard EK. Pregnancy rhinitis. *Immunol Allergy Clin North Am.* 2006;26:119–135.

67. Heinonen OP, Sloan D, Shapiro S. *Birth Defects and Drugs in Pregnancy.* Littleton, MA: PSG Publishing; 1977:1.

68. Gilbert C, Mazzotta P, Loebstein R, et al. Fetal safety of drugs used in the treatment of allergic rhinitis: a critical review. *Drug Saf.* 2005;28:707–719.

69. Einarson A, Bailey B, Jung G, et al. Prospective controlled study of hydroxyzine and cetirizine in pregnancy. *Ann Allergy Asthma Immunol.* 1997;78:183–186.

70. Weber-Schoendorfer C, Schaefer C. The safety of cetirizine during pregnancy. A prospective observational cohort study. *Reprod Toxicol.* 2008; 26:19–23.

71. Ambro BT, Scheid SC, Pribitkin EA. Prescribing guidelines for ENT medications during pregnancy. *Ear Nose Throat J.* 2003;82:565–568.

75. Gorman PJ. Hereditary angioedema and pregnancy: a successful outcome using C1 esterase inhibitor concentrate. *Can Fam Phys.* 2008;54:365–366.

76. Hermans C. Successful management with C1-inhibitor concentrate of hereditary angioedema attacks during two successive pregnancies: a case report. *Arch Gynecol Obstet.* 2007;276:271–276.

77. Bouillet L, Longhurst H, Boccon-Gibod I, et al. Disease expression in women with hereditary angioedema. *Am J Obstet Gynecol.* 2008;1:e1–e4.

78. Matz H, Orion E, Wolf R. Pruritic urticarial papules and plaques of pregnancy: polymorphic eruption of pregnancy (PUPPP). *Clin Derm.* 2006;24:105–108.

79. Aoyama Y, Asai K, Hioki K, et al. Herpes gestationis in a mother and newborn: immunoclinical perspectives based on weekly follow-up of the enzyme-linked immunosorbent assay index of a bullous pemphigoid antigen noncollagenous domain. *Arch Derm.* 2007;143:1168–1172.

80. Bork K, Barnstedt S-E. Treatment of 193 episodes of laryngeal edema with C1 inhibitor concentrate in patients with hereditary angioedema. *Arch Intern.* 2001;161:714–718.

81. Chaudhuri K, Gonzales J, Jesurun CA, et al. Anaphylactic shock in pregnancy: a case study and review of the literature. *Int J Obstet Anesth.* 2008;17(4):350–357.

83. Habek D, Cerkez-Habek J, Jalsovec D. Anaphylactic shock in response to wasp sting in pregnancy. *Zentralbl Gynakol.* 2000;122:393–394.

84. Cabestrero D, Perez-Paredes C, Fernandez-Cid R, et al. Bronchospasm and laryngeal stridor as an adverse effect of oxytocin treatment. *Crit Care.* 2003;7:392.

85. Hadar A, Holcberg G, Mazor M. Anaphylactic shock after diclofenac sodium (Voltaren). *Harefuah.* 2000; 138:211–212.

88. Cuciti C, Mayer DC, Arnette R, et al. Anaphylactoid reaction to intravenous sodium ferric gluconate complex during pregnancy. *Int J Obstet Anesth.* 2005;14:362–364.

90. Turillazzi E, Greco P, Neri M, et al. Anaphylactic latex reaction during anesthesia: the silent culprit in a fatal case. *Forensic Sci Internat.* 2008;179:e5–e8.

91. Stannard L, Bellis A. Maternal anaphylactic reaction to a general anaesthetic at emergency caesarean section for fetal bradycardia. *BJOG.* 2001;108:539–540.

CHAPTER 40

Eosinophilic Esophagitis

IKUO HIRANO, NIRMALA GONSALVES AND ANNE MARIE DITTO

■ EPIDEMIOLOGY AND DEMOGRAPHIC CHARACTERISTICS

Over the last several years, eosinophilic esophagitis (EoE) has become increasingly recognized as an important disease by allergists, internists, and gastroenterologists caring for both pediatric and adult patients. Although often abbreviated as EE in the literature, there is movement to use EoE to refer to eosinophilic esophagitis since EE has long been used by gastroenterologists to refer to erosive esophagitis. EoE may occur in isolation or in conjunction with eosinophilic gastroenteritis (1).

Previously considered a rare condition, there has been a dramatic increase in reports of EoE from North and South America, Europe, Asia, Australia, and the Middle East over the last several years (2–11). The cause for this rise is likely a combination of an increasing incidence of EoE and a growing awareness of the condition among gastroenterologists, allergists, and pathologists. Noel et al. suggest that the incidence of EoE has been rising in a population of children residing in Hamilton, Ohio. In 2000, the authors estimated the incidence to be 0.91 per 10,000 with a prevalence of 1 per 10,000 compared to 1.7 in 10,000 and a prevalence of 10.4 in 10,000 in 2007 (12). Straumann et al. studied a population of adults in Olten County, Switzerland, and found a similar trend. They estimated an incidence of 0.15 cases per 10,000 adult inhabitants with a prevalence of 3 per 10,000 inhabitants of their catchment area in Switzerland (13). These numbers are likely to underestimate the true incidence and prevalence of EoE in the general population since these data are based on patients with symptoms sufficient to warrant endoscopy. A population-based study in Sweden randomly surveyed 3,000 adult members of the population, and 1,000 healthy adults underwent endoscopy with esophageal biopsies. This group found that histologic eosinophilia meeting their criteria for definite and probable EoE was present in 1% of the population (14). These numbers suggest that EoE is becoming as common as other immunologic disorders such as inflammatory bowel disease (15). In addition, increasing publications about EoE in the last several years are contributing to

the awareness of this condition in both the gastroenterology and pathology community (9). For instance a PubMed search of articles using the term *eosinophilic esophagitis* resulted in 365 publications from 2000 to November 2008 compared to only 38 publications prior to this time.

Eosinophilic esophagitis has a male predilection. Results from 323 adult patients from 13 studies observed that 76% were males with a mean age of 38 years (range 14 to 89 years). Results from 754 pediatric patients from 16 studies found that 66% were male with a mean age of 8.6 years (range 0.5 to 21.1 years) (16). EoE has been described in patients with varied ethnicities including those of Caucasian, African American, Latin-American, and Asian descent (16). One pediatric review suggested that there was a racial predilection with 94% of the patients being Caucasian (17). A familial pattern has been recognized in the pediatric population. In a case series of 381 children with EoE, 5% of patients had siblings with EoE and 7% had a parent with either an esophageal stricture or a known diagnosis of EoE (18). One study showed that eotaxin-3, a gene encoding an eosinophil-specific chemoattractant, was the most highly induced gene in pediatric EoE patients (19). This finding supports the previous reports suggesting a potential genetic predisposition to EoE. Although formal genetic studies have not yet been pursued in adults, several case reports also suggest familial clustering of this condition in adults; therefore, a workup of patients should include a thorough family history (20–22).

■ CLINICAL FEATURES

The clinical features of EoE in both adults and children are described in Table 40.1. As with other diseases, some age-related differences in clinical presentation are noted. The most common presenting symptoms in adults include dysphagia, food impaction, heartburn, and chest pain (16,23). In one study, as many as 50% of adults presenting with food impaction were ultimately diagnosed with EoE (24). In children, the most common presenting symptoms include vomiting,

TABLE 40.1 CLINICAL FEATURES OF EOSINOPHILIC ESOPHAGITIS IN CHILDREN AND ADULTS

STUDY (REF)	N	MEAN AGE (RANGE)	MALE (%)	ATOPY BASED ON HISTORY (%)	% PATIENTS WITH PERIPHERAL EOSINOPHILIA	ENDOSCOPIC FINDINGS
Pediatric						
Boston 2002 (30)	19	8 (1 to 16)	74	84	58	ND
Philadelphia 2002 (13)	26	7 (2 to 14)	85	81	ND	ND
Australia 2003 (11)	21	10 (2 to 16)	76	67	ND	Wrinkled/thickened mucosa 67%, Mild redness 10%, Nl 33%
Philadelphia 2003 (48)	51	8 (3 to 16)	65	51	ND	Furrows 41%
Philadelphia 2005 (18)	381	9 (NA)	66	53	ND	Nl 32%, Rings 12%, Furrows 41%, Plaques 15%
Adult						
UK 2003 (29)	12	40 (22 to 64)	58	50	ND	Nl 17%, Rings 17%, Furrows 33%, Rings and Furrows 25%
Australia 2003 (2)	31	34 (14 to 77)	77	46	36	Furrows ± Furrows 97%
Mayo 2003 (87)	21	40 (28 to 55)	81	29	5	Rings 71%, Stricture 14%, Nl 14%
Switzerland 2003 (3)	30	41 (16 to 71)	73	29	50	Minimal 57%, Moderate 27%, Severe 10%, Nl 7%
Milwaukee 2004 (10)	29	35 (19 to 65)	72	48	ND	Rings 72%, Stricture 90%, Small caliber 17%, Esophagitis 14%, Nl 9%
Chicago 2005 (27)	74	38 (14 to 76)	76	70	9	Rings 81%, Furrows 74%, Strictures 31%, Plaques 15%, Small caliber 10%, Edema 8%
Australia 2006 (26)	26	36 (17 to 65)	69	77	31	Furrows 77%, Rings 62%, Small caliber 27%, Plaques 15%, Stricture 12%

ND, not done; Nl, normal

heartburn, regurgitation, emesis, and abdominal pain (16,18). While younger children rarely present with dysphagia and food impaction, these presentations were more commonly seen in older children and adolescents (12,25). In adults, this diagnosis has often been overlooked and many patients have had endoscopies with alternate diagnoses, including Schatzki rings or gastroesophageal reflux disease (GERD) prior to a diagnosis of EoE (26,27). In many cases, these patients had undergone repeated endoscopies, esophageal dilations, and a delay in the institution of appropriate medical therapy (26,27). In previous years, the presence of eosinophils in esophageal mucosal biopsies was equated with GERD and therefore some specimens may have

been classified as reflux (28). Due to this potential overlap, gastroenterologists who suspect a diagnosis of EoE should specifically request tissue eosinophil counts by the pathologist to help differentiate this diagnosis from GERD.

Endoscopic Findings

The most common endoscopic features in adults with EoE include linear or longitudinal furrows (80%), mucosal rings (64%), small caliber esophagus (28%), white plaques and/or exudates (16%), and strictures (12%) (23) (Fig. 40.1). In a large clinical series of 381 children,

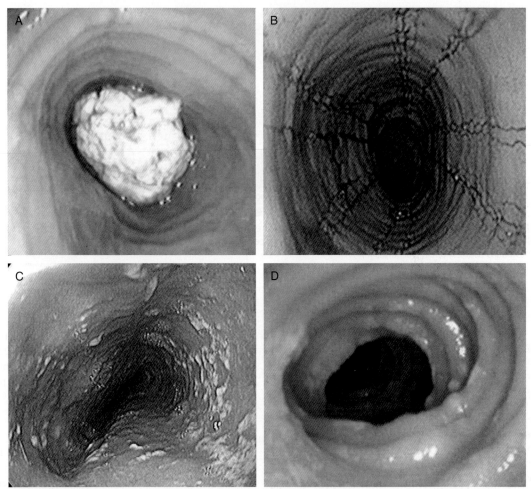

■ **FIGURE 40.1** Endoscopic photographs showing common features of eosinophilic esophagitis. **(A)** Concentric mucosal rings seen throughout the length of the esophagus in a patient presenting with a food impaction. **(B)** Linear furrows or creases in the esophageal mucosa. **(C)** White exudates/plaques which correspond to areas of eosinophilic abscess eruption through the esophageal mucosa. **(D)** Concentric mucosal rings and small caliber esophagus. (Endoscopic photos courtesy of Drs. Gonsalves and Hirano.)

the most common endoscopic features were linear furrows (41%), normal appearance (32%), esophageal rings (12%), and white plaques (15%) (18). It is important to note that the classic endoscopic features may be subtle and missed during endoscopy (16). Therefore, it is suggested that biopsies be taken for the clinical indication of unexplained dysphagia, refractory heartburn, or chest pain despite normal endoscopic findings (16).

Histologic Features

While certain endoscopic features are characteristic of EoE, this condition is ultimately diagnosed by obtaining biopsy specimens which demonstrate histologic findings of increased intramucosal eosinophils in the esophagus without concomitant eosinophilic infiltration in the stomach or duodenum (16) (Figure 40.2).

Other histologic features of this condition include superficial layering of the eosinophils, eosinophilic microabscesses (clusters of ≥4 eosinophils), intercellular edema, and degranulation of eosinophils. Other inflammatory cells such as lymphocytes, polymorphonuclear leukocytes, and mast cells may be present in the epithelium (29–31). Another histologic finding in EoE is epithelial hyperplasia, defined by papillary height elongation and basal zone proliferation (31). Epithelial hyperplasia is also a cardinal feature of the histopathology of reflux esophagitis. Studies have also shown presence of subepithelial fibrosis in biopsies of adults and children with eosinophilic esophagitis suggesting that deeper layers of the esophagus may be involved (3,32,34). Involvement of deeper layers of the esophagus has further been supported by the use of endoscopic ultrasound (35–37). It is speculated that this mucosal and submucosal fibrosis may lead to esophageal

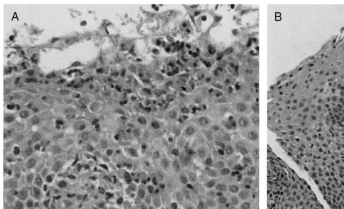
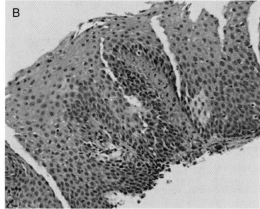

■ **FIGURE 40.2** Common histologic appearance in eosinophilic esophagitis. This image demonstrates superficial layering of eosinophils in the esophageal mucosa with presence of microabscesses seen in most patients with EoE (200×). (Histologic photographs courtesy of Dr. Gonsalves.)

remodeling and decreased compliance of the esophagus thus contributing to the symptoms of dysphagia even in the absence of an identifiable stricture.

Although a single diagnostic threshold of eosinophil density has not been determined, a recent consensus statement suggests using a threshold value of ≥ 15 eosinophils per high power field to diagnose EoE (16). It has also been demonstrated that the eosinophilic infiltration of the esophagus may not be evenly distributed within the esophagus (27). Therefore, it is suggested that biopsies be obtained from both the proximal and distal esophagus to obtain a higher diagnostic yield and perhaps increase the specificity of the diagnosis. A retrospective study of adult EoE patients found that obtaining more than five biopsies maximizes the sensitivity based on a diagnostic threshold of ≥ 15 eosinophils per high power field in the adult population (27). A follow-up study using a pediatric cohort demonstrated that 3 biopsies yielded a diagnosis of EoE in 97% of patients (38). In both the adult and pediatric studies, biopsies taken of only the proximal or distal esophagus missed the diagnosis in up to 20% of cases emphasizing the importance of taking biopsies from different locations.

Diagnostic Criteria

Recent consensus recommendations based on a systematic review of the literature and expert opinion have led to the following diagnostic criteria. EoE is a clinicopathological disease characterized by (a) the presence of symptoms including but not limited to dysphagia and food impaction in adults and feeding intolerance and GERD symptoms in children, (b) ≥ 15 eosinophils per high power field in the esophageal tissue, and (c) exclusion of other disorders associated with similar clinical, histologic, or endoscopic features such as GERD with either the use of high dose acid suppression prior to biopsy procurement or normal pH monitoring (16).

Additional Diagnostic Testing

Intraesophageal pH Testing

There have been nine adult studies and 11 pediatric studies reporting data from pH monitoring. Of 228 adult patients, 40% had pH monitoring with normal results in 82% of patients. Of 223 children, 78% had pH monitoring with normal results in 90% of patients (16).

Radiography

Radiologic studies such as barium esophagrams may be used in the workup of patients with EoE but are sometimes nondiagnostic. A recent study that correlated endoscopic and radiologic features in EoE demonstrated that both esophageal strictures as well as esophageal rings may be identified on barium studies of patients with EoE (8). In addition to identifying a stricture, the use of upper GI contrast studies may better characterize the length of a stricture as well as its caliber. This information may be helpful prior to subsequent upper endoscopy by alerting the endoscopist to use a smaller caliber endoscope or to proceed more cautiously with passage of the endoscope (16).

Manometry

Esophageal manometry was studied in 77 adults in seven studies and 14 children in three studies (16). Esophageal manometry was found to be abnormal in 41 of 77 adult patients. In the adults, the lower esophageal sphincter was normal in 66 of 77, hypotensive in 10 of 77, and hypertensive in 1 patient. Peristaltic abnormalities were seen in 30 of 77 patients and 28 of 30 patients had nonspecific peristaltic abnormalities. One patient each had diffuse esophageal spasm and nutcracker esophagus, which is defined by peristaltic pressure >180 mm Hg. Compared to these abnormalities in adults, all 14 children had a normal esophageal manometry. A recent study by Chen et al. used the newer technique of high resolution manometry in 24 adult patients with EoE (39). The most common abnormality noted was elevation in peristaltic velocity. Some patients also had failed esophageal peristalsis, repetitive simultaneous esophageal contractions, and impaired relaxation of the lower esophageal sphincter. Such manometric abnormalities may provide an explanation for the symptoms of dysphagia that occur in patients without a discernable esophageal stricture.

■ PATHOGENESIS

The pathogenesis of EoE is not known although it is thought to be allergic owing to the prominent presence of eosinophils as well as pathologic findings that share similarity with other allergic diseases such as asthma, e.g., thickened mucosa and basal layer hyperplasia. T_H2 cytokines interleukin (IL)-4, Il-5 and Il-13 have been shown to be upregulated (40) with IL-5 induced tissue specific eosinophilia causing remodeling (41,42) as well as reversibility of Il-13 induction with glucocorticoids (43). Blanchard et al. showed marked upregulation of eotaxin-3 gene expression in patients with EoE and interaction between eotaxin-3 and its receptor CCR 3 in EoE (19). Furthermore, peripheral blood eosinophils with CCR3 expression and increased $CD4^+$ cells expressing IL-5 have been demonstrated. These correlate with eosinophils in the esophagus and also with disease activity, being lower in patients whose disease is in remission (44). Kirsch et al. demonstrated increased numbers of mast cells and activation of mucosal mast cells distinguishing EoE from GERD (45). In addition, there is a high incidence of atopic disease such as allergic rhinitis, atopic dermatitis, and asthma (46).

Allergens

Although EoE is thought to be allergic, the allergen remains elusive. The concept of food as the allergenic cause was first introduced by Kelly et al. who described 10 children with severe GERD symptoms unresponsive to proton pump inhibitor (PPI) therapy (47). Eight patients had resolution and 2 had improvement in symptoms when placed on an elemental diet (ELED) for 6 weeks (Neocate One+, SHS North America, Gaithersburg, MD; EleCare, Ross Pediatrics, Abbott Laboratories, Abbott Park, IL). Histologically patients improved as well; eosinophil numbers decreased from a median of 41 per hpf (range 15 to 100) to a median of 0.5 (range 0 to 22) eos/hpf. The demonstration of recurrent symptoms on food reintroduction added credence to the role of food allergy. Markowitz et al. showed similar results in a study of 51 children diagnosed with EoE, using strict criteria to rule out GERD (48). For 3 months, 346 children

with symptoms of GERD were treated with a PPI. Those who clinically responded to empiric PPI therapy or demonstrated an abnormal 24-hour pH study after treatment were excluded from the study. The remaining 51 children were treated with an ELED for 4 weeks with marked response. Eosinophil counts per hpf decreased on average from 34 to 1. Symptoms recurred with reintroduction of food. Similar results have been reproduced in several studies in children from multiple centers with larger cohorts showing resolution of symptoms and histologic evidence of EoE (18,49,51). However, elemental diets are unpalatable and very difficult to maintain and oftentimes require tube feedings. In the study by Liacouras et al., 80% of the children were fed by nasogastric tube and eight patients were unable to tolerate the diet (18). This poor tolerability has led to trials of empiric and allergy testing directed food elimination. Kagalwalla et al. retrospectively studied children with EoE, comparing those treated with an ELED to those treated with a diet eliminating the eight (six) most common food groups involved in allergy: nuts (tree nuts and peanuts), seafood (fish and shellfish), wheat, soy, milk, and eggs. This empiric approach was termed the six food elimination diet (SFED) (49). There were 60 children studied, 35 on SFED, and 25 on ELED. Twenty five of the 35 patients (69%) on SFED and 22 of 25 (88%) on ELED showed improvement in symptoms and resultant eosinophil counts ≤ 10 per hpf.

Work has been done to try to identify culprit foods for more directed rather than empiric food elimination. However, identification of the food with traditional methods of testing for food allergy has had limited success. Since EoE patients do not have reactions that are typical of immunoglobulin E (IgE)-mediated food allergic reactions such as urticaria or anaphylaxis, and since reactions may not be immediate, it has been difficult to identify responsible foods by history. In addition, studies show that symptoms do not necessarily correlate with disease (39). Children, however, tend to have more immediate symptoms such as vomiting and it is possible that their histories and allergy test results may be more reliable. Traditional tests used for determining food allergy, skin-prick test (SPT) and ELISA ImmunoCAP, are used to detect IgE antibodies and therefore may have a limited role in predicting food allergens in EoE. Furthermore, the sensitivity, specificity, as well as positive and negative predictive values for these tests, have shown substantial variability.

Mechanisms other than an IgE-mediated food allergy may be involved in the pathogenesis of EoE such as a T cell-mediated delayed response (52). Spergel et al. have attempted to identify potential food allergens by combining allergy patch testing (APT) and SPT for foods (50,51) modeled after testing used in atopic dermatitis (53–55). One hundred forty-six children diagnosed with EoE were placed on diets eliminating foods identified by APT and SPT for 4 to 8 weeks. Foods tested were based on history. Of the 146 in the study, 112 children (77%) improved, achieving a mean of 1.1 eos/hpf. Of these 112, 40 were placed on ELED because of nutritional deficiencies that resulted from the dietary restriction. On average, five foods were eliminated. SPT identified 3.2 ± 4.3 foods with egg, milk, soy, peanut, chicken, wheat, and beef being the most common. APT identified 3.1 ± 2.6 foods with corn, soy, wheat, milk, rice, chicken, beef, and potato being most common. The causative foods were identified by elimination of a single food in 18 patients and by reintroduction of foods in 21 patients (56). Based on a cohort of children in whom the causative food could be identified, Spergel demonstrated that adding APT to SPT increases both sensitivity and specificity for most foods, with the exception of milk, which had poor sensitivity and specificity for both (56). On average, using both testing methods identified one additional food (57).

Other than for atopic dermatitis, the use of APT in evaluating food allergy remains controversial (58,59). There is no standard determined for the food preparation used (59). Finn chamber size has been shown to be critical as is interpretation of the results (60,61). Studies to standardize test interpretation are ongoing (62). In children, foods chosen for testing are based on symptoms (50,51). However in adults, whose symptoms differ, it is typically difficult to identify potential food triggers.

Food elimination has not been well studied in adults. Gonsalves et al. following the same protocol used in the aforementioned pediatric study, applied the SFED in 27 adults for 6 weeks. Median peak eos/hpf pre- and post-SFED were 36 and 3 in proximal and 41 and 9 in distal biopsies, respectively ($p < 0.05$). There was histologic improvement in 70% of patients with 33% of the patients having peak <5 eos/hpf and 52% less than 10 per hpf (63). Symptoms improved in 94% of patients. Endoscopic features of rings, furrows, and exudates showed improvement. Reintroduction of foods was completed systematically in 11 patients who responded to the SFED. In all patients, the trigger food was identified, most commonly milk and wheat. Of note, SPT correctly identified only 22% of foods that were found during reintroduction. Also, 7 of 11 patients who went through reintroduction and were found to have food triggers had negative SPT to all six foods. This suggests that further studies need to be pursued to better delineate the role of allergy testing for foods in adults with EoE. Supporting this, Simon et al. published a study in which six adults who were SPT or RAST positive to grass, rye, and wheat, eliminated rye and wheat for 6 weeks (64). Only one patient had improvement in symptoms while none of the patients demonstrated histologic improvement. These patients were not allergic to other foods commonly considered responsible in EoE such as egg and milk. These authors conclude that foods may not be the allergens responsible for EoE in adults and that the positive skin tests to wheat and rye

in these individuals may be due to cross reactivity with the grass aeroallergens. These studies call into question the utility of allergy testing directed elimination diets in adult patients with EoE that rely on IgE reactivity.

Based primarily on data from adult patients with EoE, aeroallergens are candidate allergens in the pathogenesis of EoE. Sensitization to aeroallergens is more common in adults with EoE as compared to children (65). In addition, in adults, aeroallergen sensitivity predates EoE (46,64). In a study analyzing children and adults with EoE, Sugnanam et al. noted that age correlated positively with aeroallergen sensitivity as determined by SPT although there was a negative correlation between age and food sensitivity (65). Fogg reported increased eosinophils in the esophagus of a patient during pollen season, with resolution out of the season (66). In a retrospective study of 234 children, EoE was diagnosed less often in the winter months. Although eosinophil levels in the esophagus were elevated year round, they were higher in the summer and fall months (67). Others have noted eosinophilia in the esophagus of patients with allergic rhinitis who did not have EoE (68). A recent case series of 23 adults confirms polysensitization to aeroallergens. The food-specific IgE profile in these patients suggests that aeroallergens may play a role in sensitization to at least some of the foods (69).

A causative role for aeroallergen sensitivity in EoE has also been demonstrated in an animal model. Mishra et al. noted eosinophils in both the lungs and esophagus in mice sensitized to aspergillus when they were then challenged intranasally with aspergillus (70). Aeroallergens may induce EoE via a systemic rather than local response. Nasal exposure to aeroallergens may lead to EoE just as nasal exposure has been shown to cause upregulation of activated eosinophils from the bone marrow (71–74) and deposition in the lungs (75). This may be a continuation of the "one airway" or "united airway." On the other hand, aeroallergens may act locally after being swallowed, directly causing allergic inflammation in the esophagus. Swallowed foods that share proteins with aeroallergens may affect the esophagus just as the oral mucosa can be involved in food-pollen syndrome (76–79).

■ TREATMENT

Despite being a newly recognized disease, a number of varied therapies are available that address both the symptoms and histology of eosinophilic esophagitis. Options include medical treatments such as systemic and topical corticosteroids, leukotriene-receptor antagonists, and biologic agents. High response rates to elimination of dietary allergens suggest that certain foods may serve as environmental triggers for the eosinophilic infiltration. Since many adults present with strictures, endoscopic esophageal dilation is another management modality.

The goal of therapy is not only alleviation of presenting signs and symptoms but also prevention of disease recurrence and complications. In this regard, understanding the natural history of eosinophilic esophagitis is of central importance. Unfortunately, little is known regarding the natural history, creating a challenge in managing patients, particularly those who are asymptomatic. In the longest follow-up study to date, Straumann et al. followed 30 adult patients for an average of 7.2 years in the absence of therapy (3). All patients survived the study period in good health in a stable nutritional state, but 97% continued to experience dysphagia, which increased in 23%, was stable in 37%, and improved in 37%. One patient reported a disappearance of dysphagia. Similarly, the degree of esophageal eosinophilia demonstrated an overall decline in most patients during the follow-up period. The fact that one-third of the cohort had received esophageal dilation likely affected the reported dysphagia but should not have affected the esophageal eosinophilia. The persistence of ongoing inflammatory activity may alter the elasticity of the esophagus and induce irreversible changes, raising the question as to whether treatment can prevent future stricture formation. Barrett metaplasia has been found in patients with EoE but it is unclear as to whether this is a causal relationship. No cases of esophageal malignancy related to EoE have been reported, but the follow-up period has been short.

There have not been any long-term pediatric studies that demonstrate the consequences of ongoing esophageal eosinophilia and inflammation. Currently, there is concern but no evidence that children with EoE who are left untreated will develop fibrosis or stricture formation as is common in adolescents or adults. Most studies, however, report outcomes for treated patients over a short time period. In a recent randomized, placebo-controlled trial in children, 9% of patients receiving placebo achieved histologic remission at 3-month follow-up providing evidence that a subset of patients may undergo clinical remission without therapy (80). Assa'ad et al. studied a group of 89 pediatric patients over a period of 8 years and found the disease to be both chronic and relapsing (17). Of the patients who had resolution of their EoE with therapy, 79% later relapsed with a mean follow-up of 1.4 years.

Goals of Therapy

Patients are treated for many reasons including resolution of symptoms, improvement in quality of life, and prevention of future complications. Objective treatment outcomes include endoscopic esophageal mucosal changes, radiographic presence of esophageal strictures, and histopathology. It is unclear which of the two currently used endpoints of symptom resolution and mucosal eosinophilia is the most appropriate goal of therapy. Caution is needed in the interpretation of symptom improvement as many patients modify their diets to avoid the ingestion of foods that are difficult to swallow whereas others have very sporadic symptoms that may not manifest during a short follow-up period. In many prospective studies, response is defined by a reduction in tissue eosinophilia. However, the degree of reduction is ill-defined and different endpoints have been used including <15, <10, or <5 eos/hpf. Other markers of tissue injury such as markers of eosinophil activation, basal cell hyperplasia, or subepithelial fibrosis may be as important as the actual number of eosinophils. Furthermore, histologic resolution of mucosal biopsies could be misleading. Studies have demonstrated that esophageal eosinophilia can extend to involve the submucosa as well as muscularis layers that are not sampled by esophageal mucosal biopsies (35). Fox et al. reported that children with EoE who undergo high-resolution endoscopic ultrasonography revealed significant expansion of the esophageal wall and the individual layers including the combined mucosa and submucosa, and muscularis propria compared to healthy controls (37).

Medical Therapy

Proton Pump Inhibitors

Controversy exists regarding interactions between GERD and EoE (81). Studies from the 1980s equated esophageal eosinophilia with the diagnosis of GERD. Initial reports described EoE as an entity distinct from GERD based on lack of response to PPI therapy or negative pH testing. It has become evident that EoE and GERD can coexist and that treatment of GERD may be effective in a subset of patients with symptoms, endoscopic features, and histology that are consistent with EoE. On the other hand, the presence of GERD defined by an abnormal pH study does not preclude the presence of EoE (38). Limited data on pH testing in EoE patients have demonstrated abnormal acid exposure in 5% to 41% of subjects (9,33). Two recent series of pediatric patients and an adult series reported normalization of symptoms and tissue eosinophilia after PPI therapy (82–84). An adult series reported symptomatic improvement in 19 patients with a ringed esophagus following treatment with a combination of PPI and esophageal dilation (28). Evaluation of the contribution of GERD is considered an important part of the diagnosis and management of EoE (16).

Topical Corticosteroids

Swallowed, aerosolized fluticasone propionate (FP) was first reported to be a successful treatment for EoE in 1998 by Faubion in a series of 4 children (85). Symptom resolution as well as significant reduction in eosinophils and CD3, CD8, and CD1a lymphocytes in 11 children was later demonstrated by Teitelbaum (30).

FP became a desirable option compared to systemic corticosteroids because of the low systemic bioavailability owing to first-pass hepatic metabolism. In a retrospective study by Noel et al., 20 pediatric patients with symptomatic EoE were treated with swallowed FP for a mean of 5 months (86). Half of the patients were categorized as allergic based on SPT to food and aeroallergens and had failed dietary elimination guided by SPT. After treatment, all nonallergic patients had clinical, endoscopic, and histologic resolution, but only 60% of the allergic group had complete resolution, suggesting that allergic subjects may respond less well to fluticasone.

Fluticasone has also been studied in adults and demonstrated effective symptom relief. A retrospective study by Arora et al. (87) reported resolution of dysphagia in 21 adults treated with FP for 4 months. Another retrospective study of 19 adult patients reported substantial symptom improvement in all patients and resolution in 60% treated with FP 500 µg twice per day for 4 weeks (26). The mean proximal eosinophil count fell from 25 eos/hpf to 4 eos/hpf and the mean distal count fell from 39 eos/hpf to 4 eos/hpf. Three patients developed asymptomatic esophageal candidiasis. Two-thirds of this cohort redeveloped symptoms within 3 months of discontinuing FP.

Konikoff conducted the first randomized, placebo-controlled trial in 36 children with EoE (80). FP (880 µg/day) administered for 3 months induced histologic remission defined by peak eosinophil counts of ≤ 1 eos/hpf in 50% of patients compared with 9% in the placebo arm. Peak eosinophil counts ≤ 6 were achieved in 55% with FP and 18% with placebo. Higher pretreatment esophageal eosinophilia did not predict poor responsiveness to FP. Similar to the Noel study, nonallergic individuals had a better response than did allergic individuals. Of note, the allergic individuals had failed or refused dietary elimination prior to study entry. FP responders were significantly younger, shorter, and weighed less than nonresponders.

Another topical steroid that has been described is budesonide suspension. The puff and swallow technique may be difficult for some adults and younger children. A retrospective study of 20 children treated with oral budesonide suspension, 1 mg to 2 mg daily, showed symptomatic and endoscopic improvement (88), with 65% achieving a reduction in eosinophilia to ≤ 5 eos/hpf. Improvement in basal zone hyperplasia was also noted. Morning cortisol levels were normal and only one child developed esophageal candidiasis. A randomized, double-blind, placebo controlled trial was conducted in 36 adults with EoE (89). Budesonide was swallowed during nebulized administration 1 mg orally twice a day. A reduction in tissue eosinophilia from 62 eos/hpf baseline to 4 eos/hpf after 15 days of therapy was noted with no change after placebo. Symptoms improved in 84% with budesonide and 33% with

placebo. Mast cell infiltration, tryptase, and CD3 staining improved after treatment.

Improvement in endoscopic features was reported by Lucendo in a prospective analysis of 30 adult patients treated with FP for 3 months (90). Prior to therapy, 77% had evidence of mucosal abnormalities compared with 37% after FP. Mucosal rings were evident in 57% prior to and 3% after FP.

The studies conducted to date with topical steroids have uniformly demonstrated both clinical and histologic improvement and often resolution after short course of therapy ranging from 15 days to 3 months. After withdrawal of steroids, both symptoms and esophageal eosinophilia return within 3 to 6 months (18,26). In a prospective study, a return of symptoms after steroid cessation was noted to occur gradually over the course of several weeks to months (91). It is unclear if the duration of remission is affected by any specific presenting feature, degree of response, duration of initial therapy, or possible continued allergen exposure.

The ease of administration and the favorable side effect profile make topical steroids an attractive therapy. Esophageal candidiasis occurs in the minority and is usually asymptomatic. There is concern that even topical steroids can affect long-term growth in children although greater first-pass metabolism and therefore safety would be expected with swallowed as compared to inhaled route of administration. More long-term safety data are needed as it has been shown that a majority of EoE patients will have recurrence of symptoms and eosinophilia within 6 months of discontinuing therapy (18)

Although studies have demonstrated clearance of eosinophils in the esophageal mucosa with therapy, it is unknown whether continued exposure to the offending agent may cause ongoing inflammation and fibrosis in deeper layers of the gastrointestinal tract. Studies with endoscopic ultrasonography have demonstrated increased thickening of the esophageal submucosa and muscularis layers (35,37). Topical steroid therapy may not penetrate these deeper levels. Moreover, biopsies sample only the mucosa and seldom provide adequate histology of the submucosa or muscularis.

Systemic Corticosteroids

One of the first treatment options reported for EoE was systemic corticosteroids. Liacouras et al. followed 21 pediatric patients treated with 1.5 mg/kg/day of oral methylprednisolone for 4 weeks (92). After 4 weeks, 65% became completely asymptomatic and 30% had marked improvement. All patients demonstrated histologic resolution of eosinophilia. The corticosteroids were tapered over 6 weeks and 50% of patients remained asymptomatic at 12 months. Biopsies taken 6 months after cessation of steroid therapy demonstrated a recurrence of esophageal eosinophilia to near pretreatment levels. A second pediatric study randomized 80 patients to therapy with either topical fluticasone 220 μg to 440 μg orally four times a day or prednisone 1 mg/kg twice a day (max 30 mg twice a day) for 4 weeks (91). The primary endpoint of improvement in a histologic score that combined severity of basal zone hyperplasia and eosinophilia was achieved in 94% of both groups. Likewise, secondary endpoints of symptom resolution (97% fluticasone, 100% prednisone) and reduction of tissue eosinophilia to <5 eos/hpf (67% fluticasone, 78% prednisone) were not significantly different in the two treatment arms. Normalization of the histologic score that factored in both eosinophilia and basal zone hyperplasia was significantly greater with prednisone (81%) than fluticasone (50%). Adverse effects were seen in 40% of the prednisone group that included Cushingoid features and weight gain whereas 15% of the fluticasone group developed esophageal candidiasis.

Montelukast

Montelukast, a leukotriene D4-receptor antagonist, has been studied in a small adult cohort with EoE. Attwood used montelukast in eight adult patients with an initial dose of 10 mg daily (93). Seven patients showed symptom improvement with dosages between 20 mg/day and 40 mg/day with escalation to 100 mg/day in one patient after a median of 14 months. Six patients had recurrence of symptoms within 3 weeks of discontinuing or reducing therapy. Furthermore, montelukast did not change the density of eosinophils after 4 months of treatment. Common side effects included nausea, headache, and myalgias which occurred more frequently at doses higher than 40 mg/day.

Cromolyn Sodium

Cromolyn sodium (100 mg four times per day) was used in 14 pediatric cases of EoE (18). A small and non-significant reduction of esophageal eosinophilia was observed. While cromolyn was well tolerated, symptoms did not improve.

Histamine-receptor Antagonists

Kaplan et al. reported complete symptom response in four of eight adults with EoE after treatment with a combination of H1 and H2 antagonists (94). Previous studies have shown that antihistamines can affect eosinophil activation and release of their granules (95). The results of this small, retrospective series need to be confirmed as some patients were also treated with esophageal dilation and PPI therapy.

Immunomodulators

Azathioprine and 6-mercaptopurine were used in 3 adult EoE patients who were dependent on systemic steroids (96). One patient had predominant disease of the muscularis layer whereas another patient had eosinophilic gastroenteritis as well as esophagitis. Eosinophilia normalized with the immunomodulators and allowed for steroid withdrawal. Recurrent eosinophilia was observed after cessation of the immunomodulator therapy.

Biologic Therapy

Interleukin (IL)-5 is a cytokine primarily produced by T_H2 lymphocytes that regulates the proliferation, bone marrow release, maturation, activation, and survival of eosinophils. Mepolizumab is a fully humanized monoclonal IgG antibody that selectively binds and inactivates IL-5 that demonstrated efficacy in a randomized, double-blind, placebo-controlled trial in patients with hypereosinophilic syndrome (97). Studies have also demonstrated increased expression of IL-5 in the esophageal epithelium in EoE (40). An open-label trial was conducted using anti-IL-5 for four adult EoE patients, three of whom had severe disease (98). Maximum esophageal eosinophil counts fell from 153 to 28 eos/hpf with 4 weeks of therapy. Patients reported improvement in symptoms and quality of life and therapy was generally well tolerated. Less positive results were reported in a randomized, controlled trial of 11 adults with EoE who were either unresponsive or dependent on corticosteroids. Mepolizumab was administered every 4 weeks with follow-up over 12 weeks. While a statistically significant decrease was noted in both peripheral blood and esophageal eosinophilia, remission, defined by ≤5 eos/hpf, was not achieved in any patient. A significant decrease in dysphagia occurred in two of five patients in the active treatment arm and again the therapy was well tolerated.

Anti-IgE therapy with omalizumab was used in an open-label trial of nine adults with eosinophilic gastroenteritis, of whom seven had both EoE and eosinophilic gastroenteritis (99). Significant decreases in symptoms, IgE levels (79% reduction) and peripheral eosinophilia (34% reduction) were observed. While a nonsignificant reduction in gastric and duodenal eosinophilia was noted, there was an increase in esophageal eosinophilia.

Tumor necrosis factor (TNF) expression has increased expression in EoE. Infliximab, a TNF-α monoclonal antibody, has demonstrated significant efficacy in the induction of remission and maintenance therapy of inflammatory bowel disease. In an open-label trial in three patients, treatment with two doses of infliximab 5 mg/kg at weeks 4 and 6 did not result in improvement in symptoms, esophageal eosinophilia, or tissue expression of TNF-α (100).

Dietary Therapy

Since the pivotal study by Kelly and Sampson introduced the removal of food antigens as a form of therapy for EoE (47), three types of dietary treatment of EoE have emerged primarily from pediatric centers. All three approaches have demonstrated symptomatic and histologic resolution in 70% to 97% of patients in uncontrolled studies (18,49,51). An adult study using empiric SFED demonstrated a symptom response in 94% but histologic remission in only 50% (63). Elemental formula diet has remained the "gold standard" dietary approach but in an attempt to improve tolerability, diets based on allergy skin testing and diets with empiric elimination of common food allergens have practical benefits. Based on uncontrolled observational studies, the effectiveness of the empiric SFED and allergy testing directed elimination diets appears to be lower than elemental diet therapy. The advantage of both elimination therapies is the avoidance of the generally unpalatable elemental diet that frequently necessitates nasogastric or percutaneous gastrostomy tube placement. The selective elimination approach also greatly simplifies the reintroduction phase of the dietary-based treatments. Both elimination protocols necessitate strict avoidance of specified foods and careful examination of store-bought items and restaurant food for possible contamination. The Food Allergen and Consumer Protection Act (FALCPA) passed in 2004 and in effect since 2006 requires that the products declare the presence of the most common allergens that are included in the SFED. At this time, APT administration and interpretation are not standardized, thereby limiting the widespread implementation of directed elimination diet therapy.

Endoscopic Therapy

Esophageal Dilation

Esophageal dilation is a therapeutic modality which has primarily been used in adult EoE patients with strictures. Small series have reported relief of dysphagia after dilation but the majority of patients developed recurrent symptoms in 3 to 8 months (3,10,29,101). Long mucosal tears are not uncommonly seen following esophageal dilation of EoE (Fig. 40.3). Several patients have required hospitalization for chest pain and four patients developed esophageal perforation following esophageal dilation (102,103). In these cases, the perforations have been managed conservatively without need for surgical repair. In a review of 152 dilations for EoE from a single center, one perforation was reported out of 152 dilations performed in 81 patients (104). Half of the patients who underwent dilation required repeated dilation although most patients received concomitant medical therapy. Even though esophageal dilation is effective at relieving dysphagia, it carries risks of significant complications and does not address the underlying inflammatory process. However, as it remains unclear as to whether medical or dietary

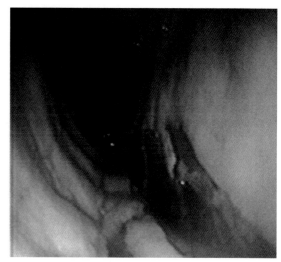

■ **FIGURE 40.3** Endoscopic photograph showing mucosal tear.

therapy can reverse the submucosal fibrosis seen in EoE, patients with strictures may benefit from esophageal dilation if they remain symptomatic following a course of medical or dietary therapy.

■ CONCLUSION

EoE is an emerging clinical problem and treatment is effective at reducing symptoms as well as tissue eosinophilia. Although the risk of not treating an asymptomatic or minimally symptomatic patient is currently unknown, sequella including fibrosis, narrow caliber esophagus, and stricture formation are well described. Furthermore, symptoms that impair quality of life as well as complications of malnutrition, food impaction, and esophageal perforation have been reported. The degree to which the structural alterations are reversible with medical or dietary therapy is uncertain. Spontaneous remission appears to occur infrequently.

A clinical approach to EoE begins with an increased awareness of the disease and its manifestations. Figure 40.4 illustrates a proposed algorithm for EoE management. The diagnosis should be considered in a child presenting with vomiting, food refusal, and abdominal pain, especially if the symptoms have not improved with empiric therapeutic trials of acid-suppression. The diagnosis should be strongly entertained in both children and adults with dysphagia and food impactions, regardless of the presence or absence of heartburn. Other presentations include atypical chest pain and heartburn that do not respond to empiric PPI therapy.

Once the presence of increased esophageal eosinophilia (generally greater than 15 eos/hpf) has been demonstrated, patients should undergo a 6- to 8-week trial of acid-suppression therapy to see if this results in

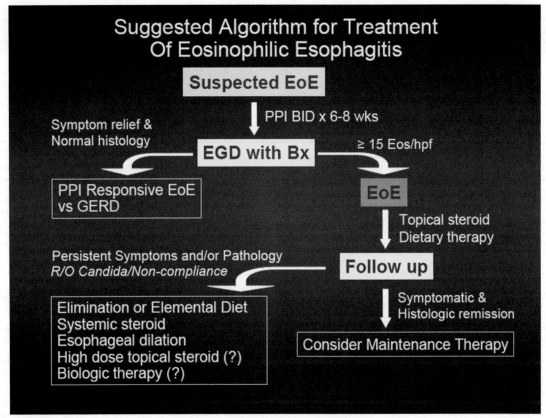

■ **FIGURE 40.4** Algorithm for the treatment and evaluation of eosinophilic esophagitis.

clinical and histologic improvement. This recommendation is based on observations that some patients with esophageal eosinophilia respond both symptomatically and histologically to PPI therapy. pH monitoring may be performed but the value of this test for predicting PPI-responsive EoE has not been clearly demonstrated. If symptoms and eosinophilia persist despite adequate acid suppression, the various treatment options for EoE are discussed with the patient and family in pediatric cases. At this time, first-line therapies for children include topical steroids, dietary elimination, and elemental diets. For adults, topical steroids are the most commonly used treatment but the preliminary results described earlier support the effectiveness of dietary therapy in some adults. Systemic corticosteroids are reserved for patients who are refractory to first-line therapy because of the side effects. Allergy testing may help to guide the choice of food elimination and reintroduction. The role of treatment of aeroallergens (e.g., allergen avoidance, nasal steroids, immunotherapy) in EoE patients remains speculative at this time. Esophageal dilation is performed cautiously for strictures that do not respond to medical or dietary treatment. Patients may benefit from maintenance therapy given the high rates of symptomatic recurrence of EoE in both children and adults.

■ **REFERENCES**

1. Rothenberg ME. Eosinophilic gastrointestinal disorders (EGID). *J Allergy Clin Immunol.* 2004;113(1):11–28;quiz 29.
2. Croese J, Fairley SK, Masson JW, et al. Clinical and endoscopic features of eosinophilic esophagitis in adults. *Gastrointest Endosc.* 2003;58(4):516–522.
3. Straumann A, Spichtin HP, Grize L, et al. Natural history of primary eosinophilic esophagitis: a follow-up of 30 adult patients for up to 11.5 years. *Gastroenterology.* 2003;125(6):1660–1669.
4. Lucendo AJ, Carrión G, Navarro M, et al. Eosinophilic esophagitis in adults: an emerging disease. *Dig Dis Sci.* 2004;49(11–12):1884–1888.
5. Esposito S, Marinetto D, Paracchini R, et al. Long-term follow-up of symptoms and peripheral eosinophil counts in seven children with eosinophilic esophagitis. *J Pediatr Gastroenterol Nutr.* 2004;38(4):452–456.
6. Khan S, Orenstein SR, Di Lorenzo C, et al. Eosinophilic esophagitis: strictures, impactions, dysphagia. *Dig Dis Sci.* 2003;48(1):22–29.
7. Fox VL, Nurko S, Furuta GT. Eosinophilic esophagitis: it's not just kid's stuff. *Gastrointest Endosc.* 2002.56(2):260–270.
8. Zimmerman SL, Levine MS, Rubesin SE, et al. Idiopathic eosinophilic esophagitis in adults: the ringed esophagus. *Radiology.* 2005; 236(1):159–165.
9. Arora AS, Yamazaki K. Eosinophilic esophagitis: asthma of the esophagus? *Clin Gastroenterol Hepatol.* 2004;2(7):523–530.
10. Potter JW, Saeian K, Staff D, et al. Eosinophilic esophagitis in adults: an emerging problem with unique esophageal features. *Gastrointest Endosc.* 2004;59(3):355–361.
11. Cheung KM, Oliver MR, Cameron DJ, et al. Esophageal eosinophilia in children with dysphagia. *J Pediatr Gastroenterol Nutr.* 2003;37(4):498–503.
12. Noel RJ, Putnam PE, Rothenberg ME. Eosinophilic esophagitis. *N Engl J Med.* 2004;351(9):940–941.
13. Straumann A, Simon HU. Eosinophilic esophagitis: escalating epidemiology? *J Allergy Clin Immunol.* 2005;115(2):418–419.

14. Ronkainen J, Talley NJ, Aro P, et al. Prevalence of oesophageal eosinophils and eosinophilic oesophagitis in adults: the population-based Kalixanda study. *Gut.* 2007;56(5):615–620.

15. Kugathasan S, Judd RH, Hoffmann RG, et al. Epidemiologic and clinical characteristics of children with newly diagnosed inflammatory bowel disease in Wisconsin: a statewide population-based study. *J Pediatr.* 2003;143(4): 525–531.

16. Furuta GT, Liacouras CA, Collins MH, et al. Eosinophilic esophagitis in children and adults: a systematic review and consensus recommendations for diagnosis and treatment. *Gastroenterology.* 2007; 133(4):1342–1363.

17. Assa'ad AH, Putnam PE, Collins MH, et al. Pediatric patients with eosinophilic esophagitis: an 8-year follow-up. *J Allergy Clin Immunol.* 2007;119(3):731–738.

18. Liacouras CA, Spergel JM, Ruchelli E, et al. Eosinophilic esophagitis: a 10-year experience in 381 children. *Clin Gastroenterol Hepatol.* 2005;3(12):1198–1206.

19. Blanchard C, Wang N, Stringer KF, et al. Eotaxin-3 and a uniquely conserved gene-expression profile in eosinophilic esophagitis. *J Clin Invest.* 2006;116(2):536–547.

20. Patel SM, Falchuk KR. Three brothers with dysphagia caused by eosinophilic esophagitis. *Gastrointest Endosc.* 2005;61(1):165–167.

21. Meyer GW. Eosinophilic esophagitis in a father and a daughter. *Gastrointest Endosc.* 2005. 61(7):932.

22. Zink DA, Amin M, Gebara S, et al. Familial dysphagia and eosinophilia. *Gastrointest Endosc.* 2007;65(2):330–334.

23. Sgouros SN, Bergele C, Mantides A. Eosinophilic esophagitis in adults: a systematic review. *Eur J Gastroenterol Hepatol.* 2006;18(2): 211–217.

24. Desai TK, Stecevic V, Chang CH, et al. Association of eosinophilic inflammation with esophageal food impaction in adults. *Gastrointest Endosc.* 2005. 61(7):795–801.

25. Gonsalves N, Kagalwalla AF, Kagalwalla A, et al. Distinct features in the clinical presentations of eosinophilic esophagitis in children and adults. *Gastroenterol Clin Biol.* 2005;128(4):S2:A7.

26. Remedios M, Campbell C, Jones DM, et al. Eosinophilic esophagitis in adults: clinical, endoscopic, histologic findings, and response to treatment with fluticasone propionate. *Gastrointest Endosc.* 2006; 63(1):3–12.

27. Gonsalves N, Policarpio-Nicolas M, Zhang Q, et al. Histopathologic variability and endoscopic correlates in adults with eosinophilic esophagitis. *Gastrointest Endosc.* 2006;64(3):313–319.

28. Morrow JB, Vargo JJ, Goldblum JR, et al. The ringed esophagus: histological features of GERD. *Am J Gastroenterol.* 2001; 96(4):984–989.

29. Attwood SE, Smyrk TC, Demeester TR, et al. Esophageal eosinophilia with dysphagia. A distinct clinicopathologic syndrome. *Dig Dis Sci.* 1993;38(1):109–116.

30. Teitelbaum JE, Fox VL, Twarog FJ, et al. Eosinophilic esophagitis in children: immunopathological analysis and response to fluticasone propionate. *Gastroenterology.* 2002;122(5):1216–1225.

31. Parfitt JR, Gregor JC, Suskin NG, et al. Eosinophilic esophagitis in adults: distinguishing features from gastroesophageal reflux disease: a study of 41 patients. *Mod Pathol.* 2006;19(1):90–96.

32. Aceves SS, Newbury RO, Dohil R, et al. Esophageal remodeling in pediatric eosinophilic esophagitis. *J Allergy Clin Immunol.* 2007;119(1): 206–212.

33. Lucendo AJ, Navarro M, Comas C, et al. Immunophenotypic characterization and quantification of the epithelial inflammatory infiltrate in eosinophilic esophagitis through stereology: an analysis of the cellular mechanisms of the disease and the immunologic capacity of the esophagus. *Am J Surg Pathol.* 2007;31(4):598–606.

34. Chehade M, Sampson M, Sampson HA, et al. Esophageal subepithelial fibrosis in children with eosinophilic esophagitis. *J Pediatr Gastroenterol Nutr.* 2007;45(3):319–328.

35. Stevoff C, Rao S, Parsons W, et al. EUS and histopathologic correlates in eosinophilic esophagitis. *Gastrointest Endosc.*2001;54(3):373–377.

36. Lusti BJ, Hirano I, Alasadi R. Manometric, endoscopic and histopathologic correlates of diffuse esophageal spasm secondary to eosinophilic esophagitis. *Am J Gastroenterol.* 2006;101(9):S394.

37. Fox VL, Nurko S, Teitelbaum JE, et al. High-resolution EUS in children with eosinophilic "allergic" esophagitis. *Gastrointest Endosc.* 2003;57(1):30–36.

38. Shah A, Kagalwalla A, Gonsalves N, et al. Histopathologic variability in children with eosinophilic esophagitis. *Am J Gastroenterol.* 2009;104(3):716–721.

39. Chen J, Pandolfino J, Kahrilas P, et al. Esophageal dysmotility in eosinophilic esophagitis: analysis using high resolution esophageal motility. *Gastroenterol.* 2007;132(4):SA6.

40. Straumann A, Bauer M, Fischer B, et al. Idiopathic eosinophilic esophagitis is associated with a T(H)2-type allergic inflammatory response. *J Allergy Clin Immunol.* 2001;108(6):954–961.

41. Mishra A, Rothenberg ME. Intratracheal IL-13 induces eosinophilic esophagitis by an IL-5, eotaxin-1, and STAT6-dependent mechanism. *Gastroenterology.* 2003;125(5):1419–1427.

42. Mishra A, Wang M, Pemmaraju VR, et al. Esophageal remodeling develops as a consequence of tissue specific IL-5-induced eosinophilia. *Gastroenterology.* 2008;134(1):204–214.

43. Blanchard C, Mingler MK, Vicario M, et al. IL-13 involvement in eosinophilic esophagitis: transcriptome analysis and reversibility with glucocorticoids. *J Allergy Clin Immunol.* 2007;120(6):1292–1300.

44. Bullock JZ, Villanueva JM, Blanchard C, et al. Interplay of adaptive th2 immunity with eotaxin-3/c-C chemokine receptor 3 in eosinophilic esophagitis. *J Pediatr Gastroenterol Nutr.* 2007;45(1):22–31.

45. Kirsch R, Marcon MA, Cutz E. Activated mucosal mast cells differentiate eosinophilic (allergic) esophagitis from gastroesophageal reflux disease. *J Pediatr Gastroenterol Nutr.* 2007;44(1):20–26.

46. Simon D, Marti H, Heer P, et al. Eosinophilic esophagitis is frequently associated with IgE-mediated allergic airway diseases. *J Allergy Clin Immunol.* 2005;115(5):1090–1092.

47. Kelly KJ, Lazenby AJ, Rowe PC, et al. Eosinophilic esophagitis attributed to gastroesophageal reflux: improvement with an amino acid-based formula. *Gastroenterology.* 1995;109(5):1503–1512.

48. Markowitz JE, Spergel JM, Ruchelli E, et al. Elemental diet is an effective treatment for eosinophilic esophagitis in children and adolescents. *Am J Gastroenterol.* 2003;98(4):777–782.

49. Kagalwalla AF, Sentongo TA, Ritz S, et al. Effect of six-food elimination diet on clinical and histologic outcomes in eosinophilic esophagitis. *Clin Gastroenterol Hepatol.* 2006;4(9):1097–1102.

50. Spergel JM, Beausoleil JL, Mascarenhas M, et al. The use of skin prick tests and patch tests to identify causative foods in eosinophilic esophagitis. *J Allergy Clin Immunol.* 2002;109(2):363–368.

51. Spergel JM, Andrews T, Brown-Whitehorn TF, et al. Treatment of eosinophilic esophagitis with specific food elimination diet directed by a combination of skin prick and patch tests. *Ann Allergy Asthma Immunol.* 2005;95(4):336–343.

52. Lucendo AJ, Bellon T, Lucendo B. The role of mast cells in eosinophilic esophagitis. *Pediatr Allergy Immunol.* 2008; Epub ahead of print Aug. 4.

53. Mehl A, Rolinck-Werninghaus C, Staden U, et al. The atopy patch test in the diagnostic workup of suspected food-related symptoms in children. *J Allergy Clin Immunol.* 2006;118(4):923–929.

54. Niggemann B. The role of the atopy patch test (APT) in diagnosis of food allergy in infants and children with atopic dermatitis. *Pediatr Allergy Immunol.* 2001;12(Suppl 14):37–40.

55. Niggemann B, Reibel S, Wahn U. The atopy patch test (APT)—a useful tool for the diagnosis of food allergy in children with atopic dermatitis. *Allergy.*2000;55(3):281–285.

56. Spergel JM, Brown-Whitehorn T, Beausoleil JL, et al. Predictive values for skin prick test and atopy patch test for eosinophilic esophagitis. *J Allergy Clin Immunol.* 2007;119(2):509–511.

57. Spergel JM, Beausoleil J, Brown-Whitehorn T, et al. Authors' response to detection of causative foods by skin prick and atopy patch tests in patients with eosinophilic esophagitis: things are not what they seem. *Ann Allergy Asthma Immunol.* 2006;96(2):376–378.

58. Osterballe M, Andersen KE, Bindslev-Jensen C. The diagnostic accuracy of the atopy patch test in diagnosing hypersensitivity to cow's milk and hen's egg in unselected children with and without atopic dermatitis. *J Am Acad Dermatol.* 2004;51(4):556–562.

59. Niggemann B. Evolving role of the atopy patch test in the diagnosis of food allergy. *Curr Opin Allergy Clin Immunol.* 2002;2(3):253–256.

60. Niggemann B, Ziegert M, Reibel S. Importance of chamber size for the outcome of atopy patch testing in children with atopic dermatitis and food allergy. *J Allergy Clin Immunol.* 2002;110(3):515–516.

61. Gefeller O, Pfahlberg A, Geier J, et al. The association between size of test chamber and patch test reaction: a statistical reanalysis. *Contact Dermatitis.* 1999;40(1):14–18.

62. Heine RG, Verdstege A, Mehl A, et al. Proposal for a standardized interpretation of the atopy patch test in children with atopic dermatitis and suspected food allergy. *Pediatr Allergy Immunol.* 2006;17(3):213–217.

63. Gonsalves N, Yang G, Doerfler B, et al. Prospective clinical trial of allergy testing and food elimination diet and food reintroduction in adults with eosinophilic esophagitis. *Gastroenterology.* 2008;134(4): A104.

64. Simon D, Straumann A, Wenk A, et al. Eosinophilic esophagitis in adults—no clinical relevance of wheat and rye sensitizations. *Allergy.* 2006;61(12):1480–1483.

65. Sugnanam KK, Collins JT, Smith PK, et al. Dichotomy of food and inhalant allergen sensitization in eosinophilic esophagitis. *Allergy.* 2007;62(11):1257–1260.

66. Fogg MI, Ruchelli E, Spergel JM. Pollen and eosinophilic esophagitis. *J Allergy Clin Immunol.* 2003;112(4):796–797.

67. Wang FY, Gupta SK, Fitzgerald JF. Is there a seasonal variation in the incidence or intensity of allergic eosinophilic esophagitis in newly diagnosed children? *J Clin Gastroenterol.* 2007;41(5):451–453.

68. Onbasi K, Sin AZ, Doganavsarqil B, et al. Eosinophil infiltration of the oesophageal mucosa in patients with pollen allergy during the season. *Clin Exp Allergy.* 2005;35(11):1423–1431.

69. Roy-Ghanta S, Larosa DF, Katzka DA. Atopic characteristics of adult patients with eosinophilic esophagitis. *Clin Gastroenterol Hepatol.* 2008;6(5):531–535.

70. Mishra A, Hogan SP, Brandt EB, et al. An etiological role for aeroallergens and eosinophils in experimental esophagitis. *J Clin Invest.* 2001;107(1):83–90.

71. Denburg J. The nose, the lung and the bone marrow in allergic inflammation. *Allergy.* 1999;54(Suppl 57):73–80.

72. Denburg JA. Bone marrow in atopy and asthma: hematopoietic mechanisms in allergic inflammation. *Immunol Today.* 1999;20(3):111–113.

73. Denburg JA, Inman MD, Leber B, et al. The role of the bone marrow in allergy and asthma. *Allergy.* 1996;51(3):141–148.

74. Dorman SC, Sehmi R, Gauvreau GM, et al. Kinetics of bone marrow eosinophilopoiesis and associated cytokines after allergen inhalation. *Am J Respir Crit Care Med.* 2004;169(5):565–572.

75. Braunstahl GJ, Overbeek SE, Kleinjan A, et al. Nasal allergen provocation induces adhesion molecule expression and tissue eosinophilia in upper and lower airways. *J Allergy Clin Immunol.* 2001;107(3):469–476.

76. Eriksson NE, Formgren H, Svenonius E. Food hypersensitivity in patients with pollen allergy. *Allergy.* 1982;37(6):437–443.

77. Ortolani C, Ispano M, Pastorello E, et al. The oral allergy syndrome. *Ann Allergy.* 1988;61(6 Pt 2):47–52.

78. Malandain H. (Allergies associated with both food and pollen). *Eur Ann Allergy Clin Immunol.* 2003;35(7):253–256.

79. Egger M, Mutschlechner S, Wopfner N, et al. Pollen-food syndromes associated with weed pollinosis: an update from the molecular point of view. *Allergy.* 2006;61(4):461–476.

80. Konikoff MR, Noel RJ, Blanchard C, et al. A randomized, double-blind, placebo-controlled trial of fluticasone propionate for pediatric eosinophilic esophagitis. *Gastroenterology.* 2006;131(5):1381–1391.

81. Spechler SJ, Genta RM, Souza RF. Thoughts on the complex relationship between gastroesophageal reflux disease and eosinophilic esophagitis. *Am J Gastroenterol.* 2007;102(6):1301–1306.

82. Dranove JE, Horn DS, Davis MA, et al. Predictors of response to proton pump inhibitor therapy among children with significant esophageal eosinophilia. *J Pediatr.* 2009;154(1):96–100.

83. Ngo P, Furuta GT, Antonioli DA, et al. Eosinophils in the esophagus–peptic or allergic eosinophilic esophagitis? Case series of three patients with esophageal eosinophilia. *Am J Gastroenterol.* 2006;101(7):1666–1670.

84. Garrean C, Gonsalves N, Hirano I. Comparison of demographic, endoscopic and histologic features in eosinophilic esophagitis patients with and without GERD. *Gastroenterology.* 2008;134 (4):A288.

85. Faubion WA Jr, Perrault J, Burgart LJ, et al. Treatment of eosinophilic esophagitis with inhaled corticosteroids. *J Pediatr Gastroenterol Nutr.* 1998;27(1):90–93.

86. Noel RJ, Putnam PE, Collins MH, et al. Clinical and immunopathologic effects of swallowed fluticasone for eosinophilic esophagitis. *Clin Gastroenterol Hepatol.* 2004;2(7):568–575.

87. Arora AS, Perrault J, Smyrk TC. Topical corticosteroid treatment of dysphagia due to eosinophilic esophagitis in adults. *Mayo Clin Proc.* 2003;78(7):830–835.

88. Aceves SS, Bastian JF, Newbury RO, et al. Oral viscous budesonide: a potential new therapy for eosinophilic esophagitis in children. *Am J Gastroenterol.* 2007; 102(10):2271–2279; quiz 2280.

89. Straumann A, Degen L, Felder S, et al. Budesonide as induction treatment for active eosinophilicesophagitis in adolescents and adults: a randomized, double-blind, placebo-controlled study (BEE-1Trial). (abstract) *Gastroenterol.* 2008.;134(4):S1:A726.

90. Lucendo AJ, Pascual-Turrión G, Navarro M, et al. Endoscopic, bioptic, and manometric findings in eosinophilic esophagitis before and after steroid therapy: a case series. *Endoscopy.* 2007;39(9):765–771.

91. Schaefer ET, Fitzgerald JF, Molleston JP, et al. Comparison of oral prednisone and topical fluticasone in the treatment of eosinophilic esophagitis: a randomized trial in children. *Clin Gastroenterol Hepatol.* 2008;6(2):165–173.

92. Liacouras CA, Wenner WJ, Brown K, et al. Primary eosinophilic esophagitis in children: successful treatment with oral corticosteroids. *J Pediatr Gastroenterol Nutr.* 1998;26(4):380–385.

93. Attwood SE, Lewis CJ, Bronder CS, et al. Eosinophilic oesophagitis: a novel treatment using Montelukast. *Gut.* 2003;52(2):181–185.

94. Kaplan M, Mutlu EA, Jakate S, et al. Endoscopy in eosinophilic esophagitis: "feline" esophagus and perforation risk. *Clin Gastroenterol Hepatol.* 2003;1(6):433–437.

95. Sedgwick JB, Busse WW. Inhibitory effect of cetirizine on cytokine-enhanced in vitro eosinophil survival. *Ann Allergy Asthma Immunol.* 1997;78(6):581–585.

96. Netzer P, et al. Corticosteroid-dependent eosinophilic oesophagitis: azathioprine and 6-mercaptopurine can induce and maintain long-term remission. *Eur J Gastroenterol Hepatol.* 2007;19(10):865–869.

97. Rothenberg ME, et al. Treatment of patients with the hypereosinophilic syndrome with mepolizumab. *N Engl J Med.* 2008;358(12):1215–1228.

98. Stein ML, Collins MH, Villanueva JM, et al. Anti-IL-5 (mepolizumab) therapy for eosinophilic esophagitis. *J Allergy Clin Immunol.* 2006;118(6):1312–1319.

99. Foroughi S, Foster B, Kim N, et al. Anti-IgE treatment of eosinophil-associated gastrointestinal disorders. *J Allergy Clin Immunol.* 2007;120(3):594–601.

100. Straumann A, Bussmann C, Conus S, et al. Anti-TNF-alpha (infliximab) therapy for severe adult eosinophilic esophagitis. *J Allergy Clin Immunol.* 2008. 122(2):425–427.

101. Schoepfer AM, Gschossmann J, Scheurer U, et al. Esophageal strictures in adult eosinophilic esophagitis: dilation is an effective and safe alternative after failure of topical corticosteroids. *Endoscopy.* 2008; 40(2):161–164.

102. Cohen MS, Kaufman AB, Palazzo JP, et al. An audit of endoscopic complications in adult eosinophilic esophagitis. *Clin Gastroenterol Hepatol.* 2007;5(10):1149–1153.

103. Eisenbach C, Merle U, Schirmacher P, et al. Perforation of the esophagus after dilation treatment for dysphagia in a patient with eosinophilic esophagitis. *Endoscopy.* 2006;38(Suppl 2):E43–44.

104. Gonsalves N, Karmali K, Hirano I. Safety and response of esophageal dilation in adults with eosinophilic esophagitis. *Gastroenterology.* 2007;132(4):S1 (T2034).

CHAPTER 41

Chronic Cough

RACHEL E. STORY AND JENNIFER S. KIM

■ INTRODUCTION

Cough is the most common complaint for which Americans see a primary care physician (1). In the United States, the cost of over-the-counter medications to treat cough is estimated to exceed two billion dollars on an annual basis (2). The differential diagnosis, diagnostic evaluation, and treatment of cough differ in children and adults. This chapter will focus on chronic cough and discuss children and adults separately.

Cough is a reflex response of the lower respiratory tract that is mediated by cough receptors of the airways. Cough receptors are present also in the pharynx, paranasal sinuses, stomach, and external auditory canal.

■ COUGH IN ADULTS

Cough in adults (patients 15 years or older) is categorized in three groups: acute cough lasting less than 3 weeks, subacute cough lasting 3 to 8 weeks, and chronic cough lasting longer than 8 weeks. Detailed discussion of each group is beyond the scope of this chapter. Acute cough is usually infectious in nature. Subacute cough is often post-infectious but can also represent the onset or exacerbation of conditions known to cause chronic cough. This chapter will focus on chronic cough in nonsmokers as it is one of the most common reasons patients seek care from a respiratory specialist.

Chronic cough occurs in 10% to 20% of adults and can be debilitating (3). Complications of cough include almost every organ system and have been shown to significantly decrease quality of life (4–7). Three conditions cause the majority of cough in nonsmoking adults who are not on an angiotensin-converting enzyme (ACE) inhibitor: upper airway cough syndrome, asthma, and gastroesophageal reflux disease (GERD). In patients with a normal chest radiograph and no symptoms suggesting a specific etiology of cough, a recent consensus document recommends investigation and treatment of upper airway cough syndrome, asthma, and GERD prior to the consideration of less common causes of cough (8). A comprehensive differential diagnosis for chronic cough in adults is included in Table 41.1.

Upper Airway Cough Syndrome

Upper airway cough syndrome (UACS) was formerly known as the postnasal drip (PND) syndrome. UACS alone or in combination with other conditions is the most common cause of chronic cough (8). PND, the drainage of secretions from the nose or paranasal sinuses into the pharynx, causes cough via mechanical stimulation of the cough reflex, increased cough receptor sensitivity, or co-existent inflammation in the lower airways (9,10). Causes of UACS include allergic rhinitis, nonallergic rhinitis, vasomotor rhinitis, nonallergic rhinitis with eosinophilia, rhinitis medimentosa, gustatory rhinitis, infectious rhinitis, infectious sinusitis, allergic fungal sinusitis, rhinitis of pregnancy, and chemical/occupational rhinitis. These conditions, their diagnosis, and specific treatments are discussed in detail in Chapters 26 and 27.

History and physical examination alone will rarely identify the cause of chronic cough. Often, patients with UACS will report the sensation of mucus dripping down their throat and frequent throat clearing. On physical examination mucoid or mucopurulent secretions may be present and cobblestone changes in the oropharynx may be noted. However, 20% of patients with cough due to UACS do not report symptoms of PND and more than 50% do not have physical examination with characteristic changes (11). A prospective study of chronic cough in adults found that medical history regarding the character and timing of cough is of little value in determining the etiology of cough (12).

Treatment of UACS depends on its etiology. If there is an apparent etiology for UACS such as chronic rhinosinusitis or allergic rhinitis, appropriate treatment with antibiotics or intranasal steroids should be instituted. However, if a specific etiology is not clear, a diagnostic/therapeutic trial with antihistamine/decongestants or nasal steroids is recommended by the American College of Chest Physicians (ACCP) prior to investigating less

TABLE 41.1 DIFFERENTIAL DIAGNOSIS OF COUGH IN ADULTS

Upper airway cough syndrome
- Allergic rhinitis
- Non-allergic rhinitis
- Vasomotor rhinitis
- Nonallergic rhinitis with eosinophilia (NARES)
- Rhinitis medimentosa
- Gustatory rhinitis
- Infectious rhinitis
- Infectious sinusitis
- Allergic fungal sinusitis
- Rhinitis of pregnancy
- Chemical/occupational rhinitis

Asthma

GERD

Nonasthmatic eosinophilic bronchitis

Tracheobronchial collapse

Irritant inhalation/occupational and environmental considerations
- Tobacco smoke (personal use or environmental exposure)
- Biomass combustion particles
- Occupational exposures (hard metal disease, asbestosis, beryllium, bioairesols—endotoxin or fungal glycans)

Medications
- ACE inhibitors
- β blockers

Pulmonary infections
- Pneumonia
- Tuberculosis
- Recurrant viral bronchitis

Chronic obstructive pulmonary disease/chronic bronchitis

Bronchiectasis

Aspiration

Interstitial Lung Disease

Cystic fibrosis

Ciliary disorder

Immunodeficiency

Sarcoidosis

Vasculitis

Respiratory tumors

Psychogenic cough

Tic (Tourette)

Vocal cord dysfunction

Increased cough receptor sensitivity

Otogenic causes (Arnold ear)

Idiopathic

common causes of cough (8). Cough due to UACS typically resolves over a period of days to weeks with treatment. If a patient's cough does not respond to empiric treatment and UACS is still suspected, the ACCP recommends a sinus CT as chronic rhinosinusitis may cause a cough without typical sinusitis symptoms.

Asthma

Asthma should be considered in all adults with chronic cough. While cough is a common symptom of asthma, most patients experience dyspnea and wheezing in addition to cough. Still, some patients with asthma have cough as their predominant symptom and this condition is referred to as cough variant asthma (CVA), also called cough equivalent asthma. Patients with CVA have a more sensitive cough reflex than healthy volunteers and patients with typical asthma (13). If reversible airflow obstruction is found on spirometry, treatment with inhaled corticosteroids and bronchodilators should be instituted. At times leukotriene antagonists, long-acting β agonists, and oral steroids may be used as discussed in Chapter 19.

In a patient with a normal physical examination and normal spirometry, a methacholine inhalation challenge (MIC) essentially rules out the diagnosis of asthma as it has a negative predictive value close to 100% (14). There is a risk of a false positive study and one prospective study of chronic cough in adults found the MIC was falsely positive 22% of the time (15). Thus, diagnosis of CVA is made only after resolution of cough with specific asthma treatment (16). A diagnostic or therapeutic trial of asthma therapy is often performed. If MIC testing is not performed, nonasthmatic eosinophilic bronchitis cannot be excluded as the etiology of the cough as discussed in detail later in this chapter.

Gastroesophageal Reflux Disease

GERD causes cough via chemical and mechanical irritation of the upper respiratory tract, irritation of the lower respiratory tract via microaspiration, and stimulating an esophageal-bronchial cough reflex (17). Intervention studies find GERD alone or in combination with other etiologies as a cause of cough in up to 41% of adults with chronic cough (18). History regarding the character and timing of cough is not sufficient to distinguish a cough due to GERD from other causes of cough. One study found that cough due to GERD occurs at night in only a minority of patients (12). In addition, GERD is "silent" with no gastrointestinal symptoms in up to 75% of patients (19). GERD is the cause of chronic cough in 91% of nonsmoking adults with a normal chest radiograph if asthma, nonasthmatic eosinophilic bronchitis, UACS, and ACE-inhibitor cough have been ruled out (18).

Empiric treatment with medical anti-reflux therapy is warranted when GERD is the likely cause of cough. This includes patients with typical symptoms of regurgitation and heartburn and those with a high likelihood of GERD-related cough, that is, patients in whom asthma, nonasthmatic eosinophilic bronchitis, and UACS have been ruled out. Medical treatment of GERD includes dietary and lifestyle modification, acid suppression therapy, and in some cases prokinetic therapy. Some experts recommend a 24-hour esophageal pH monitoring prior to treatment of GERD while the ACCP recommends empiric treatment of GERD prior to 24- hour esophageal pH monitoring (18). The 24-hour esophageal pH monitoring has limitations in that it will not detect nonacid reflux and can result in a normal study when nonacid GERD is the cause of cough (20). In addition, there is disagreement on how best to interpret test results. Diagnosis is confirmed when cough resolves with GERD therapy. Typically patients should be treated with a proton pump inhibitor for at least 3 months as cough due to GERD may take longer to resolve with treatment than cough due to other causes (21).

When UACS, asthma, and GERD have been ruled out as a cause of cough, other diagnoses should be investigated, with the workup being guided by the clinical picture.

Nonasthmatic Eosinophilic Bronchitis

Nonasthmatic eosinophilic bronchitis is a common cause of chronic cough characterized by corticosteroid responsive eosinophilic airway inflammation without variable airway obstruction or airway hyperresponsiveness. Recent studies have found that between 10% and 30% of cases of chronic cough are caused by nonasthmatic eosinophilic bronchitis (22–24). Patients with nonasthmatic eosinophilic bronchitis have chronic cough with no reversible airway obstruction on spirometry, normal airway hyperresponsiveness on MIC, and sputum eosinophilia. Because cough typically resolves with inhaled corticosteroids, this condition was likely unrecognized in the past and misdiagnosed as asthma if MIC was not performed.

Primary Pulmonary Disease

Primary pulmonary disease is a less common cause of chronic cough with varying frequency depending on the population studied. One prospective study of chronic cough found bronchiectasis and interstitial lung disease as the etiology of cough in 16% of participants (25). In this study, a productive cough and an abnormal chest radiograph were predictive of a primary pulmonary cause of cough; however, other groups have not found chest radiograph to be predictive.

Bronchiectasis

Acute and chronic infection resulting in the permanent dilation of bronchi causes most cases of bronchiectasis (26). Due to improvements in the prevention and treatment of childhood infections with immunizations and antibiotics, there is a decrease in the incidence of bronchiectasis in immunocompetent individuals (27). In developed countries, patients with bronchiectasis often have an underlying disorder that predisposes them to the development of bronchiectasis; such disorders include cystic fibrosis, allergic bronchopulmonary mycosis, hypogammaglobulinemia, HIV, primary ciliary dyskinesia, chronic mycobacterium avium complex infection, aspiration, rheumatoid arthritis, inflammatory bowel disease, and α-1 antitrypsin deficiency (26). Patients typically present with a chronic productive cough and diagnosis is made when characteristic changes are found on high-resolution computed tomography (CT) of the chest (28). Treatment includes the use of bronchodilators, chest physiotherapy, antibiotics, and mucolytics.

Interstitial Lung Disease

The interstitial lung diseases (ILDs) are a heterogeneous group of pulmonary disorders that involve the alveolar and perialveolar tissues. They can be classified into those with known causes and those without a known cause. Known causes of ILDs include environmental and occupational exposures resulting in diseases such as asbestosis, hypersensitivity pneumonitis, and berylliosis. Unknown causes of ILDs include idiopathic pulmonary fibrosis, sarcoidosis, and ILD associated with collagen vascular disease. In patients with chronic cough, ILDs should be investigated after more common causes of cough have been ruled out, especially if history or chest radiography is suggestive (29).

Tracheobronchial Collapse

One prospective study of 78 patients found that 11 patients (14.1%) had tracheobronchial collapse as a cause of chronic cough (30). Tracheobronchial collapse was diagnosed on bronchoscopy and surgical correction was recommended. In that study, asthma, GERD, and UACS, alone or in combination, were responsible for 93.6% of chronic cough cases (30).

Lung Tumors

While cough is often a presenting symptom of lung cancer, it is still a rare cause of cough (<2%) in patients presenting with chronic cough (31). A chest radiograph should be obtained in those with known risk factors for lung cancer including cigarette smokers, those with passive cigarette smoke exposure, exposure to asbestos or radon, chronic obstructive pulmonary disease, or a family history of lung cancer. Likewise, individuals with known cancer that may metastasize to the lung should have chest radiography performed. CT scans and bronchoscopy may be required if there is a high degree of suspicion and a normal chest radiograph.

Infection

Infection is not a major cause of chronic cough but it must be considered in the differential in the appropriate clinical context. Because cough is the most common symptom in active pulmonary tuberculosis (TB), it should be considered in any patient with cough lasting 2 to 3 weeks if the likelihood of active TB is high (32). High-risk groups include those living in endemic areas, HIV seropositive individuals, prisoners, and those living in nursing homes. It is important to recognize that elderly patients will present with productive cough but are less likely to have fever, diaphoresis, hemoptysis, and a positive tuberculin skin test result (33). Thus, one must have a high index of suspicion when considering TB in an elderly population. If tuberculosis is suspected, a tuberculin skin test, chest radiograph, and sputum smears and cultures for acid-fast bacilli should be obtained. Pertussis is commonly thought of as a disease of children, but can cause chronic cough in adults. In a study of adults presenting to the emergency department complaining of cough for more than 2 weeks, 21% were found to meet serologic criteria for pertussis infection (34). Endemic fungi and parasitic disease should also be considered in patients visiting or residing in endemic locations.

Aspiration

Oral-pharyngeal dysphagia resulting in aspiration can cause chronic cough. Many patients with aspiration cough when eating and drinking, but aspiration can also be "silent" with no associated cough with feeding. Aspiration is common after acute stroke with up to 38% showing aspiration on videofluoroscopic swallow evaluation (35). Other conditions in which aspiration should be suspected include neurologic impairment which occurs in Parkinson disease, anoxia, or head trauma; postoperative aspiration after cervical spine surgery; or head and neck cancer surgery (36). Elderly individuals who are bedbound and require assistance for oral care are also more likely to have aspiration and are at increased risk for cough due to aspiration (37,38). If aspiration is suspected, referral to a speech-language pathologist is recommended for an oral-pharyngeal swallow evaluation.

Angiotensin-converting Enzyme Inhibitor Cough

Cough is a clearly established side effect of angiotensin-converting enzyme inhibitor (ACE-I) medications (39). It has been reported to develop in 5% to 35% of

individuals treated with an ACE-I and is more likely in women and nonsmokers (40). Symptoms can start within hours of taking the medication or may not appear until months later. Treatment is to discontinue the medication, and cough typically resolves within days, although it has been reported to continue up to 4 weeks (39).

Psychogenic (Habit) Cough

There is no standard definition for psychogenic cough in the medical literature. While some authors equate psychogenic cough with habit cough, others consider them separate disorders. The 2006 ACCP clinical practice guidelines recommend that a diagnosis of habit or psychogenic cough only be made after an extensive evaluation rules out other disorders, including tic disorders, and when the cough improves with psychiatric therapy or behavior modification (41). If cough does not respond to psychiatric therapy or behavior modification, a diagnosis of unexplained cough should be made rather than habit or psychogenic cough.

■ APPROACH TO THE DIAGNOSIS AND MANAGEMENT OF CHRONIC COUGH IN ADULTS

Several groups have studied prospective diagnostic and treatment pathways with successful treatment of chronic cough in up to 98% of patients (11,15,25,42–44). In 9 of 12 published reports from specialist cough clinics, most using a treatment algorithm, there was a success rate of greater than 90% in the treatment of chronic cough (45). Less success was reported in patients referred to a general respiratory clinic when a treatment protocol was not used; about 43% of patients reported persistent symptoms at follow-up (46). Treatment pathways usually focus on the three leading causes of chronic cough in nonsmoking adults who are not on an ACE-I: UACS, asthma, and GERD. A significant number of patients may have multiple causes for their cough. Chronic cough was due to two or more conditions in 8% to 29% of patients in prospective studies (11,15,25,42–44).

The ACCP recommends the following approach to the management of chronic cough in adults (Fig. 41.1) (47). Patients with complaint of chronic cough should have a history, physical examination, and chest radiograph performed. If patients are smokers or being treated with an ACE-I, the offending agent should be discontinued, and if cough persists, further evaluation should occur. If a cause of cough is suggested by history, physical examination, or chest radiograph, it should be investigated and treated. If there is an inadequate response to initial treatment, investigation of UACS, asthma, nonasthmatic eosinophilic bronchitis,

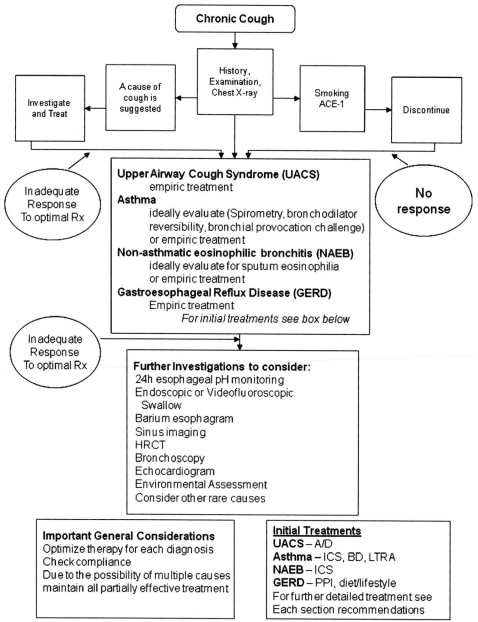

■ **FIGURE 41.1.** Management of chronic cough in adults. (Reproduced with permission of the American College of Chest Physicians, from *An Empiric Integrative Approach to the Management of Cough*, Pratter MR, Brightling CE, Boulet LP, and Irwin RS, 129(1), 2006; permission conveyed through Copyright Clearance Center, Inc.)

and GERD should occur. For UACS empiric treatment with antihistamine and/or decongestant is recommended. Asthma should be evaluated with spirometry, bronchodilator reversibility, and MIC if needed, or treated empirically with inhaled corticosteroids, bronchodilators, and/or leukotriene-receptor antagonist. Nonasthmatic eosinophilic bronchitis should be investigated with sputum eosinophils in the setting of a normal MIC or treated empirically with inhaled corticosteroids. GERD should be treated empirically with diet, lifestyle modification, and proton pump

inhibitors. If there is an inadequate response to the preceding treatment, further investigation should occur and one should consider rare causes of cough. Because cough is often multifactorial, all partially effective treatments should be maintained.

■ **PEDIATRIC COUGH**

As in adults, cough is one of the most common symptoms for which parents consult their child's primary care physician. However, based on the available published medical literature, the causes and management of cough in children differ considerably from that in adults. Overall, there is very little published research on pediatric cough despite its high prevalence.

Characterization of Cough

Cough in children can be characterized by three defining aspects: duration, quality, and potential for underlying disease (10,48).

Duration

According to the ACCP evidence-based clinical practice guidelines (49), chronic cough in children ages 15 years or younger is defined by a daily cough occurring for more than 4 weeks. The rationale for this is that cough due to acute respiratory infections resolve within 1 to 3 weeks in most children (50,51). Only approximately 5% of cough following an acute respiratory infections lasts more than 4 weeks (50,52). The focus of this chapter is primarily on chronic cough.

Quality

Characteristics such as "barking or croupy," "staccato," or paroxysmal cough are classically taught, respectively, as indicators of croup, infantile chlamydia, and pertussis. However, there are limited data on the reliability of these descriptors except for the distinction between dry and wet or moist cough, which has been validated (53). Brassy cough has been shown to be highly specific for tracheomalacia (53). In contrast, parental reports of nocturnal cough have been found to be discordant from objective measures such as recordings (54).

Potential for Underlying Disease

Cough may be expected, specific, or nonspecific. In expected cough, the presence of cough is expected (or normal), such as after an acute respiratory tract infection. Children 5 years of age or younger have 3.8 to 5 acute upper respiratory infections per year where as adults have only two (55).

In specific cough, the etiology is usually evident from coexisting symptoms or signs. Examples would include cardiac murmur (indicating cardiac disease), digital clubbing (suppurative lung disease), failure to thrive (immune deficiency or cystic fibrosis), and feeding difficulties or neurodevelopmental abnormalities (aspiration). Chronic productive purulent cough is always pathologic and must be investigated for possible bronchiectasis and evaluated for treatable causes such as cystic fibrosis and immune deficiency (49).

In contrast, nonspecific or isolated cough has been defined as usually dry cough without a serious underlying condition.

The challenge for the physician is to determine when cough is abnormal. Healthy children cough from 1 to 34 times per day (52). Cough is subject to the period effect (spontaneous resolution) (56), and the therapeutic benefit of placebo treatment for cough has been reported to be as high as 85% (57). Children also have been found to be more likely to cough under certain psychological settings (58).

A detailed clinical history is paramount in the evaluation of childhood chronic cough. Historical aspects should include frequency, severity, time course, diurnal variability, age of onset, relationship to meals, and presence of sputum, wheeze, and/or associated acute respiratory symptoms. History of passive smoke exposure should be elicited as 50% of children 2 years of age or older in families with two smokers will have significant cough (59).

Health care providers must also take into account parental perception and expectations as the reporting of cough is likely to be biased (60). Perceived severity of cough may relate closely to its effect on parents or teachers and therefore plays an important role in the parental pursuit of medical consultation.

Etiology

The three most common causes of chronic cough in adults (upper airway cough syndrome, asthma, and gastroesophageal reflux) are uncommon causes in children. In a prospective cohort of 108 children referred to a tertiary care center, less than 10% had one of these three diagnoses (61). The median age of this cohort was 2.6 years (interquartile range [IQR], 1.2 to 6.9 years) and the median duration of cough was 6 months (IQR, 3 to 12 months).

The use of isolated chronic cough in children as a marker for asthma is controversial. In fact, more recent evidence shows that in most children, cough (without wheeze or dyspnea) does not represent asthma (62–66). The diagnosis of cough-variant asthma should be one of exclusion, particularly in the absence of other IgE-mediated disease. The following diagnostic criteria have been proposed to identify which children with chronic isolated cough are more likely to have asthma (63):

- Abnormally increased cough without evidence of other nonasthma diagnoses
- Clear response to a therapeutic trial of asthma medications
- Relapse of symptoms on stopping medications with a subsequent second response after resuming them
- Presence of atopic eczema, positive aeroallergen prick tests, and/or parental (especially maternal) history of asthma

Gastroesophageal reflux (GER) is infrequently the sole cause of pediatric cough based on the little data available in the medical literature. In a study performed by Chang et al. (61), GER accounted for only 3% of primary diagnoses in their cohort. However, cough and GER can precipitate each other, and it is difficult to differentiate cause and effect (67).

Although sinusitis is commonly diagnosed in childhood, it is not associated with cough once atopy and physician-diagnosed allergic rhinitis are controlled (68). Protracted bacterial bronchitis, found in 40%, was the most common final diagnosis among the cohort mentioned above (61). The proposed clinical definition of protracted bacterial bronchitis (48) is as follows: the presence of isolated chronic moist cough, resolution of cough with appropriate antibiotics, and absence of pointers suggestive of alternative specific cough.

The other primary diagnoses among the cohort (found in more than one patient) include bronchiectasis, aspiration disorders, and *Mycoplasma pneumoniae* infection (61). Other potential causes in children (49) include a post-viral syndrome, exposure to environmental tobacco smoke or other pollutants, foreign body inhalation, airway malacia, medications (i.e., angiotensin-converting enzyme inhibitors), psychogenic disorders, and the Arnold ear-cough reflex (69).

Evaluation of Specific Cough

Specific cough should be further evaluated depending on the associated symptoms or signs present. These may include (and are not limited to) sweat chloride test, immune function studies, barium swallow, video fluoroscopy, pH probe, bronchoscopy with or without lavage, echocardiography, complex sleep polysomnography, and high resolution chest CT scan (HRCT). The risks and benefits of chest HRCT in children must be weighed as children have 10 times the increased risk of lifetime cancer mortality secondary to medical radiation compared to middle-aged adults (70). Moreover, if sedation is required, that incurs additional potential risk. However, the yield for diagnosing bronchiectasis by chest HRCT in children with chronic moist cough is very high (11).

It is important to note that after asthma, cystic fibrosis (CF) is the second most common chronic inflammatory airway disease, particularly among Caucasians. The severity and progression of airway disease can be highly variable. Classic, mild, and atypical CF has features that overlap with allergic and/or immunologic diseases. Moreover, not all patients with CF have diagnostic sweat tests. Genetic analysis should be pursued when there are equivocal levels of sweat chloride.

Evaluation of Nonspecific Cough

If the child's chronic cough is nonspecific, the initial evaluation should include chest radiography and spirometry (if school age) (49). If these yield normal results, there are two approaches to further management.

One approach would be "watch, wait, and review" (49), particularly because the placebo effect on cough has been reported to be quite high (57). One randomized controlled trial reported "parents who wanted medicine at the initial visit reported more improvement at follow-up, regardless of whether the child received drug, placebo, or no treatment" (71). Another prospective cohort study (61) revealed that 24% of children had spontaneous resolution of cough. Frequent re-evaluation should be performed as specific etiologic pointers may emerge.

The second approach would be a trial of medical therapy, depending on the quality of the cough. The ACCP clinical practice guidelines (49) suggest a trial of antibiotics (10-day course) for a **wet** cough. As noted earlier, protracted bacterial bronchitis was found to be the most common final diagnosis among a cohort of young children with chronic cough (61). Additional treatment and investigation for suppurative lung disease (including bronchiectasis) should be undertaken if a wet cough only partially resolves with antibiotics, is prolonged (more than 3 months), or is recurrent (more than two per year).

If a **dry** cough is present, particularly in a child at risk for asthma, a trial of inhaled corticosteroids is recommended (400 µg/day budesonide, 200 µg/day fluticasone, or equivalent) (49). Cough related to asthma is expected to resolve within 2 to 7 days. Therefore, a trial lasting 2 to 4 weeks would be reasonable. If unresponsive, increased doses are not indicated. Rather, the medication should be stopped and other diagnoses considered. On the other hand, given the favorable natural history of cough, a so-called positive response should not be assumed to be due to the medication tried. Once resolution of the cough has been demonstrated, it would be reasonable to wean or withhold medications.

Cough may also be voluntarily induced by older children as it has been found in adults to be cortically modulated (62), but this is unlikely to be a factor in younger children (less than 4 years of age). Absence of cough when asleep or when the child is distracted would be suspicious for habit cough. The classic presentation of habit-cough syndrome is that of a harsh, barking, repetitive cough that occurs several times per minute for hours on end, which resolves once the patient is asleep (72).

Treatment

In randomized controlled trials or systematic reviews of randomized controlled trials, the following medications have been shown to be ineffective for pediatric chronic cough (73): β2-agonists (inhaled or oral), mast cell stabilizers (cromoglycate and nedocromil), methylxanthines (theophylline), inhaled anticholinergics (ipratropium bromide), oral corticosteroids, and promotility agents. There are no relevant studies on the efficacy of proton pump inhibitors on cough and GER.

The American Academy of Pediatrics advises against the use of codeine or dextromethorphan for symptomatic treatment of any type of cough for children (74). Over-the-counter cough remedies have been associated with significant morbidity and mortality (75).

There is no supportive evidence for the use of antibiotics for chronic nonspecific dry cough. However, they may be of limited usefulness in treatment of chronic moist or wet cough, particularly in young children (younger than 7 years) (76).

■ REFERENCES

1. Schappert SM, Burt CW. Ambulatory care visits to physician offices, hospital outpatient departments, and emergency departments: United States, 2001–02. *Vital Health Stat*. 2006;13:1–66.
2. Morice AH. Epidemiology of cough. *Pulm Pharmacol Ther*. 2002;15:253–259.
3. Barbee RA, Halonen M, Kaltenborn WT, et al. A longitudinal study of respiratory symptoms in a community population sample. Correlations with smoking, allergen skin-test reactivity, and serum IgE. *Chest*. 1991;99:20–26.
4. Dicpinigaitis PV, Tso R, Banauch G. Prevalence of depressive symptoms among patients with chronic cough. *Chest*. 2006;130:1839–1843.
5. French CL, Irwin RS, Curley FJ, et al. Impact of chronic cough on quality of life. *Arch Intern Med*. 1998;158:1657–1661.
6. Irwin RS. Complications of cough: ACCP evidence-based clinical practice guidelines. *Chest*. 2006;129:54S–58S.
7. Kuzniar TJ, Morgenthaler TI, Afessa B, et al. Chronic cough from the patient's perspective. *Mayo Clin Proc*. 2007;82:56–60.
8. Pratter MR. Chronic upper airway cough syndrome secondary to rhinosinus diseases (previously referred to as postnasal drip syndrome): ACCP evidence-based clinical practice guidelines. *Chest*. 2006;129:63S–71S.
9. Irwin RS, Pratter MR, Holland PS, et al. Postnasal drip causes cough and is associated with reversible upper airway obstruction. *Chest*. 1984;85:346–352.
10. Landau LI. Acute and chronic cough. *Paediatr Respir Rev*. 2006;7(Suppl 1):S64–S67.
11. Pratter MR, Bartter T, Akers S, et al. An algorithmic approach to chronic cough. *Ann Intern Med*. 1993;119:977–983.
12. Mello CJ, Irwin RS, Curley FJ. Predictive values of the character, timing, and complications of chronic cough in diagnosing its cause. *Arch Intern Med*. 1996;156:997–1003.
13. Dicpinigaitis PV, Dobkin JB, Reichel J. Antitussive effect of the leukotriene receptor antagonist zafirlukast in subjects with cough-variant asthma. *J Asthma*. 2002;39:291–297.
14. Crapo RO, Casaburi R, Coates AL, et al. Guidelines for methacholine and exercise challenge testing-1999. This official statement of the American Thoracic Society was adopted by the ATS Board of Directors, July 1999. *Am J Respir Crit Care Med*. 2000;161:309–329.
15. Irwin RS, Corrao WM, Pratter MR. Chronic persistent cough in the adult: the spectrum and frequency of causes and successful outcome of specific therapy. *Am Rev Respir Dis*. 1981;123:413–417.
16. Irwin RS, French CT, Smyrnios NA, et al. Interpretation of positive results of a methacholine inhalation challenge and 1 week of inhaled bronchodilator use in diagnosing and treating cough-variant asthma. *Arch Intern Med*. 1997;157:1981–1987.
17. Irwin RS, Madison JM, Fraire AE. The cough reflex and its relation to gastroesophageal reflux. *Am J Med*. 2000;108(Suppl 4a): 73S–78S.
18. Irwin RS. Chronic cough due to gastroesophageal reflux disease: ACCP evidence-based clinical practice guidelines. *Chest*. 2006;129: 80S–94S.
19. Irwin RS, French CL, Curley FJ, et al. Chronic cough due to gastroesophageal reflux. Clinical, diagnostic, and pathogenetic aspects. *Chest*. 1993;104:1511–1517.
20. Irwin RS, Madison JM. Diagnosis and treatment of chronic cough due to gastro-esophageal reflux disease and postnasal drip syndrome. *Pulm Pharmacol Ther*. 2002;15:261–266.
21. Irwin RS, Zawacki JK, Curley FJ, et al. Chronic cough as the sole presenting manifestation of gastroesophageal reflux. *Am Rev Respir Dis*. 1989;140:1294–1300.
22. Ayik SO, Basoglu OK, Erdinc M, et al. Eosinophilic bronchitis as a cause of chronic cough. *Respir Med*. 2003;97:695–701.
23. Brightling CE, Pavord ID. Eosinophilic bronchitis—what is it and why is it important? *Clin Exp Allergy*. 2000;30:4–6.
24. Carney IK, Gibson PG, Murree-Allen K, et al. A systematic evaluation of mechanisms in chronic cough. *Am J Respir Crit Care Med*. 1997;156:211–216.
25. Kastelik JA, Aziz I, Ojoo JC, et al. Investigation and management of chronic cough using a probability-based algorithm. *Eur Respir J*. 2005;25:235–243.
26. Rosen MJ. Chronic cough due to bronchiectasis: ACCP evidence-based clinical practice guidelines. *Chest*. 2006;129:122S–131S.
27. Barker AF. Bronchiectasis. *N Engl J Med*. 2002;346:1383–1393.
28. McGuinness G, Naidich DP. CT of airways disease and bronchiectasis. *Radiol Clin North Am*. 2002;40:1–19.
29. Brown KK. Chronic cough due to chronic interstitial pulmonary diseases: ACCP evidence-based clinical practice guidelines. *Chest*. 2006;129:180S-5S.
30. Palombini BC, Villanova CA, Araujo E, et al. A pathogenic triad in chronic cough: asthma, postnasal drip syndrome, and gastroesophageal reflux disease. *Chest*. 1999;116:279–284.
31. Kvale PA. Chronic cough due to lung tumors: ACCP evidence-based clinical practice guidelines. *Chest*. 2006; 129:147S–153S.
32. Rosen MJ. Chronic cough due to tuberculosis and other infections: ACCP evidence-based clinical practice guidelines. *Chest*. 2006;129: 197S–201S.
33. Perez-Guzman C, Vargas MH, Torres-Cruz A, et al. Does aging modify pulmonary tuberculosis?: A meta-analytical review. *Chest*. 1999;116:961–967.
34. Wright SW, Edwards KM, Decker MD, et al. Pertussis infection in adults with persistent cough. *JAMA*. 1995;273:1044–1046.
35. Daniels SK, Brailey K, Priestly DH, et al. Aspiration in patients with acute stroke. *Arch Phys Med Rehabil*. 1998;79:14–19.
36. Smith Hammond CA, Goldstein LB. Cough and aspiration of food and liquids due to oral-pharyngeal dysphagia: ACCP evidence-based clinical practice guidelines. *Chest*. 2006;129:154S–168S.
37. Langmore SE, Terpenning MS, Schork A, et al. Predictors of aspiration pneumonia: how important is dysphagia? *Dysphagia*. 1998; 13:69–81.
38. Matsuse T, Oka T, Kida K, et al. Importance of diffuse aspiration bronchiolitis caused by chronic occult aspiration in the elderly. *Chest*. 1996;110:1289–1293.
39. Israili ZH, Hall WD. Cough and angioneurotic edema associated with angiotensin-converting enzyme inhibitor therapy. A review of the literature and pathophysiology. *Ann Intern Med*. 1992;117:234–242.
40. Dicpinigaitis PV. Angiotensin-converting enzyme inhibitor-induced cough: ACCP evidence-based clinical practice guidelines. *Chest*. 2006;129:169S–173S.
41. Irwin RS, Glomb WB, Chang AB. Habit cough, tic cough, and psychogenic cough in adult and pediatric populations: ACCP evidence-based clinical practice guidelines. *Chest*. 2006;129:174S–179S.
42. Irwin RS, Curley FJ, French CL. Chronic cough. The spectrum and frequency of causes, key components of the diagnostic evaluation, and outcome of specific therapy. *Am Rev Respir Dis*. 1990; 141:640–647.
43. Marchesani F, Cecarini L, Pela R, et al. Causes of chronic persistent cough in adult patients: the results of a systematic management protocol. *Monaldi Arch Chest Dis*. 1998;53:510–514.
44. McGarvey LP, Heaney LG, Lawson JT, et al. Evaluation and outcome of patients with chronic non-productive cough using a comprehensive diagnostic protocol. *Thorax*. 1998;53:738–743.
45. Rank MA, Kelkar P, Oppenheimer JJ. Taming chronic cough. *Ann Allergy Asthma Immunol*. 2007; 98:305–313;quiz 13-4, 48.
46. McGarvey LP, Heaney LG, MacMahon J. A retrospective survey of diagnosis and management of patients presenting with chronic cough to a general chest clinic. *Int J Clin Pract*. 1998; 52:158–161.
47. Pratter MR, Brightling CE, Boulet LP, et al. An empiric integrative approach to the management of cough: ACCP evidence-based clinical practice guidelines. *Chest*. 2006;129:222S–231S.
48. Chang AB, Landau LI, Van Asperen PP, et al. Cough in children: definitions and clinical evaluation. *Med J Aust*. 2006;184:398–403.
49. Chang AB, Glomb WB. Guidelines for evaluating chronic cough in pediatrics: ACCP evidence-based clinical practice guidelines. *Chest*. 2006;129:260S–283S.
50. Hay AD, Wilson A, Fahey T, et al. The duration of acute cough in pre-school children presenting to primary care: a prospective cohort study. *Fam Pract*. 2003;20:696–705.

51. Hay AD, Wilson AD. The natural history of acute cough in children aged 0 to 4 years in primary care: a systematic review. *Br J Gen Pract.* 2002;52:401–409.

52. Munyard P, Bush A. How much coughing is normal? *Arch Dis Child.* 1996;74:531–534.

53. Chang AB, Gaffney JT, Eastburn MM, et al. Cough quality in children: a comparison of subjective vs. bronchoscopic findings. *Respir Res.* 2005;6:3.

54. Falconer A, Oldman C, Helms P. Poor agreement between reported and recorded nocturnal cough in asthma. *Pediatr Pulmonol.* 1993;15:209–211.

55. Leder K, Sinclair MI, Mitakakis TZ, et al. A community-based study of respiratory episodes in Melbourne, Australia. *Aust N Z J Public Health.* 2003;27:399–404.

56. Evald T, Munch EP, Kok-Jensen A. Chronic non-asthmatic cough is not affected by inhaled beclomethasone dipropionate. A controlled double blind clinical trial. *Allergy.* 1989; 44:510–514.

57. Eccles R. The powerful placebo in cough studies? *Pulm Pharmacol Ther.* 2002;15:303–308.

58. Rietveld S, Van Beest I, Everaerd W. Psychological confounds in medical research: the example of excessive cough in asthma. *Behav Res Ther.* 2000;38:791–800.

59. Charlton A. Children's coughs related to parental smoking. *Br Med J (Clin Res Ed).* 1984;288:1647–1649.

60. Dales RE, White J, Bhumgara C, et al. Parental reporting of children's coughing is biased. *Eur J Epidemiol.* 1997;13:541–545.

61. Marchant JM, Masters IB, Taylor SM, et al. Evaluation and outcome of young children with chronic cough. *Chest.* 2006;129:1132–1141.

62. Chang AB. Cough, cough receptors, and asthma in children. *Pediatr Pulmonol.* 1999;28:59–70.

63. de Benedictis FM, Selvaggio D, de Benedictis D. Cough, wheezing and asthma in children: lesson from the past. *Pediatr Allergy Immunol.* 2004;15:386–393.

64. McKenzie S. Cough—but is it asthma? *Arch Dis Child.* 1994;70:1–2.

65. Tomerak AA, McGlashan JJ, Vyas HH, et al. Inhaled corticosteroids for non-specific chronic cough in children. *Cochrane Database Syst Rev.* 2005:CD004231.

66. Tomerak AA, Vyas H, Lakenpaul M, et al. Inhaled beta2-agonists for treating non-specific chronic cough in children. *Cochrane Database Syst Rev.* 2005;(4):CD005373.

67. Gilger MA. Pediatric otolaryngologic manifestations of gastroesophageal reflux disease. *Curr Gastroenterol Rep.* 2003;5:247–252.

68. Lombardi E, Stein RT, Wright AL, et al. The relation between physician-diagnosed sinusitis, asthma, and skin test reactivity to allergens in 8-year-old children. *Pediatr Pulmonol.* 1996;22:141–146.

69. Tekdemir I, Aslan A, Elhan A. A clinico-anatomic study of the auricular branch of the vagus nerve and Arnold's ear-cough reflex. *Surg Radiol Anat.* 1998;20:253–257.

70. Brenner DJ. Estimating cancer risks from pediatric CT: going from the qualitative to the quantitative. *Pediatr Radiol.* 2002;32:228–233;discussion 42–44.

71. Hutton N, Wilson MH, Mellits ED, et al. Effectiveness of an antihistamine-decongestant combination for young children with the common cold: a randomized, controlled clinical trial. *J Pediatr.* 1991;118:125–130.

72. Weinberger M, Abu-Hasan M. Pseudo-asthma: when cough, wheezing, and dyspnea are not asthma. *Pediatrics.* 2007;120:855–864.

73. Gupta A, McKean M, Chang AB. Management of chronic non-specific cough in childhood: an evidence-based review. *Arch Dis Child Educ Pract Ed.* 2007;92:33–39.

74. Berlin CM, Notterman DA, et al. Use of codeine- and dextromethorphan-containing cough remedies in children. American Academy of Pediatrics. Committee on Drugs. *Pediatrics.* 1997;99:918–920.

75. Gunn VL, Taha SH, Liebelt EL, et al. Toxicity of over-the-counter cough and cold medications. *Pediatrics.* 2001;108:E52.

76. Marchant JM, Morris P, Gaffney JT, et al. Antibiotics for prolonged moist cough in children. *Cochrane Database Syst Rev.* 2005; (4): CD004822.

CHAPTER 42

Sleep Disorders in the Allergic Patient

LISA F. WOLFE

In the fourth century biblical scholars believed that sleep was "the incomplete experience of death." The modern understanding that sleep is an active, complex, and essential behavior did not begin until the use of electroencephalography (EEG), which highlighted differences between wake and sleep (1).

■ SLEEP ARCHITECTURE

EEG has been used to identify the hallmarks of sleep and categorize stages of sleep (2,3). For ease of communication, sleep is divided first into either rapid eye movement sleep (stage REM) or nonrapid eye movement sleep (NREM). Although the eye movements of REM sleep were first discovered in 1953, it was not until 1957 that REM sleep was first described by EEG and the classic architecture of a full night's sleep was first reported (4). These papers noted that REM sleep was associated with dreaming, and heart rate variability, and the episodes recurred about three to four times per night. Ultimately, in 1968, a formal protocol was developed for scoring sleep stages combining EEG, electro-oculography (EOG), and chin electromyography (EMG) (5).

Typical, normal adult sleep architecture is demonstrated in Fig. 42.1. Sleep onset is associated with NREM sleep. NREM sleep is composed of three stages: N1, N2, and N3. N3 is also referred to as slow wave sleep (SWS). During sleep onset, N1 sleep is seen with its characteristic slow rolling eye movements and easy arousability. N2 sleep is seen soon after and is defined by a specific EEG pattern referred to as K-complexes and spindles. It becomes more difficult to awaken the sleeper. N3 follows with hallmark EEG slow waves. SWS is associated with physiologic events including endocrine changes such as growth hormone release (6). NREM sleep becomes a bridge to initiate stage REM. Reduced muscle tone and ventilatory variability are associated with REM sleep.

A complete cycle of NREM to REM sleep lasts approximately 90 minutes, and there are three to four cycles per night. SWS predominates at the beginning of the night and is virtually gone by the final cycle. Stage REM is minimal during the first cycle and concentrated in the early morning. Maturity also affects the architecture of sleep. With aging, there are significant reductions in SWS and sleep continuity. SWS decreases from 24% to 30% of the sleep period to 16% and wake after sleep onset (WASO) time increased from 2% to 4% to 17%. The percentage of REM sleep remains stable at about 20% of the total sleep time (TST) (7).

■ DETERMINATES OF SLEEP REGULATION

There are two processes that regulate the occurrence of sleep and the architecture of sleep periods. The homeostatic drive quantifies the physiologic need to sleep and the circadian pacemaker ensures proper timing of the sleep process. Additionally, the circadian pacemaker is influential in the architecture and NREM/REM distribution sleep stages throughout the night (8).

Circadian Rhythms

The word circadian is derived from Latin roots *circa*, about, and *diem*, day. The term *circadian rhythm* refers to any behavior or physiologic process that is known to vary in a predictable pattern over a 24-hour period. This internal process is governed by a three-component mechanism. First, inputs such as light and activity help synchronize (entrain) to the environment. These inputs are called zeitgebers, which is German for "time giver." Next, information from zeitgebers is transferred to an internal clock, which acts as a pacemaker—setting the rate and timing of output pathways. Examples of these output pathways include lung function (9),

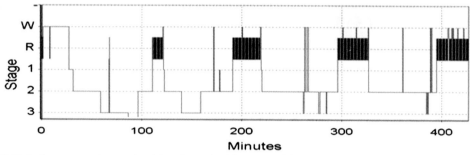

■ **FIGURE 42.1**   A representative sample of sleep from a healthy young adult without sleep complaints. *W*; wake; *1*, N1 (NREM) sleep; *2*, N2 (NREM) sleep; *3*, N3 (slow wave) sleep; *R*, REM sleep.

sympathetic tone (10), and urine production (11), all of which vary over a 24-hour period so that optimum performance occurs during the daytime.

The circadian pacemaker is focused in a hypothalamic structure, the suprachiasmatic nucleus (SCN). Genes that play a role in generating circadian rhythms were first identified in the SCN and subsequently identified in cells of every organ. There are an ever-increasing number of genes that participate in a negative feedback system to regulate the circadian processes. The mammalian circadian genes include period (*per 1, per 2,* and *per 3*), clock (*clock*), B-mal (*B-mal 1*), casein kinase 1 epsilon/1 delta (*CSNK1D* and *CSNK1E*), cryptochrome (*cry1* and *cry2*), and the nuclear hormone receptor *Rev-erba.* Less characterized components include *Timeless, Dec1, Dec2,* and *E4bp4.* These genes are highly conserved and mutations appear to impact many human conditions such as circadian rhythm disorders (advanced or delayed sleep phase), obesity, addiction, sleepiness, and bipolar disorder (12).

Sleep as a Homeostatic Process

Homeostasis is the process by which the body maintains stability. Thirst, hunger, and temperature are all processes that are carefully regulated to ensure optimum function. Sleep can be thought of as kin to these processes, and investigations in sleep deprivation have been the main tool for understanding the body's drive. Utilizing spectral analysis of EEG, slow wave activity has been shown to be a significant hallmark of sleep debt, and as that debt is repaid by sleeping, slow wave activity is reduced (13). Sleep deprivation is increasing in prevalence in western societies. The percentage of U.S. Gallup poll respondents reported sleeping 7 or more hours on weeknights decreased from 63% in 1998 to 57% in 2005. This type of partial sleep deprivation is often associated with limited insight into impairments in cognitive performance. This phenomenon contributes to increases in car accidents for those that are chronically sleep deprived. Physiologic impacts of sleep deprivation include metabolic changes. Satiety hor-

mones are altered such as decreases in Leptin and increases in Ghrelin. These findings have been associated with risk for obesity and diabetes (14).

Two Process Model

The two process model of sleep regulation has been used to explain the relationship between circadian rhythm regulation of sleep (process C) and the homeostatic drive to sleep (process S). Both processes S and C have an impact on sleep regulation, and to promote optimum sleep quality, maximum sleep debt should intersect with appropriate circadian time (15).

■ SLEEP AND THE PHYSIOLOGY OF THE IMMUNE SYSTEM

Both sleep homeostasis and circadian rhythms modulate the expression of immune molecules and cells. Cytokines such as interleukin-2 (IL-2), tumor necrosis factor-α (TNF-α), and granulocyte macrophage-colony stimulating factor (GM-CSF) cycle in a circadian manner each with a unique pattern of expression (16). IL-6 on the other hand appears to be linked more to the sleep homeostatic process, levels peak in relationship to the degree of sleep deprivation, and is associated with latency to REM, sleep efficiency, and wake-after-sleep onset time (17,18). In Table 42.1 the influence of cytokines in the generation of non-REM sleep is summarized. The sleep process influences immune cells as well; lymphocytes, monocytes, and NK cells all have a diurnal rhythm of expression but this rhythm is modified by sleep (19).

Some of the circadian influence on the immune system is mediated through the impact of melatonin. Melatonin is a hormone produced in the pineal gland as a result of dark exposure and in coordination with the central circadian clock. Binding of melatonin to specific receptors in antigen-activated T-helper cells results in an upregulation of cytokine production and immune function. Human studies demonstrate that melatonin favors a T_H1 cell response. The melatonin rhythm positively correlates with the rhythmicity of the T_H1/T_H2

TABLE 42.1 SUMMARY OF THE IMPACT OF CYTOKINES ON GENERATION OF NONRAPID EYE MOVEMENT SLEEP

CYTOKINES AND NONRAPID EYE MOVEMENT SLEEP

PROMOTERS	INHIBITORS
Low dose IL-1β	IL-4
IL-2	IL-10
IL-6	IL-13
IL-8	TGF-β
IL-18	High dose IL-1β
TNF-α	

cell ratio. This seems to be most prominent when in a state of stress or immune suppression. Melatonin may play an additional role in enhancing immunity as melatonin is produced in T-lymphocytes and acts in intracrine, autocrine, and/or paracrine fashion (20) (Table 42.2).

Immunology Impacts of Sleep Deprivation

Sleep deprivation on human immune function has many areas of impact. One night of sleep loss can induce a significant increase in E-selectin, intercellular adhesion molecule-1 (ICAM-1), IL-1β, and IL-1ra, while suppressing C-reactive protein and IL-6 (21). Sleep deprivation limits the ability of the immune system to function and respond to an influenza vaccine challenge (22). Sleep loss reduces myeloid dendritic cell precursors that produce IL-12, thereby resulting in a limit to antigen presentation due to sleep reduction (23). Overall, cellular immunity has been difficulty to evaluate as

TABLE 42.2 CYTOKINES THAT INCREASE IN RESPONSE TO NOCTURNAL ELEVATION IN MELATONIN

MELATONIN INDUCTION OF CYTOKINES

IL-1
IL-2
IFN-γ
IL-6
IL-12
IFN-γ/IL10 ratio

From Cutolo M, Maestroni GJ. The melatonin-cytokine connection in rheumatoid arthritis. *Ann Rheum Dis.* 2005;64:1109–1111.

multiple studies have shown contradictory results depending on the amount of sleep loss and the cellular immunity components studied (24). Humoral immunity is also impacted by sleep loss with increasing serum IgG, IgA, IgM, and C3, C4 (25). Sleep deprivation drives up IL-6 levels and is associated with increasing complaints of pain (26). Response to influenza vaccination is impaired in the setting of chronic partial sleep loss (22,27).

■ SLEEP DISORDERS IN THE ALLERGY PATIENT

Frequently, daytime sleepiness can persist in the face of adequate sleep and polysomnography (PSG) can be performed to assess the possible sources of poor sleep quality. During a traditional (Type 1) overnight study, EEG, electrocardiogram (EKG), chin EMG, leg EMG, EOG, respiratory effort, pulse oximetry, tracheal sound, and nasal and oral airflow are measured (28). Alternatively, limited channel portable (Type 3) devices record four to seven physiologic variables that at a minimum include two respiratory variables (airflow and effort), a cardiac signal (pulse or an EKG), and oxyhemoglobin saturation by pulse oximetry (29).

Traditionally, PSG is performed in an attended fashion, in a formal sleep laboratory. Because unattended, limited channel, home sleep studies are now approved for use and insurance reimbursement in the United States, they will become more common in the future (30). Although PSG may be used to investigate many causes of poor quality sleep, it is most frequently used in the diagnosis and treatment of sleep disordered breathing.

Snoring

Until recently, it was commonly assumed that snoring was a benign annoyance, not associated with negative health outcomes; however, snoring is associated with daytime sleepiness (31), pregnancy-induced hypertension, and intrauterine growth retardation (32). In children, it is associated with poor school performance (33), sleep problems such as parasomnias, and upper respiratory infections (34). Positive skin testing for common environmental allergens, asthma, and eczema correlate with an increased risk of snoring in pediatric populations (35,36).

Sleep Apnea

Definition

Sleep apnea is a broad diagnosis that includes many disorders of ventilation. Central sleep apnea (CSA) describes respiratory pauses that occur because of failure of the central nervous system to trigger a respiratory effort. Alternatively, when a respiratory effort has been triggered, but a partial or complete obstruction of the upper airway prevents ventilation, obstructive sleep apnea (OSA) is diagnosed. Sleep can also be disturbed by respiratory events during which an elevation of resistance through the upper airway impairs normal respiration requiring an increase in respiratory effort-related arousal (RERA) (37). The number of apneas plus hypopneas per hour is reported as the apnea hypopnea index (AHI), and more than five events per hour is abnormal in an adult and consistent with the diagnosis of obstructive sleep apnea syndrome (OSAS) when there are additional complaints of daytime sleepiness. Although not routinely measured or reported in most sleep labs, 10 or more RERAs per hour are associated with daytime sleepiness and are known as the upper airway resistance syndrome (UARS) (38).

How to Interpret a Sleep Study Report

With the introduction of limited channel monitoring, sleep study reports will significantly change. Although there are no published algorithms for evaluation of a PSG report, the following outlines one approach.

Table 42.3 compares the information gained or lost when a laboratory or portable device is used.

- Total Sleep Time (TST): TST is a marker of sample size and less than 2 to 4 hours of recording time is not adequate for a diagnostic study.
- Sleep Stages: Failing to display stage REM or SWS is not uncommon due to effects of medications or aging. Because sleep apnea may predominate or worsen in stage REM sleep, a study is not complete without it.
- Body Position: A complete study should include both supine and lateral sleeping positions. Supine sleep may worsen apnea, and isolated supine apnea may be treated with positional therapy alone (5).
- Sleep-Disturbed Breathing: When events occur between 5 to 15 times an hour, obstructive sleep apnea is mild, 15 to 30 times is moderate, and more than 30 is severe. Changing technologies for measuring flow may impact this standard in the future (39).
- Periodic Limb Movements (PLM): Events that occur at a rate greater than 15 per hour are significant and require further investigation (40).

TABLE 42.3   DIFFERENCES IN DATA RECORDED AND REPORTED IN LABORATORY (TYPE 1) AND PORTABLE (TYPE 3) DEVICES

	INTERPRETING A POLYSOMNOGRAM	
	LABORATORY STUDY	PORTABLE MONITOR
Time	EEG measures sleep time and more than 2 to 4 hours of time are adequate	Without EEG, total recording time is available but sleep time cannot be estimated
Stages	Sleep apnea may predominate or worsen in stage REM sleep	Some programs may estimate REM sleep, but they are not direct measurements
Position	Position data are available	Position data are unavailable
Respiratory events	Apnea hypopnea index as well as respiratory effort-related arousal events can be appreciated	Apnea hypopnea index is reported but frequency of respiratory effort-related arousals remains unreported
Limb movements	Events that occur at a rate greater than 15 per hour are significant and require further investigation	Events are not recorded
Cardiac	Arrhythmias are defined	If EKG is not utilized, heart rate but not rhythm may be reported

EEG, electroencephalography; EKG, electrocardiography; REM, rapid eye movement

- EEG: The EEG may have findings such as "alpha delta sleep" or "alpha intrusions." This pattern is associated with nonrestorative sleep; however, no specific treatments are available (41).
- Cardiac arrhythmias: Treatment of the underlying sleep-disturbed breathing is an important reason for treating apnea-associated arrhythmias (42).

Continuous Positive Airway Pressure Treatment and the Allergy Patient

Continuous positive airway pressure (CPAP) therapy acts as a pneumatic splint and is effective therapy for obstructive sleep apnea. Poor compliance has been an issue limiting the use of this otherwise successful therapy. Nasal complaints can contribute to noncompliance. Evaluation before initiating CPAP may not be helpful in these obstructive sleep apnea patients; subclinical nasal inflammation cannot be identified from clinical assessment or rhinomanometry. Nasal neutrophil counts before treatment predicts noncompliance because of nasal symptoms. There is a correlation between neutrophil counts and nasal bacterial scores, both before and after treatment with nasal CPAP (43). In an animal model, free of bacteria, the application of CPAP may increase nasal inflammation. Macrophage inflammatory protein-2 (MIP-2) is significantly overexpressed after only 3 hours of CPAP therapy. No significant changes were found in tumor necrosis factor-α, nerve growth factor, or tachykinin-1 receptor (44). Heated humidity can improve both CPAP compliance and peak nasal inspiratory flow in CPAP users who have nasal symptoms limiting therapy. The heated humidity has been successful even when nasal steroids and antihistamines have failed (45). Nasal resistance can also increase due to mouth leak. Mouth leak may be caused by nasal obstruction, ongoing apnea, or a poorly fitting mask (46). Although bacterial colonization, humidity, and mouth leak have been associated with nasal complaints and CPAP noncompliance, there have not been any trials evaluating specific interventions to address these issues. Table 42.4 contains some commonly used strategies to resolve these issues.

■ ALLERGY, ASTHMA, RHINITIS, AND SLEEP-DISORDERED BREATHING

Allergic conditions have an intricate relationship with OSA. Radioallergosorbent testing is positive in 40% of children that snore and 57% of children with sleep apnea (47). Nasal inflammation as assessed by polymorphonuclear cells, bradykinin, and vasoactive intestinal peptide is increased in nasal samples of patients with OSA who do not have allergic rhinitis (48). Mechanical nasal obstruction itself can induce nocturnal apneic events in individuals without underlying OSA (49). Patients with allergic rhinitis are more likely than

TABLE 42.4 SUGGESTED STRATEGIES TO ADDRESS SOME OF THE PUBLISHED CAUSES OF NASAL OBSTRUCTION FROM CONTINUOUS POSITIVE AIRWAY PRESSURE

Strategies to Improve CPAP Compliance by Reducing Nasal Symptoms

1. Increase humidity
   a. Increase temperature on the humidifier
   b. Add insulation to the tubing (socks, fabric, or run the tubing under blankets)
   c. Change to a device with heated tubing
2. Reduce mouth breathing
   a. Add a chin strap
   b. Change to a full face mask
   c. Consider re-titration, if mouth opening may be due to ongoing apnea
3. Reduce bacterial colonization
   a. Encourage proper care:
      i. Use of distilled water
      ii. Frequent cleaning with soap or vinegar
   b. Nasal saline lavage

CPAP, continuous positive airway pressure

matched controls to have snoring, disturbed sleep, sleep apnea, and daytime sleepiness (50). There is a two-fold increased risk of snoring in women with asthma (51). Occupational allergy to guar gum has been reported to cause both rhinitis and OSA which resolved after exposure ended (52).

OSA can complicate the management of asthma. By self-report, in a large nonselected population, asthma is associated with a 2.5-time increase in the prevalence of OSA, and patients with asthma and OSA may have more nocturnal hypoxemia than patients with OSA alone (53). Difficult-to-control asthma has been associated with OSA (54). Treatment of OSA can improve control of asthma symptoms (55,56) and reduce airway hyperreactivity as measured by methacholine responsiveness (57). One potential reason that OSA may worsen asthma is that OSA is associated with airway inflammation. Exhaled pentane and nitric oxide levels are increased after sleep in patients with moderate-to-severe OSA (58).

■ THE ALLERGY PATIENT AND INSOMNIA

Although sleep disturbance from asthma has classically been associated with daytime sleepiness, epidemiologic studies have found insomnia may be more common. In one study of patients with active asthma, 52% reported insomnia while only 22% reported daytime sleepiness.

Even when symptom free, 28% of asthmatics reported insomnia (59). Many factors such as medication side effects and psychologic factors may contribute to the persistence of insomnia. Medications used to treat asthma such as theophylline, pseudoephedrine, and corticosteroids are associated with insomnia and when combined the effect is magnified (60,61). Exploration of alternative medications or dosing regimens that avoid dosing late in the day should be first-line management. Psychophysiologic factors may perpetuate this insomnia. The hallmarks of psychophysiologic insomnia include chronic insomnia lasting over 1 month and although there may have been an initial trigger, the insomnia symptoms persist even though the inciting event has been resolved. These patients have anxiety about going to bed, but are able to fall asleep at other locations and times. Improvements in sleep hygiene along with behavioral and relaxation therapy may be helpful (see Table 42.5) (62). Short-term use of short-acting benzodiazapines can be a helpful adjunct but should be initiated with caution in the setting of theophylline which speeds their elimination (63).

■ SUMMARY

Sleep is a process that occurs as the result of the interaction between circadian rhythms and sleep homeostasis. An adequate amount of quality sleep is required for health and well-being. Complete care of the allergy patient requires attention to the commonly coexistent sleep disorders of asthma and rhinitis which impact the quality of life of both children and adults. Taking a routine sleep history that allows a patient to discuss issues of daytime sleepiness, snoring, apnea, or insomnia will

allow health care providers to coordinate care for these important issues.

■ REFERENCES

1. Aserinsky E, Kleitman N. Regularly occurring periods of eye motility, and concomitant phenomena, during sleep. *Science*. 1953;118:273–274.
2. Cutolo M, Maestroni GJ. The melatonin-cytokine connection in rheumatoid arthritis. *Ann Rheum Dis*. 2005;64:1109–1111.
3. Kapsimalis F, Richardson G, Opp MR, et al. Cytokines and normal sleep. *Curr Opin Pulm Med*. 2005;11:481–484.
4. Dement W, Kleitman N. Cyclic variations in EEG during sleep and their relation to eye movements, body motility, and dreaming. *Electroencephalogr Clin Neurophysiol*. 1957;9:673–690.
5. Silber MH, Ancoli-Israel S, Bonnet MH, et al. The visual scoring of sleep in adults. *J Clin Sleep Med*. 2007;3:121–131.
6. Holl RW, Hartman ML, Veldhuis JD, et al. Thirty-second sampling of plasma growth hormone in man: correlation with sleep stages. *J Clin Endocrinol Metab*. 1991;72:854–861.
7. Boselli M, Parrino L, Smerieri A, et al. Effect of age on EEG arousals in normal sleep. *Sleep*. 1998;21:351–357.
8. Borbely AA. A two process model of sleep regulation. *Hum Neurobiol*. 1982;1:195–204.
9. Spengler CM, Shea SA. Endogenous circadian rhythm of pulmonary function in healthy humans. *Am J Respir Crit Care Med*. 2000;162:1038–1046.
10. Burgess HJ, Trinder J, Kim Y, et al. Sleep and circadian influences on cardiac autonomic nervous system activity. *Am J Physiol*. 1997;273:H1761–H1768.
11. Koopman MG, Koomen GC, Krediet RT, et al. Circadian rhythm of glomerular filtration rate in normal individuals. *Clin Sci (Lond)*. 1989;77:105–111.
12. Takahashi JS, Hong HK, Ko CH, et al. The genetics of mammalian circadian order and disorder: implications for physiology and disease. *Nat Rev Genet*. 2008;9:764–775.
13. Borbely AA, Baumann F, Brandeis D, et al. Sleep deprivation: effect on sleep stages and EEG power density in man. *Electroencephalogr Clin Neurophysiol*. 1981;51:483–495.
14. Banks S, Dinges DF. Behavioral and physiological consequences of sleep restriction. *J Clin Sleep Med*. 2007;3:519–528.
15. Daan S, Beersma DG, Borbely AA. Timing of human sleep: recovery process gated by a circadian pacemaker. *Am J Physiol*. 1984;246:R161–R183.
16. Young MR, Matthews JP, Kanabrocki EL, et al. Circadian rhythmometry of serum interleukin-2, interleukin-10, tumor necrosis factor-alpha, and granulocyte-macrophage colony-stimulating factor in men. *Chronobiol Int*. 1995;12:19–27.
17. Hong S, Mills PJ, Loredo JS, et al. The association between interleukin-6, sleep, and demographic characteristics. *Brain Behav Immun*. 2005;19:165–172.
18. Vgontzas AN, Papanicolaou DA, Bixler EO, et al. Circadian interleukin-6 secretion and quantity and depth of sleep. *J Clin Endocrinol Metab*. 1999;84:2603–2607.
19. Born J, Lange T, Hansen K, et al. Effects of sleep and circadian rhythm on human circulating immune cells. *J Immunol*. 1997;158:4454–4464.
20. Carrillo-Vico A, Calvo JR, Abreu P, et al. Evidence of melatonin synthesis by human lymphocytes and its physiological significance: possible role as intracrine, autocrine, and/or paracrine substance. *FASEB J*. 2004;18:537–539.
21. Frey DJ, Fleshner M, Wright KP Jr. The effects of 40 hours of total sleep deprivation on inflammatory markers in healthy young adults. *Brain Behav Immun*. 2007;21:1050–1057.
22. Renegar KB, Floyd R, Krueger JM. Effect of sleep deprivation on serum influenza-specific IgG. *Sleep*. 1998;21:19–24.
23. Dimitrov S, Lange T, Nohroudi K, et al. Number and function of circulating human antigen presenting cells regulated by sleep. *Sleep*. 2007;30:401–411.
24. Bryant PA, Trinder J, Curtis N. Sick and tired: does sleep have a vital role in the immune system? *Nat Rev Immunol*. 2004;4:457–467.
25. Hui L, Hua F, Diandong H, et al. Effects of sleep and sleep deprivation on immunoglobulins and complement in humans. *Brain Behav Immun*. 2007;21:308–310.
26. Haack M, Sanchez E, Mullington JM. Elevated inflammatory markers in response to prolonged sleep restriction are associated with increased pain experience in healthy volunteers. *Sleep*. 2007;30:1145–1152.

TABLE 42.5 NONPHARMACOLOGIC THERAPY FOR INSOMNIA

Sleep Hygiene
1. Eliminate caffeine, alcohol, tobacco.
2. Quiet, dark, comfortable bedroom.
3. Regular sleep and rise times.
4. After exercising, allow several hours before bedtime.

Somatic Relaxation
1. Progressive muscle relaxation.
2. Cognitive relaxation—positive imagery.

Behavioral Therapies
1. Do not go to bed unless sleepy.
2. The bedroom should be used for sleep and sex only.
3. If laying in bed awake unable to sleep after 20 minutes, get out of bed until sleepy.
4. Avoid napping.

27. Spiegel K, Sheridan JF, Van Cauter E. Effect of sleep deprivation on response to immunization. *JAMA*. 2002;288:1471–1472.

28. Practice parameters for the indications for polysomnography and related procedures. Polysomnography Task Force, American Sleep Disorders Association Standards of Practice Committee. *Sleep*. 1997;20:406–422.

29. Collop NA. Portable monitoring for the diagnosis of obstructive sleep apnea. *Curr Opin Pulm Med*. 2008;14:525–529.

30. Collop NA, Anderson WM, Boehlecke B, et al. Clinical guidelines for the use of unattended portable monitors in the diagnosis of obstructive sleep apnea in adult patients. Portable Monitoring Task Force of the American Academy of Sleep Medicine. *J Clin Sleep Med*. 2007;3:737–747.

31. Gottlieb DJ, Yao Q, Redline S, et al. Does snoring predict sleepiness independently of apnea and hypopnea frequency? *Am J Respir Crit Care Med*. 2000;162:1512–1517.

32. Franklin KA, Holmgren PA, Jonsson F, et al. Snoring, pregnancy-induced hypertension, and growth retardation of the fetus. *Chest*. 2000;117:137–141.

33. Gozal D, Pope DW Jr. Snoring during early childhood and academic performance at ages thirteen to fourteen years. *Pediatrics*. 2001;107:1394–1399.

34. Ferreira AM, Clemente V, Gozal D, et al. Snoring in Portuguese primary school children. *Pediatrics*. 2000;106:E64.

35. Petry C, Pereira MU, Pitrez PM, et al. The prevalence of symptoms of sleep-disordered breathing in Brazilian schoolchildren. *J Pediatr (Rio J)*. 2008;84:123–129.

36. Marshall NS, Almqvist C, Grunstein RR, et al. Predictors for snoring in children with rhinitis at age 5. *Pediatr Pulmonol*. 2007;42:584–591.

37. Guilleminault C, Stoohs R, Clerk A, et al. A cause of excessive daytime sleepiness. The upper airway resistance syndrome. *Chest*. 1993;104:781–787.

38. Rees K, Kingshott RN, Wraith PK, et al. Frequency and significance of increased upper airway resistance during sleep. *Am J Respir Crit Care Med*. 2000;162:1210–1214.

39. Redline S, Budhiraja R, Kapur V, et al. The scoring of respiratory events in sleep: reliability and validity. *J Clin Sleep Med*. 2007;3:169–200.

40. Hening WA, Allen RP, Chaudhuri KR, et al. Clinical significance of RLS. *Mov Disord*. 2007;22(Suppl 18):S395–S400.

41. Moldofsky H, Scarisbrick P, England R, et al. Musculosketal symptoms and non-REM sleep disturbance in patients with "fibrositis syndrome" and healthy subjects. *Psychosom Med*. 1975;37:341–351.

42. Harbison J, O'Reilly P, McNicholas WT. Cardiac rhythm disturbances in the obstructive sleep apnea syndrome: effects of nasal continuous positive airway pressure therapy. *Chest*. 2000;118:591–595.

43. Shadan FF, Jalowayski AA, Fahrenholz J, et al. Nasal cytology: a marker of clinically silent inflammation in patients with obstructive sleep apnea and a predictor of noncompliance with nasal CPAP therapy. *J Clin Sleep Med*. 2005;1:266–270.

44. Almendros I, Acerbi I, Vilaseca I, et al. Continuous positive airway pressure (CPAP) induces early nasal inflammation. *Sleep*. 2008;31:127–131.

45. Winck JC, Delgado JL, Almeida J, et al. Heat it or wet it? Nasal symptoms secondary to the use of continuous positive airway pressure in sleep apnea. *Chest*. 2001;119:310–312.

46. Richards GN, Cistulli PA, Ungar RG, et al. Mouth leak with nasal continuous positive airway pressure increases nasal airway resistance. *Am J Respir Crit Care Med*. 1996;154:182–186.

47. McColley SA, Carroll JL, Curtis S, et al. High prevalence of allergic sensitization in children with habitual snoring and obstructive sleep apnea. *Chest*. 1997;111:170–173.

48. Rubinstein I. Nasal inflammation in patients with obstructive sleep apnea. *Laryngoscope*. 1995;105:175–177.

49. Zwillich CW, Pickett C, Hanson FN, et al. Disturbed sleep and prolonged apnea during nasal obstruction in normal men. *Am Rev Respir Dis*. 1981;124:158–160.

50. Young T, Finn L, Kim H. Nasal obstruction as a risk factor for sleep-disordered breathing. The University of Wisconsin Sleep and Respiratory Research Group. *J Allergy Clin Immunol*. 1997;99: S757–S762.

51. Kalra M, Biagini J, Bernstein D, et al. Effect of asthma on the risk of obstructive sleep apnea syndrome in atopic women. *Ann Allergy Asthma Immunol*. 2006;97:231–235.

52. Leznoff A, Haight JS, Hoffstein V. Reversible obstructive sleep apnea caused by occupational exposure to guar gum dust. *Am Rev Respir Dis*. 1986;133:935–936.

53. Hudgel DW, Shucard DW. Coexistence of sleep apnea and asthma resulting in severe sleep hypoxemia. *JAMA*. 1979;242:2789–790.

54. ten Brinke A, Sterk PJ, Masclee AA, et al. Risk factors of frequent exacerbations in difficult-to-treat asthma. *Eur Respir J*. 2005;26: 812–818.

55. Chan CS, Woolcock AJ, Sullivan CE. Nocturnal asthma: role of snoring and obstructive sleep apnea. *Am Rev Respir Dis*. 1988;137: 1502–1504.

56. Ciftci TU, Ciftci B, Guven SF, et al. Effect of nasal continuous positive airway pressure in uncontrolled nocturnal asthmatic patients with obstructive sleep apnea syndrome. *Respir Med*. 2005;99:529–534.

57. Lin CC, Lin CY. Obstructive sleep apnea syndrome and bronchial hyperreactivity. *Lung*. 1995;173:117–126.

58. Olopade CO, Christon JA, Zakkar M, et al. Exhaled pentane and nitric oxide levels in patients with obstructive sleep apnea. *Chest*. 1997;111:1500–1504.

59. Klink ME, Dodge R, Quan SF. The relation of sleep complaints to respiratory symptoms in a general population. *Chest*. 1994;105: 151–154.

60. Bailey WC, Richards JM Jr., Manzella BA, et al. Characteristics and correlates of asthma in a university clinic population. *Chest*. 1990;98:821–828.

61. Weinberger M, Bronsky E, Bensch GW, et al. Interaction of ephedrine and theophylline. *Clin Pharmacol Ther*. 1975;17:585–592.

62. Rakel ER, McCall WV. *A Practical Guide to Insomnia*. Minneapolis, MN: McGraw-Hill Healthcare Information;1999.

63. Henauer SA, Hollister LE, Gillespie HK, et al. Theophylline antagonizes diazepam-induced psychomotor impairment. *Eur J Clin Pharmacol*. 1983;25:743–747.

CHAPTER 43

Management of the Psychologically Complicated Patient

MICHAEL S. ZIFFRA AND JACKIE K. GOLLAN

Psychiatric and psychosocial issues complicate management of medical illness, with allergic diseases being no exception. The presence of concurrent psychiatric diagnoses or more enduring maladaptive personality traits can interfere with the physician–patient relationship and patient adherence to medical care. Even normal, expected reactions to acute and chronic medical illness can create distress and hinder care.

Who is the *psychologically* complicated patient? This term can apply to patients with a significant psychiatric illness, such as depression, bipolar disorder, or anxiety disorder. This term may also refer to individuals with problems such as substance overuse, personality disorders, and nonadherence with medical treatment. Physicians treating such patients must invest greater-than-usual amounts of time and effort to optimally manage their medical and psychiatric issues.

Balancing concurrent psychiatric and allergic diseases is challenging for patients and their health care providers. Many physicians feel they do not have sufficient experience and skill to manage these types of issues, potentially making them feel powerless or guilty about their inability to help the patient. It is essential, therefore, that all physicians develop a basic understanding of major psychiatric illnesses and clinically relevant psychosocial issues. Being able to work with psychiatrically complicated patients in an empathic manner not only leads to more compassionate care, but also enhances effective management of the primary medical diagnosis.

This chapter will highlight the clinical advances in treating individuals with allergies and comorbid psychiatric conditions, with discussion of common psychiatric disorders, treatment approaches, and clinical challenges requiring attention to promote clinical effectiveness. Common psychiatric diagnoses and other psychosocial barriers to care will first be outlined, followed by a discussion of effective, evidence-based treatments and their practical administration.

■ MOOD DISORDERS

According to the *Diagnostic and Statistical Manual of Mental Disorders* (DSM-IV) (1), a major depressive episode is defined as a period lasting 2 weeks or more of predominantly depressed mood, accompanied by other symptoms (see Table 43.1). The diagnosis of major depressive disorder (MDD) is given to an individual who has had one or more major depressive episodes (and does not meet diagnostic criteria for bipolar disorder). A devastating and recurrent disease, MDD will emerge as the second leading cause of worldwide disability by 2020 (2). Up to 20% of the general population is expected to experience major depression at least once during their lifetime. These statistics may underestimate the true prevalence of depression, since symptom complaints are often disregarded or misdiagnosed, particularly among primary care and geriatric populations (3). Also, depression recurs over the lifespan (4). Specifically, the Agency for Health Care Policy and Research has noted that the risk of recurrence increases exponentially with each successive episode. Even after treatment, 40% of patients with a history of three or more depressive episodes are likely to relapse within 7 weeks after recovery (5). Given the prevalence and chronicity of depression, innumerable people face the prospect of a lifetime struggle with depression.

MDD is more prevalent among individuals with many types of chronic illness, including hypertension, congestive heart failure, diabetes mellitus, coronary artery disease, chronic obstructive pulmonary disease, stroke, and end-stage renal disease. Depression in chronic illness has been associated with greater

TABLE 43.1   SYMPTOMS OF MAJOR DEPRESSION

- Depressed mood
- Lack of interest/pleasure
- Changes in appetite and weight
- Insomnia or hypersomnia
- Psychomotor agitation or retardation
- Fatigue
- Impaired concentration
- Feelings of worthlessness, shame, or guilt
- Thoughts about death or suicide

Adapted from American Psychiatric Association. *Diagnostic and Statistical Manual of Mental Disorders*. 4th ed., Text Revision. Washington, DC: American Psychiatric Association, 2000.

TABLE 43.2   SYMPTOMS OF MANIA

- Elevated or irritable mood
- Grandiosity
- Decreased need for sleep
- Pressured speech
- Racing thoughts
- Distractibility
- Agitation
- Impulsivity

Adapted from American Psychiatric Association. *Diagnostic and Statistical Manual of Mental Disorders*. 4th ed., Text Revision. Washington, DC: American Psychiatric Association, 2000.

symptom burden and functional impairment, higher rates of morbidity and mortality, and decreased treatment adherence. It also results in decreased productivity and greater health resource utilization (6,7).

A significant association between depression and allergic disorders has been observed. Depressed patients have higher rates of atopic illness than nondepressed individuals (8–10). Meanwhile, allergic disease may increase the risk for depression threefold (8). Psychiatric disorders are more prevalent in patients with asthma and other allergic diseases. Also, evidence has shown a correlation between the severity of depressive symptoms and that of allergic symptoms (9).

The reasons for this relationship are not completely understood and are likely very complex. Depression is associated with changes in functioning of the immune system, which could predispose individuals to atopic illness. Cytokines, leukotrienes, and other substances released during allergic reactions may have effects on neurotransmitter activity involved in the regulation of mood. Dysfunction of the hypothalamic-pituitary-adrenal axis and alterations in fatty acid metabolism are believed to occur in both depression and allergic disease (8–10). Interestingly, twin studies have suggested that the two types of illness may have a common genetic cause (8–10). Thus, the higher prevalence of depression in patients with atopic illnesses, as well as its potential effects on the severity of allergic symptoms, underscore the need for allergist-immunologists to recognize depressive disorders in their patients to ensure they receive appropriate treatment (11).

Bipolar disorder is another serious mood disorder associated with significant disability. It is characterized by the presence of both major depressive episodes and episodes of mania or hypomania. Mania is defined as a period of excessively elevated or excited mood, typically accompanied by increased energy, anger, irritability, and impulsivity. Key signs and symptoms of mania are

listed in Table 43.2. Hypomanic episodes are characterized by these same symptoms, but they are less severe and shorter in duration.

Though mood disorders can be quite disabling, they are also treatable. For this reason, it is important that treatment be initiated as soon as the disorder is identified, and sustained until remission is achieved. Increasingly, primary care physicians and other nonpsychiatrists are treating depression in their patients, typically by prescribing antidepressant medications. This practice is reasonable for patients who are reluctant to accept a referral to a mental health specialist and whose depression is not severe.

Patients with symptoms indicative of severe depression are best referred to a psychiatrist. Such symptoms include active suicidal ideation, psychotic symptoms such as hallucinations and delusions, prominent agitation or volatility, and significant decline in functioning. Other situations that warrant psychiatric consultation include treatment-resistant depression (which can be defined as failure to adequately respond to three or more antidepressants), suspicion for bipolar disorder, complicated psychiatric comorbidity, complex psychopharmacologic regimens, and concomitant substance abuse (12).

Psychotherapy is beneficial in the treatment of mood disorders, and it can be effective as the sole treatment for depressive episodes of mild-to-moderate severity. There are empirical data supporting the use of some types of psychotherapy, including cognitive-behavioral therapy and interpersonal therapy, in the treatment of depression. More severe depressions typically require a combination of concurrent psychotherapy and medication.

Bipolar disorder is best managed by mental health specialists, given the complex nature of the disease and the medications used to treat it. A variety of pharmacologic agents are used to treat bipolar disorder, including lithium, mood-stabilizing anticonvulsants, antipsychotics, and antianxiety medications.

Psychotherapy is also a key component of bipolar disorder treatment.

ANXIETY DISORDERS

Anxiety disorders are also frequently encountered in general and specialty medical practices. Like depression, anxiety disorders are highly comorbid with many types of medical illness, and they are associated with higher rates of morbidity and mortality, health care utilization, and functional disability (13). Several distinct anxiety disorders have been described in the medical literature. Among these are social phobia, an excessive fear of being scrutinized or embarrassed in social situations; obsessive-compulsive disorder, characterized by recurrent, intrusive thoughts and/or rituals and repetitive behaviors; and post-traumatic stress disorder (PTSD), in which individuals experience a number of anxiety symptoms following a life-threatening trauma (1).

There are two anxiety disorders, panic disorder and generalized anxiety disorder (GAD), that merit particular mention, given their high prevalence and the frequency with which they are encountered by nonpsychiatrists. A panic attack is an episode of intense anxiety that develops and resolves over a brief period of time and is accompanied by a number of somatic and psychologic symptoms. These symptoms can include palpitations, chest pain, shortness of breath, nausea, trembling, dizziness, and paresthesias. Because panic attacks are characterized by intense fear and uncomfortable physical symptoms, individuals in the midst of an attack may worry that they are having a heart attack or even close to dying. This may lead to their seeking medical attention (14).

Panic attacks can occur as part of many anxiety disorders. Panic disorder is specifically defined as a pattern of recurrent, unexpected panic attacks. This is accompanied by at least 1 month of the patient worrying about future attacks or changing his or her behavior because of the attacks. Panic attacks can be accompanied by agoraphobia, which is a fear of places in which escape or help might not be available if an attack were to occur (such as being on a bus or plane, or in a large crowd).

GAD, meanwhile, is characterized by uncontrollable worry about multiple topics, such as work, family, money, etc. This worry is accompanied by at least three additional physical or psychological symptoms, which include fatigue, sleep disturbance, muscle tension, restlessness, difficulty concentrating, and irritability. Just as with panic disorder, the presence of somatic symptoms in GAD may prompt patients to seek medical attention (15).

As is the case with depression, anxiety is often treated directly by patients' primary care physicians, and sometimes this can be appropriate in cases of mild-to-moderate anxiety. Most antidepressants are quite effective for treating anxiety (bupropion being a notable exception), and they actually are first-line agents for most anxiety disorders. Benzodiazepines are also commonly used, often in conjunction with an antidepressant.

Many patients with anxiety disorders, however, require treatment by a mental health specialist. Examples include patients with more serious symptoms, for example, patients whose fear of panic attacks is so severe that they rarely leave their home or avoid important activities or obligations. Other situations that would necessitate psychiatric referrals include treatment-resistant anxiety, comorbid psychiatric illness, and concomitant substance abuse. Also, obsessive-compulsive disorder and PTSD are two particularly challenging diagnoses that are best treated by mental health specialists.

Psychotherapy also plays a prominent role in the management of anxiety disorders. Many anxiety disorders of mild-to-moderate severity are very amenable to treatment with psychotherapy alone. Severe or treatment-resistant anxiety disorders are often best managed through a combination of medication and psychotherapy.

Of note, a significant correlation between anxiety and allergic disorders has been described in the literature (16–19). Anxiety is actually the most common psychiatric diagnosis in patients with allergies. The association between panic disorder and atopic illnesses, especially asthma, is particularly strong (16). Furthermore, in a series of male twins who were Vietnam War veterans, compared to subjects without asthma, the subjects with asthma had higher symptom scores on an instrument used to measure severity of PTSD (19). In veterans with mild PTSD, the prevalence of asthma was 4% compared to 7% in those veterans who had the highest scores on the PTSD instrument (19).

The reason for this correlation is unclear, and the causation may actually be bidirectional. Both acute allergic events and chronic allergic disease can be stressful, contributing to anxiety. Via classical conditioning, patients can become excessively fearful of those stimuli that cause allergic reactions. Meanwhile, anxiety can often precede (and thus possibly precipitate) allergic exacerbations, and allergic patients with anxiety have more severe physical complaints and use more medical care (17). Interestingly, there is evidence that abnormalities in the brain that contribute to anxiety may also predispose to allergic disease by disrupting the central nervous system's (CNS) regulation of the immune system (16). From these data, therefore, it seems reasonable to conclude that optimizing management of anxiety symptoms can improve allergic symptoms, and vice versa.

SOMATOFORM DISORDERS

Somatoform disorders are characterized by patients' preoccupation with physical symptoms and medical illness that cannot be fully explained by a general medical condition. Because of this, these disorders are frequently encountered by nonpsychiatrists, though they may not initially be recognized as such. Somatization and hypochondriasis are two commonly seen somatoform disorders.

Somatization occurs when a patient experiences somatic complaints that have no direct physiological cause. Psychological factors are assumed to be involved in the development and maintenance of the physical symptoms; however, the patient typically is unaware of this, and the symptoms are not consciously manufactured or feigned (20).

Patients with hypochondriasis also experience somatic complaints that are concerning to them. However, in contrast with somatization, in hypochondriasis these symptoms do in fact have some physiologic basis. Their "symptoms" are normal bodily functions and reactions that are misperceived as being signs of a serious medical illness. Hypochondriacal patients can be plagued with worry about their possibly having a dangerous disease. Even when their health care providers produce evidence of their good health, they are rarely reassured (21).

Patients with somatization and hypochondriasis usually seek medical attention to diagnose and treat their unexplained symptoms. They are typically concerned about their perceived illness, and they may become increasingly frustrated as physical exams and laboratory studies fail to reveal any identifiable medical condition. These patients can often end up seeing multiple specialists and receiving numerous expensive procedures. This experience can be just as frustrating for the physician. Feelings of incompetence, failure, and guilt can be evoked due to the inability to treat the patient's complaints and allay their worries. In cases in which the patient demands multiple visits, referrals, and studies, the physician may become angry and resentful toward the patient.

Notably, before a diagnosis of somatization or hypochondriasis is issued, a thorough investigation should occur to rule out organic medical illness. The medical literature is replete with stories of patients who were initially dismissed as being a "somatizer" or "hypochondriac" and later were found to have a genuine biological disease. Unfortunately, patients with a history of comorbid psychiatric illness in particular can be too quickly judged to have psychosomatic illness. Though a "million-dollar workup" is generally not indicated for every patient with unexplained or unusual complaints, a reasonable effort must be made to rule out likely medical causes for the patient's symptoms.

Clinical management of somatization and hypochondriasis is very similar (20,21). Mental health referral is typically helpful. Liaison with mental health specialists can also help the primary care providers appropriately understand and manage their patients.

Also, as depression and anxiety disorders are common in patients with somatoform disorders, and a psychiatrist can evaluate for, and treat, any such comorbid psychiatric illnesses. Medication helps to manage comorbid depression and anxiety, though there is less evidence that it treats somatoform disorders directly. Psychotherapy appears to be a more effective modality for treating somatization and hypochondriasis. Evidence supports the use of psychotherapeutic interventions that teach patients to cope with their physical symptoms and medical concerns in a less maladaptive manner.

Some patients may resist referral to mental health specialists, for a variety of reasons. They may see such a referral as a message that their primary treater is abandoning them, or that their problems are considered to be "all in their heads." The physician must reassure the patient that neither of these is true. Patients may be more amenable to a mental health referral if it is presented as a supplement to their existing medical treatment, or as a treatment to reduce "stress" that may be impacting on their physical complaints.

Even when psychiatric consultation is obtained, it is still necessary for the referring medical health care provider to continue to meet with the patient. In fact, denying further visits may produce a sense of abandonment, further exacerbating patients' anxiety, ultimately leading them to seek out regular medical care again. It is recommended that frequent, brief "check in" appointments be scheduled, regardless of how the patient is feeling. Such an arrangement can be reassuring to patients, even though no additional medical investigation or treatment is being performed. "As needed" visits and telephone calls should be minimized, as they can reinforce patients' maladaptive behaviors.

■ SUBSTANCE ABUSE

Substance abuse is the overuse of, and reliance on, a drug or chemical that produces specific responses that are deleterious to the well-being of the individual or others. These conditions are typically characterized by a pattern of use of a substance (medication, alcohol, drug, or toxin) that generates recurrent problems in social, occupational, academic, and personal functioning. Overuse and dependence are difficult to determine, though consideration of the DSM-IV diagnostic criteria clarify the degree of impact of use (e.g., abuse is characterized by social impairment; dependence includes behavioral and physiologic reliance, exhibited by physiologic withdrawal) (1). Patients with addiction problems may be less likely to adhere to recommended medical treatments, due to the large amount of time spent using substances and recovering from their effects. They may also avoid meeting with their physicians, due to feelings of guilt or shame, or out of fears of their addictions being discovered.

When physicians learn that a patient is actively abusing drugs or alcohol, they must remember that the patient is not necessarily ready to seek treatment for it, even if the substance use is voluntarily disclosed. The patient's readiness for change must be gauged in a non-confrontational manner, using questions that promote motivation to change (22). If the patient expresses reluctance to seek treatment, the physician should empathically explore his or her resistance. Questioning the patient aggressively and making ultimatums are likely to be counterproductive. Pointing out objective facts about the adverse consequences of the patient's substance use (such as medical problems and interpersonal difficulties) can help give him or her motivation to change. Often this process requires several conversations over multiple visits.

Once the patient expresses a desire to change, the physician must help him or her establish treatment in an appropriate setting. Patients who are at risk for complicated withdrawal—which includes those who are medically compromised and those withdrawing from alcohol, sedatives, or opiates—may need inpatient hospitalization for detoxification. Also, patients with significant active psychiatric issues (such as severe depression or suicidality) may require admission to an inpatient psychiatric unit. Other levels of care include residential treatment settings, day hospital programs, and outpatient treatment (23).

Consultation with a psychiatrist or psychologist, ideally one who specializes in addictions, may help the primary care physician refer the patient to an appropriate treatment setting. These professionals can also help to diagnose and manage any comorbid psychiatric illnesses that may be present. Ongoing mental health treatment will be necessary after any acute intervention, and participation in groups that help to maintain sobriety (such as Alcoholics Anonymous and other 12-step groups) is strongly encouraged.

■ PERSONALITY DISORDERS

The DSM-IV defines a personality disorder as "an enduring pattern of inner experience and behavior that deviates markedly from the expectations of the individual's culture" resulting in distress and social interference (1). Identifying personality disorders is particularly meaningful for medical staff working with allergy patients, as these mental disorders influence cognition, affectivity, social functioning, and impulse control. The 10 classified personality disorders in the DSM-IV are grouped into three clusters based on their prominent characteristics: cluster A, the odd or eccentric (paranoid, schizoid, schizotypal); cluster B, the dramatic, emotional, or erratic (antisocial, borderline, histrionic, narcissistic); and cluster C, the anxious or fearful (avoidant, dependent, obsessive-compulsive). The prevalence of personality disorders in the general population is 10% to 12%, though many more individuals exhibit maladaptive personality traits insufficient to merit a diagnosis of a personality disorder. These disorders are highly associated with Axis I psychiatric illness, including depression, anxiety, and substance abuse and dependence, as well as higher health care utilization (24).

We direct the interested reader to several excellent reviews for helpful treatment and management strategies for individuals with personality disorders (25,26). Generally, health care providers should, initially, construct and evaluate a differential diagnosis to ensure that patients' symptoms are unrelated to use of substances or medications, CNS disorders, or other medical problems. Then physicians should consider referral for their patients to meet with a psychologist or psychiatrist to generate a tailored treatment plan for careful and effective management of symptoms concurrent with the treatment of atopic conditions. This is essential when health care providers encounter difficulty sustaining their usual empathic neutrality and involvement, professional and personal boundaries, and interpersonal demeanor with patients and their families.

■ NONADHERENCE

Nonadherence is a significant problem, with as many as 50% of patients with persistent asthma not properly adhering to recommended pharmacologic treatments (27). Table 43.3 lists common problems that contribute to nonadherence and how they can be addressed (27–30). Many barriers to adherence are connected to problems in the delivery of care by individual physicians or the health care system as a whole. Other barriers relate to patient factors such as treatment resistance.

Treatment resistance is characterized by dimensions related to patients (e.g., behavior, thinking, and social interaction) that interfere with their abilities to utilize the treatment and learn how to handle their disease and its implications. This may manifest itself as premature termination of medical care, noncompliance with the treatment regimen, a slow learning curve, or an unequal or imbalanced therapeutic alliance. Behavioral interventions include providing psychoeducation (to eliminate treatment myths and increase realistic expectations), evaluating medication compliance between sessions, slowly integrating the assigned treatment regimen (which reduces the patient's sense of helplessness), and increasing contingencies via providing praising statements after specific behaviors. Additional strategies to address resistance include organizing the session using an agenda, making sure that the patient and physician are working collaboratively (with consistent provision of empathy, collaboration, and validation), identifying and modifying self-limiting beliefs that interfere with treatment, and responding to patients' pathological

TABLE 43.3   COMMON CAUSES OF AND REMEDIES FOR NONADHERENCE

PROBLEM	POSSIBLE SOLUTIONS
Complex medication regimen	Reduce number of medications taken. Switch to once-daily dosing. Provide clearly written instructions.
Patient forgetfulness	Provide written and telephone reminders. Instruct patient to use a pillbox. Use more convenient packaging (such as prepared blister packs).
Medication side effects	Switch to drug with fewer side effects. Add agents to treat side effects. Inquire about and address excessive worries about potential side effects.
Cost concerns	Switch to less expensive agent. Connect patient with financial assistance programs.
Language barriers	Use interpreter during visits. Provide written information in patient's primary language.
Poor understanding of disease and/or need for medication	Actively inquire about and explore patients' beliefs about their illness. Address patients' denial of severity of illness and/or concern about taking medication. Provide written educational material.
Poor relationship with physician	Engage actively with patients (ask/answer questions, provide feedback). Ensure accessibility between visits. Increase duration and/or frequency of visits. Have patient see same physician at each visit.
Patients' difficulty in making or keeping follow-up appointments	Use written/phone reminders. Assist with transportation, parking. Offer convenient clinic hours. Minimize long waits for visits.

strategies to elicit validation (such as escalating the intensity of symptom complaints or devaluing the medical provider).

■ PHARMACOLOGIC INTERVENTIONS

As noted previously, antidepressants and other psychoactive medications are commonly prescribed by physicians with minimal psychiatric training. Therefore, it is essential for clinicians to be familiar with the basic principles behind these agents' use (31). The selective serotonin reuptake inhibitors (SSRIs) are among the most commonly prescribed antidepressants. This class of antidepressants, which includes fluoxetine, paroxetine, sertraline, citalopram, and escitalopram, is effective in treating depression and anxiety and has a favorable side effect profile. The SSRIs tend to not cause serious drug interactions, though fluoxetine, paroxetine, and

sertraline have the potential to cause some interactions via action at the hepatic P450 system.

Other newer antidepressants commonly prescribed include venlafaxine, duloxetine, bupropion, and mirtazapine. Like the SSRIs, they are all considered to be efficacious and relatively safe agents, though each has a unique mechanism of action and side effect profile.

Tricyclic antidepressants (TCAs) and monoamine oxidase inhibitors (MAOIs) are older classes of antidepressants that are used less frequently, though they can be effective medications in patients with treatment-resistant depression. The primary reason for their less frequent use is their potential to cause more severe side effects and more dangerous drug interactions. Thus, these agents are best prescribed by clinicians who are familiar with their use and aware of the potential for adverse events.

After prescribing an antidepressant, it is important to schedule regular follow-up. This step is necessary to ensure that patients are responding to treatment and to make any necessary adjustments. Regular follow-up also enables the physician to quickly identify and address any adverse side effects. For example, antidepressants can trigger agitation or mania in patients with undiagnosed bipolar disorder. Therefore, it is crucial to screen for bipolar disorder before prescribing an antidepressant.

Regarding the use of these medications in patients with atopic illness, most of them are safe and well tolerated. An exception is MAOIs. In conjunction with the administration of sympathomimetics like epinephrine, hypertensive crisis has been reported. Before prescribing any medication, the potential for drug interactions must be considered. In those who are significantly medically compromised or are taking several other medications, the TCAs and MAOIs may be best avoided.

As mentioned previously, benzodiazepines are commonly used antianxiety agents, and unlike antidepressants, they have the benefit of producing immediate effect. Because of the risk for tolerance and dependence, these medications should be used judiciously. Using the smallest amount necessary for the shortest amount of time necessary is a wise practice.

Although the most commonly prescribed psychoactive medications are unlikely to exacerbate allergic diseases, several medications used to treat allergic disorders can worsen psychiatric disorders. Allergists thus need to be aware of these potential reactions in patients with comorbid psychiatric illness.

Corticosteroids are particularly notorious for the potential to cause neuropsychiatric side effects. Such effects can manifest in multiple ways, including mania, depression, memory impairment, delirium, and psychosis. The risk for these adverse events is dose-dependent, with those patients taking less than 40 mg/day at minimal risk, and those receiving 80 mg/day at significant risk. The most effective management of these side effects is to lower the dose of the corticosteroid, or discontinue it completely. As this approach may not be feasible, addition of a psychoactive medication (the particular medication depending on the specific type of side effect) can be helpful (33).

β-Adrenergic agonists used in the treatment of asthma can produce several physiologic effects shared with panic attacks, including elevated heart rate, palpitations, tremor, and CNS stimulation. Thus, among patients prescribed such medications, those with preexisting panic attacks may experience worsened anxiety symptoms, and those without may report panic-like episodes. If avoiding β agonists is impractical, patients may benefit from a mental health referral to help manage their anxiety symptoms (34).

Both prescription and over-the-counter antihistamines are used to treat a variety of illnesses and are in general quite safe. Because of the potential for sedation, primarily from first-generation antihistamines, they should be used with caution when combined with sedating psychoactive medications such as benzodiazepines. In addition, first-generation antihistamines have the potential to cause delirium, which is generally attributable to their anticholinergic effects. Thus these medications should be used judiciously in older patients and others whose illnesses and pharmacologic regimens may predispose them to delirium. Second- and third-generation antihistamines that do not cross the blood–brain barrier are much less likely to produce these adverse events (34).

■ COGNITIVE AND BEHAVIORAL THEORIES AND THERAPIES

Evidence-based psychotherapy, specifically cognitive and behavioral therapies, assist in the management and treatment of psychiatric issues among patients presenting with allergic conditions. These approaches underwent intense empirical scrutiny in the 1980s, and the application of these models is producing a variety of effective psychosocial treatments (e.g., psychological therapies with demonstrated efficacy in comparison to pill placebos or active medications). Such empirically-validated approaches to psychotherapy are exemplified by cutting-edge therapies for depression, anxiety disorders, eating disorders, personality disorders, and substance use disorders (35).

Behavioral psychotherapy focuses on changing behavior by helping individuals "unlearn" previously acquired associations that linked stimuli and maladaptive behaviors. This type of therapy is especially indicated for the treatment of anxiety disorders. Effective treatment of anxiety includes, initially, anxiety management techniques, including breathing retraining and progressive muscle relaxation, followed by exposure and response prevention (e.g., step-wise introduction to feared situations that rely on habituation and systematic desensitization). Behavioral therapy is also used to modify behaviors by conditioning them with negative or positive feedback. The targeted application of positive feedback from a physician, for example, is an effective strategy for enhancing treatment compliance. Exemplar techniques include modifying behavior with contingency contracts (e.g., formal written agreements between two individuals that outline the behaviors that are to be modified and the rewards that follow the performance of those behaviors).

Cognitive psychotherapy focuses on conscious thought processes. It is primarily based on two principles: first, cognitive processes are a primary determinant of behavior; and second, cognitive restructuring (i.e., modifying assumptions and beliefs) may produce behavioral and emotional change and alleviate illness. The cognitive model views psychiatric symptoms as being produced by inappropriate patterns of thought or

TABLE 43.4   COGNITIVE DISTORTIONS IN DEPRESSION

DISTORTION	DESCRIPTION
All-or-nothing thinking	Seeing things in black-and-white categories. If performance or situation is less than expected, then it is perceived as a total failure, unacceptable, etc.
Overgeneralization	Seeing a single negative event, no matter how minor, as part of a never-ending pattern of defeat.
Mental filter	Exclusively focusing on one negative to the exclusion of others so that your vision of reality becomes entirely centered on this one issue.
Disqualifying the positive	Rejecting positive experiences by insisting that they do not count for some reason or another. You can then maintain a consistent negative self-bias even though everyday experiences contradict your perception.
Jumping to conclusions	Making a negative interpretation even through there are no definite facts that convincingly support the conclusion.
(a) Mind-reading	Creating arbitrary conclusions that people, situations, and things are reacting to you negatively.
(b) Fortune-telling error	Anticipating that situations will not turn out well, you feel convinced that your prediction is already an established fact.
Magnification	Exaggerating the importance or relevance of things (such as failure, incompletion, another person's achievements).
Catastrophizing	Amplifying the consequences of ambiguous or negative events or situations.
Minimization	Inappropriately reducing your (or someone else's) skills and strengths until they are negligible factors.
Emotional reasoning	Issuing greater importance to negative feelings than is realistic: "I feel bad, therefore it must be true."
Should statements	Statements about self and others that reflect expectations of behavior or situations ("I *should* be more competent; I *need* to be happy all the time"). Should statements directed at the self usually produce feelings of guilt. Similar statements directed at others often generate feelings of anger and resentment.
Labeling and mislabeling	An extreme form of overgeneralization. Rather than describing the situation, labels are assigned to the person or self ("I am a terrible person not worthy of love from another"). This often includes using colorful language expressing strong emotions.
Personalization	Viewing yourself as the origin or cause of a problem. Assuming someone's opinion is more valuable or more correct than your own.

cognitive distortions. For example, most depressed people automatically interpret situations in negative ways (refer to Table 43.4 for examples). If individuals recognize and change these illogical thought patterns, symptoms improve. Cognitive psychotherapy is indicated for depressed or anxious patients who demonstrate the ability for self-insight. Cognitive-behavioral therapy is time-limited, generally occurring weekly, and it follows specific published protocols (36).

■ CONCLUSIONS

Empirical research and clinical management of psychiatric conditions among allergy patients have dramatically advanced in the past decade. A variety of effective pharmacologic and psychotherapeutic interventions are available for treatment of the many psychiatric illnesses seen in individuals with atopic diseases. With more recent attention to clinical demands for responsiveness, the treatment of mental illness is beginning to close the gulf between research and clinical practice.

■ REFERENCES

1. American Psychiatric Association. *Diagnostic and Statistical Manual of Mental Disorders*. 4th ed., Text Revision. Washington, DC: American Psychiatric Association; 2000.
2. Murray CJL, Lopez AD, eds. *The Global Burden of Disease. A Comprehensive Assessment of Mortality and Disability from Diseases, Injuries and Risk Factors in 1990 and Projected to 2020*. Cambridge, MA: Harvard School of Public Health on behalf of the World Health Organization and the World Bank; 1996.
3. Wells KB, Burnam MA, Rogers W, et al. The course of depression in adult outpatients. Results from the Medical Outcomes Study. *Arch Gen Psychiatry*. 1992;49:788–794.

4. Thase ME. Long-term treatments of recurrent depressive disorders. *J Clin Psychiatry*. 1992;53 (Suppl):32–44.

5. Jarrett RB, Kraft D, Doyle J, et al. Preventing recurrent depression using cognitive therapy with and without a continuation phase. A randomized clinical trial. *Arch Gen Psychiatry*. 2001;58:381–388.

6. Egede LE. Major depression in individuals with chronic medical disorders: prevalence, correlates and association with health resource utilization, lost productivity and functional disability. *Gen Hosp Psychiatry*. 2007;29:409–416.

7. Katon WJ. Clinical and health services relationships between major depression, depressive symptoms, and general medical illness. *Biol Psychiatry*. 2003;54:216–226.

8. Timonen M, Jokelainen J, Herva A, et al. Presence of atopy in first-degree relatives as a predictor of a female proband's depression: results from the Northern Finland 1966 Birth Cohort. *J Allergy Clin Immunol*. 2003;111:1249–1254.

9. Kovacs M, Stauder A, Szedmak S. Severity of allergic complaints: the importance of depressed mood. *J Psychosom Res*. 2003;54:549–557.

10. Wamboldt MZ, Hewitt JK, Schmitz S, et al. Familial association between allergic disorders and depression in adult Finnish twins. *Am J Medi Genet*. 2000;96:146–153.

11. Kuehn BM. Asthma linked to psychiatric disorders. *JAMA*. 2008;299:158–160.

12. Ziffra MS, Gilmer WS. STAR*D: lessons learned for primary care. *Primary Psychiatry*. 2007;14:51-58.

13. Scott KM, Bruffaerts R, Tsang A, et al. Depression-anxiety relationships with chronic physical conditions: results from the World Mental Health Surveys. *J Affect Disord*. 2007;103:113–120.

14. Katon WJ. Panic Disorder. *N Engl J Med*. 2006;354:2360–2367.

15. Allgulander, C. Generalized anxiety disorder: what are we missing? *Eur Neuropsychopharmacol*. 2006;16:S101–S108.

16. Kovalenko PA, Hoven CW, Wu P, et al. Association between allergy and anxiety disorders in youth. *AustN Z J Psychiatry*. 2001;35: 815–821.

17. Stauder A, Kovacs M. Anxiety symptoms in allergic patients: identification and risk factors. *Psychosom Med*. 2003;65:816–823.

18. Hashizume H, Takigawa M. Anxiety in allergy and atopic dermatitis. *Curr Opin Allergy Clin Immunol*. 2006;6:335–339.

19. Goodwin RD, Fischer ME, Goldberg J. A twin study of post-traumatic stress disorder symptoms and asthma. *Am J Respir Crit Care Med*. 2007;176:983–987.

20. Mai F. Somatization disorder: a practical review. *Can J Psychiatry*. 2004;49:652–661.

21. Barsky AJ. The patient with hypochondriasis. *N Engl J Med*. 2001;345:1395–1399.

22. Miller WR, Rollnick S. *Motivational Interviewing: Preparing People for Change*. 2nd ed. New York: Guilford Press; 2002.

23. Weaver MF, Jarvis MAE, Schnoll SH. Role of the primary care physician in problems of substance abuse. *Arch Intern Med*. 1999;159:913–924.

24. Dhossche DM, Shevitz SA. Assessment and importance of personality disorders in medical patients: an update. *South Med J*. 1999;92:546–556.

25. Oldham JM, Skodol AE, Bender DS, eds. *The American Psychiatric Publishing Textbook of Personality Disorders*. Arlington, VA: American Psychiatric Publishing; 2005.

26. Gunderson JG, Gabbard GO, eds. *Psychotherapy for Personality Disorders*, Washington, DC: American Psychiatric Press; 2000.

27. Cochrane GM, Horne R, Chanez P. Compliance in asthma. *Respir Med*. 1999;93:763–769.

28. Osterberg L, Blaschke T. Adherence to medication. *N Engl J Med*. 2005:353;487–497.

29. Bender BG. Overcoming barriers to nonadherence in asthma treatment. *J Allergy Clin Immunol*. 2002;109:S554–S559.

30. Vermeire E, Hearnshaw H, Van Royen P, et al. Patient adherence to treatment: three decades of research. A comprehensive review. *J Clin Pharm Ther*. 2001;26:331–342.

31. Schatzberg AF, Cole JO, DeBattista C. *Manual of Clinical Psychopharmacology*. 6th ed. Arlington,VA: American Psychiatric Publishing, Inc.; 2007.

32. Nieuwstraten C, Labiris NR, Holbrook A. Systematic overview of drug interactions with antidepressant medication. *Can J Psychiatry*. 2006 51:300–316.

33. Warrington TP, Bostwick JM. Psychiatric adverse effects of corticosteroids. *Mayo Clin Proc*. 2006;81:1361–1367.

34. Bender B, Milgrom H. Neuropsychiatric effects of medications for allergic diseases. *J Allergy Clin Immunol*. 1995;95:523–528.

35. Barlow DS ed. *Clinical Handbook of Psychological Disorders, a Step-by-Step Treatment Manual*. 3rd ed. New York: Guilford Press; 2001.

36. Schnurr PP, Friedman MJ, Engel CC, et al. Cognitive behavioral therapy for posttraumatic stress disorder in women. *JAMA*. 2007; 297:820–830.

CHAPTER 44

Controversial and Unproved Methods in Allergy Diagnosis and Treatment

ABBA I. TERR, MD

Unconventional and unproved theories, procedures, and practices are often referred to as "complementary and alternative medicine" (CAM) (1). Many of these practices are offered to patients with actual or suspected allergy (2), even though there is no evidence that they are either alternative or complementary to rational scientifically-based medical practice.

Accurate diagnosis and effective therapy of allergic disorders can be achieved by relying on sound theory and the results of scientific clinical research. This evidence-based medicine can be accomplished efficiently, safely, and cost effectively. There is little if any justification today for an empirical approach to allergy. However, the clinician who treats allergic patients should be sufficiently knowledgeable about both accepted and unproved theories and techniques in order to counsel their patients.

■ DEFINITIONS

A number of terms have been used to describe different forms of medical practice (Table 44.1).

Standard practice is generally defined as the methods of diagnosis and treatment used by reputable physicians in a particular subspecialty or primary care practice. Standard practice usually involves a range of options. Procedures should be tailored to the individual patient's clinical status. In general, physicians who are knowledgeable, trained, and experienced in allergy may prefer certain accepted diagnostic and therapeutic methods while at the same time recognizing that other methods are equally acceptable.

Acceptable methods are based on, or consistent with, currently established mechanisms of allergy. In addition, they have "stood the test of time" through a sufficient period of usage and evaluations by properly conducted scientifically based clinical trials that demonstrate efficacy and safety.

Experimental procedures are potentially new methods of practice arising from the results of scientific studies or from chance empiric observation. Experimental methods of diagnosis and treatment are those undergoing clinical trials on subjects who are informed of the experimental nature of the procedure, their potential risks, and their potential benefits. Subjects must give informed consent to participate in experimental trials.

Controversial methods refer to those procedures that lack scientific credibility and have not been shown to have clinical efficacy, even though they may be used by a few physicians in their practices. They are not used by the majority of allergists. Most of the controversial methods discussed in this chapter have been tested in clinical trials. The published results show either ineffectiveness or insufficient data to establish effectiveness. In some cases only anecdotal testimonies are available. The term *unproved* is also used for those procedures that are controversial, as defined above.

The terms *alternative* and *complementary* are not appropriate, because they tend to obscure the real issue of whether or not a particular procedure has been validated for clinical use by proper scientific scrutiny. *Fraud* and *quackery* generally refer to medical practices performed by those individuals who knowingly, deliberately, and deceitfully use unproven and controversial methods for profit. Many physicians who use controversial procedures in allergy practice, however, do so because they sincerely believe that these practices are worthwhile and are unwilling to accept evidence to the contrary.

Standard of care is the terminology usually used in the course of litigation. The definition will vary according to jurisdiction.

TABLE 44.1 TERMINOLOGY

- Standard Practice
- Accepted Practice
- Conventional (or unconventional) methods
- Proven (or unproven) methods
- Controversial methods
- Experimental (investigational) procedures
- Alternative medicine
- Complementary medicine
- Fraud
- Quackery
- Standard of care

■ CONTROVERSIAL THEORIES ABOUT ALLERGY

Current allergy practice is based on a foundation of scientifically based immunologic and physiologic principles, thoroughly discussed elsewhere in this book. Some unconventional methods of diagnosis and treatment seemingly derive from these theories, others are based on unsubstantiated theories arising from empirical observations, and still others appear to lack any theoretical foundation. Some of these unconventional theories are discussed in this section.

Allergic Toxemia

Allergic diseases are characterized by focal inflammation in certain target organs. These include the bronchi in asthma; the nasal mucosa and conjunctivae in allergic rhinitis; the gastrointestinal mucosa in allergic gastroenteropathy; the skin in atopic dermatitis, urticaria, and allergic contact dermatitis; and alveolae and lung interstitium in hypersensitivity pneumonitis. Multiple target organs are involved in systemic anaphylaxis and in serum sickness. During the course of illness of any of these localized diseases, the allergic patient may experience systemic symptoms such as fatigue or other focal symptoms in parts of the body not directly involved in the allergic inflammation. These collateral symptoms are sometimes explainable pathophysiologically, for example, as secondary effects of hypoxemia and hyperventilation in asthma or from cranial and neck muscle tension from excessive sneezing in rhinitis. Locally released inflammatory mediators and cytokines may produce systemic effects, although direct proof is lacking.

On the other hand, certain practitioners have proposed that a variety of systemic complaints, especially fatigue, drowsiness, weakness, body aching, nervousness, irritability, mental confusion, sluggishness, and poor memory—in the absence of any clinical sign of allergic inflammation–are caused by exposure to environmental allergens. The allergens most often implicated are foods, food additives, environmental chemicals, and

drugs. This has been referred to as allergic toxemia, allergic tension fatigue syndrome (3), or cerebral allergy (4). The literature on this subject is largely anecdotal. No definitive controlled studies have yet shown the existence of such a syndrome (5). Patients often claim dramatic improvement from eliminating certain foods or chemicals, but this is not supported by scientific evidence.

The allergic toxemia concept is also used to explain allergy as the cause of certain psychiatric conditions. Attention deficit disorder and attention deficit hyperactivity disorder (ADD, ADHD) in children are attributed to food coloring and preservatives (6). Several controlled studies, however, do not support this concept (7). The claim that ingestion of wheat and certain other foods cause or contribute to adult schizophrenia (8,9) has not been confirmed.

Idiopathic Environmental Intolerances (Multiple Chemical Sensitivities)

For years a small group of physicians have accepted a concept that environmental chemicals cause a variety of physical and psychological illnesses. This concept was applied to patients with a host of nonspecific complaints without objective physical signs of disease. These patients also attribute their symptoms to multiple food sensitivities.

This practice is known as clinical ecology (10–12), which postulates disease from failure of the human species to adapt to synthetic chemicals (13). One theory proposes that symptoms represent an exhaustion of normal homeostasis from ingestion of foods and inhalation of chemicals. An alternative theory is that common environmental substances are toxic to the human immune system (14). These and other clinical ecology theories rely on certain unique and unscientific concepts, such as a maximum total body load of antigen, masked food hypersensitivity, and a "spreading phenomenon" whereby the presence of one specific allergy induces others of different specificities.

Clinical ecology practitioners diagnose "environmental illness," also called multiple chemical sensitivities, ecologic illness, chemical hypersensitivity syndrome, total allergy syndrome, and 20th century disease. The term *idiopathic environmental intolerances* (IEI) is the most appropriate one, because it avoids unproved mechanisms (15). Patients with this diagnosis generally have a wide range of symptoms that are often compatible with conversion reactions, anxiety and depression, or psychosomatic illness. The diagnosis is subjective with no requirement for any specific physical findings or abnormal laboratory test results.

Lacking a characteristic history or pathognomonic physical signs or laboratory abnormalities (16–18), the diagnosis usually depends on the provocation-neutralization procedure described below. Some clinical ecologists also measure serum immunoglobulins, complement components, blood level of lymphocyte subsets, and blood or tissue level of environmental chemicals to supplement provocation-neutralization testing. It is not clear, however, how these test results indicate the presence of environmental illness. The few published reports show variable and often conflicting abnormalities of dubious clinical significance, because they lack proper controls or evidence of reproducibility (5).

The primary treatments advocated by clinical ecologists are avoidance and neutralization therapy. Avoidance of foods believed to cause or aggravate illness is accomplished by a rotary diversified diet, because multiple food "sensitivities" are believed to occur in this illness. Avoidance of all food additives, environmental synthetic chemicals, and even some natural chemicals is recommended, but the extent of avoidance varies with the enthusiasm of the patient and physician and not on scientific evidence of efficacy. Patients often avoid scented household products, synthetic fabrics and plastics, and pesticides. They generally try to limit exposure to air pollutants, gasoline fumes, and vehicle exhaust fumes. Several isolated rural communities have been established for these patients.

Neutralization therapy with food and chemical extracts, megadose vitamin therapy, mineral or amino acid supplements, and antioxidants are commonly recommended. Drug therapy is generally condemned as a form of chemical exposure, although oxygen, mineral salts, and antifungal drugs are frequently prescribed. None of these forms of treatment—either singly or in combination—have been evaluated in properly controlled trials to determine efficacy or potential adverse effects.

Candida Hypersensitivity Syndrome

Environmental illness is also alleged to be caused by *Candida albicans* normally resident in the microflora of the gastrointestinal and female genitourinary mucous membranes. Many persons with no clinical evidence of Candida infection and no evidence of defective local or systemic immunity, pregnancy, diabetes mellitus, endocrine diseases, or medications known to cause opportunistic candidiasis are said to suffer an illness known as Candida hypersensitivity syndrome (19,20). Clinically, the syndrome is indistinguishable from environmental illness. *C. albicans* also has been claimed to cause behavioral and emotional diseases and a variety of physical illnesses and symptomatic states. Individuals who have ever received antibiotics, corticosteroids, birth control pills, or have ever been pregnant, even in the remote past, are said to be susceptible to this syndrome. Diagnosis is made by history and not by diagnostic testing. The recommended treatment is avoidance of sugar, yeast, and mold in the diet, and the

use of a rotary diversified diet. Nystatin, ketoconazole, caprylic acid, and vitamin–mineral supplements are recommended. This syndrome is reminiscent of the concept of autointoxication that was popular in the early 20th century. In the opinion of some practitioners of that era, the bacterial component of the normal intestinal flora was considered to cause numerous physical and psychologic disabilities (21).

Disease from Indoor Molds

Atmospheric mold sensitivity has recently replaced environmental chemical sensitivity as causing a variety of subjective complaints or illnesses in persons living in homes or working in buildings that have sustained water damage from flooding or excessive humidity, promoting indoor mold growth (22). Fungi are a major component of the environment, and fungal spores are almost always present in the atmosphere. In contrast to well-recognized infectious and allergic diseases caused by molds, a combined toxicity/hypersensitivity theory is often invoked (23) as in the case of environmental illness.

One particular fungus, Stachybotrys atra (chartarum), has created considerable publicity because of the suspicion that Stachybotrys mycotoxin was the causative agent in cases of pulmonary hemorrhage/hemosiderosis in young infants living in water-damaged homes (24). The role of the mycotoxin in these cases has been called into question (25), but there remains unsubstantiated fear of the presence of any indoor mold spores as pathogenic. This unproved theory should not be confused with allergic diseases caused by fungal allergy, especially asthma, some cases of hypersensitivity pneumonitis, allergic bronchopulmonary aspergillosis, and allergic fungal sinusitis. These can be identified by localized symptomatology, objective physical findings, functional and imaging studies that confirm pathology, and the presence of the relevant immune response by the patient.

Other Unconventional Practices

Acupuncture, Chinese herbal therapy, homeopathy, naturopathy, and similar alternative practices have all been used for allergy treatment. None of these are based on accepted scientific principles of physiology, immunology, or pharmacology. Reasonably acceptable clinical trials have failed to show benefit (26–28).

■ UNCONVENTIONAL DIAGNOSTIC METHODS

Experienced allergists recognize that a thorough history and physical examination are essential for diagnosis. Laboratory testing is used selectively to supplement the clinical findings, especially when objective measurement

TABLE 44.2   CATEGORIES OF INAPPROPRIATE PROCEDURES

- Ineffective
- Effective but misused
- Effective but misinterpreted

of a functional abnormality such as airway obstruction is desired, or when alternative diagnoses must be considered. *In vivo* allergy tests such as skin-prick or intradermal tests, patch tests, or *in vitro* serum antibody tests are procedures that detect the presence of an immune response of a particular type (e.g., immunoglobulin E (IgE) antibody or cell-mediated immunity) to a specific allergen. These tests alone do not diagnose or necessarily predict a clinical allergic disease; however, they assist the clinician in diagnosis when the results are correlated with the patient's history.

Inappropriate diagnostic tests fall into three categories (Table 44.2): (a) procedures of no possible diagnostic value under any circumstances, (b) procedures that are intrinsically capable of a valid measurement but not appropriate for the diagnosis of allergic disorders, and (c) procedures that are intrinsically capable of being used in allergy diagnosis but are not appropriate for general clinical use because of low sensitivity or specificity, lack of general availability, or expense. For example, the *in vitro* histamine release test has been widely used in allergy research, where it has been invaluable in furthering knowledge of disease, but it cannot be recommended for clinical use at this time. It may eventually be modified to assume a place in allergy practice in the future.

"Diagnostic" Procedures of No Value under Any Circumstances

The procedures included in this category are not based on sound scientific principles, and they have not been shown by proper controlled clinical trials to be capable of assisting in the diagnosis of any condition.

The Cytotoxic Test

This is also known as the leukocytotoxic test or Bryan test (29,30). It consists of the microscopic examination of an unstained wet mount of whole blood or buffy coat on a slide that had been previously coated with a food extract. Subjective impressions of leukocyte swelling, vacuolation, crenation, or other changes in morphology are designated as a "positive" test result. This is diagnosed as evidence of allergy to the food. The procedure has not been standardized for time of incubation, pH, osmolarity, temperature, or other conditions that may be responsible for the observed changes (30). Test reproducibility has not been established. The procedure is advertised as a test for allergy to both foods and drugs.

There are currently no allergic diseases known to be caused by leukocyte cytotoxicity from foods, either directly or immunologically. Some drugs do occasionally cause immunologically mediated cytotoxicity (e.g., immune granulocytopenia from cephalothin), but there have been no studies to show that this can be detected *in vitro* by the Bryan test.

Several controlled clinical trials have reported that the cytotoxic test is not reproducible and does not correlate with clinical evidence of food allergy (31,32).

The Antigen Leukocyte Cellular Antibody Test

A modification of the cytotoxic test, the antigen leukocyte cellular antibody test (ALCAT) uses electronic instrumentation and computerized data analysis to examine and monitor changes in cell volumes. Like the cytotoxic test, it also has been promoted as a screening procedure for diagnosing food allergy or intolerance in a host of conditions, including arthritis, urticaria, bronchitis, gastroenteritis, childhood hyperactivity, rhinitis, and atopic dermatitis. Results are used to recommend elimination diets for these diseases. There are no proper controlled trials to establish diagnostic efficacy (33).

Provocation–Neutralization

This is a procedure that is claimed by its proponents to diagnose "allergy" to foods, inhalant allergens, environmental chemicals, hormones, and microorganisms, such as *Candida albicans*. The patient is given a small dose of an extract of one of these substances by either intracutaneous injection, subcutaneous injection, or by sublingual drop. Any subjective "sensations" (i.e., symptoms) during the next 10 minutes are recorded as a positive test result, diagnosed as allergy to that substance. If the test is negative (i.e., no recorded sensations), it is repeated at higher concentrations until the patient reports a sensation. Progressively lower concentrations are then administered, and if fewer or no symptoms are reported, the reaction is said to be "neutralized" (34–41). The neutralizing dose is then used as ongoing therapy. The test result is graded as positive regardless of whether or not the reported sensations are the same as those in the patient's initial history. When the test is performed by intradermal injection, increasing wheal diameter with increasing dose is considered corroborative evidence of a positive test result. Some proponents measure change in pulse rate during the test, but there is disagreement about its significance.

Published reports of provocation–neutralization testing yield conflicting results (5). Studies have included subjects with varying clinical manifestations, different testing methods, and variable criteria for a positive test result. Many lack relevant controls, reflecting the absence of standardization and the subjective nature of provocation–neutralization.

Current knowledge of immunologic disease provides no rationale for the provocation of subjective symptoms and their immediate neutralization under the conditions used in this procedure (16). A placebo-controlled double-blind evaluation of provocation–neutralization for diagnosis of food allergy in 18 patients concluded that symptoms were provoked with equal frequency by food extracts and by placebo (42), showing that results are based on suggestion (43). Furthermore, there is a potential danger of buccal angioedema or even a systemic reaction (44) in testing with an allergen to which the patient has significant IgE sensitivity. The procedure is time-consuming, because only a single concentration of one allergen can be "tested" at one time.

Electrodermal Diagnosis

This procedure purports to measure changes in skin resistance after the patient is exposed to an allergen (45). The allergen extract, usually a food, is placed in a glass vial on a metal plate in an electrical circuit between two electrodes on the skin. A galvanometer is used to detect a decrease in skin electrical resistance compared to an empty vial, indicating allergy to the food.

There is no rational basis for such a test and no publications to support its use. Proponents use acupuncture points on the skin when performing this bizarre procedure, often referred to as electroacupuncture. A recent controlled study reported that it was incapable of detecting specific allergic sensitivities (46,47).

Applied Kinesiology

In applied kinesiology, the muscle strength of a limb is measured before and after the patient is exposed to a test allergen (48). Exposure to the allergen, usually a food, is done by placing a glass vial of the allergen in the patient's hand (or elsewhere on the skin), and muscle strength of the arm is estimated subjectively. A loss or weakening is considered a positive test result, indicating allergy to the tested food.

There is no scientific rationale behind the concept that allergy to a food or to any other allergen changes the function of skeletal muscle, and the belief that any exposure to the allergen could occur through a glass vial on contact with the skin is clearly untenable.

Diagnostic Procedures Misused for Allergy "Diagnosis"

The procedures included in this category are ineffective for allergy diagnosis, although they may be useful for diagnosis of other medical conditions. They are considered under two categories: nonimmunologic tests and immunologic tests.

Nonimmunologic Tests That Are Inappropriate for Allergy Diagnosis

Certain procedures are valid diagnostic tests for certain conditions, although not when used for allergy. Those discussed here are the pulse test and quantitation of chemicals in body fluids and tissues. These tests have been promoted for allergy diagnosis based on erroneous concepts of the pathogenesis of allergy.

Pulse Test

Measuring a change in pulse rate, either an increase or decrease after a test substance is ingested or injected, has been used by some as indication of allergy (49). A change in pulse rate occurs from a variety of physiologic conditions and during the course of many other diseases. There is no rationale or documentation that an increase or decrease in heart rate by itself can diagnose allergy.

Testing for Environmental Chemicals in the Body

Some physicians subscribe to the unsubstantiated belief that all synthetic chemicals, regardless of dose, are toxic to the human immune system, resulting in "sensitivities" to numerous chemicals, foods, drugs, and other agents (50,51). Samples of whole blood, erythrocytes, serum, urine, fat, and hair are analyzed for the presence of environmental chemicals. The tested chemicals are typically organic solvents, other hydrocarbons, and pesticides. Analytical methods and instrumentation are available for quantifying almost any chemical at the level of parts per billion, and indeed many environmental chemicals are found at this low level in almost everyone because of the ubiquitous presence of these substances in today's environment. Under some circumstances, it may be appropriate to detect toxic quantities of a suspected chemical where poisoning is suspected, but the presence of such chemicals in the body, regardless of quantity, bears no relationship to allergic disease. The concept of an immunotoxic cause of allergic "sensitivity" is unproved.

Immunologic Tests That Are Inappropriate for Allergy Diagnosis

The immunologic pathogenesis of allergy is firmly established. The mechanisms of allergy caused by IgE antibodies, immune complexes, or cell-mediated hypersensitivity are discussed elsewhere in this book. The clinical manifestations of diseases mediated through these pathways and the appropriate immunologic tests for diagnosis are explained in detail. Clinical laboratories offer valid tests for detecting immunoglobulins, complement components, circulating immune complexes, blood levels of lymphocyte subsets, and other measurements of immune function. These tests may be highly sensitive and specific and the resulting measurement valid and relevant for the clinical evaluation of immunologic and other diseases. However, their use in allergy diagnosis is not appropriate for this purpose.

Serum Immunoglobulin G Antibodies

Immunoglobulin G (IgE) antibodies to allergens such as foods or inhalants are not involved in the pathogenesis of atopic diseases. Although some allergists have speculated that adverse delayed reactions to foods may be caused by circulating immune complexes containing IgG or IgE antibodies to foods (52–54), this concept is unproved. In fact, IgG antibodies and postprandial circulating immune complexes to foods are probably normal phenomena and not indicative of disease (55). They are found in very low concentrations in serum compared to the quantity of antibody and immune complex required to evoke inflammation in serum sickness. Circulating IgG antibodies to the common injected allergens can usually be detected in the serum of patients receiving allergen immunotherapy (hyposensitization). Although referred to as "blocking antibodies," their protective role in injection therapy of atopic respiratory disease and Hymenoptera insect venom anaphylaxis is uncertain. Therefore, measurement of serum IgG antibodies or immune complexes has no diagnostic value in the management of atopic patients. Detecting serum IgG antibody to the relevant antigen may be diagnostic for those immune complex diseases where the immunogenic antigen is known or suspected, i.e., serum sickness or allergic bronchopulmonary aspergillosis.

Total Serum Immunoglobulin Concentrations

Quantifying the total serum concentrations of IgG, IgA, IgM, and IgE can be accomplished easily and accurately. Significant reductions of one or more of these define the immunoglobulin deficiency diseases, wherein deficient antibody production may lead to susceptibility to certain infections (56). Polyclonal increases in the serum concentrations of these immunoglobulins occur in certain chronic infections and autoimmune diseases. Monoclonal hyperproduction occurs in multiple myeloma and Waldenstrom macroglobulinemia. Alterations in the total serum concentration of IgG, IgA, and/or IgM, are not found in allergic disorders.

Total serum IgE concentrations are generally higher in atopic than in nonatopic individuals. It is higher in allergic asthma than in allergic rhinitis and very high in some patients with atopic dermatitis. In allergic bronchopulmonary aspergillosis, the total serum IgE concentration has prognostic significance because it correlates with disease activity (57). However, the total serum IgE is not a useful "screen" for the atopic diseases, because a significant number of such patients have concentrations that fall within the range of nonatopic controls, and it gives no information about antibody specificity that is necessary for allergy diagnosis.

Lymphocyte Subset Counts

Lymphocyte subsets are identified by specific cell surface markers, termed *clusters of differentiation* (CD). Quantifying lymphocyte subsets in blood is useful in the diagnosis of lymphocyte cellular immunodeficiencies and lymphocytic leukemias, but not in allergy. The "normal" range of circulating levels for many of these subsets is wide and fluctuates under physiologic conditions.

Food Immune Complex Assay

Some commercial clinical laboratories offer tests that detect circulating immune complexes containing specific food antigens purportedly for the diagnosis of food allergy. The method involves a two-site recognition system in which a heterologous antibody to the food is bound to a solid-phase immunosorbent medium (58,59). When incubated with the test serum, the reagent antibody detects the antigen within the immune complex which is then detected and quantified by a labeled anti-immunoglobulin.

A portion of ingested food protein is normally absorbed intact across the gastrointestinal mucosal barrier, permitting the formation of an immune response and low levels of circulating antibody to these food proteins (55–57). It has been suggested that certain allergic reactions may be caused by circulating immune complexes that contain food antigens complexed with IgE or IgG antibodies (58,59). Such immune complexes, however, are more likely to be a normal physiologic mechanism for clearing the food antigens from the circulation and not pathogenic (60).

To date there is no clinical evidence that circulating food immune complexes cause any form of human disease. Patients with IgA deficiency may have abnormally high concentrations of circulating immune complexes to bovine albumin, but the pathophysiologic role of these complexes is unknown (60,61). No support exists for the use of assays for food immune complexes in the diagnosis of allergic disease.

■ UNCONVENTIONAL TREATMENT METHODS

Effective management of the patient with allergic disease requires an accurate diagnosis of both the disease itself and the causative allergen(s). Once this is accomplished, the three principal forms of treatment are (a) allergen avoidance, (b) medications to reverse the symptoms and pathophysiologic abnormalities, and (c) specific allergen immunotherapy. Nonspecific immunomodulation using monoclonal anti-IgE therapy has been shown to be effective in some cases of atopic asthma (62). Management of allergy also must take into account the physical, emotional, and social conditions of the patient, and therefore the program must be individualized in each case. All forms of treatment, including allergen avoidance, are subject to undesired adverse effects. Treatment should be monitored for both efficacy and complications.

This section discusses controversial therapies that are ineffective or inappropriate for allergy. These methods are considered in two categories: (a) treatments that have not been shown to be effective for any disease, and (b) treatments that are not appropriate for allergy but may be effective in other conditions.

Treatment Methods of No Value

This section discusses treatments directed specifically toward allergy as well as others promoted for allergy and other chronic conditions. All are without proven therapeutic benefit, even though in some cases they may result in temporary symptomatic improvement or sense of well-being. Such placebo effect accompanies any therapeutic maneuver, whether effective or not.

Neutralization

Neutralization (also called symptom-relieving) therapy (34,63,65) is an extension of provocation–neutralization testing, discussed previously. It consists of self-treatment with extracts of inhalant allergens, foods, or chemicals at a concentration determined from the prior symptom-neutralizing testing by the injection or sublingual methods. The goal is to relieve or prevent symptoms of environmental exposure. An ongoing maintenance program is sometimes recommended. There is no rational mechanism based on currently-accepted immunologic theory to account for immediate symptom neutralization by this method. Published studies are either anecdotal or inadequate, suggesting that any beneficial effect is based on suggestion (43). The treatment is usually prescribed for chemical and food hypersensitivity.

Acupuncture

The ancient Chinese procedure of acupuncture has been used over the centuries to treat virtually every disease. It is popular in Western culture as well, although modern medical science offers little theoretical support for its continued use. It is employed exclusively by some practitioners or as an adjunct to pharmacotherapy, herbal therapy, homeopathy, naturopathy, and psychotherapy. It is likely that a significant number of allergic patients in the United States have tried acupuncture at some time for relief of asthma, allergic rhinitis, and allergic dermatoses. It is also used by patients

who have other nonallergic symptoms or medical conditions incorrectly diagnosed as allergic. Although some patients report temporary benefit, there have been no reported studies documenting either symptomatic improvement or long-term alteration in the course of allergic disease (66,67). Furthermore, acupuncture is not always free from side effects (68).

Homeopathic Remedies

Homeopathy is an alternative form of "healing" based on treating "like with like," i.e., the causative agent of a disease is administered therapeutically in exceedingly small amounts. Homeopathic remedies consist of extracts of a number of natural substances, including plants, animal products, and insects. These extracts are diluted in a serial fashion through a process known as succussion, which is merely the violent shaking of a container of diluted extract. Homeopathists also prescribe "natural" hormones in the form of orally administered extracts of animal adrenal cortex, thyroid, thymus, pancreas, and spleen. There is no evidence that homeopathic remedies have any therapeutic benefit for any disease, including allergy (69,70). There is no scientific theory to support homeopathic practice, despite its popularity. Because this procedure has a superficial resemblance to immunotherapy or desensitization, it is not surprising that homeopathic practitioners offer their remedies for the treatment of allergic diseases.

Detoxification

Detoxification for allergy treatment is recommended by those who subscribe to the unfounded theory that an allergic state can be induced by toxic damage to the immune system from exposure to environmental chemicals (50,51). Supporters of this concept believe that immunotoxic lipid-soluble chemicals may be stored in body fat for long periods of time.

The method consists of a program of exercise and sauna. High-dose niacin is given to induce erythema. Body fluids are replenished with water and electrolytes. Certain "essential" oils are prescribed, presumably to help replace fat-soluble chemical contaminants. This procedure takes about 5 hours and is repeated daily for 20 to 30 days.

The theory of immunotoxicity as a cause of allergic disease is unproved and contrary to an extensive body of clinical experience. The concept that augmenting blood circulation, vasodilatation, and oral ingestion of vegetable oils can mobilize "toxins" from fat into sweat is untested. The potential dangers of this program have not been adequately studied.

Injection of Food Extracts

Anaphylaxis and urticaria can result from food ingestion if IgE antibody to the relevant food exists in the patient.

Fatal or life-threatening anaphylactic reactions can occur from eating minute quantities of the food, especially in peanut allergy. The only accepted method to prevent food anaphylaxis is avoidance. Specific allergen immunotherapy to eliminate or reduce the anaphylactic sensitivity in IgE-mediated food allergy is currently undergoing investigational controlled clinical trials.

However, some practitioners routinely prescribe food extract injections, often because of (a) positive food skin or radioallergosorbent test results in the absence of clinical allergic reactions to those foods, or (b) nonallergic intolerance to foods without evidence of specific IgE antibodies. There is no evidence in either case that immunotherapy with food extracts is clinically beneficial.

Urine Injections

The drinking of urine was an ancient healing practice. The modern medical literature contains a single paper on "urine therapy," published in 1947, in which intramuscular injections of the patient's own urine was recommended for a long list of symptoms and illnesses, including allergy (71). In recent years, a small number of medical and "alternative" practitioners have revived this bizarre procedure, claiming that urine contains unspecified chemicals produced by the patient during an allergic reaction and that injections of these chemicals inhibit or neutralize future allergic reactions. There is no scientific evidence to support autogenous urine injections, nor are there clinical reports that the treatment is effective.

The risk of injecting urine is potentially serious, because soluble renal tubular and glomerular antigens are normally excreted in the urine. Repeated injections of these antigens could theoretically induce autoimmune nephritis.

Enzyme-potentiated Desensitization

A modification of conventional allergen immunotherapy by mixing β-glucuronidase with an exceedingly low dose of allergen is known as enzyme-potentiated desensitization (EPD) (72). It is recommended as a single preseasonal intradermal injection for seasonal pollen allergies or every 2 to 6 months for patients with perennial symptoms. For unexplained reasons, practitioners who use this procedure advise the patient to avoid common food allergens, food additives, and all medications for 3 days before and 3 weeks after each injection; to avoid allergen exposure for 1 to 2 days before and after the injection; and to consume a special "EPD diet." It is recommended for not only atopic and anaphylactic diseases, but also for ulcerative colitis, irritable bowel syndrome, rheumatoid arthritis, migraine headaches, petit mal seizures, chronic fatigue syndrome, "immune dysfunction syndrome," food-induced depression and anxiety, and childhood hyperactivity.

Several controlled short-term clinical trials claim to show improved symptoms of allergic rhinitis or asthma, but objective measures of disease activity are either absent or were not measured (73,74). No trial has compared enzyme-potentiated desensitization treatment with either the allergen or enzyme alone. There is no information about possible chemical or biological alteration of the allergen when mixed with the enzyme.

Inappropriate Treatment Methods

Each of the forms of therapy discussed below has a specific role in the management of certain diseases, but not for treatment of allergy.

Vitamin, Mineral, and Nutrient Supplementation

"Supplements" have been recommended to relieve symptoms or as a cure for patients with allergies. Most often, these include vitamins, minerals, and amino acids. There are various theories to rationalize their use. The usual explanation is a deficiency of these nutrients as a cause of allergy. There is no scientific basis for this, nor have there been controlled clinical trials demonstrating that replacement by dietary supplementation is efficacious for any allergic disease. Fortunately, most patients are not harmed by taking supplements, although excessive intake of fat-soluble vitamins could result in toxicity. Proponents of therapy with antioxidants, such as vitamin C and E and glutathione, justify the practice by citing evidence that allergic inflammation generates free radicals that cause oxidative damage to tissues (75). Although toxic oxygen metabolites are activated during the course of certain inflammatory reactions, the kinetics and localization of these events and the normal activation of endogenous antioxidants make it unlikely that ingestion of these dietary supplements would be effective.

Diets

Avoidance is the only certain method for managing food allergy. Although any food has the potential for being allergenic, food allergy in adults is relatively uncommon, and in each case it is usually limited to one or at most a few foods. Food allergy is more common among allergic infants and young children. Except in rare instances, avoidance therapy does not require an extensive elimination diet, and adequate food substitutes are available.

Numerous subjective symptoms, behavioral problems, and emotional illness are often attributed to multiple food allergies. This unsubstantiated concept can result in the unnecessary restriction of large numbers of foods. The risk of nutritional deficiency is obvious, although in practice many patients abandon highly restrictive diets because of the lack of any long-term benefit.

Proponents of the concept of multiple food allergies sometimes recommend a "rotary diversified diet," in which the patient rotates foods so that the same food is eaten only once every 4 to 5 days (76). To do this, it is necessary to keep extensive and accurate records, causing further unnecessary and time-consuming attention to diet and symptoms (77).

Environmental Chemical Avoidance

Allergists recommend a reasonable and cost-effective program of allergen avoidance for patients with respiratory allergy. The usual advice is to reduce house dust and dust mite exposure by using special casings for the bedding and by removing bedroom carpeting. Similar measures can be taken to lessen indoor levels of airborne mold spores and other allergens. Occupational exposure to proven workplace allergens and irritants, such as animals, isocyanate fumes, acid anhydrides, wood dusts, and grain dusts, are mandatory for patients with documented occupational asthma or hypersensitivity pneumonitis caused by these agents. Proven clinical allergy to foods can be managed by selective food elimination.

In contrast, the concept of multiple food and chemical sensitivities discussed above carries with it a recommendation for extensive avoidance of environmental "chemicals." Typically, patients diagnosed by unproved methods—usually provocation–neutralization—have unexplained multiple chronic vague symptoms. They are advised to avoid any exposure, even minute amounts, to chemicals (10,78,79) such as pesticides, organic solvents, vehicle exhaust fumes, gasoline fumes, household cleaners, glue and adhesives, new carpets, and many others. There is no proof that these drastic measures are helpful; on the contrary, there is evidence for significant psychologic harm (80).

Antifungal Medications

The unsubstantiated theories of "*Candida* hypersensitivity syndrome" and disease caused by indoor molds, both discussed above, have prompted some physicians to recommend a treatment program of antifungal medications and a special "mold-free" diet. Although some antifungal drugs are effective in the treatment of cutaneous and systemic candidiasis, their use in the unsubstantiated "*Candida* syndrome" cannot be justified. A controlled clinical trial showed that nystatin did not differ from placebo in its effect on such patients (81).

Immunologic Manipulation

Allergic diseases affect a minority of the population who are exposed to allergens. Allergen avoidance prevents disease but without altering the underlying immunologically-induced hypersensitive state. It is not currently possible to manipulate the immune system in such a way to remove a patient's specific allergic sensitivities completely and predictably without also inhibiting other necessary immune functions. Specific allergen immunotherapy and monoclonal anti-IgE therapy, both discussed elsewhere in this book, do not achieve this goal, although they are clinically beneficial in most carefully selected cases.

Immunosuppressive drugs, immunostimulating drugs, therapeutic monoclonal antibodies to certain components of the immune system, and immunoregulatory cytokines are now standard treatment for other diseases, particularly autoimmunity and cancer, but not at this time for allergic diseases.

Therapeutic gammaglobulin injections are a standard treatment for documented IgG antibody deficiency, and they have proved effective for this purpose. They also have been used empirically for other diseases, although the mechanism of efficacy is unknown. Gammaglobulin injections have been recommended by some practitioners for allergy, but until effectiveness is shown by proper double-blind studies, such treatment should be considered experimental.

■ REMOTE PRACTICE OF ALLERGY

In allergy practice, the proper diagnosis and treatment for each patient is based on a thorough history and physical examination by a physician knowledgeable about allergic diseases. In many cases, testing for specific sensitivities by skin or *in vitro* tests, other laboratory tests, imaging studies, and other diagnostic procedures may be indicated to supplement the findings from the history and physical examination. Accurate diagnoses and therapy require knowledge of the patient's current and past symptomatology, physical findings, and physiological and biochemical tests (where indicated). The results of allergy skin tests and *in vitro* tests for IgE antibodies do not distinguish whether the patient has current, present, or future symptomatic disease; therefore, these test results alone reveal only potential, but not necessarily clinical, sensitivities. They therefore cannot be used alone as the basis for recommending drug therapy or allergy immunotherapy.

Skin and *in vitro* testing for IgE antibody sensitivities are readily available. Therefore, some practitioners do in fact diagnose and recommend treatment for allergy solely from these test results. This is known as the remote practice of allergy (82). It is clearly unacceptable, because allergic disease occurs through a complex interplay of constitutional, environmental, and allergic factors, all of which must be known to the treating physician prior to recommending effective management and to avoid unnecessary, inappropriate, and potentially dangerous treatment.

■ REFERENCES

1. Owen OK, Lewith G, Stephens CR. Can doctors respond to patients' increasing interest in complementary and alternative medicine? *BMJ.* 2001;322:154–158.

2. Gershwin ME, Terr A. Introduction: alternative and complementary therapy for asthma. *Clin Rev Allergy Immunol.* 1996;14:241.

3. Speer F. The allergic tension-fatigue syndrome. *Pediatr Clin North Am.* 1954;1:1029–1057.

4. Miller JB. *Food Allergy: Provocative Testing and Injection Therapy.* Springfield, IL: Charles C Thomas; 1972.

5. American College of Physicians. Position paper: clinical ecology. *Ann Intern Med.* 1989;111:104–106.

6. Feingold B. *Why your child is hyperactive.* New York: Random House; 1975.

7. Consensus Conference. Defined diets and childhood hyperactivity. *JAMA.* 1982;248:290–292.

8. Dohan FC, Grasberger JC. Relapsed schizophrenics: earlier discharge from the hospital after cereal-free, milk-free diet. *Am J Psychiatry.* 1973;130:685–688.

9. Singh MM, Na SR. Wheat gluten as a pathogenic factor in schizophrenia. *Science.* 1976;191:401–402.

10. Dickey LD. *Clinical Ecology.* Springfield, IL: Charles C Thomas; 1976.

11. Bell JR. *Clinical Ecology: A New Medical Approach to Environmental Illness.* Bolinas, CA: Common Knowledge Press; 1982.

12. Randolph TG, Moss RW. *An Alternative Approach to Allergies.* New York: Lippincott and Cromwell; 1980.

13. Randolph TG. Sensitivity to petroleum including its derivatives and antecedents (Abstract). *J Lab Clin Med.* 1952;40:931.

14. Levin AS, Byers VS. Environmental illness: a disorder of immune regulation. *Occup Med.* 1987;2:669–681.

15. American Academy of Allergy, Asthma and Immunology. Position statement: idiopathic environmental intolerances. *J Allergy Clin Immunol.* 1999;103:36.

16. Terr AI. Multiple chemical hypersensitivities: immunologic critique of clinical ecology theories and practice. *Occup Med.* 1987;2:683–694.

17. Terr AI. Environmental illness: clinical review of 50 cases. *Arch Intern Med.* 1986;146:145.

18. Terr AI. Clinical ecology in the workplace. *J Occup Med.* 1989;31:257.

19. Truss CO. The role of Candida albicans in human illness. *J Orthomol Psychiatry.* 1981;10:228.

20. Truss CO. Tissue injury induced by Candida albicans: mental and neurologic manifestations. *J Orthomol Psychiatry.* 1978;7:17.

21. Bassler A. *Intestinal Toxemia (Autointoxication) Biologically Considered.* Philadelphia: FA Davis; 1930.

22. Johanning E, Landsbergis P, Gareis M, et al. Clinical experience and results of a sentinel health investigation related to indoor fungal exposure. *Environ Health Perspect.* 1999;107(suppl 3):489.

23. Bush RK, Portnoy JM, Saxon A, et al. The medical effects of mold exposure. *J Allergy Clin Immunol.* 2006;117:326–333.

24. Etzel RA, Montana E, Sorenson WG, et al. Acute pulmonary hemorrhage in infants associated with exposure to Stachybotrys atra and other fungi. *Arch Pediatr Adolesc Med.* 1998;152:757.

25. Centers for Disease Control and Prevention. Update: pulmonary hemorrhage/hemosiderosis among infants-Cleveland, Ohio, 1993–1996. *MMWR.* 2000;49:180–184.

26. Kleijnen J, ter Riet G, Knipschild P. Acupuncture and asthma: a review of controlled trials. *Thorax.* 1991:46:799–802.

27. Reilly DT, Taylor MA, McSharry C, et al. Is homoeopathy a placebo response? Controlled trial of homoeopathic potency, with pollen in hayfever as model. *Lancet.* 1985;2:881–886.

28. Brien S, Lewith G, Bryant T: Ultramolecular homeopathy has no observable clinical effects. A randomized, double-blind, placebo-controlled proving trial of Belladonna 30C. *Br J Clin Pharmacol.* 2003;56:562–568.

29. Bryan WTK, Bryan M. The application of in vitro cytotoxic reactions to clinical diagnosis of food allergy. *Laryngoscope.* 1960;70:810.

30. Bryan MP, Bryan WTK. Cytologic diagnosis of allergic disorders. *Otolaryngol Clin North Am.* 1974;7:637–666.

31. Lieberman P, Crawford L, Bjelland J, et al. Controlled study of the cytotoxic food test. *JAMA.* 1974;231:728–730.

32. Lehman CW. The leukocytic food allergy test: a study of its reliability and reproducibility; effect of diet and sublingual food drops on this test. *Ann Allergy.* 1980;45:150–158.

33. Potter PC, Mullineux J, Weinberg EG, et al. The ALCAT test-inappropriate in testing for food allergy in clinical practice [Letter]. *S Afr Med J.* 1992;81:384.

34. Lee CH, Williams RI, Binkley EL. Provocative inhalant testing and treatment. *Arch Otolaryngol.* 1969;90:173–177.

35. Lehman CW. A double-blind study of sublingual provocative food testing: a study of its efficacy. *Ann Allergy.* 1980;45:144–149.

36. Draper LW. Food testing in allergy: intradermal provocative vs. deliberate feeding. *Arch Otolaryngol.* 1972:95:169–171.

37. Crawford LV, Lieberman P, Hanfi HA, et al. A double-blind study of subcutaneous food testing sponsored by the Food Committee of the American Academy of Allergy [Abstract]. *J Allergy Clin Immunol.* 1976;57:236.

38. King DS. Can allergic exposure provoke psychological symptoms? A double-blind test. *Biol Psychiatry.* 1981;16:3–19.

39. Willoughby JW. Provocative food test technique. *Ann Allergy.* 1965;23:543.

40. Rinkel RH, Lee CH, Brown DW, et al. The diagnosis of food allergy. *Arch Otolaryngol.* 1964;79:71.

41. Lee CH, William RI, Binkley EL. Provocative inhalation testing and treatment. *Arch Otolaryngol.* 1969;90:173–177.

42. Jewett DL, Fein G, Greenberg MH. A double-blind study of symptom provocation to determine food sensitivity. *N Engl J Med.* 1990;323:429–433.

43. Ferguson A. Food sensitivity or self-deception? *N Engl J Med.* 1990;323:476.

44. Green M. Sublingual provocative testing for food and FD and C dyes. *Ann Allergy.* 1974;32:274–281.

45. Tsuei JJ, Lehman CW, Lam FMK, et al. A food allergy study utilizing the EAV acupuncture technique. *Am J Acupuncture.* 1984;12:105.

46. Lewith GT, Kenyon JF, Broomfield PP, et al. Is electrodermal testing as effective as skin prick tests for diagnosing allergies? A double blind, randomized block design study. *BMJ.* 2001;332:131–134.

47. Lewith GT. Can we evaluate electrodermal testing? *Complement Ther Med.* 2003; 11:115–117.

48. Garrow JS. Kinesiology and food allergy. *Lancet.* 1988;296:1573–1574.

49. Coca A. *The Pulse Test.* New York: University Books; 1956.

50. Laseter JL, DeLeon IR, Rea WJ, et al. Chlorinated hydrocarbon pesticides in environmentally sensitive patients. *Clin Ecol.* 1983;2:3.

51. Rousseaux CG. Immunologic responses that may follow exposure to chemicals. *Clin Ecol.* 1987;5:33.

52. Paganelli R, Levinsky RJ, Brostoff J, et al. Immune complexes containing food proteins in normal and atopic subjects after oral challenge and effect of sodium cromoglycate on antigen absorption. *Lancet.* 1979;1:1270–1272.

53. Delire M, Cambiaso CL, Masson PL. Circulating immune complexes in infants fed on cow's milk. *Nature.* 1978;272:632.

54. Paganelli R, Atherton DJ, Levinsky R. The differences between normal and milk allergic subjects in their immune response after milk ingestion. *Arch Dis Child.* 1983;58:201–206.

55. Husby S, Oxelius V-A, Teisner B, et al. Humoral immunity to dietary antigens in healthy adults. Occurrence, isotype and IgG subclass distribution of serum antibodies to protein antigens. *Int Arch Allergy Appl Immunol.* 1985;77:416–422.

56. Roberts RI, Stiehm R. Antibody (B cell) immunodeficiency disorders. In: Parslow TG, Stites DP, Terr AI, eds. *Human Immunology.* 10th ed. New York: Lange Medical Books; 2001:299.

57. Greenberger PA, Patterson R. Allergic bronchopulmonary aspergillosis and the evaluation of the patient with asthma. *J Allergy Clin Immunol.* 1988;81:646–650.

58. Haddad ZH, Vetter M, Friedman J. et al. Detection and kinetics of antigen-specific IgE and IgG immune complexes in food allergy. *Ann Allergy.* 1983;51:255.

59. Leary HL, Halsey JF. An assay to measure antigen-specific immune complexes in food allergy patients. *J Allergy Clin Immunol.* 1984;74:190–195.

60. Cunningham-Rundels C, Brandeis WE, Good RA, et al. Milk precipitins, circulating immune complexes and IgA deficiency. *Proc Natl Acad Sci USA.* 1978;75:3387–3389.

61. Cunningham-Rundels C, Brandies WE, Good RA, et al. Bovine proteins and the formation of circulating immune complexes in selective IgA deficiency. *J Clin Invest.* 1979;64:272–279.

62. Fahy JV. Anti-IgE: lessons from effects on airway inflammation and asthma exacerbation. *J Allergy Clin Immunol.* 2006;117:1230–1232.

63. Rea WJ, Podell RN, Williams ML, et al. Intracutaneous neutralization of food sensitivity: a double-blind evaluation. *Arch Otolaryngol.* 1984;110:248.

64. Kailin EW, Collier R. "Relieving" therapy for antigen exposure [Letter]. *JAMA.* 1971;217:78.

65. Golbert TM. Sublingual desensitization. *JAMA*. 1971;217:1703–1704.
66. Chanez P, Bousquet J, Godard P, et al. Controversial forms of treatment for asthma. *Clin Rev Allergy Immunol*. 1996;14:247.
67. Stockert K, Schneider B, Porenta G, et al. Laser acupuncture and probiotics in school age children with asthma: a randomized, placebo-controlled pilot study of therapy guided by principles of Traditional Chinese Medicine. *Pediatr Allergy Immunol*. 2007;18:160–166.
68. Ernst E, White AR. Acupuncture may be associated with serious adverse events. *BMJ*.2000;320:513–514.
69. Brien S, Lewith G, Bryant T. Ultramolecular homeopathy has no observable clinical effects. A randomized, double-blind, placebo-controlled proving trial of Belladonna 30C. *Br J Clin Pharmacol*. 2003;56:562–568.
70. McCarney RW, Lasserson TJ, Linde K, et al. An overview of two Cochrane systematic reviews of complementary treatments for chronic asthma: acupuncture and homeopathy. *Respir Med*. 2004;98:687–696.
71. Plesch J. Urine therapy. *Med Press*. 1947;218:128.
72. McEwen LM. Enzyme potentiated desensitization: V. Five case reports of patients with acute food allergy. *Ann Allergy*.1975;35:98–103.
73. Cantani A, Ragno V, Monteleone MA, et al. Enzyme-potentiated desensitization in children with asthma and mite allergy: a double-blind study. *J Invest Allergol Clin Immunol*. 1996;6:270–276.
74. Astarita C, Scala G, Sproviero S, et al. Effects of enzyme-potentiated desensitization in the treatment of pollinosis: a double-blind placebo-controlled trial. *J Invest Allergol Clin Immunol*.1996;6:248–255.
75. Levine SA, Reinhardt JH. Biochemical-pathology initiated by free radicals, oxidant chemicals, and therapeutic drugs in the etiology of chemical hypersensitivity disease. *Orthomol Psychiatry*. 1983;12:166–183.
76. Rinkel HJ. Food allergy: function and clinical application of the rotary diversified diet. *J Pediatr*. 1948;32:266.
77. Terr AI. Editorial: clinical ecology. *J Allergy Clin Immunol*. 1987;79:423–426.
78. Rea WJ, Bell IR, Suits CW, et al. Food and chemical susceptibility after environmental chemical overexposure: case histories. *Ann Allergy*. 1978;41:101–109.
79. Randolph TG. *Human Ecology and Susceptibility to the Chemical Environment*. Springfield, IL: Charles C Thomas; 1962.
80. Brodsky CM. Allergic to everything: a medical subculture. *Psychosomatics*. 1983;24:731–742.
81. Dismukes WE, Wade JS, Lee JY, et al. A randomized double-blind trial of nystatin therapy for the candidiasis hypersensitivity syndrome. *N Engl J Med*. 1990;323:1717–1723.
82. American Academy of Allergy and Immunology. Position statement: the remote practice of allergy. *J Allergy Clin Immunol*. 1986;77:651–652.

Index

Page numbers followed by "f" denote figures; those followed by "t" denote tables